# TEXTBOOK OF WOMEN'S REPRODUCTIVE MENTAL HEALTH

EDITED BY

**Lucy A. Hutner, M.D.**
**Lisa A. Catapano, M.D., Ph.D.**
**Sarah M. Nagle-Yang, M.D.**
**Katherine E. Williams, M.D.**
**Lauren M. Osborne, M.D.**

AMERICAN PSYCHIATRIC ASSOCIATION PUBLISHING

**Note:** The authors have worked to ensure that all information in this book is accurate at the time of publication and consistent with general psychiatric and medical standards, and that information concerning drug dosages, schedules, and routes of administration is accurate at the time of publication and consistent with standards set by the U.S. Food and Drug Administration and the general medical community. As medical research and practice continue to advance, however, therapeutic standards may change. Moreover, specific situations may require a specific therapeutic response not included in this book. For these reasons and because human and mechanical errors sometimes occur, we recommend that readers follow the advice of physicians directly involved in their care or the care of a member of their family.



First Edition

Manufactured in the United States of America on acid-free paper
25 24 23 22 21 5 4 3 2 1

American Psychiatric Association Publishing
800 Maine Avenue SW, Suite 900
Washington, DC 20024-2812
www.appi.org

Library of Congress Cataloging-in-Publication Data

Names: Hutner, Lucy A., editor. | Catapano, Lisa A., editor. | Nagle-Yang, Sarah M., editor. | Williams, Katherine E. (Professor of psychiatry) editor. | Osborne, Lauren M., editor. | American Psychiatric Association Publishing, issuing body.
Title: Textbook of women's reproductive mental health / edited by Lucy A. Hutner, Lisa A. Catapano, Sarah M. Nagle-Yang, Katherine E. Williams, Lauren M. Osborne.
Description: First edition. | Washington, DC : American Psychiatric Association Publishing, [2022] | Includes bibliographical references and index.
Identifiers: LCCN 2021033778 (print) | LCCN 2021033779 (ebook) | ISBN 9781615373062 (hardcover ; alk. paper) | ISBN 9781615373864 (ebook)
Subjects: MESH: Mental Health | Reproductive Health | Women's Health | Mental Disorders | Pregnant Women—psychology | Pregnancy Complications—psychology
Classification: LCC RG101 (print) | LCC RG101 (ebook) | NLM WA 309.1 | DDC 618.1—dc23
LC record available at https://lccn.loc.gov/2021033778
LC ebook record available at https://lccn.loc.gov/2021033779

**British Library Cataloguing in Publication Data**
A CIP record is available from the British Library.

# Contents

## PART II
## Pregnancy and the Postpartum Period

# Contributors

**Elizabeth Albertini, M.D.**
Assistant Professor of Psychiatry, Icahn School of Medicine, New York, New York

**Jaina Amin, M.D.**
Assistant Professor of Clinical Psychiatry, Department of Psychiatry, Case Western Reserve University/University Hospitals of Cleveland, Cleveland, Ohio

**Priyanka Amin, M.D.**
Assistant Professor of Psychiatry, University of Pittsburgh Medical Center Western Psychiatric Hospital, Pittsburgh, Pennsylvania

**Lauren Augello, M.D.**
Instructor of Psychiatry/Addiction Psychiatrist, Boston University/Boston Medical Center, Cambridge, Massachusetts

**Vanessa Babineau, Ph.D.**
Clinical Psychologist and Postdoctoral Fellow, Columbia University Irving Medical Center, New York, New York

**Nina T. Ballone, M.D.**
Consultation-Liaison Psychiatry Fellow, Department of Psychiatry, The George Washington University Medical Center/Inova Fairfax Hospital, Falls Church, Virginia

**Erin Murphy Barzilay, M.D.**
Health Sciences Assistant Professor, Department of Psychiatry and Behavioral Sciences; Co-Director, The Women's Life Center; and Medical Director, Maternal Mental Health Program, UCLA Semel Institute and Resnick Neuropsychiatric Hospital, The David Geffen School of Medicine at UCLA, Los Angeles, California

**Brittney Bastow, M.D., M.Sc.**
Physician, Department of Obstetrics and Gynecology, Colorado Permanente Medical Group, Aurora, Colorado

**Madeleine A. Becker, M.D., M.A., FACLP**
Professor, Department of Psychiatry and Human Behavior and Department of Integrative Medicine and Nutritional Sciences, Marcus Institute of Integrative Health–Jefferson Health; Director, Graduate Medical Education, Associate Director, Fellowship, Integrative Medicine, Sidney Kimmel Medical College at Thomas Jefferson University, Philadelphia, Pennsylvania

**Catherine Birndorf, M.D.**
Chief Executive Officer and Medical Director, The Motherhood Center, New York, New York

**Lisa A. Catapano, M.D., Ph.D.**
Associate Professor of Psychiatry and Behavioral Sciences, Department of Psychiatry, George Washington University, Washington, DC

**Jessica L. Coker, M.D.**
Assistant Professor, Psychiatric Research Institute, University of Arkansas for Medical Sciences, Little Rock, Arkansas

**Jeanne Coulehan, C.N.M., M.P.H.**
Midwife/Clinical Practice Manager, Division of Maternal Fetal Medicine, Department of Obstetrics-Gynecology, Columbia University Medical Center, New York, New York

**Maureen Curley, Ph.D.**
Clinical Assistant Professor of Psychiatry, University of Cleveland Medical Center/ Case Western Reserve University, Cleveland, Ohio

**Sarah A. DeBrunner, M.D.**
Clinical Assistant Professor of Psychiatry, University of Pittsburgh Medical Center, Pittsburgh, Pennsylvania

**Marley Doyle, M.D.**
Assistant Professor of Psychiatry, University of Nebraska Medical Center, Omaha, Nebraska

**C. Neill Epperson, M.D.**
Robert Freedman Endowed Professor and Chair, Department of Psychiatry, School of Medicine, University of Colorado Anschutz Medical Campus, Aurora, Colorado

**Courtney Erdly, B.A.**
Project Manager, National Curriculum in Reproductive Psychiatry, Johns Hopkins School of Medicine, Johns Hopkins Hospital, Baltimore, Maryland

**Andrea Favini, M.D.**
Psychiatrist, Allegheny Health Network, Women's Behavioral Health, Pittsburgh, Pennsylvania

**Elizabeth M. Fitelson, M.D.**
Associate Professor, Department of Psychiatry, Columbia University Irving Medical Center; Director, The Women's Program, Columbia University Department of Psychiatry, New York, New York

**Julia Frew, M.D.**
Assistant Professor of Psychiatry, Obstetrics and Gynecology, and Medical Education, Geisel School of Medicine at Dartmouth/Dartmouth-Hitchcock Medical Center, Lebanon, New Hampshire

**Soudabeh Givrad, M.D.**
Assistant Professor of Clinical Psychiatry, Director of Maternal-Infant Psychiatry Program, and Associate Director of Sackler Infant Psychiatry Fellowship, Weill Cornell Medicine, New York, New York

**Jody Glance, M.D.**
Associate Professor of Psychiatry, University of Pittsburgh Medical Center Western Psychiatric Hospital, Pittsburgh, Pennsylvania

**Priya Gopalan, M.D.**
Assistant Professor of Psychiatry, University of Pittsburgh Medical Center Western Psychiatric Hospital, Pittsburgh, Pennsylvania

**Alyson Gorun, M.D.**
Assistant Professor of Clinical Psychiatry, Department of Psychiatry, Weill Cornell Medicine; Assistant Attending Psychiatrist, New York Presbyterian Hospital, New York, New York

**Gioia M. Guerrieri, D.O.**
Founder and Director, Well-Minded, LLC; Special Volunteer, Clinical Research Physician, NIH/NIMH Section of Behavioral Endocrinology, Bethesda, Maryland

**Constance Guille, M.D.**
Professor of Psychiatry and Behavioral Science and Obstetrics and Gynecology, Medical University of South Carolina, Charleston, South Carolina

**Caitlin Hasser, M.D.**
Portland VA Health Care System, Portland, Oregon

**Susan Hatters Friedman, M.D.**
The Phillip Resnick Professor of Forensic Psychiatry, Professor of Reproductive Biology and Pediatrics, and Adjunct Professor of Law, Case Western Reserve University, Cleveland, Ohio; Honorary Associate Professor of Psychological Medicine, University of Auckland, Auckland, New Zealand

**M. Camille Hoffman, M.D., M.Sc.**
Associate Professor, Maternal Fetal Medicine, Department of Obstetrics and Gynecology and Department of Psychiatry, University of Colorado, Aurora, Colorado

**Neha S. Hudepohl, M.D.**
Clinical Assistant Professor, Department of Psychiatry, University of South Carolina School of Medicine–Greenville, Greenville, South Carolina

**Lucy A. Hutner, M.D.**
Co-founder and Chief Medical Officer, Phoebe, New York, New York

**Allyce K. Jones, DNP, MSN, PMHNP-BC, APRN**
Associate Professor, College of Nursing, Rocky Mountain University of Health Professions, Provo, Utah

**Premala Jones, Ph.D.**
Mental Health Consultant, Life Perspectives, San Diego, California

**Aimee Kaempf, M.D.**
Clinical Associate Professor, Department of Psychiatry, University of Arizona College of Medicine Tucson, Tucson, Arizona

**Saira Kalia, M.D.**
Assistant Professor of Psychiatry, University of Arizona College of Medicine, Tucson, Arizona

**Susan Karabell, M.D.**
Assistant Professor of Clinical Psychiatry, Weill Cornell Medical College; Assistant Attending Psychiatrist, New York Presbyterian Hospital, Collaborative Care Center, New York, New York

**Sarah M. Kauffman, M.D.**
Reproductive Psychiatrist, The Motherhood Center of New York, New York; Staff Psychiatrist, California Department of Corrections, San Diego; and Physician Director, Maternal Mental Health Program, Hoag Hospital, Newport Beach, California

**Erika Kelley, Ph.D.**
Clinical Psychologist, Department of Obstetrics and Gynecology, University Hospitals Cleveland Medical Center; Assistant Professor, Department of Reproductive Biology, Case Western Reserve University, Cleveland, Ohio

**Sheryl A. Kingsberg, Ph.D.**
Chief, Division of Behavioral Medicine, Department of Obstetrics and Gynecology, MacDonald Women's Hospital/University Hospitals Cleveland Medical Center; Professor, Departments of Reproductive Biology and Psychiatry, Case Western Reserve University School of Medicine, Cleveland, Ohio

**Pooja Lakshmin, M.D.**
Clinical Assistant Professor, Department of Psychiatry and Behavioral Sciences, George Washington University School of Medicine and Health Sciences, Washington, DC

**Jacqueline Landess, M.D., J.D.**
Clinical Assistant Professor, Associate Training Director, Forensic Psychiatry Fellowship, Department of Psychiatry and Behavioral Medicine, Medical College of Wisconsin, Madison, Wisconsin

**Nicole Leistikow, M.D.**
Assistant Professor, Department of Psychiatry, University of Maryland, Baltimore, Maryland

**Mimi Levine, M.D.**
Clinical Assistant Professor of Psychiatry, Department of Psychiatry, New York University/Langone Medical Center, New York, New York

**Joanna V. MacLean, M.D.**
Attending Psychiatrist, Women's Behavioral Medicine, Women's Medicine Collaborative; Assistant Professor, Clinician Educator, Department of Psychiatry and Human Behavior and Department of Medicine, Alpert Medical School of Brown University, Providence, Rhode Island

**Jovana Martinovic, M.D.**
Lecturer, Department of Psychiatry, Women's College Hospital, University of Toronto, Toronto, Ontario, Canada

**Samantha Meltzer-Brody, M.D., M.P.H.**
Assad Meymandi Distinguished Professor and Chair, Department of Psychiatry, The University of North Carolina at Chapel Hill, Chapel Hill, North Carolina

**Joy E. Moel, Ph.D.**
Clinical Assistant Professor, Department of Psychiatry, University of Iowa Hospitals and Clinics; Women's Wellness and Counseling Service, Iowa City, Iowa

**Catherine Monk, Ph.D.**
Professor of Medical Psychology, Departments of Obstetrics and Gynecology, and Psychiatry Director, Women's Mental Health @Ob/Gyn, Columbia University Irving Medical Center; Research Scientist VI, New York State Psychiatric Institute, New York

**Ashley Mulvihill, M.D.**
Assistant Professor of Clinical Psychiatry, University of Illinois at Chicago, Chicago, Illinois

**Mireya Nadal-Vicens, M.D., Ph.D.**
Chief, Department of Behavioral Health, Harvard University Health Services, Cambridge, Massachusetts

**Madhavi-Latha Nagalla, M.D.**
Assistant Professor, Department of Psychiatry, Michigan State University/Pine Rest Christian Mental Health Services, Grand Rapids, Michigan

**Sarah M. Nagle-Yang, M.D.**
Associate Professor of Psychiatry, University of Colorado–Anschutz Medical Campus, Aurora, Colorado

**Margo Nathan, M.D.**
Clinical Assistant Professor, Department of Psychiatry, University of North Carolina School of Medicine, Chapel Hill, North Carolina

**Andrew M. Novick, M.D., Ph.D.**
Assistant Professor, Department of Psychiatry, University of Colorado—Anschutz Medical Campus, Aurora, Colorado

**Laura Obler, M.D.**
Resident, Department of Psychiatry, UCLA Semel Institute, Los Angeles, California

**Melisa Olgun, B.A.**
J.D. Candidate, Yale Law School, New Haven, Connecticut

**Lauren M. Osborne, M.D.**
Associate Professor of Psychiatry and Behavioral Sciences and of Gynecology and Obstetrics; Director, The Johns Hopkins Center for Women's Reproductive Mental Health; and Fellowship Director, Advanced Specialty Training Program in Reproductive Psychiatry, Johns Hopkins University School of Medicine, Baltimore, Maryland

**Jennifer J. Paul, Ph.D.**
Assistant Professor of Psychiatry; Clinical Director, Healthy Expectations Perinatal Mental Health Program; and Associate Director of Clinical Services, Connections Program for High-Risk Infants and Families, University of Colorado School of Medicine, Anschutz Medical Campus, Aurora, Colorado

**Jennifer L. Payne, M.D.**
Associate Professor, Departments of Psychiatry and Behavioral Sciences and Gynecology and Obstetrics, and Director, The Johns Hopkins Women's Mood Disorders Center, Johns Hopkins University School of Medicine, Baltimore, Maryland

**Chandni Prakash, M.D.**
Consultant Psychiatrist, Auckland District Health Board, Epsom, Auckland, New Zealand

**Madhumathi Rao, M.D.**
Attending Psychiatrist, MedStar Georgetown University Hospital, Washington, DC

**Eric Reed, M.D.**
Senior Clinical Instructor, University Hospitals, Case Western Reserve University College of Medicine, Cleveland, Ohio

**Surya Sabhapathy, M.D., M.P.H.**
Assistant Professor of Clinical Psychiatry, and Director, Gender and Sexuality Clinic in Psychiatry, University of Illinois at Chicago, Chicago, Illinois

**Jyoti Sachdeva, M.D.**
Associate Professor of Clinical Psychiatry, Department of Psychiatry and Behavioral Neuroscience, and Associate Professor of Clinical Obstetrics and Gynecology–Secondary Appointment, University of Cincinnati, Cincinnati, Ohio

**Ripal Shah, M.D., M.P.H.**
Clinical Assistant Professor, Department of Psychiatry and Behavioral Sciences, Stanford University School of Medicine; Attending Physician, Women's Wellness Clinic; Director of Integrative Mental Health, Stanford Center for Integrative Medicine, Stanford, California

**Neeta Shenai, M.D.**
Assistant Professor of Psychiatry, University of Pittsburgh Medical Center Western Psychiatric Hospital, Pittsburgh, Pennsylvania

**Sharvari P. Shivanekar, M.D.**
Clinical Assistant Professor, Department of Psychiatry, University of Pittsburgh School of Medicine, Pittsburgh, Pennsylvania

**Milena H. Smith, M.D., Ph.D.**
Instructor, Department of Psychiatry and Behavioral Sciences, The Johns Hopkins University School of Medicine, Baltimore, Maryland

**Lindsay R. Standeven, M.D.**
Assistant Professor of Psychiatry and Behavioral Sciences, and Assistant Director, Women's Mood Disorders Center, Johns Hopkins University School of Medicine, Baltimore, Maryland

**Celeste St. John-Larkin, M.D.**
Anschutz Chair in Perinatal Mental Health and Assistant Professor, Department of Psychiatry, University of Colorado School of Medicine; Medical Director, Healthy Expectations Program, Children's Hospital Colorado, Aurora, Colorado

**Lea Takács, Ph.D.**
Postdoctoral Research Scientist, Columbia University Irving Medical Center, New York, New York; Faculty of Arts, Department of Psychology, Charles University, Prague, Czech Republic

**Katherine Unverferth, M.D.**
Clinical Instructor, Department of Psychiatry, UCLA Resnick Neuropsychiatric Institute, The David Geffen School of Medicine at UCLA, Los Angeles, California

**Robin Valpey, M.D.**
Assistant Professor of Clinical Psychiatry, Department of Psychiatry, University of Pittsburgh Medical Center, Pittsburgh Pennsylvania

**Alexis Lighten Wesley, M.D.**
Child and Adolescent Psychiatry Fellow, Division of Psychiatry, Children's National Medical Center, Washington, DC

**Katherine E. Williams, M.D.**
Clinical Professor of Psychiatry, and Director, Women's Wellness Clinic, Stanford University School of Medicine, Stanford, California

**Katherine L. Wisner, M.D., M.S.**
Norman and Helen Asher Professor of Psychiatry and Behavioral Sciences and Obstetrics and Gynecology; Director, Asher Center for the Study and Treatment of Depressive Disorders, Northwestern University Feinberg School of Medicine, Chicago, Illinois

**Christine Wittmann, M.D.**
Assistant Professor of Psychiatry, Harvard Medical School; Associate Program Director, BIDMC Harvard Psychiatry Residency Training Program, Beth Israel Deaconess Medical Center, Boston, Massachusetts

**Mira Zein, M.D.**
Clinical Assistant Professor, Department of Psychiatry and Behavioral Sciences, Stanford University School of Medicine, Stanford, California

**Lulu Zhao, M.D.**
Assistant Professor, Department of Obstetrics and Gynecology; Clinical Assistant Professor, Department of Psychiatry, University Hospitals/Case Western Reserve University, School of Medicine, Cleveland, Ohio

## Disclosure of Interests

The following contributors have indicated financial interest in or other affiliation with a commercial supporter, manufacturer of commercial products, provider of commercial services, nongovernmental organization, and/or government agency, as listed.

**Catherine Birndorf, M.D.**
*Owner, CEO, and Medical Director:* Glenbervie Healthcare (d/b/a The Motherhood Center).

**Jessica L. Coker, M.D.**
Brain and Behavior Research Foundation; National Institute on Drug Abuse; Janssen Pharmaceuticals; Arkansas Children's Research Institute.

**C. Neill Epperson, M.D.**
*Consultant, Research, Speaker:* Sage Therapeutics. *Advisory Boards:* Asarina Pharma, Sage Therapeutics.
**Soudabeh Givrad, M.D.**
*Consultant:* Sage Therapeutics.
**Lucy A. Hutner, M.D.**
*Co-Founder:* Phoebe, Inc.
**Sheryl A. Kingsberg, Ph.D.**
*Consultant/Investigator/Scientific Advisory Board:* AMAG, Astellas, Daré, Duchesney, Ovoca, Lupin, Materna Medica, Mitsubishi Tanaba NA, Palatin Technologies, Pfizer, Sprout, Strategic Science Technologies. *Stock Options:* Materna Medica and Viveve. *Physician Education Group Board:* Ms. Medicine.
**Lauren M. Osborne, M.D.**
*Speaker:* Psychopharmacology Institute, March 2020.
**Jennifer L. Payne, M.D.**
*Patent:* "DNA Methylation Biomarkers of Postpartum Depression Risk" (No. 13851897.2-1403 PCT/US2013068241).
**Lea Takács, Ph.D.**
*Grants:* Fulbright Commission (Czech Republic); European Regional Development Fund-Project "Creativity and Adaptability as Conditions of the Success of Europe in an Interrelated World" (No. CZ.02.1.01/0.0/0.0/16_019/0000734).

# Foreword

Katherine L. Wisner, M.D., M.S.
Samantha Meltzer-Brody, M.D., M.P.H.

This book is a timely and much-needed contribution to the literature. Our most sincere thanks are due to these industrious and talented editors—Drs. Lauren Osborne, Lucy Hutner, Lisa Catapano, Sarah Nagle-Yang, and Katherine Williams—who have constructed this long-awaited and urgently needed *Textbook of Women's Reproductive Mental Health*. The commitment and passion of this group is inspiring! For far too long, this area of medical practice has fallen between the specialties of psychiatry, obstetrics and gynecology, and pediatrics. The result? Today, more than 20 years after the establishment of postresidency training in reproductive psychiatry, a comprehensive textbook of the field has yet to be published. This work was inspired by the National Curriculum on Reproductive Psychiatry (NCRP), a comprehensive educational resource that is free of charge and funded by the American Board of Psychiatry and Neurology (www.ncrptraining.org).

Why is this book important? Women develop mental health problems at significantly higher rates than men. The prevalence of any mental illness is higher among women (22.3%) than men (15.1%) (National Institute of Mental Health 2020). Young adults ages 18–25 years have the highest prevalence (25.8%) compared with adults ages 26–49 (22.2%) and 50+ years (13.8%). More women (47.6%) receive mental health services compared with men (34.8%). Women are twice as likely as men to develop major depressive disorder. Furthermore, 10%–15% of women experience depression during the perinatal period, which makes depression one of the most common complications of childbirth (Gaynes et al. 2005). These statistics illustrate that psychiatric disorders in women are common during the reproductive years and that the hormonal fluctuations associated with the reproductive life cycle contribute to the etiology of mental illness in women. Medical practitioners in all fields will encounter female patients with mental illness across the lifespan, particularly major depressive and anxiety disorders. Consequently, there is a great imperative for high-quality educational materials that increase the competency of providers.

Over the past decade, increasing advocacy, research, and health policy changes have underscored the need for clinicians with expertise in women's reproductive health. The shortage of psychiatrists in general and specifically those with expertise in reproductive mental health is a major public health concern. For example, most women with perinatal depression do not receive adequate screening nor treatment (Cox et al. 2016).

Few residency programs require any training in reproductive psychiatry. No consensus set of competencies or formal certification process exists. Given these significant gaps, The National Task Force on Women's Reproductive Mental Health was formed and subsequently urged residency training program directors to ensure that all psychiatrists acquire basic knowledge and skills in reproductive psychiatry (Osborne et al. 2015). This book is the resulting compendium of excellent up-to-date information to address that goal.

Reproductive events in women's lives are powerful experiences that change the course of health in both biological and psychosocial domains. As health care professionals, we must view these events as opportunities for engagement to improve short- and long-term health. They also compose a "natural longitudinal laboratory of women's reproductive health" (Wisner 2007) for hypothesis generation and research. The physiological noise that menstrual cycling, pregnancy, lactation, and menopause create in the interpretation of research data has been reconceptualized as an opportunity for elucidating the impact of reproductive function on brain health.

This outstanding work is divided into two parts. Part I provides a comprehensive overview of the reproductive life cycle and covers mental health concerns across the lifespan, including the relationship between gynecological and sexual health and mental health as well as infertility, the premenstrual period, and perimenopause. Part II is devoted to the perinatal period and offers a conceptual framework for a clinical approach to the pregnant and postpartum patient, followed by evidence-based reviews of the management of psychiatric disorders (by diagnostic category), as well as covering stress in pregnancy, infant mental health, and legal/forensic issues. The individual chapters are structured logically for continuity and consistency in information presentation. Critical summaries of the epidemiology, risk factors, screening methods, and clinical features are presented. Expert views of the impact of reproductive events on the clinical presentation are particularly salient.

This book must be required reading for all faculty and trainees who will care for women. This information must be part of the education of *all* mental health professionals. We strongly endorse this outstanding textbook. It is an overdue and very welcome tool to use in our training programs.

## References

Cox EQ, Sowa NA, Meltzer-Brody SE, Gaynes BN: The perinatal depression treatment cascade: baby steps toward improving outcomes. J Clin Psychiatry 77(9):1189–1200, 2016 27780317

Gaynes BN, Gavin N, Meltzer-Brody S, et al: Perinatal depression: prevalence, screening accuracy, and screening outcomes. Evid Rep Technol Assess (Summ) (119):1–8, 2005 15760246

National Institute of Mental Health: Mental illness, in Mental Health Information: Statistics. Bethesda, MD, National Institute of Mental Health, 2020. Available at: https://www.nimh.nih.gov/health/statistics/mental-illness.shtml. Accessed March 17, 2020.

Osborne LM, Hermann A, Burt V, et al: Reproductive psychiatry: the gap between clinical need and education. Am J Psychiatry 172(10):946–948, 2015 26423479

Wisner KL: The longitudinal laboratory of women's reproductive health, in Age and Gender Considerations in Psychiatric Diagnosis: A Research Agenda for DSM-V. Edited by Narrow WN, First MB, Regier D, Sirovatka P, et al. Washington, DC, American Psychiatric Publishing, 2007, pp 101–112

# Preface

This is a textbook of women's reproductive mental health. It is not meant to be a comprehensive look at all aspects of women's mental health but, rather, a look at the somewhat narrower field of reproductive psychiatry—the branch of medicine that encompasses the science and practice of treating mental, emotional, and behavioral disturbances related to female reproductive stages. It is the product of a remarkable volunteer effort representing the work of 83 specialists, including reproductive psychiatrists, obstetrician-gynecologists, and other specialists in women's health. Together, these authors represent more than 30 institutions across the United States and Canada.

This textbook is the first specifically in reproductive psychiatry, although it follows in the footsteps of the foundational text in women's mental health edited by Susan Kornstein and Anita Clayton nearly 20 years ago (Kornstein and Clayton 2004). This book appears at a moment when women's reproductive mental health is coming into its own as a discipline, with (at current count) 17 postresidency training programs and an extraordinary blossoming of interest among current psychiatry trainees. However, this textbook could not have come about without the changes in the research and clinical landscape that have occurred over the past 30+ years, changes that have removed women's health from the fringes of our profession. These changes can be charted back to 1985, when the Public Health Service called for the expansion of medical and behavioral research into conditions that were more prevalent in, or unique to, women (Kirschstein and Merritt 1985). The National Institutes of Health (1987) responded with a policy—later upgraded to a mandate in 1993—to include women in clinical research. These early landmark policies and the refinements that have occurred to them since (including a 2001 requirement that data be reported by sex and a 2014 requirement that preclinical research include animals of both sexes) (Arnegard et al. 2020; National Institutes of Health 2011) have resulted in a dramatic expansion of our knowledge base about how reproductive cycle transitions affect women's mental health.

Alongside this expansion of research, our field has seen the founding and growth of professional societies devoted to women's mental health or reproductive psychiatry. These include the International Society of Psychosomatic Obstetrics and Gynecology (founded in 1962), the International Marcé Society (founded in 1980), and the International Association for Women's Mental Health (founded in 2001), along with numerous national branches of these societies and independent local and regional groups. This time has also seen a number of key public policy initiatives in the United States, including statewide projects to combat perinatal depression (Schade et al. 2011) and requirements that all pregnant and postpartum women be screened for depression (Rhodes and Segre 2013). Clinical programs devoted to the field have burgeoned as well, with specialized inpatient units, mother–baby day hospitals, and numerous specialty outpatient practices in both academic centers and the community.

This growth in research, policy, and clinical programs has been gratifying, but it has been dismaying to realize that most psychiatrists receive no education, either during their training or afterward, in reproductive mental health. More than 50% of psychiatric patients are women, and more than 80% of women will experience at least one pregnancy (and nearly all will have menstrual cycles and go through menopause), yet most psychiatrists lack the knowledge of how these transitions affect mental health.

This textbook offers one tool for improving that knowledge base, and the textbook would not exist if not for the efforts of another extraordinary volunteer effort, the National Curriculum in Reproductive Psychiatry (www.ncrptraining.org), or NCRP. The NCRP was conceived at the Biennial Perinatal Mental Health meeting in 2013, when a group of academic psychiatrists came together to present a symposium on the current state of education in reproductive psychiatry. In the wake of that symposium, the presenters formed the National Task Force on Women's Reproductive Mental Health, with an agenda to research the current state of education in reproductive psychiatry and to move toward national standards. Informed by surveys of residency and fellowship directors, the task force identified six core knowledge areas for specialists in the field of reproductive psychiatry:

1. Relationship between reproductive cycle stages and psychopathology
2. Epidemiology, pathophysiology, and phenomenology of psychiatric disorders during pregnancy and the postpartum period, including pharmacokinetic changes
3. Treatment of perinatal disorders, including but not limited to psychopharmacology
4. Psychiatric symptoms related to infertility, pregnancy loss, birth trauma, and delivery of offspring with major health problems
5. Premenstrual mood disorders
6. Symptoms related to perimenopause

As we explored whether these topics were being covered in current residency training, it became apparent that most were not—and that the major barriers to teaching included lack of qualified faculty and lack of time (because reproductive psychiatry is not a specialty required by the Accreditation Council for Graduate Medical Education [ACGME]). It also became clear that residency programs would be unlikely to pay for the curriculum for a non-ACGME specialty and that other groups of learners (advanced-practice nurses, psychiatrists in general practice, obstetrician-gynecologists, and residents in other fields such as pediatrics and family medicine) would also benefit from this training. We therefore set out to create an interactive Web-based national curriculum, based on our competency guide, that could serve three purposes:

- To provide materials to be used in the classroom by nonexpert facilitators that could be freely adopted by any residency program in any specialty
- To provide self-study materials for trainees or doctors in general practice to learn materials on their own

- To provide rigorous continuing medical education assessments that, if taken together, could represent an examination of a trainee's knowledge in the entire field of reproductive psychiatry, with an eye toward certification and eventual subspecialty recognition

In 2017, the task force merged its curriculum efforts with those of Marcé of North America (formerly the Perinatal Mental Health Society, sponsor of the original conference where this idea was hatched), which had simultaneously been working on a fellowship-level curriculum. Together, we have created a curriculum that can be used in a modular fashion for residency education and in its entirety as a fellowship curriculum. The NCRP has won numerous educational awards, including the Educational Innovator Award from the Johns Hopkins Institute for Excellence in Education (2018) and the Scholarship in Teaching Award from Case Western Reserve University (2019), and has been funded by a Faculty Innovation in Education Award from the American Board of Psychiatry and Neurology.

## Structure

This textbook is a direct outgrowth of the NCRP. Many of its chapters have a parallel module in the curriculum, and lead authors of the curriculum were offered the first opportunity for lead authorship of the textbook chapters. We begin the book with a prefatory comment about the name (why we have chosen to focus on women). Thereafter, the book is divided into two parts. Part I covers reproductive mental health across the lifespan. It begins with a refresher chapter on the reproductive life cycle and then has chapters on the relationship between mental health and gynecological conditions, sexual health, contraception, and infertility and loss. The section concludes with chapters on premenstrual mood syndromes and perimenopause, which represent the two main reproductive transitions of women's lives outside of pregnancy. Part II, which comprises the bulk of the book, covers mental health in pregnancy and postpartum. We begin with two chapters that cover the clinical approach to women in these periods (one each for pregnancy and postpartum), and a short chapter on handling psychiatric emergencies. We then have chapters focusing on stress in pregnancy and attachment, two key concepts that undergird much of our understanding about the importance of treating mental health conditions in the perinatal period. Following are 11 chapters devoted to particular disorders in the perinatal period; each of these covers epidemiology, clinical presentation, pathophysiology, and treatment. We end with an overview of forensic issues as they apply to perinatal psychiatry. The Appendix contains a table with brief prescribing information for commonly used drugs, including information about pregnancy and lactation.

## Future Directions

It was only as we began to write and edit this book that we realized that, for every topic we included, we could have easily included two or three others. In our field of reproductive psychiatry, we are building the plane as we fly it. In that spirit, we hope that readers will consider this book a work in progress—a living document—much like our evolving specialty. At times, we were not able to include a topic that we recognize is important because we were unable to identify an expert to serve as lead author (personality disorders in the perinatal period is one example). We referenced—but were not able to expand upon—other topics, such as cognition, systems of care, policy and public health, psychology and specific psychotherapies, and resilience and coping. With yet other topics, we are witnessing a dynamic evolution in real time—such as the role of fathers and partners, LBGTQ+ families, racial and socioeconomic disparities, definitions of sex and gender, and even the basic neuroscience of pregnancy and the postpartum period. Any omission of a particular topic is our responsibility (and regret) entirely. We look forward to continuing to build on and consolidate our knowledge in the future. In particular, we hope to expand the reach of our efforts to other communities and the place of reproductive mental health within psychiatry. We are currently working with a group of obstetricians, for example, to adapt our curricular materials specifically for the obstetrics audience. We are working with national groups to advocate for awareness of, and policies that advance, women's mental health. We hope that, in the future, reproductive psychiatry will be included in the Milestones of psychiatric education and that our field will be officially recognized by the ACGME as a subspecialty of psychiatry.

## Acknowledgments

As an editing team, we are extraordinarily grateful to have had the chance to create this book. Our first and foremost thanks go to our patients and their loved ones. We have the honor of witnessing their resilience during some of the most deeply transformative moments of their lives. Their experiences form the heart and soul of this book.

We are also deeply grateful to the leadership of Laura Roberts, Erika Parker, and everyone on the team at American Psychiatric Association Publishing. They took an enormous leap of faith to support us in creating a comprehensive textbook in this emerging field. Jennifer Gilbreath was an outstanding manuscript editor who not only ensured that our grammar and style were consistent but also engaged with us intellectually and improved the book in many ways. We are also grateful to the original leadership of the task force that began this journey, which, along with Drs. Osborne and Nagle-Yang, included Laura Miller, Samantha Meltzer-Brody, Vivian Burt, Elizabeth Fitelson, Erin Murphy Barzilay, Alison Hermann, and Kara Driscoll. The leadership of Marcé of North America, and in particular Katherine Wisner and Crystal Clark, worked with us to incorporate our task force and curriculum within the organization and cheered our work. We are so thankful for the efforts of all of the authors of the NCRP. Many of them are represented in these pages, but some were unable to contribute; their work nevertheless served as an inspiration. We are especially grateful to the American Board of Psychiatry and Neurology for the funding that supported that curriculum.

We want to thank all the authors of this textbook and our incredible colleagues around the country and the world who joined us in this labor of love. Whether we are clinicians, researchers, educators, or policy advocates, we are drawn together by our commitment to improving the health and well-being of women and their loved ones throughout the reproductive lifespan. It would have been impossible to create this book but for the collaborative spirit of our colleagues in the field. Several individuals offered peer reviews of sections, including Bob Davies and Liisa Hantsoo, and we appreciate their contributions.

Although this text was created by authors across the country, Dr. Osborne's office at Johns Hopkins served as the coordinating center, and that staff deserves special thanks. Everyone at the Women's Mood Disorders Center helped at some point: Jennifer Payne, Liisa Hantsoo, Gina Grinstead, Samantha Meilman, Lindsay Standeven, Allison Craig, Meeta Pangtey, Joshua Kleiner, Amitoj Brar, and Jamie Archibong. We want to single out two people in particular at Johns Hopkins: David Rini created our beautiful illustrations, and Courtney Erdly—well, we cannot offer enough praise of and thanks for Courtney. Courtney joined Johns Hopkins as a research assistant when this project was in its infancy and quickly took on the project management of both the curriculum and the textbook. Without her incredible organizational skills, this book would still be in disparate parts scattered over redundant, vaguely named shared drives and on coffee-stained pages somewhere on our desks. She does it all with a smile (and whatever eyerolling she does, she keeps entirely to herself). We cannot thank her enough.

We all became specialists in reproductive psychiatry through a combination of scientific and clinical interests, but none of us would have completed that journey without the encouragement of those who came before us in this field. Beginning with Louis-Victor Marcé, who presented the first case series in modern times of mental illness in pregnant and postpartum women, several generations of women and men have led the advancement of knowledge in this field. We cannot name them all here, but we would like to single out those who had particular influences on each of us by serving as our individual mentors (most in women's mental health, but some in other fields): Theodore Stern, Felicia Smith, Peter Shapiro, Philip Muskin, Janis Cutler, Adam Brenner, Miriam Rosenthal, Laura Miller, Katherine Wisner, Maria Muzik, C. Neill Epperson, Catherine Birndorf, Elizabeth Fitelson, Kristen Leight, Catherine Monk, Jennifer Payne, Meg Chisolm, Samantha Meltzer-Brody, Regina Casper, and Natalie Rasgon.

Our field is all about giving women and their loved ones a voice. We also recognize the many voices throughout time and in this present day that have been silenced. We recognize the privilege and responsibility that comes with being able to put our words to paper—to have our voices count. In the words of Katherine Min (2018):

> Think of all the people who have lived and died without comment: prehistoric people who left behind no record beyond their own bones; millions of slaves, across all cultures and civilizations, who built the ego palaces of the rich, and the glory mansions to Gods that were no help to them in their lifetimes; peasants, laborers, servants; tillers of the soil, and cogs in the machinery of industry; indigenous peoples before there were non-indigenous: Native Americans, Aborigines, Aleuts and Inuits, Nubians and Berbers, Ainus and Ugyhurs.... It's hard not to feel humble before so many silent and inscrutable forebears. What can one possibly say to put up against the dignity of their mute passage? (Used with permission of Kollin Min. Full article available at https://therumpus.net/2018/11/writing-when-your-life-depends-on-it.)

Finally, we give our deepest thanks to our families, friends, and loved ones—in other words, our village. All of us took on this project while caring for small children, ill parents, or both, and our families have suffered from our absences and cheered our achievements. This book is dedicated to mothers and children everywhere, all of whom can be represented by our children:

Simeon Hutner
Julia Hutner
Benjamin Lieberman
Martha Lieberman
Aaron Lieberman
George Thabit
William Thabit
Peppin Thomas
Jasper Thomas
Chetty Thomas
Samson Yang
Franklin Yang
Walton Yang

*Lucy A. Hutner, M.D.*

*Lisa Catapano, M.D., Ph.D.*

*Sarah Nagle-Yang, M.D.*

*Katherine E. Williams, M.D.*

*Lauren M. Osborne, M.D.*

## References

Arnegard ME, Whitten LA, Hunter C, Clayton JA: Sex as a biological variable: a 5-year progress report and call to action. J Womens Health (Larchmt) 29(6):858–864, 2020 31971851

Kirschstein RL, Merritt DH: Women's health: report of the Public Health Service Task Force on Women's Health Issues. Public Health Rep 100(1):73–106, 1985 3918328

Kornstein SG, Clayton AH (eds): Women's Mental Health: A Comprehensive Textbook. New York, Guilford, 2004

Min K: Writing when your life depends on it. The Rumpus, November 6, 2018. Available at: https://therumpus.net/2018/11/writing-when-your-life-depends-on-it. Accessed September 15, 2020.

National Institutes of Health: NIH Guide for Grants and Contracts, Vol 16, No 3. Washington, DC, U.S. Department of Health and Human Services, 1987

National Institutes of Health: Inclusion of women and minorities in clinical research, in Title 42: The Public Health and Welfare. Washington, DC, Government Printing Office, 2011. Available at: https://www.govinfo.gov/app/details/USCODE-2010-title42/USCODE-2010-title42-chap6A-subchapIII-partH-sec289a-2/summary. Accessed September 15, 2020

NIH Revitalization Act of 1993 (Pub L 103-43)

Rhodes AM, Segre LS: Perinatal depression: a review of U.S. legislation and law. Arch Women Ment Health 16(4):259–270, 2013 23740222

Schade M, Miller L, Borst J, et al: Statewide innovations to improve services for women with perinatal depression. Nurs Womens Health 15(2):128–136, 2011 21504547

# Introduction

## What's in a Name? Why We Use "Women's Reproductive Mental Health," and Toward a Future of Different Names

Lucy A. Hutner, M.D.
Lisa A. Catapano, M.D., Ph.D.
Erika Kelley, Ph.D.
Sheryl A. Kingsberg, Ph.D.
Sarah M. Nagle-Yang, M.D.
Katherine E. Williams, M.D.
Lauren M. Osborne, M.D.

When we first proposed this textbook to the American Psychiatric Association, we editors (all of whom call ourselves reproductive psychiatrists or perinatal psychiatrists) were adamant that the title be reflective of the subject—mental illness that arises at moments of female reproductive transitions. This is not the same as women's mental health—women's mental health is a broader definition that includes our subject, the intersection of mental illness with female reproductive cycles—but also includes other categories, such as female sex (e.g., brain sexual dimorphism, female-specific comorbidities, pharmacokinetic sex differences) and female gender (e.g., gender roles, gender-linked trauma). "Reproductive psychiatry" or "reproductive mental health" alone would not do because this book does not address mental illness related to reproduction in men. "Women's reproductive mental health" seemed the most accurate term, but we are conscious of the fact that it may not long remain so. Definitions of "woman" are evolving rapidly in our society, and we recognize that many people assigned female sex at birth do not identify as women, that many people assigned male sex at birth DO identify as women, and that many people of both biological sexes identify as neither (Stroumsa and Wu 2018). The view that gender and sex can be categorized into two genetically fixed, nonoverlapping constructs has been swept away, and increasingly, our reliance on two culturally constructed categories is misleading and outdated (Hyde et al. 2019). As of the writing of this book, the data concerning mental illness at times of reproductive transition in people who are not cisgender women are extremely limited. We know little about either the biological or psychological effects on mental health of hormonal transitions for transgender men who choose to become pregnant, for example, or whether premenstrual mood symptoms present or are interpreted differently in nonbinary individuals than in cisgender women.

Although we are thus conscious that the resulting book is therefore focused primarily on the reproductive mental health of cisgender women, we are also confident that this will not always be the case. We hope and expect that subsequent editions will be able to incorporate more about people with gender-diverse identities and that one day there will be enough data for an additional book. Physicians have been writing about mental health associated with female reproductive transitions since the time of Hippocrates, and in the United States, it has been just over 20 years since the establishment of the first postdoctoral fellowship position in women's mental health, yet *this* is the first comprehensive textbook on the subject. It may be another 20 years before enough data accumulate for a whole textbook on reproductive mental health in people with gender-diverse identities, but we do not think it will be another *2,500* years.

That said, we have tried whenever possible to incorporate available data in the appropriate chapters and to use inclusive language and case examples. In addition, we would like to outline here some special considerations for those living with gender-diverse identities and for sexual minorities who face challenges not shared by other groups, as well as some basic definitions that may not be familiar to all readers and may be useful in understanding the subsequent chapters.

Research indicates that LGBTQ+ individuals may experience increased barriers to health care, including discrimination, stigmatization, and lack of provider knowledge about the health care needs for this population (Baptiste-Roberts et al. 2017; Chapman et al. 2012; Institute of Medicine 2011). Psychiatry providers should be familiar with guidelines for the health care of LGBTQ+ patients, such as those published by the Gay and Lesbian Medical Association (2005), The Joint Commission (2014), and the American Academy of Child and Adolescent Psychiatry (Adelson and American Academy of Child and Adolescent Psychiatry Committee on Quality Issues 2012).

The term *gender roles* refers to society's expectations regarding behaviors, traits, and attitudes according to one's sex assigned at birth. A patient's (or their partner's) expectations and attitudes toward gender roles may affect their sexual functioning (e.g., traditional gender norms reflect expectations that women should be sexually subservient to men). *Gender identity* reflects how one identifies one's own gender, such as male, female, transgender, or nonbinary. It is influenced by socially defined constructs, and it is increasingly apparent that there may be a heritable biological component as well (Polderman et al. 2018). *Sexual orientation* refers to one's pattern of emotional and physical arousal and the gender(s) of persons to whom one is sexually or physically attracted. *Sexual identity* refers to individuals' assessment of their own sexual orientation (e.g., lesbian, gay, bisexual, questioning or queer) (Levine and Committee on Adolescence 2013). Sexual orientation and sexual identity are unrelated to gender identity.

Providers working with transgender individuals should be familiar with the World Professional Association for Transgender Health (2012) standards of care. Transgender individuals seeking gender-affirming therapy (e.g., feminizing or masculinizing hormone therapy, surgery) require referrals from mental health providers, which is described further in the standards of care document. Psychotherapy is not an absolute requirement for hormone therapy and surgery, although it is highly recommended. Mental health professionals working with individuals seeking or undergoing gender-affirming therapy (e.g., hormone therapy, surgery) should be aware of the benefits and risks of these therapies on mental health and sexual function.

Part of the criteria for recommendation for gender-affirming therapy is persistent, well-documented gender dysphoria (World Professional Association for Transgender Health 2012). *Gender dysphoria* in adolescents and adults is typically defined as a distressing, marked incongruence or discrepancy between one's gender identity and one's sex assigned at birth and the gender role, primary sex characteristics, or secondary sex characteristics associated with that sex (American Psychiatric Association 2013; Knudson et al. 2010). DSM-5 (American Psychiatric Association 2013) includes specific criteria for the diagnosis of gender dysphoria. Despite some controversy regarding gender dysphoria as a diagnosis (e.g., potential stigmatizing or overpathologizing effect) (Davies and Davies 2020), the diagnostic label was changed from *gender identity disorder* to reduce the potential stigmatizing effect, and the diagnosis was retained in part to acknowledge the full impact of dysphoria and to increase access to gender-affirming services (e.g., billing requirements) (Byne et al. 2018).

Sexual identity can be fluid and dynamic across time (Diamond 2008). Thus, clinicians should be careful not to make assumptions about patients' sexual behavior or about their family planning or reproductive health care needs based on their described gender or sexual identity. For example, many women who have sex with women also report having had sex with men (Diamond 2008). Discussion of issues such as contraception, risk for pregnancy and sexually transmitted infections, and accessing services for third-party involvement in reproduction (e.g., gestational carrier) or adoption is still relevant to women who have sex with women, as well as for trans men (who may continue to have vaginal intercourse with men) and for trans women, who have disproportionately high rates of HIV (Baral et al. 2013). Research regarding rates and phenomenology of sexual dysfunction among LGBTQ+ persons is scarce, although it remains important to assess sexual functioning in this population with consideration of the biopsychosocial model. Notably, LGBTQ+ individuals experience greater rates of victimization and mental health concerns (e.g., depression, anxiety) (Institute of Medicine 2011), which can negatively affect sexual function. Additional sexuality considerations across female reproductive milestones are outlined in the following discussion.

## Puberty

Approximately 8% of U.S. teenagers identify as lesbian, gay, or bisexual (Kann et al. 2016). Uncertainty about sexual orientation decreases with age. As noted, sexual identity can be fluid across time, and many adolescents engage in sexual experimentation with same-sex and opposite-sex partners (Diamond 2008; McCabe et al. 2011). Moreover, females ages 16–20 years are at greatest risk for dating violence, including sexual victimization, and gender-nonconforming individuals are at greater risk for victimization (Coker et al. 2010).

## Pregnancy and Postpartum

Individuals with minority identities are at greater risk for preterm birth and lower birth weight babies (Institute of Medicine 2011). Pregnancy history and health should not be overlooked in women who identify as LGBTQ+; a meta-analysis indicated that although lesbian women have lower rates of pregnancies than heterosexual women, estimates of pregnancy rates (including via assisted reproductive technology) among lesbian women range from 9.9% (previous births in women who exclusively have sex with women) to 37% (lesbian women who were ever pregnant) (Hodson et al. 2017). Transgender individuals who are going through gender-affirming therapy would also likely benefit from counseling on its potential effects on reproductive health, which may affect decision making regarding gender-affirming therapy or family building (World Professional Association for Transgender Health 2012). Transgender individuals who are pregnant may experience fluidity of gender identity or experience dysphoria with bodily changes in pregnancy. Transgender individuals may also benefit from counseling and resources for chest (breast) feeding (Obedin-Maliver and Makadon 2016).

## Menopause

The fluidity of sexual identity spans time and age, including in the postmenopausal stage. Providers should take care not to make assumptions about sexuality due to age and should be aware of the intersections of LGBTQ+ identity and aging (Garnets and Peplau 2006). For transgender individuals, the menopausal transition may be met with experiences of dysphoria associated with physiological and hormonal changes. Individuals who are interested in gender-affirming hormone therapy would benefit from education regarding the role of aging in such therapy. For example, trans women may experience decreased effectiveness of hormone therapy either due to long-term masculinizing effects of testosterone or when lower doses of feminizing therapy are indicated due to increased medical contraindications associated with age (Dahl et al. 2006). For trans men, the initiation of gender-affirming testosterone therapy is associated with some symptoms of menopause at any age (although trans men receiving testosterone therapy may also remain fertile) (Moravek 2018).

Although the challenges noted here for the LGBTQ+ population at different reproductive stages are distinct, this population is, of course, subject to many of the same mental health concerns as cisgender heterosexual women, and we therefore hope that what follows will be useful to providers treating all people who undergo reproductive transitions associated with female reproductive hormones, no matter how they identify themselves.

## References

Adelson SL, American Academy of Child and Adolescent Psychiatry Committee on Quality Issues: Practice parameter on gay, lesbian, or bisexual sexual orientation, gender nonconformity, and gender discordance in children and adolescents. J Am Acad Child Adolesc Psychiatry 51(9):957–974, 2012

American Psychiatric Association: Diagnostic and Statistical Manual of Mental Disorders, 5th Edition. Arlington, VA, American Psychiatric Association, 2013

Baptiste-Roberts K, Oranuba E, Werts N, Edwards LV: Addressing health care disparities among sexual minorities. Obstet Gynecol Clin North Am 44(1):71–80, 2017 28160894

Baral SD, Poteat T, Strömdahl S, et al: Worldwide burden of HIV in transgender women: a systematic review and meta-analysis. Lancet Infect Dis 13(3):214–222, 2013 23260128

Byne W, Karasic DH, Coleman E, et al: Gender dysphoria in adults: an overview and primer for psychiatrists. Transgend Health 3(1):57–70, 2018 29756044

Chapman R, Wardrop J, Zappia T, et al: The experiences of Australian lesbian couples becoming parents: deciding, searching and birthing. J Clin Nurs 21(13–14):1878–1885, 2012 22554189

Coker TR, Austin SB, Schuster MA: The health and health care of lesbian, gay, and bisexual adolescents. Annu Rev Public Health 31:457–477, 2010 20070195

Dahl M, Feldman JL, Goldberg JM, Jaberi A: Physical aspects of transgender endocrine therapy. International Journal of Transgenderism 9(3–4):111–134, 2006

Davies RD, Davies ME: The (slow) depathologizing of gender incongruence. J Nerv Ment Dis 208(2):152–154, 2020 31977826

Diamond LM: Sexual Fluidity: Understanding Women's Love and Desire. Cambridge, MA, Harvard University Press, 2008

Garnets L, Peplau LA: Sexuality in the lives of aging lesbian and bisexual women, in Lesbian, Gay, Bisexual, and Transgender Aging: Research and Clinical Perspectives. Edited by Kimmel D, Rose T, David S. New York, Columbia University Press, 2006, pp 70–90

Gay and Lesbian Medical Association: Guidelines for Care of Lesbian, Gay, Bisexual, and Transgender Patients. Washington, DC, Gay and Lesbian Medical Association, 2005. Available at: http://www.glma.org/_data/n_0001/resources/live/GLMA%20guidelines%202006%20FINAL.pdf. Accessed October 31, 2019.

Hodson K, Meads C, Bewley S: Lesbian and bisexual women's likelihood of becoming pregnant: a systematic review and meta-analysis. BJOG 124(3):393–402, 2017 27981741

Hyde JS, Bigler RS, Joel D, et al: The future of sex and gender in psychology: five challenges to the gender binary. Am Psychol 74(2):171–193, 2019 30024214

Institute of Medicine: The Health of Lesbian, Gay, Bisexual, and Transgender People: Building a Foundation for Better Understanding. Washington, DC, National Academies Press, 2011

The Joint Commission: Advancing Effective Communication, Cultural Competence, and Patient- and Family-Centered Care for the Lesbian, Gay, Bisexual, and Transgender (LGBT) Community: A Field Guide. Oak Brook, IL, The Joint Commission, 2014. Available at: https://www.jointcommission.org/lgbt. Accessed October 31, 2019.

Kann L, Olsen EO, McManus T, et al: Sexual identity, sex of sexual contacts, and health-related behaviors among students in grades 9–12—United States and selected sites, 2015. MMWR Surveill Summ 65(9):1–202, 2016 27513843

Knudson G, De Cuypere G, Bockting W: Recommendations for revision of the DSM diagnoses of gender identity disorders: consensus statement of The World Professional Association for Transgender Health. International Journal of Transgenderism 12(2):115–118, 2010

Levine DA, Committee on Adolescence: Office-based care for lesbian, gay, bisexual, transgender, and questioning youth. Pediatrics 132(1):e297–e313, 2013 23796737

McCabe J, Brewster KL, Tillman KH: Patterns and correlates of same-sex sexual activity among U.S. teenagers and young adults. Perspect Sex Reprod Health 43(3):142–150, 2011 21884381

Moravek MB: Gender-affirming hormone therapy for transgender men. Clin Obstet Gynecol 61(4):687–704, 2018 30285972

Obedin-Maliver J, Makadon HJ: Transgender men and pregnancy. Obstet Med 9(1):4–8, 2016

Polderman TJC, Kreukels BPC, Irwig MS, et al: The biological contributions to gender identity and gender diversity: bringing data to the table. Behav Genet 48(2):95–108, 2018 29460079
Stroumsa D, Wu JP: Welcoming transgender and nonbinary patients: expanding the language of "women's health." Am J Obstet Gynecol 219(6):585.e1–585.e5, 2018 30267652
World Professional Association for Transgender Health: Standards of care for the health of transsexual, transgender, and gender-nonconforming people. International Journal of Transgenderism 13(4):165–232, 2012

# PART I

## Reproductive Health Across the Lifespan

# CHAPTER 1

# The Reproductive Life Cycle

Alexis Lighten Wesley, M.D.
Mira Zein, M.D.
Melisa Olgun, B.A.
Lisa A. Catapano, M.D., Ph.D.

Most of the chapters in this textbook are focused on the bidirectional relationship between mental health and reproductive hormone transitions. Readers already familiar with such transitions can proceed directly to those chapters. For readers who are not familiar, this chapter offers an overview of the physiology of the reproductive life cycle, an understanding of which is critical to the overall understanding of women's mental health. This chapter focuses on the basic physiology of reproductive transitions, including descriptions of the menstrual cycle, the stages of pregnancy, labor and delivery, the postpartum period, lactation, and menopause. Each subsection covers the biological changes that define these physiological stages and their clinical impact.

## Menstrual Cycle

### Menarche

*Menarche*, defined as the first occurrence of menstruation, plays an integral role in women's health. Menarche is achieved through regulated coordination between the hypothalamus, pituitary systems, and female reproductive structures.

### Hypothalamic-Pituitary-Gonadal Axis

The hypothalamus plays a critical role in the production and regulation of reproductive hormones. Gonadotropin-releasing hormone (GnRH), produced and released in a pulsatile fashion by the hypothalamus, stimulates the anterior pituitary to release the gonadotropins—luteinizing hormone (LH) and follicle-stimulating hormone (FSH)—that are instrumental in the production of two ovarian hormones, estrogen and progesterone (Figure 1–1).

With the exception of brief periods in early embryonic and postnatal stages of life, during which it is thought to be active, the hypothalamic-pituitary-gonadal (HPG) axis is quiescent throughout childhood, likely through a primarily inhibitory mechanism (Abreu and Kaiser 2016). Pubertal maturation is initiated first by *adrenarche*, which is the reemergence of adrenal production, and subsequently by the reactivation of the HPG axis through a sustained increase in the pulsatile release of GnRH (Hoyt and Falconi 2015). Although the mechanism underlying the reactivation of the HPG axis is still under investigation, the inhibitory neurotransmitter GABA is thought to play a role, in conjunction with stimulatory and nutrition-dependent factors such as neuropeptide Y, kisspeptin, and glutamate (Emans and Laufer 2011).

GnRH, also known as the pulse generator, is formed in the preoptic area of the hypothalamus and is secreted from the axon terminal in the median eminence in the aforementioned pulsatile fashion required for pituitary-gonadal activation (Abreu and Kaiser 2016). LH and FSH are subsequently released in similar fashion. The significance of the pulsatile nature of GnRH release is evident because gonadotropin secretion is restored to persons lacking endogenous GnRH only when it is administered in a pulsatile fashion (Ferin 2008). GnRH administered continuously, without pulsatile release, results in decreased levels of LH and FSH (Ferin 2008).

The primary effect of FSH and LH in the menstrual cycle is the development of follicles in the ovaries (Figure 1–2) (Gabbe et al. 2017). Theca cells in the ovary produce androgen precursors when stimulated by LH, whereas granulosa cells in the ovary stimulated by FSH increase the production of the enzyme aromatase, which converts androgen precursors into estrogen. The ovaries additionally produce peptides that, in addition to the androgens, trigger a feedback loop that targets both the hypothalamus and the pituitary, affecting the frequency and amplitude of GnRH release and the amount of gonadotropins released (Emans and Laufer 2011).

## Phases of the Menstrual Cycle

The ovarian cycle occurs, on average, every 28 days, and sequentially follows the patterns of follicular growth (the follicular phase), ovulation, and the successive formation and degeneration of the corpus luteum (the luteal phase) (Goodman 2003) (Figure 1–3).

### Follicular Phase

The process of follicular growth in the ovary begins before birth; by midgestation, the female fetus already has close to 7 million germ cells, which regress to 1–2 million primordial follicles by the time of birth. More than half of these will degenerate during the quiescent phase prior to puberty. After puberty, follicles gradually develop into primary, secondary, and tertiary (early antral) follicles, each over the course of about 1 year (Cox and Takov 2020). During the follicular phase, a subset of tertiary follicles during each menstrual cycle is recruited to evade the atretic process, further develop, and potentially ovulate (Ferin 2008) (Figure 1–4).

FSH levels begin to rise toward the end of the previous cycle and are at their highest during the first week of the follicular phase (which begins on the first day of menses).

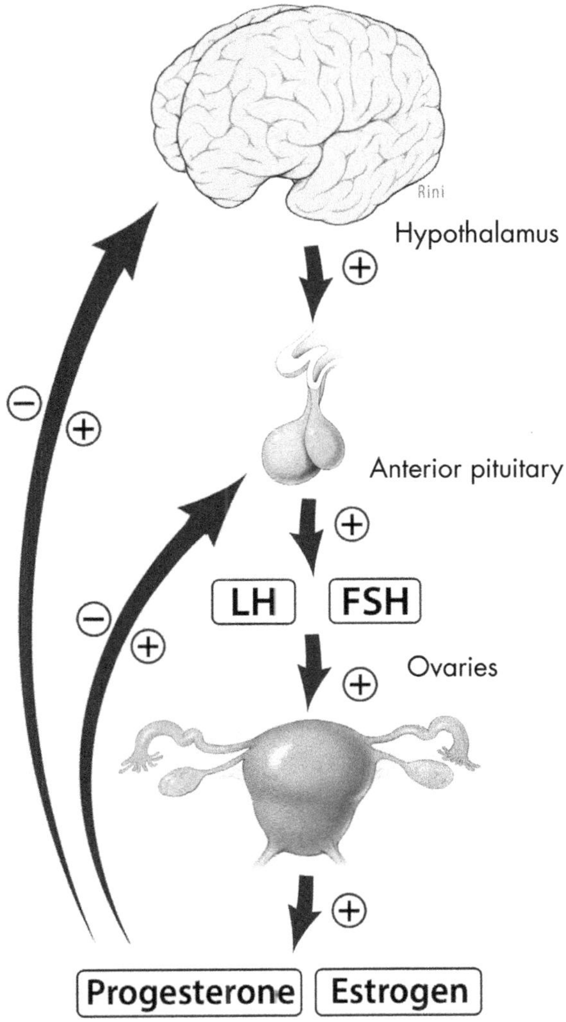


**FIGURE 1–1. The hypothalamic-pituitary-gonadal axis.**
FSH=follicle-stimulating hormone; LH=luteinizing hormone.
*Source.* Image by David Rini.

Estrogen and progesterone are at low levels during the early follicular phase; this means a lack of negative feedback to the hypothalamus, which thus increases pulsatile release of GnRH, resulting in increasing levels of FSH (Chou et al. 2021). With the presence of FSH, granulosa cells hypertrophy and divide, increasing estrogen; FSH also induces the aromatase enzyme to convert androgens to estradiol (Goodman 2003). Estradiol further amplifies the effects of FSH by increasing the number of FSH receptors; meanwhile, LH promotes androgen synthesis through induction of the theca cells.

By days 5–7 of the menstrual cycle, a dominant follicle emerges and exerts negative feedback on the other developing follicles (Emans and Laufer 2011). Meanwhile, elevated estrogen levels stimulate the growth of the endometrium in the uterus by increased production of glandular and stroma cells. This process is known as the *proliferative phase* of the uterine cycle and coincides with the follicular phase of the ovar-

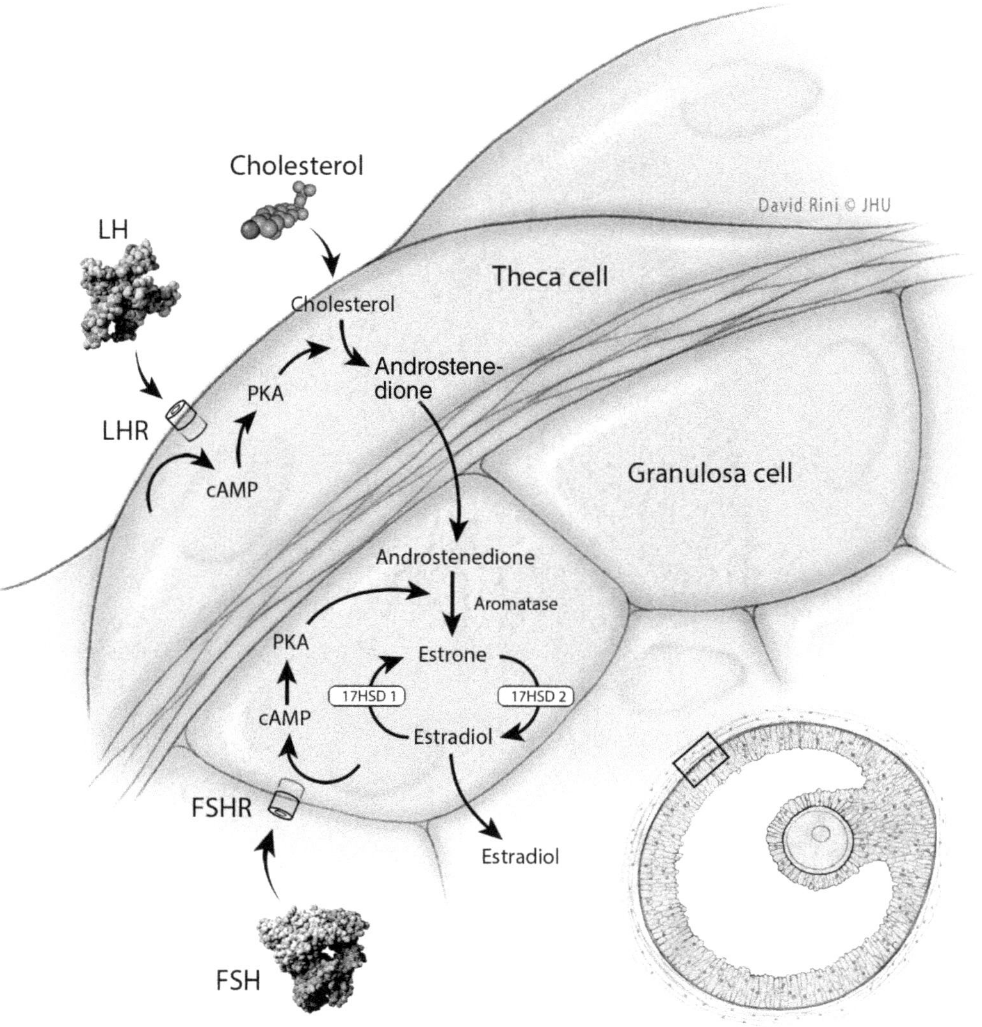


**FIGURE 1–2. Actions provoked by luteinizing hormone (LH) and follicle stimulating hormone (FSH) during the follicular phase.**
cAMP=cyclic adenosine monophosphate; FSHR=follicle-stimulating hormone receptor; LHR=luteinizing hormone receptor; PKA=protein kinase A.
*Source.* Image by David Rini.

ian cycle. Additional changes to the reproductive tract triggered by elevated estrogen levels include increased cilia formation and muscular wall contractility in the oviducts; increased growth of the myometrium and watery secretions from the cervical glands; and increased epithelial proliferation and glycogen deposition of the vagina (Goodman 2003).

By mid–follicular phase, FSH is beginning to decline, partially due to negative feedback by estradiol and inhibin on the hypothalamus and pituitary (Chou et al. 2021). By the late follicular phase, estradiol makes a sudden switch from negative to positive feedback, promoting increased release of FSH and LH by the anterior pituitary (Chou et al. 2021). LH rises 10-fold during the "LH surge" that triggers ovulation (Gabbe et al. 2017).

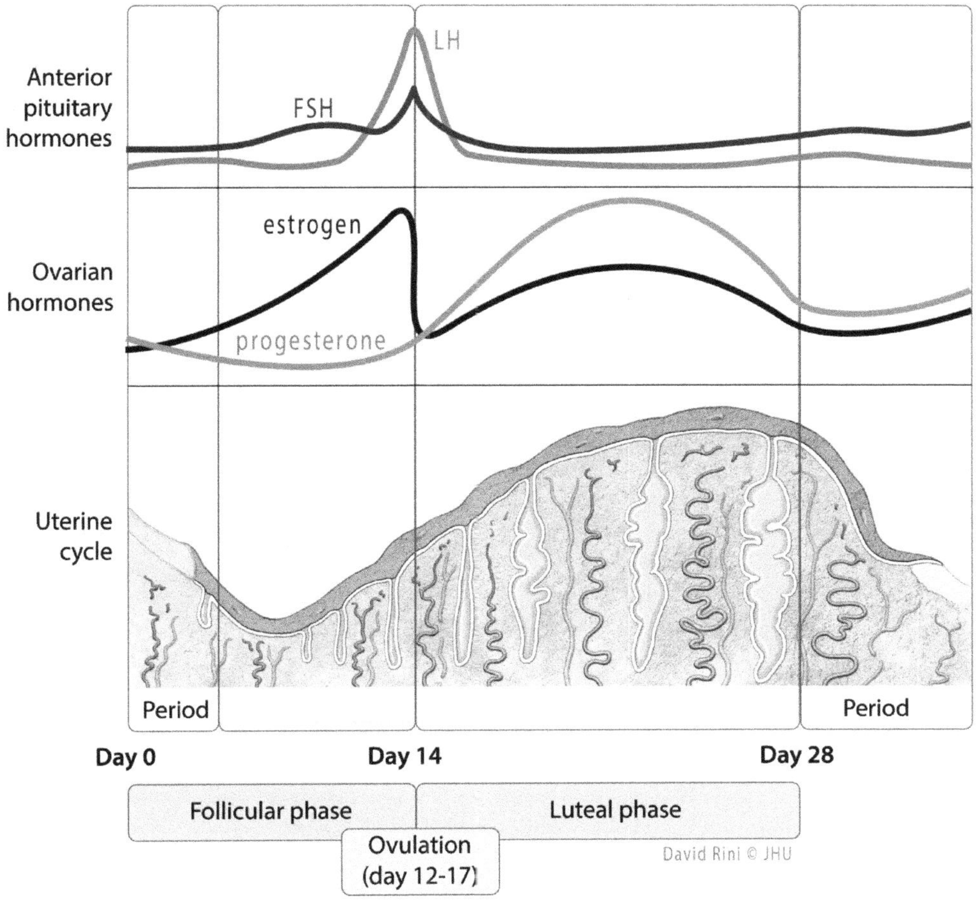


**FIGURE 1–3. The menstrual and uterine cycles.**
FSH=follicle-stimulating hormone; LH=luteinizing hormone.
*Source.* Image by David Rini.

## Ovulation

The mechanism underlying ovulation is thought to be related to the activation of proteolytic enzymes and prostaglandins that digest the collagen within the follicular wall, leading to follicular rupture and expulsion of the ovum (Reed and Carr 2018). This process is initiated by the downstream cascade of the intracellular second messenger cyclic adenosine monophosphate in the theca and granulosa cells as a result of elevated LH (Goodman 2003).

## Luteal Phase

The luteal phase immediately follows ovulation and is characterized by the formation of the corpus luteum from the dominant follicle after it releases the ovum. The dominant follicle is transformed into the corpus luteum, whose purpose is to prepare the uterine lining for pregnancy and relax uterine smooth muscle. The primary product of the corpus luteum in the luteal phase is progesterone. The corpus luteum typically achieves maturity by 8–9 days after ovulation (day 22–23 of the ovarian cycle) (Ferin 2008). Progesterone, and estrogen to a lesser degree, produced by the corpus luteum

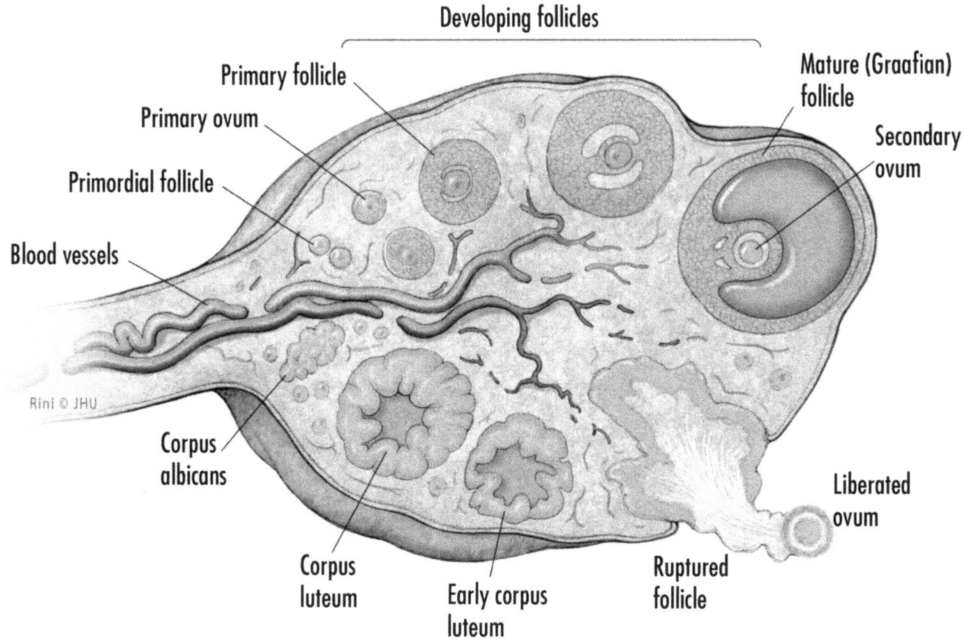


**FIGURE 1–4.** Follicle maturation.
*Source.* Image by David Rini.

promotes vascularization and thickening of the endometrial lining (called the *secretory phase* of the uterine cycle) in preparation for pregnancy.

When fertilization and implantation do not occur in the luteal phase, progesterone and inhibin reach their peak and inhibit further release of FSH and LH from the anterior pituitary. In the absence of FSH and LH, the corpus luteum begins to atrophy, and progesterone levels fall off. This triggers shedding of the endometrial lining, represented by day 1 of the next cycle (Gabbe et al. 2017). The endometrium releases prostaglandins that induce uterine smooth muscle contraction and sloughing of the endometrial tissue. Falling levels of progesterone and estrogen lead to a rise in FSH during the last few days of the menstrual cycle in preparation for follicle recruitment in the next cycle (Reed and Carr 2018).

## Pregnancy

The three trimesters of pregnancy are delineated as the first trimester (0–12 weeks), second trimester (13–27 weeks), and third trimester (28–40 weeks). These 40 weeks are counted from the first day of the last menstrual period; thus, on the day that a woman's next period is due, she is considered 4 weeks pregnant even though she is only 2 weeks past ovulation (and thus 2 weeks past the likely date of conception) (Chou et al. 2021).

During the three trimesters of pregnancy, a number of physiological changes occur that have profound effects on the woman, including on her mental health. Some of these physical changes can induce or mimic psychiatric symptoms (described later). Importantly, many of these changes also affect the pharmacokinetics of psychiatric medications. Considerable evidence of such effects is available for some drug classes, but for other classes almost no information is available. Moreover, little is known about whether such changes impact drug efficacy or side effects, and no guidelines exist for altering psychiatric drug dosages in pregnancy (Pariente et al. 2016). (Further details about known drug effects can be found in the specific sections that follow, as well as in Chapter 8, "A Clinical Approach to Psychiatric Diagnosis and Treatment During Pregnancy," and the individual disorder chapters.)

## Systemic Physiological Changes

### Weight Gain

The mean gestational weight gain for a woman of normal weight carrying a full-term infant is typically 22–36 lb. Although recommendations have fluctuated over the past several decades, current recommendations are based on BMI. For instance, women considered underweight prior to pregnancy (BMI $<18.5$ kg/m$^2$) are recommended to gain between 28 and 40 lb, whereas women considered obese prior to pregnancy (BMI $>30$ kg/m$^2$) are recommended to gain between 11 and 20 lb (Gabbe et al. 2017).

High pre-pregnancy BMI and too much or too little weight gain during pregnancy have been correlated with preterm birth (Mitanchez and Chavatte-Palmer 2018). The correlation between obesity and preterm birth may differ according to race or ethnicity, and such differences may explain some of the racial disparity in preterm birth and maternal morbidity rates (Liu et al. 2019). For some women, changes in weight and shape across pregnancy are associated with feelings of low self-worth and low mood.

### Sleep

Most pregnant women (66%–94%; Gabbe et al. 2017) report experiencing alterations in sleep patterns that lead to a subjective perception of poor sleep quality. Sleep-disordered breathing, insomnia, and sleep apnea all occur at elevated rates in pregnant women, and these may contribute to pregnancy complications such as hypertensive disorders and fetal growth restriction (Gabbe et al. 2017). Pregnant women experience varying changes in sleep patterns across the three trimesters of pregnancy. In the first trimester, women tend to experience an increase in total sleep time, including the time spent taking naps. Women can also expect an increase in daytime sleepiness and increased nocturnal insomnia during this trimester. In the second trimester, although total sleep time normalizes overall, women may experience increased awakenings. Finally, in the third trimester, total sleep time declines; women experience increases in insomnia, nocturnal awakenings, and daytime sleepiness (Gabbe et al. 2017; Santiago et al. 2001).

Sleep difficulties during pregnancy often extend through the first 2 months postpartum (Cunningham et al. 2014), when they are further complicated by a newborn's erratic sleep patterns. Various studies have provided data on racial disparities in sleep in the general population. Black adults in the United States show significantly shorter duration and poorer-quality sleep than other racial or ethnic groups, and literature links sleep disruption to the disparity in cardiometabolic disease (Curtis et al. 2017). In pregnancy, Black women have been found to have higher short sleep prevalence compared with white women (Feinstein et al. 2020). Black women may also have different patterns of inflammation related to poor sleep than white women (Carroll et al. 2020), and poor sleep and associated inflammation may mediate the relationship between race and preterm birth (Blair et al. 2015). Significant evidence is available about the relationship between disrupted sleep and psychiatric symptoms in the perinatal period. For details, see Chapter 9, "A Clinical Approach to Psychiatric Diagnosis and Treatment in the Postpartum Period," and Chapter 19, "Anxiety Disorders and Insomnia in the Perinatal Period."

# Physiological Changes by Organ System

## Endocrine System

**Reproductive hormones.** Human chorionic gonadotropin (hCG) levels remain high throughout pregnancy, returning to nonpregnant values at about 2–4 weeks postpartum, although they can take longer (Betz and Fane 2020; Reyes et al. 1985). Estrogen (in the form of estradiol) is produced first by the corpus luteum and subsequently by the placenta, and the level overall rises throughout pregnancy. Consequences of increased estrogen include suppression of the hypothalamic-pituitary-adrenal (HPA) axis and of menstruation. Concurrently, progesterone promotes pregnancy in numerous ways, including preparing the endometrial lining, modifying the maternal immune system, decreasing contractility of the smooth muscle, and inhibiting lactation (Gabbe et al. 2017). The neuroactive metabolites of progesterone, 5α-dihydroprogesterone and allopregnanolone, act centrally on $GABA_A$ receptors (McEvoy et al. 2018). Clinically, by amplifying the actions of GABA, the neuroactive metabolites play a role in suppressing oxytocin, a hormone involved in lactation and parturition (Russell and Brunton 2009). Levels of estrogen and progesterone decrease dramatically immediately after delivery but may not return completely to normal levels until about 6 months after delivery.

The high levels of estrogen and progesterone keep LH, FSH, and gonadotropins low throughout pregnancy, and they remain low for the first few weeks postpartum. The return of ovulation generally occurs 4–6 weeks after delivery, but in breastfeeding women, ovulation is inhibited by elevated prolactin stimulated by the newborn's suckling mechanism. Increased levels of prolactin suppress the pulsatile release of GnRH, which in turn suppresses LH and contributes to inhibition of ovulation and amenorrhea (Cunningham et al. 2014; Gabbe et al. 2017). Estrogen levels are also decreased for a longer period of time postpartum in lactating women (Gabbe et al. 2017).

The extent to which GnRH is suppressed, delaying the resumption of both ovulation and menstruation, is affected by the intensity of breastfeeding and the maternal metabolic or nutritional integrity (World Health Organization Task Force on Methods for the Natural Regulation of Fertility 1998). When the frequency of breastfeeding is maintained at more than eight episodes per day, along with suckling episodes lasting longer than 7 minutes, prolactin levels are likely to remain elevated, and ovarian function continues to be inactive. For breastfeeding women with poor nutritional status, lactational energy demands may not be met, which can prolong GnRH suppression (World Health Organization Task Force on Methods for the Natural Regulation of Fertility 1998).

The mean reinstitution of ovulation for breastfeeding women is approximately 6 months, but menstruation can be delayed as long as 36 months (Gabbe et al. 2017). Maternal biological variations can also contribute to the onset of ovulation and men-

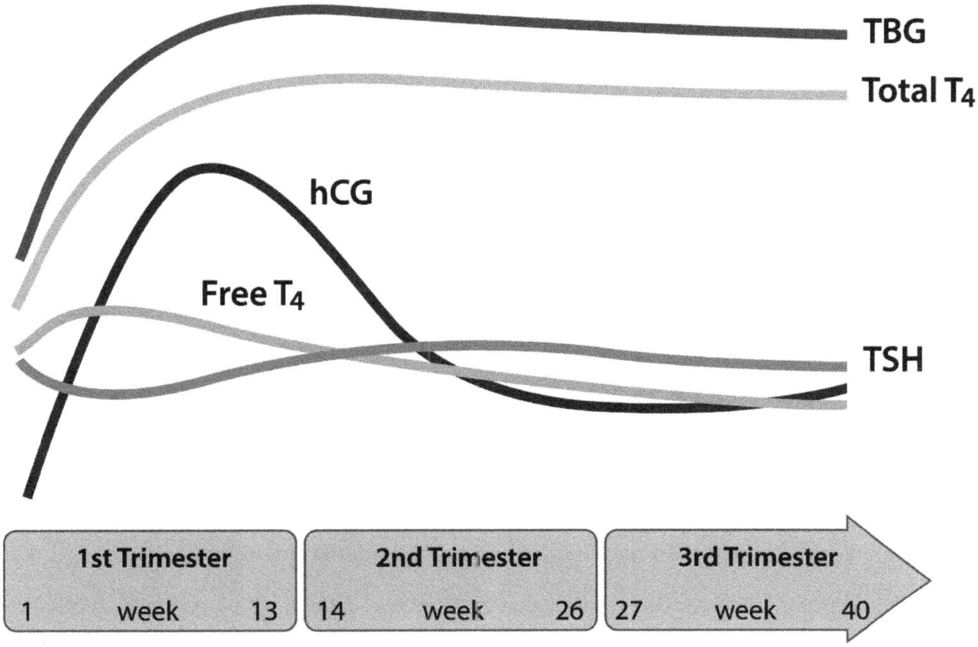


**FIGURE 1–5. Changes in the thyroid system across pregnancy.**
hCG=human chorionic gonadotropin; $T_4$=thyroxine; TBG=thyroid-binding globulin; TSH=thyroid-stimulating hormone.

struation postpartum; therefore, it is important to emphasize the variability of both ovulation and postpartum bleeding (bleeding can occur without ovulation, and ovulation can occur without menstruation). These fluctuations in reproductive hormones during the postpartum period may contribute to affective dysregulation, most likely associated with the period immediately following delivery or with weaning (Burke et al. 2019; Schiller et al. 2015).

**Thyroid gland.** Pregnancy induces significant changes in the thyroid gland and its function (Gabbe et al. 2017). Normal pregnancy-related changes include an increase in renal iodine excretion (resulting in recommendations for increased iodine supplementation in developed countries), an increase in thyroid-binding globulin, an increase in the production of the thyroid hormones triiodothyronine ($T_3$) and thyroxine ($T_4$), and suppression of thyroid-stimulating hormone (TSH) (Alexander et al. 2017; Glinoer et al. 1990). Such physiological changes ultimately result in increased levels of total $T_4$ and total $T_3$ during pregnancy, whereas levels of free $T_4$ and free $T_3$ remain relatively normal (Glinoer et al. 1990). Remarkably, these myriad physiological changes occur effortlessly in healthy pregnant women (Figure 1–5); however, thyroid dysfunction can occur during pregnancy, and its evaluation is complicated by challenges in the accurate assessment of laboratory testing in the pregnant patient (Alexander et al. 2017; Gabbe et al. 2017).

Although routine screening for thyroid dysfunction has been debated in the literature, it is not currently endorsed by the American College of Obstetricians and Gynecologists, the American Thyroid Association, or the Endocrine Society (Committee on Patient Safety and Quality Improvement and Committee on Professional Liability

2007; Stagnaro-Green et al. 2011; Surks et al. 2004). Presently, the recommended approach is a targeted screening process that considers risk factors for thyroid dysfunction, including family or personal history of thyroid disease, morbid obesity, use of lithium, age >30 years, and prior head or neck radiation (Melmed et al. 2019).

Psychiatrists may want to measure thyroid function to rule out thyroid dysfunction in patients with depressive or anxiety symptoms or previously known thyroid disease. It is important to use population-based, trimester-specific reference ranges for TSH and free or total $T_4$ (Alexander et al. 2017). The first choice is a laboratory-specific pregnancy range that accounts for the characteristics of the population (Korevaar 2018). If that is not available, the upper and lower reference limits for both TSH and free $T_4$ can be estimated using the American Thyroid Association's clinical guidelines, which provide reference ranges for different populations found in the literature (Alexander et al. 2017).

Thyroid function generally returns to prepartum levels by about 4 weeks postpartum; however, thyroid dysfunction can occur in the postpartum period and may be an important contributor to postpartum mental illness (Bergink et al. 2011, 2018). Postpartum autoimmune thyroiditis is an important diagnosis to rule out in evaluating postpartum depression, anxiety, and other psychological disorders.

**Adrenal gland.** Pregnancy is associated with marked changes in adrenocortical function, characterized by increased serum levels of aldosterone, deoxycorticosterone, corticosteroid-binding globulin, adrenocorticotropic hormone, cortisol, and free cortisol, ultimately leading to a state of physiological hypercortisolism. By the end of pregnancy, the levels of total cortisol are nearly three times higher than nonpregnant values, reaching levels equivalent to those seen in Cushing's syndrome. These increased cortisol levels are thought to play some role in the weight gain, stretch marks, insulin resistance, and fatigue experienced in pregnancy (Gabbe et al. 2017). The degree to which pregnancy-related physiological hypercortisolemia causes clinically significant psychiatric symptoms is unknown. However, there is a theoretical correlation with depression, mood dysregulation, sleep disturbance, and cognitive dysfunction (Tang et al. 2013).

**Pituitary gland.** Maternal levels of FSH and LH are decreased to undetectable amounts as a result of feedback inhibition from elevated levels of estrogen, progesterone, and inhibin during pregnancy. Serum prolactin levels begin to rise at approximately 5–8 weeks' gestation and by full term are elevated 10-fold, which allows the body to prepare for lactation (Gabbe et al. 2017). It is not certain to what degree prolactin in pregnancy may cause psychiatric symptoms, but animal studies suggest that prolactin is an important modulator in both lactation and maternal behavior (Babb et al. 2014; Larsen and Grattan 2012).

**Insulin and glucose metabolism.** During pregnancy, an increase in available glucose is required to promote fetal development while simultaneously maintaining adequate maternal nutrition. Such an increase in available glucose is associated with at least a mild peripheral insulin resistance, which develops later in pregnancy (Gabbe et al. 2017; Soma-Pillay et al. 2016). In early pregnancy, the increases in insulin secretion by insulin-secreting pancreatic $\beta$ cells are met with increased insulin sensitivity. Progesterone and estrogen, in conjunction with other diabetogenic hormones (e.g., human placental lactogen, growth hormone, cortisol), are thought to play a role in mediating the insulin resistance that peaks in the third trimester. In general, standard pregnancy glucose metabolism results in slight fasting hypoglycemia, postprandial hyperglycemia, and hyperinsulinemia. Insulin resistance and relative hypoglycemia—in conjunction with increased concentrations of free fatty acids, triglycerides, and cholesterol—promote lipolysis, which allows pregnant women to preferentially metabolize fat for fuel, preserving glucose metabolism for the fetus (Cunningham et al. 2014; Soma-Pillay et al. 2016). In about 6%–9% of women, these changes in glucose and insulin will result in gestational diabetes (Centers for Disease Control and Prevention 2018). Data have shown an increased risk for gestational diabetes in Asian American and Hispanic women as compared with non-Hispanic white women, and Hispanic women have a greatly increased risk of progression to type 2 diabetes within 5 years of having had gestational diabetes (Chou et al. 2021; Pu et al. 2015).

## Central Nervous System

The CNS undergoes profound changes during pregnancy and the postpartum period, utilizing significant plasticity to adapt to motherhood (Hillerer et al. 2014). For example, a functional imaging study noted that pregnancy was associated with profound and specific changes in the structure of the brain, especially in areas specific to social cognition (Hoekzema et al. 2017). During pregnancy, there is a reduction in total brain volume that reverses within 6 months of parturition (Oatridge et al. 2002); postpartum regional reductions are also seen, some of which are positively related to levels of maternal attachment (Hoekzema et al. 2017). Specific postpartum anatomical changes also occur, such as gray matter changes in the hypothalamus, amygdala, and prefrontal cortex (Kim et al. 2010).

## Cardiovascular System

Profound changes occur in the cardiovascular system during pregnancy. Cardiac output increases throughout pregnancy and peaks at 30%–50% above preconception values (Chou et al. 2021). This is secondary to an increase in both heart rate and stroke volume (Pacheco et al. 2013). The increase in cardiac output is disproportionally directed to the uterus, placenta, and breasts and diminishes over time in the postpartum period, remaining above pre-pregnancy levels up to 1 year later. Maternal blood volume also increases by the second half of pregnancy and is mostly attributed to an increase in plasma volume (Gabbe et al. 2017). The compensatory experience of increased heart rate (approaching 90 bpm in the third trimester) may sometimes induce anxiety or panic attacks in women with underlying anxiety disorders.

Maternal blood pressure falls somewhat in the first and second trimesters because increased progesterone causes a decrease in systemic vascular resistance (Chou et al. 2021). As pregnancy advances, the heart is physically displaced upward and toward the left. Eccentric cardiac hypertrophy, which is a physiological phenomenon, is common in pregnancy and thought to result from expanded blood volume. This is likely an adaptive process, as seen in athletes, that enables the pregnant woman's heart to work more efficiently. As a result of these and other physiological changes of pregnancy (e.g., drop in albumin concentration), plasma levels of medications may be diluted, creating the possibility for a decrease in efficacy (Gabbe et al. 2017).

Cardiovascular complications are the most common cause of pregnancy-related mortality (Creanga et al. 2017) and predict cardiovascular disease later in life (Margerison et al. 2019). Black women have higher rates of cardiovascular diseases such as preeclampsia in pregnancy, as well as higher associated fatality rates (Bibbins-Domingo et al. 2017). This increased risk is likely to have both physiological and socioeconomic determinants.

## Hematological System

Pregnancy is considered a hypercoagulable state, in preparation for hemostasis following delivery. There are overall increases in most proclotting factors and decreases in fibrinolysis and inhibitors of coagulation. These adaptations are thought to infer protection against excessive blood loss during delivery, but they also incur risk. The risk of thromboembolic disease is increased five- to sixfold, and pulmonary embolus is a leading cause of maternal mortality in the developed world (Petersen et al. 2019). The duration of this elevated risk lasts until at least 12 weeks postpartum (Soma-Pillay et al. 2016).

Additionally, the significant increases in plasma volume with only a slight increase in red blood cell mass result in a decrease in hemoglobin concentration, hematocrit, and red blood cell count (Figure 1–6) (Soma-Pillay et al. 2016), with Black women generally experiencing lower hematocrit and hemoglobin concentration than white women (Chou et al. 2021). This phenomenon, sometimes termed "physiological anemia of pregnancy," may contribute to fatigue, shortness of breath, and exercise intolerance in pregnant women (Pacheco et al. 2013). It also results in decreased concentration of drug-binding proteins, altering the apparent volume of distribution and, in some cases, drug clearance (Pariente et al. 2016). Hemoglobin and hematocrit fluctuate in the first few days postpartum and return to pre-pregnancy levels by 8 weeks postpartum.

Finally, iron requirements during pregnancy increase by two- to threefold, attributable not only to hemoglobin synthesis but also to fetal needs, including enzyme production. There is also a 10- to 20-fold increase in the requirements for folate and a twofold increase in vitamin $B_{12}$ requirements (Soma-Pillay et al. 2016).

## Pulmonary System

During pregnancy, the nasopharynx mucosa becomes edematous due to increased estrogen, leading to marked nasal stuffiness and decreased nasal patency. Regarding lung volume and pulmonary function, alterations in the diaphragm and chest wall configurations lead to reduced total lung capacity and functional residual capacity. Finally, increasing progesterone levels lead to chronic hyperventilation, low maternal $PaCO_2$, and chronic respiratory alkalosis (Gabbe et al. 2017). From a psychiatric perspective, decreased lung capacity and changes in $PaCO_2$ may lead to increased anxiety and risk of panic attacks, particularly in patients with a history of panic disorder (Wilhelm et al. 2001).

## Gastrointestinal System

Nausea and vomiting, also known as "morning sickness," complicate up to 80% of pregnancies and can occur at any time of day. For most women, symptoms resolve by about 18 weeks of gestation, but 15%–20% of women will continue to have symptoms in the third trimester. The most severe form of nausea and vomiting is hyperemesis gravidarum, which affects 0.5%–3% of women and often leads to weight loss, dehydration, and electrolyte imbalance (Chou et al. 2021; Soma-Pillay et al. 2016).

During pregnancy, elevated levels of progesterone affect several organs, including the stomach and gallbladder. The smooth muscle tone of the stomach and the tone of

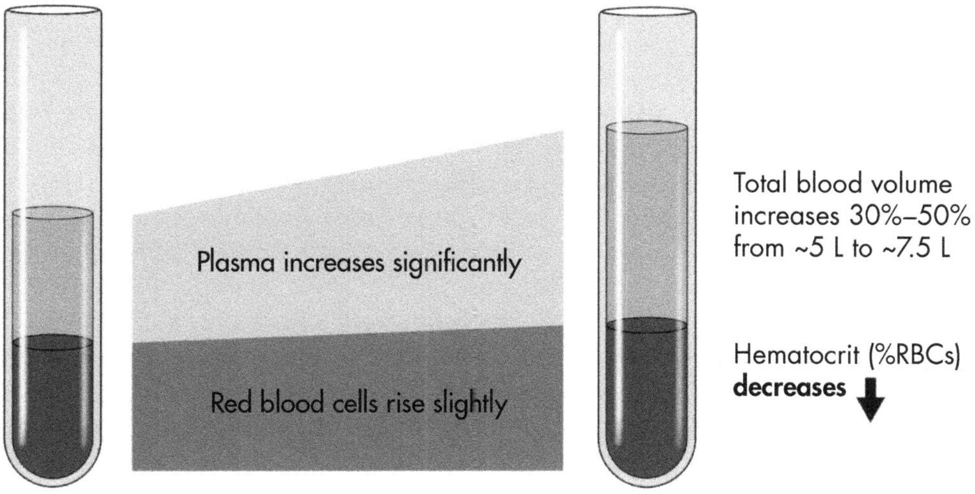


**FIGURE 1–6.** **Hematological changes in pregnancy.**

the lower esophageal sphincter are both decreased, leading to increased rates of gastroesophageal reflux disease, affecting 30%–50% of pregnant women (Chou et al. 2021). The rate at which the gallbladder empties is slowed due to higher progesterone levels, increasing the risk of gallstones. In the small intestines and colon, perturbations in motility are common in pregnancy and result in an increased incidence of constipation in some women and diarrhea in others.

In the liver, total body protein increases, but serum albumin and total protein levels fall during gestation as a result of hemodilution (Gabbe et al. 2017). Pregnancy also leads to changes in both cytochrome P450 enzyme activity and glucuronidation, with corresponding implications for medication metabolism (Dallmann et al. 2018). I particular, the activity of the following is affected: the uridine 5′-diphospho-glucuronosyltransferase (UGT) isoenzymes UGT1A4 and UGT2B7 and the CYP450 isoenzymes CYP3A4, CYP2D6, CYP2C9, CYP1A2, and CYP2C19 (Pariente et al. 2016).

## Genitourinary System

Physiological changes in the vagina interact with the vaginal microbiome to protect against infection and promote pregnancy maintenance. The kidneys enlarge during pregnancy, with dilation of the ureters and renal pelvis. These anatomical changes are mediated by progesterone (Soma-Pillay et al. 2016). Renal plasma flow rises 50%–80% in pregnancy, with a resulting increase in glomerular filtration rate, which reaches 40%–50% above pre-pregnancy levels by the end of the first trimester (Chou et al. 2021). This hyperfiltration leads to urinary frequency and renal excretion of various nutrients, vitamins, and renally excreted medications (e.g., lithium, risperidone, gabapentin, topiramate) (Cunningham et al. 2014). Glomerular filtration rate returns to pre-pregnancy levels by 8 weeks' gestation, which is important to consider if medication changes were made due to physiological changes of pregnancy (Gabbe et al. 2017).

### Immune System

Pregnancy is a time of dramatic changes in the immune system. It was once thought that pregnancy must be a time of total immune suppression to prevent fetal rejection. Later, evidence arose for a shift from proinflammatory to anti-inflammatory forces across pregnancy. The reality is much more complex, because the body works both to keep out foreign pathogens and to dampen cytotoxic activity (Mor and Cardenas 2010; Osborne and Monk 2013). The result is increased susceptibility to some viral and bacterial pathogens (e.g., influenza) and decreased activity for some autoimmune diseases (e.g., systemic lupus erythematosus). Some of these immune changes are still evident at 6 months postpartum and perhaps longer (Osborne et al. 2019b). In the postpartum period, an increased risk of "flare-ups" of autoimmune diseases and latent infections is associated with the return of normal immune function. In addition, increasing evidence indicates that mood and anxiety disorders experienced during the peripartum period may be related to these changes in immune functioning (Osborne et al. 2019a, 2020).

# Parturition and the Postpartum Period

## Phases of Parturition

The four phases of parturition, more commonly known as labor and delivery, are described in the following subsections. Figure 1–7 provides a brief synopsis.

### Phase 0: Quiescence

Throughout most of pregnancy, the uterus is maintained in a state of quiescence, distinguished by uterine smooth muscle tranquility and cervical structural preservation (Behrman and Butler 2007). This process is mediated by inhibitory hormones, including (but not limited to) progesterone, nitric oxide, relaxin, prostacyclin, and parathyroid-related hormone. During quiescence, the uterus undergoes significant vascular and dimensional changes in preparation for contractions. Although this phase precedes uterine activation, women may nevertheless experience low-intensity myometrial (Braxton Hicks) contractions; these are not accompanied by cervical change and wane over time. During most of the quiescent phase, cervical structural integrity remains intact to support progression of the pregnancy to full term. Toward the end of this phase, the cervix undergoes a progressive remodeling, known as *cervical softening*, in preparation for labor (Cunningham et al. 2014).

### Phase 1: Activation

The onset of the uterine activation phase typically occurs during the last 6–8 weeks of pregnancy and is defined by a series of uterine changes driven by estrogen. These include increased expression of contraction-associated proteins, including myometrial receptors for oxytocin and prostaglandin. There is also activation of certain ion channels and amplification of key proteins within gap junctions (e.g., connexin-43), which promote electrical synchrony between adjacent myometrial cells and allow for efficient uterine contractions (Challis and Gibb 1996; MacDonald 1993).

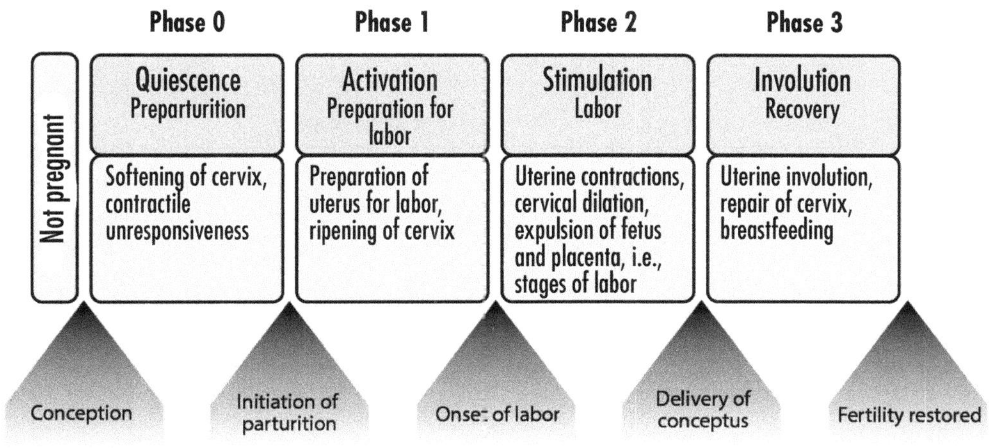


**FIGURE 1–7.** The phases of parturition.

Concurrently during this phase, the cervix undergoes continued remodeling and transitions from cervical softening to *cervical ripening*. Cervical ripening occurs days or weeks before the onset of contractions and is characterized by degradation of cervical collagen in preparation for cervical dilation. Prostaglandins likely play a role in this process (Cunningham et al. 2014; Keirse 1979).

## Phase 2: Stimulation

Following the activation phase, the uterus is prepared for stimulation by uterotonic agents, primarily prostaglandins and oxytocin, which promote uterine contractions. This process of regular uterine contractions occurs over days to weeks (Gabbe et al. 2017). The stimulation phase of parturition is typically recognized as active labor. Labor is divided into three sequential stages: cervical effacement and dilation, fetal descent and delivery, and placental separation and delivery (Figure 1–8) (Cunningham et al. 2014).

**Stage 1: Cervical effacement and dilation.** The first stage begins at the onset of labor and continues until cervical dilation is achieved. Onset of labor is typically characterized by regular painful contractions. Consistent contractions, with sufficient intensity and duration, lead to cervical thinning and shortening, also known as *cervical effacement*. This stage of labor is further divided into the latent and active phases. The *latent phase* is characterized by a slow rate of cervical change. This is followed by rapid acceleration of cervical dilation, known as the *active phase*. Although variable in the literature, historically, active labor requires 80% effacement and dilation of at least 4 cm, but it has recently been recognized that it may not begin until dilation of 6 cm (Chou et al. 2021). The cervix is considered fully dilated when it reaches approximately 10 cm (Cunningham et al. 2014).

Historically (based on the "Friedman criteria"), the mean time (95th percentile) for cervical dilation from 4 cm to 10 cm was 4.6 hours (11.7) in nulliparous women and 2.4 hours (5.2) in multiparous women (Friedman 1978). More recently, Zhang et al. (2010) observed the median times (95th percentile) to be 5.3 hours (16.4) in nulliparous women and 3.8 hours (15.7) in multiparous women (Zhang et al. 2010). In general, in-

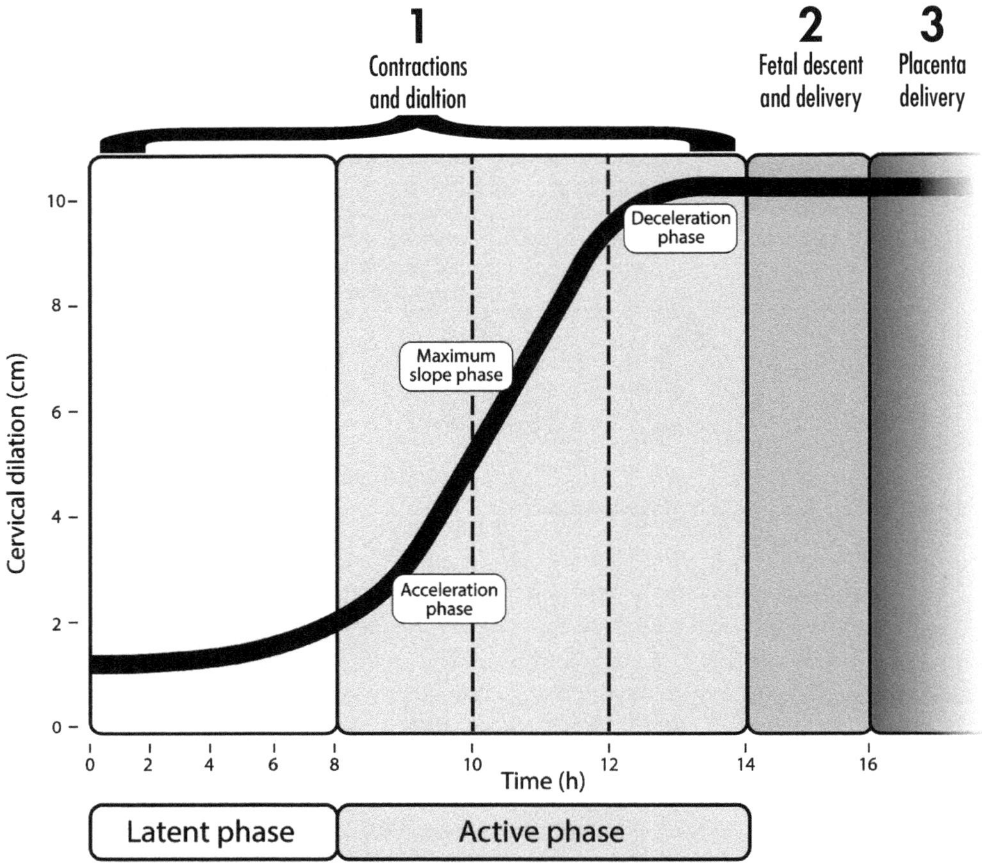


**FIGURE 1–8.** The stages of labor (Cunningham et al. 2014).

creased maternal BMI, older maternal age, and nonoptimal fetal position correlate with longer labor times (Gabbe et al. 2017).

**Stage 2: Fetal descent and delivery.** The second stage of labor begins once cervical dilation is complete and continues until the fetus is delivered. Although engagement with the fetal head (most neonates are delivered head first) can occur before labor begins, active fetal descent typically occurs after the progression of cervical dilation. As such, increased rates of fetal descent correlate with the maximal phase of cervical dilation. The increased rates are maintained until the observed fetal head reaches the perineal floor (Cunningham et al. 2014). According to Zhang et al. (2010), for nulliparous and parous women with epidural anesthesia, the median duration (95th percentile) of the second stage was 1.1 hours (3.6) and 0.4 hours (2.0), respectively. For nulliparous and parous women without epidural anesthesia, the median duration (95th percentile) was 0.6 hours (2.8) and 0.2 hours (1.3), respectively.

**Stage 3: Placental separation and delivery.** The third stage of labor is defined as the time following fetal delivery until placental expulsion. Placental separation occurs as a result of the inevitably reduced size of the uterine cavity following fetal delivery creating a tension with the unchanged placental size. Once separation is achieved, the placenta is expelled through increased abdominal pressure. This is typically accomplished by compressing the fundus of the uterus while placing minimal traction on the umbilical cord (Cunningham et al. 2014).

### Phase 3: Involution

Involution of the uterus takes place after fetal and placental delivery and is mediated primarily by oxytocin. Immediately following delivery, the uterus undergoes persistent contraction and retraction. Such rigidity allows compression of large uterine vessels to the point of thrombosis, with the goal of preventing hemorrhage. Uterine involution and cervical repair are components of the postdelivery remodeling processes, with the goal of restoring female organs to their nonpregnant state. These processes help protect the female reproductive tract from infection and restore endometrial responses to hormonal activity (Asgari Safdar et al. 2013; Behrman and Butler 2007).

## Postpartum Period

The postpartum period, also called the *puerperium*, is the period following delivery of the placenta and lasts for the first several weeks after delivery. During this period, maternal anatomy and physiology return to nonpregnant states. Classically, this period is thought to last 4–6 weeks, but some body systems may not return to the nonpregnant state for up to 12 months (Porter 2013). Timing of the return to the nonpregnant state for most body systems was discussed earlier (see "Pregnancy" section); here we cover changes to the pelvic anatomy and body shape. Breast changes are discussed in greater detail later.

### Pelvic Anatomy

Immediately following delivery, the fundus of the uterus is typically firm and nontender, and it lies slightly below the umbilicus. The uterus and endometrium return to nonpregnant size by approximately 8 weeks postpartum (Chou et al. 2021); however, this baseline can be affected by several factors, including uterine overdistention predelivery, multiparity, cesarean section delivery, and breastfeeding (Negishi et al. 1999). The cervix after delivery may have small lacerations. For the first few days postpartum, the cervix remains slightly dilated (width ~2–4 cm), but by about 1 week postpartum, the opening narrows and the cervix thickens. The external os, the opening of the uterine cervix into the vagina, never resumes its original shape. The vagina slowly contracts postpartum but does not return to its nulligravid size (Cunningham et al. 2014).

### Weight and Shape

The expulsion of the fetus, placenta, and amniotic fluid combined represents a mean weight loss of approximately 10–13 lb; however, this weight loss is not immediately observed due to fluid retention postpartum, and this delay can be anxiety provoking for some women (Gabbe et al. 2017). During the first 6 weeks postdelivery, approximately one-half of the gestational weight gained during pregnancy is lost, and only approximately one-fourth of women return to their pre-pregnancy weight by 6 weeks postpartum. A slower rate of weight loss occurs during the subsequent months, for up to 6 months postpartum (Gunderson et al. 2001). If the amount of weight gained during pregnancy exceeds recommended amounts (e.g., >35 lb in a woman with normal BMI), women are likely to have an approximate net weight gain of 11 lb. Breastfeeding does not have a significant impact on postpartum weight loss (Gabbe et al. 2017). Notable racial disparities have been shown in postpartum weight loss, with Black women demonstrating significantly greater postpartum weight retention 1 year after delivery compared with white women (Headen et al. 2012).

## Breast Development and Lactation

### Anatomy

The adult female breast is made up of specialized glandular tissue and adipose tissue. The glandular tissue is organized into 15–20 lobes, which are further divided into small lobules in which breastmilk is produced (the lobules themselves are clusters of secretory epithelial cells called *acini*). Breastmilk is secreted through a network of ducts that arise from smaller lobular units, which then converge and eventually exit the skin via duct orifices in the nipple (Sriraman 2017). Figure 1–9 depicts the anatomical structure of a breast.

### Breast Development

The mammary gland first develops during embryogenesis. A mammary bud forms in the developing epidermis and extends into the subepidermal mesenchyme, while an adipose pad precursor develops underneath. A rudimentary mammary duct system then develops, canalizing and spreading through the adipose pad precursor. After birth until puberty, the mammary gland remains small, with existing ducts growing in parallel with child growth (Macias and Hinck 2012; Sriraman 2017).

*Mammogenesis* refers to the growth and development of the mammary glands in preparation for milk production. The process begins in puberty, with estrogen and growth factors stimulating the proliferation and branching of ducts into a treelike pattern throughout the developing adipose tissue. Initial lobular and alveolar development also occurs, which is further spurred by changes in estrogen and progesterone levels during menstruation. By the end of puberty, various lobules with a complex duct system have formed. No further changes occur until pregnancy, when further alveolar development and epithelial maturation occur in response to higher progesterone levels, leading to secretory tissue proliferation and breast enlargement. These changes are accompanied by a marked increase in vascular supply to the breast. In early pregnancy, larger, complex lobules form (Alex et al. 2020; Sriraman 2017).

### Lactation

The term *lactogenesis* refers to the physiological changes that allow a woman to produce and secrete breastmilk. These changes begin during pregnancy and direct the alveolar epithelium to differentiate. Lactogenesis occurs in three stages: secretory initiation, secretory activation, and ongoing milk production (Pillay and Davis 2020).

#### Stage I: Secretory Initiation

Secretory initiation begins during the second half of pregnancy, at which point the mammary glands have become sufficiently differentiated to produce small quantities

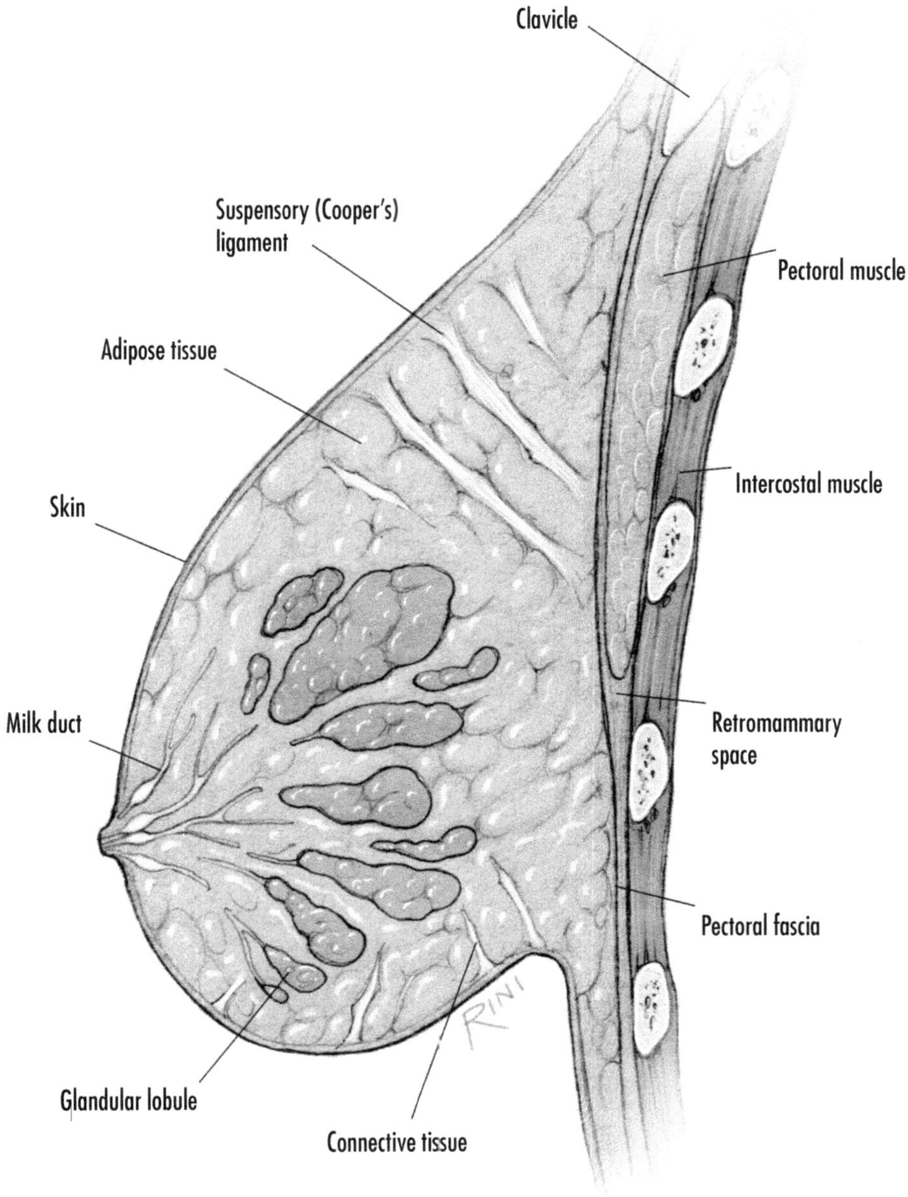


**FIGURE 1–9.** Anatomy of the breast.
*Source.* Image by David Rini.

of milk components such as casein and lactose. High levels of plasma progesterone (secreted by the placenta) inhibit further secretion and gland differentiation.

## Stage II: Secretory Activation

Secretory activation occurs after delivery. With the removal of the placenta, the rapid drop in progesterone and the elevated levels of prolactin, cortisol, and insulin stimulate milk secretion. Usually, at day 2 or 3 postpartum, women experience swelling of the breast along with copious milk production. In primiparous women, the secretory activation stage is slightly delayed, and early milk volume is lower. Lower milk volume is also observed in women who had cesarean births compared with those who delivered vaginally. Late onset of milk production has also been seen in women who have had retained placental fragments, diabetes, and stressful vaginal deliveries. With retained placental fragments, stage II could be inhibited by the continued secretion of progesterone and would continue to be inhibited until the remaining placental fragments are removed (Alex et al. 2020; Wagner et al. 2018).

### Stage III: Galactopoiesis

The term *galactopoiesis* refers to ongoing milk production, which is maintained by regular removal of milk and stimulation of the nipple, which trigger prolactin release from the anterior pituitary gland and oxytocin from the posterior pituitary gland. For the ongoing synthesis and secretion of milk, the mammary gland must receive hormonal signals from both prolactin and oxytocin. Prolactin stimulates mammary gland ductal growth and epithelial cell proliferation and induces milk protein synthesis through binding to receptors on the alveolar epithelium of the mammary gland. Nipple stimulation leads to sensory transmission through the spinothalamic tracks; the hypothalamus is then stimulated, leading to decreased tonic prolactin inhibition and resulting in prolactin surges within 15 minutes of nursing (Sriraman 2017).

Oxytocin governs the milk ejection, or let-down, reflex (Svennersten-Sjaunja and Olsson 2005). The tactile stimulation of the nipple-areolar complex by suckling sends afferent signals to the hypothalamus, triggering release of oxytocin from the posterior pituitary. Oxytocin travels to the mammary glands and binds to G-protein-coupled oxytocin receptors located on the myoepithelial cells, causing the cells to contract. The myoepithelial cell contraction releases milk into the ducts from the alveolar lumens and through the nipple. The release of oxytocin becomes a conditioned response in the lactating woman, requiring only visual stimulation or conscious thought (Leng et al. 2005; Sriraman 2017). Figure 1–10 summarizes the let-down reflex.

Once lactation is established and maintained, both physical and biochemical factors regulate milk production. If milk is not removed, intramammary pressure increases and leads to vascular stasis and accumulation of a lactation feedback inhibitor (thought to be whey protein in breastmilk); milk production consequently stops and mammary involution is initiated. Conversely, breastmilk removal decreases pressure, improves blood flow to the mammary glands, and removes the inhibitor, leading to resumed production (Institute of Medicine Committee on Nutritional Status During Pregnancy and Lactation 1991; Macias and Hinck 2012; Sriraman 2017).

## Menopause

*Menopause* is defined as the absence of menstrual periods for a full year, and it is caused by reduced secretion of ovarian hormones, including estrogen and progesterone (Bacon 2017). An estimated 1 billion women worldwide have experienced menopause (Hoga et al. 2015). The average age of menopause in the United States is 51.5 years (Hoffman et al. 2020).

Menopause is a normal event for women and generally signals the end of a woman's reproductive capacity. It may be experienced as a liberating end to anxieties about child-

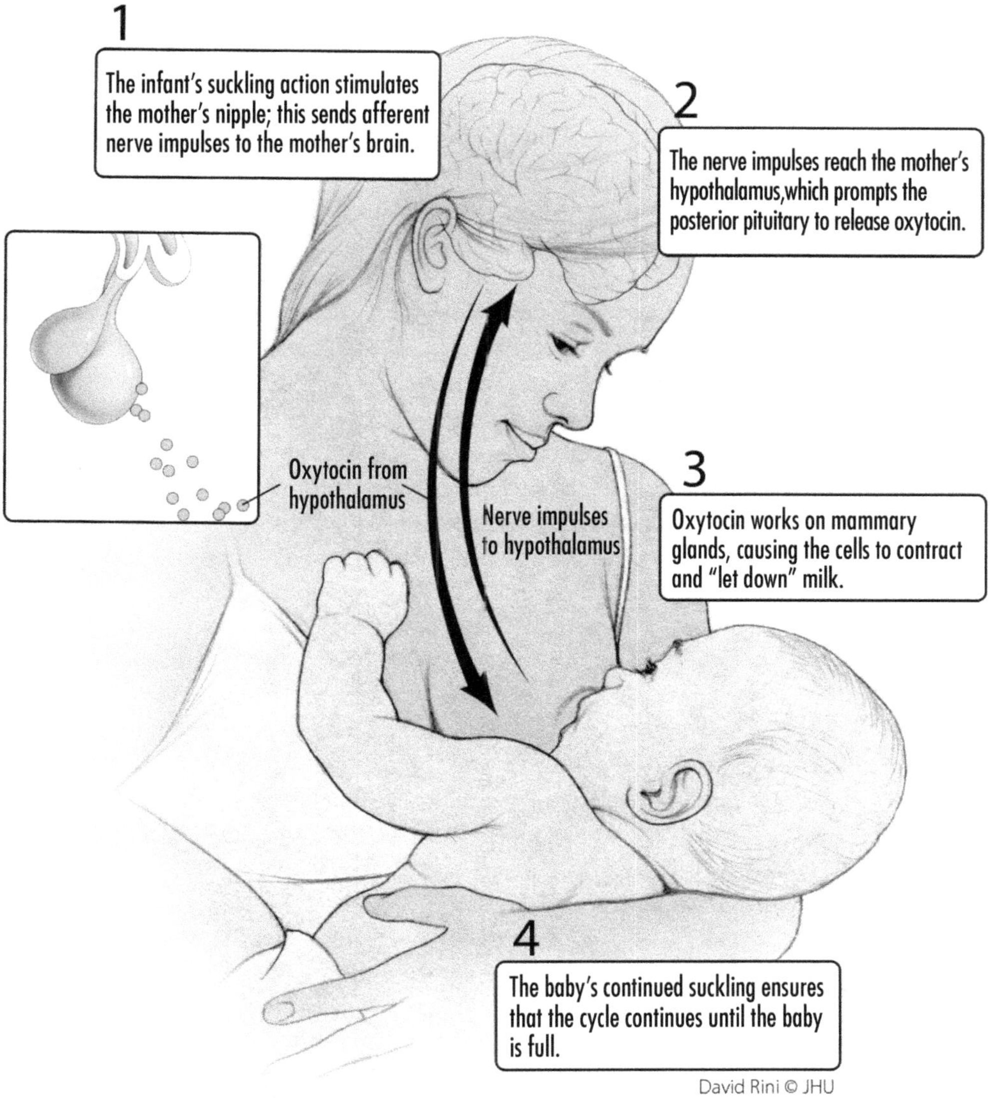


**FIGURE 1–10. The milk let-down reflex.**
*Source.* Image by David Rini.

birth and to discomfort related to one's reproductive life, or it may be viewed negatively—particularly in Western cultures—through its association with aging (Minkin 2019). (Some women might experience a combination or neither of these reactions.) Individual experiences of menopause vary, and at times women will seek medical or mental health attention for the management of symptoms (Nelson 2008). In this section, we review the physiology of the menopausal transition. See Chapter 7, "Perimenopause," for a review of the relationship between the menopausal transition and mental health.

Menopause can be a naturally occurring event, or it can be brought about either medically or surgically as a result of—or for the prevention of—disease. Medical menopause is beyond the scope of this chapter, but it is worth noting that women with medical or surgical menopause, particularly prior to age 45 years, may have more severe and prolonged menopausal symptoms (Rodriguez and Shoupe 2015). In addition, women experiencing medical menopause have an increased risk of depression, heart disease, osteopenia or osteoporosis, sexual dysfunction, and cognitive decline compared with women in the general population (Rodriguez and Shoupe 2015).

The menopausal transition has several phases: perimenopause, menopause, and postmenopause. *Perimenopause*, characterized by estrogen decline and irregular menstrual cycle length, is the interval of time preceding the onset of menopause (Dutton and Rymer 2015). On average, perimenopause begins 4 years prior to the final menstrual cycle—on average, age 47—and lasts for several years (Hoffman et al. 2020). *Menopause* reflects the process of ovarian follicular depletion. Ovarian senescence begins in utero with programmed oocyte atresia and then continues after birth by way of follicular maturation and regression (Hoffman et al. 2020). Beginning in a woman's later 30s to early 40s, ovarian follicles are depleted at a more rapid rate until the eventual loss of ovarian activity by the time menopause is reached; loss of ovarian function before age 40 is termed *premature ovarian insufficiency* (Hoffman et al. 2020).

In the early perimenopausal transition stage, the length of time between menstrual cycles increases from the typical 25–35 days during reproductive years to approximately 40–50 days (Dutton and Rymer 2015). During this time, FSH levels vary, but generally this hormone is on the rise. Estradiol levels are initially maintained steadily or, like FSH levels, are increased (Dutton and Rymer 2015). Such changes reflect diminished ovarian reserve: fewer follicles are present to secrete inhibin, a hormone that exerts negative feedback on FSH secretion (Dutton and Rymer 2015; Hoffman et al. 2020). Initially, increased FSH levels result in greater follicle recruitment and therefore an increase in estradiol; this transition period correlates with a variability in menstrual cycle length, increased amenorrhea, and more frequent anovulatory cycles (Dutton and Rymer 2015). Eventually, cycle lengths shorten and anovulatory cycles become more frequent, although unpredictably so (Hoffman et al. 2020). In addition to changes in estrogen levels, progesterone levels start to decline (Hoffman et al. 2020). As the perimenopausal period progresses and menopause is reached, FSH continues to rise and estradiol levels fall, whereas in the postmenopausal period, FSH and estradiol levels initially stabilize and eventually both decline (Dutton and Rymer 2015).

The most common physical symptom of menopause is the development of hot flashes, reported by up to 50% of menopausal women (Hoffman et al. 2020). Classically, hot flashes last 2–4 minutes and are described as a sudden sensation of heat beginning on the chest and face and then progressively spreading throughout the body. They can occur several times in a day and can be associated with perspiration, palpitations, chills, anxiety, and irritability (Hoffman et al. 2020). The proposed physiology surrounding both hot flashes and night sweats (vasomotor symptoms) reported by menopausal women is related to changes in central thermoregulatory functioning due to decreased estradiol (Dutton and Rymer 2015). Skin temperatures can increase, particularly in the fingers and toes, due to peripheral vasodilation, whereas core temperatures may slightly decrease (Hoffman et al. 2020). Recent studies estimate that hot flashes last for 7 years on average (Hoffman et al. 2020). Significant differences in the prevalence of vasomotor symptoms in women of different racial backgrounds have been reported, with Black women experiencing the highest prevalence and longest duration of all groups studied (El Khoudary et al. 2019).

Additional symptoms noted during menopause include vaginal dryness and an increase in urinary tract infections, which are functions of decreased estradiol and progesterone in the urogenital tract (Dutton and Rymer 2015). Specifically, depleted estrogen levels lead to the thinning of the epithelial lining of the vagina and subsequently, in the long term, to vaginal atrophy (the vagina shortens, narrows, and becomes less flexible) (Hoffman et al. 2020). Women may first notice a decline in vaginal lubrication during sexual activity; however, as the decreased estrogen state progresses, discomfort may be noticed during daily activities. Vaginal dryness and associated discomfort are likely among several factors in the decreased sexual function associated with menopause. Studies have shown racial differences in postmenopausal sexual functioning; compared with white women, Asian women report lower sexual desire and lower importance of sex, and Black women report lower levels of arousal and greater importance of sex (El Khoudary et al. 2019).

Estrogen depletion can also affect other organ systems and can be associated with cardiovascular disease, metabolic syndromes, and osteopenia or osteoporosis. Estrogen deficiency is proposed to play a role in the increased risk of cardiovascular disease after menopause and may be impacted in part by shifts in lipid profiles during perimenopause (Derby et al. 2009). There are also proposed shifts in body composition in the postmenopausal period, including increased fat content and decreased lean muscle. In terms of bone health, it is postulated that decreased estrogen levels lead to excessive bone resorption (Hoffman et al. 2020). Ultimately, this results in osteopenia (a condition that occurs when the body does not make new bone as quickly as it reabsorbs old bone), which is the precursor to osteoporosis, a progressive reduction in bone mass and strength that contributes to fractures (Hoffman et al. 2020). Approximately 40%–50% of postmenopausal women will experience a fracture related to osteoporosis in their lifetime (Hoffman et al. 2020). Racial differences in postmenopausal fractures have been described—rates among Black and Asian women are approximately half of those in white women—however, the physiological differences that underlie this pattern are not well understood (El Khoudary et al. 2019). For a detailed discussion of these clinical features and their relationship to mental health, see Chapter 7, "Perimenopause."

## Conclusion

Clinicians treating women for mental health conditions at times of reproductive transition must have a firm understanding of the hormonal and other physiological changes that accompany such transitions. This chapter offered an overview of the physical changes that accompany the menstrual cycle, pregnancy, parturition and the postpartum period, lactation, and menopause. The mental health sequelae of these changes are the subject of the remaining chapters of this book.

## Key Points

- Women's reproductive years begin with menarche, when reproductive hormones initiate the menstrual cycle and the development of primary and secondary sexual characteristics.
- The first half of the menstrual cycle is the follicular phase (days 1–14), when follicle-stimulating hormone (FSH) and luteinizing hormone (LH) spur the development of a dominant follicle, and estrogen and progesterone levels rise gradually.
- Ovulation occurs at approximately day 14 and is followed by the luteal phase, when the uterine lining is prepared for implantation and the dominant follicle develops into the progesterone-producing corpus luteum.
- When pregnancy does not occur, the uterine lining is shed, and the next cycle begins with menses.
- The enormous changes of pregnancy are not confined to the reproductive system; they include changes in other endocrine systems as well as the central nervous, cardiovascular, hematological, pulmonary, gastrointestinal, genitourinary, and immune systems.
- There are four phases to parturition: quiescence (most of pregnancy), activation (beginning of contractions), stimulation (active labor), and involution (return of the uterus to pre-pregnancy size).
- The three stages of active labor are cervical dilation, delivery of the fetus, and delivery of the placenta.
- Changes in breast anatomy and physiology in pregnancy prepare for lactation, which is regulated by prolactin and oxytocin.
- Menopause, which represents the end of a woman's reproductive life, is induced by changes in reproductive hormones, with a decrease in estrogen and progesterone and an increase in LH and FSH.

## References


Abreu AP, Kaiser UB: Pubertal development and regulation. Lancet Diabetes Endocrinol 4(3):254–264, 2016 26852256

Alex A, Bhandary E, McGuire KP: Anatomy and physiology of the breast during pregnancy and lactation. Adv Exp Med Biol 1252:3–7, 2020 32816256

Alexander EK, Pearce EN, Brent GA, et al: 2017 guidelines of the American Thyroid Association for the diagnosis and management of thyroid disease during pregnancy and the postpartum. Thyroid 27(3):315–389, 2017 28056690

Asgari Safdar AH, Daghigh Kia H, Farhadi R: Physiology of parturition. International Journal of Advanced Biological and Biomedical Research 1(3):214–221, 2013

Babb JA, Carini LM, Spears SL, Nephew BC: Transgenerational effects of social stress on social behavior, corticosterone, oxytocin, and prolactin in rats. Horm Behav 65(4):386–393, 2014 24657520

Bacon JL: The menopausal transition. Obstet Gynecol Clin North Am 44(2):285–296, 2017 28499537

Behrman RE, Butler AS (eds): Preterm Birth: Causes, Consequences, and Prevention. Washington, DC, National Academies Press, 2007

Bergink V, Kushner SA, Pop V, et al: Prevalence of autoimmune thyroid dysfunction in postpartum psychosis. Br J Psychiatry 198(4):264–268, 2011 21343331
Bergink V, Pop VJM, Nielsen PR, et al: Comorbidity of autoimmune thyroid disorders and psychiatric disorders during the postpartum period: a Danish nationwide register-based cohort study. Psychol Med 48(8):1291–1298, 2018 28929982
Betz D, Fane K: Human Chorionic Gonadotropin (hCG). Treasure Island, FL, StatPearls Publishing, 2020
Bibbins-Domingo K, Grossman DC, Curry SJ, et al: Screening for preeclampsia: U.S. Preventive Services Task Force Recommendation Statement. JAMA 317(16):1661–1667, 2017 28444286
Blair LM, Porter K, Leblebicioglu B, et al: Poor sleep quality and associated inflammation predict preterm birth: heightened risk among African Americans. Sleep (Basel) 38(8):1259–1267, 2015 25845693
Burke CS, Susser LC, Hermann AD: GABAA dysregulation as an explanatory model for late-onset postpartum depression associated with weaning and resumption of menstruation. Arch Women Ment Health 22(1):55–63, 2019 29968131
Carroll JE, Rentscher KE, Cole SW, et al: Sleep disturbances and inflammatory gene expression among pregnant women: differential responses by race. Brain Behav Immun 88:654–660, 2020 32360438
Centers for Disease Control and Prevention: Diabetes during pregnancy. CDC.gov, June 12, 2018. Available at: https://www.cdc.gov/reproductivehealth/maternalinfanthealth/diabetes-during-pregnancy.htm. Accessed December 30, 2020.
Challis JRG, Gibb W: Control of parturition. Prenat Neonatal Med 1:283, 1996
Chou B, Bienstock JL, Satin AJ (eds): Johns Hopkins Manual of Gynecology and Obstetrics, 6th Edition. Baltimore, MD, Wolters Kluwer, 2021
Committee on Patient Safety and Quality Improvement, Committee on Professional Liability: ACOG Committee Opinion No. 381: subclinical hypothyroidism in pregnancy. Obstet Gynecol 110(4):959–960, 2007 17906045
Cox E, Takov V: Embryology, Ovarian Follicle Development. Treasure Island, FL, StatPearls Publishing, 2020
Creanga AA, Syverson C, Seed K, et al: Pregnancy-related mortality in the United States, 2011–2013. Obstet Gynecol 130(2):366–373, 2017 28697109
Cunningham FH, Leveno KJH, Bloom SL, et al: Williams Obstetrics, 24th Edition. New York, McGraw-Hill Education, 2014
Curtis DS, Fuller-Rowell TE, El-Sheikh M, et al: Habitual sleep as a contributor to racial differences in cardiometabolic risk. Proc Natl Acad Sci USA 114(33):8889–8894, 2017 28760970
Dallmann A, Ince I, Coboeken K, et al: A physiologically based pharmacokinetic model for pregnant women to predict the pharmacokinetics of drugs metabolized via several enzymatic pathways. Clin Pharmacokinet 57(6):749–768, 2018 28924743
Derby CA, Crawford SL, Pasternak RC, et al: Lipid changes during the menopause transition in relation to age and weight: the Study of Women's Health Across the Nation. Am J Epidemiol 169(11):1352–1361, 2009 19357323
Dutton PJ, Rymer JM: Physiology of the menstrual cycle and changes in perimenopause, in Managing the Menopause: 21st Century Solution. Cambridge, UK, Cambridge University Press, 2015, pp 1–10
El Khoudary SR, Greendale G, Crawford SL, et al: The menopause transition and women's health at midlife: a progress report from the Study of Women's Health Across the Nation (SWAN). Menopause 26(10):1213–1227, 2019 31568098
Emans S, Laufer M: Emans, Laufer, Goldstein's Pediatric and Adolescent Gynecology. Philadelphia, PA, Wolters Kluwer Health/Lippincott Williams & Wilkins Health, 2011
Feinstein L, McWhorter KL, Gaston SA, et al: Racial/ethnic disparities in sleep duration and sleep disturbances among pregnant and non-pregnant women in the United States. J Sleep Res 29(5):e13000, 2020 32112620

Ferin M: The hypothalamic-hypophyseal-ovarian axis and the menstrual cycle, in Global Library of Women's Medicine. London, The Foundation for the Global Library of Women's Medicine, 2008. Available at: www.glowm.com/section_view/heading/the-hypothalamic-hypophyseal-ovarian-axis-and-the-menstrual-cycle/item/282. Accessed December 30, 2020.
Friedman EA: Labor: Clinical Evaluation and Management, 2nd Edition. New York, Appleton-Century-Crofts, 1978
Gabbe S, Niebyl J, Simpson J: Obstetrics: Normal and Problem Pregnancies, 7th Edition. Philadelphia, PA, Elsevier, 2017
Glinoer D, de Nayer P, Bourdoux P, et al: Regulation of maternal thyroid during pregnancy. J Clin Endocrinol Metab 71(2):276–287, 1990 2116437
Goodman HM: Basic Medical Endocrinology, 3rd Edition. New York, Academic Press, 2003
Gunderson EP, Abrams B, Selvin S: Does the pattern of postpartum weight change differ according to pregravid body size? Int J Obes Relat Metab Disord 25(6):853–862, 2001 11439300
Headen IE, Davis EM, Mujahid MS, et al: Racial-ethnic differences in pregnancy-related weight. Adv Nutr 3(1):83–94, 2012 22332106
Hillerer KM, Jacobs VR, Fischer T, Aigner L: The maternal brain: an organ with peripartal plasticity. Neural Plast 574159:2014, 2014 24883213
Hoekzema E, Barba-Müller E, Pozzobon C, et al: Pregnancy leads to long-lasting changes in human brain structure. Nat Neurosci 20(2):287–296, 2017 27991897
Hoffman B, Schorge J, Halvorson L, et al: Williams Gynecology, 4th Edition. New York, McGraw-Hill, 2020
Hoga L, Rodolpho J, Gonçalves B, et al: Women's experience of menopause: a systematic review of qualitative evidence. JBI Database Syst Rev Implement Reports 13(8):250–337, 2015 26455946
Hoyt LT, Falconi AM: Puberty and perimenopause: reproductive transitions and their implications for women's health. Soc Sci Med 132:103–112, 2015 25797100
Institute of Medicine Committee on Nutritional Status During Pregnancy and Lactation: Nutrition During Lactation. Washington, DC, National Academies Press, 1991
Keirse MJNC: Endogenous prostaglandins in human parturition, in Human Parturition. Edited by Keirse MJNC, Anderson ABM, Bennebroek-Gravenhorstm J. Leiden, The Netherlands, Leiden University Press, 1979, pp 101–142
Kim P, Leckman JF, Mayes LC, et al: The plasticity of human maternal brain: longitudinal changes in brain anatomy during the early postpartum period. Behav Neurosci 124(5):695–700, 2010 20939669
Korevaar TIM: The upper limit for TSH during pregnancy: why we should stop using fixed limits of 2.5 or 3.0 mU/L. Thyroid Res 11:5, 2018 29942352
Larsen CM, Grattan DR: Prolactin, neurogenesis, and maternal behaviors. Brain Behav Immun 26(2):201–209, 2012 21820505
Leng G, Caquineau C, Sabatier N: Regulation of oxytocin secretion. Vitam Horm 71:27–58, 2005 16112264
Liu B, Xu G, Sun Y, et al: Association between maternal pre-pregnancy obesity and preterm birth according to maternal age and race or ethnicity: a population-based study. Lancet Diabetes Endocrinol 7(9):707–714, 2019 31395506
MacDonald PC: Parturition: Biomolecular and physiologic process, in Williams Obstetrics, 19th Edition. Edited by Cunningham FG, MacDonald PC, Gant NF, et al. Norwalk, CT, Appleton & Lange, 1993, p 297–361
Macias H, Hinck L: Mammary gland development. Wiley Interdiscip Rev Dev Biol 1(4):533–557, 2012 22844349
Margerison CE, Catov J, Holzman C: Pregnancy as a window to racial disparities in hypertension. J Womens Health (Larchmt) 28(2):152–161, 2019 29927696
McEvoy K, Payne JL, Osborne LM: Neuroactive steroids and perinatal depression: a review of recent literature. Curr Psychiatry Rep 20(9):78, 2018 30094520
Melmed S, Koenig R, Rosen C, et al: Williams Textbook of Endocrinology, 14th Edition. New York, Elsevier, 2019
Minkin MJ: Menopause: hormones, lifestyle, and optimizing aging. Obstet Gynecol Clin North Am 46(3):501–514, 2019 31378291

Mitanchez D, Chavatte-Palmer P: Review shows that maternal obesity induces serious adverse neonatal effects and is associated with childhood obesity in their offspring. Acta Paediatr 107(7):1156–1165, 2018 29421859

Mor G, Cardenas I: The immune system in pregnancy: a unique complexity. Am J Reprod Immunol 63(6):425–433, 2010 20367629

Negishi H, Kishida T, Yamada H, et al: Changes in uterine size after vaginal delivery and cesarean section determined by vaginal sonography in the puerperium. Arch Gynecol Obstet 263(1–2):13–16, 1999 10728621

Nelson HD: Menopause. Lancet 371(9614):760–770, 2008 18313505

Oatridge A, Holdcroft A, Saeed N, et al: Change in brain size during and after pregnancy: study in healthy women and women with preeclampsia. AJNR Am J Neuroradiol 23(1):19–26, 2002 11827871

Osborne LM, Monk C: Perinatal depression: the fourth inflammatory morbidity of pregnancy? Theory and literature review. Psychoneuroendocrinology 38(10):1929–1952, 2013 23608136

Osborne LM, Brar A, Klein SL: The role of Th17 cells in the pathophysiology of pregnancy and perinatal mood and anxiety disorders. Brain Behav Immun 76:7–16, 2019a 30465878

Osborne LM, Yenokyan G, Fei K, et al: Innate immune activation and depressive and anxious symptoms across the peripartum: an exploratory study. Psychoneuroendocrinology 99:80–86, 2019b 30195110

Osborne LM, Gilden J, Kamperman AM, et al: T-cell defects and postpartum depression. Brain Behav Immun 87:397–403, 2020 31926288

Pacheco LD, Costantine MM, Hankins GD: Physiologic changes during pregnancy. Obstet Gynecol 1:5–16, 2013

Pariente G, Leibson T, Carls A, et al: Pregnancy-associated changes in pharmacokinetics: a systematic review. PLoS Med 13(11):e1002160, 2016 27802281

Petersen EE, Davis NL, Goodman D, et al: Vital signs: pregnancy-related deaths, United States, 2011–2015, and strategies for prevention, 13 states, 2013–2017. MMWR Morb Mortal Wkly Rep 68(18):423–429, 2019 31071074

Pillay J, Davis TJ: Physiology, Lactation. Treasure Island, FL, StatPearls Publishing, 2020

Porter SB (ed): Tidy's Physiotherapy, 15th Edition. New York, Churchill Livingstone Elsevier, 2013

Pu J, Zhao B, Wang EJ, et al: Racial/Ethnic differences in gestational diabetes prevalence and contribution of common risk factors. Paediatr Perinat Epidemiol 29(5):436–443, 2015 26201385

Reed BG, Carr BR: The Normal Menstrual Cycle and the Control of Ovulation. Edited by Feingold KR, Anawalt B, Boyce A. South Dartmouth, MA, Endotext, MDText.com, 2018

Reyes FI, Winter JS, Faiman C: Postpartum disappearance of chorionic gonadotropin from the maternal and neonatal circulations. Am J Obstet Gynecol 153(5):486–489, 1985 4061509

Rodriguez M, Shoupe D: Surgical Menopause. Endocrinol Metab Clin North Am 44(3):531–542, 2015 26316241

Russell JA, Brunton PJ: Oxytocin (peripheral/central actions and their regulation), in Encyclopedia of Neuroscience. New York, Elsevier, 2009

Santiago JR, Nolledo MS, Kinzler W, et al: Sleep and sleep disorders in pregnancy. Ann Intern Med 134(5):396–408, 2001 11242500

Schiller CE, Meltzer-Brody S, Rubinow DR: The role of reproductive hormones in postpartum depression. CNS Spectr 20(1):48–59, 2015 25263255

Soma-Pillay P, Nelson-Piercy C, Tolppanen H, et al: Physiological changes in pregnancy. Cardiovasc J Afr 27(2):89–94, 2016 27213856

Sriraman NK: The nuts and bolts of breastfeeding: anatomy and physiology of lactation. Curr Probl Pediatr Adolesc Health Care 47(12):305–310, 2017 29246381

Stagnaro-Green A, Abalovich M, Alexander E, et al: Guidelines of the American Thyroid Association for the diagnosis and management of thyroid disease during pregnancy and postpartum. Thyroid 21(10):1081–1125, 2011 21787128

Surks MI, Ortiz E, Daniels GH, et al: Subclinical thyroid disease: scientific review and guidelines for diagnosis and management. JAMA 291(2):228–238, 2004 14722150

Svennersten-Sjaunja K, Olsson K: Endocrinology of milk production. Domest Anim Endocrinol 29(2):241–258, 2005 15876512

Tang A, O'Sullivan AJ, Diamond T, et al: Psychiatric symptoms as a clinical presentation of Cushing's syndrome. Ann Gen Psychiatry 12(1):23, 2013 23866099

Wagner CL, Baatz JE, Newton D, et al: Analytical considerations and general diagnostic and therapeutic ramifications of milk hormones during lactation. Best Pract Res Clin Endocrinol Metab 32(1):5–16, 2018 29549960

Wilhelm FH, Gevirtz R, Roth WT: Respiratory dysregulation in anxiety, functional cardiac, and pain disorders: assessment, phenomenology, and treatment. Behav Modif 25(4):513–545, 2001 11530714

World Health Organization Task Force on Methods for the Natural Regulation of Fertility: The World Health Organization Multinational Study of Breast-feeding and Lactational Amenorrhea. II. Factors associated with the length of amenorrhea. Fertil Steril 70(3):461–471, 1998 9757874

Zhang J, Landy HJ, Branch DW, et al: Contemporary patterns of spontaneous labor with normal neonatal outcomes. Obstet Gynecol 116(6):1281–1287, 2010 21099592

CHAPTER 2

# Gynecological Conditions and Mental Health

Brittney Bastow, M.D., M.Sc.
Pooja Lakshmin, M.D.

Health care guidelines from the American College of Obstetricians and Gynecologists (ACOG) recommend an annual well-woman visit. This visit presents an excellent opportunity to screen, evaluate, and counsel women about their current health, as well as to provide anticipatory guidance for upcoming life changes, including contraception, preconception counseling, menopause, and so forth. During these visits, gynecologists and primary care providers often diagnose other gynecological conditions, such as chronic pelvic pain (CPP), endometriosis, polycystic ovary syndrome (PCOS), or sexual dysfunction (genito-pelvic pain/penetration disorder [GPPPD]). Gynecological care is aimed at treating the physical symptoms that women experience; however, significant comorbidity is known to exist between gynecological issues and psychiatric disorders. Patients with such comorbidities are typically referred to a psychiatrist or psychotherapist for further workup and treatment of their mental health conditions. Mental health professionals working with women with gynecological conditions can benefit from having a basic understanding of these medical conditions. This chapter includes sections on four common classes of gynecological conditions. Each section offers a brief overview of epidemiology, clinical features, pathophysiology, and treatment options, with a focus on gynecological basics and treatment from a psychiatric lens.

## Chronic Pelvic Pain

Ms. A presents to her gynecologist reporting 3 years of pain. She had first noticed her pain after coming back from a cruise, where she assumed she had "overdone it" with exercise. She first had lower back and hip pain but then developed pain in her lower abdomen, rectum, and vagina. She has daily pain that is worse when she is sitting, and she describes it as a gnawing, annoying pain. Increased activity and driving for a long time exacerbate her pain, and resting and reclining improve it. She initially had improvement with pelvic floor physical therapy (PT), amitriptyline, and rectal valium, but she has hit a wall in her improvement. She has no issues with her bowel or bladder, and neither voiding nor having a bowel movement worsens her pelvic pain. Her goal of seeking care is to "get back to my normal life with hiking, fishing, and golfing." She is postmenopausal but reports no issues with vaginal dryness. A pelvic examination reproduces her pain with palpation of her pelvic floor musculature. Her lumbar spine is also tender to palpation in her paraspinal muscles, as were her sacroiliac joints.

Ms. A reports a long-standing history of anxiety, as well as some relationship dissatisfaction with her same-sex partner of 9 years. She reports feeling anxiety about her chronic pain, which includes worries about whether she will ever be pain free and anxiety about how her chronic pain impacts her partner. She also worries about the amount of sick leave she has had to take for her medical issues and often ruminates about whether her family and friends find her to be a burden. There have been periods of time when she has trouble getting out of bed and lacks the motivation to do much of anything. Ms. A has never felt suicidal, but she does reveal that at times she wonders if everyone else would be better off if she were not here.

### Impression

Ms. A has vulvodynia with high-tone pelvic floor muscle dysfunction. Her pain treatment plan included pelvic floor PT with biofeedback and dry needling techniques, as well as pharmacological intervention with amitriptyline to treat the neuropathic component of her vulvodynia. She was also referred to a psychiatrist for evaluation and treatment of her generalized anxiety and depressive symptoms. Her psychiatrist prescribed duloxetine for treatment of her anxiety disorder and referred Ms. A to a psychotherapist who specialized in chronic medical conditions. With her therapist, she learned tools from cognitive-behavioral therapy (CBT), guided imagery, and mindfulness to reduce her anxiety and pain symptoms. She was encouraged to engage in aerobic exercise, but this was difficult in the setting of her pain.

### Outcome

Ms. A has continued to work with her gynecological pain doctor, physical therapist, and psychiatry team. Her pain has improved, and she is now able to sit more comfortably and was able to travel for a golf vacation. As her anxiety improved, she and her partner became motivated to start couples therapy, where they learned communication skills training. Ms. A says that their relationship has improved, and she feels more confident in communicating with her partner about her pain and mental health. Through CBT and mindfulness, she has much better awareness about her pain and her triggers. She reports an improvement in her pain to a consistent 2/10 rating from her previous rating of at least 4/10 with exacerbations of 8/10.

# Epidemiology

## Rates/Incidence

In 2006, the World Health Organization recognized CPP as the most common reason for referral to a women's health specialist, representing 20% of all referrals (Latthe et al. 2006a, 2006b). Prevalence data are limited due to the multifactorial and multidimensional characteristics of CPP, as well as limitations in pelvic pain research. Most sources put the prevalence around 15%, which would make it as common as asthma in the general population (Ahangari 2014; Allaire et al. 2018).

### Risk Factors

Reviewing patient history for risk factors can improve diagnosis of CPP. An important risk factor for the development of both pain and psychiatric distress related to pain is a history of physical or sexual abuse. An estimated 45%–65% of patients experiencing pelvic pain have such a history (As-Sanie et al. 2014). It is important to clarify two points: 1) that a history of abuse is not necessary for the diagnosis of CPP and 2) that a history of abuse does not mean that the abuse survivor will automatically develop CPP. Instead, there is merely an association between abuse and CPP, with several theories of how abuse could lead to pain. One theory is that chronic psychological stress from abuse can dampen immune response, which can predispose the patient to gynecological disorders, including pain (Schliep et al. 2016). Another theory involves chronic sensitization of the limbic system by chronic pain stimuli. Sensitization of the limbic system has been shown to correlate with higher depression scores in women with pain, and the depression in turn increases the morbidity from chronic pain and leads to more pain-related disability (As-Sanie et al. 2014). An additional risk factor to consider is genetics, although twin studies have shown only a 14% correlation between twins with CPP (Vehof et al. 2014).

## Screening Methods

Screening during routine care visits can help providers care for patients with CPP. The first step is to ask patients about symptoms of pain with menses, urination, bowel movements, intercourse, and so on. Pain scales and questionnaires can be useful adjuncts to the clinician interview and can allow the clinician to assess severity, effect of functioning, and type of pain (nociceptive vs. neuropathic). A visual analog scale can be a good first step in assessing severity of perceived pain; ask the patient to record her highest level of pain, her lowest level, and the level experienced on the day of evaluation. Multidimensional pain scales, such as the McGill Pain Questionnaire (Melzack 1975), can help also to assess the nature and location of pain, and neuropathic-specific questionnaires can further clarify the nature of the patient's pain. Several questionnaires are designed specifically for pelvic pain, some focusing on urological complaints and others focusing on a wider variety of complaints. The Pelvic Pain and Urgency/Frequency Patient Symptom Scale (Parsons et al. 2002) is widely used to assess pain, urinary symptoms of frequency and urgency, and sexual dysfunction. The International Pelvic Pain Society (IPPS; www.pelvicpain.org) has developed an integrated Pelvic Pain Assessment Form that is specific to women and includes all of the above types of pain assessments along with relevant clinical history (Passavanti et al. 2017).

## Clinical Features

### Diagnostic Criteria

CPP is defined as noncyclic pain in the pelvis present for >6 months with pain sufficient to interfere with normal activities and quality of life (QoL) (Ahangari 2014). The Royal College of Obstetricians and Gynecologists defines CPP as "intermittent or constant pain in the lower abdomen or pelvis of at least 6 months duration, not occurring exclusively with menstruation or intercourse and not associated with pregnancy" (Ahangari 2014, p. 2). The IPPS developed a publicly available form on their website (www.pelvicpain.org) that can help patients and providers synthesize pertinent information about a patient's history and physical examination. The intake form is available in English, French, Spanish, and Portuguese. The patient fills out her full medical and surgical history along with a pain history, including exacerbating and relieving factors. The provider uses the form to document the extensive physical examination. Additional documents include a health care assessment form and a patient follow-up form to monitor and record the patient's progress in her pain management plan. Again, forms are available on the IPPS website.

### Clinical Presentation

Presentation of symptoms can be variable because CPP is multifactorial, with contributions from structures that are not only gynecological but also urological, gastrointestinal, musculoskeletal, and psychological. CPP is an overlapping pain syndrome and can be thought of as a complex neuromuscular-psychosocial disorder (Speer et al. 2016). Patients often report other somatic pain syndromes, such as irritable bowel syndrome and chronic fatigue syndrome, in addition to mental health disorders such as PTSD and depression (Speer et al. 2016). Patients with CPP report higher rates of depression than do their pain-free counterparts, which can also lead to functional impairments with sleep, household activities, absences from work, and difficulties with sexual relationships, among others (Miller-Matero et al. 2016).

### Course and Prognosis

The course and prognosis of CPP are also variable and dependent on underlying etiologies. For patients with primarily gynecological etiologies, pain can persist even after standard gynecological management of underlying conditions (Allaire et al. 2018). A multidisciplinary approach can improve patient outcomes, but even in that setting the prognosis can be variable. Factors associated with higher pain severity even after starting a multidisciplinary treatment protocol include greater pain catastrophizing ($P=0.02$), abdominal wall pain ($P=0.02$), history of sexual assault ($P=0.04$), total number of comorbidities ($P=0.02$), and patients discharged from a pain clinic who require re-referral to return to treatment ($P=0.008$) (Allaire et al. 2018).

### Differential Diagnosis

The differential diagnosis of CPP is broad, with patients often reporting pain in multiple organ systems. For example, in a study of patients with interstitial cystitis, 93% had concurrent pelvic pain, 70% had dyspareunia, 60% had vulvodynia, 52% had constipation, 49% had irritable bowel syndrome, and 17% had fibromyalgia (Hoffman 2011). Clearly, the diagnosis of CPP requires a thorough approach with consideration of the entire person and not merely the location of the reported pain.

## Pathophysiology

### Biological Factors

The multifactorial nature of CPP means that it has various causes. For patients with underlying gynecological conditions, an inciting event can lead to pain. For example, a hemorrhagic ovarian cyst can lead to pain with hemoperitoneum. Similarly, patients experiencing pregnancy and delivery can have acute pain after delivery that persists into CPP. The process of acute pain transitioning to chronic pain is related to several neurobiological factors. Through convergence of afferent nerves at the level of the dorsal root ganglion in the spinal cord, pain can propagate through viscerovisceral convergence, viscerosomatic convergence, and somatovisceral convergence (Hoffman 2011). Nociceptive stimulation can travel along afferent nerves to the CNS and lead to efferent stimulation, allowing inflammatory mediators to be released into viscera. In *viscerovisceral convergence*, nerves from painful viscera converge on the dorsal horn with nerves from nonpainful viscera, which can lead to pain separate from the organ of origin. A good example of this type of convergence is endometriosis, in which pain from endometrial implants in the pelvis or on the ovaries can lead to bladder voiding dysfunction and pain. In *viscerosomatic convergence*, noxious afferent signals from a visceral pain source converge with somatic afferents in the spinal cord, which leads to areas of the body that are seemingly unconnected but share a dermatome for experiencing pain. For example, noxious stimuli from dysmenorrhea (painful periods) converge with somatic afferents and lead to abdominal wall pain and hyperalgesia. Finally, in *somatovisceral convergence*, noxious afferents from muscle and somatic structures converge with visceral afferents in the spinal cord and lead to pain in an end organ. This is seen when pelvic floor dysfunction and muscle hypertonicity lead to constipation with painful bowel movements or incomplete bladder emptying and pain (Hoffman 2011).

The plasticity of the CNS can also lead to worsening pain and pain that is distant from the initial nidus. Central sensitization causes expanded areas of pain beyond the original noxious stimuli due to long-term changes in perception from repeated stimuli of pain (Hoffman 2011). When nociceptive stimuli enter the spinal column at the dorsal horn, stimuli can spread to segments above, below, and contralateral to the site of origin. The persistent aberrant stimuli lead to a maladaptive response in the CNS, which causes hyperalgesia, allodynia, and pain remote from the site of origin (Hoffman 2011). Concurrent to the abnormal spread of the painful stimuli, central sensitization can cause de novo pain without any noxious stimuli. Studies have shown that these central changes with chronic pain are not specific to any specific pain etiology but are common to all disease states that cause chronic pain (Hoffman 2011; Morotti et al. 2017).

## Psychological Factors

Patients with CPP have been found to have higher rates of depression and anxiety than those without CPP, with rates as high as 40% and 73%, respectively (Miller-Matero et al. 2016; Walker et al. 1988). The psychological profile of patients with CPP includes high levels of psychological distress and related increased pain severity (Gomide et al. 2012). There is also a positive correlation between depression symptoms and pain interference, pain catastrophizing, and limiting self-efficacy beliefs (Bryant et al. 2016). Pain catastrophizing is associated with higher pain levels and decreased QoL (Sewell et al. 2018). One theory for the presence of depressive symptoms in patients with CPP is dysregulation of the hypothalamic-pituitary-adrenal (HPA) axis. Patients with CPP who also have depression have demonstrated enhanced cortisol response to adrenocorticotropic hormone stimulation testing (Wingenfeld et al. 2009).

Although sexual abuse itself is unlikely to be a specific etiological factor in the pathogenesis of CPP, the literature shows an association between CPP and sexual abuse in some subset groups (Fry et al. 1993; Randolph and Reddy 2006). Studies have found that patients with CPP who also experienced childhood sexual abuse have higher scores on psychological distress, somatization, and dissociation measures.

### Social Considerations

Patients who have CPP experience considerable deficits in social and professional functioning (Cox et al. 2007; Miller-Matero et al. 2016; Walker et al. 1988). The relationship between functional impairment, CPP, and mood symptoms is complex, with research finding that some areas of functional impairment were not associated with pain but rather with the higher levels of depression and anxiety that accompany chronic pain (Miller-Matero et al. 2016). Similarly, although rates of sexual dysfunction are elevated in patients with CPP, it appears that in some cases the sexual dysfunction is mediated by childhood sexual abuse, depression symptoms, and lack of relationship support rather than by pain itself (Randolph and Reddy 2006; ter Kuile et al. 2010).

A lifetime history of drug or alcohol abuse is associated with increased risk of CPP (Latthe et al. 2006b). Patients experiencing intimate partner violence are at higher risk for developing CPP, as well as other gynecological conditions (Campbell and Lewandowski 1997). Social factors independently associated with a higher severity of CPP include higher BMI, current smoking, and family history of CPP (Yosef et al. 2016).

When considering social support factors, qualitative research has found the most common problems with social support included perceived lack of engagement and a lack of empathy. Patients reported that tangible support was most helpful when coming from clinicians and preferred emotional and informational support when coming from their wider social networks. Patients with CPP reported anger and anxiety around the trauma they experienced in dealing with CPP and wished for external support that also bolstered their personal autonomy (Warwick et al. 2004).

## Treatment

### Psychopharmacology

Pharmacological treatment of patients with CPP is targeted toward minimizing pain symptomatology and treating associated mood and anxiety disorders. In general, psychopharmacological agents that increase the availability of serotonin and norepinephrine benefit patients who experience chronic pain and depression, whereas agents that increase the availability of norepinephrine alone benefit patients who have CPP without depressive symptoms (Atkinson et al. 1998).

Tricyclic antidepressants (TCAs), which elevate levels of norepinephrine and serotonin by inhibiting reuptake, are some of the most common medications used to treat chronic pain conditions, including CPP. Although few empirical studies have looked at the efficacy of TCAs for CPP, the efficacy of TCAs as analgesics is well established for chronic pain in general (Lynch 2001). Clinically, pain tends to respond more quickly to TCAs than do mood symptoms and requires lower doses than needed for treatment of mood or anxiety disorders (Carey et al. 2017; Guay 2001). These medications have considerable side effects, however, including sedation, dizziness, blurry vision, dry mouth, and other anticholinergic effects. Side effects are typically worse with tertiary amines, such as amitriptyline and imipramine, leading to poor adherence and early discontinuation, although amitriptyline is recommended by consensus guidelines for treatment of CPP (Gunter 2003; Rees et al. 2015). Secondary amines, such as nortriptyline and desipramine, tend to be better tolerated (Carey et al. 2017).

Gabapentin, an antiepileptic drug believed to have an effect on voltage-dependent calcium ion channels leading to relief of neuropathic pain sensations, is also recommended by consensus guidelines for treatment of CPP (Rees et al. 2015). Considering CPP in particular, a randomized controlled trial (RCT) found gabapentin, alone or in combination with amitriptyline, to be more effective than amitriptyline monotherapy, with treatment up to 24 months (Sator-Katzenschlager et al. 2005). An additional multicenter pilot RCT also supported the efficacy of gabapentin for patients with CPP (Lewis et al. 2016). Unfortunately, this follow-up study, which randomized 300 women with CPP for at least 3 months with negative laparoscopy for pelvic pathology causing pain, did not demonstrate improvement in pain based on a numerical rating scale (Horne et al. 2020). At this time, use of gabapentin would still be considered off-label and should be done with caution in select patients.

Serotonin-norepinephrine reuptake inhibitors are also thought to have an analgesic effect, and duloxetine in particular is recommended by consensus guidelines for treatment of CPP in women (Rees et al. 2015). That said, the data supporting duloxetine are limited, with one prospective trial of 48 women with interstitial cystitis failing to find a significant improvement in symptoms (Giannantoni et al. 2014). Small studies have found venlafaxine to be effective for depression symptoms and pain relief in fibromyalgia, neuropathic pain, and pain related to mood and anxiety symptoms, although no studies have examined its use in patients with CPP (Grothe et al. 2004).

The literature examining the use of selective serotonin reuptake inhibitors (SSRIs) as analgesics is mixed, with one randomized double-blind crossover study of 23 women with CPP finding no significant improvements in pain or functioning from taking sertraline (Engel et al. 1998; Lynch 2001). Despite these findings, an empirical trial of SSRIs for the treatment of mood or anxiety symptoms may be warranted in a subset of patients, given the high prevalence of psychiatric comorbidity in patients with CPP (Walker et al. 1993). Other adjuvant medications that can be useful include antihistamines, such as hydroxyzine, and the $\alpha_2$-adrenergic agonist clonidine; antihistamines are thought to be helpful for interstitial cystitis because they counteract the mast cell activation in this specific disorder, whereas clonidine works synergistically with morphine (Gunter 2003). Anticonvulsants such as carbamazepine, lamotrigine, and topiramate are also used for neuropathic pain disorders, although no data are available regarding the use of these medications for CPP (Carey et al. 2017). Trazodone may be used, primarily due to the absence of sexual dysfunction side effects; however, small placebo-controlled trials have not shown consistent efficacy for analgesia, and larger-scale studies are warranted (Bossini et al. 2012). Table 2–1 summarizes the psychopharmacological treatments for CPP.

## Other Medical Interventions

CPP is multifactorial, with many gynecological and nongynecological etiologies. As such, the treatment options vary based on the underlying causes. Dysmenorrhea will respond to menstrual suppression through various hormones, such as oral contraceptive pills (OCPs), hormonal intrauterine devices, or progestin implants. Pelvic pain is a common diagnosis leading to hysterectomy, with 10%–32% of all hysterectomies being performed for CPP (Mowers et al. 2016). Interstitial cystitis requires dietary changes, medications, and even procedures such as bladder instillations and cystoscopy. High-tone pelvic floor dysfunction, defined as hypertonic pelvic floor muscles with pain on penetration, squeeze, or palpation of the musculature, can be a musculoskeletal cause of CPP (Jia et al. 2019). PT focusing on myofascial release techniques,

TABLE 2–1. **Psychopharmacological treatment for chronic pelvic pain (CPP)**

| Psychotropic medication | Considerations |
|---|---|
| **Tricyclic antidepressants** | |
| Amitriptyline | Recommended by consensus guidelines for treatment of CPP; considerable anticholinergic side effects |
| Nortriptyline, desipramine | May have fewer anticholinergic effects than amitriptyline |
| **Serotonin-norepinephrine reuptake inhibitors** | |
| Duloxetine | Limited data supporting use, but recommended by consensus guidelines for treatment of CPP |
| Venlafaxine | Small studies showing efficacy for pain in fibromyalgia and neuropathic pain |
| **Selective serotonin reuptake inhibitors** | |
| Sertraline | Literature on efficacy for CPP is mixed, with at least one negative randomized controlled trial; however, given high prevalence of psychiatric comorbidity in patients with CPP, empirical trial can be considered |
| Trazodone | Primarily useful as sleep aid but has been used for analgesia for CPP, although small placebo-controlled trials have not shown efficacy |
| **Anticonvulsants** | |
| Gabapentin | Recommended by consensus guidelines for treatment of CPP; can be used in combination with amitriptyline |
| Carbamazepine, lamotrigine, topiramate | No data regarding use for CPP, but useful for neuropathic pain disorders |
| **$\alpha_2$-Adrenergic agonist** | |
| Clonidine | Works synergistically with morphine for chronic pain |
| **Antihistamine** | |
| Hydroxyzine | Helpful in CPP for interstitial cystitis due to neutralization of mast cell response |

biofeedback, and electrical stimulation is an effective treatment modality (Jia et al. 2019). One study of PT for CPP showed improvement on a visual numerical pain rating scale after approximately 7 weeks of treatment (Zoorob et al. 2015).

Determining the best therapies requires trial and error and a multidisciplinary team. One prospective study on the management of CPP and endometriosis at an interdisciplinary tertiary referral center demonstrated improvement in both pain and QoL (Allaire et al. 2018). The team provided minimally invasive gynecological surgery, pain education, physiotherapy, and psychological therapies. In this program, participants received pain education with validation of their pain. They were taught breathing techniques, postural adjustments, graded exercise, manual therapy, and dietary modifications. Finally, mindfulness-based strategies were implemented with meditation, guided breathing, progressive muscle relaxation, and CBT. After 1 year, participants had decreased severity of pain and improved QoL. Significantly fewer patients presented to the emergency department for pain in the last 3 months of the study period. Although approximately one-third of the participants ultimately had

**TABLE 2–2. Chronic pelvic pain: important points**

| | |
|---|---|
| Screening | Provider-initiated history |
| | Validated questionnaires (e.g., visual analog scale, McGill Pain Questionnaire, Pelvic Pain and Urgency/Frequency Questionnaire, Pelvic Pain Assessment Form) |
| | Addressing concerns at each screening examination, annual examination, or well-woman visit |
| Risk factors | History of sexual or physical abuse |
| | Genetic factors |
| Clinical presentation | Variable depending on organ system(s) involved (e.g., gynecological, urological, gastrointestinal) |
| | Higher rates of depression and anxiety |
| | Social and functional impairments |
| Differential diagnosis | Variable depending on organ system(s) involved (e.g., gynecological, urological, gastrointestinal) |
| Clinical points | Higher rates of depression and anxiety, as high as 40% and 73%, respectively, than patients without chronic pelvic pain |
| | Higher risk in patients with a lifetime history of drug or alcohol abuse and those experiencing intimate partner violence |
| | Amitriptyline, gabapentin, and duloxetine recommended by consensus guidelines for treatment |
| | Multidisciplinary evaluation and care essential for optimal outcomes |

surgery, those who had surgery at this center within this model had improvement in their pain ($P=0.008$), whereas those who had surgery outside of the center did not have improvement ($P=0.84$). This speaks to the importance of the additional services offered in this pain program over surgery alone for treatment of CPP.

Interpersonal psychotherapy has been found to be effective for women with CPP and depression, specifically for reducing depressive symptoms and improving social adjustment (Poleshuck et al. 2010, 2014). It has not been found to be effective in reducing pain interference in this population. With the complexity of CPP, evaluation and treatment require a team approach and patience. Important points to consider during work up and treatment can be seen in Table 2–2.

## Endometriosis

Ms. B is a 26-year-old woman who presents to the gynecologist with 4 years of pelvic pain related to biopsy-proven endometriosis. Her past surgical history includes a hemorrhage following delivery that required a dilation and curettage. A complication during that surgery resulted in uterine perforation with bowel injury. She was emergently taken to the operating room, where she had a partial bowel resection and colostomy formation. She was ultimately able to have the colostomy reversed. Ms. B also underwent a hysterectomy for endometriosis pain 2 years prior to this visit, and all of her surgeries have resulted in significant adhesive disease in her abdomen and pelvis.

Ms. B describes her pain as a constant burning with a dull pain in her lower abdomen that is exacerbated by her periods. Although she no longer experiences bleeding, she experiences cyclic changes of her hormones with ovulation. She continues to have constant, daily, noncyclic pain. She is unable to take OCPs with estrogen due to a personal history of blood clots when taking them previously. She reports bladder dysfunction with the sensation of incomplete emptying and an exacerbation of her pain after she finishes voiding. She also has a history of irritable bowel syndrome with alternating diarrhea and constipation. Bowel movements are painful, but she does get some relief afterward.

Ms. B is happily married, with a daughter. She reports good support from her husband, but sexual intimacy is difficult due to dyspareunia that she experiences with deeper penetration. She describes decreased sexual desire and inability to achieve orgasm with penetration but no issues with nonpenetrative intercourse. She feels like she has to "force herself" to have intercourse with her husband. Ms. B works as a massage therapist and has had to significantly cut back on her work due to her pain. She voices a goal of trying to get back to work full time.

### Impression

Ms. B has CPP due to her endometriosis. She also has musculoskeletal pain in her abdomen and pelvis. She has been taking a gonadotropin-releasing hormone (GnRH) antagonist to treat her endometriosis and deep dyspareunia. Norethindrone was also added to her hormone regimen to further suppress her ovaries to prevent cyst formation. Because of her extensive surgical history, she was told that she was not a good candidate for further surgeries. She also has been taking gabapentin for her neuropathic pain associated with her multiple abdominal surgeries and endometriosis. Ms. B previously had pelvic floor PT and returned to her therapist for further pelvic floor musculoskeletal treatments, including biofeedback and pelvic musculature downtraining. She was referred to a psychiatrist with a trauma-focused practice, and they are using guided imagery to help with muscle relaxation. Additionally, she is working through the trauma of her delivery and subsequent surgeries, as well as the experience of having a hysterectomy at such a young age. Through psychotherapy, Ms. B has been able to process her feelings about infertility and is exploring advanced reproductive technology options to enlarge her family, including oocyte retrieval with use of a gestational carrier.

## Epidemiology

### Rates/Incidence

Endometriosis is a chronic gynecological condition in which endometrial glands and stroma are found in aberrant locations outside the uterus. The cyclic stimulation of these implants with the normal menstrual cycle results in release of inflammatory mediators and can result in worsening pain. Women with endometriosis represent 7%–15% of the general population, about 200 million women worldwide, and upward of one-third of women with CPP (Howard 2009; Morotti et al. 2017). Of women undergoing pelvic laparoscopy for pelvic pain, at least 33% will ultimately be diagnosed with endometriosis (Howard 2009). The ACOG reports that 38% of infertile women are ultimately diagnosed with endometriosis (American College of Obstetricians and Gynecologists 2010).

### Risk Factors

Risk factors for endometriosis include white race, lower BMI, painful periods, and a family history of endometriosis (Mowers et al. 2016). In fact, monozygotic twin studies have demonstrated that having a first-degree relative with endometriosis increases the risk of endometriosis diagnosis by a factor of 7–10 (Mowers et al. 2016). Other risk factors include early menarche, with the first period occurring before age 11 years, short cycles of <27 days, and heavy periods (American College of Obstetricians and Gynecologists 2010).

## Screening Methods

Most women with endometriosis present with pelvic pain or infertility, and thus, screening is not needed; a high index of suspicion can alert providers to the possibility of endometriosis in women presenting with pelvic pain and infertility. Collaboration with a gynecologist can lead to early surgical intervention with diagnosis and treatment to prevent progression. The best outcomes are seen for those patients who receive early diagnosis and intervention.

## Clinical Features

### Diagnostic Criteria

Endometriosis is diagnosed by surgical confirmation of ectopic growths of endometrial glands and stroma (Howard 2009). Neither serum markers nor imaging studies are able to replace surgical evaluation. Endometriosis implants have been described as "powder-burn" black, red, or white lesions (American College of Obstetricians and Gynecologists 2010). At the time of surgery, histological evaluation with excision of endometrial implants is the preferred way to confirm diagnosis. Findings consistent with endometriosis as visualized by surgeons are often used to make the diagnosis; however, due to the variable patterns of intraoperative presentation, research has shown a discrepancy between visual diagnosis and histological diagnosis (American College of Obstetricians and Gynecologists 2010). Imaging studies are not sufficient for diagnosis but can be useful if any adnexal or pelvic masses are present, and in this setting, transvaginal ultrasound is the imaging modality of choice.

### Clinical Presentation

Several theories have been formed about the etiology of the ectopic endometrial growths, including retrograde menstruation, hematogenous or lymphatic spread, or stem cells from bone marrow (American College of Obstetricians and Gynecologists 2010). No matter the underlying etiology of the ectopic endometrium, endometriosis is characterized as a chronic condition. Although most patients report pain and some have difficulty conceiving, a proportion of patients with endometriosis do not have any pain or fertility manifestations. Their disease is typically diagnosed incidentally at the time of surgery for a different indication, such as a tubal ligation. Endometriosis is much more commonly diagnosed in women presenting with "classic symptoms," including abdominal and pelvic pain (OR 5.2), dysmenorrhea (OR 8.1), menorrhagia or heavy periods (OR 4.0), and dyspareunia (OR 6.0) (American College of Obstetricians and Gynecologists 2010; Howard 2009). Dysmenorrhea in this case is pain starting *prior to* menses, typically around ovulation, and continuing through the period.

### Course and Prognosis

With endometriosis, the pain progresses with each cycle and often changes from cyclic pain with periods into a chronic, noncyclic pelvic pain. Additionally, endometriosis implants on nongynecological organs can lead to dysfunction and pain, such as premenstrual tenesmus and dyschezia as a result of bowel implants or bladder pain and dysfunction as a result of bladder implants. However, bowel and bladder symptoms can occur even without direct implants on those organs due to neural convergence at the level of the spinal cord, similar to that seen with CPP (American College of Obstetricians and Gynecologists 2010). If left untreated, the disease can progress, with patients experiencing worsening pain and increased difficulty with infertility. Patients with symptomatic endometriosis report poorer QoL and worse mental health outcomes than those with pain-free endometriosis (Facchin et al. 2015; Souza et al. 2011).

# Pathophysiology

## Biological Factors

The principal manifestations of endometriosis include pain and infertility. As discussed by Howard (2009) and Morotti et al. (2017), endometriosis-related pelvic pain is established through well-understood mechanisms: inflammatory, nociceptive, and neuropathic. Inflammatory mediators (tumor necrosis factor-α, cytokines, interleukin-1β, interleukin-6) and nerve growth factor are increased in the peritoneal fluid in women with endometriosis. The inflammatory markers in the peritoneal fluid lower the threshold of sensory nerves and lead to de novo pain generation. Nerve growth factor causes neuroangiogenesis at the sites of ectopic endometriosis implants with increased nerve growth. Noxious stimuli travel through these sensory nerves to the dorsal root ganglion, where they converge with visceral nerves and carry nociceptive signals to the brain. Once these nerves are damaged or dysfunctional, they cause neuropathic pain with sensitization in the CNS (Howard 2009; Morotti et al. 2017). At this point in the chronic pain cycle, pain generation can be independent of ongoing peripheral stimuli.

The mechanisms whereby endometriosis leads to infertility are less well understood, but the increased inflammatory milieu of the peritoneum is a likely contributor to both sperm and oocyte dysfunction (American College of Obstetricians and Gynecologists 2010).

## Psychological Factors

Women with endometriosis have a higher risk of developing major depression and anxiety disorders. It is unclear, however, whether that risk exists because of the CPP associated with endometriosis or is etiologically related to endometriosis or another factor, such as chronic inflammation (Chen et al. 2016; Pope et al. 2015). Women with endometriosis-related pelvic pain have higher rates of depression and poorer QoL in comparison with those with endometriosis and no chronic pain (Facchin et al. 2015; Lorençatto et al. 2006). Additionally, high levels of depressive or anxiety symptoms can increase pain severity, and higher levels of pain intensity have been associated with increased anxiety (Laganà et al. 2017; Sepulcri and do Amaral 2009). In comparison with healthy control subjects, women living with endometriosis demonstrate higher levels of somatization, phobic anxiety, depression, and emotional sensitivity and lower QoL scores (Laganà et al. 2015). An association between endometriosis stage and psychiatric symptoms has not been found (Sepulcri and do Amaral 2009).

Several small studies have examined whether an association exists between endometriosis and bipolar disorder, with mixed results (Lewis et al. 1987; Walker et al. 1989). A 2011 study compared 27 women with endometriosis with 12 women with CPP unrelated to endometriosis and found that significantly more women in the endometriosis group met criteria for bipolar disorder (Kumar et al. 2011). Moreover, a 2020 population-based cohort study found that patients with endometriosis have increased risk for bipolar disorder (Chen et al. 2020). Given this evidence, a critical component of comprehensive care for women with endometriosis is a thorough psychiatric screening and review of systems (Pope et al. 2015).

Researchers are looking to identify how the experience of living with endometriosis may or may not differ from that of living with other types of CPP. On the one hand, a cross-sectional study of 138 women compared women with endometriosis with women with CPP due to either myofascial pelvic pain or pelvic adhesions and found no difference in pain-related symptoms, disability, frequency of depressive symptoms, level of psychological distress, or satisfaction with relationships. These findings suggest the power of the overarching experience of chronic pain (Roth et al. 2011). On the other hand, some studies suggest that women with endometriosis have more difficulty with social functioning, higher pain scores, and lower QoL than women with other types of CPP (Kumar et al. 2011; Peveler et al. 1996). In a 2018 meta-analysis, Gambadauro et al. (2019) pooled data from nearly 100,000 women and found the association between endometriosis and depression to be largely mediated by CPP. This study found no significant difference in depressive symptoms between patients with CPP related to endometriosis and those with CPP related to other causes.

## Social Considerations

Women with endometriosis consistently score lower on QoL ratings than women without the condition and may have more difficulty in interpersonal relationships than women with unexplained CPP (Laganà et al. 2015; Peveler et al. 1996; Sepulcri and do Amaral 2009). Extended treatment duration is associated with lower QoL scores (Sepulcri and do Amaral 2009).

Women living with endometriosis report a decreased capacity to maintain intimate relationships and report that their chronic pain condition leads to feeling isolated from friends and family. Focus group data from women living with endometriosis suggest that social isolation is a pervasive problem for patients partially because women perceive their relatives and friends as lacking understanding about the condition and the impairments it can cause. Women who experienced social isolation also felt resignation in the face of chronic pain and poor understanding about their symptoms (Mellado et al. 2016). Avoidance of intimate relationships and isolation from family and friends were both aspects of overall social isolation.

Endometriosis affects women's sexual functioning across multiple domains, and although dyspareunia is a major reported sexual symptom in patients with endometriosis, it is not the only factor implicated in sexual dysfunction. Women with endometriosis report being afraid of pain before or during sexual intercourse, and when pain with sex is present, women have fewer episodes of intercourse per month and report greater fear that their partner will separate from them because of their coital pain (Fritzer et al. 2013). Factors that influence sexual functioning include CPP, advanced stage of disease, comorbid psychiatric conditions, and personality traits (Pluchino et al. 2016). Endometriosis affects women's functioning in relationships, with one study finding that 34% of women experienced significant problems with a partner due to their disease, and 10% of women considered endometriosis as a cause of their divorce (De Graaff et al. 2013).

## Treatment

The goals of treatment for endometriosis are multifactorial, meaning that treatment should include pain control, improvement in QoL, reduction of psychiatric symptoms and psychological distress, prevention of disease recurrence and tissue damage, and fertility preservation. Given this complicated set of goals, a multidisciplinary team is required.

### Psychopharmacology

Treatment of psychiatric disorder in patients with endometriosis requires two main considerations: the symptoms related to endometriosis and the symptoms related to the use of GnRH agonists, which are effective in reducing endometriosis symptoms (Laganà et al. 2017; Pope et al. 2015; Warnock et al. 1998a). Trials of psychotropic medications, such as antidepressants and anticonvulsants, are commonly used for both of these indications; however, limited data are available on efficacy in this patient population. The combination of gabapentin, which is a GABA analogue, and amitriptyline has been found to be effective, along with regional anesthesia techniques for managing pain specifically in patients with endometriosis who continue to have symptoms after surgical intervention (Malec-Milewska et al. 2015). Animal studies indicate that the molecular makeup of gabapentin supports its use for chronic pain in endometriosis patients (Bellessort et al. 2018).

It is also important to evaluate existing psychiatric comorbidities that could increase the risk of decompensation related to hormonal therapy (Pope et al. 2015). One retrospective study considered the use of sertraline in patients receiving GnRH agonist therapy. Warnock et al. (1998b) retrospectively studied 42 women with endometriosis who were treated with 24 weeks of GnRH agonist therapy, with or without sertraline. Participants also receiving sertraline reported significantly fewer depressive symptoms, as measured by the Hamilton Depression Rating Scale, but these patients did not differ in reporting of physical symptoms compared with those receiving only the GnRH agonist.

### Other Medical Interventions

Endometriosis is a lifelong disease that requires ongoing management. The use of hormones, such as OCPs, hormonal intrauterine devices, and even leuprolide injections, has been a mainstay of treatment in endometriosis due to the hormonally mediated and cyclic pain seen in the early stages of the disease. Providers prescribe birth control and other hormones to induce anovulation and amenorrhea. The FDA has specifically approved oral norethindrone acetate and subcutaneous depot-medroxyprogesterone acetate (DMPA) for use with endometriosis, with DMPA being as effective as GnRH agonists but without the concurrent bone loss (American College of Obstetricians and Gynecologists 2010). The use of an intrauterine progesterone, such as the levonorgestrel intrauterine system, is not approved by the FDA for endometriosis, but studies have demonstrated improvement in endometriosis-related pelvic pain (American College of Obstetricians and Gynecologists 2010). Medications that affect the hypothalamic-pituitary-ovarian (HPO) axis include GnRH agonists, GnRH antagonists, and aromatase inhibitors. The GnRH agonist leuprolide can be administered monthly or every 3 months in a depot injection. The agonist activity decreases GnRH pulsatility and leads to suppression of the HPO axis and thus anovulation. Elagolix, a medication acting as a GnRH antagonist, has a similar goal of suppressing the HPO axis (Taylor et al. 2017). The long-term use of these medications is limited by side effects, including vasomotor symptoms of menopause and bone health. Aromatase inhibitors are another route to decreasing systemic estrogen and can be used for the management of endometriosis. Aromatase inhibitors prevent the conversion of circulating androgens into estrogen. Aromatase is expressed at higher levels in endometrial implants versus the normal endometrium (American College of Obstetricians and Gynecologists 2018a). Use of an aromatase inhibitor with norethindrone acetate was shown to be more effective at managing pain symptoms than norethindrone acetate alone (American College of Obstetricians and Gynecologists 2018a).

### Nonpharmacological Somatic Treatments

Endometriosis can also be managed surgically. Excision or destruction (fulguration) of the endometriosis can reduce the perception of pain and speaks to the theory that the ectopic endometriotic implant serves as a noxious stimulus leading to nociceptive pain (Howard 2009). When performed in infertile patients, surgical destruction or removal can also improve pregnancy rates (American College of Obstetricians and Gynecologists 2010). Definitive surgical management for endometriosis-related pain is accomplished by hysterectomy with removal of ovaries. The retention of ovarian tissue can lead to recurrent symptoms in 62% of patients and additional surgery in 31% (American College of Obstetricians and Gynecologists 2010). Approximately 5%–19% of all hysterectomies are performed because of endometriosis (Mowers et al. 2016).

Additional therapies include nonsteroidal anti-inflammatory drugs and PT. Progressive muscle relaxation was studied in women with endometriosis who were undergoing GnRH agonist therapy. At 12 weeks, the group receiving progressive muscle relaxation had significantly better improvement in anxiety, depression, and QoL than the control group (Zhao et al. 2012). Moreover, mindfulness-based stress reduction interventions have been found to have long-term effects on QoL in this population (Hansen et al. 2017). A 2016 study that investigated psychotherapy with somatosensory stimulation (e.g., acupuncture techniques) found improvement in QoL and lowered pain scores in treated subjects compared with waitlist subjects, with improvements holding at 24-month follow-up (Meissner et al. 2016). Minimally invasive laparoscopic surgery is associated with improved QoL and emotional well-being when compared with medical therapies (Deguara et al. 2012). A high index of suspicion can alert providers to the possibility of endometriosis, which has both immediate and long-lasting effects on pain, fertility, and mental health. See Table 2–3 for important points to consider for these patients.

## Polycystic Ovary Syndrome

Ms. C is a 34-year-old woman with a past medical history of PCOS. She is referred to a reproductive psychiatrist by her infertility doctor for concern about her depressed mood, which is impairing her ability to lose weight and to become a candidate for in vitro fer-

**TABLE 2–3. Endometriosis: important points**

| | |
|---|---|
| Screening | Patient history<br>Gynecological referral for possible surgical intervention and diagnosis |
| Risk factors | White race<br>Low BMI<br>Painful periods (dysmenorrhea)<br>Genetics |
| Clinical presentation | Cyclic and noncyclic pelvic pain<br>Dysmenorrhea<br>Dyspareunia<br>Infertility<br>Depression and anxiety |
| Differential diagnosis | Chronic pelvic pain |
| Clinical points | Early diagnosis leads to early intervention<br>Higher risk of developing major depression and anxiety disorders<br>Higher levels of somatization, phobic anxiety, depression, and emotional sensitivity, and lower quality of life scores vs. healthy control subjects<br>Affects sexual functioning across multiple domains; dyspareunia major reported sexual symptom<br>Multidisciplinary evaluation and care essential for optimal outcomes |

tilization. During her intake, the patient says that she was diagnosed with PCOS when she was 23 years old after reporting irregular periods and difficulty with excessive hair growth, acne, and her attempts to lose weight. Her doctor prescribed metformin, which helped her lose weight initially, but she has more recently seen a plateau of her weight and even some weight gain.

While describing her psychiatric history, Ms. C describes clear episodes of recurrent, moderate depression during which "I don't have the energy to do any of the things I usually love." She also notes symptoms of increased sensitivity, increased need for sleep, anhedonia, increased appetite, poor concentration, and fleeting hopelessness. She has a long history of binge-eating behaviors, followed by a few days when she restricts calories and feels excessively guilty about overeating and is distracted by thoughts about her body weight.

Ms. C and her husband have been trying to conceive for 2 years and began seeing a reproductive endocrinologist 6 months ago. She has attempted four cycles using letrozole. At this time, the fertility clinic is recommending that she consider in vitro fertilization, but she is not a candidate due to her BMI. The clinic has provided her with a nutrition referral, and she has attempted to implement the suggestions but has not seen improvement. On further evaluation, Ms. C admits that in addition to the stress she feels about ongoing infertility treatment, she has felt very depressed over the past 2 months. She has been having more thoughts about wanting to give up on trying to conceive and thinks that this is "proof" that she will be a bad mother.

## Impression

Ms. C is currently experiencing an episode of severe depression and would benefit from a combination of psychotherapy and psychotropic medications. The psychiatrist ultimately has the patient start taking sertraline 50 mg/day and over several weeks increases the dose to 175 mg/day. Ms. C continues outpatient psychotherapy, which she finds helpful for managing thoughts related to her low self-esteem, issues related to her weight loss struggles, and concerns about fertility.

### Outcome

When Ms. C returns 2 months later, she reports improvement in her mood and is particularly proud because she has been involved in an exercise program that has helped her lose 5 lb. She is feeling more optimistic about her future fertility and the possibility of conceiving through in vitro fertilization.

## Epidemiology

### Rates/Incidence

PCOS is a disease characterized by irregular menstrual bleeding, hyperandrogenism, hyperandrogenemia, and polycystic-appearing ovaries. It is part of the spectrum of diseases leading to normogonadotropic normoestrogenic anovulation, and PCOS is diagnosed in 55%–91% of women with this anovulatory bleeding pattern (American College of Obstetricians and Gynecologists 2018b; Fauser 2004). Women with hyperandrogenic anovulation/oligoovulation make up 7% of reproductive-aged women, and PCOS represents one of the most common endocrinopathies among this patient population (Bednarska and Siejka 2017). Because PCOS is a diagnosis of exclusion, the exact prevalence varies depending on the diagnostic criteria used.

### Risk Factors

PCOS has no known genetic or environmental risk factors, but insulin resistance and obesity may play a role because increased circulating insulin can lead to a decrease in sex hormone–binding globulin and thus increased androgens (American College of Obstetricians and Gynecologists 2018b). PCOS is diagnosed with a higher frequency in Hispanic and Native American women (Bednarska and Siejka 2017).

## Screening Methods

According to the ACOG's Practice Bulletin, at the time of diagnosis, patients should be screened for insulin resistance or diabetes with a 2-hour oral glucose tolerance test (American College of Obstetricians and Gynecologists 2018b). Due to unopposed estrogen exposure at the level of the endometrium from anovulation, women with PCOS are at risk of developing metabolic syndrome and insulin resistance, type 2 diabetes, nonalcoholic fatty liver, obesity-related obstructive sleep apnea, and endometrial cancer (American College of Obstetricians and Gynecologists 2018b; Fauser 2004). They have a three- to sevenfold increased risk of developing type 2 diabetes (Fauser 2004). Upon diagnosis of PCOS, whether made by a gynecologist or primary care physician, the patient should be counseled about implications related to her obstetric and gynecological health, as well as her overall health and well-being. The ACOG recommends serial blood pressure measurements, monitoring and documentation of BMI, measurement of waist circumference, and evaluation for stigmata of PCOS, including hirsutism, acne, and acanthosis nigricans (American College of Obstetricians and Gynecologists 2018b). Although the physiological changes are important to evaluate, treat, and follow, the psychological changes associated with PCOS are also essential to evaluate and treat.

# Clinical Features

## Diagnostic Criteria

No single set of criteria has yet been accepted for PCOS, and providers must first rule out other causes of symptoms. Patients who present with symptoms consistent with PCOS should first be evaluated with thyroid hormone testing, a serum prolactin to rule out hyperprolactinemia, and other studies, including follicle-stimulating hormone (FSH) and estradiol, to rule out a hypothalamic or pituitary etiology for their oligomenorrhea (Fauser 2004). Hyperandrogenic symptoms could be related to an androgen-secreting tumor, intake of exogenous androgens, Cushing syndrome, nonclassic congenital adrenal hyperplasia, or acromegaly (American College of Obstetricians and Gynecologists 2018b). Screening with serum androgens (free and total testosterone and dehydroepiandrosterone sulfate) and serum 17α-hydroxyprogesterone can assist with making the diagnosis. The level of 17α-hydroxyprogesterone will be elevated in patients with nonclassic congenital adrenal hyperplasia (American College of Obstetricians and Gynecologists 2018b). Several diagnostic algorithms are used, including the National Institutes of Health criteria developed in 1990 (Zawadski and Dunaif 1992), the Rotterdam criteria developed in 2003 (Fauser 2004), and the Androgen Excess Society criteria developed in 2006 (Azziz et al. 2006) (Table 2–4).

## Clinical Presentation

Patients typically present with menstrual disorders or infertility (American College of Obstetricians and Gynecologists 2018b; Bednarska and Siejka 2017; Fauser 2004). Abdominal obesity is diagnosed in 30%–70% of patients with PCOS (Bednarska and Siejka 2017). Hyperandrogenism is also a common finding that can be expressed through clinical features, such as hirsutism and acne, or as hyperandrogenemia (American College of Obstetricians and Gynecologists 2018b; Fauser 2004). Comorbid insulin resistance and type 2 diabetes are often diagnosed in these patients; up to 50% of both obese and nonobese women with PCOS demonstrate insulin resistance (Fauser 2004). Finally, there is a close correlation between PCOS and mental health disorders, including an increased risk of depression, anxiety, bipolar disorder, bulimia, and anorexia (Bednarska and Siejka 2017).

# Pathophysiology

## Biological Factors

The underlying pathophysiology of the development of PCOS is unknown (American College of Obstetricians and Gynecologists 2018b). No certain genetic condition or environmental substance has been identified as a causative agent. Obesity is a common comorbidity, but it is not required for diagnosis. Insulin resistance may play a role because hyperinsulinemia may be linked to decreased levels of sex hormone–binding globulin; however, hyperandrogenism, which is central to PCOS, can be due to causes other than hyperinsulinemia.

## Psychological Factors

PCOS, historically conceptualized as an endocrine disorder, is a condition with profound impact on emotional life, psychology, and social functioning. Although many

**TABLE 2–4. Diagnostic criteria for polycystic ovary syndrome**

| National Institutes of Health criteria[a] | Rotterdam criteria[b] | Androgen Excess Society criteria[c] |
|---|---|---|
| 1. Hyperandrogenism and<br>2. Oligomenorrhea or amenorrhea | Must have at least two of three:<br>1. Polycystic appearance to ovaries*<br>2. Hyperandrogenism or hyperandrogenemia<br>3. Oligomenorrhea or amenorrhea | Hyperandrogenism with<br>1. Polycystic appearance to ovaries* and/or<br>2. Oligomenorrhea or amenorrhea |

*Defined as ≥12 follicles (defined as a cyst measuring 2–9 mm in diameter) or ovarian volume ≥10 mL (Fauser 2004).

*Source.* [a]Zawadski and Dunaif 1992; [b]Fauser 2004; [c]Azziz et al. 2006.

conditions associated with PCOS, such as infertility, hirsutism, acne, and obesity, can cause psychological distress and affect women's sense of self (Kitzinger and Willmott 2002), researchers have identified that women with PCOS are at higher risk for psychiatric comorbidities independent of these factors. For example, meta-analysis data show a fourfold increased prevalence of depressive symptoms in women with well-defined PCOS compared with control subjects (Dokras et al. 2011). Researchers have not yet been able to identify a specific neurobiological cause for depressive symptoms (Himelein and Thatcher 2006b). Hormone studies have been inconclusive, with one study showing that higher levels of free testosterone are associated with improved mood (Rasgon and Elman 2005; Weiner et al. 2004). The increased prevalence of depression has been found to be independent of BMI or infertility (Dokras et al. 2011; Hollinrake et al. 2007). A systematic review and meta-analysis study reported an increased prevalence of generalized anxiety disorder and higher mean anxiety scores in women with PCOS compared with control groups (Dokras et al. 2011). Hirsutism in particular is associated with higher levels of social fears (Keegan et al. 2003; Kitzinger and Willmott 2002; Sonino et al. 1993).

Given the association with metabolic syndrome and obesity, PCOS often affects women's body images. One study looking at body image compared 40 women with PCOS with women with infertility but not PCOS and women with neither PCOS nor infertility; women with PCOS had increased body dissatisfaction and depression scores (Himelein and Thatcher 2006a). Women with PCOS report higher rates of disordered eating, with a 2017 cross-sectional study demonstrating that the risk is four times that of healthy control subjects (Lee et al. 2017). Even when controlling for weight, women with PCOS were at higher risk for disordered eating, as well as comorbid anxiety symptoms, indicating the importance of screening for eating disorders regardless of BMI.

## Social Considerations

PCOS significantly decreases QoL; women with PCOS report decreased satisfaction across domains including family relationships, professional life, leisure, and physical activity (Elsenbruch et al. 2003). Given that women with PCOS report high levels of concern with appearance-related issues (i.e., "growth of visible hair on face," "difficulties staying at the weight you would like"), it has been suggested that the way in which women with PCOS perceive themselves affects their social interactions (Cronin et al. 1998).

In terms of intimate relationships, PCOS negatively affects sexual functioning. Compared with women without PCOS, women with PCOS report lower levels of sexual satisfaction and view themselves as less attractive to their partners (Elsenbruch et al. 2003). Studies looking at hormone levels and sexual functioning in women with PCOS have not shown correlations; ultimately, women with PCOS likely struggle with sexual functioning as a result of the physical manifestations of the condition, which ultimately lead to concerns about sexual attractiveness (Himelein and Thatcher 2006a).

# Treatment

## Psychopharmacology

No RCTs have yet assessed antidepressants for psychiatric symptoms in women with PCOS. A 2013 Cochrane Review on antidepressants for PCOS found no studies reporting on antidepressants' effects on mood disorders, QoL, and adverse events in these women (Zhuang et al. 2013). A 2003 pilot study of 16 women found an association among depression, insulin resistance, and BMI, indicating that hormone dysregulation and underlying metabolic disorder are implicated in the psychiatric symptoms of these patients (Rasgon et al. 2003). Some studies support that some patients with PCOS see improvement in depression with treatment of the underlying hormonal pathophysiology, such as metformin targeting insulin resistance, spironolactone for high testosterone levels, and healthy diet plus exercise to improve glycemic control (Rasgon and Elman 2005).

The decision whether to treat with antidepressants depends on the severity of the depressive symptoms and whether the underlying PCOS is being treated when the patient presents for psychiatric evaluation. If the patient is displaying mild to moderate depression and is not yet being treated for PCOS, and the clinician suspects this diagnosis, the patient should be referred to a gynecologist or endocrinologist for treatment with insulin-sensitizing medication. At least one small non-placebo-controlled study found a reduction in depressive symptoms when patients with unipolar or bipolar depression were treated with an insulin-sensitizing medication (Rasgon et al. 2010); however, this effect has yet to be studied in placebo-controlled trials. Spironolactone's antiandrogenic effects may also help improve depressive symptoms. If the patient is already taking an antidepressant prior to starting treatment for PCOS or is exhibiting severe symptoms of depression, it is reasonable to continue the antidepressant medication or, if not, to prescribe one and refer the patient for PCOS workup and management. When evaluating whether the antidepressant should be continued in conjunction with the initiation of PCOS treatment, the clinician should consider the severity of the patient's psychiatric symptoms. For example, if the patient presents with severe depression or in an acutely decompensated clinical state, stopping the antidepressant would confer added risk.

The relationship between OCPs and mood in women with PCOS requires further research. Studies on this topic have been equivocal, with one observational study reporting improved depressive symptoms in women with PCOS who were taking an OCP (Rasgon et al. 2003) and another study reporting no mood benefits with OCP for women with PCOS (Cinar et al. 2012). The current literature suggests that there may be a subset of women with PCOS for whom an OCP can affect mood symptoms (Robakis et al. 2019); however, more research is needed to further investigate this relationship.

## Other Medical Interventions

When deciding on a treatment plan for a woman with PCOS, the clinician should take into account the woman's clinical presentation and desired clinical effect (Bednarska and Siejka 2017). A common early decision-making concern is whether the patient is trying to conceive. According to the ACOG Practice Bulletin, for women hoping for menstrual regularity, combined OCPs are helpful in restoring normal cycles, decreasing hyperandrogenism, and reducing the risk of endometrial hyperplasia (American College of Obstetricians and Gynecologists 2018b). OCPs are the most commonly used and recommended first-line treatment option for PCOS because of their ability to suppress luteinizing hormone, increase sex hormone–binding globulin, and decrease ovarian androgen secretion. For patients who cannot or will not use OCPs, oral progestins, injection with DMPA, or progestin-secreting intrauterine devices can also be used to protect the endometrium from developing hyperplasia or malignancy.

For women who wish to conceive, providers must focus on inducing ovulation in anovulatory patients. A first-line treatment recommendation, per the ACOG (American College of Obstetricians and Gynecologists 2018b), is lifestyle modification with weight loss and exercise. Pharmacological management in the form of either clomiphene citrate or letrozole can induce ovulation as well. Clomiphene is a selective estrogen receptor modulator that acts centrally in the pituitary gland as an antagonist, increasing FSH and leading to ovulation. Letrozole is an aromatase inhibitor that decreases circulating estrogen levels and increases FSH production in the pituitary gland, with subsequent increases in ovulation. Clomiphene was once the first-line ovulation induction agent, but more recent studies demonstrate that letrozole leads to improved ovulation rates (61.7% with letrozole vs. 48.3% with clomiphene; $P<0.001$), clinical pregnancy rates (OR 1.4; 95% CI 1.18–1.65), and live birth rates (OR 1.64; 95% CI 1.32–2.04). Metformin is another medication commonly used to treat PCOS. When used for infertility, it can improve ovulation rates by increasing sex hormone–binding globulin and decreasing circulating androgens (American College of Obstetricians and Gynecologists 2018b).

Patients presenting with complaints of hirsutism have medical options for treatment, including OCPs and antiandrogens (Bednarska and Siejka 2017); OCPs have FDA approval for this indication (American College of Obstetricians and Gynecologists 2018b). Antiandrogen therapies have FDA approval for the treatment of women with hyperandrogenism. These medications have different mechanisms of action but are all teratogenic because they pose a risk of developing ambiguous genitalia in the fetus and should thus be used only in combination with effective contraception. Spironolactone is a diuretic and aldosterone antagonist that acts as an antiandrogen, but it can take up to 6 months to show full clinical effect. Flutamide is an androgen receptor antagonist and has been shown to be effective in small trials, but patients also reported issues with dry skin. Finally, finasteride inhibits 5α-reductase as its mechanism of antiandrogen action. According to Bednarska and Siejka (2017), patients not desiring medical management have the option of local therapies, including hair removal or destruction techniques such as laser destruction of the follicles or electrolysis. Eflornithine is an inhibitor of the enzyme ornithine decarboxylase that, when applied twice daily for 6 months, can reduce hair growth; it is more effective when used in combination with laser epilation (Bednarska and Siejka 2017).

The other medical comorbidities associated with PCOS, including the stigmata of metabolic syndrome, should be evaluated and treated. As noted, metformin can regulate ovulation and improve menstrual regularity, but it will reduce insulin resistance and improve lipid profiles and thus can also help reduce body weight (American College of Obstetricians and Gynecologists 2018b; Bednarska and Siejka 2017). Weight loss alone can improve multiple fundamental aspects of PCOS by decreasing circulating androgens and can even lead to spontaneous resumption of menses (American College of Obstetricians and Gynecologists 2018b). Therefore, it is important to consider all women with PCOS as being at risk of an unintended pregnancy, so counseling about contraception is important. A PCOS diagnosis has implications for the patient's gynecological health, general health and well-being, and mental health. Table 2–5 has important points to consider when making the diagnosis, treating, and following up with women with PCOS.

## Genito-Pelvic Pain/Penetration Disorder

Ms. D, a 39-year-old married woman with a history of vaginismus, dyspareunia, and generalized anxiety disorder, presents for initial psychiatric evaluation. She has been taking sertraline 50 mg/day on and off for the past 10 years, with good effect. She has never been able to use a tampon due to pain, pelvic examinations have always been painful, and she typically drinks several glasses of wine before intercourse to make herself feel "more comfortable." As a teenager, she remembers having frequent urinary tract infections. In her 20s, when she became serious with a long-term partner and was having increased anxiety as the relationship progressed, she went to a sex therapist and completed a course of vaginal dilator therapy. Ms. D says that this took her pain and avoidance symptoms from a rating of 8 to about a 3–4 on a 10-point scale. She continued to require alcohol to have vaginal intercourse, but she was able to lead a satisfying sex life through nonpenetrative intercourse with her partner.

Three months ago, she married her partner, who is age 45. They would like to start a family, and Ms. D is concerned that she will have trouble conceiving. Since marriage, she has noticed a recurrence of her avoidance behaviors. She and her husband have had penetrative sex only twice in the past 3 months. Ms. D reports feeling as though she is "failing" at her duties as a wife and expresses frustration that her body "doesn't work the way it should." She is panicked that she will not be able to get pregnant. She also notes that although her husband is supportive, she has a hard time communicating with him about sex. Ms. D reports that her libido is intact, and she is able to get aroused when participating in nonpenetrative sexual activities. She is able to achieve orgasm without problem. Ms. D screens negative for depressive symptomatology and does not have a history of trauma. She denies panic attacks but does report an increase in generalized anxiety related to her performance at work and her worries about being able to become pregnant.

### Impression

Ms. D has several factors in her history that are associated with a genito-pelvic pain disorder, including an inability to use tampons, history of pain with pelvic examinations, and chronic urinary tract infections. Dyspareunia can have a relapsing and remitting course. With the couple's new goal of starting a family and the additional concerns about

**TABLE 2–5. Polycystic ovary syndrome (PCOS): important points**

| | |
|---|---|
| Screening | Menstrual history<br>Glucose intolerance testing<br>Evaluation for metabolic syndrome<br>Evaluation for hyperandrogenism/hyperandrogenemia |
| Risk factors | Insulin resistance<br>Obesity<br>Ethnicity (higher among Hispanic and Native American women) |
| Clinical presentation | Amenorrhea or oligomenorrhea<br>Abdominal obesity<br>Hyperandrogenism<br>Insulin resistance<br>Depression<br>Anxiety<br>Bipolar disorder<br>Eating disorders |
| Differential diagnosis | Anovulatory bleeding<br>Thyroid disease or prolactinoma |
| Clinical points | Associated conditions (e.g., infertility, hirsutism, acne, obesity) may cause psychological distress and affect sense of self; patients at higher risk for psychiatric comorbidities independent of these factors<br>Given association with metabolic syndrome and obesity, PCOS often affects body image; patients report higher rates of disordered eating<br>Negatively affects sexual functioning; patients reporting lower levels of sexual satisfaction and viewing themselves as less attractive to partners compared with women without PCOS |

her fertility, Ms. D's condition has flared, causing increased generalized anxiety. Her workup should consist of a referral to a sexual medicine specialist, a pelvic floor physical therapist, and a couples' therapist. She would also benefit from individual psychotherapy to address her generalized anxiety symptoms and to cope with the transition to motherhood. Given that her history puts her at elevated risk for perinatal mood and anxiety disorders, an increase of sertraline would be reasonable; the fact that her orgasm and libido are intact indicates that her sexual dysfunction is not related to the SSRI.

## Outcome

Ms. D is diagnosed with provoked vulvodynia by a sexual medicine specialist and given education about her condition and treatment options. She is taught strategies such as mindfulness, progressive muscle relaxation, and deep breathing. In her work with a pelvic floor physical therapist, she learns exercises to complete at home for pelvic floor muscle downtraining, as well as desensitization techniques using vaginal dilators. Her husband is asked to attend sessions and participate in her exercises at home. Through couples therapy, they are able to learn more helpful communication techniques around sex and desire. They also decide to concurrently pursue fertility treatment to reduce the pressure on penetrative sex and increase the chances of conception. Through individual psychotherapy and an increase of sertraline to 150 mg/day, Ms. D's generalized anxiety returns to baseline levels. Within 6 months, she and her husband are having more regular penetrative sex, and she becomes pregnant after her second fertility treatment.

# Epidemiology

## Rates/Incidence

Although the prevalence of GPPPD is unknown, more is understood about specific dimensions of the disorder (dimensions that were considered separate disorders prior to being combined into one disorder in DSM-5 [American Psychiatric Association 2013]). Vulvodynia—chronic pain or discomfort around the vulva with no identifiable cause—is the most common cause of pain with sex. It is estimated to affect 5%–17% of women in the general population, but both vulvodynia and the related genito-pelvic pain condition vestibulodynia (a more localized form of vulvodynia) are underdiagnosed and undertreated (Lahaie et al. 2010). Dyspareunia (painful or difficult intercourse) affects between 14% and 34% of younger women and between 6.5% and 45.0% of older women. Vaginismus (painful spasmodic contraction of the vagina in response to physical contact or pressure) is less commonly researched, and prevalence ranges from 1% to 6% (see van Lankveld et al. 2010 for a discussion of women's sexual pain disorders). The prevalence of persistent genital arousal disorder (PGAD), a genital pain condition characterized by unwanted genital arousal, is currently unknown (Squibb et al. 2019). Although most of the literature studying genital pain has reported on heterosexual women, one survey of more than 1,000 lesbian and heterosexual women looking at the prevalence of sexual problems found that sexual pain was the most frequent sexual problem reported by both groups (Peixoto and Nobre 2015).

## Risk Factors

The correlation between sexual or physical abuse and GPPPD remains unclear. Although abuse is a commonly cited predictor of dyspareunia and vaginismus as defined in DSM-IV (American Psychiatric Association 1994), Lahaie et al. (2010) found relatively few good-quality research studies investigating this issue, and five of the six studies found no evidence of a higher prevalence of sexual and physical abuse in women with these disorders. The medical literature frequently reports that women with dyspareunia and vaginismus more often endorse negative sexual attitudes; however, only one study has used a control group and standardized measures, and the results did not support this notion (Biswas and Ratnam 1995). Women with genito-pelvic pain report fewer sexual relationships and increased avoidance of sexual activity when compared with control subjects, yet it is unclear whether these findings are consequences or causes of vaginismus and sexual dysfunction. A community-based epidemiological study found that women with prior mood or anxiety disorders were four times more likely to develop vulvodynia. This work also demonstrated that vulvodynia was associated with recurrent or new-onset anxiety or mood disorders (Khandker et al. 2011). A more recent study found that women with PGAD are also more likely to report depressive symptoms, panic attacks, and obsessive-compulsive symptoms; however, no causal relationship has been identified (Squibb et al. 2019).

# Screening Methods

Screening for and diagnosing GPPPD and related sexual dysfunction are difficult because of the stigma surrounding sex. Furthermore, because women often present for treatment only after they experience sexual dysfunction, earlier clinical signs (e.g., difficulty with the use of tampons) might not be appreciated (American Psychiatric Association 2013). When asking about libido, the clinician should ask directly about pain with sex, because it is not uncommon for women to report decreased interest in sex without disclosing that sex is, in fact, painful. Evaluation of GPPPD must include a thorough evaluation of the onset of sexual activity and sexual experiences, childhood experiences and trauma history, reproductive history and infertility concerns, and partner violence. Mental health professionals should pay close attention to mood, anxiety, posttraumatic stress symptoms, and substance use issues (Brotto et al. 2016).

# Clinical Features

## Diagnostic Criteria

DSM-5 collapses the DSM-IV concepts of dyspareunia and vaginismus into the single diagnostic category, GPPPD (Box 2–1), based on the fact that the literature and clinical practice suggest that differentiating these conditions may not be possible (Sungur and Gündüz 2014). This expanded DSM-5 category includes four commonly comorbid symptom dimensions and requires the presence of only one of these for a duration of 6 months for the diagnosis: 1) difficulty with vaginal penetration during intercourse, 2) marked vulvovaginal or pelvic pain during vaginal penetration or attempts at penetration, 3) fear or anxiety about pain with vaginal penetration, or 4) pelvic floor tightening when vaginal penetration is attempted. Some experts in the field propose a disease spectrum, with vaginismus accompanied by anxiety and avoidance at one end and pain with intercourse and hypertonic pelvic floor muscles at the other (Derogatis et al. 2010). Current conceptualizations of vaginismus integrate pelvic floor muscle tension, genital pain, and fear (Lahaie et al. 2010).

### Box 2–1. DSM-5 Criteria for Genito-Pelvic Pain/Penetration Disorder

A. Persistent or recurrent difficulties with one (or more) of the following:
   1. Vaginal penetration during intercourse.
   2. Marked vulvovaginal or pelvic pain during vaginal intercourse or penetration attempts.
   3. Marked fear or anxiety about vulvovaginal or pelvic pain in anticipation of, during, or as a result of vaginal penetration.
   4. Marked tensing or tightening of the pelvic floor muscles during attempted vaginal penetration.

B. The symptoms in Criterion A have persisted for a minimum duration of approximately 6 months.

C. The symptoms in Criterion A cause clinically significant distress in the individual.

D. The sexual dysfunction is not better explained by a nonsexual mental disorder or as a consequence of a severe relationship distress (e.g., partner violence) or other significant stressors and is not attributable to the effects of a substance/medication or another medical condition.

*Specify* whether:

**Lifelong:** The disturbance has been present since the individual became sexually active.

**Acquired:** The disturbance began after a period of relatively normal sexual function.

*Specify* current severity:

**Mild:** Evidence of mild distress over the symptoms in Criterion A.

**Moderate:** Evidence of moderate distress over the symptoms in Criterion A.

**Severe:** Evidence of severe or extreme distress over the symptoms in Criterion A.

*Source.* Reprinted from American Psychiatric Association: *Diagnostic and Statistical Manual of Mental Disorders*, 5th Edition. Arlington, VA, 2013, p. 437. Copyright © 2013 American Psychiatric Association. Used with permission.

## Clinical Considerations

The prevalence of postpartum genito-pelvic pain in women has been found to be as high as 27% at 3 months postpartum, with the literature reporting rates as high as 33% at 1 year postpartum. The prevalence of postpartum dyspareunia is higher; studies report that up to 62% of women report pain with sex at 3 months postpartum, with rates as high as 33% lasting through 18 months postpartum. Perineal trauma increases the risk for CPP in the short term; however, the results are equivocal when looking at mode of delivery or parity status. Women who had deliveries requiring vaginal instrumentation are at a higher risk of experiencing pelvic pain after childbearing (Rosen and Pukall 2016).

When looking at conception and pregnancy patterns for women with preexisting GPPPD, clinicians should be aware that trying to conceive and the childbearing process may trigger a worsening of mood or anxiety symptoms. The concerns for women with sexual pain disorders include managing pain during intercourse, the use of lubricants or pain medications to allow for penetration and the women's safety in pregnancy, the need to pursue advanced reproductive technologies for conception when intercourse is not possible, and fears around pelvic examination during pregnancy and around the delivery itself (Rosenbaum and Padoa 2012).

Research looking at this population is limited, but the existing data indicate that women with GPPPD are more likely to have cesarean sections, with one study of almost 200,000 deliveries finding that women with vaginismus also have higher rates of labor induction and vacuum extraction but no differences in birth outcomes (Goldsmith et al. 2009). Women with vulvodynia have been found to be just as likely to carry a pregnancy to term but experience higher rates of cesarean section (Nguyen et al. 2012). Qualitative data analyzing how women with vulvodynia regarded conception, pregnancy, and delivery indicate that dyspareunia itself plays an important role in a couple's physical and emotional ability to conceive. To deal with pain around pregnancy, women report utilizing coping mechanisms including pain minimization, planning pregnancy-safe treatment, and timing intercourse around ovulation. These women report experiencing anxiety around how pregnancy may change pain symptoms, as well as having a mistrustful attitude toward dealing with the health care system and clinicians in the context of prenatal care and delivery (Johnson et al. 2015).

# Pathophysiology

## Biological Factors

Current understanding of chronic pain syndromes such as GPPPD suggest that chronic pain often has both peripheral and central nervous system contributions to pain signaling. These can include local response to tissue injury and abnormal central processing of pain. Pain response and signaling are known to be modulated by psychiatric disorders such as depression and anxiety, as well as by environmental stress and trauma (Carey et al. 2017). Little research has been done on biological pathways that contribute to GPPPD specifically.

## Psychological Factors

Women presenting with sexual complaints are likely to report mood or anxiety concerns. Conversely, women presenting with mood or anxiety concerns are likely to report difficulty in their sex lives. Meta-analysis data support a bidirectional relationship between sexual dysfunction and depressive disorders (Atlantis and Sullivan 2012). For women with GPPPD, fear plays a critical role (Lahaie et al. 2010). Fear of pain has been reported as the primary reason that women with these conditions abstain from or avoid sexual intercourse (Reissing et al. 2003). Moreover, women with vulvodynia describe the emotional burden associated with their vulvar pain, as well as the negotiation of sexual intercourse within heterosexual relationships, as causing them to feel inadequate as women and as partners (Ayling and Ussher 2008). Women with vulvar pain report higher rates of depression and affective distress (Pukall et al. 2007); one study found that one-fourth of women experiencing vulvar pain reported considering suicide (Gordon et al. 2003). A 2019 survey of 51 women with PGAD found that depressive symptoms significantly predicted sexual distress, but anxiety and stress measures did not (Squibb et al. 2019).

## Social Considerations

GPPPD and related conditions have a pervasive impact on women's interpersonal relationships and QoL. Studies show that most women with vulvodynia report at least a moderate impact on their sex life; in one study, 40% of women reported an extreme effect (Arnold et al. 2006). Although some women abstain from intercourse altogether, others who continue to be sexually active have reported experiencing emotional or physical pleasure that outweighs the pain (Gordon et al. 2003). The impact on relationship functioning for these women is somewhat variable, with some couples developing a problematic cycle of pain, avoidance, conflict, and distress (Pukall et al. 2007). Some women with vulvodynia, however, reported that an understanding partner helped them cope with pain (Gordon et al. 2003). Although most research on GPPPD and related conditions has involved heterosexual women, one survey of more than 800 lesbian, bisexual, and heterosexual women investigated associations between relationship qualities and the influence of women's perceptions of pain on their relationships. This study noted that the quality of genital pain reported by all three groups was similar. Women who were in relationships with men, or those who had the potential to be in relationships with men, reported more pain than women who were less likely to be in a relationship with men. Among same-sex couples, better communication between partners was associated with the perception that chronic pain had less of an effect on relationship functioning (Blair et al. 2015). Research on GPPPD in transgender and nonbinary individuals is lacking.

**Table 2–6. Best practices in preparation for delivery in patients with genito-pelvic pain disorders**

| |
|---|
| Childbirth education classes |
| Perineal massage and stretching |
| Positioning that encourages control and autonomy |
| Doula support |
| Trauma-sensitive obstetrical care |
| Discouraging rigid birth plan |
| Encouraging mindfulness-based practices and acceptance |

# Treatment

## Psychopharmacology

Treatment options for GPPPD should target the presenting symptoms (American College of Obstetricians and Gynecologists 2019). Patients with genito-pelvic pain benefit from local therapy. Topical low-dose estrogen is the first-line treatment for women who are able to use estrogen products. For women who are unable to use estrogen products, ospemifene (a selective estrogen receptor modulator) with agonist activity in the vagina can be an alternate. Intravaginal prasterone (a dehydroepiandrosterone preparation) can also be of use for women with dyspareunia. When compared with placebo, prasterone improved all domains of the female sexual function index (American College of Obstetricians and Gynecologists 2019).

## Other Medical Interventions

Patients with GPPPD may benefit from pelvic floor PT. They also may benefit from using lubricants, topical anesthesia, and vaginal moisturizers for symptomatic treatment of dyspareunia (American College of Obstetricians and Gynecologists 2019).

## Nonpharmacological Somatic Treatments

A woman with GPPPD requires an interdisciplinary treatment team, such as a gynecologist, sex therapist, and pelvic floor physical therapist, to achieve symptom remission. Thus, in addition to pharmacological treatments, treatment options should include patient education about anatomy and sexual health, psychological interventions including CBT or exposure therapy and pelvic floor PT (American College of Obstetricians and Gynecologists 2019). For further details on these treatments, see Chapter 3, "Sexual Health and Reproductive Psychiatry."

Given the fear associated with pelvic examinations and childbirth for women with sexual pain disorders, some practices can be put in place to reduce anxiety for these women. Childbirth education and preexposure to the labor and delivery ward can be helpful. Doula support and trauma-sensitive obstetrical practices are also recommended, when available. Women with sexual pain disorders may also benefit from mindfulness-based approaches to childbirth, such as letting go of rigid goals or birth plans and instead cultivating self-acceptance and being in the moment (Rosenbaum and Padoa 2012). Table 2–6 summarizes recommended practices for helping patients with sexual pain disorders prepare for delivery. Important points regarding GPPPD are presented in Table 2–7.

TABLE 2–7. **Genito-pelvic pain/penetration disorder: important points**

| | |
|---|---|
| Screening | Provider-initiated full sexual history, including questions about libido and discomfort or pain during vaginal intercourse, pelvic examinations, or tampon insertion |
| | Inquire about avoidance behaviors |
| | Obstetrical history, including inquiries about birth trauma |
| Risk factors | Prior mood or anxiety disorders |
| | History of abuse, relationship factors, negative sexual attitudes, and lack of sexual education |
| | In postpartum women, perineal trauma and deliveries requiring instrumentation |
| Clinical presentation | Avoidance of sexual activity |
| | Intentionally limited sexual relationships |
| | Avoidance or fear of vaginal penetration (may not volunteer this information without provider-initiated questions) |
| | Reduced sexual interest during pregnancy and postpartum |
| | Symptoms that overlap with those of postpartum depression |
| | Abstaining from or avoiding sexual intercourse out of fear of pain |
| Differential diagnosis | Genito-pelvic pain disorder (including vaginismus and dyspareunia) |
| | Female sexual interest and arousal disorder |
| | Female orgasmic disorder |
| | Vulvodynia/Vestibulodynia |
| | Persistent genital arousal disorder |
| | Infection or vulvar dermatological condition |
| Clinical points | Genito-pelvic pain conditions common postpartum; women with perinatal trauma at higher risk |
| | Provoked vestibulodynia most common cause of dyspareunia; symptoms include burning or itching sensations and can be localized to vestibule region (in which case condition is vestibulodynia) |
| | Persistent genital arousal disorder is relatively newly described condition characterized by unwanted genital arousal in absence of subjective desire or interest; has been associated with selective serotonin reuptake inhibitor initiation and discontinuation syndrome |
| | Trying to conceive and the childbearing process may trigger a worsening of mood or anxiety symptoms for patients |
| | Patient often presents with more than one type of female sexual dysfunction and will require an interdisciplinary team, such as a gynecologist, sex therapist, and pelvic floor physical therapist, to achieve symptom remission |

# Conclusion

The perinatal period is one in which reproductive health comes to the forefront; however, it is important for mental health professionals to remember that gynecological conditions affect women at all stages of life. The majority of women who are referred to a mental health professional secondary to a gynecological condition arrive in the clinician's office due to sequelae of their conditions (e.g., CPP, fertility issues, sexual dysfunction secondary to genito-pelvic pain). The role of a mental health professional is not only to diagnose and treat concurrent psychiatric or psychological conditions but also to provide support for the patient who is navigating a complicated and often confusing medical system. It is important that patients feel validated, because they have often heard, "It's all in your head." Moreover, given that women with many of these conditions must see multiple clinicians to arrive at a diagnosis, they may feel considerable distrust toward the medical system. Mental health professionals are uniquely poised to support women who find themselves with uncertain diagnoses or who have experienced treatment options that still leave them with residual symptoms.

## Key Points

- No single diagnosis or treatment can be used for all patients with any one of these gynecological conditions.
- The multiple underlying causes, diagnostic techniques, and treatments require providers to take additional time with each patient to get to the root of the problem(s) and find helpful treatments.
- When supporting the mental health of a woman experiencing gynecological conditions, clinicians should work together with the patient and a multidisciplinary team to reach the best outcome.
- Mental health professionals should be sensitive to the complex nature of the physical experiences of pain, infertility, abnormal bleeding, and sexual dysfunction, as well as the psychological toll that these gynecological conditions take on women and their families.

## References


Ahangari A: Prevalence of chronic pelvic pain among women: an updated review. Pain Physician 17(2):E141–E147, 2014 24658485

Allaire C, Williams C, Bodmer-Roy S, et al: Chronic pelvic pain in an interdisciplinary setting: 1-year prospective cohort. Am J Obstet Gynecol 218(1):114.e1–114.e12, 2018 29031895

American College of Obstetricians and Gynecologists: Practice Bulletin No. 114: management of endometriosis. Obstet Gynecol 116(1):223–236, 2010 20567196

American College of Obstetricians and Gynecologists: ACOG committee opinion No. 738: aromatase inhibitors in gynecologic practice. Obstet Gynecol 131(6):e194–e199, 2018a 29794680

American College of Obstetricians and Gynecologists: ACOG Practice Bulletin No. 194: polycystic ovary syndrome. Obstet Gynecol 131(6):e157–e171, 2018b 29794677

American College of Obstetricians and Gynecologists: Female sexual dysfunction: ACOG Practice Bulletin Summary, Number 213. Obstet Gynecol 134(1):203–205, 2019 31241595

American Psychiatric Association: Diagnostic and Statistical Manual of Mental Disorders, 4th Edition. Washington, DC, American Psychiatric Association, 1994

American Psychiatric Association: Diagnostic and Statistical Manual of Mental Disorders, 5th Edition. Arlington, VA, American Psychiatric Association, 2013

Arnold LD, Bachmann GA, Rosen R, et al: Vulvodynia: characteristics and associations with comorbidities and quality of life. Obstet Gynecol 107(3):617–624, 2006 16507933

As-Sanie S, Clevenger LA, Geisser ME, et al: History of abuse and its relationship to pain experience and depression in women with chronic pelvic pain. Am J Obstet Gynecol 210(4):317.e1–317.e8, 2014 24412745

Atkinson JH, Slater MA, Williams RA, et al: A placebo-controlled randomized clinical trial of nortriptyline for chronic low back pain. Pain 76(3):287–296, 1998 9718247

Atlantis E, Sullivan T: Bidirectional association between depression and sexual dysfunction: a systematic review and meta-analysis. J Sex Med 9(6):1497–1507, 2012 22462756

Ayling K, Ussher JM: "If sex hurts, am I still a woman?" the subjective experience of vulvodynia in hetero-sexual women. Arch Sex Behav 37(2):294–304, 2008 17876696

Azziz R, Carmina E, Dewailly D, et al: Criteria for defining polycystic ovary syndrome as a predominantly hyperandrogenic syndrome: an Androgen Excess Society guideline. J Clin Endocrinol Metab 91(11):4237–4245, 2006

Bednarska S, Siejka A: The pathogenesis and treatment of polycystic ovary syndrome: what's new? Adv Clin Exp Med 26(2):359–367, 2017 28791858

Bellessort B, Bachelot A, Grouthier V, et al: Comparative analysis of molecular signatures suggests the use of gabapentin for the management of endometriosis-associated pain. J Pain Res 11:715–725, 2018 29692624

Biswas A, Ratnam SS: Vaginismus and outcome of treatment. Ann Acad Med Singapore 24(5):755–758, 1995 8579326

Blair KL, Pukall CF, Smith KB, et al: Differential associations of communication and love in heterosexual, lesbian, and bisexual women's perceptions and experiences of chronic vulvar and pelvic pain. J Sex Marital Ther 41(5):498–524, 2015 24918840

Bossini L, Casolaro I, Koukouna D, et al: Off-label uses of trazodone: a review. Expert Opin Pharmacother 13(12):1707–1717, 2012 22712761

Brotto L, Atallah S, Johnson-Agbakwu C, et al: Psychological and interpersonal dimensions of sexual function and dysfunction. J Sex Med 13(4):538–571, 2016 27045257

Bryant C, Cockburn R, Plante AF, et al: The psychological profile of women presenting to a multidisciplinary clinic for chronic pelvic pain: high levels of psychological dysfunction and implications for practice. J Pain Res 9:1049–1056, 2016 27895510

Campbell JC, Lewandowski LA: Mental and physical health effects of intimate partner violence on women and children. Psychiatr Clin North Am 20(2):353–374, 1997 9196919

Carey ET, Till SR, As-Sanie S: Pharmacological management of chronic pelvic pain in women. Drugs 77(3):285–301, 2017 28074359

Chen LC, Hsu JW, Huang KL, et al: Risk of developing major depression and anxiety disorders among women with endometriosis: a longitudinal follow-up study. J Affect Disord 190:282–285, 2016 26544610

Chen S-F, Yang Y-C, Hsu C-Y, Shen Y-C: Risk of bipolar disorder in patients with endometriosis: a nationwide population-based cohort study. J Affect Disord 270:36–41, 2020

Cinar N, Harmanci A, Demir B, et al: Effect of an oral contraceptive on emotional distress, anxiety and depression of women with polycystic ovary syndrome: a prospective study. Hum Reprod 27(6):1840–1845, 2012 22473394

Cox L, Ayers S, Nala K, Penny J: Chronic pelvic pain and quality of life after laparoscopy. Eur J Obstet Gynecol Reprod Biol 132(2):214–219, 2007 16730874

Cronin L, Guyatt G, Griffith L, et al: Development of a health-related quality-of-life questionnaire (PCOSQ) for women with polycystic ovary syndrome (PCOS). J Clin Endocrinol Metab 83(6):1976–1987, 1998 9626128

De Graaff AA, D'Hooghe TM, Dunselman GAJ, et al: The significant effect of endometriosis on physical, mental and social wellbeing: results from an international cross-sectional survey. Hum Reprod 28(10):2677–2685, 2013 23847114

Deguara CS, Pepas L, Davis C: Does minimally invasive surgery for endometriosis improve pelvic symptoms and quality of life? Curr Opin Obstet Gynecol 24(4):241–244, 2012 22729092

Derogatis LR, Laan E, Brauer M, et al: Responses to the proposed DSM-V changes. J Sex Med 7(6):1998–2014, 2010 20929516

Dokras A, Clifton S, Futterweit W, et al: Increased risk for abnormal depression scores in women with polycystic ovary syndrome: a systematic review and meta-analysis. Obstet Gynecol 117(1):145–152, 2011 21173657

Elsenbruch S, Hahn S, Kowalsky D, et al: Quality of life, psychosocial well-being, and sexual satisfaction in women with polycystic ovary syndrome. J Clin Endocrinol Metab 88(12):5801–5807, 2003 14671172

Engel CC Jr, Walker EA, Engel AL, et al: A randomized, double-blind crossover trial of sertraline in women with chronic pelvic pain. J Psychosom Res 44(2):203–207, 1998 9532549

Facchin F, Barbara G, Saita E, et al: Impact of endometriosis on quality of life and mental health: pelvic pain makes the difference. J Psychosom Obstet Gynaecol 36(4):135–141, 2015 26328618

Fauser BCJM, Rotterdam ESHRE/ASRM-Sponsored PCOS Consensus Workshop Group: Revised 2003 consensus on diagnostic criteria and long-term health risks related to polycystic ovary syndrome. Fertil Steril 81(1):19–25, 2004 14711538

Fritzer N, Haas D, Oppelt P, et al: More than just bad sex: sexual dysfunction and distress in patients with endometriosis. Eur J Obstet Gynecol Reprod Biol 169(2):392–396, 2013 23642970

Fry RP, Crisp AH, Beard RW, et al: Psychosocial aspects of chronic pelvic pain, with special reference to sexual abuse: a study of 164 women. Postgrad Med J 69(813):566–574, 1993 8415346

Gambadauro P, Carli V, Hadlaczky G: Depressive symptoms among women with endometriosis: a systematic review and meta-analysis. Am J Obstet Gynecol 220(3):230–241, 2019 30419199

Giannantoni A, Porena M, Gubbiotti M, et al: The efficacy and safety of duloxetine in a multidrug regimen for chronic prostatitis/chronic pelvic pain syndrome. Urology 83(2):400–405, 2014 24231216

Goldsmith T, Levy A, Sheiner E, et al: Vaginismus as an independent risk factor for cesarean delivery. J Matern Fetal Neonatal Med 22(10):863–866, 2009 19701866

Gomide L, Lima de Souza Montenegro ML, Nogueira AA: Lower pain thresholds in women with chronic pelvic pain: recognizing the role of anxiety and depression as part of person-centered approaches to treatment. International Journal of Person Centered Medicine 2(2):271–278, 2012

Gordon AS, Panahian-Jand M, Mccomb F, et al: Characteristics of women with vulvar pain disorders: responses to a Web-based survey. J Sex Marital Ther 29(suppl 1):45–58, 2003 12735088

Grothe DR, Scheckner B, Albano D: Treatment of pain syndromes with venlafaxine. Pharmacotherapy 24(5):621–629, 2004 15162896

Guay DRP: Adjunctive agents in the management of chronic pain. Pharmacotherapy 21(9):1070–1081, 2001 11560197

Gunter J: Chronic pelvic pain: an integrated approach to diagnosis and treatment. Obstet Gynecol Surv 58(9):615–623, 2003 12972837

Hansen KE, Kesmodel US, Kold M, et al: Long-term effects of mindfulness-based psychological intervention for coping with pain in endometriosis: a six-year follow-up on a pilot study. Nordic Psychol 69(2):100–109, 2017

Himelein MJ, Thatcher SS: Depression and body image among women with polycystic ovary syndrome. J Health Psychol 11(4):613–625, 2006a 16769740

Himelein MJ, Thatcher SS: Polycystic ovary syndrome and mental health: a review. Obstet Gynecol Surv 61(11):723–732, 2006b 17044949

Hoffman D: Understanding multisymptom presentations in chronic pelvic pain: the interrelationships between the viscera and myofascial pelvic floor dysfunction. Curr Pain Headache Rep 15(5):343–346, 2011 21739128

Hollinrake E, Abreu A, Maifeld M, et al: Increased risk of depressive disorders in women with polycystic ovary syndrome. Fertil Steril 87(6):1369–1376, 2007 17397839

Horne AW, Vincent K, Hewitt CA, et al: Gabapentin for chronic pelvic pain in women (GaPP2): a multicentre, randomised, double-blind, placebo-controlled trial. Lancet 396(10255):909–917, 2020

Howard FM: Endometriosis and mechanisms of pelvic pain. J Minim Invasive Gynecol 16(5):540–550, 2009 19835795

Jia X, Rana N, Crouss T, Whitmore KE: Gynecological associated disorders and management. Int J Urol 26(Suppl 1):46–51, 2019 31144734

Johnson NS, Harwood EM, Nguyen RHN: "You have to go through it and have your children": reproductive experiences among women with vulvodynia. BMC Pregnancy Childbirth 15(1):114, 2015 25976086
Keegan A, Liao LM, Boyle M: 'Hirsutism': a psychological analysis. J Health Psychol 8(3):327–345, 2003 14670212
Khandker M, Brady SS, Vitonis AF, et al: The influence of depression and anxiety on risk of adult onset vulvodynia. J Womens Health (Larchmt) 20(10):1445–1451, 2011 21823918
Kitzinger C, Willmott J: 'The thief of womanhood': women's experience of polycystic ovarian syndrome. Soc Sci Med 54(3):349–361, 2002 11824912
Kumar V, Khan M, Vilos GA, et al: Revisiting the association between endometriosis and bipolar disorder. J Obstet Gynaecol Can 33(11):1141–1145, 2011 22082788
Laganà AS, Condemi I, Retto G, et al: Analysis of psychopathological comorbidity behind the common symptoms and signs of endometriosis. Eur J Obstet Gynecol Reprod Biol 194:30–33, 2015 26319653
Laganà AS, La Rosa VL, Rapisarda AMC, et al: Anxiety and depression in patients with endometriosis: impact and management challenges. Int J Womens Health 9:323–330, 2017 28553145
Lahaie MA, Boyer SC, Amsel R, et al: Vaginismus: a review of the literature on the classification/diagnosis, etiology and treatment. Womens Health (Lond) 6(5):705–719, 2010 20887170
Latthe P, Latthe M, Say L, et al: WHO systematic review of prevalence of chronic pelvic pain: a neglected reproductive health morbidity. BMC Public Health 6(1):177, 2006a 16824213
Latthe P, Mignini L, Gray R, et al: Factors predisposing women to chronic pelvic pain: systematic review. BMJ 332(7544):749–755, 2006b 16484239
Lee I, Cooney LG, Saini S, et al: Increased risk of disordered eating in polycystic ovary syndrome. Fertil Steril 107(3):796–802, 2017 28104244
Lewis DO, Comite F, Mallouh C, et al: Bipolar mood disorder and endometriosis: preliminary findings. Am J Psychiatry 144(12):1588–1591, 1987 3688284
Lewis SC, Bhattacharya S, Wu O, et al: Gabapentin for the management of chronic pelvic pain in women (GaPP1): a pilot randomised controlled trial. PLoS One 11(4):e0153037, 2016 27070434
Lorençatto C, Petta CA, Navarro MJ, et al: Depression in women with endometriosis with and without chronic pelvic pain. Acta Obstet Gynecol Scand 85(1):88–92, 2006 16521687
Lynch ME: Antidepressants as analgesics: a review of randomized controlled trials. J Psychiatry Neurosci 26(1):30–36, 2001 11212591
Malec-Milewska M, Horosz B, Sekowska A, et al: Pharmacological treatment and regional anesthesia techniques for pain management after completion of both conservative and surgical treatment of endometriosis and pelvic adhesions in women with chronic pelvic pain as a mandated treatment strategy. Ann Agric Environ Med 22(2):353–356, 2015 26094538
Meissner K, Schweizer-Arau A, Limmer A, et al: Psychotherapy with somatosensory stimulation for endometriosis-associated pain: a randomized controlled trial. Obstet Gynecol 128(5):1134–1142, 2016 27741200
Mellado BH, Falcone ACM, Poli-Neto OB, et al: Social isolation in women with endometriosis and chronic pelvic pain. Int J Gynaecol Obstet 133(2):199–201, 2016 26873129
Melzack R: The McGill Pain Questionnaire: major properties and scoring methods. Pain 1:277–299, 1975
Miller-Matero LR, Saulino C, Clark S, et al: When treating the pain is not enough: a multidisciplinary approach for chronic pelvic pain. Arch Women Ment Health 19(2):349–354, 2016 25941014
Morotti M, Vincent K, Becker CM: Mechanisms of pain in endometriosis. Eur J Obstet Gynecol Reprod Biol 209:8–13, 2017 27522645
Mowers EL, Lim CS, Skinner B, et al: Prevalence of endometriosis during abdominal or laparoscopic hysterectomy for chronic pelvic pain. Obstet Gynecol 127(6):1045–1053, 2016 27159755
Nguyen RHN, Stewart EG, Harlow BL: A population-based study of pregnancy and delivery characteristics among women with vulvodynia. Pain Ther 1(1):2, 2012 25134931
Parsons CL, Dell J, Stanford EJ, et al: Increased prevalence of interstitial cystitis: previously unrecognized urologic and gynecologic cases identified using a new symptom questionnaire and intravesical potassium sensitivity. Urology 60(4):573–578, 2002 12385909

Passavanti MB, Pota V, Sansone P, et al: Chronic pelvic pain: assessment, evaluation, and objectivation. Pain Res Treat 9472925:2017, 2017 29359045
Peixoto MM, Nobre P: Prevalence of sexual problems and associated distress among lesbian and heterosexual women. J Sex Marital Ther 41(4):427–439, 2015 24794229
Peveler R, Edwards J, Daddow J, et al: Psychosocial factors and chronic pelvic pain: a comparison of women with endometriosis and with unexplained pain. J Psychosom Res 40(3):305–315, 1996 8861127
Pluchino N, Wenger JM, Petignat P, et al: Sexual function in endometriosis patients and their partners: effect of the disease and consequences of treatment. Hum Reprod Update 22(6):762–774, 2016 27591248
Poleshuck EL, Talbot NE, Zlotnick C, et al: Interpersonal psychotherapy for women with comorbid depression and chronic pain. J Nerv Ment Dis 198(8):597–600, 2010 20699727
Poleshuck EL, Gamble SA, Bellenger K, et al: Randomized controlled trial of interpersonal psychotherapy versus enhanced treatment as usual for women with co-occurring depression and pelvic pain. J Psychosom Res 77(4):264–272, 2014 25280823
Pope CJ, Sharma V, Sharma S, et al: A systematic review of the association between psychiatric disturbances and endometriosis. J Obstet Gynaecol Can 37(11):1006–1015, 2015 26629721
Pukall CF, Smith KB, Chamberlain SM: Provoked vestibulodynia. Womens Health (Lond) 3(5):583–592, 2007 19804035
Randolph ME, Reddy DM: Sexual functioning in women with chronic pelvic pain: the impact of depression, support, and abuse. J Sex Res 43(1):38–45, 2006 16817066
Rasgon N, Elman S: When not to treat depression in PCOS with antidepressants. Current Psychiatry 4(2):47–60, 2005
Rasgon NL, Rao RC, Hwang S, et al: Depression in women with polycystic ovary syndrome: clinical and biochemical correlates. J Affect Disord 74(3):299–304, 2003 12738050
Rasgon NL, Kenna HA, Williams KE, et al: Rosiglitazone add-on in treatment of depressed patients with insulin resistance: a pilot study. ScientificWorldJournal 10:321–328, 2010 20191245
Rees J, Abrahams M, Doble A, et al: Diagnosis and treatment of chronic bacterial prostatitis and chronic prostatitis/chronic pelvic pain syndrome: a consensus guideline. BJU Int 116(4):509–525, 2015 25711488
Reissing ED, Binik YM, Khalifé S, et al: Etiological correlates of vaginismus: sexual and physical abuse, sexual knowledge, sexual self-schema, and relationship adjustment. J Sex Marital Ther 29(1):47–59, 2003 12519667
Robakis T, Williams KE, Nutkiewicz L, et al: Hormonal contraceptives and mood: review of the literature and implications for future research. Curr Psychiatry Rep 21(7):57, 2019 31172309
Rosen NO, Pukall C: Comparing the prevalence, risk factors, and repercussions of postpartum genito-pelvic pain and dyspareunia. Sex Med Rev 4(2):126–135, 2016 27872022
Rosenbaum TY, Padoa A: Managing pregnancy and delivery in women with sexual pain disorders. J Sex Med 9(7):1726–1735, quiz 1736, 2012 22759362
Roth RS, Punch M, Bachman JE: Psychological factors in chronic pelvic pain due to endometriosis: a comparative study. Gynecol Obstet Invest 72(1):15–19, 2011 21606636
Sator-Katzenschlager SM, Scharbert G, Kress HG, et al: Chronic pelvic pain treated with gabapentin and amitriptyline: a randomized controlled pilot study. Wien Klin Wochenschr 117(21–22):761–768, 2005 16416358
Schliep KC, Mumford SL, Johnstone EB, et al: Sexual and physical abuse and gynecologic disorders. Hum Reprod 31(8):1904–1912, 2016 27334336
Sepulcri RdeP, do Amaral VF: Depressive symptoms, anxiety, and quality of life in women with pelvic endometriosis. Eur J Obstet Gynecol Reprod Biol 142(1):53–56, 2009 19010584
Sewell M, Churilov L, Mooney S, et al: Chronic pelvic pain: pain catastrophizing, pelvic pain and quality of life. Scand J Pain 18(3):441–448, 2018 29794266
Sonino N, Fava GA, Mani E, et al: Quality of life of hirsute women. Postgrad Med J 69(809):186–189, 1993 8497431
Souza CA, Oliveira LM, Scheffel C, et al: Quality of life associated to chronic pelvic pain is independent of endometriosis diagnosis: a cross-sectional survey. Health Qual Life Outcomes 9:41, 2011 21663624

Speer LM, Mushkbar S, Erbele T: Chronic pelvic pain in women. Am Fam Physician 93(5):380–387, 2016 26926975

Squibb L, Stepleman L, Goldstein I, et al: Predictors and moderators of sexually related distress in women with persistent genital arousal disorder. International Journal of Sexual Health 31(4):426–438, 2019

Sungur MZ, Gündüz A: A comparison of DSM-IV-TR and DSM-5 definitions for sexual dysfunctions: critiques and challenges. J Sex Med 11(2):364–373, 2014 24251541

Taylor HS, Giudice LC, Lessey BA, et al: Treatment of endometriosis-associated pain with elagolix, an oral GnRH antagonist. N Engl J Med 377(1):28–40, 2017 28525302

ter Kuile MM, Weijenborg PTM, Spinhoven P: Sexual functioning in women with chronic pelvic pain: the role of anxiety and depression. J Sex Med 7(5):1901–1910, 2010 19678881

van Lankveld JJ, Granot M, Weijmar Schultz WC, et al: Women's sexual pain disorders. J Sex Med 7(1 Pt 2):615–631, 2010 20092455

Vehof J, Zavos HMS, Lachance G, et al: Shared genetic factors underlie chronic pain syndromes. Pain 155(8):1562–1568, 2014 24879916

Walker E, Katon W, Harrop-Griffiths J, et al: Relationship of chronic pelvic pain to psychiatric diagnoses and childhood sexual abuse. Am J Psychiatry 145(1):75–80, 1988 3337296

Walker E, Katon W, Jones LM, Russo J: Relationship between endometriosis and affective disorder. Am J Psychiatry 146(3):380–381, 1989 2784036

Walker EA, Sullivan MD, Stenchever MA: Use of antidepressants in the management of women with chronic pelvic pain. Obstet Gynecol Clin North Am 20(4):743–751, 1993 8115088

Warnock JK, Bundren JC, Morris DW: Depressive symptoms associated with gonadotropin-releasing hormone agonists. Depress Anxiety 7(4):171–177, 1998a 9706454

Warnock JK, Bundren JC, Morris DW: Sertraline in the treatment of depression associated with gonadotropin-releasing hormone agonist therapy. Biol Psychiatry 43(6):464–465, 1998b 9532352

Warwick R, Joseph S, Cordle C, Ashworth P: Social support for women with chronic pelvic pain: what is helpful from whom? Psychology and Health 19(1):117–134, 2004

Weiner CL, Primeau M, Ehrmann DA: Androgens and mood dysfunction in women: comparison of women with polycystic ovarian syndrome to healthy controls. Psychosom Med 66(3):356–362, 2004 15184695

Wingenfeld K, Hellhammer DH, Schmidt I, et al: HPA axis reactivity in chronic pelvic pain: association with depression. J Psychosom Obstet Gynaecol 30(4):282–286, 2009 19922402

Yosef A, Allaire C, Williams C, et al: Multifactorial contributors to the severity of chronic pelvic pain in women. Am J Obstet Gynecol 215(6):760.e1–760.e14, 2016 27443813

Zawadski JK, Dunaif A: Diagnostic criteria for polycystic ovary syndrome: towards a rational approach, in Polycystic Ovary Syndrome. Edited by Dunaif A, Givens JR, Haseltine F. Boston, MA, Blackwell Scientific, 1992, pp 377–384

Zhao L, Wu H, Zhou X, et al: Effects of progressive muscular relaxation training on anxiety, depression and quality of life of endometriosis patients under gonadotrophin-releasing hormone agonist therapy. Eur J Obstet Gynecol Reprod Biol 162(2):211–215, 2012 22455972

Zhuang J, Wang X, Xu L, et al: Antidepressants for polycystic ovary syndrome. Cochrane Database Syst Rev 2013(5):CD008575, 2013 23728677

Zoorob D, South M, Karram M, et al: A pilot randomized trial of levator injections versus physical therapy for treatment of pelvic floor myalgia and sexual pain. Int Urogynecol J Pelvic Floor Dysfunct 26(6):845–852, 2015 25527482

CHAPTER 3

# Female Sexual Dysfunctions and Reproductive Psychiatry

Erika Kelley, Ph.D.
Brittney Bastow, M.D., M.Sc.
Pooja Lakshmin, M.D.
Sheryl A. Kingsberg, Ph.D.

Sexual health comprises a broad range of experiences, behaviors, and concepts and is an important part of women's health and well-being (World Health Organization 2006). This chapter focuses on sexual functioning and female sexual dysfunctions (FSDs) in the context of female reproductive milestones (i.e., puberty, pregnancy and the postpartum period, and menopause). Additional information about specific causes of sexual dysfunction can be found in Chapter 2, "Gynecological Conditions and Mental Health." Research indicates that sexual functioning concerns have a bidirectional relationship with mental health concerns and are often underreported by patients and underassessed by medical providers. Although patients prefer these conversations to be provider initiated, research indicates that medical education on women's sexual functioning is limited, and adequate knowledge about this topic is a reported provider-based barrier to addressing these concerns with women (Kingsberg 2006; Kingsberg et al. 2019b; Parish et al. 2019). Increased understanding of female sexual response and the nature of FSDs may help fill this gap in health care. A majority (62%) of women ages 25–74 years reported engaging in sex in the previous 6 months, according to a U.S. nationally representative survey, and around 60% of women older than 60 years reported being sexually active (Thomas et al. 2015). Despite general decreases in frequency of sexual activity with age, sexual activity, function, and satisfaction remain an important part of well-being across the lifespan.

## Female Sexual Functioning

Female sexual functioning incorporates multiple domains of sexual response, including sexual desire (i.e., sexual "hunger," interest, or drive), cognitive arousal (i.e., mental excitement associated with sexual activity, feeling "turned on"), genital arousal (i.e., vulvovaginal lubrication, genital engorgement, and sensitivity associated with sexual activity), and orgasm (i.e., transient peak of pleasure sensation and release of sexual tension, usually accompanied by involuntary muscle contractions). Female sexual functioning is thought to be multifactorial, affected by biological/physiological, psychological, interpersonal, and sociocultural factors.

## Biopsychosocial Model of Female Sexual Functioning

Classic sexual response models, such as that by Masters and Johnson (1970), described a linear model of sexual response progressing from excitement, through plateau and orgasm, to resolution. Contemporary models of female sexual functioning describe a more dynamic, circular model of female sexual response that involves an interplay of emotional and physical intimacy, relationship satisfaction, sexual stimuli, and psychological factors. These models indicate that some women are likely to begin from a place of "sexual neutrality" and seek out, or are receptive to, sexual stimuli for reasons other than spontaneous sexual desire (e.g., emotional intimacy with a partner) (Basson 2000, 2001; Kaplan 1974). Thus, desire may be "responsive," because sexual stimuli and arousal may precede sexual desire. These models also indicate that both the emotional and physical aspects of satisfaction are important outcomes of sexual activity.

Disruptions in any part of the sexual response cycle may contribute to diminished sexual functioning and FSDs. Furthermore, it has been proposed that sexual response is determined by neurochemical and hormonal underpinnings, including excitatory factors (e.g., dopamine, norepinephrine, testosterone) and inhibitory factors (e.g., serotonin, prolactin) (Kingsberg et al. 2015). According to dual-control biopsychosocial models (Bancroft et al. 2009; Perelman 2007), an imbalance in these factors (e.g., diminished excitatory or excessive inhibitory factors) can result in sexual dysfunction, including disruptions in desire and orgasm (Kingsberg et al. 2015; Parish et al. 2016; Portman et al. 2017).

Studies have shown higher levels of the inhibitory neurotransmitters (e.g., serotonin, endocannabinoids) versus excitatory neurotransmitters (e.g., norepinephrine, oxytocin, dopamine, the melanocortins) in women diagnosed with hypoactive sexual desire disorder (HSDD) (Portman et al. 2017). Other neurochemical and hormonal factors, such as the estrogen deficiency associated with genitourinary syndrome of menopause (GSM) contributing to vulvovaginal atrophy and the sexual pain and vaginal dryness associated with lactation in postpartum women, may determine sexual response. The neurobiology of women's pleasure has historically been understudied and poorly understood, but recent attempts have been made to elucidate the neuronal basis of sexual response in women. Functional MRI data show a gradual increase in brain activity leading up to and during orgasm in women. The brain regions activated include sensory, motor, reward, frontal cortical, and brain stem regions, specifically including areas such as the genital sensory cortex, secondary somatosensory cortex, insula, hippocampus, amygdala, cerebellum, ventral tegmental area, hypothalamus, and prefrontal cortex (Wise et al. 2017).

These contemporary models are consistent with the biopsychosocial approach to female sexual functioning and FSDs, which delineates multiple variables that can affect sexual response, including biological (e.g., endocrine functioning, use of medications, overall physical health, and neurobiological factors), psychological (e.g., mental health symptoms such as depression and anxiety, cognitions or thoughts about sexual function/activity, sexual performance anxiety, body image concerns), interpersonal (e.g., intimate relationship functioning, partner's sexual functioning, life stressors, past relationship or sexual experiences such as sexual abuse), and sociocultural (e.g., religious beliefs about sexual activity and reproduction, family upbringing, other cultural norms and expectations about women and relationships) (Althof et al. 2005; Rosen and Barsky 2006). A thorough understanding of a woman's sexual functioning requires taking these components into account.

## Female Sexual Dysfunctions

FSDs are the experience of a persistent, distressing impairment in a domain of sexual response (i.e., desire, cognitive and genital arousal, orgasm) or the experience of sexual pain that is not otherwise accounted for by other medical or psychiatric conditions, the effects of medication or other substance use, other psychosocial stressors, or relationship distress or problems (American Psychiatric Association 2013; Parish et al. 2019). Although specific definitions vary, dysfunction can be distinguished from normal variations in sexual functioning based on the persistence (e.g., minimum of 3–6 months) and frequency (e.g., impairment occurs in 75% or more of sexual experiences) of symptoms and the experience of distress (Parish et al. 2019; Simon and Lukas 2017). *Sexual distress* can refer to personal distress (e.g., concern, anger, frustration) or be related to the impact on the partner or relationship.

DSM-IV-TR (American Psychiatric Association 2000) included diagnoses of HSDD (persistent lack of sexual desire or motivation), sexual aversion disorder (persistent aversive reaction to and avoidance of genital sexual contact with a sexual partner), female sexual arousal disorder (FSAD; persistent lack of genital lubrication-swelling response of sexual excitement), female orgasmic disorder (persistent lack of orgasm following excitement and adequate stimulation), vaginismus (persistent involuntary muscle spasm or contraction of muscles around the vagina with penetration or intercourse that is often experienced as painful or impossible), and dyspareunia (persistent genital pain before, during, or after penetration or intercourse, often classified as superficial or deep in terms of location of pain). (For further discussion of genito-pelvic pain/penetration disorder, specifically dyspareunia and vaginismus, please see Chapter 2.) DSM-5 (American Psychiatric Association 2013) includes diagnoses of female sexual interest/arousal disorder (integrating DSM-IV-TR's HSDD and FSAD), female orgasmic disorder, and female genito-pelvic pain/penetration disorder (integrating DSM-IV-TR's dyspareunia and vaginismus). However, the International Society for the Study of Women's Sexual Health (ISSWSH) and the International Consultation on

Sexual Medicine (ICSM) support retaining the DSM-IV-TR approach of separating arousal and desire, in part to inform characterization and assessment of functioning and in part because treatment often focuses on one (primary) domain of impaired sexual function (Parish et al. 2019). This recommendation also reflects the equivocal nature of research supporting the combined disorders in DSM-5 (DeRogatis et al. 2011; Pyke and Clayton 2015).

The ISSWSH process of care model for identification of sexual concerns and problems in women presents an overview of evidence-based and expert consensus–based nomenclature for FSDs in line with ISSWSH and ICSM recommendations (Parish et al. 2019). This document includes further specification of arousal and orgasmic disorders beyond those delineated in DSM, such as persistent genital arousal disorder (i.e., the distressing experience of genital arousal or dysesthesia not associated with sexual desire). Table 3–1 lists the ISSWSH and ICSM nomenclature and definitions of FSDs, and Table 3–2 summarizes guidance documents, including the ISSWSH process of care model and additional documents for the assessment and treatment of FSDs.

Estimates of the prevalence of FSDs vary, in part due to variations in the diagnostic classification used, methodology used to assess conditions (e.g., some studies do not assess distress, which can result in overestimates of dysfunction), and sample characteristics. Notably, comorbidity of FSDs is common (e.g., prolonged experience of sexual pain can reduce sexual desire), and it is important to determine which dysfunction is primary when planning treatment (Hayes et al. 2008). Research indicates that disorders of desire and sexual pain are the most common. To date, the largest prevalence survey on FSDs among U.S. women found that 10% experienced distressing low desire, 5.5% reported distressing low arousal, and 4.7% reported distressing lack of orgasm (Shifren et al. 2008). Middle-aged women more commonly reported distressing sexual concerns (14.8% of women ages 45–65 years) compared with younger (10.8%) and older (8.9%) women. Sexual pain disorders were not assessed in that survey.

## Sexual Functioning Across the Reproductive Lifespan

Specific biopsychosocial factors and changes associated with three reproductive stages—puberty, pregnancy and the postpartum period, and menopause—may help determine women's sexual functioning or contribute to FSDs. In this section, we discuss each stage and present rates of and risk factors for FSDs.

### Puberty

Limited research is available on normal sexual functioning and rates of FSDs in girls during puberty, in part due to ethical concerns about assessing sexual function in minor populations. Also, the measures typically used to assess female sexual functioning are validated with adult populations. Much of the extant research focuses on sexual behavior and sexual health risk rather than function. However, understanding of normative sexual behaviors may help guide psychiatry providers in assessing and counseling their young patients.

**TABLE 3–1. ISSWSH and ICSM female sexual dysfunctions nomenclature and definitions**

| | |
|---|---|
| Hypoactive sexual desire disorder | Lack of motivation for sexual activity<br>Reduced or absent spontaneous desire (sexual thoughts or fantasies)<br>Reduced or absent responsive desire to erotic cues and stimulation or inability to maintain desire or interest throughout sexual activity<br>Loss of desire to initiate or participate in sexual activity, including behavioral responses such as avoidance of situations that could lead to sexual activity, not secondary to sexual pain disorders<br>Any of the above, experienced for at least 6 months and combined with clinically significant personal distress that includes frustration, grief, incompetence, loss, sadness, sorrow, or worry |
| Female sexual (cognitive) arousal disorder | Distressing difficulty or inability to attain or maintain adequate mental excitement associated with sexual activity<br>Problems feeling engaged or mentally turned on or sexually aroused |
| Female genital arousal disorder | Distressing difficulty or inability to attain or maintain adequate genital response<br>Vulvovaginal lubrication<br>Engorgement of the genitalia<br>Sensitivity of the genitalia associated with sexual activity |
| Persistent genital arousal disorder | Persistent, unwanted, or intrusive distressing feelings of genital arousal or being on the verge of orgasm, not associated with co-occurring sexual interest, thoughts, or fantasies |
| Female orgasmic disorders | Persistent, distressing compromise of orgasm frequency, intensity, timing, or pleasure associated with sexual activity<br>Orgasm frequency is reduced or absent<br>Orgasm intensity is reduced (muted)<br>Orgasm timing is too late or too early than desired<br>Orgasm pleasure is reduced or absent |
| Female orgasmic illness syndrome | Peripheral or central aversive symptoms that occur before, during, or after orgasm not related to a compromise of orgasm quality |
| Genito-pelvic pain/penetration dysfunction | Persistent difficulties with one or more of the following:<br>Vaginal penetration during intercourse<br>Marked vulvovaginal or pelvic pain during genital contact<br>Marked fear or anxiety about vulvovaginal or pelvic pain in anticipation of, during, or as a result of genital contact<br>Marked hypertonicity or overactivity of pelvic floor muscles with or without genital contact |

ICSM=International Consultation on Sexual Medicine; ISSWSH=International Society for the Study of Women's Sexual Health.

*Source.* Adapted from Parish et al. 2019.

**TABLE 3–2. Guidance documents for assessment and management of female sexual dysfunctions (FSDs) and genitourinary syndrome of menopause (GSM)**

| Reference | Focus of guidance |
|---|---|
| "The International Society for the Study of Women's Sexual Health Process of Care for the Identification of Sexual Concerns and Problems in Women" (Parish et al. 2019) | Process of care for assessment and management of FSDs |
| "The International Society for the Study of Women's Sexual Health Process of Care for Management of Hypoactive Sexual Desire Disorder in Women" (Clayton et al. 2018) | Process of care for assessment and management of HSDD |
| "Global Consensus Position Statement on the Use of Testosterone Therapy for Women" (Davis et al. 2019) | Consensus recommendations regarding off-label use of testosterone therapy (with specific indication for HSDD in postmenopausal women) |
| "The Role of Androgens in the Treatment of Genitourinary Syndrome of Menopause (GSM): International Society for the Study of Women's Sexual Health (ISSWSH) Expert Consensus Panel Review" (Simon et al. 2018) | Consensus document regarding management of GSM, including treatments involving androgens |
| "Management of Genitourinary Syndrome of Menopause in Women With or at High Risk for Breast Cancer: Consensus Recommendations from The North American Menopause Society and The International Society for the Study of Women's Sexual Health" (Faubion et al. 2018) | Guidance on treatment for GSM in women with or at high risk for breast cancer |
| "The 2020 Genitourinary Syndrome of Menopause Position Statement of the North American Menopause Society" (North American Menopause Society 2020) | Guidance on treatment for GSM |
| "International Society for the Study of Women's Sexual Health Clinical Guideline for the Use of Systemic Testosterone for Hypoactive Sexual Desire Disorder in Women" (Parish et al. 2021) | Guidance document regarding off-label use of testosterone therapy for HSDD in postmenopausal women |

HSDD=hypoactive sexual desire disorder.

In general, puberty is seen as the time of onset for sexual thoughts and behavior. Important developmental tasks of adolescence include acquiring a mature sexual identity, expressing responsible sexual behavior, and developing capacity for intimate relationships. Sexual experimentation, either through masturbation or partnered sexual activity, can begin in early adolescence (ages 10–14 years). The physiological changes associated with puberty are typically experienced in middle adolescence (15–18 years) and accompanied by increased engagement in intimate relationships. Middle adolescence is associated with increased engagement in sexual risk-taking behaviors. The prefrontal cortex is still developing into age 22 among females, and decision making and abstract thinking (which may affect sexual decision making and understanding of risks) are not fully formed among adolescent girls (Tulloch and Kaufman 2013).

Research indicates that youth become aware of their sexual orientation between ages 8 and 11 years. LGBTQ+ youth who experience victimization and lack of social support are at greatest risk for mental health concerns, and those who are early in their sexual identity development and who have not yet fully disclosed their orientation are at highest risk for suicide (Scott and Walsh 2014). For most individuals, gender identity will be consolidated by adolescence, although there is evidence of sexual fluidity (dynamic changes in one's same-sex or other-sex desire) across time (Diamond 2008). Thus, psychiatry practitioners should validate adolescents' gender identities and normalize experiences with fluidity in sexual orientation and exploration.

### Rates

As noted, research into FSDs during puberty is scarce. However, a Canadian study of 144 sexually active female adolescents, ages 16–21 years, found that 49.3% reported a sexual problem, with difficulties in desire and orgasm reported most often. Furthermore, 53.5% reported sexual distress associated with the sexual problem. Orgasm complaints appear negatively associated with age (perhaps as a result of increased understanding of sexual activity or increased sexual "skill"), whereas other complaints, including dyspareunia, may be positively associated with age (O'Sullivan et al. 2014).

### Risk Factors

Specific biopsychosocial factors in the context of puberty may determine female sexual functioning (Fortenberry 2013; O'Sullivan et al. 2016; Tulloch and Kaufman 2013). For example, puberty can be experienced as a social role transition associated with the onset of sexual activity. Hormonal changes associated with puberty can initiate feelings of sexual desire that may feel unfamiliar to girls. Physiological and bodily changes may increase vulnerability to body image or self-esteem concerns that can negatively affect sexual function. Young women may be vulnerable to social and peer pressures regarding engaging in sexual activity. Education about sexual activity and health may shape adolescents' perceptions and affect functioning. Further research is needed to examine risk factors for impaired sexual function among LGBTQ+ youth and specific racial or ethnic groups, given evidence in health disparities among minority populations. It may also be difficult to establish risk factors for FSDs in adolescents, especially those who have not yet had sufficient sexual activity experiences to evaluate sexual problems. Assessment of risk factors that are established in adult populations is likely relevant to adolescents. For example, assessment of abuse exposure (especially given that girls in late adolescence and early adulthood are at greatest risk for sexual victimization) and history of medical conditions (e.g., childhood cancer), including those that may affect body image, is warranted.

## Pregnancy and the Postpartum Period

Compared with research on the menopausal transition, relatively less research is available on sexuality during pregnancy or the postpartum period. Research indicates that temporary declines in sexual activity occur during pregnancy, especially in the first and third trimesters, and into the postpartum period. Although most women remain sexually active during pregnancy, this number declines in the third trimester (Lowenstein et al. 2013; Wallwiener et al. 2017). Pregnant women's or partners' concerns about preterm labor, harm to fetus, and vaginal infections (which have largely been proved unjustified) may contribute to lack of sexual activity. Most women are not sexually active immediately following childbirth, and perineal trauma can determine the timing of resumption of sexual intercourse. However, most women (~90%) resume sexual activity within 3–6 months postpartum (Barrett et al. 2000; De Souza et al. 2015; Wallwiener et al. 2017). Overall, research regarding sexual behavior and function in pregnancy and the postpartum period among sexual minority women is limited, but assessment of these variables in this population remains warranted.

## Rates

Rates of FSDs in pregnant and postpartum women are not well documented and are likely overestimated, because researchers often do not consider sexual inactivity or distress. Most studies also do not assess pre-pregnancy sexual functioning, and mixed methodologies and sampling characteristics (e.g., mixed parities) make it difficult to draw generalizations from research. Motivations to abstain from sexual activity in late pregnancy or the early postpartum period may not be associated with lowered sexual function; thus, providers should take care to assess motivations and reasons for lack of sexual activity, when reported.

Research indicates a decline in sexual functioning, including desire, arousal, and orgasmic functioning, across pregnancy but especially in the third trimester (Leeman and Rogers 2012; Serati et al. 2010). Research also indicates temporary decreases in sexual desire and orgasm functioning into 3–6 months postpartum. Typically, these decreases in sexual functioning resolve within 1 year postpartum (Barrett et al. 2000; Brubaker et al. 2008). Reports of postpartum sexual pain that reduces with time appear to have a similar trajectory, such that 42% of women experience perineal pain immediately after delivery, 22% at 8 weeks postpartum, and 10% at 12 weeks postpartum (Abdool et al. 2009). Thus, women who are pregnant or intending to become pregnant may benefit from counseling about normative declines in sexual functioning in pregnancy and the early to middle postpartum period.

## Risk Factors

Despite changes in hormonal levels during pregnancy, research has not demonstrated consistent associations between domains of sexual function and hormonal changes (Serati et al. 2010). However, lactation status is associated with vulvovaginal atrophy (i.e., dyspareunia, dryness, and itching/irritability), which can contribute to decreased sexual functioning and sexual pain. It is thought that elevated prolactin levels in lactating women result in lowered androgens (which may lower desire) and estrogens (which may reduce vaginal lubrication) due to suppressed ovarian activity (Leeman and Rogers 2012; Wallwiener et al. 2017). Thus, lactating women should be encouraged to use a lubricant to address vaginal dryness and may benefit from education explaining that a lack of lubrication does not necessarily reflect a lack of desire for sexual activity or of arousal or attraction toward a partner.

High-quality evidence to support an association between mode of delivery (vaginal vs. cesarean) and sexual functioning (Serati et al. 2010; Viswanathan et al. 2006) is scarce. Cross-sectional research examining early postpartum sexual functioning is somewhat mixed, with some research showing no difference in rates of FSDs and other research showing that vaginal delivery is associated with greater risk of FSDs (Serati et al. 2010). However, longitudinal data suggest no long-term (e.g., 12 months postpartum) impact of mode of delivery on sexual functioning (De Souza et al. 2015; Wallwiener et al. 2017). Similar trends for lack of evidence of long-term negative impacts on sexual function are demonstrated for perineal injury (De Souza et al. 2015), although some data suggest that short-term dyspareunia and perineal pain are associated with perineal trauma and instrumental delivery (Abdool et al. 2009).

Psychiatric concerns in the context of pregnancy and the postpartum period may also affect sexual function. Perinatal depression is associated with a greater likelihood of reported sexual problems (Abdool et al. 2009; Morof et al. 2003), and antidepressant medications can negatively affect sexual function (American College of Obstetricians and Gynecologists 2011; Balon 2006). It is important to consider the pregnancy and lactation status of women in the postpartum period who present with depression and sexual functioning concerns. Compared with other antidepressants, selective serotonin reuptake inhibitors (SSRIs) are most often associated with sexual dysfunctions and have a more robust body of evidence regarding their safety in pregnancy and lactation. Some alternative or adjunctive medications for depression (e.g., bupropion) have more limited data on pregnancy and lactation safety, so clinicians must consider how to balance the potential risks of any medication with the risk to the patient's mental health or sexual dysfunction. (For a complete discussion of the use of antidepressants in pregnancy, see Chapter 13, "Depressive Disorders.")

Additional biopsychosocial changes associated with pregnancy and the postpartum period may affect sexual function. Bodily changes with pregnancy and during the postpartum period may lower body image (e.g., breasts that used to be perceived as sexual are now used for feeding, stretch marks developed during pregnancy) or otherwise negatively affect sexual functioning. Overall physical discomfort and physical complications associated with pregnancy or the postpartum period (e.g., increased urination, pain, pelvic floor dysfunction or changes), decreased sleep, and increased fatigue can affect sexual function (Read 2004). Women and their partners are commonly navigating role transitions that may negatively affect their intimate relationship, and demands of caring for the infant can limit opportunities for sexual activity with a partner.

## Menopause

Sexual activity and sexual functioning tend to decline with age, although sex remains an important area of health and well-being for most midlife women (Schick et al. 2010). (See Chapter 1, "The Reproductive Life Cycle," for an explanation of the physiology of perimenopause and postmenopause, and Chapter 7, "Perimenopause," for mental health concerns related to this stage.)

In perimenopause, declines in estrogen contribute to physiological changes that affect sexual functioning. Androgens decline gradually with age; in women in their late 40s or early 50s, testosterone levels are approximately half what they were when the women were in their early 20s. Decreased lubrication with arousal is often the first noticeable change with menopause (North American Menopause Society 2021). Subsequent vascular, connective tissue, and muscular changes occur over time that also affect sexual function (e.g., decreased vascularization affects genital arousal). For some women, declining levels of free testosterone, associated with declining ovarian function, cause decreased sexual drive.

In postmenopausal women, the clitoris may be less sensitive, which can negatively affect orgasm functioning. GSM results from postmenopausal estrogen deficiency, resulting in bothersome symptoms, including sexual (e.g., dyspareunia), genital (e.g., vaginal dryness, burning, itching), and urinary (e.g., frequency and urgency concerns, recurrent urinary tract infections) symptoms (North American Menopause Society 2020; see also Chapter 7). GSM affects about 50% of postmenopausal women, is considered a chronic condition if left untreated, and can significantly impair sexual functioning and satisfaction. Decreased desire and orgasm functioning may be secondary to vulvovaginal atrophy in this context; thus, treatment of GSM may potentially resolve sexual concerns for these women (North American Menopause Society 2013, 2020; Parish et al. 2013). Research is needed to better understand the phenomenology of GSM in transgender individuals; for example, given that high testosterone levels are aromatized to estrogen, it is possible that circulating estradiol is sufficient to maintain the vaginal mucosa in these patients.

## Rates

According to a study of U.S. women (Shifren et al. 2008), distressing difficulties with desire (12.3% in midlife women) and arousal (7.5% in midlife women) tend to be highest among midlife women compared with younger women, and difficulties in orgasm (5.7% in midlife women) are more prevalent in midlife women than younger women.

## Risk Factors

Perimenopause is often associated with specific psychosocial stressors, including role transitions such as retirement, that may affect female sexual function. With age, women become more likely to be affected by partner variables that can impair sexual function, such as decreased partner availability or a partner's own diminished sexual function (Thomas and Thurston 2016; Thomas et al. 2015). However, many women experience improvement in sexual function with perimenopause (e.g., due to changes such as children moving out of the home) and effectively adapt to physical changes with age and menopausal transition to maintain sexual activity (e.g., by placing more emphasis on emotional closeness aspects of sex). Research on factors specifically contributing to sexual functioning resilience in midlife women is scarce. However, several psychosocial and interpersonal variables, including self-esteem, general life satisfaction, optimism, emotional support, absence of psychiatric conditions such as depression and anxiety, and higher general satisfaction with one's partner and quality of relationship communication, are likely protective for midlife women's sexual health (Brotto et al. 2016; Mernone et al. 2019).

Research indicates that early menopause is associated with greater impairments in sexual function, and that rates of HSDD are higher among women with surgical menopause, which results in more abrupt reduction in circulating ovarian hormone levels than does natural menopause (Kingsberg et al. 2020). After surgical menopause, women's androgen levels are approximately one-third those of women with natural menopause. Providers should be mindful of the increased risk with age of chronic diseases (e.g., hypertension, diabetes) and use of medication(s) that can negatively impact women's sexual functioning. Reduced physical function and activity that may occur with age (particularly in women with obesity or osteoarthritis) can negatively affect both body image and sexual activity. Moreover, vasomotor symptoms (e.g., hot flashes, night sweats) may indirectly impair sexual functioning (Thomas and Thurston 2016; Thomas et al. 2015). Assessment of depressive symptoms in the context of assessing sexual functioning is warranted in perimenopausal women, given their increased risk for depressive symptoms and the relationship between depression and lowered sexual function. Evidence indicates that, compared with premenopause, perimenopause is associated with a three times greater risk for a major depressive episode (Santoro et al. 2015).

## Assessment of Female Sexual Dysfunctions

As noted previously, the ISSWSH published a document outlining a process of care for the identification and management of FSDs (Parish et al. 2019). This document describes core and advanced levels of assessment and treatment. Similarly, the ISSWSH published a process-of-care document specifically for the identification and management of HSDD (Clayton et al. 2018), and a recent guide provides an overview of causes, diagnosis, and treatment of HSDD (Kingsberg and Simon 2020). These documents outline options for providers to adjust interventions to their level of comfort, experience, skill, and resources available and to identify opportunities to refer patients to specialists for assessment or treatment when indicated. See Table 3–2 for relevant guidance documents for assessment and treatment of FSDs.

Universal screening for FSDs is recommended across subspecialties because it can reduce the burden placed on the patient to initiate disclosure of a sensitive concern and normalize the importance of this aspect of health for women (Kingsberg et al. 2019b; Parish et al. 2019). Assessment across subspecialties is essentially the same, but the timing may differ within the review of systems according to each subspecialty. For example, in obstetrics and gynecology settings, a review of systems and medical history would include sexual health and function, and in psychiatry settings, sexual function assessment could be included within a checklist of basic mental health and psychosocial history (e.g., when inquiring about mood, situational, and relationship factors). Psychiatrists prescribing psychotropic medications should assess for baseline sexual function and concerns prior to initiating treatment and then screen for sexual side effects of medications at follow-up appointments. When time is limited, providers can briefly assess sexual functioning using open-ended questions with a calm, nonjudgmental, and patient-oriented demeanor (see the brief three-item screener in Table 3–3). Also, if time is limited, practitioners should schedule a follow-up appointment for further assessment and treatment of FSDs (if indicated and within the skill and scope of practice of the provider) or provide referral to a specialist. Table 3–3 presents brief screening options (Hatzichristou et al. 2004; Kingsberg 2006; Parish et al. 2019).

According to the ISSWSH process of care, core-level assessment of FSDs includes thorough assessment of sexual response domains and sexual pain, distress associated with the sexual problem(s), and relationship variables. Several validated self-report measures can be used to assess sexual functioning in research or clinical settings (Table 3–4). Patients may complete these measures in the waiting room or during a session. The Female Sexual Function Index (Rosen et al. 2000) has an empirically derived clinical cut point; a full-scale score ≤26.55 indicates FSDs. Some measures assess a range of sexual function domains (e.g., Brief Profile of Female Sexual Dysfunction), whereas others focus on specific domains, such as distress (Female Sexual Distress Scale–Revised; Derogatis et al. 2002) or desire (Decreased Sexual Desire Screener; Clayton et al. 2009).

TABLE 3–3. **Brief sexual function screening questions**

| | |
|---|---|
| Single item[a]: | "Do you have questions or concerns about your sexual functioning?" |
| Ubiquity statements framed in the context of other health or psychosocial factors (e.g., reproductive stage, other health conditions, relationship with partner)[b]: | "Women who are breastfeeding often experience vaginal dryness and pain. What changes in sexual functioning have you noticed?" |
| Three-item screener[c]: | "Are you currently involved in a relationship?" and/or "Are you sexually active?" |
| If yes: | "Have your partners included men, women, or both?" |
| | "Any sexual concerns or pain with sex?" |
| If no: | "Do you have sexual concerns that you would like to discuss or that have contributed to lack of sexual behavior?" |

*Source.* [a]Hatzichristou et al. 2004; [b]Parish et al. 2019; [c]Kingsberg 2006.

For some FSD conditions (although not typically to assess HSDD), a critical part of assessment might be referral to an expert in obstetrics and gynecology or sexual health for a physical examination (Parish et al. 2019). For example, assessment of sexual pain may include examination of external genitalia consisting of pressure-point testing, visual inspection, and palpation. The vagina and cervix might be evaluated (e.g., via speculum examination), and abdominal, bimanual, and rectovaginal examinations may be included (Kingsberg 2006; Parish et al. 2019; Sorensen et al. 2018). Laboratory evaluation (e.g., assessment of vaginal pH) or imaging studies (e.g., transvaginal ultrasound) may also be indicated, depending on patient symptoms and physical examination findings (Hatzichristou et al. 2004; Kingsberg 2006; Parish et al. 2019). It is important to note that no cutoff blood level for any measured circulating androgen can be used to differentiate women with and without FSDs (Davis et al. 2019).

Psychiatry practitioners may be well positioned to conduct an advanced level of FSD assessment, which includes more detailed assessment of the biopsychosocial factors that can affect sexual function. Specific attention should be paid to the identification of modifiable contributing factors. Table 3–5 presents the ISSWSH process-of-care list of medical conditions and medications that may be contributing to FSDs. Sexual functioning may be negatively affected by a number of psychiatric conditions, including mood and anxiety disorders, PTSD, substance use disorders, eating disorders, and somatic symptom–related disorders (Atlantis and Sullivan 2012; Basson and Schultz 2007; Palha and Esteves 2008; Pinheiro et al. 2010; Solmaz et al. 2016; Yehuda et al. 2015), as well as some of the treatments for these disorders.

When assessing relationship factors, providers should screen for current partner violence and history of interpersonal violence exposure because psychological, physical, or sexual assault victimization is associated with greater risk of disruptions in sexual functioning. Abuse may negatively affect sexual functioning in pathways consistent with the biopsychosocial model, including negative impacts on interpersonal functioning and sexual self-esteem, lack of positive emotions toward sexuality, and increased risk for mental and physical health conditions associated with FSDs (e.g., depression, anxiety) (Campbell 2002; Pulverman et al. 2018; Weaver 2009). Although specific rates of the association

**TABLE 3–4. Validated self-report measures assessing female sexual function**

| |
|---|
| Brief Profile of Female Sexual Dysfunction (Rust et al. 2007) |
| Brief Sexual Symptom Checklist–Women's Version (Hatzichristou et al. 2004) |
| Decreased Sexual Desire Screener (Clayton et al. 2009) |
| Female Sexual Distress Scale–Revised (Derogatis et al. 2002) |
| Female Sexual Function Index (Rosen et al. 2000) |
| McGill Pain Questionnaire (Melzack 1975) and Short Form (Goldstein et al. 2016) |

**TABLE 3–5. Contributing factors to sexual dysfunction from the International Society for the Study of Women's Sexual Health Process of Care for the Identification of Sexual Concerns and Problems in Women**

| Medical conditions | Medications |
|---|---|
| Cardiovascular disorders | Anticonvulsants |
| Endocrine disorders | Carbamazepine |
| Diabetes | Phenytoin |
| Thyroid disease | Primidone |
| Neurological disorders | Cardiovascular medications |
| Multiple sclerosis | Amiodarone |
| Neuromuscular disorders | β-Blockers |
| Prolactinoma | Calcium channel blockers |
| Oncological disorders/treatment | Clonidine |
| Gynecological/Colorectal surgery | Digoxin |
| Mastectomy | Hydrochlorothiazide |
| Pelvic radiation treatment | Methyldopa |
| | Statins |
| Gynecological disorders | Hormonal agents |
| Endometriosis | Antiandrogens (flutamide, spironolactone) |
| Fibroids | Aromatase inhibitors |
| Pelvic organ prolapse | Combined hormonal contraceptives |
| Vulvar dermatoses | Gonadotropin-releasing hormone agonists |
| Vulvodynia/vestibulodynia | Tamoxifen |
| Psychiatric disorders | Pain medications |
| Chronic pain | Nonsteroidal anti-inflammatory drugs |
| Urinary incontinence | Opioids |
| Spinal cord injury | Psychotropic medications |
| | Antipsychotics |
| | Benzodiazepines |
| | Lithium |
| | Selective serotonin reuptake inhibitors |
| | Serotonin and norepinephrine reuptake inhibitors |
| | Tricyclic antidepressants |

*Source.* Adapted from Parish et al. 2019.

between specific traumatic events and FSD are difficult to estimate, screening for other history of trauma more common to women, including reproductive coercion, child abuse, and childbirth trauma, is likely warranted when assessing sexual function, given existing research on different types of trauma and impaired sexual function and satisfaction (O'Malley et al. 2018; Pulverman et al. 2018). Research and theory point to overlapping biological and psychological mechanisms between PTSD and sexual dysfunctions that may help explain comorbidities between FSDs and trauma (O'Driscoll and Flanagan 2016; Yehuda et al. 2015). (For further discussion of trauma and reproductive function, see Chapter 18, "Trauma and Reproductive Health.")

## Treatment of Female Sexual Dysfunctions

Treatment of FSDs is often best approached in a multidisciplinary manner. The ISSWSH process-of-care model also outlines management and treatment strategies (Clayton et al. 2018; Parish et al. 2019). Across FSD types, core-level treatment approaches include education on normal sexual functioning and modification of biopsychosocial factors affecting sexual function (e.g., cognitive therapy to alter negative beliefs or guilt about sexuality; reducing performance anxiety; addressing relationship conflict; education regarding use of vaginal lubricants to address dryness; addressing GSM). Advanced-level treatments may require referral to one or more specialists. Table 3–6 provides a summary of evaluations of treatment interventions for FSDs.

### Flibanserin and Bremelanotide

Two medications have FDA approval to treat FSDs. The medications are not indicated for lifelong HSDD but rather for acquired, generalized (loss of desire in all situations) HSDD in premenopausal women that is not better accounted for by a coexisting medical or psychiatric condition, problems within the relationship, or effects of a medication or other drug substance. Flibanserin is a multifunctional serotonin 1A ($5\text{-HT}_{1A}$) receptor agonist and type 2A ($5\text{-HT}_{2A}$) receptor antagonist that is administered orally at bedtime daily. There is a risk evaluation and mitigation strategy related to the risk for hypotension and syncope (Sprout Pharmaceuticals 2016). Patients should be counseled to discontinue alcohol use 2 hours prior to taking flibanserin at bedtime, avoid consuming alcohol until the following day after taking the medication, and skip the daily dose if they consume three or more standard drinks. Full response to flibanserin may take up to 8–12 weeks (Joffe et al. 2016).

Bremelanotide consists of seven amino acids and is a cyclic melanocortin receptor agonist. It is self-administered, as needed, via an autoinjector (29-gauge needle) into the skin of the thigh or abdomen at least 45 minutes prior to anticipated sexual activity and has approximately 12–16 hours of effect. Recommended maximums are one dose per 24 hours and eight doses per month (Kingsberg et al. 2019a). No existing data examine the safety and risk of flibanserin or bremelanotide in pregnant or lactating women, and these medications are not currently recommended for use by these women.

### Testosterone

A global consensus position statement summarizes the efficacy and safety evidence, as well as guidance, for the off-label use of testosterone therapy to treat HSDD in post-

TABLE 3–6. **Summary of evaluation of treatment interventions for female sexual dysfunctions**

| Intervention | Level of evidence |
|---|---|
| Psychological interventions for hypoactive sexual desire disorder | |
| Cognitive-behavioral therapy | 2 |
| Mindfulness+cognitive-behavioral therapy | 2 |
| Sex therapy | 2 |
| Pharmacological interventions for hypoactive sexual desire disorder | |
| Bremelanotide | 1 |
| Bupropion | 2 |
| Buspirone | 2 |
| Flibanserin | 1 |
| Lybrido/Lybridos | 2 |
| Testosterone therapy | 1 |
| Psychological intervention for female sexual arousal disorder | |
| Mindfulness + cognitive-behavioral therapy | 2 |
| Pharmacological interventions for female sexual arousal disorder | |
| Bupropion | 2 |
| Phosphodiesterase type 5 inhibitors | 2 |
| Testosterone therapy | 1 |
| Tibolone | 2 |
| Psychological intervention for female orgasmic disorder | |
| Directed masturbation | 2 |

*Note.* Level 1=evidence from a systematic review or meta-analysis of all relevant randomized controlled trials (RCTs) or evidence-based clinical practice guidelines based on systematic reviews of RCTs or three or more RCTs of good quality that have similar results. Level 2=evidence obtained from at least one well-designed RCT (e.g., large multisite RCT).

*Source.* Adapted from Kingsberg et al. 2017.

menopausal women (Davis et al. 2019). If a trial of testosterone therapy for postmenopausal HSDD is initiated, women should have their testosterone level checked at baseline and then again at 3–6 weeks after initiation of treatment, with the goal that serum testosterone should not exceed the level of a reproductive-aged female (American College of Obstetricians and Gynecologists 2019; Davis et al. 2019). Women should be monitored for clinical response to testosterone, and serum total testosterone level should be measured for signs of androgen excess every 6 months, per expert opinion (Davis et al. 2019). All testosterone products should be discontinued at 6 months if the patient shows no signs of improvement. No data are available regarding use in premenopausal women (American College of Obstetricians and Gynecologists 2019).

According to the consensus documents regarding use of testosterone treatment for postmenopausal women with HSDD (Davis et al. 2019; Parish et al. 2021), it is reasonable to use a male formulation at approximately one-tenth of the male dose as an off-label treatment for HSDD in postmenopausal women. Commonly used preparations for women include transdermal delivery of FDA-approved male topical gel (1%–2%)

at one-tenth the standard male dose and applied to a skin surface, typically the back of the calf, buttock, or upper outer thigh. Pellets, intramuscular injections, oral formulations, and compounded formulations are not recommended to treat postmenopausal HSDD. Systemic testosterone administered according to these recommendations carries the risk of androgenic effects, such as mild increases in acne and body and facial hair growth in some women.

Oral testosterone is associated with adverse effects on lipid profiles, whereas nonoral testosterone therapies (in dosing just described) have not shown to have significant adverse short-term effects on lipid profiles, although recommendations regarding cardiovascular health effects of physiological doses of testosterone are not generalizable to longer-term therapy or higher-risk populations (Davis et al. 2019). The only recommended indication for testosterone therapy is HSDD in postmenopausal women; however, research also indicates positive effects of testosterone therapy on arousal, orgasm, and sexual distress in this population (Davis et al. 2019).

The ISSWSH process-of-care guidance document provides a summary of additional off-label pharmacological (e.g., bupropion, buspirone) and nonpharmacological treatments with evidence of efficacy for FSDs and GSM in postmenopausal women (Parish et al. 2019). Table 3–2 lists that document, as well as others. Lybrido and lybridos are in development but not approved for the treatment of HSDD. Lybrido is a combination of oral sildenafil and sublingual testosterone for lack of desire due to lack of excitation, and lybridos is a combination of oral buspirone and sublingual testosterone for lack of desire due to excess inhibition. Bupropion, although sometimes used to increase desire or as a possible antidote for SSRI-induced sexual desire or arousal problems, does not have an indication for the treatment of any sexual dysfunction.

## Behavioral and Somatic Treatments

A variety of nonpharmacological treatment approaches are used for FSDs. Pelvic floor physical therapy is a widely used approach for treatment of sexual pain, although research examining the efficacy of specific protocols is limited. This approach includes manual therapy, psychoeducation, relaxation and breathing (re)training, local tissue sensitization, electromyographic biofeedback, and instructed, progressive use of vaginal dilators (Bergeron et al. 2010, 2015). Small pilot studies have demonstrated improvement in arousal and achieving orgasm by increasing blood flow and engorgement with the use of a small, FDA-approved clitoral suction device (American College of Obstetricians and Gynecologists 2019).

Research provides some limited support for sex therapy (for treatment of HSDD), cognitive-behavioral therapy (CBT; for treatment of HSDD and sexual pain disorders), mindfulness combined with CBT (for treatment of HSDD, FSAD, and sexual pain disorders), therapist-aided exposure therapy (for treatment of sexual pain disorders), and directed masturbation (for treatment of female orgasmic disorder). Psychotherapy to treat FSDs may be facilitated in individual, couples, or group format.

Sex therapy typically includes psychoeducation on sexual functioning and sensate focus exercises. Sensate focus consists of a progressive series of exercises intended to increase one's attention to sensations and understanding of their physical response (Althof 2011). Typically, couples are instructed to begin with nongenital touching, without the expectation of intercourse, to focus on a nonjudgmental and nonevaluative awareness of the sensations of touch with one partner touching the other. Exclusion of intercourse allows the couple to focus more mindfully on the sensation of the current exercise without worrying about the "outcome." These touching exercises progress until eventually the couple experiences sensual intercourse. CBT includes psychoeducation on sexual functioning in addition to techniques to modify maladaptive cognitions related to sexual activity and functioning and maladaptive behaviors, such as avoidance of sexual contact due to anxiety (Nobre and Pinto-Gouveia 2008). Mindfulness+CBT focuses on improving nonjudgmental awareness of sexual response and sensation and improving the ability to be aware of the present moment (Brotto and Goldmeier 2015).

Exposure therapy for sexual pain includes psychoeducation and a graded series of in-vivo exposure exercises to sexual contact and penetration via a dilator (van Lankveld et al. 2006). Various dilator devices exist, including plastic dilator kits with a range of dilator sizes and expanding dilators that can increase or decrease in size. Collaboration with a pelvic floor physical therapist for such exposure treatment may be useful when available. Directed masturbation for orgasm dysfunction is a series of progressive exercises that the patient engages in (at home) to build awareness of sexual stimulation and response, focusing first on self-stimulation to explore one's body and genitals and progressing to partner-based activity (if desired) (Heiman and LoPiccolo 1988).

## Management of FSDs in the Context of Comorbid Psychiatric Illness or Treatment

As noted earlier (see "Assessment of Female Sexual Dysfunctions"), diagnosis of FSDs requires consideration of other conditions, including any psychiatric conditions, that might be associated with the sexual problems. Due to the significant strength of the bidirectional relationship between depression and sexual dysfunctions (Atlantis and Sullivan 2012), screening for depression in women presenting with sexual problems, particularly low desire, is recommended (Clayton et al. 2018). Psychotropic medications used to treat psychiatric conditions, most commonly antidepressants (Clayton and Montejo 2006; Montejo et al. 2019; Serretti and Chiesa 2009), often have sexual side effects. Unfortunately, these side effects can contribute to nonadherence and discontinuation of treatment and decreased recovery. However, it is difficult to clearly identify whether sexual problems are specifically due to depression, primary FSDs, or medication side effects. Moreover, for some individuals, sexual functioning improves with psychotropic treatment, particularly for those whose depression is effectively improved.

Specific rates of sexual problems due to psychotropic medications (i.e., treatment-emergent sexual dysfunctions) vary, with rates ranging between 26% and 80% (Clayton et al. 2016; Montejo et al. 2019; Serretti and Chiesa 2009). Identifying medications' differential effects on sexual function is difficult, in part due to limited availability of randomized controlled trials and variations in methodology (e.g., patient spontaneous report vs. assessment with a validated measure) and in part due to confounding by indication (i.e., that depression also results in sexual dysfunctions).

Evidence indicates that adverse sexual effects of antidepressants are most commonly in domains of desire and arousal, followed by orgasm, whereas evidence of effects on pain are mixed (Lorenz et al. 2016). Studies indicate that sexual side effects are more likely when the medication's mechanism of action is on the blockade of serotonin reuptake at 5-HT receptors (particularly 5-$HT_2$), whereas medications that increase norepinephrine or dopamine uptake or that block 5-$HT_2$ receptors may have fewer sexual side effects. It is thought that serotonin plays a multifaceted role in hypothalamic and cortical regulation of sexual response and is an inhibitory factor affecting sexual response. In general, medications affecting inhibitory factors (e.g., serotonin, which regulates satiety; opioids, which mediate sexual rewards; endocannabinoids, which induce sedation) or excitatory factors (e.g., norepinephrine and oxytocin, which stimulate sexual arousal; melanocortins and dopamine, which stimulate desire and attention) can affect sexual function (Kingsberg et al. 2015).

Consistent evidence suggests that bupropion, compared with SSRIs, is associated with lower rates of sexual side effects, perhaps due to its noradrenergic-dopaminergic effects, and that paroxetine tends to have higher rates of sexual side effects compared with other antidepressants. Emerging evidence also indicates that medications with multimodal serotonin modulation, including mirtazapine, vilazodone, and vortioxetine, have less potential than SSRIs for adversely affecting sexual function in women treated for depression (Clayton et al. 2016; Montejo et al. 2019; Serretti and Chiesa 2009). Research regarding differential sexual side effects of antipsychotics is limited and variable. Antipsychotics, particularly first-generation antipsychotics and risperidone, followed by olanzapine, appear to have higher rates of sexual dysfunctions. Antipsychotics with lesser sexual side effects appear to be ziprasidone, quetiapine, and aripiprazole (Basson and Gilks 2018; Clayton et al. 2016). Specifically, aripiprazole appears to have the strongest evidence of a favorable sexual side effect profile (Clayton et al. 2016).

Research regarding treatment-emergent FSDs with lithium, mood stabilizers, and anxiolytics is limited and mixed (Montejo et al. 2019; Reisman 2017; Serretti and Chiesa 2009). Table 3–7 summarizes the relative frequency of sexual side effects that can occur with antidepressants, and Table 3–8 summarizes evidence of sexual side effects related to drugs' mechanisms of action.

Strategies to address antidepressant-emergent sexual dysfunctions have been suggested, yet research evaluating the efficacy or comparative efficacy of each approach is limited. Prior to initiating treatment, providers should consider proactively assessing baseline sexual function in order to assess and monitor medication-related changes. Women should be counseled about the potential for sexual side effects when an antidepressant is initiated, and preventive strategies for women with concerns about sexual side effects should be considered, including psychotherapy, physical activity prior to sexual activity to improve sexual desire, and selecting a medication with evidence of less impact on sexual function when indicated (Basson and Gilks 2018).

Some research indicates limited success with dose reduction in the management of antidepressant-emergent FSDs (Balon 2006), although other research suggests dose reduction may be effective (Clayton et al. 2016). Sexual side effects may be dose related for some antidepressants (Clayton et al. 2016); however, dose reduction should be considered only for individuals whose depression is in full remission, given the potential for worsening of depressive symptoms with this approach (Balon 2006). "Drug holidays," or temporary cessation of psychotropic treatment to allow improvement in sexual function, are relatively uncommon in clinical practice, in part due to concerns related to discontinuation symptoms, treatment dropout, and worsening of depressive symptoms (Balon 2006; Clayton et al. 2016).

TABLE 3–7. **Relative frequency of sexual dysfunctions by antidepressant drug**

| Drug | Impact on sexual desire | Impact on sexual arousal | Impact on orgasm |
|---|---|---|---|
| Bupropion | <10%, or <5% relative to placebo | <10%, or <5% relative to placebo | <10%, or <5% relative to placebo |
| Citalopram | >25% | >25% | >25% |
| Fluoxetine | >25% | 10%–25% | >25% |
| Fluvoxamine | >25% | 10%–25% | >25% |
| Mirtazapine | 10%–25% | 10%–25% | 10%–25% |
| Nefazodone | <10%, or <5% relative to placebo | <10%, or <5% relative to placebo | <10%, or <5% relative to placebo |
| Paroxetine | >25% | >25% | >25% |
| Sertraline | >25% | >25% | >25% |
| Venlafaxine | >25% | >25% | >25% |
| Vilazodone | <10%, or <5% relative to placebo | <10%, or <5% relative to placebo | <10%, or <5% relative to placebo |

*Source.* Adapted from Clayton et al. 2014.

Available evidence of the efficacy of adjunctive therapy is overall limited (Balon 2006; Taylor et al. 2005), although Table 3–9 presents an overview of options to address sexual side effects. Bupropion has the strongest evidence base to support its use in diminishing the sexual side effects of other psychiatric medications (Safarinejad 2011; Taylor et al. 2005), likely due to its dopaminergic properties. Given that the cause of sexual dysfunctions with SSRIs is thought to be related to stimulation of the serotonin system, strategies to counteract this effect include adding the 5-$HT_2$ antagonist cyproheptadine on a standing or as-needed basis prior to sexual activity, a strategy with limited evidence from case studies (Aizenberg et al. 1995; Javanbakht 2015), or adding the partial 5-$HT_{1A}$ agonist buspirone (Landén et al. 1999), a strategy that is more commonly used in clinical practice. Side effects of the alternative medication or adjunctive therapy should be taken into consideration when treatment planning. Weight gain (e.g., with mirtazapine) and anxiety (e.g., with bupropion) may subsequently negatively impair sexual function. Furthermore, potential antiserotonergic effects that might interfere with an antidepressant effect (e.g., daily administration of cyproheptadine) should be considered with adjunctive therapies. Finally, some evidence suggests efficacy of nonpharmacological approaches (e.g., adjunctive sex therapy, complementary and integrative approaches such as acupuncture) to address treatment-emergent sexual dysfunctions (Basson and Gilks 2018).

Options for treating antipsychotic-induced sexual problems and available research on this topic are more limited, although recommendations generally include dose reduction, switching to an antipsychotic with fewer side effects (e.g., aripiprazole), or concurrent psychotherapy and psychoeducation to target modifiable factors affecting sexual dysfunctions. In general, evidence indicates that the propensity of these drugs to affect sexual function is associated with their propensity to increase prolactin; thus, selection of antipsychotics with less impact on prolactin (e.g., quetiapine) and moni-

TABLE 3–8. **Mechanisms of action and risk of treatment-induced sexual dysfunctions**

| Drug | Main relevant mechanisms | Psychotropic-induced sexual dysfunction risk |
|---|---|---|
| **Antidepressants** | | |
| Vilazodone | Blocks 5-HT reuptake, stimulates 5-$HT_{1A}$ (partial agonist) | Negligible, more study needed |
| Vortioxetine | Blocks 5-HT reuptake; stimulates 5-$HT_{1A}$ (agonist) and 5-$HT_{1B}$ (partial agonist); blocks 5-$HT_7$, 5-$HT_{1D}$, 5-$HT_3$; increases 5-HT, norepinephrine, and acetylcholine neurotransmission | Negligible, more study needed |
| Bupropion | Blocks norepinephrine and dopamine reuptake, increases norepinephrine and dopamine neurotransmission | Very low |
| Trazodone | Blocks 5-$HT_{2A}$ receptors, weakly blocks 5-HT reuptake | Very low |
| Mirtazapine | Blocks 5-$HT_{2A}$, 5-$HT_{2C}$, 5-$HT_3$, $H_1$, and $\alpha_2$-adrenergic presynaptic receptors; increases serotonin and norepinephrine neurotransmission | Low |
| SNRIs | Block 5-HT and norepinephrine reuptake; weakly block dopamine reuptake; desensitize 5-HT and β-adrenergic receptors; increase 5-HT, dopamine, and norepinephrine neurotransmission | Medium |
| SSRIs | Block 5-HT reuptake, desensitize 5-HT receptors, increase 5-HT neurotransmission | High |
| **Mood stabilizers/antipsychotics** | | |
| Aripiprazole | Partial agonist $D_2$, 5-$HT_{1A}$; agonist 5-$HT_{2A}$; spares prolactin | Negligible, more study needed |
| Lithium | Unclear | Medium, more study needed |
| Quetiapine | Dopaminergic, noradrenergic but serotoninergic | Medium |

D=dopamine; 5-HT=serotonin; SNRI=serotonin-norepinephrine reuptake inhibitor; SSRI= selective serotonin reuptake inhibitor.

*Source.* Adapted from Basson and Gilks 2018; Schwartz et al. 2011; Stahl 2015.

toring of prolactin levels may be beneficial in reducing impact on sexual function (Clayton et al. 2016; Knegtering et al. 2008).

## Conclusion

Sexual functioning remains an important part of women's health and well-being across the lifespan, and women prefer that their providers inquire about their sexual

**TABLE 3–9. Medications to address treatment-emergent sexual dysfunctions**

| | |
|---|---|
| Medications with evidence to improve SSRI-related sexual dysfunctions (see Basson and Gilks 2018; Clayton et al. 2016; Fooladi et al. 2014; Lorenz et al. 2016; Montejo et al. 2019; Nurnberg et al. 2008) | Bupropion (strongest available evidence)<br>Mirtazapine<br>Olanzapine<br>Testosterone gel<br>Sildenafil<br>Buspirone<br>Adjunctive aripiprazole<br>Adjunctive phosphodiesterase type 5 inhibitors |
| Medication to improve SSRI- or SNRI-related sexual desire dysfunction (Fooladi et al. 2014) | Transdermal testosterone 300 μg |
| Medication to improve SSRI-related sexual dysfunctions, in individuals with depression in remission (Jacobsen et al. 2015) | Vortioxetine (compared with escitalopram) |

SNRI=serotonin-norepinephrine reuptake inhibitor; SSRI=selective serotonin reuptake inhibitor.

functioning. Increased awareness of the importance of this aspect of women's health and knowledge of the phenomenology, assessment, and treatment of female sexual function and FSDs would help fill this gap in health care. Psychiatry practitioners are well positioned to help address women's sexuality or to refer women to helpful resources to address FSDs, which is often best addressed in a multidisciplinary manner given the biopsychosocial components of female sexual function.

## Key Points

- Sexual functioning concerns in women are underassessed and underreported.
- Female sexual response is determined by a multitude of biopsychosocial variables and includes domains of desire, arousal, lubrication, and orgasm.
- Female sexual dysfunctions (FSDs) are classified as a persistent, distressing impairment in one or more specific domains of sexual response, or the experience of pain during sexual activity.
- Specific biopsychosocial variables associated with reproductive milestones may affect women's sexual functioning.
- Universal screening for sexual concerns is recommended.
- Evidence-based approaches to treating FSDs exist, and treatment for FSDs is often approached in an interdisciplinary manner.

## References

Abdool Z, Thakar R, Sultan AH: Postpartum female sexual function. Eur J Obstet Gynecol Reprod Biol 145(2):133–137, 2009 19481858

Aizenberg D, Zemishlany Z, Weizman A: Cyproheptadine treatment of sexual dysfunction induced by serotonin reuptake inhibitors. Clin Neuropharmacol 18(4):320–324, 1995 8665544
Althof SE: Sex therapy and combined (sex and medical) therapy. J Sex Med 8(6):1827–1828, 2011 21631735
Althof SE, Leiblum SR, Chevret-Measson M, et al: Psychological and interpersonal dimensions of sexual function and dysfunction. J Sex Med 2(6):793–800, 2005 16422804
American College of Obstetricians and Gynecologists: ACOG Practice Bulletin No. 119: female sexual dysfunction. Obstet Gynecol 117(4):996–1007, 2011 21422879
American College of Obstetricians and Gynecologists: Female sexual dysfunction: ACOG Practice Bulletin Summary, Number 213. Obstet Gynecol 134(1):203–205, 2019 31241595
American Psychiatric Association: Diagnostic and Statistical Manual of Mental Disorders, 4th Edition, Text Revision. Washington, DC, American Psychiatric Association, 2000
American Psychiatric Association: Diagnostic and Statistical Manual of Mental Disorders, 5th Edition. Arlington, VA, American Psychiatric Association, 2013
Atlantis E, Sullivan T: Bidirectional association between depression and sexual dysfunction: a systematic review and meta-analysis. J Sex Med 9(6):1497–1507, 2012 22462756
Balon R: SSRI-associated sexual dysfunction. Am J Psychiatry 163(9):1504–1509, 2006 16946173
Bancroft J, Graham CA, Janssen E, et al: The dual control model: current status and future directions. J Sex Res 46(2–3):121–142, 2009 19308839
Barrett G, Pendry E, Peacock J, et al: Women's sexual health after childbirth. BJOG 107(2):186–195, 2000 10688502
Basson R: The female sexual response: a different model. J Sex Marital Ther 26(1):51–65, 2000 10693116
Basson R: Female sexual response: the role of drugs in the management of sexual dysfunction. Obstet Gynecol 98(2):350–353, 2001 11506856
Basson R, Gilks T: Women's sexual dysfunction associated with psychiatric disorders and their treatment. Womens Health (Lond) 14:1745506518762664, 2018 29649948
Basson R, Schultz WW: Sexual sequelae of general medical disorders. Lancet 369(9559):409–424, 2007 17276781
Bergeron S, Morin M, Lord MJ: Integrating pelvic floor rehabilitation and cognitive-behavioral therapy for sexual pain: what have we learned and where do we go from here? Sexual and Relationship Therapy 25(3):304–313, 2010
Bergeron S, Corsini-Munt S, Aerts L, et al: Female sexual pain disorders: a review of the literature on etiology and treatment. Current Sexual Health Reports 7(3):159–169, 2015
Brotto LA, Goldmeier D: Mindfulness interventions for treating sexual dysfunctions: the gentle science of finding focus in a multitask world. J Sex Med 12(8):1687–1689, 2015 26289539
Brotto L, Atallah S, Johnson-Agbakwu C, et al: Psychological and interpersonal dimensions of sexual function and dysfunction. J Sex Med 13(4):538–571, 2016 27045257
Brubaker L, Handa VL, Bradley CS, et al: Sexual function 6 months after first delivery. Obstet Gynecol 111(5):1040–1044, 2008 18448733
Campbell JC: Health consequences of intimate partner violence. Lancet 359(9314):1331–1336, 2002 11965295
Clayton AH, Montejo AL: Major depressive disorder, antidepressants, and sexual dysfunction. J Clin Psychiatry 67(suppl 6):33–37, 2006 16848675
Clayton AH, Goldfischer ER, Goldstein I, et al: Validation of the Decreased Sexual Desire Screener (DSDS): a brief diagnostic instrument for generalized acquired female hypoactive sexual desire disorder (HSDD). J Sex Med 6(3):730–738, 2009 19170868
Clayton AH, Croft HA, Handiwala L: Antidepressants and sexual dysfunction: mechanisms and clinical implications. Postgrad Med 126(2):91–99, 2014 24685972
Clayton AH, Alkis AR, Parikh NB, et al: Sexual dysfunction due to psychotropic medications. Psychiatr Clin North Am 39(3):427–463, 2016 27514298
Clayton AH, Goldstein I, Kim NN, et al: The International Society for the Study of Women's Sexual Health process of care for management of hypoactive sexual desire disorder in women. Mayo Clin Proc 93(4):467–487, 2018 29545008

Davis SR, Baber R, Panay N, et al: Global consensus position statement on the use of testosterone therapy for women. Climacteric 22(5):429–434, 2019 31474158
Derogatis LR, Rosen R, Leiblum S, et al: The Female Sexual Distress Scale (FSDS): initial validation of a standardized scale for assessment of sexually related personal distress in women. J Sex Marital Ther 28(4):317–330, 2002 12082670
Derogatis LR, Clayton AH, Rosen RC, et al: Should sexual desire and arousal disorders in women be merged? Arch Sex Behav 40(2):217–219, author reply 221–225, 2011 20945084
De Souza A, Dwyer PL, Charity M, et al: The effects of mode delivery on postpartum sexual function: a prospective study. BJOG 122(10):1410–1418, 2015 25752211
Diamond LM: Sexual Fluidity: Understanding Women's Love and Desire. Cambridge, MA, Harvard University Press, 2008
Faubion SS, Larkin LC, Stuenkel CA, et al: Management of genitourinary syndrome of menopause in women with or at high risk for breast cancer: consensus recommendations from The North American Menopause Society and The International Society for the Study of Women's Sexual Health. Menopause 25(6):596–608, 2018 29762200
Fooladi E, Bell RJ, Jane F, et al: Testosterone improves antidepressant-emergent loss of libido in women: findings from a randomized, double-blind, placebo-controlled trial. J Sex Med 11(3):831–839, 2014 24433574
Fortenberry JD: Puberty and adolescent sexuality. Horm Behav 64(2):280–287, 2013 23998672
Goldstein AT, Pukall CF, Brown C, et al: Vulvodynia: assessment and treatment. J Sex Med 13(4):572–590, 2016 27045258
Hatzichristou D, Rosen RC, Broderick G, et al: Clinical evaluation and management strategy for sexual dysfunction in men and women. J Sex Med 1(1):49–57, 2004 16422983
Hayes RD, Dennerstein L, Bennett CM, Fairley CK: What is the "true" prevalence of female sexual dysfunctions and does the way we assess these conditions have an impact? J Sex Med 5(4):777–787, 2008 18266650
Heiman JR, LoPiccolo J: Becoming Orgasmic: A Sexual and Personal Growth Program for Women (Revised and Expanded Edition). New York, Simon and Schuster; 1988
Jacobsen PL, Mahableshwarkar AR, Chen Y, et al: Effect of vortioxetine vs. escitalopram on sexual functioning in adults with well-treated major depressive disorder experiencing SSRI-induced sexual dysfunction. J Sex Med 12(10):2036–2048, 2015 26331383
Javanbakht A: As-needed use of cyproheptadine for treatment of selective serotonin reuptake inhibitor-related female anorgasmia. J Clin Psychopharmacol 35(1):91–93, 2015 25502486
Joffe HV, Chang C, Sewell C, et al: FDA approval of flibanserin: treating hypoactive sexual desire disorder. N Engl J Med 374(2):101–104, 2016 26649985
Kaplan HS: The New Sex Therapy. New York, Brunner-Routledge, 1974
Kingsberg SA: Taking a sexual history. Obstet Gynecol Clin North Am 33(4):535–547, 2006 17116499
Kingsberg SA, Simon JA: Female hypoactive sexual desire disorder: a practical guide to causes, clinical diagnosis, and treatment. J Womens Health (Larchmt) 29(8):1101–1112, 2020 32460605
Kingsberg SA, Clayton AH, Pfaus JG: The female sexual response: current models, neurobiological underpinnings and agents currently approved or under investigation for the treatment of hypoactive sexual desire disorder. CNS Drugs 29(11):915–933, 2015 26519340
Kingsberg SA, Althof S, Simon JA, et al: Female sexual dysfunction: medical and psychological treatments, Committee 14. J Sex Med 14(12):1463–1491, 2017 29198504
Kingsberg SA, Clayton AH, Portman D, et al: Bremelanotide for the treatment of hypoactive sexual desire disorder: two randomized phase 3 trials. Obstet Gynecol 134(5):899–908, 2019a 31599840
Kingsberg SA, Schaffir J, Faught BM, et al: Female sexual health: barriers to optimal outcomes and a roadmap for improved patient-clinician communications. J Womens Health (Larchmt) 28(4):432–443, 2019b 30714849
Kingsberg SA, Larkin LC, Liu JH: Clinical effects of early or surgical menopause. Obstet Gynecol 135(4):853–868, 2020 32168205
Knegtering H, van den Bosch R, Castelein S, et al: Are sexual side effects of prolactin-raising antipsychotics reducible to serum prolactin? Psychoneuroendocrinology 33(6):711–717, 2008 18395353

Landén M, Eriksson E, Agren H, et al: Effect of buspirone on sexual dysfunction in depressed patients treated with selective serotonin reuptake inhibitors. J Clin Psychopharmacol 19(3):268–271, 1999 10350034
Leeman LM, Rogers RG: Sex after childbirth: postpartum sexual function. Obstet Gynecol 119(3):647–655, 2012 22353966
Lorenz T, Rullo J, Faubion S: Antidepressant-induced female sexual dysfunction. Mayo Clin Proc 91(9):1280–1286, 2016 27594188
Lowenstein L, Mustafa S, Burke Y: Pregnancy and normal sexual function: are they compatible? J Sex Med 10(3):621–622, 2013 23458213
Masters WH, Johnson VE: Human Sexual Inadequacy. Boston, MA, Little, Brown, 1970
Melzack R: The McGill Pain Questionnaire: major properties and scoring methods. Pain 1(3):277–299, 1975 1235985
Mernone L, Fiacco S, Ehlert U: Psychobiological factors of sexual functioning in aging women: findings from the Women 40+ Healthy Aging Study. Front Psychol 10:546, 2019 30918494
Montejo AL, Prieto N, de Alarcón R, et al: Management strategies for antidepressant-related sexual dysfunction: a clinical approach. J Clin Med 8(10):1640, 2019 31591339
Morof D, Barrett G, Peacock J, et al: Postnatal depression and sexual health after childbirth. Obstet Gynecol 102(6):1318–1325, 2003 14662221
Nobre PJ, Pinto-Gouveia J: Cognitions, emotions, and sexual response: analysis of the relationship among automatic thoughts, emotional responses, and sexual arousal. Arch Sex Behav 37(4):652–661, 2008 17960474
North American Menopause Society: Management of symptomatic vulvovaginal atrophy: 2013 position statement of The North American Menopause Society. Menopause 20(9):888–902, quiz 903–904, 2013 23985562
North American Menopause Society: The 2020 genitourinary syndrome of menopause position statement of The North American Menopause Society. Menopause 27(9):976–992, 2020 32852449
North American Menopause Society: Decreased arousal. Menopause.org, 2021. Available at: http://menopause.org/for-women/sexual-health-menopause-online/sexual-problems-at-midlife/decreased-arousal. Accessed January 6, 2021.
Nurnberg HG, Hensley PL, Heiman JR, et al: Sildenafil treatment of women with antidepressant-associated sexual dysfunction: a randomized controlled trial. JAMA 300(4):395–404, 2008 18647982
O'Driscoll C, Flanagan E: Sexual problems and post-traumatic stress disorder following sexual trauma: a meta-analytic review. Psychol Psychother 89(3):351–367, 2016 26449962
O'Malley D, Higgins A, Begley C, et al: Prevalence of and risk factors associated with sexual health issues in primiparous women at 6 and 12 months postpartum: a longitudinal prospective cohort study (the MAMMI study). BMC Pregnancy Childbirth 18(1):196, 2018 29855357
O'Sullivan LF, Brotto LA, Byers ES, et al: Prevalence and characteristics of sexual functioning among sexually experienced middle to late adolescents. J Sex Med 11(3):630–641, 2014 24418498
O'Sullivan LF, Byers ES, Brotto LA, et al: A longitudinal study of problems in sexual functioning and related sexual distress among middle to late adolescents. J Adolesc Health 59(3):318–324, 2016 27320034
Palha AP, Esteves M: Drugs of abuse and sexual functioning. Adv Psychosom Med 29:131–149, 2008 18391561
Parish SJ, Nappi RE, Krychman ML, et al: Impact of vulvovaginal health on postmenopausal women: a review of surveys on symptoms of vulvovaginal atrophy. Int J Womens Health 5:437–447, 2013 23935388
Parish SJ, Goldstein AT, Goldstein SW, et al: Toward a more evidence-based nosology and nomenclature for female sexual dysfunctions-Part II. J Sex Med 13(12):1888–1906, 2016 27843072
Parish SJ, Hahn SR, Goldstein SW, et al: The International Society for the Study of Women's Sexual Health process of care for the identification of sexual concerns and problems in women. Mayo Clin Proc 94(5):842–856, 2019 30954288

Parish SJ, Simon JA, Davis SR: International Society for the Study of Women's Sexual Health clinical practice guideline for the use of systemic testosterone for hypoactive sexual desire disorder in women. Climacteric 2021 33792440 Epub ahead of print
Perelman MA: Clinical application of CNS-acting agents in FSD. J Sex Med 4(suppl 4):280–290, 2007 17958620
Pinheiro AP, Raney TJ, Thornton LM, et al: Sexual functioning in women with eating disorders. Int J Eat Disord 43(2):123–129, 2010 19260036
Portman DJ, Brown L, Yuan J, et al: Flibanserin in postmenopausal women with hypoactive sexual desire disorder: results of the PLUMERIA Study. J Sex Med 14(6):834–842, 2017 28583342
Pulverman CS, Kilimnik CD, Meston CM: The impact of childhood sexual abuse on women's sexual health: a comprehensive review. Sex Med Rev 6(2):188–200, 2018 29371141
Pyke RE, Clayton A: Models vs. realities in female sexual dysfunction. J Sex Med 12(9):1977–1978, 2015 26272595
Read J: Sexual problems associated with infertility, pregnancy, and ageing. BMJ 329(7465):559–561, 2004 15345632
Reisman Y: Sexual consequences of post-SSRI syndrome. Sex Med Rev 5(4):429–433, 2017 28642048
Rosen RC, Barsky JL: Normal sexual response in women. Obstet Gynecol Clin North Am 33(4):515–526, 2006 17116497
Rosen R, Brown C, Heiman J, et al: The Female Sexual Function Index (FSFI): a multidimensional self-report instrument for the assessment of female sexual function. J Sex Marital Ther 26(2):191–208, 2000 10782451
Rust J, Derogatis L, Rodenberg C, et al: Development and validation of a new screening tool for hypoactive sexual desire disorder: the Brief Profile of Female Sexual Function (B-PFSF). Gynecol Endocrinol 23(11):638–644, 2007 17926163
Safarinejad MR: Reversal of SSRI-induced female sexual dysfunction by adjunctive bupropion in menstruating women: a double-blind, placebo-controlled and randomized study. J Psychopharmacol 25(3):370–378, 2011 20080928
Santoro NC, Epperson N, Mathews SB: Menopausal symptoms and their management. Endocrinol Metab Clin North Am 44(3):497–515, 2015 26316239
Schick V, Herbenick D, Reece M, et al: Sexual behaviors, condom use, and sexual health of Americans over 50: implications for sexual health promotion for older adults. J Sex Med 7(suppl 5):315–329, 2010 21029388
Schwartz TL, Siddiqui UA, Stahl SM: Vilazodone: a brief pharmacological and clinical review of the novel serotonin partial agonist and reuptake inhibitor. Ther Adv Psychopharmacol 1(3):81–87, 2011
Scott SM, Walsh AM: Adolescent sexual development: an overview of recent research. Can J Commun Ment Health 33:21–29, 2014
Serati M, Salvatore S, Siesto G, et al: Female sexual function during pregnancy and after childbirth. J Sex Med 7(8):2782–2790, 2010 20626601
Serretti A, Chiesa A: Treatment-emergent sexual dysfunction related to antidepressants: a meta-analysis. J Clin Psychopharmacol 29(3):259–266, 2009 19440080
Shifren JL, Monz BU, Russo PA, et al: Sexual problems and distress in United States women: prevalence and correlates. Obstet Gynecol 112(5):970–978, 2008 18978095
Simon JA, Lukas VA: Distressing sexual function at midlife: unmet needs, practical diagnoses, and available treatments. Obstet Gynecol 130(4):889–905, 2017 28885410
Simon JA, Goldstein I, Kim NN, et al: The role of androgens in the treatment of genitourinary syndrome of menopause (GSM): International Society for the Study of Women's Sexual Health (ISSWSH) expert consensus panel review. Menopause 25(7):837–847, 2018 29870471
Solmaz V, Ceviz A, Aksoy D, et al: Sexual dysfunction in women with migraine and tension-type headaches. Int J Impot Res 28(6):201–204, 2016 27654031
Sorensen J, Bautista KE, Lamvu G, et al: Evaluation and treatment of female sexual pain: a clinical review. Cureus 10(3):e2379, 2018 29805948
Sprout Pharmaceuticals: Addyi (Flibanserin) Tablets, for Oral Use (package insert). Bridgewater, NJ, Sprout Pharmaceuticals, 2016

Stahl SM: Modes and nodes explain the mechanism of action of vortioxetine, a multimodal agent (MMA): blocking 5HT3 receptors enhances release of serotonin, norepinephrine, and acetylcholine. CNS Spectr 20(5):455–459, 2015 26122791
Taylor MJ, Rudkin L, Hawton K: Strategies for managing antidepressant-induced sexual dysfunction: systematic review of randomised controlled trials. J Affect Disord 88(3):241–254, 2005 16162361
Thomas HN, Thurston RC: A biopsychosocial approach to women's sexual function and dysfunction at midlife: a narrative review. Maturitas 87:49–60, 2016 27013288
Thomas HN, Hess R, Thurston RC: Correlates of sexual activity and satisfaction in midlife and older women. Ann Fam Med 13(4):336–342, 2015 26195678
Tulloch T, Kaufman M: Adolescent sexuality. Pediatr Rev 34(1):29–37, quiz 38, 2013 23281360
van Lankveld JJ, ter Kuile MM, de Groot HE, et al: Cognitive-behavioral therapy for women with lifelong vaginismus: a randomized waiting-list controlled trial of efficacy. J Consult Clin Psychol 74(1):168–178, 2006 16551154
Viswanathan M, Visco AG, Hartmann K, et al: Cesarean delivery on maternal request. Evid Rep Technol Assess (Full Rep) 133(133):1–138, 2006 17627329
Wallwiener S, Müller M, Doster A, et al: Sexual activity and sexual dysfunction of women in the perinatal period: a longitudinal study. Arch Gynecol Obstet 295(4):873–883, 2017 28251311
Weaver TL: Impact of rape on female sexuality: review of selected literature. Clin Obstet Gynecol 52(4):702–711, 2009 20393422
Wise NJ, Frangos E, Komisaruk BR: Brain activity unique to orgasm in women: an fMRI analysis. J Sex Med 14(11):1380–1391, 2017 28986148
World Health Organization: Defining Sexual Health: Report of a Technical Consultation on Sexual Health, 28–31 January 2002, Geneva. Geneva, World Health Organization, 2006. Available at: https://www.who.int/reproductivehealth/publications/sexual_health/defining_sexual_health.pdf?ua=1. Accessed October 31, 2019.
Yehuda R, Lehrner A, Rosenbaum TY: PTSD and sexual dysfunction in men and women. J Sex Med 12(5):1107–1119, 2015 25847589

CHAPTER 4

# Contraception

## Implications for Mental Health

Lulu Zhao, M.D.

Few medical inventions have changed the lives of women as much as the advent of reliable, accessible contraception. In 1973, about a decade after the introduction of the birth control pill, 70% of married American women (to whom the pill was available legally) were using some form of contraception (Gibson 2015). Today, almost 90% of women at risk for unintended pregnancy use some form of contraception, with almost 75% of these women choosing modern methods of high or moderate efficacy (Kavanaugh and Jerman 2018).

Reliable contraceptive methods such as hormonal birth control, long-acting reversible contraceptives, or permanent sterilization effectively uncouple the act of sexual intercourse from the consequence of childbearing. Women who use contraception correctly and consistently account for only 5% of all unintended pregnancies in the United States; 95% of all unintended pregnancies result from women using contraception inconsistently, incorrectly, or not at all (Sonfield et al. 2014). Unplanned birth negatively affects women's educational and economic opportunities, and these losses often have downstream adverse effects on their mental health (Johnston et al. 2017). Children born from unplanned pregnancies may be subject to greater environmental adversity and have increased risks for both physical and psychological health conditions (Sonfield et al. 2011).

Women with mental health disorders are at higher risk for unplanned pregnancy for various reasons, including disease-related sexual behaviors, environmental influences that decrease contraceptive access or uptake, lowered contraceptive efficacy due to medication interactions, and disease-related medical comorbidities that limit contraceptive choice (Dietz et al. 1999; Hall et al. 2013a, 2014; Judge-Golden et al. 2018; Marengo et al. 2015). A broad understanding of the biological mechanism of modern contraceptive methods, and of the interplay between psychiatric illness and contraceptive efficacy, should be part of psychiatrists' armamentarium in providing high-quality, competent care. Inattention to reproductive health may lead to undesirable outcomes such as unintended pregnancy or medication interactions, all of which have significant biological and psychosocial ramifications for female patients.

# Physiology

## Female Reproductive Cycle

The female reproductive cycle is controlled by interwoven processes within the brain, ovaries, and uterus—a signaling pathway referred to as the hypothalamic-pituitary-gonadal (HPG) axis. The ormation of a mature oocyte starts with pulsatile releases of gonadotropin-releasing hormone (GnRH) by the hypothalamus. This stimulates the anterior pituitary gland to release two gonadotropins, follicle-stimulating hormone (FSH) and luteinizing hormone (LH). These gonadotropins stimulate the ovary to begin the process of *folliculogenesis*. The ovary, under the influence of FSH, produces a mature oocyte each cycle and, under the influence of LH, releases it toward the uterus for fertilization and implantation in a process called *ovulation*. During folliculogenesis, the maturing oocyte produces the sex steroid estradiol, which builds up the lining of the uterus in preparation for implantation. After ovulation, a dynamic endocrine gland called the *corpus luteum* forms within the empty space left by the ovulated oocyte. The corpus luteum produces the sex steroid progesterone, which stabilizes and supports the thickened uterine lining while awaiting implantation. If pregnancy does not occur, ovarian sex steroid production ceases, and the now unsupported uterine lining sheds in a process called *menstruation*.

Contraception blocks the reproductive cycle at critical points (see Figure 4–1). Reproduction would not be possible without the release of a mature oocyte capable of being fertilized. As with any endocrine system, the HPG axis is influenced by external factors, including but not limited to exogenous sex steroids, inflammation from acute or chronic illness, environmental stress, and hyper- or hypoglycemia. Modern contraception works via one of four main routes:

1. Inhibition of folliculogenesis and ovulation via negative feedback on the HPG axis. Exogenous estrogen suppresses the FSH secretion necessary for folliculogenesis, and exogenous progestin suppresses the LH surge necessary for ovulation.
2. Thickening of the cervical mucus, making it less penetrable by sperm. This is produced with low doses of progestins; at higher doses, progestin produces the negative feedback noted in item 1.
3. Creation of a sterile inflammatory environment that is toxic to the sperm or ova and unfavorable for implantation.
4. Prevention of the physical union of sperm and oocyte by creation of a physical (e.g., condoms) or physiological (e.g., mucus plug) barrier.

Chronic exposure to progestins can also create other fertility-inhibiting effects, such as atrophy of the endometrium, which creates a less favorable environment for implantation, or impairment of tubal peristalsis and motility. These additional effects explain why progestin-only methods can be effective for contraception even without the syner-

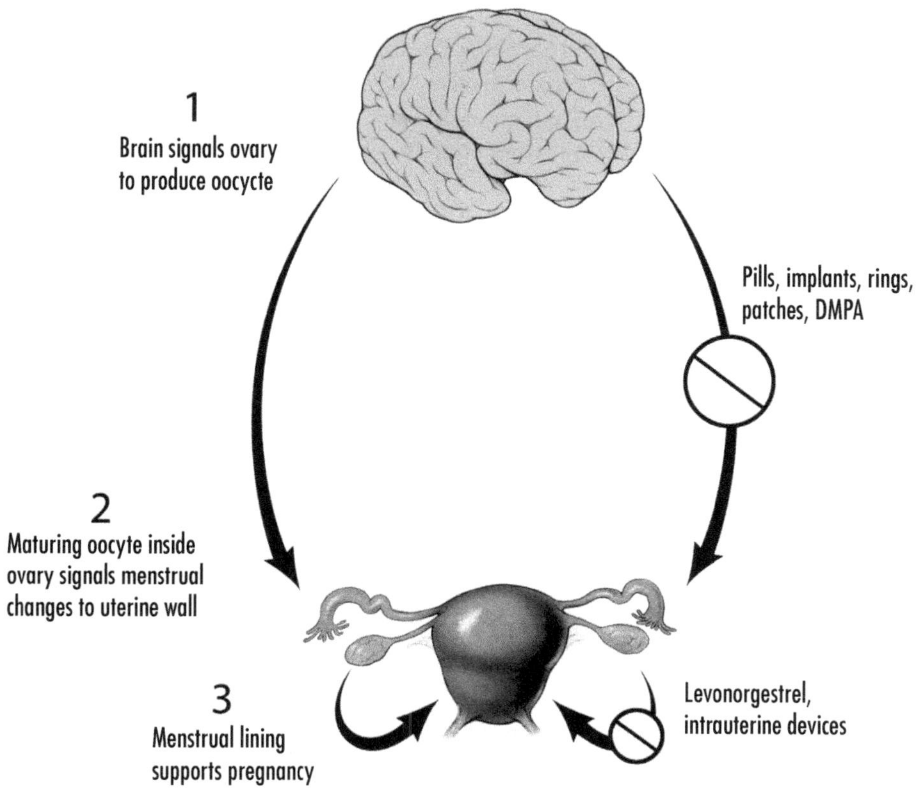


**FIGURE 4–1.** Where contraceptives act.

gistic inhibitory actions from estrogen on folliculogenesis. Meanwhile, no estrogen-only contraceptive options exist because the dose of estrogen required to suppress the HPG axis would cause unacceptably high levels of thrombotic risk and endometrial growth.

Systemic methods such as combined hormonal contraception (e.g., pills, patches, vaginal rings), depot medroxyprogesterone acetate (DMPA) injections, and the etonogestrel arm implant all work by inhibiting folliculogenesis and ovulation. Contraceptive methods such as an intrauterine device (IUD) or low-dose progestin-only pill produce low doses of progestin and primarily work by thickening cervical mucus (Regidor 2018). The nonhormonal IUD works by releasing copper ions, which are toxic to sperm, and induces a sterile inflammatory environment.

## Physiological Effects of Ovulation Suppression

Suppression of ovulation via systemic contraception causes distinct changes to female sex hormones. During a physiological cycle, levels of estradiol fluctuate across the month. During a cycle when a woman is using systemic contraception, levels of estradiol are low and relatively constant, mimicking those seen in early folliculogenesis (prior to the maturation of a dominant follicle) but much higher than those that occur in postmenopausal women (Mishell et al. 1972). The stabilization of estradiol levels may have salutary effects for individuals with disorders that are exacerbated by sex hormone fluctuation, such as women with premenstrual dysphoric disorder (PMDD) (Halbreich et al. 2012; Schmidt et al. 2017; Yonkers et al. 2017; also see Chapter 6, "Premenstrual Mood Syndromes," in this text). For other women, long-term ovarian suppression may produce adverse effects, such as decreased libido related to increased production of sex hormone–binding globulin, which decreases circulating levels of free and total testosterone (Zimmerman et al. 2014).

## Clinical Considerations

### Choosing a Contraceptive Method: Shared Decision Making

The contraceptive choice will depend on each patient's needs, limitations, and goals. For example, patients who have difficulty adhering to a frequent contraceptive dosing schedule may best be served with a long-acting reversible contraceptive, such as the IUD or arm implant, or with a quarterly injectable contraceptive, such as DMPA. Studies have shown that these options have superior rates of pregnancy prevention (99.5% for arm implant, 99% for IUD, and 97% for depot injection) compared with daily oral contraceptives, whose success rates range from 92% to 98% depending on the reliability of the patient's use (Centers for Disease Control and Prevention 2020). It is not uncommon for patients, especially those who are afraid of adverse medication reactions, to desire a contraceptive that they can easily start and stop. For these patients, the increased risk of unintended pregnancy with the daily methods must be balanced by the principle of patient autonomy. Providers may offer contraceptive pills with shorter or less frequent placebo periods, the contraceptive patch, or the contraceptive ring as a way to increase contraceptive effectiveness without taking away the patient's locus of control.

Contraceptive choice may also vary based on which noncontraceptive goals the patient wishes to achieve. For example, the combined hormonal methods will provide the best suppression of androgenic manifestations, such as hirsutism and acne. Women hoping to decrease menstrual flow and its associated discomforts would benefit most from methods that produce good ovarian suppression, endometrial atrophy, or both. Contraceptive methods with high rates of amenorrhea include DMPA injections (50%–60% at 1 year), IUDs containing 52 mg progestin (50% at 1 year), and continuous combined hormonal contraception (70% at 1 year) (Hillard 2014).

Some studies have found that women with mood disorders have higher rates of contraceptive discontinuation due to experienced side effects, such as weight changes and moodiness (Hall et al. 2012, 2013a). Providers should discuss potential side effects up front both to allow for effective management and to build patient–provider trust. Moreover, efforts should be made to arrange follow-up visits so that adverse side effects and other patient concerns may be addressed promptly. Reports of adverse side effects, even if not common or expected, should be taken seriously to build trust and to avoid retraumatization of patients who have experienced invalidating power relationships in their lives. Plans should be made to address any reported side effects, and the patient should be allowed to switch contraceptive method if she desires. Emergency contraception should also be offered if there is a risk that the patient might self-discontinue contraception.

## Contraception and Psychotropic Drug Interactions

In patients with psychiatric diagnoses, some contraceptive methods will be preferred due to drug-drug interactions. The estrogen and progestin components of common contraceptive methods are metabolized by intestinal and hepatic oxidation, glucuronidation, and sulfation. Cytochrome (CY) P450 3A4, in particular, appears to play a large role in the oxidative metabolism of ethinyl estradiol, the major estrogen component in most combined hormonal contraceptives. Meanwhile, combined hormonal contraceptives may moderately inhibit CYP1A2 and weakly inhibit CYP3A4, CYP2C19, and CYP2D6 enzymes. Because these enzymes are implicated in the metabolism of psychotropic drugs, drug-drug interactions may exist (Berry-Bibee et al. 2016).

In general, there is low concern that hormonal contraception interferes with the efficacy of selective serotonin reuptake inhibitors or serotonin-norepinephrine reuptake inhibitors, or vice versa. Tricyclic antidepressants and combined hormonal contraceptives are also not expected to have any clinically significant interactions. One good-quality pharmacokinetic study showed a modest decrease in bupropion serum levels in users of combined hormonal contraception, but whether this clinically produces a change in depression symptoms is unknown (Palovaara et al. 2003). The data for antipsychotics and hormonal contraception are limited but overall reassuring that these medications have no clinically significant drug-drug interactions. Benzodiazepine levels may be modestly affected (with some increased and some decreased) by hormonal contraception, but these interactions are unlikely to have much clinical significance (Berry-Bibee et al. 2016; Osborne and Payne 2017).

Of the psychotropic drugs, antiepileptic drugs have the most evidence of interactions with hormonal contraceptives (Reddy 2010). Specifically, estrogen-containing contraceptives are known to decrease the serum concentration of both lamotrigine and valproate, and doses may need to be uptitrated to effect in women newly initiated in combined hormonal contraception. The reverse is not true, however: use of lamotrigine or valproate does not decrease the contraceptive efficacy of hormonal contraception (Reimers 2019; Wegner et al. 2014). Fortunately, serum levels of both drugs are readily available in most laboratory results. Serum levels may be used to guide medication adjustments in patients who seem to demonstrate mood changes when beginning to use hormonal contraception. It may be prudent to draw a "reference serum level" prior to contraception initiation to create a target, assuming the patient was symptomatically stable prior to initiation. When the patient appears clinically stable, antiepileptic drug levels should not be adjusted based on serum levels alone. Clinical response is still considered the most reliable indicator of dose adequacy (Jacob and Nair 2016; Paulzen et al. 2015). Finally, most combined hormonal contraceptives include a placebo phase during which withdrawal bleeding occurs. Because this phase has no estrogen, the patient may temporarily experience a surge in lamotrigine levels and experience medication-related side effects. To prevent this, it is recommended that women taking antiepileptic drugs skip the placebo phase of their combined hormonal contraceptives and use the medications in a continuous fashion.

Other psychotropic drugs, again mostly in the antiepileptic class, may decrease the effectiveness of hormonal contraception by lowering serum concentrations of either its estrogen or progestin components. Carbamazepine, oxcarbazepine, topiramate, and modafinil are among those included in this class. Studies have shown breakthrough ovulation and bleeding when these drugs are combined with hormonal contraception, although studies have not directly assessed accidental pregnancy (American College of Obstetricians and Gynecologists Committee on Practice Bulletins 2019). If an estrogen-containing contraceptive is strongly desired in this population, a preparation containing at least 35 μg of ethinyl estradiol should be chosen, and the medication should be used continuously to decrease the risk of escape ovulation. Moreover, patients should be encouraged to utilize an additional layer of contraception, such as condoms (Centers for Disease Control and Prevention 2016). The etonogestrel implant, although somewhat affected by antiepileptic drugs, may be a better choice than other methods because it is so effective at preventing pregnancy that even the slightly lowered effectiveness in this population is still better than other methods (e.g., barrier methods). Preferred contraceptives for women who are taking antiepileptic drugs include DMPA injections and IUDs, neither of which interacts with these drugs (American College of Obstetricians and Gynecologists 2020a). Table 4–1 provides a comprehensive list of interactions.

Finding an appropriate method of contraception for women taking antiepileptic drugs is especially important given the teratogenic nature of some of these drugs. Although lamotrigine can be used safely in pregnancy, valproate (and to a lesser extent carbamazepine) is associated with a substantial risk of neural tube defects and cognitive deficits in the child (Veroniki et al. 2017). (For further details on the use of these drugs in pregnancy, see Chapter 15, "Bipolar Disorder and Related Disorders.") No woman of childbearing age should begin taking an antiepileptic drug without a solid contraceptive plan in place.

Ms. E is a 27-year-old single (gravida 0 para 0) graduate student with a long history of mood fluctuation, "rage," and impulsive behavior, along with several documented episodes of depression characterized by irritability, sadness, anhedonia, social withdrawal, poor appetite, and suicidal ideation. She reports that her mood symptoms fluctuate mildly with her menstrual cycle, with increased irritability starting a week before her menses. She has also had several discrete episodes of increased energy and productivity, during each of which she felt fully rested on 3–4 hours of sleep a night. During these times, she successfully submitted 12 applications for graduate school (although she had initially planned on submitting only 4), planned an elaborate family vacation that was not realistic for her family and resulted in the loss of some nonrefundable deposits, and spontaneously got in the car and drove 8 hours to pay a surprise visit to her college roommate. Her medical history is noncontributory, she has no allergies, and her family history is significant for a fraternal twin sister who has PMDD, a mother with a history of postpartum depression, and a paternal uncle with bipolar I disorder.

Upon first meeting Ms. E, you decide to start her on lamotrigine. She tolerates the medication well, and you successfully titrate the dose to 300 mg/day. She is stable on this dose for 9 months, with a level of 7.7. Her mood is stable, and she reports no premenstrual irritability. She decreases the frequency of her visits to once every 3 months, and you congratulate yourself on your expert diagnostic and treatment skills.

Today, however, Ms. E presents in clinic wearing garish lipstick and expressing rapid speech and is convinced that she has some "fantastic" ideas about how to fix the perennial scheduling issues in your office. Upon questioning, she reports that she has been sleeping only 3–4 hours a night for the past month, but "this is good, I'm not tired at all." She reports that she has recently started an oral contraceptive, and you decide to check her lamotrigine level again; you find that it has decreased to 5.8. What might account for her change in status, and what treatment recommendations might you make?

**TABLE 4–1. Interactions between oral contraceptives and psychiatric medications**

| Psychiatric medication | Interactions |
|---|---|
| **Antidepressants** | |
| Selective serotonin reuptake inhibitors | No interactions |
| Serotonin-norepinephrine reuptake inhibitors | No interactions |
| Monoamine oxidase inhibitors | No interactions |
| Tricyclic antidepressants (TCAs) | Monitor blood level; TCA level will be increased |
| Other antidepressants (bupropion, mirtazapine, trazodone, vilazodone) | No interactions |
| **Mood stabilizers and antiepileptics** | |
| Carbamazepine | OCP efficacy will be reduced |
| Gabapentin | No interactions |
| Lamotrigine | Lamotrigine levels will be reduced; no change in OCP efficacy |
| Lithium | No interactions |
| Oxcarbazepine | OCP efficacy will be reduced |
| Topiramate | OCP efficacy will be reduced |
| Valproic acid | No interactions |
| **Antianxiety medications** | |
| Alprazolam | Alprazolam effect will be increased |
| Barbiturates | OCP efficacy will be reduced |
| Chlordiazepoxide | Chlordiazepoxide effect will be increased |
| Diazepam | Diazepam effect will be increased |
| Flurazepam | Flurazepam effect will be increased |
| Lorazepam | Lorazepam effect will be increased |
| Oxazepam | Oxazepam effect will be increased |
| Temazepam | Temazepam effect will be increased |
| Triazolam | Triazolam effect will be increased |
| **Antipsychotics** | |
| Chlorpromazine | Chlorpromazine blood level (and adverse effects) will be increased |
| Clozapine | Clozapine blood level (and adverse effects) will be increased |
| Other typical and atypical antipsychotics | No interactions |
| **Biologically based therapies** | |
| Melatonin | Melatonin effect will be increased |
| Phytoestrogens and soy | Adverse effects of OCPs may be increased (theoretical) |
| St. John's wort | OCP efficacy will be reduced |
| Vitex agnus-castus | OCP efficacy will be reduced |

OCP=oral contraceptive pill.

*Source.* Adapted from Osborne and Payne 2017.

- There is no specific therapeutic window for lamotrigine, so we cannot say what the level should be for effectiveness. However, the decrease from a level at which the patient was stable may mean that her new symptoms have something to do with that decrease.
- Lamotrigine is metabolized by glucuronidation (uridine diphosphate glucuronosyltransferase [UGT] 1A4) and is renally excreted; estrogen is a known inducer of UGTs and is also glucuronidated by 1A4. The interaction has resulted in increased renal excretion of lamotrigine. Evidence supports increased clearance of lamotrigine due to exogenous, but not endogenous, estrogens, but thus far there is little evidence about the clinical effect of this increased excretion.
- If the patient wishes to continue the oral contraceptive, it will be important to increase the dose of lamotrigine to achieve remission. The patient may benefit from continuous dosing of the contraceptive to minimize fluctuations in lamotrigine level.
- The patient may also choose to switch to a progestin-only method or a method acting locally at the level of the uterus.

## Mood Effects of Contraception

Recent studies analyzing the relationship between hormonal contraception and mood disorders are overall reassuring, with adverse mood effects being possible but infrequent (Böttcher et al. 2012; Schaffir et al. 2016). A few studies have found an association between hormonal contraception use and lifetime diagnoses of depression, particularly among adolescents (Gregory et al. 2018; Skovlund et al. 2016; Zettermark et al. 2018). Some studies suggest that the mood effects of hormonal contraception are related to individual sensitivity to the progestin component (Merki-Feld et al. 2017; Svendal et al. 2012). However, multiple other studies have not found such an effect (McKetta and Keyes 2019; Pagano et al. 2016; Worly et al. 2018). In fact, some studies have found that current use of combined hormonal contraception *improves* mood, a finding that may relate to the benefits of contraception, which include reproductive and menstrual control, decrease in premenstrual symptoms, and improvement in conditions such as acne and gynecological pain (Svendal et al. 2012; Toffol et al. 2012).

The risk of contraception producing adverse mood effects must be weighed against the possibility that unintended pregnancy itself may lead to psychological distress or clinical depression. A large percentage of pregnancies in the United States are unplanned or mistimed. An analysis of more than 100,000 mothers between 2009 and 2011 found that only 32% of the women in the sample were desiring pregnancy at the time of conception (Gauthreaux et al. 2017). Among individuals with mental health disorders, up to 92% of pregnancies may be unplanned, because individuals with affective disorders may be more prone to risky sexual behaviors with ineffective contraceptive use (Adan Sanchez et al. 2019; Cunningham et al. 2016; Hall et al. 2012, 2013a, 2014). Several studies have found that mothers with unplanned pregnancies, even if the pregnancy is ultimately accepted, experience higher rates of postpartum depression (Abajobir et al. 2016; Barton et al. 2017; Gauthreaux et al. 2017). Most of these studies cite a two- or threefold increase in postpartum depression risk. Preexisting affective disorders, social support, and race may all influence the strength of this association (Barton et al. 2017; Suh et al. 2016).

Finally, patients concerned about mood changes should be aware that hormonal contraception has been used to improve mood in some patients with PMDD. For this subset of women, changes in estrogen and progesterone levels trigger a cascade of neuroendocrine changes, resulting in often debilitating changes in mood and affect (Schmidt et al. 1998, 2017). Thus, maintenance of steady levels of sex steroids via ovulation suppression can improve PMDD symptoms (Reid and Soares 2018). The extensive literature on PMDD and perinatal depression indicates that some women are vulnerable to *fluctuating* hormones rather than to decreased or increased levels, and for such women the constant low levels of hormones in systemic contraceptives stabilizes hormone levels and has a beneficial effect on mood (Schiller et al. 2014).

Studies have endorsed the efficacy of combined hormonal contraception with drospirenone as a treatment for PMDD (Rapkin and Mikacich 2013), particularly when it is accompanied by short or nonexistent hormone-free intervals (Lopez et al. 2012; Pearlstein et al. 2005; Yonkers et al. 2005). Other combined oral contraceptives, particularly when used continuously (without a hormone-free interval), may also be effective for the treatment of PMDD, although the results tend to be more mixed and show a potential placebo effect (Freeman et al. 2012; Halbreich et al. 2012). Any oral contraceptive can be used continuously (without a placebo period), regardless of how the drug is packaged or marketed. Relatedly, women with binge-eating and other disordered eating behaviors in the luteal phase of the menstrual cycle may also benefit from ovarian suppression with hormonal contraception (Dahlgren and Qvigstad 2018; Ko et al. 2015).

## Psychiatrist's Role in Contraceptive Access

For many women with mental health disorders, the psychiatrist will be the most consistent point of medical contact in their lives. For this reason, psychiatrists play a crucial role in helping women understand the interplay of reproductive health and mental health and are positioned to be an active force in enabling reproductive choice.

Although the placement of IUDs and administration of contraceptive injections may be out of the purview of the general psychiatrist, most psychiatrists should be able to prescribe combined hormonal contraception with some basic education. Table 4–2 lists some common contraindications for using combined hormonal contraception. The psychiatrist should prescribe contraception if the patient desires it, lacks contraindications, and is likely not pregnant (a useful Quick Start Algorithm for determining the likelihood of pregnancy is available from the Reproductive Health Access Project at www.reproductiveaccess.org/resource/quick-start-algorithm). The risks of unintended pregnancy generally outweigh the risk of taking oral contraception when already pregnant. These medications are neither teratogens nor abortifacients. Their main risk when used during early pregnancy is delaying the diagnosis of pregnancy. Table 4–3 lists several examples of combined hormonal contraception that the psychiatrist may want to consider, as well as emergency contraceptive options.

For women who are not candidates for combined hormonal contraception, or those who struggle with medication adherence, psychiatrists should strongly encourage the use of highly reliable forms of contraception. For many women, an IUD may be the best option in terms of contraceptive efficacy and longevity, lack of medication interactions, and lack of systemic side effects. These devices can be placed quickly in the office by an experienced provider and are usually well tolerated by patients. Some women will not want any medications or implants. Options for these women include menstrual cycle

**TABLE 4–2. Common contraindications for combined hormonal contraception**

| |
|---|
| Current pregnancy |
| Postpartum period (within 6 weeks after giving birth) |
| History of a thromboembolism |
| Migraine headaches with aura |
| Hypertension |
| Smoking after age 35 years |
| Carcinoma of the breast or endometrium |
| Hepatic disease or impairment |

*Note.* This table lists frequently encountered contraindications. For a complete list, see Centers for Disease Control and Prevention (2016).

tracking (valid only for women with regular menses), barrier methods such as diaphragms and condoms, spermicides, vaginal pH modulators, and permanent sterilization. Lastly, for women who decline all contraceptive options, psychiatrists should offer emergency contraception as a layer of protection against unintended pregnancy.

Ms. F is a 20-year-old college student who sees you for a diagnosis of major depressive disorder and borderline personality disorder. Her symptoms have been staying well controlled with fluoxetine, which she remembers to take most of the time. Today, Ms. F seems happy; she states that she is doing well in class and hopes to pursue graduate school in psychology after graduating. Upon further interviewing, she tells you that she has also started a new relationship with "someone who I never thought would even look at me!" She states that they are planning to go on vacation together tomorrow, and she is a little bummed because she started her period today and they will not be able to have sex. When you ask if she is using anything to prevent unintended pregnancy or sexually transmitted infections, she seems nonplussed. "Don't worry—he always pulls out." You know it usually takes 2 months for patients to get an appointment with the campus gynecologist at your institution. What advice do you provide?

- Sexually active healthy women who are not using contraception are at high risk for pregnancy. Women with borderline personality disorder, bipolar disorder, and substance use disorders, in particular, demonstrate high rates of unintended pregnancy.
- Barrier methods, such as condoms, are the best way to protect against sexually transmitted infections. If she is unable to use these methods, Ms. F should undergo screening for sexually transmitted infections at regular intervals; screening is typically performed via urine and blood tests. Untreated infections may lead to complications such as infertility and chronic pelvic pain.
- Because Ms. F is having unprotected sex, she is at risk for unintended pregnancy. She does not have ready access to a gynecologist, so you should strongly consider prescribing and starting her on contraception today. As long as pregnancy is reasonably excluded, and no contraindications to using contraceptives exist, oral contraception may be initiated at any point in the menstrual cycle. Some studies have shown that women are less likely to start oral contraception if asked to wait until their next menstrual period.
- Because she has forgotten doses of her fluoxetine in the past, Ms. F may struggle with pill compliance with oral contraceptives. Therefore, a patch or a ring would be preferred, and either can be prescribed by any physician. Ultimately, she may be a good candidate for a long-acting reversible method, such as an

**TABLE 4–3. Select list of contraceptive options**

| Contraceptive formulation | Notes | Consider for |
|---|---|---|
| Drospirenone/Ethinyl estradiol 3 mg/0.02 mg (Beyaz) | 24 days of active pills; decreases risk of accidental ovulation with a shorter placebo period | Women with premenstrual dysphoric disorder |
| Norethindrone acetate/Ethinyl estradiol 0.4 mg/0.035 mg chewable tablets (Femcon Fe) | Chewable tablets | Women who report trouble swallowing pills |
| Levonorgestrel/Ethinyl estradiol 0.15 mg/0.03–0.01 mg (Seasonique) | Packaged as a 3-month supply of 84 active pills + 7 days of inactive pills; placebo week has ethinyl estradiol 10 μg | Women desiring periods every 3 months; women with estrogen withdrawal headaches, those taking lamotrigine, and those particularly sensitive to premenstrual symptoms may benefit from the continued estradiol in the placebo week |
| Norelgestromin/Ethinyl estradiol 0.15/0.035 mg patch (Xulane) | Weekly topical patch; may be relatively less effective in obese women | Women weighing ≤198 lb with poor pill compliance |
| Etonogestrel/Ethinyl estradiol 0.12/0.015 mg ring (NuvaRing) | Monthly vaginal ring | Women with poor pill compliance |
| Levonorgestrel 1.5 mg (Plan B); ullipristal acetate 30 mg (Ella) | Emergency contraception; can be used within 72 hours and 120 hours of unprotected intercourse, respectively<br>Ullipristal not available at all pharmacies<br>Levonorgestrel emergency contraception may be relatively less effective in obese women | Any woman who is having unprotected intercourse or who may be nonadherent to contraception |

IUD or arm implant, which you can encourage her to consider when she sees the gynecologist. These methods are well tolerated and have an extremely low rate of failure (~1%).

- If Ms. F declines to start a contraceptive method, you should at least offer her emergency contraception, such as levonorgestrel 1.5 mg, which can be taken within 72 hours of unprotected intercourse, or ullipristal 30 mg, which can be taken within 5 days of unprotected intercourse.

## Special Considerations: Voluntary Termination of Pregnancy

Not all women want to carry a pregnancy to birth. This makes voluntary termination of pregnancy (VTOP) a medical reality, regardless of societal or legal support. In 2014, almost 20% of pregnancies in the United States ended in VTOP (Jones and Jerman 2017). Most women seeking VTOP are poor or have low income (Jerman et al. 2016). Reasons commonly cited for obtaining VTOP include feeling unable to raise a child based on personal or economic circumstances, believing that a child would interfere with the woman's obligations to herself or others, or lack of a supportive partner with whom to share the responsibility of parenthood (Finer et al. 2005). The decision to terminate a pregnancy is rarely an eagerly made choice, even when a woman thinks it is the right choice. Accordingly, some women do experience negative feelings following a VTOP, and some experience clinically significant disorders such as depression and VTOP-specific PTSD.

In examining the causal relationship of VTOP with mental health, however, methodology is vitally important. Historical studies that have compared rates of depression among women seeking VTOPs with those of women in the general population who have live births fail to account for the mediating factors of patient choice and psychosocial context (Steinberg et al. 2012; Stotland 2019). A more appropriate comparison would be women with unwanted pregnancies who chose VTOP, live birth with parenting, or live birth with adoption. Nonpregnant women are never an appropriate control group for women who have had VTOPs. Relatedly, in examining prevalence rates for women's mental health disorders following VTOP, the comparison should be made with women's mental health disorders after giving birth; postpartum rates of disorders such as anxiety and depression are commonly cited at 15%–20% in the literature (Kendig et al. 2017). Finally, investigators should strive to delineate whether the mood symptoms arose from the act of VTOP itself or from the circumstances that led the woman to contemplate VTOP in the first place.

The American Psychological Association (2008), the American Psychiatric Association (2018), and the American College of Obstetricians and Gynecologists (2020b) all refute a causal relationship between the act of VTOP and mental health disorders such as depression, anxiety, or PTSD. These position statements arise from several methodologically appropriate studies examining large, longitudinal data sets (Coleman et al. 2009; Cougle et al. 2003; Steinberg et al. 2018; van Ditzhuijzen et al. 2018). Other studies have shown that external and internal stigma play a large role in the meaning that women attribute to their VTOPs, and their subsequent emotional sequelae are informed by that narrative (Cozzarelli et al. 2000; Hanschmidt et al. 2018; Steinberg et al. 2016). Choice also informs whether VTOP is considered traumatic, and women who are denied VTOPs or are coerced into VTOPs experience adverse psychological outcomes (Biggs et al. 2017; Hunter et al. 2017; Rue et al. 2004). Among women with unwanted pregnancies, VTOPs and live births have similar rates of depressive symptoms, and the most important prognostic factor for a woman's postpartum mood is her mental state prior to undergoing the VTOP itself (Gomez 2018; Reardon 2018).

In working with women contemplating VTOP, mental health providers should be mindful not to contribute to stigma and to support the woman psychologically, whatever her ultimate choice may be. Women with a prior history of psychiatric comorbidities, unsupportive environments, substance use, and exposure to violence are at elevated risk for psychiatric symptoms with an unwanted pregnancy and may benefit from proactive mental health engagement.

## Conclusion

Although contraceptive care has not traditionally been within the scope of mental health care, the documented interplay between reproductive health and mental health clearly indicates that clinical excellence in psychiatric care includes competency in contraceptive counseling and management. Psychiatrists and other mental health providers are well positioned to educate women about the risks and benefits of contraception and the ways in which mood symptoms may be influenced by various methods. At a minimum, prevention of unwanted pregnancy should be a core component of comprehensive psychiatric care.

## Key Points

- Contraception drastically alters a woman's reproductive destiny, which has downstream effects on her physical and mental health.
- Negative effects on mood are not seen in the vast majority of women using contraception.
- Contraception has noncontraceptive benefits, including but not limited to improvement in mental well-being for women who experience menstrual-related mood changes.
- With the exception of antiepileptic medications, most psychotropic medications do not demonstrate clinically significant drug-drug interactions with hormonal contraception.
- Mental health providers can optimize psychological functioning by playing an active role in contraceptive access, including but not limited to treatment referral and medication initiation.
- Contraceptive decision making is often nuanced, and shared decision-making best respects the autonomy of the woman while maximizing opportunities for contraceptive benefit and satisfaction.

# References


Abajobir AA, Maravilla JC, Alati R, et al: A systematic review and meta-analysis of the association between unintended pregnancy and perinatal depression. J Affect Disord 192:56–63, 2016 26707348

Adan Sanchez AY, McMillan E, Bhaduri A, et al: High-risk sexual behaviour in young people with mental health disorders. Early Interv Psychiatry 13(4):867–873, 2019 29920952

American College of Obstetricians and Gynecologists Committee on Practice Bulletins: Committee Opinion #206: use of hormonal contraception in women with coexisting medical conditions. Obstet Gynecol 133(2):e128–e150, 2019 30681544

American College of Obstetricians and Gynecologists: Gynecologic management of adolescents and young women with seizure disorders. ACOG Committee Opinion Summary, number 806. Obstet Gynecol 135(5):1242–1243, 2020a

American College of Obstetricians and Gynecologists: Increasing access to abortion. ACOG Committee Opinion Number 815. Obstet Gynecol 136(6):e107–e115, 2020b

American Psychiatric Association: Position Statement on Abortion. Washington, DC, American Psychiatric Association, 2018. Available at: https://www.psychiatry.org/File%20Library/About-APA/Organization-Documents-Policies/Policies/Position-2018-Abortion.pdf. Accessed June 2021.

American Psychological Association: Report of the APA Task Force on Mental Health and Abortion. Washington, DC, American Psychological Association, 2008

Barton K, Redshaw M, Quigley MA, et al: Unplanned pregnancy and subsequent psychological distress in partnered women: a cross-sectional study of the role of relationship quality and wider social support. BMC Pregnancy Childbirth 17(1):44, 2017 28122585

Berry-Bibee EN, Kim MJ, Simmons KB, et al: Drug interactions between hormonal contraceptives and psychotropic drugs: a systematic review. Contraception 94(6):650–667, 2016 27444984

Biggs MA, Upadhyay UD, McCulloch CE, et al: Women's mental health and well-being 5 years after receiving or being denied an abortion: a prospective, longitudinal cohort study. JAMA Psychiatry 74(2):169–178, 2017 27973641

Böttcher B, Radenbach K, Wildt L, et al: Hormonal contraception and depression: a survey of the present state of knowledge. Arch Gynecol Obstet 286(1):231–236, 2012 22467147

Centers for Disease Control and Prevention: U.S. Medical Eligibility Criteria for Contraceptive Use. Atlanta, GA, Centers for Disease Control and Prevention, 2016. Available at: https://www.cdc.gov/reproductivehealth/contraception/mmwr/mec/summary.html. Accessed August 20, 2019.

Centers for Disease Control and Prevention: Reproductive Health: Contraception (online). Atlanta, GA, Centers for Disease Control and Prevention, 2020. Available at: https://www.cdc.gov/reproductivehealth/contraception/index.htm. Accessed June 2021.

Coleman PK, Coyle CT, Shuping M, et al: Induced abortion and anxiety, mood, and substance abuse disorders: isolating the effects of abortion in the National Comorbidity Survey. J Psychiatr Res 43(8):770–776, 2009 19046750

Cougle JR, Reardon DC, Coleman PK: Depression associated with abortion and childbirth: a long-term analysis of the National Longitudinal Survey of Youth cohort. Med Sci Monit 9:105–112, 2003

Cozzarelli C, Major B, Karrasch A: Women's experiences of and reactions to antiabortion picketing. Basic Appl Soc 22:265–275, 2000

Cunningham SD, Smith A, Kershaw T, et al: Prenatal depressive symptoms and postpartum sexual risk among young urban women of color. J Pediatr Adolesc Gynecol 29(1):11–17, 2016 26165914

Dahlgren CL, Qvigstad E: Eating disorders in premenstrual dysphoric disorder: a neuroendocrinological pathway to the pathogenesis and treatment of binge eating. J Eat Disord 6:35, 2018 30386599

Dietz PM, Spitz AM, Anda RF, et al: Unintended pregnancy among adult women exposed to abuse or household dysfunction during their childhood. JAMA 282(14):1359–1364, 1999 10527183

Finer LB, Frohwirth LF, Dauphinee LA, et al: Reasons U.S. women have abortions: quantitative and qualitative perspectives. Perspect Sex Reprod Health 37(3):110–118, 2005 16150658
Freeman EW, Halbreich U, Grubb GS, et al: An overview of four studies of a continuous oral contraceptive (levonorgestrel 90 mcg/ethinyl estradiol 20 mcg) on premenstrual dysphoric disorder and premenstrual syndrome. Contraception 85(5):437–445, 2012 22152588
Gauthreaux C, Negron J, Castellanos D, et al: The association between pregnancy intendedness and experiencing symptoms of postpartum depression among new mothers in the United States, 2009 to 2011: a secondary analysis of PRAMS data. Medicine (Baltimore) 96(6):e5851, 2017 28178128
Gibson M: The long, strange history of birth control. TIME, February 2, 2015. Available at: https://www.time.com/3692001/birth-control-history-djerassi. Accessed May 28, 2019.
Gomez AM: Abortion and subsequent depressive symptoms: an analysis of the National Longitudinal Study of Adolescent Health. Psychol Med 48(2):294–304, 2018 28625180
Gregory ST, Hall K, Quast T, et al: Hormonal contraception, depression, and academic performance among females attending college in the United States. Psychiatry Res 270:111–116, 2018 30245373
Halbreich U, Freeman EW, Rapkin AJ, et al: Continuous oral levonorgestrel/ethinyl estradiol for treating premenstrual dysphoric disorder. Contraception 85(1):19–27, 2012 22067793
Hall KS, White KO, Rickert VI, et al: Influence of depressed mood and psychological stress symptoms on perceived oral contraceptive side effects and discontinuation in young minority women. Contraception 86(5):518–525, 2012 22673038
Hall KS, Moreau C, Trussell J, et al: Young women's consistency of contraceptive use: does depression or stress matter? Contraception 88(5):641–649, 2013a 23850075
Hall KS, Kusunoki Y, Gatny H, et al: The risk of unintended pregnancy among young women with mental health symptoms. Soc Sci Med 100:62–71, 2014 24444840
Hanschmidt F, Treml J, Klingner J, et al: Stigma in the context of pregnancy termination after diagnosis of fetal anomaly: associations with grief, trauma, and depression. Arch Womens Ment Health 21(4):391–399, 2018 29288285
Hillard PA: Menstrual suppression: current perspectives. Int J Womens Health 6:631–637, 2014 25018654
Hunter A, Tussis L, MacBeth A: The presence of anxiety, depression and stress in women and their partners during pregnancies following perinatal loss: a meta-analysis. J Affect Disord 223:153–164, 2017 28755623
Jacob S, Nair AB: An updated overview on therapeutic drug monitoring of recent antiepileptic drugs. Drugs R D 16(4):303–316, 2016 27766590
Jerman J, Jones RK, Onda T: Characteristics of U.S. abortion patients in 2014 and changes since 2008. May 2016 Report. New York, Guttmacher Institute, 2016. Available at: https://www.guttmacher.org/report/characteristics-us-abortion-patients-2014. Accessed January 7, 2021.
Johnston EM, Courtot B, Fass F, et al: Prevalence and perceptions of unplanned births. Urban Institute Health Policy Center, March 2017. Available at: http://www.urban.org/sites/default/files/publication/88801/prevalence_and_perceptions_of_unplanned_births.pdf. Accessed July 27, 2019.
Jones RK, Jerman J: Abortion incidence and service availability in the United States, 2014. Perspect Sex Reprod Health 49(1):17–27, 2017 28094905
Judge-Golden CP, Borrero S, Zhao X, et al: The association between mental health disorders and history of unintended pregnancy among women veterans. J Gen Intern Med 33(12):2092–2099, 2018 30187377
Kavanaugh ML, Jerman J: Contraceptive method use in the United States: trends and characteristics between 2008, 2012 and 2014. Contraception 97(1):14–21, 2018 29038071
Kendig S, Keats JP, Hoffman MC, et al: Consensus bundle on maternal mental health: perinatal depression and anxiety. Obstet Gynecol 129(3):422–430, 2017 28178041
Ko CH, Yen CF, Long CY, et al: The late-luteal leptin level, caloric intake and eating behaviors among women with premenstrual dysphoric disorder. Psychoneuroendocrinology 56:52–61, 2015 25800149

Lopez LM, Kaptein AA, Helmerhorst FM: Oral contraceptives containing drospirenone for premenstrual syndrome. Cochrane Database Syst Rev (2):CD006586, 2012 22336820
Marengo E, Martino DJ, Igoa A, et al: Unplanned pregnancies and reproductive health among women with bipolar disorder. J Affect Disord 178:201–205, 2015 25827504
McKetta S, Keyes KM: Oral contraceptive use and depression among adolescents. Ann Epidemiol 29:46–51, 2019 30674431
Merki-Feld GS, Apter D, Bartfai G, et al: ESC expert statement on the effects on mood of the natural cycle and progestin-only contraceptives. Eur J Contracept Reprod Health Care 22(4):247–249, 2017 28728451
Mishell DR Jr, Thorneycroft IH, Nakamura RM, et al: Serum estradiol in women ingesting combination oral contraceptive steroids. Am J Obstet Gynecol 114(7):923–928, 1972 4645131
Osborne LM, Payne JL: Clinical updates in women's health care summary: mood and anxiety disorders: primary and preventive care review. Obstet Gynecol 130(3):674, 2017 28832483
Pagano HP, Zapata LB, Berry-Bibee EN, et al: Safety of hormonal contraception and intrauterine devices among women with depressive and bipolar disorders: a systematic review. Contraception 94(6):641–649, 2016 27364100
Palovaara S, Pelkonen O, Uusitalo J, et al: Inhibition of cytochrome P450 2B6 activity by hormone replacement therapy and oral contraceptive as measured by bupropion hydroxylation. Clin Pharmacol Ther 74(4):326–333, 2003 14534519
Paulzen M, Lammertz SE, Veselinovic T, et al: Lamotrigine in pregnancy—therapeutic drug monitoring in maternal blood, amniotic fluid, and cord blood. Int Clin Psychopharmacol 30(5):249–254, 2015 26086711
Pearlstein TB, Bachmann GA, Zacur HA, et al: Treatment of premenstrual dysphoric disorder with a new drospirenone-containing oral contraceptive formulation. Contraception 72(6):414–421, 2005 16307962
Rapkin AJ, Mikacich JA: Premenstrual dysphoric disorder and severe premenstrual syndrome in adolescents. Paediatr Drugs 15(3):191–202, 2013 23529867
Reardon DC: The abortion and mental health controversy: a comprehensive literature review of common ground agreements, disagreements, actionable recommendations, and research opportunities. SAGE Open Med 6:2050312118807624, 2018 30397472
Reddy DS: Clinical pharmacokinetic interactions between antiepileptic drugs and hormonal contraceptives. Expert Rev Clin Pharmacol 3(2):183–192, 2010 20369030
Regidor PA: Clinical relevance in present day hormonal contraception. Horm Mol Biol Clin Investig 37(1), 2018 30367791
Reid RL, Soares CN: Premenstrual dysphoric disorder: contemporary diagnosis and management. J Obstet Gynaecol Can 40(2):215–223, 2018 29132964
Reimers A: Lamotrigine, bipolar disorder, and the pill-free week. Bipolar Disord 21(4):372–373, 2019 30920110
Rue VM, Coleman PK, Rue JJ, et al: Induced abortion and traumatic stress: a preliminary comparison of American and Russian women. Med Sci Monit 10(10):SR5–SR16, 2004 15448616
Schaffir J, Worly BL, Gur TL: Combined hormonal contraception and its effects on mood: a critical review. Eur J Contracept Reprod Health Care 21(5):347–355, 2016 27636867
Schiller CE, Schmidt PJ, Rubinow DR: Allopregnanolone as a mediator of affective switching in reproductive mood disorders. Psychopharmacology (Berl) 231(17):3557–3567, 2014 24846476
Schmidt PJ, Nieman LK, Danaceau MA, et al: Differential behavioral effects of gonadal steroids in women with and in those without premenstrual syndrome. N Engl J Med 338(4):209–216, 1998 9435325
Schmidt PJ, Martinez PE, Nieman LK, et al: Premenstrual dysphoric disorder symptoms following ovarian suppression: triggered by change in ovarian steroid levels but not continuous stable levels. Am J Psychiatry 174(10):980–989, 2017 28427285
Skovlund CW, Mørch LS, Kessing LV, et al: Association of hormonal contraception with depression. JAMA Psychiatry 73(11):1154–1162, 2016 27680324
Sonfield A, Kost K, Gold RB, et al: The public costs of births resulting from unintended pregnancies: national and state-level estimates. Perspect Sex Reprod Health 43(2):94–102, 2011 21651708

Sonfield A, Hasstedt K, Gold RB: Moving forward: family planning in the era of health reform. March 2014 Report. New York, Guttmacher Institute, 2014. Available at: https://www.guttmacher.org/report/moving-forward-family-planning-era-health-reform. Accessed July 27, 2019.
Steinberg JR, Trussell J, Hall KS, et al: Fatal flaws in a recent meta-analysis on abortion and mental health. Contraception 86(5):430–437, 2012 22579105
Steinberg JR, Tschann JM, Furgerson D, et al: Psychosocial factors and pre-abortion psychological health: the significance of stigma. Soc Sci Med 150:67–75, 2016 26735332
Steinberg JR, Laursen TM, Adler NE, et al: Examining the association of antidepressant prescriptions with first abortion and first childbirth. JAMA Psychiatry 75(8):828–834, 2018 29847626
Stotland NL: Update on reproductive rights and women's mental health. Med Clin North Am 103(4):751–766, 2019 31078205
Suh EY, Ma P, Dunaway LF, et al: Pregnancy intention and post-partum depressive affect in Louisiana Pregnancy Risk Assessment Monitoring System. Matern Child Health J 20(5):1001–1013, 2016 26649877
Svendal G, Berk M, Pasco JA, et al: The use of hormonal contraceptive agents and mood disorders in women. J Affect Disord 140(1):92–96, 2012 22537684
Toffol E, Heikinheimo O, Koponen P, et al: Further evidence for lack of negative associations between hormonal contraception and mental health. Contraception 86(5):470–480, 2012 22465115
van Ditzhuijzen J, Ten Have M, de Graaf R, et al: Long-term incidence and recurrence of common mental disorders after abortion: a Dutch prospective cohort study. J Psychiatr Res 102:132–135, 2018 29649722
Veroniki AA, Cogo E, Rios P, et al: Comparative safety of anti-epileptic drugs during pregnancy: a systematic review and network meta-analysis of congenital malformations and prenatal outcomes. BMC Med 15(1):95, 2017 28472982
Wegner I, Wilhelm AJ, Lambrechts DA, et al: Effect of oral contraceptives on lamotrigine levels depends on comedication. Acta Neurol Scand 129(6):393–398, 2014 24571554
Worly BL, Gur TL, Schaffir J: The relationship between progestin hormonal contraception and depression: a systematic review. Contraception 97(6):478–489, 2018 29496297
Yonkers KA, Brown C, Pearlstein TB, et al: Efficacy of a new low-dose oral contraceptive with drospirenone in premenstrual dysphoric disorder. Obstet Gynecol 106(3):492–501, 2005 16135578
Yonkers KA, Cameron B, Gueorguieva R, et al: The influence of cyclic hormonal contraception on expression of premenstrual syndrome. J Womens Health (Larchmt) 26(4):321–328, 2017 27854559
Zettermark S, Perez Vicente R, Merlo J: Hormonal contraception increases the risk of psychotropic drug use in adolescent girls but not in adults: a pharmacoepidemiological study on 800,000 Swedish women. PLoS One 13(3) e0194773, 2018 29566064
Zimmerman Y, Eijkemans MJ, Coelingh Bennink HJ, et al: The effect of combined oral contraception on testosterone levels in healthy women: a systematic review and meta-analysis. Hum Reprod Update 20(1):76–105, 2014 24082040

CHAPTER 5

# Infertility and Perinatal Loss

Neha S. Hudepohl, M.D.
Jessica L. Coker, M.D.
Sharvari P. Shivanekar, M.D.
Madhavi-Latha Nagalla, M.D.
Soudabeh Givrad, M.D.
Lindsay R. Standeven, M.D.
Courtney Erdly, B.A.
Premala Jones, Ph.D.
Katherine E. Williams, M.D.

For many women, pregnancy and becoming a parent represent major life milestones. However, the journey at times can be a challenging one—one that contains loss, grief, and unexpected hardship. Infertility and perinatal loss represent two such challenges. Collectively termed *reproductive trauma,* these issues can significantly affect mental health (Bhat and Byatt 2016). In this chapter, we review the fundamentals of infertility and perinatal loss, with a particular focus on their intersection with mental health.

## Infertility

Infertility is common, and it is physically and emotionally challenging (Patel et al. 2018). Its impact on a woman's mental health can be profound. Additionally, psychiatric conditions may be related to infertility and its treatment in a bidirectional but complex manner. In the sections that follow, we review the epidemiology, pathophysiology, evaluation, and management of infertility. We summarize the use of assisted reproductive technology (ART). Of note, the use of ART in populations with infertility has different mental health implications than the use of ART in populations for whom it offers an important opportunity to build a family, such as with LGBTQ+ families. (Although ART for family building in same-sex couples is now routine, and there is a good evidence base for fertility preservation for both transgender men and women, little evidence is available about actual pregnancy in transgender individuals.) This section also reviews the mental health components of infertility and its treatment and the impact of ART on mental health.

## Definitions

*Infertility* is defined as the failure to establish a clinical pregnancy after 12 months of regular, unprotected sexual intercourse or the impairment of a person's capacity to reproduce, either as an individual or with a partner (Zegers-Hochschild et al. 2017). *Primary infertility* refers to meeting criteria for infertility with no prior clinical pregnancy; *secondary infertility* refers to meeting criteria for infertility but with a prior pregnancy in the past (Zegers-Hochschild et al. 2017). An infertility evaluation is recommended for women younger than age 35 years who have failed to conceive after 12 months of unprotected intercourse and for women age 35 years or older who have failed to conceive after 6 months of unprotected intercourse (American College of Obstetricians and Gynecologists 2019). Women age 40 and older and those who have a condition associated with infertility should be offered an immediate evaluation (American College of Obstetricians and Gynecologists 2019).

## Epidemiology

### Rates/Incidence

Infertility is estimated to affect 8%–12% of couples of reproductive age, and the prevalence among women of reproductive age ranges across the world (Mascarenhas et al. 2012; Ombelet et al. 2008). It is estimated that primary infertility occurs in one in every seven couples in the Western world and one in every four couples in developing countries. Primary infertility rates may reach as high as 30% in some countries of South Asia, Sub-Saharan Africa, the Middle East, North Africa, Central and Eastern Europe, and Central Asia (Mascarenhas et al. 2012). In the United States, some studies find no difference in infertility across racial, ethnic, or economic categories, whereas others find increased rates of infertility among Black women and American Indian/Alaskan Native women (Lynch 2019; Shirazi and Rosinger 2020).

The way infertility is defined is, in itself, racially biased, because many definitions of infertility depend on a women's cohabitation status, and rates of cohabiting differ across racial and ethnic groups. Regardless of whether there are discrepancies in rates of infertility, however, there are certainly discrepancies in access to infertility treatment (which is expensive and often not covered by insurance) and in success of treatment (Insogna and Ginsburg 2018; Janitz et al. 2019). Numerous studies have found that Black, Hispanic, and Asian women have lower clinical pregnancy rates and live birth rates after in vitro fertilization (IVF) compared with white women (Humphries et al. 2016). This is also true for pregnancies after oocyte donation (Zhou et al. 2020).

### Risk Factors

Approximately 40% of infertility cases are due to female factors, 40% are due to male factors, and 20% are a combination or unexplained (Practice Committee of the Amer-

TABLE 5–1. **Female factors in infertility**

| | |
|---|---|
| Ovarian factors | Ovulatory dysfunction<br>  Polycystic ovary syndrome<br>  Functional hypothalamic amenorrhea<br>  Maternal age |
| Tubal factors | Blockage of fallopian tubes |
| Uterine factors | Endometriosis<br>Uterine fibroids<br>Endometrial polyps<br>Congenital malformations |
| Immune factors | Thyroid autoimmune disorders<br>  Hashimoto's thyroiditis<br>  Graves' disease<br>  Autoimmune thyroiditis |

ican Society for Reproductive Medicine 2015). Table 5–1 summarizes the most common identified female factors in infertility.

Of the medical causes of infertility, several conditions also commonly have associated psychiatric symptoms. For example, polycystic ovary syndrome (PCOS) is the most common endocrine disorder of women, affecting 6%–10% of women of reproductive age, with a prevalence of infertility of 70%–80% (Bozdag et al. 2016; Joham et al. 2015). Higher rates of psychiatric symptoms, including anxiety, depression, sexual dysfunction, eating disorders (in particular, binge-eating disorder), and sleep disturbances are common in women with PCOS. For additional information on PCOS, see Chapter 2, "Gynecological Conditions and Mental Health." Endometriosis is another common disorder associated with both infertility and mood symptoms (Macer and Taylor 2012). Endometriosis is associated with an increased risk of developing anxiety and depressive disorders, and higher levels of pelvic pain are associated with higher levels of depressive symptoms (Chen et al. 2016; Gambadauro et al. 2019). Similarly, autoimmune thyroid disorders, such as Hashimoto's thyroiditis, Graves' disease, and autoimmune thyroiditis, are associated with difficulty conceiving, increased rates of miscarriage, and mood, energy, and anxiety symptoms (Demartini et al. 2014; Fukao et al. 2019; Khizroeva et al. 2019; Samuels 2014).

Functional hypothalamic amenorrhea (FHA) is the failure of ovulation and menstruation in women, often associated with extreme physical exercise, disordered eating, or emotional stress. The condition is associated with increased cortisol levels and hypoestrogenism, leading to medical complications such as bone loss and impaired cardiovascular function (Shufelt et al. 2017). Certain temperamental traits may be associated with FHA, including perfectionism, low self-esteem, high need for social approval, and preoccupation with weight and body image (Giles and Berga 1993; Pentz and Rados 2017). In recognition of this association, the Endocrine Society's clinical practice guidelines recommend screening for these traits, as well as anxiety and depressive symptoms, in all women with FHA (Gordon et al. 2017).

## Evaluation

The evaluation of infertility involves a history and physical examination and targeted laboratory testing (including but not limited to follicle-stimulating hormone [FSH], luteinizing hormone [LH], testosterone, estradiol, and prolactin levels), as well as studies to assess for structural abnormalities and ovarian function (American College of Obstetricians and Gynecologists 2019). One commonly performed study is hysterosalpingography, a procedure used to view the uterus and fallopian tubes by injecting radiopaque contrast through the cervix during fluoroscopy (American College of Obstetricians and Gynecologists 2019; Graupera et al. 2015). Male factor infertility is most often assessed with semen analysis, which evaluates sperm volume, total sperm count, concentration, motility, and morphology. Other tests that may be performed under specific circumstances include genetic analysis, chromosomal analysis, and testicular biopsy (Pathak et al. 2020).

## Assisted Reproductive Technology

The ART process is time intensive and involves exposure to a number of medications at specific points in the menstrual cycle. The most common ART procedures, intrauterine insemination (IUI) and IVF, are described in the following discussion.

### Intrauterine Insemination

IUI cycles typically involve ovarian stimulation with oral medications (clomiphene citrate, aromatase inhibitors, or metformin), serial ultrasounds to evaluate and follow follicular development, an injection of human chorionic gonadotropin (hCG) to induce follicular maturation and ovulation, and timed insemination with sperm. Some women are then prescribed progesterone supplementation, either oral or vaginal, for endometrial support (van der Linden et al. 2015).

### In Vitro Fertilization

IVF cycles are significantly more intensive than IUI protocols, requiring daily visits for monitoring, additional procedures and medications (often injectable), and sedation/anesthesia for the outpatient surgical egg retrieval procedure. The IVF cycle often begins with at least 1 month of hypothalamic-pituitary-gonadal (HPG) axis suppression with oral birth control pills, with or without gonadotropin-releasing hormone (GnRH) agonists. The stimulation phase follows, which is typically 5–7 days of controlled ovarian stimulation with injected gonadotropins, with daily assessment of follicle growth and laboratory testing. When several follicles are mature, an injection of hCG triggers ovulation. Retrieval of mature oocytes is then done within the next 2 days under twilight anesthesia in a dedicated operating room. The oocytes are then fertilized with partner or donor sperm, and embryos are cultivated in the laboratory for several days, often until the blastocyst stage. Embryos may then be transferred into the uterus (a "fresh" transfer) or may be frozen and transferred later (Wang and Sauer 2006). Some patients choose to test the embryos for genetic abnormalities, a process that requires frozen embryos. In most cycles, luteal phase support is added with progesterone—typically an intramuscular injection—and/or estrogen (van der Linden et al. 2015).

## Neuropsychiatric Effects

The ART process involves the use of many medications that have potential psychiatric side effects, as discussed here and summarized in Table 5–2. In the assessment of patients undergoing ART, clinicians should clarify whether patients have a history of psychiatric symptoms at times of hormonal change, such as in the premenstrual period, with oral contraceptive use, or in the postpartum period. Patients who have such symptoms may be at greater risk for mood destabilization during the ART process.

**Oral contraceptives.** Most IVF cycles begin with at least 1 month of combined oral contraceptive pills (OCPs) in order to suppress the HPG axis prior to controlled ovarian stimulation. As described in Chapter 4, "Contraception," most women do not experience mood changes with oral contraceptives. If women have a previous history of mood destabilization with OCPs, they should be counseled to discuss their history with their reproductive endocrinologist (Williams 2015).

**Clomiphene citrate.** Clomiphene citrate is a selective estrogen receptor modulator with mixed agonist-antagonist properties. Taken orally on days 3–7 of the menstrual cycle, it creates a central perception of low estradiol, which leads to increased FSH and LH via negative feedback and then to ovarian stimulation and increased follicular development (Kousta et al. 1997). Clomiphene citrate is associated with mood lability, often characterized as "super PMS" (premenstrual syndrome), as well as insomnia and decreased libido (Aussedat et al. 2017; Blenner 1991; Choi et al. 2005). It has been associated with case reports of transient psychosis occurring in patients with and without a previous psychiatric history (Altmark et al. 1987; Seeman 2015; Siedentopf et al. 1997). In these case reports, sleeplessness and agitation were early symptoms, followed by auditory hallucinations, paranoia, delusions, and ideas of reference. Treatment with neuroleptics, electroconvulsive therapy, or a combination of both resolved the symptoms (Siedentopf et al. 1997; Sinha and Garg 2014).

**Gonadotropins.** Gonadotropins are used for controlled ovarian stimulation. These medications increase the number of ovarian follicles and are associated with extremely high serum estradiol levels (Usadi and Merriam 2015). As with clomiphene citrate, women exposed to these medications frequently describe mood lability (Choi et al. 2005). Carefully controlled studies of women undergoing IVF with gonadotropins and progesterone supplementation showed increased depressive symptoms as they moved from the estrogen-dominant ("follicular") phase to the progesterone-dominant ("luteal") phase, suggesting that changing levels rather than absolute levels of these hormones were associated with symptoms (Bloch et al. 2011). Furthermore, women who had a previous Axis I diagnosis of anxiety or major depressive disorder (MDD) had even greater shifts in mood symptoms (Zaig et al. 2013).

**Aromatase inhibitors.** Letrozole is an oral, highly potent, and selective aromatase inhibitor. Aromatase inhibition decreases the peripheral conversion of androgens to estrogen; consequently, this drug is used primarily in the treatment of hormone receptor–positive breast cancer (Goldvaser et al. 2017). Letrozole is also used in fertility treatment because its production of a low-estrogen state ultimately leads to an increase in FSH and LH (via negative feedback), leading to ovarian follicle stimulation. Although used mainly in women with PCOS (Legro 2016), it has been increasingly used in women with

**TABLE 5–2. Neuropsychiatric effects of assisted reproductive technology medications**

| Medication | Use | Mood effects |
|---|---|---|
| Oral contraceptives | Suppression of the HPG axis prior to controlled ovarian stimulation | Women with history of mood destabilization should be counseled to discuss oral contraceptive use |
| Clomiphene citrate | Ovarian stimulation and increased follicular development | Associated with mood lability ("super PMS"), insomnia, decreased libido, and transient psychosis |
| Gonadotropins | Control of ovarian stimulation | Associated with frequent mood lability and increased depressive symptoms |
| Aromatase inhibitor (letrozole) | Decrease of the peripheral conversion of androgens to estrogen | No data on psychiatric side effects in women using letrozole for fertility cycles; neuropsychiatric side effects (e.g., hot flashes, night sweats, arthralgias, depression, anxiety, memory/concentration problems) reported in patients using letrozole for cancer treatment |
| GnRH agonists and antagonists | Prevention of premature ovulation during in vitro fertilization cycles | Agonists: Anxiety and depression symptoms increase as estrogen levels rapidly increase; associated with increased daily mood lability in women with elevated baseline mood lability and neuroticism<br>Antagonists: no evidence of significant mood changes |
| Progesterone | Endometrial support of implantation and early embryo development | Micronized progesterone: no evidence of CNS effects<br>Synthetic progestins: associated with depression and anxiety symptoms |
| Metformin | Decrease of insulin for ovulation induction in women with PCOS | Associated with improved depressive symptoms |
| Bromocriptine and cabergoline | Dopamine agonist medications used in patients with hyperprolactinemia | Associated with hypomania and psychotic symptoms; patients with preexisting affective or psychotic illnesses at greatest risk<br>Associated with increased risk of impulse-control disorders; women with personal or family history of mania or psychosis should be counseled regarding risks |
| Corticosteroids (prednisone and prednisolone) | Enhancement of uterine receptivity | Well-established associations with insomnia, irritability, anxiety, new onset of mania and psychosis, and acute depressive symptoms with suicidality |

GnRH=gonadotropin-releasing hormone; HPG=hypothalamic-pituitary-gonadal; PCOS=polycystic ovary syndrome; PMS=premenstrual syndrome.

unexplained subfertility (Diamond et al. 2015). To date, no studies have been published of psychiatric side effects in women using letrozole for fertility cycles, but patients who are using it for cancer treatment have experienced neuropsychiatric side effects, such as hot flashes, night sweats, arthralgias, depression and anxiety symptoms, and memory/concentration problems (Beckwée et al. 2017; Rosenfeld et al. 2018).

**GnRH agonists and antagonists.** GnRH agonists and antagonists are used frequently in IVF cycles to prevent premature ovulation; these medications lead to a temporary hypogonadal state similar to menopause (Copperman and Benadiva 2013). Most studies of psychiatric side effects from GnRH agonists have included women who take the medications for fibroids and are thus exposed for prolonged periods. In these women, hot flashes, sleep disturbance, irritability, depressed mood, and difficulty with memory/concentration are common side effects (Warnock et al. 1998). Women receiving fertility treatment are likely to be exposed to these medications for a shorter period of time and thus may experience fewer side effects.

In a prospective study, patients did not have increased mood or anxiety symptoms during pretreatment with GnRH agonists. Instead, increased anxiety and depression symptoms emerged as estrogen levels were rapidly rising (Bloch et al. 2011). In a randomized trial of the mood effects of GnRH agonist and antagonist treatments in women undergoing IVF, neither treatment was associated with significant mood changes. However, pretreatment neuroticism was related to mental distress throughout treatment, independent of protocol (Stenbæk et al. 2015). GnRH agonist treatment has also been associated with increased daily mood lability in women with elevated baseline mood lability and neuroticism (Stenbæk et al. 2015, 2019).

**Progesterone.** Progesterone is used in ART for endometrial support of implantation and early embryo development. Although most ART cycles use micronized progesterone, which does not appear to have CNS effects, some cycles use synthetic progestins, such as medroxyprogesterone acetate, which have been associated with depression and anxiety symptoms in some women (Skovlund et al. 2016; Wang et al. 2016).

**Metformin.** Metformin is an oral insulin-sensitizing medication prescribed to women with PCOS to decrease insulin resistance for ovulation induction (Practice Committee of the American Society for Reproductive Medicine 2017). Interestingly, metformin may be associated with *improved* depression symptoms in women with PCOS. In a pilot study of 19 adolescents and 25 adults with PCOS, treatment with metformin for 90 days was associated not only with decreased insulin resistance but also with decreased depression and anxiety scores (Erensoy et al. 2019).

**Bromocriptine and cabergoline.** Bromocriptine and cabergoline are ergot-derived dopamine $D_2$ agonist medications that are used in patients with hyperprolactinemia (Usadi and Merriam 2015). Dopamine agonists have been associated with psychiatric side effects, including hypomania and psychotic symptoms; patients with preexisting affective or psychotic illnesses appear to be at greatest risk (Seeman 2015; Snellen et al. 2016). Dopamine agonists can also increase the risk of impulse-control disorders (Grall-Bronnec et al. 2016; Thondam et al. 2013). All infertile women with a personal or family history of mania or psychosis, if prescribed these medications, should be counseled regarding the relatively rare but serious risk for psychiatric side effects and monitored for early symptoms, such as insomnia, racing thoughts, or impaired impulse control.

**Corticosteroids.** Prednisone and prednisolone are oral corticosteroids prescribed in some ART cycles to enhance uterine receptivity, especially in women with a history of recurrent pregnancy losses or multiple failed IVF cycles. It is well established that these medications may have a range of mental health effects, including insomnia, irritability, anxiety, new onset of mania and psychosis, and acute depressive symptoms with suicidality (Kenna et al. 2011). Mood and psychotic disorders associated with corticosteroids are treated with mood stabilizers, including lithium, valproic acid, and atypical antipsychotics (Brown and Suppes 1998).

## Impact of Mental Health Conditions on Fertility

### Depression and Anxiety

It is difficult to determine the role of psychiatric illnesses as the primary risk factors for infertility because many of the biological processes thought to underlie increased risk for infertility, such as inflammation, are also found in mood and anxiety disorders. Most studies of fertility rates in women with mood disorders have not controlled for important confounding variables, such as subclinical hypothyroidism or obesity (Williams et al. 2007). When studies report higher rates of stress, anxiety, and mood disorders in patients undergoing infertility evaluation and treatment, it may not be specified whether the fertility problems themselves led to psychiatric symptoms and disorders or the psychiatric disorders affected fertility (Rooney and Domar 2018). Proposed mechanisms through which MDD could directly affect fertility involve physiological changes in the depressed state, such as thyroid dysfunction and disruptions in the HPG and hypothalamic-pituitary-adrenal (HPA) axes. For instance, results from one small study of 10 women with and 13 women without depression suggest that women with MDD may have changes in LH pulsatility, leading to subtle menstrual changes and subfertility (Grambsch et al. 2004). Changes in immune function associated with stress and depression may also adversely affect reproductive function (Haimovici and Hill 1998). Further studies are needed to distinguish the direct effects of MDD from symptoms and behaviors associated with these disorders, such as low libido, smoking, and alcohol use, which may also interfere with reproductive success.

### Eating Disorders

Studies have shown high rates of current or past histories of eating disorders in women in infertility clinic populations. Anorexia nervosa is typically associated with ovulatory dysfunction; amenorrhea is estimated to occur in 66%–84% of patients and oligomenorrhea in 6%–11% (Kimmel et al. 2016). Fertility problems may persist even after recovery because ovulatory dysfunction may persist. Women with a history of bulimia nervosa also report high rates of amenorrhea (7%–40%) and oligomenorrhea (36%–64%) (Kimmel et al. 2016), and they are more likely than women without psychiatric disorders to undergo fertility treatment (Micali et al. 2014). Both anorexia nervosa and bulimia nervosa are also associated with higher rates of miscarriage (Boutari et al. 2020). Binge-eating disorder can also be related to infertility because of its association with a high BMI (McCuen-Wurst et al. 2018), a risk factor for infertility (Silvestris et al.

2018). Women with PCOS are at particular risk of binge-eating disorder, with rates of 4%–15%, and have high rates of other types of disordered eating (Krug et al. 2019). Finally, eating disorders that do not meet the threshold for anorexia nervosa, bulimia nervosa, or binge-eating disorder have also been associated with infertility; one study demonstrated that 16%–20% of infertility patients met criteria for an eating disorder when eating disorder not otherwise specified was included (Freizinger et al. 2010).

Notably, women often do not disclose their current or past eating disorders to their fertility providers (Freizinger et al. 2010), and many fertility clinics do not routinely screen for eating disorders (Rodino et al. 2017). Historically, no consensus has been found among reproductive endocrinologists regarding deferring ovulation induction in patients with these disorders. Increasingly, however, specialists recommend screening and referral for treatment of eating disorders prior to initiating fertility medications and interventions (Paslakis and de Zwaan 2019). For a thorough discussion of the impact of eating disorders on reproductive mental health, see Chapter 22, "Eating Disorders."

## Substance Use Disorders

To date, few studies have examined the prevalence of substance use disorders in women undergoing infertility treatment. In one large, retrospective cohort study of 98,320 Danish women who had been evaluated for infertility, women who did not go on to give birth had twice the risk of alcohol and intoxicant abuse as women who had given birth (Baldur-Felskov et al. 2013). Heavy alcohol use (binge drinking ≥5 days in past month) is associated with decreased fecundity in women, because heavy drinking is associated with decreased ovarian reserve and a rise in estrogens, leading to decreased FSH secretion and impaired ovulation (Van Heertum and Rossi 2017). Cigarette smoking has a negative effect on follicular development, embryo transport, and endometrial receptivity (Dechanet et al. 2011). In some studies, frequent marijuana consumption is associated with ovulatory dysfunction, although several large observational studies have not found that marijuana use is associated with longer time to conceive (Dunne 2019; Kasman et al. 2018).

## Psychosocial Stress

The role of psychosocial stress as a risk factor for infertility in women remains controversial (Rooney and Domar 2018). Part of the complexity is due to the fact that, despite extensive study, psychosocial stress itself remains challenging to define. *Stress* is often defined as a process whereby a stimulus imposes demands on or overwhelms an organism's ability to cope, causing physiological and psychological responses (Koolhaas et al. 2011). However, the magnitude, duration, and quality of these responses are contingent on individual interpretation of the stressor and how well the person adapts to or copes with it (Cohen et al. 2007; King and Hegadoren 2002; Lazarus and Folkman 1984; Wosu et al. 2013).

Psychosocial stress can exert effects on many biological systems related to fertility. One example is its impact on follicular development and ovulation. During a physical or emotional stressor, the hypothalamus secretes corticotropin-releasing hormone and arginine vasopressin, which act on the pituitary gland to increase adrenocorticotropic hormone release, which in turn stimulates the production of cortisol from the adrenal cortical cells. Elevated corticotropin-releasing hormone and cortisol levels inhibit the HPG axis through decreasing hypothalamic GnRH secretion, leading to decreased LH. This deprives the ovarian follicles of adequate gonadotropin support, leading to reduced estradiol production and immature follicular development (Prasad et al. 2016).

Excessive stress may also affect fertilization, implantation, and maintenance of pregnancy, in particular through the effects of cytokines (Haimovici et al. 2018). Cytokines produced in the CNS and periphery in response to stress may influence gonadal function by changing hormone production and responsiveness within the HPA axis or directly through brain-gonadal input. CNS cytokines may also cause changes in peripheral leukocyte activation and function and may provoke cytokine cascades in the periphery that can modulate specific functions related to reproduction (Altun et al. 2011; Capuron and Miller 2011; Ozkan et al. 2014). Proinflammatory cytokines have been found to be elevated in both infertile men and women, and they may modulate uterine receptivity and embryo survival in women (Havrylyuk et al. 2015). Of note, elevated levels of cytokines have also been found in women with repeat implantation failures (Liang et al. 2015). However, cytokines are elevated in response to a variety of conditions, and it can be challenging to discern whether this response is related to stress or other factors that contribute to the presence of infertility.

Although it is accepted that stress can increase rates of depression and anxiety symptoms, which can have an impact on fertility rates, it is less clear whether stress alone has a similar impact (Domar et al. 1993; Rooney and Domar 2018). From a patient perspective, this question can set the stage for a cycle of perceived "victim blaming" and guilt, whereby a patient undergoing the stressful process of ART may blame her own stress if the ART is unsuccessful. Some studies report an impact of subjective distress on ART outcomes, whereas others do not (Rooney and Domar 2018). Reviews of the literature have reported that depressive symptoms, anxiety, distress, and certain coping strategies are linked to reduced chances of pregnancy during ART (Eugster and Vingerhoets 1999; Homan et al. 2007; Klonoff-Cohen 2005; Rooney and Domar 2018). However, data have been mixed. Some studies show that higher levels of distress during ART are correlated with lower pregnancy rates (Matthiesen et al. 2011; Purewal et al. 2018), but other studies report that stress levels have no effect on fertility treatment outcome (Boivin et al. 2011; Nicoloro-SantaBarbara et al. 2018). Two meta-analyses also reported conflicting results (Boivin et al. 2011; Matthiesen et al. 2011). Thus, the relationship among stress, psychiatric illness, and success of infertility treatments remains unclear. What is clear is that infertility can create substantial distress in those affected, and interventions aimed at addressing this distress can be beneficial in overall treatment outcomes (Rooney and Domar 2018). Future studies must control for important fertility variables such as age, ovarian reserve, sperm quality, lifestyle factors, and medication use (Williams et al. 2007).

## Lifestyle Factors

Excessive exercise can lead to a reduction in the frequency of ovulation, poor endometrial development (luteal phase deficiency), and amenorrhea. Recreational or moderate levels of activity also can induce abnormalities of gonadotropin secretion and ovulatory disorders, even without inducing amenorrhea (Harrison et al. 2016; Hart 2016). Other lifestyle factors, such as the frequency of coitus, may affect the chances of conception. Regular sexual intercourse two to three times per week, beginning soon after menses, is an important determinant for the occurrence of pregnancy (Wilcox et al. 1995). Various factors can affect the frequency of coitus, including frequent travel, erratic work schedules, age, and other social considerations. Gaskins et al. (2018) reported that male age, female rotating shift work schedule, and male exercise frequency had the strongest impact on sexual intercourse frequency. Weight status can have an impact as well: obesity is associated with sexual dysfunction and decreased rates of sexual intercourse in both men and women (Oliveira et al. 2019; Wekker et al. 2018; Xu et al. 2019). The presence of depression or anxiety symptoms in an individual also affects the frequency of intercourse and is known to affect libido (Gaskins et al. 2018).

## Impact of Treatment for Mental Health Disorders on Fertility

Psychopharmacological treatment for MDD can increase the risk for infertility, primarily through effects on hormonal processes, such as prolactin levels, thyroid function, and insulin resistance. For example, several categories of psychiatric medications, such as antipsychotics and selective serotonin reuptake inhibitors (SSRIs), are associated with increased prolactin levels (Ajmal et al. 2014). Prolactin has an important role in fertility. It directly decreases the sensitivity of the LH and FSH receptors in the gonads and indirectly reduces GnRH secretion, which suppresses LH and FSH secretion and thereby inhibits ovulation. Women with elevated prolactin levels generally present with oligomenorrhea or amenorrhea, anovulatory cycles, galactorrhea, and infertility (Patel and Bamigboye 2007). The risk of elevated prolactin levels has been reported to be highest with first-generation antipsychotics and the second-generation antipsychotic risperidone (Smith 2003). Elevated prolactin levels with SSRIs are rare but can occur (Ajmal et al. 2014).

Many psychiatric medications, such as antidepressants and antipsychotics, are associated with weight gain and insulin resistance, both of which are associated with infertility (Arterburn et al. 2016; Barton et al. 2020; Blumenthal et al. 2014). These medications also may be associated with decreased libido and sexual dysfunction, which may affect sexual frequency and thus the frequency of conception events (Elnazer et al. 2015; Montejo et al. 2015). Individual medications need to be considered as potentially having an impact on fertility. For example, lithium is associated with hypothyroidism, which is a clear risk factor for infertility (Dosiou 2020; Gitlin 2016). Thus, all patients taking lithium should have thyroid levels carefully assessed when they attempt to conceive.

## Impact of Infertility on Mental Health

Ms. G is a 36-year-old overweight woman who reports a long history of "irregular menstrual cycles" and who has recently begun undergoing evaluation for infertility. She and her partner decided to discontinue birth control more than 3 years ago, and they have been actively trying to get pregnant for 2 years, using timed intercourse and ovulation prediction methods, including basal body temperature and ovulation predictor kits. Ms. G describes feeling increasingly discouraged about her fertility, a loss of energy, and a desire to escape all the physician visits and diagnostic testing that she knows lie ahead. Her partner complains that they have become increasingly isolated because Ms. G has lost interest in socializing and does not want to go with him to events with friends. She complains that the future looks very "bleak," but she does not have suicidal ideation. She has been sleeping more than 10 hours a day and overeating, causing her to be even more overweight. Her partner is alarmed at how self-critical she has become.

Initial workup for Ms. G should include a thorough psychiatric evaluation to determine whether she meets criteria for MDD, as well as a thorough medical workup to determine whether her irregular periods and obesity are related to PCOS.

## Psychiatric Conditions

The incidence rates of MDD in women undergoing infertility evaluation and treatment range from 20% to 40%, which are higher than rates in women of reproductive age in the general population (Williams et al. 2007). Previous history of MDD predicts its development during ART; therefore, all patients should be screened for past history and current depressive symptoms (Holley et al. 2015). Higher rates of MDD are associated with lower levels of social support in women experiencing infertility (Lund et al. 2009). When women attending infertility clinics are screened for depression, high scores have been associated with both a decreased likelihood of initiating fertility treatment and an increased likelihood of stopping treatment (Crawford et al. 2017; Domar et al. 2018).

Anxiety disorders are also more common in women undergoing infertility evaluation and treatment than in women in the general population. Studies have suggested the prevalence of any anxiety disorder as ranging from 15% to 30% in women undergoing ART (Chen et al. 2004; Omani-Samani et al. 2018; Volgsten et al. 2008). Some anxiety disorders, such as needle or injection phobias, may interfere with the patient's ability to complete infertility treatment.

Although many studies demonstrate high rates of depressive and anxiety symptoms in women experiencing infertility, few studies have examined rates of completed suicide in this population. In a large study of more than 50,000 Danish women with no prior history of psychiatric hospitalizations, women with primary infertility who remained childless had more than twice the rate of suicide compared with women who had at least one child after fertility evaluation (Kjaer et al. 2011). In a small study of 106 women undergoing infertility treatment, 9.4% were identified as being at risk for suicide based on the Suicidal Behaviors Questionnaire–Revised (Osman et al. 2001), and women at risk were found to have higher levels of depression symptoms, self-blame, social withdrawal, and the use of denial as a coping strategy (Shani et al. 2016).

## Psychological Reactions

The experience of infertility is associated with significant personal distress (Rooney and Domar 2018). Childlessness is often perceived as a life crisis, and the emotional strain is equal to that of traumatic events (Cousineau and Domar 2007; Greil 1997; Mahlstedt 1985; Oddens et al. 1999; Schmidt et al. 2005). Grieving infertility often involves shock, disbelief, anger, blame, shame, and guilt (Mahlstedt 1985; Rooney and Domar 2018). Loss of control is a central theme in women and their partners who are experiencing infertility (Greil et al. 2011). The affected woman's sense of identity may be challenged, and infertility can lead to feelings of worthlessness and guilt (Greil et al. 2016). Achieving a pregnancy can become a singular focus, and professional goals and social connections are often placed on hold or dismissed altogether (Cousineau and Domar 2007; Thorn 2009).

Couples struggling with infertility often experience a wide range of emotional reactions, including guilt and a sense of isolation, due to perceived or real social unacceptability (El Kissi et al. 2013; Péloquin et al. 2018). Given the invasive nature of the process of infertility workup and treatments, sexual dysfunction can be common (Tao et al. 2011). Marital discord may also occur (Tabong and Adongo 2013). Nevertheless, some studies indicate that couples who remain childless are as satisfied with their lives as those who have conceived, and many couples report that their relationship has strengthened as a result of having managed the crisis together (Amiri et al. 2016; Masoumi et al. 2016; Schmidt et al. 2005).

Notably, several facets of ART itself can be associated with distress (Boivin et al. 2011). The process of decision making can be complicated and contribute to distress for couples. The diagnosis of "unexplained infertility" can be especially challenging because it may cause feelings of both hope and distress (Greil et al. 2011). The lack of a clear cause can set couples on what feels like an endless pursuit of additional examinations and procedures. The option of third-party assisted reproduction (gamete donation or surrogacy) may confront the couple with further complex decisions. ART is time consuming and logistically complicated, and the expense of infertility treatments can also contribute to stress and may strain the financial resources of the couple or individual (Cousineau and Domar 2007). Finally, there is a dearth of information on long-term effects of ART, either physical or emotional.

## Treatment of Psychiatric Conditions in the Context of Infertility

### Psychopharmacology

Women struggling with infertility may be reluctant to take medications for depression and anxiety for fear that the medication might present risks to fertility or pregnancy (Walton et al. 2014). Women already taking antidepressants at the time of ART should be cautioned that even with continued medication, they are at risk for relapse of depression symptoms (Freeman et al. 2018). In the only existing systematic review of the effects of SSRIs on pregnancy and live birth rates in women undergoing ART, no SSRI effect was found on any parameters studied in IVF success, including mean number of oocytes retrieved, number of embryos transferred, implantation rates, live births, and spontaneous abortions (Akioyamen et al. 2016). A nationwide cohort study in Sweden evaluated the odds of success of three IVF cycle outcomes (i.e., pregnancy, live birth, and miscarriage) (Cesta et al. 2016). The study found slightly reduced odds of pregnancy and live birth for women taking non-SSRI antidepressants compared with healthy women, but no difference between women taking SSRIs and healthy women. However, women with untreated anxiety or depression also exhibited reduced odds of pregnancy and live birth, indicating perhaps that the effect found for non-SSRI antidepressants may be a marker for the underlying illness.

### Psychotherapy

Psychotherapy remains the first-line treatment for infertile women with mild to moderate depressive symptoms and anxiety. Individual studies have demonstrated significant decreases in both anxiety and depression symptom scores for infertility patients as a result of psychotherapy treatment. Mindfulness-based group cognitive-behavioral therapy (CBT) programs that have been adapted to focus on important concerns for infertility patients appear especially promising (Domar et al. 1992; Kalhori et al. 2020). Interpersonal therapy (IPT) and brief supportive therapy have also shown effectiveness in the treatment of MDD among infertile women (Koszycki et al. 2012). Data are mixed, however, as to the efficacy of psychotherapy in this population (Boivin 2003; Frederiksen et al. 2015; Hämmerli et al. 2009; Rooney and Domar 2018; Verkuijlen et al. 2016; Ying et al. 2016). In one meta-analysis including only randomized controlled trials of psychological interventions, in 4 of 14 studies (28.6%) psychotherapy was found to have a moderate effect size for anxiety, whereas 0 of 9 studies showed that the interventions had effects on depression in IVF patients (Ying et al. 2016).

Mindfulness-based CBT programs have been adapted to focus on the important themes and concerns for infertility patients (Rooney and Domar 2018). Additionally, relaxation techniques have been shown to reduce anxiety scores in women undergoing infertility treatment (Domar et al. 2000; Gaitzsch et al. 2020; Rooney and Domar 2018). In a randomized controlled trial of 89 women with MDD who were struggling with infertility, group CBT was compared with fluoxetine and with no treatment (Faramarzi et al. 2008). CBT was superior to fluoxetine at reducing infertility stress scores (social, sexual, and marital concerns), and both interventions were superior to the control (Faramarzi et al. 2013). Mindfulness-based interventions are associated with an increase in self-compassion, meaning-based coping strategies, and higher pregnancy rates (Li et al. 2016). IPT and brief supportive therapy are also effective in the treatment of MDD among infertile women (Koszycki et al. 2012).

## Special Considerations

Ms. H and Ms. I have been married for 3 years and in a romantic relationship for more than 5 years. Ms. H, who is 32, has an 8-year-old son from a previous heterosexual relationship in which she conceived with her male partner without fertility interventions and carried to term without complications. Ms. I, who is 42 years old, has never been pregnant and is eager to experience having a baby. Ms. H has struggled with bipolar disorder since her teens, but she has been stable since she started taking lithium 3 years ago. The couple meets with a reproductive psychiatrist for preconception counseling. Ms. H reports that she is not eager to become pregnant again because she does not want to risk destabilizing her mood and wants her wife to have the opportunity to carry a child. Ms. I, who does not have a psychiatric illness, agrees that mood stabilization for Ms. H is of paramount importance, but she is concerned about the potentially low quality of her own eggs due to her age. The two decide that Ms. H will undergo ovarian stimulation and have her oocytes fertilized with donor sperm; they will then transfer embryos to Ms. I.

### Third-Party Assisted Reproduction With Gamete Donation (Ovum and Sperm Donation)

ART with donor sperm is common. Between 2015 and 2017, an estimated 440,986 women used donor sperm for either IUI or IVF procedures (Arocho et al. 2019). Common reasons for conception through sperm donation include male factor infertility, single motherhood, and family building for lesbian couples. Although some of these individuals suffer the stresses and psychological consequences associated with infertility, others approach ART without infertility and may have different experiences.

Ovum donation is much less common, because it requires time-intensive ovarian stimulation protocols; it is estimated that 10% of IVF cycles in the United States use ovum donation (American Society for Reproductive Medicine 2018). Common reasons for egg donation include advanced maternal age, premature menopause, infertility due to previous treatments with toxic medications such as chemotherapy, or creation of an embryo in same-sex couples. Cumulative live birth rates in ART cycles with ovum donation decrease with increasing age of the donor: 33.6% when donors are between ages 33 and 35 years, 22.5% when they are between ages 38 and 40 years, and only 5.1% when they are older than 41 years (Hogan et al. 2019). Pregnancies from ovum donation are associated with an increased risk of obstetrical complications, regardless of the recipient's age (Storgaard et al. 2017).

The American Society for Reproductive Medicine (ASRM) and the Society for Assisted Reproductive Technology recommend that all couples who choose to pursue pregnancy through gamete donation meet with an experienced mental health professional to discuss the psychological issues associated with donation (Practice Committee of the American Society for Reproductive Medicine and the Society for Assisted Reproductive Technology 2013). During this meeting, the mental health professional evaluates whether the couple is in agreement regarding several key issues, such as the choice of an anonymous versus an identified donor. Psychological and financial coercion must be ruled out, including coercion within the couple's relationship and within the relationship between the couple and the donor. The mental health professional should counsel the donor and the couple about the importance of mutually agreed upon boundaries, and all should agree regarding issues of disclosure with family members and friends.

The ASRM publishes guidelines regarding disclosure with gamete donor–conceived children and acknowledges that although the ultimate decision to tell children of their origins is up to the couple, disclosure is recommended (Ethics Committee of the American Society for Reproductive Medicine 2018). No specific optimal age of disclosure has been identified, but studies suggest that telling the children prior to adolescence is preferred (Ethics Committee of the American Society for Reproductive Medicine 2018). Couples who choose to tell their children should be counseled that several preschool and early childhood books are available that describe the ways in which families are created and may help in explaining their family building to children. Follow-up studies of heterosexual couples who chose gamete donation showed no significant differences in maternal–child relationships between donor-conceived and natural-conception families who disclosed origins to the child (Bracewell-Milnes et al. 2016; Imrie and Golombok 2018). Children conceived through gamete donation, from both heterosexual and same-sex couple families, do not appear to have increased rates of psychiatric disorders compared with children not conceived via gamete donation (Imrie and Golombok 2018).

The ASRM also publishes guidelines for the evaluation of ovum donors. Relative contraindications to participating in an ovum donor program include active psychiatric illness or substance abuse, high-risk sexual practices, and a history of sexual or physical abuse without a history of professional counseling (Practice Committee of the American Society for Reproductive Medicine and the Society for Assisted Reproductive Technology 2013). Evaluation of ovum donors should include assessment of the donor's ability to understand the potential medical risks associated with the ovarian stimulation procedure, as well as the potential psychological reactions. Most follow-up studies report that ovum donors have favorable experiences, with few short- or long-term medical or psychological sequelae, and that they would choose to do it again, recommend the process to a friend, or both (Bracewell-Milnes et al. 2016).

## Ovum Cryopreservation

Cryopreservation of oocytes, also known as "egg freezing," has become an increasingly viable option for fertility preservation (Milman et al. 2017; Practice Committee of the American Society for Reproductive Medicine and the Society for Assisted Reproductive Technology 2013). In this procedure, patients undergo ovarian stimulation procedures followed by egg retrieval and vitrification.

Cryopreservation of oocytes can offer some advantages to several populations. First, women may choose to undergo elective egg freezing to preserve oocytes from a chronologically younger age for use in a future pregnancy. Second, premenopausal women who are diagnosed with cancer and planning to undergo treatments should be counseled regarding fertility preservation options and offered psychological counseling in order to decide about these options (Lawson et al. 2015; Loren et al. 2013). Third, transgender men may choose to cryopreserve mature ooctyes prior to gender affirmation surgery, whereas transgender women may choose to freeze their sperm (Armuand et al. 2020; Ethics Committee of the American Society for Reproductive Medicine 2015; Hembree et al. 2009). Evidence indicates that ovarian stimulation and oocyte retrieval have excellent rates of success in transgender men, even if undertaken after testosterone therapy has been initiated, and this path to fertility preservation is increasingly undertaken in adolescence prior to gender affirmation surgery (Adeleye et al. 2019; Amir et al. 2020).

## Surrogacy

Surrogacy is used when there is a need for a person with a healthy uterus to act as a gestational carrier of a pregnancy—for example, a woman unable to carry a child in her own uterus, a male same-sex couple, or some transgender individuals. *Gestational surrogacy* refers to implantation of an embryo created from the fertility patient's or donor's eggs into the gestational carrier, whereas "traditional" surrogacy uses the carrier's own eggs. Gestational surrogacy ART cycles are uncommon, but increasing, in the United States, comprising 2.5% of all ART cycles in 2013 (Perkins et al. 2016).

ART with surrogacy requires careful legal, medical, and psychosocial planning. The ASRM has extensive guidelines for mental health counseling for both intended parents and potential gestational carriers. Unlike gamete donation, in which the third party may be either anonymous or identified, surrogacy requires some form of relationship between the parties. The ASRM recommends that couples participating in a gestational surrogacy program recognize the importance of the intended parents' ability to manage the interpersonal complexity of the surrogate relationship. Contraindications include not only current untreated psychiatric illnesses and substance abuse but also inability to maintain a "respectful and caring relationship with the surrogate" or to comply with the gestational carrier's desire about number of embryos to transfer (Practice Committee of the American Society for Reproductive Medicine and Practice Committee of the Society for Assisted Reproductive Technology 2017). Studies of children born from gestational surrogacy report no increased rates of medical or psychological disturbances compared with children born naturally or from other forms of ART (Söderström-Anttila et al. 2016). See Chapter 24, "Forensic Issues in Perinatal Psychiatry," for the legal issues involved in surrogacy.

## Infertility Summary

Infertility is a common problem in women, and mental health professionals serve in a wide variety of roles in the evaluation and treatment of psychiatric conditions in this population. They perform individual psychotherapy in the private practice setting and take on consultation-liaison and embedded mental health roles within fertility clinics. Mental health professionals need to be aware of the unique relationships between common causes of infertility in women and comorbid psychiatric conditions. Unique aspects of these conditions need to be integrated into psychological and psychiatric treatment approaches. Mental health professionals also need to be aware of the potential for fertility medications to destabilize mood in women. Future research should focus on the identification of patients at greatest risk for this mood destabilization, as well as the adaptation and development of evidence-based psychotherapy and psychopharmacology treatments for mood and anxiety disorders in this population. Psychopharmacology research should continue the investigation of effects of psychiatric medications on the menstrual cycle; fertility treatments, including egg and sperm quality; implantation physiology; and pregnancy outcomes.

# Perinatal Loss

Perinatal loss is a common and distressing experience for many women, and it can be associated with significant psychological and psychiatric sequelae. The goals of this section are to review the epidemiology, clinical features, mental health impacts, and treatment of perinatal loss.

Ms. J is a 38-year-old Black nurse who has experienced recurrent pregnancy loss. Initially, she was able to conceive without fertility treatments; however, at ages 32 and 34 years she experienced spontaneous abortions at 10 and 12 weeks of pregnancy, respectively. She says that she decided to "take a break" from trying to have a child after the second miscarriage because, although she had "coped well" after the first miscarriage, after the second she experienced her "first depression." She had loss of interest in activities, experienced problems with memory and concentration, and found her work extremely challenging for several months because of a "foggy head." Although she did not have suicidal ideation, she did feel hopelessness and helplessness. Ms. J did not seek treatment for her MDD, and she says that the symptoms slowly resolved over 2 years.

When she turned 38, Ms. J and her husband pursued IVF, and she became pregnant after the first cycle. She was anxious throughout the first trimester, but when she reached week 14 of her pregnancy, she began "to have a little hope" that this pregnancy would go smoothly. However, at week 22, she experienced the sudden onset of intense back pain followed by the passing of bright red blood. She was rushed to the hospital, where an ultrasound revealed placental abruption and intrauterine fetal demise, and she subsequently underwent an emergency cesarean section. In the months that followed, Ms. J experienced a return of her symptoms of depression. She says she "could have handled that because I had it before," but this time the loss of energy and interest were accompanied by intense irritability. She had difficulty sleeping, with nightmares about the blood loss. During the day she experienced repeated flashbacks of the day of the placental abruption. Always known for her calm demeanor in the past, she reported having severe anxiety, with racing heart, shortness of breath, and sweating.

Ms. J took a month to recover physically from her surgery, but her psychiatric symptoms persisted. She constantly blamed herself for her baby's death and felt no pleasure

**TABLE 5–3. Perinatal loss definitions**

| |
|---|
| Spontaneous abortion: <20 weeks' gestation |
| Stillbirth: >20 weeks' gestation |
| Fetal demise: 7–28 days after birth |
| Infant mortality: occurring from 1 to 11 months of life |
| Voluntary termination of pregnancy: termination for fetal anomalies, multiple fetal reduction, risk to mother's health, psychosocial factors |

in her usual activities. She thought that returning to work would help, but at 6 weeks she still could not bring herself to go into the hospital—the same place where she had lost her baby. She took a medical leave of absence, her first leave of her career.

## Definitions

*Perinatal loss* is defined as the nonvoluntary end of pregnancy or death of an infant from the time of conception until postpartum day 28 (Table 5–3) (Bhat and Byatt 2016). In the United States, *spontaneous abortion,* also termed *miscarriage,* is defined as pregnancy loss prior to 20 weeks' gestation. *Intrauterine fetal demise* (IUFD), or *stillbirth,* is defined as loss after 20 weeks' gestation or after the fetus reaches 14 oz in weight. *Early neonatal death* is defined as death of an infant prior to 7 days of life, and *late neonatal death* is defined as death between 7 and 28 days of life (Barfield 2011). Termination of pregnancy for fetal abnormalities or genetic indications is included in the definition of perinatal loss, whereas termination for elective reasons is not. *Recurrent perinatal loss* (RPL) is defined by the ASRM as two or more losses, and it can be further subdivided into *primary RPL,* defined as pregnancy loss in women who have never had a viable pregnancy, and *secondary RPL* in women who have had a previous live birth (Barfield 2011; Bhat and Byatt 2016).

## Epidemiology

### Rates/Incidence

Approximately 12%–20% of pregnancies end in loss prior to 20 weeks' gestation (Hemels et al. 2005; Hemminki and Forssas 1999; Robinson 2014; Wilcox et al. 1988). Maternal age is a determinant for overall incidence of different types of perinatal loss. For instance, 27% of women ages 25–29 experience spontaneous abortion, compared with 75% of women ages 45 and older (Robinson 2014). Many early first-trimester losses are never recognized as a pregnancy, and thus spontaneous abortion may occur in up to one-third of all pregnancies (Wilcox et al. 1988). Approximately 50%–80% of all women who experience perinatal loss will have a subsequent pregnancy. Recurrent perinatal loss occurs in 2%–3% of pregnancies (Bhat and Byatt 2016; Kolte et al. 2014). In contrast, IUFD after 20 weeks' gestation is rare, affecting an estimated 4.6 per 1,000 births, whereas neonatal death occurs in approximately 6.2 per 1,000 births (Bhat and Byatt 2016). The risk of IUFD is highest in teenagers (0.07%–0.13%) and in women older than 40 years (0.11%–0.21%) (American College of Obstetricians and Gynecologists and Society for Maternal-Fetal Medicine 2020).

TABLE 5–4. **Risk factors for perinatal loss**

| | |
|---|---|
| Risk factors for spontaneous abortion | Age: >40 years<br>Previous history of miscarriage<br>Medical conditions (e.g., hypothyroidism)<br>Parental cytogenic abnormalities<br>Infertility treatment |
| Risk factors for intrauterine fetal demise | Age: <20 years or >35 years<br>Black race<br>Obesity<br>Medical conditions (e.g., hypertension, diabetes, thrombophilias)<br>Infertility treatment<br>>40 weeks' gestation<br>Cigarette smoking<br>Poverty |

### Risk Factors

The main risk factors for perinatal loss are listed in Table 5–4 (Maconochie et al. 2007). Although research on racial disparities in spontaneous abortion is surprisingly scarce, some studies indicate higher rates of loss among Black women compared with white women (Price 2006). Because lower socioeconomic status, lower education, and income below poverty level are also risk factors for recurrent loss, this racial difference may be due in part to socioeconomic differences. Non-Hispanic Black women have the highest risks for IUFD and early infant death as compared with other populations (MacDorman and Gregory 2015; Muglu et al. 2019; Mukherjee et al. 2013). Some of this difference is likely attributable to the higher rates of preterm birth and pregnancy morbidities in the Black population, while some of it may also represent disparity in access to quality health care (Martin et al. 2019).

## Clinical Features

### Clinical Presentation

Miscarriage typically presents as acute vaginal bleeding and pain. The loss is confirmed by ultrasound (Robinson 2014). Later in pregnancy, pregnancy loss may present with decreased or absent fetal movement and may be identified by ultrasound at a routine prenatal visit, or it may occur despite management of conditions that are known to be related to late pregnancy loss, such as incompetent cervix or maternal infection (Michels and Tiu 2007).

### Pathophysiology

The most common etiologies of perinatal loss include chromosomal abnormalities, fetal anomalies, death of a fetus during labor and delivery, preterm labor, hypertensive disorders in the mother, umbilical cord abnormalities, infection, and other medical conditions (Murphy et al. 2017). However, no clear cause is identified in up to 50% of cases (Wilcox et al. 1988).

## Medical Management of Perinatal Loss

The management of perinatal loss varies based on timing. Management of early pregnancy loss is based on a variety of factors, including the length of gestation, and medical or surgical intervention may be indicated based on the clinical presentation (Jurkovic et al. 1998; Nielsen and Hahlin 1995). Medical management—with mifepristone (an antiglucocorticoid medication administered intravaginally or orally), misoprostol (a synthetic prostaglandin analogue), or both—is used to shorten the time for expulsion of pregnancy tissue in women without current infections or bleeding disorders (American College of Obstetricians and Gynecologists 2018; Henshaw et al. 1993). Surgical evacuation of uterine contents is needed in the case of an incomplete miscarriage (Jurkovic et al. 1998), as well as molar pregnancy (Elias et al. 2019).

## Impact of Mental Health on Perinatal Loss

Although studies have not conclusively demonstrated that MDD, anxiety, or other mental illnesses are risk factors for spontaneous abortion or perinatal loss, a bidirectional relationship may exist between psychiatric disorders and perinatal loss. Women with a history of depressive or anxiety disorders may have an increased risk of perinatal loss, and perinatal loss clearly increases the risk for mood and anxiety disorders (Farren et al. 2018; Gold et al. 2007; Klock et al. 1997). The mechanism of action between mental illness and pregnancy loss is unclear. One hypothesis involves the impact of mental illness, specifically MDD, on the functioning of the HPA axis and the sympathetic nervous system. The release of maternal glucocorticoids with stress response can promote placental prostaglandins, increase the effect of oxytocin on the uterus, and upregulate proinflammatory cytokines, which may be associated with the pathophysiology of pregnancy loss (Li et al. 2012).

Although some meta-analyses and systematic reviews report an increase in spontaneous abortions in women taking SSRI antidepressants in pregnancy (Hemels et al. 2005), others have not shown a significant association (Ross et al. 2013). Studies have generally not adequately controlled for important confounding variables, such as maternal age, BMI, thyroid disorders, or previous history of spontaneous abortion, nor have most been able to separate the role of MDD or depression severity in early pregnancy loss (Hemels et al. 2005). In a large population-based cohort study, SSRIs were not associated with an increased risk of stillbirth, neonatal death, or postnatal infant death (Stephansson et al. 2013).

## Impact of Perinatal Loss on Mental Health

Many women and their partners experience the period immediately following a perinatal loss as an emotionally difficult time that includes a range of depressive, anxiety, and stress-related symptoms. Researchers have different perspectives regarding the assessment of severity and course of these symptoms, with some viewing the symptoms as normal emotional reactions and others characterizing symptoms within a framework of psychiatric illness once symptoms pass a certain threshold or disrupt functioning (Gold et al. 2016). The risk of psychiatric illness is elevated in the first year following loss, particularly after IUFD (Lewkowitz et al. 2019).

## Grief

**Epidemiology.** Grief reactions are common after perinatal loss (Cassaday 2018). The incidence is difficult to assess because studies use different psychological measures and definitions of grief and investigate different types and timing of perinatal loss and different time periods since the loss. When grief is prolonged and so intense that it is disabling, it has historically been termed "complicated grief." It is estimated that complicated grief occurs in up to 30% of patients after perinatal loss (Kersting and Wagner 2012).

**Risk factors.** Risk factors for the development of complicated grief after perinatal loss include a history of a prior mental illness, poor social support, ambivalent attitude toward the pregnancy, and a preloss neurotic personality, and it is more likely to happen in women experiencing sudden or traumatic loss (Badenhorst and Hughes 2007; Kersting and Wagner 2012; Lasker and Toedter 1991). In contrast, studies have not shown a correlation between the severity of grief and greater maternal age, sex of the baby, socioeconomic status, or religious observance (Badenhorst and Hughes 2007). Some studies have shown the presence of other children to be a protective factor (deMontigny et al. 2017; Janssen et al.1997; Kersting and Wagner 2012). The quality of the relationship between partners and the concordance between their grieving processes can be protective factors (Badenhorst and Hughes 2007; Kersting and Wagner 2012; Scheidt et al. 2012). Lack of perceived social support, including dissatisfaction with the health care system during the pregnancy and after the loss, has also been associated with more intense grief and longer duration of grief (deMontigny et al. 2017; Kersting and Wagner 2012).

**Screening.** The most common screening instrument for grief is the Perinatal Grief Scale (Toedter et al. 1988). This 33-item scale has high convergent validity and reliability, has been translated into multiple languages, and is used worldwide.

**Diagnostic criteria.** Although there are no formal diagnostic criteria for perinatal grief, there are recognized descriptions and definitions of the normative experience of grief in general (Shear 2012). Similar to grief at other times in life, perinatal grief is a psychobiological reaction to a loss (Brier 2008; Shear 2012). It is the loss of a developing infant and the expectation, hope, and vision of that child and thus is considered a prospective loss (Leon 2018). Perinatal grief is considered an expected and normative process associated with time-limited sadness and yearning for and preoccupation with thoughts of the lost baby (Rowland and Goodnight 2009). When grief is unusually intense, more disruptive, or lasts longer than the timeline anticipated, it can evolve into complicated grief. Complicated grief is described in DSM-5 as persistent complex bereavement disorder, which is included in the section "Conditions for Further Study" (American Psychiatric Association 2013).

**Clinical features.** Grief reactions can include disruption in daily functioning, feelings of yearning, numbness, isolation, retreat from usual activities, and intrusive thoughts (Kersting and Wagner 2012). In perinatal grief, parents can have feelings of guilt, shame, inadequacy, failure, sadness, irritability, and anger (Kersting and Wagner 2012).

**Course and differential diagnosis.** Grief following a perinatal loss can last from 1 month to 2 years (Badenhorst and Hughes 2007) but typically declines by 6 months following the loss (Bhat and Byatt 2016). For many parents, however, grief can last for years in a more subdued form, often referred to as "shadow grief," intensifying around anniversaries such as the due date, birth date, or death date (Leon 2018; Peppers and Knapp 1980).

The primary differential diagnoses for grief and complicated grief/complex bereavement disorder are MDD and acute stress disorder. Although grieving patients may have complaints of sleep disturbance and other vegetative symptoms seen in depressive disorders, they should not experience anhedonia. Their loss of interest should be focused on the loss of the child, and they should experience positive emotions as well as negative ones (Shear 2012). Their preoccupation with thinking about their loss should not lead to inability to care for themselves or others or be associated with suicidal ideation (Kavan and Barone 2014). The existence of any of these factors may indicate the presence of a depressive disorder rather than (or in addition to) grief.

**Pathophysiology.** To date, no studies have been published investigating the neurobiology of perinatal grief. From the few extant studies regarding grief in patients responding to other forms of attachment loss, such as loss of a marriage partner, it appears that when compared with patients who are adapting well, patients with complicated grief demonstrate greater activity in the nucleus accumbens (O'Connor et al. 2008). This increased activity is associated with greater self-reported yearning as well, suggesting that the experience of grief-related yearning is associated with a specific area of the basal ganglia (O'Connor et al. 2008). Grief associated with other forms of loss is also associated with immunological changes, including changes to proinflammatory interleukin-6, which may play a role in the mood changes seen in complicated grief because proinflammatory cytokines have been found to be elevated in MDD (Cohen et al. 2015; Knowles et al. 2019).

Throughout pregnancy, parents often develop future ideas about their child and the child's characteristics and about themselves as parents. These mental representations are influenced by many factors, including personality structure, past experiences of parenting, past trauma, and cultural differences (Stern 1995). These mental representations are further elaborated through medical technology, which has made it possible for parents to visualize the fetus at various points during pregnancy. These experiences contribute to increasing emotional attachment to the fetus, starting early in the prenatal period. Research has shown that prenatal parental representations and attachment to the infant are associated with postpartum parent–infant attachment (Dubber et al. 2015; Petri et al. 2018). Perinatal loss is a major disruption in these mental representations, leaving parents with immense grief for the relationship they had dreamed about but did not get to experience (Leon 2018).

A primary factor that affects the course and trajectory of grief is how the person makes meaning out of the loss. The process starts with a set of preexisting beliefs about oneself, the world, and the future; the death of the child shatters or alters these beliefs in significant ways (Keesee et al. 2008). When a discrepancy exists between the meaning of loss and one's beliefs, one starts a process of adaptation to make sense of the experience; if one is unable to assimilate the loss successfully, one may experience more intense grief (Keesee et al. 2008). Schema, or core beliefs about the world, comprise three major components: benevolence, meaningfulness of the world, and worthiness of the self (Krosch and Shakespeare-Finch 2017). Perinatal loss can alter or shake any of these components. Parents grieving a perinatal loss have reported themes of unfairness, guilt, and loss of control

(Krosch and Shakespeare-Finch 2017). For many women, perinatal loss can undermine feelings about themselves and their bodies. In a woman with long-standing feelings of self-doubt, shame, and low self-worth, perinatal loss can be seen as a confirmation of those feelings. Some women may conclude that they have not been able to do one of the main jobs of a parent: protect their child. Cultural and societal factors can deeply affect the bereavement and meaning-making processes. Grief is also affected by the person's attachment style, religious beliefs, the presence of other living children, the quality of one's relationship with one's partner, and other support structures (Scheidt et al. 2012).

## Depressive Disorders

**Epidemiology.** Following a perinatal loss, 10%–54% of women report depressive symptoms severe enough to meet criteria for MDD within 6 months of the loss (deMontigny et al. 2017; Farren et al. 2018). Up to 20% of women have symptoms that are of moderate or greater severity at 6 weeks postloss (Farren et al. 2018).

**Risk factors.** Women with recurrent miscarriage have an especially elevated risk for MDD, with prevalence rates of 30% (Lok and Neugebauer 2007). Women with a previous history of MDD are at especially increased risk for recurrence after a perinatal loss, with prevalence rates of 54% (Neugebauer et al. 1997). Other risk factors for MDD following a perinatal loss include younger age, history of infertility and infertility treatments, history of trauma and abuse, history of PTSD, being single, marital discord, feeling of lack of control over one's life, or feeling responsible for the loss (Table 5–5) (Bhat and Byatt 2016; Farren et al. 2018). The highest risk of MDD following pregnancy loss is for IUFD or pregnancy loss after 20 weeks' gestation (Bhat and Byatt 2016; Hogue et al. 2015).

**Screening.** Screening for MDD in patients with perinatal loss should be completed with validated scales used to screen for depression at other times in a woman's life. The Patient Health Questionnaire–9 (Kroenke et al. 2001), Center for Epidemiologic Studies–Depression Scale (Radloff 1977), Beck Depression Inventory (Beck et al. 1996), and Edinburgh Postnatal Depression Scale (Cox et al. 1987) are all validated screening tools that can be used to screen for MDD in the setting of perinatal loss. Diagnostic criteria are the same as those for MDD at other times. (See Chapter 13, "Depressive Disorders," for further details.)

**Clinical features.** MDD after a perinatal loss includes all the same clinical features of MDD at other times of a woman's life (see Chapter 13). Her ruminations often include themes and concerns related to pregnancy, such as unreasonable guilt regarding engagement or lack of engagement in activities that preceded the miscarriage or self-critical thoughts focused on her own body (Cassaday 2018).

**Course and differential diagnosis.** Studies show both high prevalence and high severity of depressive symptoms in the first 2–6 weeks following perinatal loss, but for many women the severity of these symptoms decreases with the passage of time, with a return to baseline 1 year following loss (Farren et al. 2018). In a large population study, Gold et al. (2016) reported that bereaved mothers had four times higher odds of depressive symptoms and seven times higher odds of PTSD symptoms at 9 months postpartum as compared with nonbereaved mothers. Symptoms can often be triggered when trying to conceive or during a subsequent pregnancy (Farren et al. 2018; Hamama et al. 2010).

**TABLE 5–5. Risk factors for depressive disorders after perinatal loss**

| |
|---|
| Pregnancy loss after 20 weeks' gestation or intrauterine fetal demise |
| Recurrent pregnancy loss |
| History of infertility and/or infertility treatments |
| Younger age |
| Being single or having marital problems |
| History of trauma or abuse |
| History of major depressive disorder or PTSD |
| Psychological factors: feelings of loss of control, feelings of responsibility for the loss |

## Acute Stress Disorder and PTSD

**Epidemiology.** Acute stress disorder and PTSD are common after a perinatal loss and are distinguishable from grief and complicated grief (Horsch 2009; Lee and Slade 1996). Rates of PTSD have been shown to be up to 45% at 3 months after loss in those with frequent miscarriages (Farren et al. 2016, 2018). Many studies do not separate out types of perinatal loss when looking at rates of acute stress and PTSD. In one large cohort study, criteria for PTSD were met by 29% of women at 1 month after an early miscarriage and by 18% at 9 months after the loss (Farren et al. 2016).

**Risk factors.** Risk factors for developing PTSD in the context of a perinatal loss include maternal age (with younger age conveying higher risk), gestational age, lower educational level, a history of previous physical or sexual trauma, prior history of mental health problems, and current depression, anxiety, or perinatal grief symptoms (Dauggirdaite et al. 2015). Length of gestational age is correlated with the intensity of reported PTSD symptoms, with later perinatal losses, such as stillbirth or neonatal death, associated with more severe intensity of reported symptoms (Dauggirdaite et al. 2015).

**Screening.** The most common screening tool for PTSD following perinatal loss is the Perinatal Post-Traumatic Stress Disorder Questionnaire. This 14-item self-report screening tool measures symptoms of hyperarousal, reexperiencing, and avoidance behaviors (Callahan et al. 2006).

**Course and differential diagnosis.** It is unclear whether the clinical course of acute stress disorder and PTSD associated with perinatal loss differs from the clinical course of these disorders related to other times in a woman's reproductive life (see Chapter 18, "Trauma and Reproductive Health" for greater detail). No comparison studies have looked at symptom cluster frequency or intensity between women experiencing the trauma of perinatal loss and those experiencing other types of trauma or between perinatal loss subgroups. In a prospective study of women recruited in early pregnancy who suffered a perinatal loss, 25% met criteria for PTSD at 1 month following loss, and the most common symptoms were reexperiencing (77%), hyperarousal (42%), and avoidance (40%) (Engelhard et al. 2001). Longitudinal studies report that the frequency and intensity of symptoms of acute stress disorder and PTSD after perinatal loss decrease over time in most studies (Engelhard et al. 2001). PTSD associated with perinatal loss can be differentiated from MDD by the presence of prominent flashbacks, reexperiencing, and avoidance specific to stimuli related to the loss. As in the general population, PTSD frequently co-occurs with MDD in women after a perinatal loss (Engelhard et al. 2001).

## Anxiety Disorders

Most scholarly work on perinatal loss focuses more on bereavement, depression symptoms, and trauma-related disorders and less on the development of specific anxiety disorders in the aftermath of loss (Armstrong and Hutti 1998; Blackmore et al. 2011). In a large prospective cohort study of 537 women who miscarried and 111 who had an ectopic pregnancy, moderate or severe anxiety occurred in 25% of patients (Farren et al. 2016). Although most studies look at anxiety symptoms in general, a few studies have examined specific disorders. Most have included OCD among the anxiety disorders, as it was classified prior to DSM-5. Geller et al. (2004) compared 227 women who miscarried with 230 matched community control subjects and found that 3% of those who miscarried met criteria for OCD, an eight times greater risk than for women in the community. In contrast, in a study comparing 399 women with perinatal loss and 232 women with live births at 9 months post-loss or postpartum, women with perinatal loss had higher odds of screening positive for generalized anxiety disorder and social phobia, but not panic disorder and OCD, when adjusting for confounding variables (Gold et al. 2014). Rates of generalized anxiety disorder and social phobia were 19% and 44%, respectively, in bereaved women compared with 7% and 22%, respectively, in nonbereaved women (Gold et al. 2014).

## Mania

The literature includes case reports of acute mania following a pregnancy loss, primarily in those with a history of bipolar disorder (Sharma et al. 2013). One hypothesis links the incidence of post-loss mania to fluctuations in estrogen levels at the end of the pregnancy (Sharma et al. 2013). Further research is required to elucidate this link; please see Chapter 15, "Bipolar Disorder and Related Disorders," and Chapter 16, "Postpartum Psychosis," for full descriptions of postpartum mania and the closely related postpartum psychosis.

## Suicide

Multiple studies show an increased risk of suicide following perinatal loss, particularly immediately after the loss. The mean annual suicide rate in the first year following pregnancy loss is 18.1 of 100,000, compared with 5.9 of 100,000 following live birth (Bhat and Byatt 2016; Hvidtjørn et al. 2016). Perinatal loss or neonatal death can increase the rate of psychiatric hospitalization for suicide attempts up to threefold in the year following loss (Schiff and Grossman 2006). Mothers who lose a child often describe ambivalence about their own mortality. Suicide can serve a dual purpose: release from the pain of the loss and reunion with the deceased child. Obligations to other living children may serve as a protective factor (Gissler et al. 1996).

## Mental Health Impact of Perinatal Loss in Subsequent Pregnancies

Approximately 86% of women experiencing perinatal loss become pregnant again within 18 months following the loss (Lee et al. 2017). A meta-analysis (Hunter et al. 2017) showed an association between perinatal loss and depression and anxiety symptoms during subsequent pregnancies, a finding that has been replicated in many other studies (Chojenta et al. 2014; Gong et al. 2013; Gravensteen et al. 2018). Previous spontaneous abortion has also been linked to an increased risk of posttraumatic stress during a subsequent pregnancy, a risk that is increased by a history of sexual trauma and the desire for a subsequent pregnancy sooner (Hamama et al. 2010). The emotional effects of perinatal loss can last into a subsequent successful pregnancy, increasing levels of stress, anxiety, and emotional vulnerability (Armstrong and Hutti 1998; Mills et al. 2014).

The burden of depression and anxiety does not remit following the birth of a healthy child. For instance, Gravensteen et al. (2018) showed higher prevalence of anxiety (22.5%) and depression (19.7%) in pregnant women with a history of stillbirth compared with nulliparous women or women with a history of live birth; moreover, these symptoms could persist up to 6–18 months after the birth of a live infant. Perceived low levels of support can increase the risk of depression and anxiety in a subsequent pregnancy, as can pregnancy within the first year following the loss (Armstrong et al. 2009). Parents also report decreased attachment to the infant in pregnancies subsequent to perinatal loss (Armstrong 2002; Armstrong and Hutti 1998).

The timing of assessment of mood and anxiety in a subsequent pregnancy is important, because anxiety varies depending on the gestational age and time of assessment in relation to timing and circumstances of the previous loss. Anxiety may abate after the mother gets reassurance through routine testing and screenings (Hunter et al. 2017). The anxiety often increases when the mother gets closer to the gestational age at which the previous perinatal loss occurred (Mills et al. 2014). In a subsequent pregnancy, parents often experience isolation related to societal expectations to recover from the previous loss (Mills et al. 2014). It is common for parents not to share news of their pregnancy after a previous perinatal loss. Some might be emotionally detached from the pregnancy, whereas others might experience intrusive levels of anxiety and mental preoccupation with the pregnancy (Armstrong 2002).

Although many studies show an increased rate of stress, anxiety, and depression symptoms in a subsequent pregnancy, not all results are similar (Armstrong 2004; Bergner et al. 2008; Blackmore et al. 2011; Hughes et al. 1999). These variations might be due to a broader definition of perinatal loss, differing uses of the term across studies, and the impact of cultural beliefs and practices in emotional outcomes for women and their partners.

## Treatment of Perinatal Loss and Grief

### Psychopharmacology

To date, no psychopharmacology treatment studies of psychiatric conditions associated with perinatal loss have been published, despite the finding in one study that 37.5% of parents were prescribed a medication—usually an antidepressant—in the year following perinatal or neonatal loss (Lacasse and Cacciatore 2014). Medication management of MDD and PTSD related to perinatal loss should follow the same principles and practices as treatment of these conditions at other times of a woman's life (see Chapters 13 and 18 for more information). Because many women do attempt another pregnancy after perinatal loss, clinicians should follow guidelines for prescribing medication in pregnancy and the postpartum period.

## Psychotherapy

**General approach.** Perinatal loss, especially spontaneous abortion, is a very personal loss that is often not shared with others, so grieving patients often feel alone in their suffering (Markin and Zilcha-Mano 2018). Reproductive loss is a type of "disenfranchised grief"—a grief that occurs when a loss is not generally recognized by society (Doka 1989)—so a major part of the corresponding treatment is the establishment of a strong therapeutic alliance with other individuals, couples, or families navigating through such loss. Alliance can be fostered by assisting those experiencing the loss through validation of their seeking treatment (Jaffe and Diamond 2011).

By setting therapeutic goals, providing psychoeducation on reproductive loss, and helping those experiencing reproductive loss to identify their strengths, clinicians can facilitate patient empowerment to navigate through the grief and mourning process. Worden (2009) provided a framework for facilitating adjustment to grief. He listed four tasks of grieving: 1) accepting the reality of the loss, 2) processing the pain of grief, 3) adjusting to a world without the deceased, 4) and finding an enduring connection with the deceased in the midst of embracing a new life. It is important to stress to those obtaining mental health services pertaining to reproductive loss that these tasks are not linear but rather more like "messy circles." Exploring what is known as one's "reproductive story" may help with the grieving process. These narratives are internalized images of what parents hope for their children, and most are not fully realized until the parents experience a reproductive loss (Jaffe 2017). Psychoeducation should be provided to patients to reinforce individualized methods and timelines for grief.

Engagement in mental health treatment appears to be influenced by racial, cultural, and economic factors. For instance, studies of Black women in the United States have found that many grieving women chose not to utilize perinatal loss support groups due to the groups' lack of racial diversity (Boyden et al. 2014; Van and Meleis 2003). Outreach to high-risk groups, research regarding barriers to care, and culturally sensitive treatment approaches are needed.

**Specific psychotherapy interventions.** Despite the well-established association of perinatal loss with psychiatric sequelae, a systematic review of psychotherapy treatment studies published in 2012 did not find demonstrated superiority of psychological treatments over no treatment (Murphy et al. 2012). Since that publication, more studies using evidence-based treatments have been completed, and a new systematic review is in process (Charrois et al. 2020). Still, very few randomized controlled trials for specific psychiatric symptoms and disorders associated with specific forms of perinatal loss have been conducted to date. IPT, which is evidence based for the treatment of perinatal depression, has been adapted to perinatal loss (Sockol 2018). Early trials that used a manualized phone approach reported significantly decreased depressive symptoms in treated subjects over the six to nine sessions (Neugebauer et al. 2006, 2007). In a pilot randomized controlled trial of women with MDD after miscarriage, stillbirth, or early neonatal death, in-person IPT was found to be feasible, acceptable to patients, and associated with reduced depressive symptoms (Johnson et al. 2016). For women after miscarriage, both in-person and internet-based CBT have been found to reduce depression and anxiety symptoms from pretreatment to posttreatment in small studies (Kersting et al. 2011; Séjourné et al. 2010).

# Special Considerations

## Perinatal Loss in LGBTQ+ Families

Most studies on the psychological and psychiatric aspects of perinatal loss include cisgender women, typically in heterosexual relationships. Very few studies exist examining the experience of perinatal loss in LGBTQ+ families. For these families, pregnancy is often achieved through ART, and these pregnancies often require a high degree of effort and planning. Consequently, loss of these pregnancies is experienced as highly distressing (Peel 2010; Wojnar 2007). A concept of double disenfranchisement has been proposed (Cacciatore and Raffo 2011): because historically many LGBTQ+ families have been devalued by the wider society, their perinatal loss represents a "double loss," and their isolation in their grief represents a "double disenfranchisement."

## Gender Differences

To date, all studies of men's responses to perinatal loss have focused on cisgender heterosexual men, and studies are needed that focus on the unique experience of miscarriage, IUFD, or neonatal death for men who have chosen to become parents through surrogacy or adoption (Obst et al. 2020). In heterosexual couples, perinatal loss has been found to have varied effects on men, and these effects are important to clarify because they may affect couples' relationships, which can have downstream effects on a woman's functioning. In their systematic review of 19 quantitative and 26 qualitative studies, Obst et al. (2020) found that men are likely to engage in active coping styles and invest in both emotional and instrumental supportive behaviors for their partners. In turn, this may leave the men feeling less able to express their grief or to seek help from family and other supports for their own psychological distress, leading them to also feel a sense of disenfranchisement (Obst et al. 2020). They are also more likely to engage in avoidance behaviors during grief, including excessive attention to work outside the home and substance abuse (Obst et al. 2020).

# Perinatal Loss Summary

Perinatal loss is associated with many psychological and psychiatric reactions in women. Most women experience grief reactions, and due to the unexpected nature of perinatal loss, many also develop acute stress disorder and PTSD. MDD is especially common in women who have experienced recurrent miscarriages and in women with IUFD or pregnancy loss after 20 weeks' gestation. Mental health practitioners can play a critical role in helping women recover from the despair associated with the loss of a pregnancy through psychotherapy and the use of reproductive loss–related informed grief counseling.

# Key Points

- Polycystic ovary syndrome, endometriosis, autoimmune conditions, and hypothalamic amenorrhea are associated with increased rates of mood and anxiety disorders as well as infertility.

- Infertility medications may be associated with significant mood and anxiety symptoms.
- Most studies of the psychiatric issues in infertility patients include heterosexual cisgender women; more research is needed in diverse populations.
- Assisted reproductive technology (ART) is emotionally and physically demanding, and ART with third parties—such as surrogates—is especially challenging.
- The American Society for Reproductive Medicine publishes guidelines for evaluation and treatment of third-party ART participants; mental health clinicians should consult these guidelines.
- Perinatal loss is a common complication of pregnancy and is divided into loss prior to 20 weeks' gestation, loss after 20 weeks' gestation, and early and late neonatal death.
- Grief is a common reaction following perinatal loss but in some cases can evolve into a more complex process with prolonged, intense physical and emotional symptoms.
- Perinatal loss increases the risk of various psychiatric disorders, and it is possible that psychiatric illness increases the risk of perinatal loss.
- Certain risk factors are found in all forms of perinatal loss, including lack of social support, previous psychiatric disorders, and previous history of trauma.
- Treatment of the psychological consequences of perinatal loss revolves around psychotherapy and psychosocial support for the woman and the couple (where applicable).

## References

Adeleye AJ, Cedars MI, Smith J, et al: Ovarian stimulation for fertility preservation or family building in a cohort of transgender men. J Assist Reprod Genet 36(10):2155–2161, 2019 31435820

Ajmal A, Joffe H, Nachtigall LB: Psychotropic-induced hyperprolactinemia: a clinical review. Psychosomatics 55(1):29–36, 2014 24140188

Akioyamen LE, Minhas H, Holloway AC, et al: Effects of depression pharmacotherapy in fertility treatment on conception, birth, and neonatal health: a systematic review. J Psychosom Res 84:69–80, 2016 27095162

Altmark D, Tomer R, Sigal M: Psychotic episode induced by ovulation-initiating treatment. Isr J Med Sci 23(11):1156–1157, 1987 3436800

Altun T, Jindal S, Greenseid K, et al: Low follicular fluid IL-6 levels in IVF patients are associated with increased likelihood of clinical pregnancy. J Assist Reprod Genet 28(3):245–251, 2011 21046223

American College of Obstetricians and Gynecologists: ACOG Practice Bulletin No. 200: early pregnancy loss. Obstet Gynecol 132(5):e197–e207, 2018 30157093

American College of Obstetricians and Gynecologists: Infertility workup for the women's health specialist: ACOG Committee Opinion Summary, Number 781. Obstet Gynecol 133(6):1294–1295, 2019 31135761

American College of Obstetricians and Gynecologists, Society for Maternal-Fetal Medicine: Management of stillbirth: Obstetric Care Consensus No. 10. Obstet Gynecol 135(3):e110–e132, 2020 32080052

American Psychiatric Association: Diagnostic and Statistical Manual of Mental Disorders, 5th Edition. Arlington, VA, American Psychiatric Association, 2013
American Society for Reproductive Medicine: Infertility: An Overview. Washington, DC, American Society for Reproductive Medicine, 2015. Available at: https://www.reproductivefacts.org/globalassets/rf/news-and-publications/bookletsfact-sheets/english-fact-sheets-and-info-booklets/infertility-an_overview_booklet2.pdf. Accessed June 13, 2020.
American Society for Reproductive Medicine: Assisted Reproductive Technologies. Washington, DC, American Society for Reproductive Medicine, 2018. Available at: https://www.reproductivefacts.org/globalassets/rf/news-and-publications/bookletsfact-sheets/english-fact-sheets-and-info-booklets/art-booklet2.pdf. Accessed June 13, 2020.
Amir H, Oren A, Klochendler Frishman E, et al: Oocyte retrieval outcomes among adolescent transgender males. J Assist Reprod Genet 37(7):1737–1744, 2020 32430731
Amiri M, Sadeqi Z, Hoseinpoor MH, et al: Marital satisfaction and its influencing factors in fertile and infertile women. J Family Reprod Health 10(3):139–145, 2016 28101115
Armstrong DS: Emotional distress and prenatal attachment in pregnancy after perinatal loss. J Nurs Scholarsh 34(4):339–345, 2002 12501737
Armstrong DS: Impact of prior perinatal loss on subsequent pregnancies. J Obstet Gynecol Neonatal Nurs 33(6):765–773, 2004 15561665
Armstrong D, Hutti M: Pregnancy after perinatal loss: the relationship between anxiety and prenatal attachment. J Obstet Gynecol Neonatal Nurs 27(2):183–189, 1998 9549704
Armstrong DS, Hutti MH, Myers J: The influence of prior perinatal loss on parents' psychological distress after the birth of a subsequent healthy infant. J Obstet Gynecol Neonatal Nurs 38(6):654–666, 2009 19930279
Armuand G, Dhejne C, Olofsson JI, et al: Attitudes and experiences of health care professionals when caring for transgender men undergoing fertility preservation by egg freezing: a qualitative study. Ther Adv Reprod Health 14:2633494120911036, 2020 32518917
Arocho R, Lozano EB, Halpern CT: Estimates of donated sperm use in the United States: National Survey of Family Growth 1995–2017. Fertil Steril 112(4):718–723, 2019 31371048
Arterburn D, Sofer T, Boudreau DM, et al: Long-term weight change after initiating second generation antidepressants. J Clin Med 5(4):48, 2016 27089374
Aussedat M, Jean-Louis J, Djahangirian O, et al: Clomiphene for the treatment of male infertility: a case report of mood change and a literature overview. Curr Drug Saf 12(3):208–215, 2017 28625145
Badenhorst W, Hughes P: Psychological aspects of perinatal loss. Best Pract Res Clin Obstet Gynaecol 21(2):249–259, 2007 17196434
Baldur-Felskov B, Kjaer SK, Albieri V, et al: Psychiatric disorders in women with fertility problems: results from a large Danish register-based cohort study. Hum Reprod 28(3):683–690, 2013 23223399
Barfield WD, Committee on Fetus and Newborn: Standard terminology for fetal, infant, and perinatal deaths. Pediatrics 128(1):177–181, 2011 21708807
Barton BB, Segger F, Fischer K, et al: Update on weight-gain caused by antipsychotics: a systematic review and meta-analysis. Expert Opin Drug Saf 19(3):295–314, 2020 31952459
Beck AT, Steer RA, Brown GK: Beck Depression Inventory, 2nd Edition. Bloomington, MN, Pearson Assessments, 1996
Beckwée D, Leysen L, Meuwis K, et al: Prevalence of aromatase inhibitor-induced arthralgia in breast cancer: a systematic review and meta-analysis. Support Care Cancer 25(5):1673–1686, 2017 28204994
Bergner A, Beyer R, Klapp BF, et al: Pregnancy after early pregnancy loss: a prospective study of anxiety, depressive symptomatology and coping. J Psychosom Obstet Gynaecol 29(2):105–113, 2008 17943588
Bhat A, Byatt N: Infertility and perinatal loss: when the bough breaks. Curr Psychiatry Rep 18(3):31, 2016 26847216
Blackmore ER, Côté-Arsenault D, Tang W, et al: Previous prenatal loss as a predictor of perinatal depression and anxiety. Br J Psychiatry 198(5):373–378, 2011 21372060

Blenner JL: Clomiphene-induced mood swings. J Obstet Gynecol Neonatal Nurs 20(4):321–327, 1991 1941294
Bloch M, Azem F, Aharonov I, et al: GnRH-agonist induced depressive and anxiety symptoms during in vitro fertilization-embryo transfer cycles. Fertil Steril 95(1):307–309, 2011 20801439
Blumenthal SR, Castro VM, Clements CC, et al: An electronic health records study of long-term weight gain following antidepressant use. JAMA Psychiatry 71(8):889–896, 2014 24898363
Boivin J: A review of psychosocial interventions in infertility. Soc Sci Med 57(12):2325–2341, 2003 14572840
Boivin J, Griffiths E, Venetis CA: Emotional distress in infertile women and failure of assisted reproductive technologies: meta-analysis of prospective psychosocial studies. BMJ 342:d223, 2011 21345903
Boutari C, Pappas PD, Mintziori G, et al: The effect of underweight on female and male reproduction. Metabolism 107:154229, 2020 32289345
Boyden JY, Kavanaugh K, Issel LM, et al: Experiences of African American parents following perinatal or pediatric death: a literature review. Death Stud 38(6–10):374–380, 2014 24666143
Bozdag G, Mumusoglu S, Zengin D, et al: The prevalence and phenotypic features of polycystic ovary syndrome: a systematic review and meta-analysis. Hum Reprod 31(12):2841–2855, 2016 27664216
Bracewell-Milnes T, Saso S, Bora S, et al: Investigating psychosocial attitudes, motivations and experiences of oocyte donors, recipients and egg sharers: a systematic review. Hum Reprod Update 22(4):450–465, 2016 27016289
Brier N: Grief following miscarriage: a comprehensive review of the literature. J Womens Health (Larchmt) 17(3):451–464, 2008 18345996
Brown ES, Suppes T: Mood symptoms during corticosteroid therapy: a review. Harv Rev Psychiatry 5(5):239–246, 1998 9493946
Cacciatore J, Raffo Z: An exploration of lesbian maternal bereavement. Soc Work 56(2):169–177, 2011 21553580
Callahan JL, Borja SE, Hynan MT: Modification of the Perinatal PTSD Questionnaire to enhance clinical utility. J Perinatol 26(9):533–539, 2006 16826190
Capuron L, Miller AH: Immune system to brain signaling: neuropsychopharmacological implications. Pharmacol Ther 130(2):226–238, 2011 21334376
Cassaday TM: Impact of pregnancy loss on psychological functioning and grief outcomes. Obstet Gynecol Clin North Am 45(3):525–533, 2018 30092926
Cesta CE, Viktorin A, Olsson H, et al: Depression, anxiety, and antidepressant treatment in women: association with in vitro fertilization outcome. Fertil Steril 105(6):1594–1602, 2016 26920258
Charrois EM, Bright KS, Wajid A, et al: Effectiveness of psychotherapeutic interventions on psychological distress in women who have experienced perinatal loss: a systematic review protocol. Syst Rev 9(1):125, 2020 32487235
Chen LC, Hsu JW, Huang KL, et al: Risk of developing major depression and anxiety disorders among women with endometriosis: a longitudinal follow-up study. J Affect Disord 190:282–285, 2016 26544610
Chen TH, Chang SP, Tsai CF, et al: Prevalence of depressive and anxiety disorders in an assisted reproductive technique clinic. Hum Reprod 19(10):2313–2318, 2004 15242992
Choi SH, Shapiro H, Robinson GE, et al: Psychological side-effects of clomiphene citrate and human menopausal gonadotrophin. J Psychosom Obstet Gynaecol 26(2):93–100, 2005 16050534
Chojenta C, Harris S, Reilly N, et al: History of pregnancy loss increases the risk of mental health problems in subsequent pregnancies but not in the postpartum. PLoS One 9(4):e95038, 2014 24733508
Cohen M, Granger S, Fuller-Thomson E: The association between bereavement and biomarkers of inflammation. Behav Med 41(2):49–59, 2015 24266503
Cohen S, Janicki-Deverts D, Miller GE: Psychological stress and disease. JAMA 298(14):1685–1687, 2007 17925521
Copperman AB, Benadiva C: Optimal usage of the GnRH antagonists: a review of the literature. Reprod Biol Endocrinol 11:20, 2013 23496864

Cousineau TM, Domar AD: Psychological impact of infertility. Best Pract Res Clin Obstet Gynaecol 21(2):293–308, 2007 17241818
Cox JL, Holden JM, Sagovsky R: Detection of postnatal depression: development of the 10-item Edinburgh Postnatal Depression Scale. Br J Psychiatry 150:782–786, 1987
Crawford NM, Hoff HS, Mersereau JE: Infertile women who screen positive for depression are less likely to initiate fertility treatments. Hum Reprod 32(3):582–587, 2017 28073974
Dauggirdaite V, van den Akker O, Purewal S: Posttraumatic stress and posttraumatic stress disorder after termination of pregnancy and reproductive loss: a systematic review. J Pregnancy 646345:2015, 2015
Dechanet C, Anahory T, Mathieu Daude JC, et al: Effects of cigarette smoking on reproduction. Hum Reprod Update 17(1):76–95, 2011 20685716
Demartini B, Ranieri R, Masu A, et al: Depressive symptoms and major depressive disorder in patients affected by subclinical hypothyroidism: a cross-sectional study. J Nerv Ment Dis 202(8):603–607, 2014 25010109
deMontigny F, Verdon C, Meunier S, et al: Women's persistent depressive and perinatal grief symptoms following a miscarriage: the role of childlessness and satisfaction with healthcare services. Arch Women Ment Health 20(5):655–662, 2017 28623418
Diamond MP, Legro RS, Coutifaris C, et al: Letrozole, gonadotropin, or clomiphene for unexplained infertility. N Engl J Med 373(13):1230–1240, 2015 26398071
Doka KJ (ed): Disenfranchised Grief: Recognizing Hidden Sorrow. Lexington, MA, Lexington Books/DC Heath and Com, 1989
Domar AD, Zuttermeister PC, Seibel M, et al: Psychological improvement in infertile women after behavioral treatment: a replication. Fertil Steril 58(1):144–147, 1992 1623995
Domar AD, Zuttermeister PC, Friedman R: The psychological impact of infertility: a comparison with patients with other medical conditions. J Psychosom Obstet Gynaecol 14(suppl):45–52, 1993 8142988
Domar AD, Clapp D, Slawsby E, et al: The impact of group psychological interventions on distress in infertile women. Health Psychol 19(6):568–575, 2000 11129360
Domar AD, Rooney K, Hacker MR, et al: Burden of care is the primary reason why insured women terminate in vitro fertilization treatment. Fertil Steril 109(6):1121–1126, 2018 29935647
Dosiou C: Thyroid and fertility: recent advances. Thyroid 30(4):479–486, 2020 31903865
Dubber S, Reck C, Müller M, et al: Postpartum bonding: the role of perinatal depression, anxiety and maternal-fetal bonding during pregnancy. Arch Women Ment Health 18(2):187–195, 2015 25088531
Dunne C: The effects of cannabis on female and male reproduction. BC Med J 61(7):282–285, 2019
El Kissi Y, Romdhane AB, Hidar S, et al: General psychopathology, anxiety, depression and self-esteem in couples undergoing infertility treatment: a comparative study between men and women. Eur J Obstet Gynecol Reprod Biol 167(2):185–189, 2013 23298895
Elias KM, Berkowitz RS, Horowitz NS: State-of-the-art workup and initial management of newly diagnosed molar pregnancy and postmolar gestational trophoblastic neoplasia. J Natl Compr Canc Netw 17(11):1396–1401, 2019
Elnazer HY, Sampson A, Baldwin D: Lithium and sexual dysfunction: an under-researched area. Hum Psychopharmacol 30(2):66–69, 2015 25619161
Engelhard IM, van den Hout MA, Arntz A: Posttraumatic stress disorder after pregnancy loss. Gen Hosp Psychiatry 23(2):62–66, 2001 11313072
Erensoy H, Niafar M, Ghafarzadeh S, et al: A pilot trial of metformin for insulin resistance and mood disturbances in adolescent and adult women with polycystic ovary syndrome. Gynecol Endocrinol 35(1):72–75, 2019 30182764
Ethics Committee of the American Society for Reproductive Medicine: Access to fertility services by transgender persons: an Ethics Committee opinion. Fertil Steril 104(5):1111–1115, 2015 26363388
Ethics Committee of the American Society for Reproductive Medicine: Informing offspring of their conception by gamete or embryo donation: an Ethics Committee opinion. Fertil Steril 109(4):601–605, 2018

Eugster A, Vingerhoets AJ: Psychological aspects of in vitro fertilization: a review. Soc Sci Med 48(5):575–589, 1999 10080360
Faramarzi M, Kheirkhah F, Esmaelzadeh S, et al: Is psychotherapy a reliable alternative to pharmacotherapy to promote the mental health of infertile women? A randomized clinical trial. Eur J Obstet Gynecol Reprod Biol 141(1):49–53, 2008 18848381
Faramarzi M, Pasha H, Esmailzadeh S, et al: The effect of the cognitive behavioral therapy and pharmacotherapy on infertility stress: a randomized controlled trial. Int J Fertil Steril 7(3):199–206, 2013 24520487
Farren J, Jalmbrant M, Ameye L, et al: Post-traumatic stress, anxiety and depression following miscarriage or ectopic pregnancy: a prospective cohort study. BMJ Open 6(11):e011864, 2016 27807081
Farren J, Mitchell-Jones N, Verbakel JY, et al: The psychological impact of early pregnancy loss. Hum Reprod Update 24(6):731–749, 2018 30204882
Frederiksen Y, Farver-Vestergaard I, Skovgård NG, et al: Efficacy of psychosocial interventions for psychological and pregnancy outcomes in infertile women and men: a systematic review and meta-analysis. BMJ Open 5(1):e006592, 2015 25631310
Freeman MP, Lee H, Savella GM, et al: Predictors of depressive relapse in women undergoing infertility treatment. J Womens Health (Larchmt) 27(11):1408–1414, 2018 30067141
Freizinger M, Franko DL, Dacey M, et al: The prevalence of eating disorders in infertile women. Fertil Steril 93(1):72–78, 2010 19006795
Fukao A, Takamatsu J, Arishima T, et al: Graves' disease and mental disorders. J Clin Transl Endocrinol 19:100207, 2019 31763175
Gaitzsch H, Benard J, Hugon-Rodin J, et al: The effect of mind-body interventions on psychological and pregnancy outcomes in infertile women: a systematic review. Arch Women Ment Health 23(4):479–491, 2020 31897607
Gambadauro P, Carli V, Hadlaczky G: Depressive symptoms among women with endometriosis: a systematic review and meta-analysis. Am J Obstet Gynecol 220(3):230–241, 2019 30419199
Gaskins AJ, Sundaram R, Buck Louis GM, et al: Predictors of sexual intercourse frequency among couples trying to conceive. J Sex Med 15(4):519–528, 2018 29523477
Geller PA, Kerns D, Klier CM: Anxiety following miscarriage and the subsequent pregnancy: a review of the literature and future directions. J Psychosom Res 56(1):35–45, 2004 14987962
Giles DE, Berga SL: Cognitive and psychiatric correlates of functional hypothalamic amenorrhea: a controlled comparison. Fertil Steril 60(3):486–492, 1993 8375531
Gissler M, Hemminki E, Lönnqvist J: Suicides after pregnancy in Finland, 1987–94: register linkage study. BMJ 313(7070):1431–1434, 1996 8973229
Gitlin M: Lithium side effects and toxicity: prevalence and management strategies. Int J Bipolar Disord 4(1):27, 2016 27900734
Gold KJ, Dalton VK, Schwenk TL, et al: What causes pregnancy loss? Preexisting mental illness as an independent risk factor. Gen Hosp Psychiatry 29(3):207–213, 2007 17484937
Gold KJ, Boggs ME, Muzik M, Sen A: Anxiety disorders and obsessive compulsive disorder 9 months after perinatal loss. Gen Hosp Psychiatry 36(6):650–654, 2014 25305711
Gold KJ, Leon I, Boggs ME, et al: Depression and posttraumatic stress symptoms after perinatal loss in a population-based sample. J Womens Health (Larchmt) 25(3):263–269, 2016 26258870
Goldvaser H, AlGorashi I, Ribnikar D, et al: Efficacy of extended adjuvant therapy with aromatase inhibitors in early breast cancer among common clinicopathologically defined subgroups: a systematic review and meta-analysis. Cancer Treat Rev 60:53–59, 2017 28881223
Gong X, Hao J, Tao F, et al: Pregnancy loss and anxiety and depression during subsequent pregnancies: data from the C-ABC study. Eur J Obstet Gynecol Reprod Biol 166(1):30–36, 2013 23146315
Gordon CM, Ackerman KE, Berga SL, et al: Functional hypothalamic amenorrhea: an Endocrine Society clinical practice guideline. J Clin Endocrinol Metab 102(5):1413–1439, 2017 28368518
Grall-Bronnec M, Sauvaget A, Perrouin F, et al: Pathological gambling associated with aripiprazole or dopamine replacement therapy: do patients share the same features? A review. J Clin Psychopharmacol 36(1):f63–f70, 2016 26658263

Grambsch P, Young EA, Meller WH: Pulsatile luteinizing hormone disruption in depression. Psychoneuroendocrinology 29(7):825–829, 2004 15177697
Graupera B, Pascual MA, Hereter L, et al: Accuracy of three-dimensional ultrasound compared with magnetic resonance imaging in diagnosis of Müllerian duct anomalies using ESHRE-ESGE consensus on the classification of congenital anomalies of the female genital tract. Ultrasound Obstet Gynecol 46(5):616–622, 2015 25690307
Gravensteen IK, Jacobsen EM, Sandset PM, et al: Anxiety, depression and relationship satisfaction in the pregnancy following stillbirth and after the birth of a live-born baby: a prospective study. BMC Pregnancy Childbirth 18(1):41, 2018 29361916
Greil AL: Infertility and psychological distress: a critical review of the literature. Soc Sci Med 45(11):1679–1704, 1997 9428088
Greil AL, McQuillan J, Lowry M, et al: Infertility treatment and fertility-specific distress: a longitudinal analysis of a population-based sample of U.S. women. Soc Sci Med 73(1):87–94, 2011 21645954
Greil AL, Schmidt L, Peterson BD: Understanding and treating the psychosocial consequences of infertility, in The Oxford Handbook of Perinatal Psychology. Edited by Wenzel A. New York, Oxford University Press, 2016, pp 524–547
Haimovici F, Hill JA (eds): Cytokines in Reproduction. Austin, TX, Landes Bioscience, 1998
Haimovici F, Anderson JL, Bates GW, et al: Stress, anxiety, and depression of both partners in infertile couples are associated with cytokine levels and adverse IVF outcome. Am J Reprod Immunol 79(4):e12832, 2018 29528174
Hamama L, Rauch SA, Sperlich M, et al: Previous experience of spontaneous or elective abortion and risk for posttraumatic stress and depression during subsequent pregnancy. Depress Anxiety 27(8):699–707, 2010 20577979
Hämmerli K, Znoj H, Barth J: The efficacy of psychological interventions for infertile patients: a meta-analysis examining mental health and pregnancy rate. Hum Reprod Update 15(3):279–295, 2009 19196795
Harrison CL, Brown WJ, Hayman M, et al: The role of physical activity in preconception, pregnancy and postpartum health. Semin Reprod Med 34(2):e28–e37, 2016 27169984
Hart RJ: Physiological aspects of female fertility: role of the environment, modern lifestyle, and genetics. Physiol Rev 96(3):873–909, 2016 27252278
Havrylyuk A, Chopyak V, Boyko Y, et al: Cytokines in the blood and semen of infertile patients. Cent Eur J Immunol 40(3):337–344, 2015 26648778
Hembree WC, Cohen-Kettenis P, Delemarre-van de Waal HA, et al: Endocrine treatment of transsexual persons: an Endocrine Society clinical practice guideline. J Clin Endocrinol Metab 94(9):3132–3154, 2009 19509099
Hemels MEH, Einarson A, Koren G, et al: Antidepressant use during pregnancy and the rates of spontaneous abortions: a meta-analysis. Ann Pharmacother 39(5):803–809, 2005 15784808
Hemminki E, Forssas E: Epidemiology of miscarriage and its relation to other reproductive events in Finland. Am J Obstet Gynecol 181(2):396–401, 1999 10454690
Henshaw RC, Cooper K, el-Refaey H, et al: Medical management of miscarriage: non-surgical uterine evacuation of incomplete and inevitable spontaneous abortion. BMJ 306(6882):894–895, 1993 8490413
Hogan RG, Wang AY, Li Z, et al: Oocyte donor age has a significant impact on oocyte recipients' cumulative live-birth rate: a population-based cohort study. Fertil Steril 112(4):724–730, 2019 31248619
Hogue CJ, Parker CB, Willinger M, et al: The association of stillbirth with depressive symptoms 6–36 months post-delivery. Paediatr Perinat Epidemiol 29(2):131–143, 2015 25682858
Holley SR, Pasch LA, Bleil ME, et al: Prevalence and predictors of major depressive disorder for fertility treatment patients and their partners. Fertil Steril 103(5):1332–1339, 2015 25796319
Homan GF, Davies M, Norman R: The impact of lifestyle factors on reproductive performance in the general population and those undergoing infertility treatment: a review. Hum Reprod Update 13(3):209–223, 2007 17208948

Horsch A: Post-traumatic stress disorder following childbirth and pregnancy loss, in Clinical Psychology in Practice. Edited by Beinart H, Kennedy P, Llewelyn S. West Sussex, UK, Blackwell, 2009, pp 274–287
Hughes PM, Turton P, Evans CDH: Stillbirth as risk factor for depression and anxiety in the subsequent pregnancy: cohort study. BMJ 318(7200):1721–1724, 1999 10381705
Humphries LA, Chang O, Humm K, et al: Influence of race and ethnicity on in vitro fertilization outcomes: systematic review. Am J Obstet Gynecol 214(2):212.e1–212.e17, 2016 26363483
Hunter A, Tussis L, MacBeth A: The presence of anxiety, depression and stress in women and their partners during pregnancies following perinatal loss: a meta-analysis. J Affect Disord 223:153–164, 2017 28755623
Hvidtjørn D, Wu C, Schendel D, et al: Mortality in mothers after perinatal loss: a population-based follow-up study. BJOG 123(3):393–398, 2016 25565567
Imrie S, Golombok S: Long-term outcomes of children conceived through egg donation and their parents: a review of the literature. Fertil Steril 110(7):1187–1193, 2018 30503104
Insogna IG, Ginsburg ES: Infertility, inequality, and how lack of insurance coverage compromises reproductive autonomy. AMA J Ethics 20(12):E1152–E1159, 2018 30585578
Jaffe J: Reproductive trauma: Psychotherapy for pregnancy loss and infertility clients from a reproductive story perspective. Psychotherapy (Chic) 54(4):380–385, 2017 29251957
Jaffe J, Diamond MO: Reproductive Trauma: Psychotherapy With Infertility and Pregnancy Loss Clients. Washington, DC, American Psychological Association, 2011
Janitz AE, Peck JD, Craig LB: Racial/ethnic differences in the utilization of infertility services: a focus on American Indian/Alaska Natives. Matern Child Health J 23(1):10–18, 2019 29998430
Janssen HJEM, Cuisinier MCJ, de Graauw KPH, et al: A prospective study of risk factors predicting grief intensity following pregnancy loss. Arch Gen Psychiatry 54(1):56–61, 1997 9006401
Joham AE, Teede HJ, Ranasinha S, et al: Prevalence of infertility and use of fertility treatment in women with polycystic ovary syndrome: data from a large community-based cohort study. J Womens Health (Larchmt) 24(4):299–307, 2015 25654626
Johnson JE, Price AB, Kao JC, et al: Interpersonal psychotherapy (IPT) for major depression following perinatal loss: a pilot randomized controlled trial. Arch Women Ment Health 19(5):845–859, 2016 27003141
Jurkovic D, Ross JA, Nicolaides KH: Expectant management of missed miscarriage. Br J Obstet Gynaecol 105(6):670–671, 1998 9647160
Kalhori F, Masoumi SZ, Shamsaei F, et al: Effect of mindfulness-based group counseling on depression in infertile women: randomized clinical trial study. Int J Fertil Steril 14(1):10–16, 2020 32112629
Kasman AM, Thoma ME, McLain AC, et al: Association between use of marijuana and time to pregnancy in men and women: findings from the National Survey of Family Growth. Fertil Steril 109(5):866–871, 2018 29555335
Kavan MG, Barone EJ: Grief and major depression: controversy over changes in DSM-5 diagnostic criteria. Am Fam Physician 90(10):690, 694, 2014 25403033
Keesee NJ, Currier JM, Neimeyer RA: Predictors of grief following the death of one's child: the contribution of finding meaning. J Clin Psychol 64(10):1145–1163, 2008 18698614
Kenna HA, Poon AW, de los Angeles CP, et al: Psychiatric complications of treatment with corticosteroids: review with case report. Psychiatry Clin Neurosci 65(6):549–560, 2011 22003987
Kersting A, Wagner B: Complicated grief after perinatal loss. Dialogues Clin Neurosci 14(2):187–194, 2012 22754291
Kersting A, Kroker K, Schlicht S, et al: Efficacy of cognitive behavioral internet-based therapy in parents after the loss of a child during pregnancy: pilot data from a randomized controlled trial. Arch Women Ment Health 14(6):465–477, 2011 22006106
Khizroeva J, Nalli C, Bitsadze V, et al: Infertility in women with systemic autoimmune diseases. Best Pract Res Clin Endocrinol Metab 33(5):101369, 2019 31837981
Kimmel MC, Ferguson EH, Zerwas S, et al: Obstetric and gynecologic problems associated with eating disorders. Int J Eat Disord 49(3):260–275, 2016 26711005

King SL, Hegadoren KM: Stress hormones: how do they measure up? Biol Res Nurs 4(2):92–103, 2002 12408215
Kjaer TK, Jensen A, Dalton SO, et al: Suicide in Danish women evaluated for fertility problems. Hum Reprod 26(9):2401–2407, 2011 21672927
Klock SC, Chang G, Hiley A, et al: Psychological distress among women with recurrent spontaneous abortion. Psychosomatics 38(5):503–507, 1997 9314720
Klonoff-Cohen H: Female and male lifestyle habits and IVF: what is known and unknown. Hum Reprod Update 11(2):179–203, 2005 15708968
Knowles LM, Ruiz JM, O'Connor MF: A systematic review of the association between bereavement and biomarkers of immune function. Psychosom Med 81(5):415–433, 2019 30950921
Kolte AM, van Oppenraaij RH, Quenby S, et al: Non-visualized pregnancy losses are prognostically important for unexplained recurrent miscarriage. Hum Reprod 29(5):931–937, 2014 24603132
Koolhaas JM, Bartolomucci A, Buwalda B, et al: Stress revisited: a critical evaluation of the stress concept. Neurosci Biobehav Rev 35(5):1291–1301, 2011 21316391
Koszycki D, Bisserbe JC, Blier P, et al: Interpersonal psychotherapy versus brief supportive therapy for depressed infertile women: first pilot randomized controlled trial. Arch Women Ment Health 15(3):193–201, 2012 22526405
Kousta E, White DM, Franks S: Modern use of clomiphene citrate in induction of ovulation. Hum Reprod Update 3(4):359–365, 1997 9459281
Kroenke K, Spitzer R, Williams J: The PHQ-9: validity of a brief depression severity measure. Gen Intern Med 16:606–613, 2001
Krosch DJ, Shakespeare-Finch J: Grief, traumatic stress, and posttraumatic growth in women who have experienced pregnancy loss. Psychol Trauma 9(4):425–433, 2017 27607765
Krug I, Giles S, Paganini C: Binge eating in patients with polycystic ovary syndrome: prevalence, causes, and management strategies. Neuropsychiatr Dis Treat 15:1273–1285, 2019 31190833
Lacasse JR, Cacciatore J: Prescribing of psychiatric medication to bereaved parents following perinatal/neonatal death: an observational study. Death Stud 38(6–10):589–596, 2014 24588074
Lasker JN, Toedter LJ: Acute versus chronic grief: the case of pregnancy loss. Am J Orthopsychiatry 61(4):510–522, 1991 1746627
Lawson AK, Klock SC, Pavone ME, et al: Psychological counseling of female fertility preservation patients. J Psychosoc Oncol 33(4):333–353, 2015 25996581
Lazarus R, Folkman S: Stress, Appraisal, and Coping. New York, Springer, 1984
Lee C, Slade P: Miscarriage as a traumatic event: a review of the literature and new implications for intervention. J Psychosom Res 40(3):235–244, 1996 8861119
Lee L, McKenzie-McHarg K, Horsch A: The impact of miscarriage and stillbirth on maternal-fetal relationships: an integrative review. J Reprod Infant Psychol 35(1):32–52, 2017 29517293
Legro RS: Ovulation induction in polycystic ovary syndrome: current options. Best Pract Res Clin Obstet Gynaecol 37:152–159, 2016 27866938
Leon I: Reproductive loss and its impact on the next pregnancy, in Motherhood in the Face of Trauma. Edited by Muzik M, Rosenblum KL. New York, Springer, 2018, pp 69–81
Lewkowitz AK, Rosenbloom JI, Keller M, et al: Association between stillbirth ≥23 weeks gestation and acute psychiatric illness within 1 year of delivery. Am J Obstet Gynecol 221(5):491.e1–491.e22, 2019 31226297
Li J, Long L, Liu Y, et al: Effects of a mindfulness-based intervention on fertility quality of life and pregnancy rates among women subjected to first in vitro fertilization treatment. Behav Res Ther 77:96–104, 2016 26742022
Li W, Newell-Price J, Jones GL, et al: Relationship between psychological stress and recurrent miscarriage. Reprod Biomed Online 25(2):180–189, 2012 22687324
Liang PY, Diao LH, Huang CY, et al: The pro-inflammatory and anti-inflammatory cytokine profile in peripheral blood of women with recurrent implantation failure. Reprod Biomed Online 31(6):823–826, 2015 26371706
Lok IH, Neugebauer R: Psychological morbidity following miscarriage. Best Pract Res Clin Obstet Gynaecol 21(2):229–247, 2007 17317322

Loren AW, Mangu PB, Beck LN, et al: Fertility preservation for patients with cancer: American Society of Clinical Oncology clinical practice guideline update. J Clin Oncol 31(19):2500–2510, 2013 23715580
Lund R, Sejbaek CS, Christensen U, et al: The impact of social relations on the incidence of severe depressive symptoms among infertile women and men. Hum Reprod 24(11):2810–2820, 2009 19625314
Lynch CD: There are racial and ethnic disparities in infertility, indeed, but we need better data. Paediatr Perinat Epidemiol 33(2):126–128, 2019 30920007
MacDorman MF, Gregory EC: Fetal and perinatal mortality: United States, 2013. Natl Vital Stat Rep 64(8):1–24, 2015 26222771
Macer ML, Taylor HS: Endometriosis and infertility: a review of the pathogenesis and treatment of endometriosis-associated infertility. Obstet Gynecol Clin North Am 39(4):535–549, 2012 23182559
Maconochie N, Doyle P, Prior S, et al: Risk factors for first trimester miscarriage: results from a U.K.-population-based case-control study. BJOG 114(2):170–186, 2007 17305901
Mahlstedt PP: The psychological component of infertility. Fertil Steril 43(3):335–346, 1985 3979571
Markin RD, Zilcha-Mano S: Cultural processes in psychotherapy for perinatal loss: breaking the cultural taboo against perinatal grief. Psychotherapy (Chic) 55(1):20–26, 2018 29565619
Martin JA, Hamilton BE, Osterman MJK, et al: Births: final data for 2018. Natl Vital Stat Rep 68(13):1–47, 2019 32501202
Mascarenhas MN, Flaxman SR, Boerma T, et al: National, regional, and global trends in infertility prevalence since 1990: a systematic analysis of 277 health surveys. PLoS Med 9(12):e1001356, 2012 23271957
Masoumi SZ, Garousian M, Khani S, et al: Comparison of quality of life, sexual satisfaction and marital satisfaction between fertile and infertile couples. Int J Fertil Steril 10(3):290–296, 2016 27695611
Matthiesen SM, Frederiksen Y, Ingerslev HJ, et al: Stress, distress and outcome of assisted reproductive technology (ART): a meta-analysis. Hum Reprod 26(10):2763–2776, 2011 21807816
McCuen-Wurst C, Ruggieri M, Allison KC: Disordered eating and obesity: associations between binge-eating disorder, night-eating syndrome, and weight-related comorbidities. Ann N Y Acad Sci 1411(1):96–105, 2018 29044551
Micali N, dos-Santos-Silva I, De Stavola B, et al: Fertility treatment, twin births, and unplanned pregnancies in women with eating disorders: findings from a population-based birth cohort. BJOG 121(4):408–416, 2014 24206173
Michels TC, Tiu AY: Second trimester pregnancy loss. Am Fam Physician 76(9):1341–1346, 2007 18019878
Mills TA, Ricklesford C, Cooke A, et al: Parents' experiences and expectations of care in pregnancy after stillbirth or neonatal death: a metasynthesis. BJOG 121(8):943–950, 2014 24589119
Milman LW, Senapati S, Sammel MD, et al: Assessing reproductive choices of women and the likelihood of oocyte cryopreservation in the era of elective oocyte freezing. Fertil Steril 107(5):1214.e3–1222.e3, 2017 28476182
Montejo AL, Montejo L, Navarro-Cremades F: Sexual side-effects of antidepressant and antipsychotic drugs. Curr Opin Psychiatry 28(6):418–423, 2015 26382168
Muglu J, Rather H, Arroyo-Manzano D, et al: Risks of stillbirth and neonatal death with advancing gestation at term: a systematic review and meta-analysis of cohort studies of 15 million pregnancies. PLoS Med 16(7):e1002838, 2019 31265456
Mukherjee S, Velez Edwards DR, Baird DD, et al: Risk of miscarriage among black women and white women in a U.S. Prospective Cohort Study. Am J Epidemiol 177(11):1271–1278, 2013 23558353
Murphy FA, Lipp A, Powles DL: Follow-up for improving psychological well being for women after a miscarriage (review). Cochrane Database Syst Rev 3(3):CD008679, 2012 22419336
Murphy SL, Mathews TJ, Martin JA, et al: Annual summary of vital statistics: 2013–2014. Pediatrics 139(6):e20163239, 2017 28814547
Neugebauer R, Kline J, Shrout P, et al: Major depressive disorder in the 6 months after miscarriage. JAMA 277(5):383–388, 1997 9010170

Neugebauer R, Kline J, Markowitz JC, et al: Pilot randomized controlled trial of interpersonal counseling for subsyndromal depression following miscarriage. J Clin Psychiatry 67(8):1299–1304, 2006 16965211
Neugebauer R, Kline J, Bleiberg K, et al: Preliminary open trial of interpersonal counseling for subsyndromal depression following miscarriage. Depress Anxiety 24(3):219–222, 2007 16988939
Nicoloro-SantaBarbara J, Busso C, Moyer A, et al: Just relax and you'll get pregnant? Meta-analysis examining women's emotional distress and the outcome of assisted reproductive technology. Soc Sci Med 213:54–62, 2018 30056327
Nielsen S, Hahlin M: Expectant management of first-trimester spontaneous abortion. Lancet 345(8942):84–86, 1995 7815886
Obst KL, Due C, Oxlad M, et al: Men's grief following pregnancy loss and neonatal loss: a systematic review and emerging theoretical model. BMC Pregnancy Childbirth 20(1):11, 2020 31918681
O'Connor MF, Wellisch DK, Stanton AL, et al: Craving love? Enduring grief activates brain's reward center. Neuroimage 42(2):969–972, 2008 18559294
Oddens BJ, den Tonkelaar I, Nieuwenhuyse H: Psychosocial experiences in women facing fertility problems: a comparative survey. Hum Reprod 14(1):255–261, 1999 10374131
Oliveira CFA, Dos Santos PO, de Oliveira RA, et al: Changes in sexual function and positions in women with severe obesity after bariatric surgery. Sex Med 7(1):80–85, 2019 30509513
Omani-Samani R, Ghaheri A, Navid B, et al: Prevalence of generalized anxiety disorder and its related factors among infertile patients in Iran: a cross-sectional study. Health Qual Life Outcomes 16(1):129, 2018 29914527
Ombelet W, Cooke I, Dyer S, et al: Infertility and the provision of infertility medical services in developing countries. Hum Reprod Update 14(6):605–621, 2008 18820005
Osman A, Bagge CL, Gutierrez PM, et al: The Suicidal Behaviors Questionnaire–Revised (SBQ-R): validation with clinical and nonclinical samples. Assessment 8(4):443–454, 2001
Ozkan ZS, Deveci D, Kumbak B, et al: What is the impact of Th1/Th2 ratio, SOCS3, IL17, and IL35 levels in unexplained infertility? J Reprod Immunol 103:53–58, 2014 24368037
Paslakis G, de Zwaan M: Clinical management of females seeking fertility treatment and of pregnant females with eating disorders. Eur Eat Disord Rev 27(3):215–223, 2019 30848019
Patel A, Sharma PSVN, Kumar P: Role of mental health practitioner in infertility clinics: a review on past, present and future directions. J Hum Reprod Sci 11(3):219–228, 2018 30568350
Patel SS, Bamigboye V: Hyperprolactinaemia. J Obstet Gynaecol 27(5):455–459, 2007 17701788
Pathak UI, Gabrielsen JS, Lipshultz LI: Cutting-edge evaluation of male infertility. Urol Clin North Am 47(2):129–138, 2020 32272984
Peel E: Pregnancy loss in lesbian and bisexual women: an online survey of experiences. Hum Reprod 25(3):721–727, 2010 20023293
Péloquin K, Brassard A, Arpin V, et al: Whose fault is it? Blame predicting psychological adjustment and couple satisfaction in couples seeking fertility treatment. J Psychosom Obstet Gynaecol 39(1):64–72, 2018 28635527
Pentz I, Rados NS: Functional hypothalamic amenorrhea and its psychological correlates: a controlled comparison. J Reprod Infant Psychol 35(2):137–149, 2017 29517358
Peppers LG, Knapp RJ: Maternal reactions to involuntary fetal/infant death. Psychiatry 43(2):155–159, 1980 7189892
Perkins KM, Boulet SL, Jamieson DJ, et al: Trends and outcomes of gestational surrogacy in the United States. Fertil Steril 106(2):435–442.e2, 2016 27087401
Petri E, Palagini L, Bacci O, et al: Maternal-foetal attachment independently predicts the quality of maternal-infant bonding and post-partum psychopathology. J Matern Fetal Neonatal Med 31(23):3153–3159, 2018 28783985
Practice Committee of the American Society for Reproductive Medicine: Diagnostic evaluation of the infertile female: a committee opinion. Fertil Steril 103(6):e44–e50, 2015 25936238
Practice Committee of the American Society for Reproductive Medicine: Role of metformin for ovulation induction in infertile patients with polycystic ovary syndrome (PCOS): a guideline. Fertil Steril 108(3):426–441, 2017 28865539

Practice Committee of the American Society for Reproductive Medicine, Practice Committee of the Society for Assisted Reproductive Technology: Recommendations for practices utilizing gestational carriers: a committee opinion. Fertil Steril 107(2):e3–e10, 2017 28069181
Practice Committees of the American Society for Reproductive Medicine and the Society for Assisted Reproductive Technology: Mature oocyte cryopreservation: a guideline. Fertil Steril 99(1):37–43, 2013 23083924
Prasad S, Tiwari M, Pandey AN, et al: Impact of stress on oocyte quality and reproductive outcome. J Biomed Sci 23:36, 2016 27026099
Price SK: Prevalence and correlates of pregnancy loss history in a national sample of children and families. Matern Child Health J 10(6):489–500, 2006 16802189
Purewal S, Chapman SCE, van den Akker OBA: Depression and state anxiety scores during assisted reproductive treatment are associated with outcome: a meta-analysis. Reprod Biomed Online 36(6):646–657, 2018 29622404
Radloff LS: The CES-D scale: a self report depression scale for research in the general population. Applied Psychological Measurements 1:385–401, 1977
Robinson GE: Pregnancy loss. Best Pract Res Clin Obstet Gynaecol 28(1):169–178, 2014 24047642
Rodino IS, Byrne SM, Sanders KA: Eating disorders in the context of preconception care: fertility specialists' knowledge, attitudes, and clinical practices. Fertil Steril 107(2):494–501, 2017 27889099
Rooney KL, Domar AD: The relationship between stress and infertility. Dialogues Clin Neurosci 20(1):41–47, 2018 29946210
Rosenfeld CS, Shay DA, Vieira-Potter VJ: Cognitive effects of aromatase and possible role in memory disorders. Front Endocrinol (Lausanne) 9:610, 2018 30386297
Ross LE, Grigoriadis S, Mamisashvili L, et al: Selected pregnancy and delivery outcomes after exposure to antidepressant medication: a systematic review and meta-analysis. JAMA Psychiatry 70(4):436–443, 2013 23446732
Rowland A, Goodnight WH: Fetal loss: addressing the evaluation and supporting the emotional needs of parents. J Midwifery Womens Health 54(3):241–248, 2009 19410217
Samuels MH: Psychiatric and cognitive manifestations of hypothyroidism. Curr Opin Endocrinol Diabetes Obes 21(5):377–383, 2014 25122491
Scheidt CE, Hasenburg A, Kunze M, et al: Are individual differences of attachment predicting bereavement outcome after perinatal loss? A prospective cohort study. J Psychosom Res 73(5):375–382, 2012 23062812
Schiff MA, Grossman DC: Adverse perinatal outcomes and risk for postpartum suicide attempt in Washington state, 1987–2001. Pediatrics 118(3):e669–e675, 2006 16950958
Schmidt L, Holstein B, Christensen U, et al: Does infertility cause marital benefit? An epidemiological study of 2250 women and men in fertility treatment. Patient Educ Couns 59(3):244–251, 2005 16310331
Seeman MV: Transient psychosis in women on clomiphene, bromocriptine, domperidone and related endocrine drugs. Gynecol Endocrinol 31(10):751–754, 2015 26291819
Séjourné N, Callahan S, Chabrol H: The utility of a psychological intervention for coping with spontaneous abortion. J Reprod Infant Psychol 28(3):287–296, 2010
Shani C, Yelena S, Reut BK, et al: Suicidal risk among infertile women undergoing in-vitro fertilization: Incidence and risk factors. Psychiatry Res 240:53–59, 2016 27084991
Sharma V, Sommerdyk C, Sharma S: Post-abortion mania. Arch Women Ment Health 16(2):167–169, 2013 23381493
Shear MK: Grief and mourning gone awry: pathway and course of complicated grief. Dialogues Clin Neurosci 14(2):119–128, 2012 22754284
Shirazi TN, Rosinger AY: Reproductive health disparities in the USA: self-reported race/ethnicity predicts age of menarche and live birth ratios, but not infertility. J Racial Ethn Health Disparities May 6, 2020 [Epub ahead of print] 32378159
Shufelt CL, Torbati T, Dutra E: Hypothalamic amenorrhea and the long-term health consequences. Semin Reprod Med 35(3):256–262, 2017 28658709
Siedentopf F, Horstkamp B, Stief G, et al: Clomiphene citrate as a possible cause of a psychotic reaction during infertility treatment. Hum Reprod 12(4):706–707, 1997 9159429

Silvestris E, de Pergola G, Rosania R, et al: Obesity as disruptor of the female fertility. Reprod Biol Endocrinol 16(1):22, 2018 29523133

Sinha P, Garg A: Could clomiphene kindle acute manic episode in a male patient? A case report. Gen Hosp Psychiatry 36(5):549.e5–549.e6, 2014 24950916

Skovlund CW, Mørch LS, Kessing LV, et al: Association of hormonal contraception with depression. JAMA Psychiatry 73(11):1154–1162, 2016 27680324

Smith S: Effects of antipsychotics on sexual and endocrine function in women: implications for clinical practice. J Clin Psychopharmacol 23(3 suppl 1):S27–S32, 2003 12832947

Snellen M, Power J, Blankley G, et al: Pharmacological lactation suppression with D2 receptor agonists and risk of postpartum psychosis: a systematic review. Aust NZ J Obstet Gynaecol 56(4):336–340, 2016 27297803

Sockol LE: A systematic review and meta-analysis of interpersonal psychotherapy for perinatal women. J Affect Disord 232:316–328, 2018 29501991

Söderström-Anttila V, Wennerholm UB, Loft A, et al: Surrogacy: outcomes for surrogate mothers, children and the resulting families-a systematic review. Hum Reprod Update 22(2):260–276, 2016 26454266

Stenbæk DS, Toftager M, Hjordt LV, et al: Mental distress and personality in women undergoing GnRH agonist versus GnRH antagonist protocols for assisted reproductive technology. Hum Reprod 30(1):103–110, 2015 25398970

Stenbæk DS, Budtz-Jørgensen E, Pinborg A, et al: Neuroticism modulates mood responses to pharmacological sex hormone manipulation in healthy women. Psychoneuroendocrinology 99:251–256, 2019 30390443

Stephansson O, Kieler H, Haglund B, et al: Selective serotonin reuptake inhibitors during pregnancy and risk of stillbirth and infant mortality. JAMA 309(1):48–54, 2013 23280224

Stern DN: The Motherhood Constellation: A Unified View of Parent-Infant Psychotherapy. New York, Basic Books, 1995

Storgaard M, Loft A, Bergh C, et al: Obstetric and neonatal complications in pregnancies conceived after oocyte donation: a systematic review and meta-analysis. BJOG 124(4):561–572, 2017 27592694

Tabong PTN, Adongo PB: Understanding the social meaning of infertility and childbearing: a qualitative study of the perception of childbearing and childlessness in Northern Ghana. PLoS One 8(1):e54429, 2013 23342158

Tao P, Coates R, Maycock B: The impact of infertility on sexuality: a literature review. Australas Med J 4(11):620–627, 2011 23386877

Thondam SK, Alusi S, O'Driscoll K, et al: Impulse control disorder in a patient on long-term treatment with bromocriptine for a macroprolactinoma. Clin Neuropharmacol 36(5):170–172, 2013 24045609

Thorn P: Understanding infertility: psychological and social considerations from a counseling perspective. Int J Fertil Steril 3(2):48–51, 2009

Toedter LJ, Lasker JN, Alhadeff JM: The Perinatal Grief Scale: development and initial validation. Am J Orthopsychiatry 58(3):435–449, 1988 3407734

Usadi RS, Merriam KS: On-label and off-label drug use in the treatment of female infertility. Fertil Steril 103(3):583–594, 2015 25660647

Van P, Meleis AI: Coping with grief after involuntary pregnancy loss: perspectives of African American women. J Obstet Gynecol Neonatal Nurs 32(1):28–39, 2003 12570179

van der Linden M, Buckingham K, Farquhar C, et al: Luteal phase support for assisted reproduction cycles. Cochrane Database Syst Rev 2015(7):CD009154, 2015 26148507

Van Heertum K, Rossi B: Alcohol and fertility: how much is too much? Fertil Res Pract 3:10, 2017 28702207

Verkuijlen J, Verhaak C, Nelen WL, et al: Psychological and educational interventions for subfertile men and women. Cochrane Database Syst Rev 31:3, 2016 27031818

Volgsten H, Skoog Svanberg A, Ekselius L, et al: Prevalence of psychiatric disorders in infertile women and men undergoing in vitro fertilization treatment. Hum Reprod 23(9):2056–2063, 2008 18583334

Walton GD, Ross LE, Stewart DE, et al: Decisional conflict among women considering antidepressant medication use in pregnancy. Arch Women Ment Health 17(6):493–501, 2014 25104244
Wang J, Sauer MV: In vitro fertilization (IVF): a review of 3 decades of clinical innovation and technological advancement. Ther Clin Risk Manag 2(4):355–364, 2006 18360648
Wang Y, Chen Q, Wang N, et al: Controlled ovarian stimulation using medroxyprogesterone acetate and hMG in patients with polycystic ovary syndrome treated for IVF: a double-blind randomized crossover clinical trial. Medicine (Baltimore) 95(9):e2939, 2016 26945402
Warnock JK, Bundren JC, Morris DW: Sertraline in the treatment of depression associated with gonadotropin-releasing hormone agonist therapy. Biol Psychiatry 43(6):464–465, 1998 9532352
Wekker V, Karsten MDA, Painter RC, et al: A lifestyle intervention improves sexual function of women with obesity and infertility: a 5 year follow-up of a RCT. PLoS One 13(10):e0205934, 2018 30352059
Wilcox AJ, Weinberg CR, O'Connor JF, et al: Incidence of early loss of pregnancy. N Engl J Med 319(4):189–194, 1988 3393170
Wilcox AJ, Weinberg CR, Baird DD: Timing of sexual intercourse in relation to ovulation: effects on the probability of conception, survival of the pregnancy, and sex of the baby. N Engl J Med 333(23):1517–1521, 1995 7477165
Williams KE: Evaluation and treatment of mood and anxiety disorders in infertility patients and their partners, in Fertility Counseling: Clinical Guide and Case Studies. Edited by Covington S. Cambridge, UK, Cambridge University Press, 2015
Williams KE, Marsh WK, Rasgon NL: Mood disorders and fertility in women: a critical review of the literature and implications for future research. Hum Reprod Update 13(6):607–616, 2007 17895237
Wojnar D: Miscarriage experiences of lesbian couples. J Midwifery Womens Health 52(5):479–485, 2007 17826711
Worden JW: Grief Counseling and Grief Therapy: A Handbook for the Mental Health Practitioner. New York, Springer, 2009
Wosu AC, Valdimarsdóttir U, Shields AE, et al: Correlates of cortisol in human hair: implications for epidemiologic studies on health effects of chronic stress. Ann Epidemiol 23(12):797–811.e2, 2013 24184029
Xu J, Wu Q, Zhang Y, et al: Effect of bariatric surgery on male sexual function: a meta-analysis and systematic review. Sex Med 7(3):270–281, 2019 31302076
Ying L, Wu LH, Loke AY: The effects of psychosocial interventions on the mental health, pregnancy rates, and marital function of infertile couples undergoing in vitro fertilization: a systematic review. J Assist Reprod Genet 33(6):689–701, 2016 26979745
Zaig I, Azem F, Schreiber S, et al: Psychological response and cortisol reactivity to in vitro fertilization treatment in women with a lifetime anxiety or unipolar mood disorder diagnosis. J Clin Psychiatry 74(4):386–392, 2013 23656846
Zegers-Hochschild F, Adamson GD, Dyer S, et al: The international glossary on infertility and fertility care. Hum Reprod 32(9):1786–1801, 2017 29117321
Zhou X, McQueen DB, Schufreider A, et al: Black recipients of oocyte donation experience lower live birth rates compared with white recipients. Reprod Biomed Online 40(5):668–673, 2020 32278673

CHAPTER 6

# Premenstrual Mood Syndromes

Erin Murphy Barzilay, M.D.
Katherine Unverferth, M.D.
Laura Obler, M.D.

The menstrual cycle is the reproductive hormonal transition that occurs most often in women's lives, with the average woman experiencing approximately 480 menstrual periods in a lifetime (minus any periods of pregnancy) (National Health Service 2019). Up to 90% of women report experiencing undesirable premenstrual physical and emotional symptoms that vary from mild to severe and can be classified into three types (Mishell 2005; O'Brien et al. 2011).

First, for most women, these symptoms take the form of the commonly known premenstrual syndrome (PMS). PMS is a pattern of physical and emotional/behavioral symptoms that occurs in the 5 days prior to menses in at least three consecutive cycles and resolves with menstruation. Affective symptoms of PMS include depression, angry outbursts, irritability, anxiety, confusion, and social withdrawal, and physical symptoms include breast tenderness, abdominal bloating, headache, and swelling of the extremities (American College of Obstetricians and Gynecologists 2014). Women can have emotional symptoms, physical symptoms, or both. Although it affects most women, no formal psychiatric diagnosis is associated with PMS.

Second, in the case of women with psychiatric illness, PMS symptoms may take the form of a premenstrual exacerbation (PME) of their underlying illness (Haley et al. 2013). In PME, which is not well studied, women have a luteal-phase worsening of their typical affective symptoms; more than 50% of women with a mood disorder experience premenstrual worsening (Haley et al. 2013).

Finally, a small minority of women (with or without other psychiatric illness) may meet criteria for premenstrual dysphoric disorder (PMDD), which is the primary focus of this chapter. From a historical standpoint, the formal recognition of PMDD is in its infancy, having joined the DSM diagnostic class of depressive disorders in 2013 with the publication of DSM-5 (American Psychiatric Association 2013). Previously, patients with PMDD were diagnosed with a mood disorder not otherwise specified or, prior to that, "late luteal phase dysphoric disorder." Fortunately, what has previously been a potentially overlooked condition is now a formal diagnosis and an area of active research and study. Because PMDD has been so recently accepted as a formal diagnosis, much of the existing evidence mixes individuals with PMS and those with PMDD and may sometimes merge either of these with PME. In this chapter, we attempt to indicate when evidence is specific to one syndrome or the other whenever possible, while acknowledging that there are many gaps in the literature and opportunities for further research that may better elucidate the differences among these syndromes.

## Epidemiology

Premenstrual disorders, by definition, occur only in women who experience a menstrual cycle. They therefore do not occur in those who have not undergone menarche, are pregnant, or are postmenopausal. Women who have had a hysterectomy without oophorectomy may continue to experience premenstrual symptoms because they continue to ovulate and experience hormonal change. Transgender men may also continue to experience some premenstrual symptoms, either prior to initiation of gender-affirming therapy or even after, because a delay often occurs between the initiation of testosterone and the cessation of menses (and some individuals may continue to ovulate) (Pradhan and Gomez-Lobo 2019).

Although many studies on the incidence and prevalence of PMDD and associated risk factors have been published, their results vary. Reasons for this variance in findings include differing symptom criteria for diagnosis of PMS and PMDD (ranging from more inclusive to more exclusive criteria), differing thresholds of the severity and timing of symptoms, and differing study designs (O'Brien et al. 2011). Many studies measuring prevalence are conducted via retrospective data collection, a method that appears to measure the pattern of symptoms reasonably well when compared with prospective studies; this method, however, introduces recall bias that can overestimate the number and intensity of symptoms (Rapkin et al. 1988; Rubinow and Roy-Byrne 1984).

### Rates/Incidence

Premenstrual symptoms are quite common in menstruating women, with an estimated 80%–95% of women experiencing some physical or emotional symptoms (O'Brien et al. 2011). Far fewer women have symptoms severe enough to meet DSM-5 criteria for diagnosis of PMDD (Box 6–1). According to studies that have collected prospective data in women, PMS has an estimated prevalence of 20%–30% (Borenstein et al. 2007; Qiao et al. 2012), and a meta-analysis of 15 prevalence studies (covering both prospective and retrospective data collection) reported a pooled prevalence of 47.8% (95% CI 32.6–62.9). PMDD, by contrast, is much less common, with an estimated prevalence of 1.3%–7.7% (Cohen et al. 2002; Gehlert et al. 2009; Hussein Shehadeh and Hamdan-Mansour 2018). In a large community sample investigation, the Harvard Study of

Moods and Cycles studied 4,164 women ages 36–44 years, of whom 513 agreed to participate in prospective evaluation with daily records over a menstrual cycle. PMDD was confirmed in 6.4% of women (Cohen et al. 2002). Both PMS and PMDD occur in menstruating women of all ages; one retrospective study showed that onset is near the age of menarche in most studies (Steiner et al. 2011b). Adolescents appear to have PMS and PMDD at rates similar to those of adults (Parker et al. 2010; Steiner et al. 2011b).

## Box 6–1. DSM-5 Criteria for Premenstrual Dysphoric Disorder

A. In the majority of menstrual cycles, at least five symptoms must be present in the final week before the onset of menses, start to *improve* within a few days after the onset of menses, and become *minimal* or absent in the week postmenses.

B. One (or more) of the following symptoms must be present:

1. Marked affective lability (e.g., mood swings; feeling suddenly sad or tearful, or increased sensitivity to rejection).
2. Marked irritability or anger or increased interpersonal conflicts.
3. Marked depressed mood, feelings of hopelessness, or self-deprecating thoughts.
4. Marked anxiety, tension, and/or feelings of being keyed up or on edge.

C. One (or more) of the following symptoms must additionally be present, to reach a total of *five* symptoms when combined with symptoms from Criterion B above.

1. Decreased interest in usual activities (e.g., work, school, friends, hobbies).
2. Subjective difficulty in concentration.
3. Lethargy, easy fatigability, or marked lack of energy.
4. Marked change in appetite; overeating; or specific food cravings.
5. Hypersomnia or insomnia.
6. A sense of being overwhelmed or out of control.
7. Physical symptoms such as breast tenderness or swelling, joint or muscle pain, a sensation of "bloating," or weight gain.

**Note:** The symptoms in Criteria A–C must have been met for most menstrual cycles that occurred in the preceding year.

D. The symptoms are associated with clinically significant distress or interference with work, school, usual social activities, or relationships with others (e.g., avoidance of social activities; decreased productivity and efficiency at work, school, or home).

E. The disturbance is not merely an exacerbation of the symptoms of another disorder, such as major depressive disorder, panic disorder, persistent depressive disorder (dysthymia), or a personality disorder (although it may co-occur with any of these disorders).

F. Criterion A should be confirmed by prospective daily ratings during at least two symptomatic cycles. (**Note:** The diagnosis may be made provisionally prior to this confirmation.)

G. The symptoms are not attributable to the physiological effects of a substance (e.g., a drug of abuse, a medication, other treatment) or another medical condition (e.g., hyperthyroidism).

*Source.* Reprinted from American Psychiatric Association: *Diagnostic and Statistical Manual of Mental Disorders,* 5th Edition. Arlington, VA, 2013, pp. 171–172. 

PMS and PMDD occur in menstruating people worldwide (de Carvalho et al. 2018; Hong et al. 2012; Hussein Shehadeh and Hamdan-Mansour 2018; Padhy et al. 2015; Qiao et al. 2012). Studies conducted in some countries report much higher prevalence than studies in the United States. For instance, one study in Jordan reported a prevalence of PMS of 92.3% (Hussein Shehadeh and Hamdan-Mansour 2018), and another study in Brazil reported a prevalence of PMDD of 17.6% (de Carvalho et al. 2018). Making conclusions about varying prevalence in differing countries is challenging due to differences in PMS and PMDD definitions and study methodologies. PME also affects a large majority of women with mood disorders, from 50% to 66% (Haley et al. 2013; Kornstein et al. 2005).

## Risk Factors

Most studies that identify risk factors for PMDD are either cross-sectional or post hoc in design, which limits their ability to determine causal links to the development of PMDD. Despite these limitations, some interesting associations have been observed. The development of premenstrual disorders has a heritable component, with monozygotic twins having more overlap of PMS symptoms than dizygotic twins (Condon 1993). One modeling study suggested that genetic factors account for 95% of the development of PMS (Jahanfar et al. 2011). PMDD and PMS both appear to occur at higher rates in white women than in Black women (Pilver et al. 2011a). Researchers have investigated numerous candidate genes, often without finding a connection; those that have at least one positive finding include brain derived neurotrophic factor (*BDNF*), estrogen receptors 1 and 2 (*ESR1*, *ESR2*), and the serotonin transporter (*SERT*) (Comasco et al. 2014; Dhingra et al. 2007; Gingnell et al. 2010; Huo et al. 2007; Marrocco et al. 2020; Praschak-Rieder et al. 2002; Takeo et al. 2005; Yen et al. 2014). Recent evidence has also implicated ESC/E(Z) complex genes (an ovarian steroid-regulated gene silencing complex), with more than half the genes in this complex being overexpressed in women with PMDD when compared with healthy control subjects (Dubey et al. 2017).

There is a positive correlation between increasing PMS scores and increased prevalence of metabolic syndrome (Hashemi et al. 2016). This may be related to adiposity, as one study showed a linear relationship between BMI at baseline and the risk of developing PMS (1 kg/m$^2$ resulted in 3% increased risk of developing PMS). In that sample, subjects with BMI ≥27.5 kg/m$^2$ had a significantly higher risk of PMS (Bertone-Johnson et al. 2010).

Certain lifestyle choices are also associated with risk of premenstrual disorders. Diet may play a role; high-potassium diets may increase risk, whereas diets high in nonheme iron, zinc, thiamine, and riboflavin may lower risk (Chocano-Bedoya et al. 2011, 2013). Nicotine use increases the risk (Bertone-Johnson et al. 2010; Cohen et al. 2002). Women with lower education status have higher rates of premenstrual disorders, and working from home (vs. outside the home) is associated with lower rates of PMS (Cohen et al. 2002).

Several studies have investigated the relationship between history of traumatic events, PTSD, and premenstrual disorders. These studies have varying results, but many have found a positive correlation between trauma and increased risk of developing PMS or PMDD. Having experienced childhood abuse appears to increase the risk of PMS (Bertone-Johnson et al. 2014). Another study showed that a history of trauma, either with or without accompanying PTSD, increases the odds of PMDD (Pilver et al. 2011b), but not all studies have found the same correlation (Segebladh et al. 2011). One

**TABLE 6–1. Common screening tools for premenstrual dysphoric disorder**

| Screening tool | Number of items |
|---|---|
| **Retrospective** | |
| Premenstrual Assessment Form (pre-DSM-5) (Halbreich et al. 1982) | 96 (short version, 10) |
| Premenstrual Symptoms Screening Tool (Steiner et al. 2003) | 19 |
| **Prospective** | |
| Daily Record of Severity of Problems (Endicott et al. 2006) | 21 |
| Carolina Premenstrual Assessment Scoring System (Eisenlohr-Moul et al. 2017) | 24 |

study, which followed participants prospectively for several years, showed that having experienced a traumatic event increased the odds of developing PMDD during the time period of the study (Perkonigg et al. 2004).

## Screening

Multiple screening and symptom inventories have been developed over the past several decades to assist in research, evaluation, and treatment of PMDD (Table 6–1) (Bosman et al. 2016; Hall and Steiner 2015; Haywood et al. 2002). Retrospective reports provide the most time-efficient method for screening, but accurate diagnosis is based on prospective symptom tracking tools. The Premenstrual Assessment Form (Halbreich et al. 1982), one of the oldest methods, is a retrospective self-report questionnaire that has demonstrated validity and reliability. The original 96-item form is lengthy and time consuming; a shortened 10-item version has also been shown to be reliable and valid (Allen et al. 1991). The Premenstrual Symptoms Screening Tool (Steiner et al. 2003) is another short 19-item retrospective tool that can be used in both adults and adolescents with PMDD. The 21-item Daily Record of Severity of Problems (DRSP; Endicott et al. 2006) was developed to aid in the diagnosis and evaluation of DSM-IV PMDD (included in DSM-IV's "Criteria Sets and Axes Provided for Further Study"; American Psychiatric Association 1994). The DRSP is the most widely used screening and diagnostic tool and should be prospectively completed for at least two consecutive menstrual cycles. It includes 11 of the symptoms of the DSM-5 criteria for PMDD, which are rated on a severity scale from 1 (none at all) to 6 (extreme). The Carolina Premenstrual Assessment Scoring System (Eisenlohr-Moul et al. 2017) is a new diagnostic tool based on DSM-5 PMDD criteria that uses items from the DRSP to create a diagnostic algorithm; this standardized method of scoring can be completed manually or via computer and is available for SAS and Excel macros.

Other older mood rating scales that have been used for the diagnosis of PMDD include the Calendar of Premenstrual Experiences (Mortola et al. 1990), the Visual Analogue Scales for Premenstrual Mood Symptoms (Steiner and Streiner 2005), and the Premenstrual Tension Syndrome Rating Scales (Steiner et al. 2011a). Many cellphone symptom trackers also exist, but these are not validated screening tools.

TABLE 6–2. **Diagnostic criteria for premenstrual syndrome**

| Affective symptoms | Somatic symptoms |
|---|---|
| Angry outbursts | Abdominal bloating |
| Anxiety | Breast tenderness or swelling |
| Confusion | Headache |
| Depression | Joint or muscle pain |
| Irritability | Swelling of extremities |
| Social withdrawal | Weight gain |

Patient must report at least one of the symptoms above from each category during the 5 days before menses in each of her three previous menstrual cycles.

Symptoms must be relieved within 4 days of the onset of menses, without recurrence until at least day 13 of the cycle.

Symptoms must be present in the absence of pharmacological treatment, hormone ingestion, or drug or alcohol use.

Patient must exhibit functional impairment in social, academic, or work performance.

*Source.* Adapted from American College of Obstetricians and Gynecologists 2014.

# Clinical Features

## Diagnostic Criteria

PMS is not listed in DSM-5; however, a useful definition is provided by the American College of Obstetricians and Gynecologists (ACOG) (Table 6–2). PMS is defined as more than one physical or emotional symptom associated with either economic or social dysfunction occurring during 5 days before menses in three consecutive cycles.

The DSM-5 diagnostic criteria for PMDD (see Box 6–1 earlier in chapter) emphasize mood symptoms that cause functional impairment. To meet criteria, the person must have five of these symptoms, at least one of which is a mood symptom. Symptoms must be accompanied by either behavioral or physical symptoms that begin during the luteal phase of the menstrual cycle, start to decrease after menstrual flow, and are minimal or absent during the early follicular phase (American Psychiatric Association 2013).

An accurate diagnosis of PMDD requires prospective mood charting of at least one but preferably two menstrual cycles. A mood chart consistent with PMS or PMDD will demonstrate symptoms that begin in the premenstrual period and resolve at the beginning or shortly after the onset of menses. Ongoing symptoms during the follicular phase that worsen during the premenstrual phase are more consistent with the PME of another disorder, such as depression or anxiety. Although no consensus exists regarding the necessary percentage of change, a 30%–50% change in symptoms between luteal and follicular phases of the cycle is generally considered an important diagnostic guideline (Hall and Steiner 2015).

## Clinical Presentation

Ms. K is a 40-year-old married lesbian woman with no significant past medical or gynecological history who presents with complaints of monthly "outbursts" that are interfering with her relationship with her partner. She says that she has very regular menstrual cycles, and in the week before the onset of her menstrual flow, she feels like she is constantly going to "explode." She says that "the littlest things" annoy her, such as her wife not putting her clothes in the hamper, and these same things are easily overlooked earlier in the month. She says she has trouble at work during this week every month because she is easily annoyed by coworkers and has trouble concentrating. She has been put on probation at work as a result of one of her outbursts. She feels "like a train hit her" and wants to sleep for longer than 10 hours a day. Ms. K blames her steady weight gain over the years on this time of her cycle because she craves carbohydrates and always eats more cookies before her menstrual flow. Her mood is consistently low, and although she has never been actively suicidal, she has thought often in the luteal phase that she would be better off dead.

The physician asks Ms. K to chart her symptoms prospectively over two menstrual cycles using the DRSP. Her daily symptom ratings, ranging from 1 to 6, are shown in Table 6–3. The physician concludes that Ms. K meets criteria for PMDD and prescribes a low-dose selective serotonin reuptake inhibitor (SSRI) for luteal-phase dosing.

PMDD is a cyclical disorder in which symptoms begin after ovulation and remit early in the follicular phase of the menstrual cycle. The cardinal mood features include marked mood lability, irritability, anxiety, or tension (feeling "keyed up or on edge"), feelings of depression, and feeling "overwhelmed" and hopeless (American College of Obstetricians and Gynecologists 2014; American Psychiatric Association 2013). Women with PMDD complain of many of the vegetative symptoms seen in a major depressive episode, including changes in sleep (hypersomnia or insomnia), loss of energy, and problems with concentration. Hyperphagia in the luteal phase is a common symptom in PMDD, and women may have specific food cravings, often for highly sweet foods (Reed et al. 2008; Yen et al. 2018). Women with PMS also have distress from the emotional and physical symptoms that occur premenstrually, but they do not have as many symptoms as women with PMDD (i.e., more than five symptoms, including at least one emotional symptom). In addition, women with PMS may have physical symptoms alone. Women with PME may have symptoms during the premenstrual period that are similar to those in women with PMDD, but they also have symptoms outside the luteal phase. For women with a mood disorder whose symptoms in the premenstrual period differ in severity but not quality from those in other periods, PME is likely. In this case, fully treating the underlying mood disorder may also treat the PME (Osborne and Payne 2017). In contrast, women whose premenstrual symptoms are markedly different in quality from their symptoms at other times are likely to have PMDD.

## Course and Prognosis

PMDD is a stable condition that has low overall spontaneous remission rates. One study reported <10% remission over 2 years (Wittchen et al. 2002). PMDD does not occur during anovulatory cycles or pregnancy but may return in the postpartum period when women resume menstrual cycles (Takayama et al. 2020). For some women the disorder begins in adolescence, whereas for others it may begin later in adulthood.

**TABLE 6–3. Daily Record of Severity of Problems for the case of Ms. K**

| Symptoms | Day of menstrual cycle (Day 1 should be the start of the menstrual period) | | | | | | | | | | | | | | | | | | | | | | | | | | | |
|---|---|---|---|---|---|---|---|---|---|---|---|---|---|---|---|---|---|---|---|---|---|---|---|---|---|---|---|---|
| | 1 | 2 | 3 | 4 | 5 | 6 | 7 | 8 | 9 | 10 | 11 | 12 | 13 | 14 | 15 | 16 | 17 | 18 | 19 | 20 | 21 | 22 | 23 | 24 | 25 | 26 | 27 | 28 |
| Felt depressed, sad, down, or blue | 3 | 2 | 1 | 1 | 1 | 1 | 1 | 1 | 1 | 1 | 1 | 1 | 1 | 2 | 1 | 2 | 4 | 3 | 5 | 4 | 5 | 4 | 4 | 5 | 5 | 4 | 5 | 6 |
| Felt hopeless | 2 | 1 | 1 | 1 | 1 | 1 | 1 | 1 | 1 | 1 | 1 | 1 | 1 | 1 | 1 | 2 | 3 | 5 | 4 | 6 | 5 | 5 | 6 | 5 | 6 | 6 | 6 | 6 |
| Felt worthless or guilty | 2 | 1 | 1 | 1 | 1 | 1 | 1 | 1 | 1 | 1 | 1 | 1 | 1 | 2 | 2 | 3 | 5 | 4 | 5 | 6 | 5 | 5 | 6 | 5 | 6 | 6 | 4 | 5 |
| Felt anxious, tense, keyed up, or on edge | 3 | 2 | 1 | 1 | 1 | 1 | 1 | 1 | 1 | 1 | 1 | 1 | 1 | 2 | 1 | 3 | 5 | 4 | 6 | 5 | 4 | 6 | 4 | 6 | 5 | 5 | 5 | 6 |
| Had mood swings (e.g., suddenly felt sad or tearful) | 3 | 1 | 1 | 1 | 1 | 1 | 1 | 1 | 1 | 1 | 1 | 1 | 1 | 1 | 2 | 4 | 3 | 5 | 4 | 6 | 5 | 5 | 4 | 6 | 5 | 4 | 6 | 5 |
| Was more sensitive to rejection or feelings were more easily hurt | 2 | 1 | 1 | 1 | 1 | 1 | 1 | 1 | 1 | 1 | 1 | 1 | 1 | 2 | 2 | 3 | 2 | 5 | 4 | 5 | 3 | 5 | 6 | 5 | 5 | 5 | 4 | 5 |
| Felt angry, irritable | 3 | 2 | 1 | 1 | 2 | 1 | 1 | 1 | 1 | 1 | 1 | 1 | 1 | 2 | 2 | 2 | 3 | 4 | 5 | 4 | 5 | 5 | 5 | 6 | 6 | 6 | 6 | 6 |
| Had conflicts or problems with people | 3 | 1 | 1 | 1 | 1 | 1 | 1 | 1 | 1 | 1 | 1 | 1 | 1 | 1 | 2 | 1 | 3 | 4 | 3 | 5 | 5 | 5 | 6 | 5 | 6 | 6 | 5 | 5 |
| Had less interest in usual activities (e.g., work, school, friends, hobbies) | 2 | 2 | 1 | 1 | 1 | 1 | 1 | 1 | 1 | 1 | 1 | 1 | 1 | 1 | 2 | 1 | 3 | 4 | 3 | 4 | 5 | 3 | 4 | 5 | 4 | 4 | 5 | 4 |
| Had difficulty concentrating | 1 | 1 | 1 | 1 | 1 | 1 | 1 | 1 | 1 | 1 | 1 | 1 | 1 | 1 | 2 | 3 | 2 | 4 | 3 | 4 | 5 | 5 | 4 | 5 | 4 | 5 | 6 | 5 |
| Felt lethargic, tired, fatigued, or had a lack of energy | 2 | 1 | 1 | 1 | 1 | 1 | 1 | 1 | 1 | 1 | 1 | 1 | 1 | 1 | 1 | 3 | 2 | 3 | 4 | 4 | 3 | 4 | 3 | 4 | 4 | 4 | 4 | 3 |
| Had increased appetite or overate | 1 | 1 | 1 | 1 | 1 | 1 | 1 | 1 | 1 | 1 | 1 | 1 | 1 | 1 | 1 | 1 | 1 | 4 | 5 | 4 | 3 | 3 | 4 | 3 | 4 | 4 | 3 | 5 |

**TABLE 6–3. Daily Record of Severity of Problems for the case of Ms. K *(continued)***

| | Day of menstrual cycle (Day 1 should be the start of the menstrual period) | | | | | | | | | | | | | | | | | | | | | | | | | | | |
|---|---|---|---|---|---|---|---|---|---|---|---|---|---|---|---|---|---|---|---|---|---|---|---|---|---|---|---|---|
| **Symptoms** | **1** | **2** | **3** | **4** | **5** | **6** | **7** | **8** | **9** | **10** | **11** | **12** | **13** | **14** | **15** | **16** | **17** | **18** | **19** | **20** | **21** | **22** | **23** | **24** | **25** | **26** | **27** | **28** |
| Had cravings for specific foods | 1 | 1 | 1 | 1 | 1 | 1 | 1 | 1 | 1 | 1 | 1 | 1 | 1 | 1 | 1 | 1 | 2 | 3 | 2 | 3 | 4 | 4 | 3 | 4 | 3 | 4 | 4 | 5 |
| Slept more, took naps, found it hard to get up when intended | 1 | 1 | 1 | 1 | 1 | 1 | 1 | 1 | 1 | 1 | 1 | 1 | 1 | 1 | 2 | 1 | 3 | 2 | 3 | 4 | 4 | 4 | 3 | 4 | 3 | 4 | 5 | 3 |
| Had trouble getting to sleep or staying asleep | 1 | 1 | 1 | 1 | 1 | 1 | 1 | 1 | 1 | 1 | 1 | 1 | 1 | 2 | 3 | 3 | 4 | 5 | 6 | 5 | 6 | 6 | 5 | 6 | 5 | 6 | 6 | 5 |
| Felt overwhelmed or that I could not cope | 2 | 1 | 1 | 1 | 1 | 1 | 1 | 1 | 1 | 1 | 1 | 1 | 1 | 3 | 2 | 3 | 4 | 6 | 6 | 6 | 6 | 5 | 6 | 5 | 6 | 6 | 5 | 5 |
| Felt out of control | 1 | 1 | 1 | 1 | 1 | 1 | 1 | 1 | 1 | 1 | 1 | 1 | 1 | 3 | 3 | 5 | 6 | 4 | 6 | 5 | 6 | 5 | 6 | 6 | 6 | 6 | 5 | 6 |
| Had breast tenderness | 2 | 2 | 2 | 1 | 1 | 1 | 1 | 1 | 1 | 1 | 1 | 1 | 1 | 1 | 1 | 1 | 1 | 1 | 1 | 1 | 1 | 2 | 3 | 4 | 5 | 5 | 6 | 5 |
| Had breast swelling, felt bloated, or had weight gain | 2 | 2 | 2 | 1 | 1 | 1 | 1 | 1 | 1 | 1 | 1 | 1 | 1 | 1 | 1 | 1 | 1 | 1 | 1 | 1 | 1 | 2 | 3 | 5 | 4 | 5 | 5 | 4 |
| Had headache | 2 | 2 | 1 | 1 | 2 | 1 | 1 | 1 | 1 | 1 | 1 | 1 | 1 | 1 | 1 | 1 | 1 | 1 | 1 | 1 | 1 | 2 | 2 | 2 | 3 | 3 | 4 | 3 |
| Had joint or muscle pain | 2 | 2 | 1 | 1 | 1 | 1 | 1 | 1 | 1 | 1 | 1 | 1 | 1 | 1 | 1 | 1 | 1 | 1 | 1 | 1 | 1 | 2 | 2 | 2 | 4 | 3 | 4 | 3 |
| At work, school, home, or in daily routine, at least one of the problems noted above caused reduced productivity or inefficiency | 1 | 1 | 1 | 1 | 1 | 1 | 1 | 1 | 1 | 1 | 1 | 1 | 1 | 1 | 1 | 1 | 2 | 1 | 2 | 3 | 3 | 5 | 6 | 5 | 4 | 5 | 4 | 5 |

**TABLE 6–3. Daily Record of Severity of Problems for the case of Ms. K *(continued)***

| | Day of menstrual cycle (Day 1 should be the start of the menstrual period) | | | | | | | | | | | | | | | | | | | | | | | | | | | |
|---|---|---|---|---|---|---|---|---|---|---|---|---|---|---|---|---|---|---|---|---|---|---|---|---|---|---|---|---|
| **Symptoms** | **1** | **2** | **3** | **4** | **5** | **6** | **7** | **8** | **9** | **10** | **11** | **12** | **13** | **14** | **15** | **16** | **17** | **18** | **19** | **20** | **21** | **22** | **23** | **24** | **25** | **26** | **27** | **28** |
| At least one of the problems noted above interfered with hobbies or social activities (e.g., avoided or did less) | 1 | 1 | 1 | 1 | 1 | 1 | 1 | 1 | 1 | 1 | 1 | 1 | 1 | 1 | 1 | 1 | 2 | 1 | 1 | 3 | 5 | 4 | 6 | 4 | 5 | 5 | 3 | 5 |
| At least one of the problems noted above interfered with relationships with others | 1 | 1 | 1 | 1 | 1 | 1 | 1 | 1 | 1 | 1 | 1 | 1 | 1 | 1 | 1 | 1 | 1 | 2 | 3 | 3 | 4 | 4 | 5 | 6 | 6 | 4 | 4 | 5 |
| Menstrual flow: H=heavy; M=medium, L=light or spotting; leave blank for no bleeding | H | H | M | M | L | L | | | | | | | | | | | | | | | | | | | | | | |

More studies investigating the course of PMDD over the reproductive lifespan are needed; however, cross-sectional studies of PMDD during perimenopause do exist, and it is clear that the disorder persists through this time period (Chung et al. 2014). PMS and PMDD may worsen during the perimenopausal transition, when cyclicity becomes disjointed (Baker and O'Brien 2012; Pinkerton et al. 2010). Notably, women with a history of PMDD also appear to be at greater risk for other mood disorders during the perimenopausal transition (Freeman and Lewis 2004). PMDD ceases after natural, surgical, and medically induced menopause, as long as no add-back hormonal replacement is utilized (Reid 2012; Wyatt et al. 2004).

Comorbidity with other psychiatric illnesses is high in individuals with premenstrual disorders. In one study, only 26.5% of women with PMDD in a community sample did *not* have another psychiatric diagnosis (Wittchen et al. 2002). Comorbid affective disorders are common in women with PMDD; comorbid major depression rates range from 30% to 50% (Endicott 1993). Comorbidity of PMDD and bipolar disorder is also common, ranging from 10% to 27% depending on study populations and methodologies (Teatero et al. 2014; Wittchen et al. 2002). Women with comorbid PMDD and bipolar disorder have an earlier onset of bipolar disorder, increased frequency of mood cycling, and more lifetime depressive episodes (Slyepchenko et al. 2017; Wittchen et al. 2002). Suicide risk may also be affected by PMDD diagnosis; one study found that women admitted to the psychiatric hospital for a suicide attempt were more likely to have PMDD (Shams-Alizadeh et al. 2018).

Anxiety disorders also are common in women with PMDD. Comorbid panic disorder is common, occurring in 25% of women with PMDD, whereas rates of comorbid OCD range from 11% to 13% and social phobia from 19% to 23% (Kim et al. 2004). Rates of comorbid generalized anxiety disorder are more varied across studies, ranging from 4% to 38% (Kim et al. 2004). Nicotine and alcohol use are also common (Fernández et al. 2019a; Hong et al. 2012; Marks et al. 1994). PMDD is also highly comorbid with bulimia nervosa. In a large epidemiological study of 8,693 participants, women with PMDD were seven times as likely as women without PMDD to have a comorbid diagnosis of bulimia nervosa (OR 7.2; 95% CI 2.3–22.4) (Nobles et al. 2016). Due to limitations in study design, it is unclear whether PMDD makes individuals more susceptible to developing comorbid psychiatric disorders (e.g., major depression) or vice versa. However, having premenstrual depressive symptoms appears to increase the risk of having a future major depressive episode (Graze et al. 1990).

Untreated PMDD has a significant impact on a woman's life, and the burden of illness is related both to the number of days per cycle that she suffers and to the severity of her symptoms. Women with PMDD report impairment in interpersonal relationships and roles, including more hours absent from work and decreased productivity (Dahlgren and Qvigstad 2018). When one adds up the days a woman with PMDD suffers over her reproductive lifetime, it totals approximately 3.8 years (Halbreich et al. 2003).

## Differential Diagnosis

Ms. L is a 26-year-old woman referred to a psychiatrist by the local inpatient unit, where she has been on a 72-hour involuntary hold after an overdose of an SSRI. She had been prescribed the medication by her gynecologist after she complained of PMS. At the time of the overdose, she had taken the medication for 4 days and was experiencing insomnia, extreme anxiety, and irritability, despite being at cycle day 10. For these 4 days, she

**TABLE 6–4. Differential diagnosis for premenstrual dysphoric disorder**

| |
|---|
| Bipolar disorder |
| Borderline personality disorder |
| Major depressive disorder |
| Premenstrual exacerbation of major depressive disorder |
| Premenstrual syndrome |
| Thyroid disorders |

had slept only a few hours each night and felt "revved up" and full of energy. The day of the overdose, she had gone to the store to buy three new shelves and had stayed up until 3 A.M. assembling them. She says that she was so discouraged that the medication was not helping her and "seemed to make her worse" that she impulsively decided to end her life by taking the entire bottle.

Ms. L states that she has had severe depressive episodes since her teenage years, which interfered with her ability to complete high school. When depressed, she would be unable to get out of bed, would sleep 14 hours per day, and had excessive appetite with weight gain. The loss of energy was extreme, and she had problems with concentration. During the depressive episodes, she had suicidal ideation and "came close" at times to driving her car off the road.

Ms. L's menstrual cycles began when she was 12 years old and have been regular almost from the beginning. She says that her depressive symptoms worsen "at the end of every month" and that that is when her suicidal ideation increases. She describes having had a difficult childhood because her mother had bipolar disorder and was "constantly hospitalized" for suicidal ideation and suicide attempts. She states that she has previously avoided going to a psychiatrist because "I don't want to be like my mother," but she told her gynecologist about her mood worsening before her menstrual cycle and her suicidal ideation, and the doctor prescribed an SSRI.

A diagnosis of PMDD requires a careful psychiatric, gynecological, and medical history. It is crucial to differentiate a primary diagnosis of PMDD from that of another mood disorder with premenstrual exacerbation (Table 6–4), and especially from bipolar disorder, as well as from other cycling mood disorders. Because certain symptoms such as sleep and energy disturbance, irritability, and dysphoria may occur not only in PMDD but also in other disorders with a cyclical course, caution must be exercised in the appropriate prescription of psychotropic medications. For example, SSRI antidepressants are first-line treatments for PMDD but not for bipolar disorder. This is further discussed later in "Treatment Strategies." Finally, certain personality disorders, such as borderline personality disorder, may also present with variability and what may appear to be a cyclical nature in the severity of symptoms; therefore, careful attention is also recommended for appropriate diagnosis and subsequent referrals to psychotherapy resources. Prospective mood charting is necessary to confirm that the symptoms always begin in the luteal phase and remit in the follicular phase. Women with bipolar disorder will have sustained periods of depression that are not confined to the luteal phase. Women with bipolar I disorder may also have frank mania and psychosis, neither of which is present in PMDD. Cyclical premenstrual psychosis is a rare disorder that is believed to be part of the bipolar spectrum (Brockington 2011).

It is also important to differentiate PMDD from PME of major depression. Again, mood charts are critical to make the correct diagnosis. In other primary mood disorders, the depressive symptoms will be found in the follicular phase as well as the luteal phase. PME is common, as demonstrated by the fact that 66% of women in the large Sequenced Treatment Alternatives to Relieve Depression study (Haley et al. 2013) reported PME of depression at baseline, and this condition was associated with longer index episodes, more medical conditions, more anxious features, and shorter time to relapse than was major depressive disorder without PME.

Abnormalities in thyroid function may contribute to symptoms of depression, anxiety, and irritability, similar to those seen in PMDD. Because thyroid disorders are common in reproductive-age women, thyroid function should be tested in women presenting for a PMDD assessment. In the presence of abnormal test results, the thyroid condition should be treated as a first step, followed by prospective assessment of mood and physical symptoms to determine whether the woman has a PMDD diagnosis independent of the thyroid condition. Note, however, that thyroid dysfunction alone would not explain the cyclicity of symptoms seen in PMDD (i.e., symptoms that occur solely in the luteal phase) (Yonkers and Simoni 2018).

### Sociodemographic Considerations

PMDD appears to be more common among white women in the United States than among other groups. In one large study of 2,590 English-speaking premenopausal American women (Pilver et al. 2011a), ages 18–40 years, the prevalence of PMDD was 2.9% in Black women and 4.4% in white women. There is little research on variations in prevalence among people of different ethnicities in the United States.

Notably, most studies on premenstrual disorders have included individuals who self-identify as women. Little information is available regarding PMDD in persons who identify as male or nonbinary. As described earlier (see "Epidemiology"), PMDD can only occur in individuals who are having menstrual cycles (with or without menstrual bleeding), but this group could include individuals who identify as male or nonbinary. Studies show that individuals who have undergone bilateral oophorectomy, cycle suppression with gonadotropin-releasing hormone (GnRH) agonists, and hormone (e.g., estrogen) replacement can have improvement or remission of premenstrual symptoms (Reid 2012; Schmidt et al. 2017; Studd 2014). This may be relevant in future investigations of individuals with nonfemale gender identification who experience PMDD.

## Pathophysiology

### Biological Factors

Sex steroids are believed to be intimately involved in the etiopathology of PMDD. Because PMDD does not occur before menarche or after menopause, exposure to cycling levels of sex steroids is obligatory. In women with PMDD, symptoms are not precipitated by an excess or deficit of a specific hormone but, rather, by the individual's response to fluctuating levels of sex hormones. This has been clearly demonstrated in the literature; women who have undergone ovarian suppression have reemergence of their PMS or PMDD symptoms when add-back hormone is utilized but not once steady-state levels have been reached (Schmidt et al. 2017).

Exposure to or withdrawal from allopregnanolone may contribute to PMS or PMDD symptoms in a certain subset of women. Allopregnanolone (along with its breakdown products allopregnanediol and 3β, 5α-tetrahydroprogesterone) is a downstream neuroactive metabolite of progesterone and is active at the $GABA_A$ receptor (Figure 6–1). The GABA system is the major inhibitory system in the CNS. Positive modulators active at the $GABA_A$ receptor lead to sedative, anxiolytic, and antiepileptic effects (Bäckström et al. 2011). Medications and substances that are active at the $GABA_A$ receptor include barbiturates, benzodiazepines, alcohol, and $GABA_A$ receptor modulators (e.g., allopregnanolone) (Bäckström et al. 2011).

Although allopregnanolone would be expected to exert a calming effect due to its positive modulation of $GABA_A$, it may also exert a paradoxical disinhibitory effect similar to that of alcohol and benzodiazepines. Estimates of a strongly negative paradoxical response occur in 3%–6% of human subjects, with an additional 2%–30% exhibiting moderate symptoms characterized by anxiety, irritability, or aggression (Bäckström et al. 2011). In keeping with this paradoxical response, and similar to other $GABA_A$ positive modulators, allopregnanolone demonstrates a biphasic relationship between negative mood symptoms and blood concentrations (Bäckström et al. 2011) in sensitive individuals. As such, at moderate levels, some women may experience a paradoxical anxiogenic effect, whereas at higher doses, allopregnanolone would be expected to produce a more anxiolytic effect. Therefore, it is believed that rising allopregnanolone levels (concomitant with rising progesterone) during the menstrual cycle in sensitive women may contribute to PMS and PMDD symptoms during the luteal phase.

Two main studies have demonstrated that blockage of this rise (via a 5α-reductase inhibitor [Martinez et al. 2016] and via $GABA_A$ modulating steroid antagonist sepranolone [Bixo et al. 2017]) in women with PMDD ameliorates core symptoms. An alternative view is that withdrawal from (rather than exposure to) allopregnanolone may precipitate premenstrual symptoms in sensitive populations. One study found that although women with PMDD overall had elevated levels of allopregnanolone compared with control subjects, those who were most symptomatic had lower levels than less symptomatic women, and those with PMDD had lower levels compared with those with PMS (Bicíková et al. 1998; Girdler et al. 2001; Lovick 2013; Monteleone et al. 2000; Rapkin et al. 1997). SSRIs, a mainstay of treatment for PMDD, may directly influence the formation of allopregnanolone and increase $GABA_A$ receptor sensitivity to allopregnanolone via the mechanism shown in Figure 6–2 (Raffi and Freeman 2017). Furthermore, SSRIs have this effect at levels well below the half maximal effective concentration required for serotonin inhibition (Lovick 2013). Additionally, treatment of PMDD with SSRIs has been demonstrated to modulate allopregnanolone levels (Devall et al. 2015; Fry et al. 2014).

Serotonin is also involved in the pathogenesis of PMS and PMDD. Gonadal steroids are known to cause behaviors such as aggression and increased sexual behavior and are located in areas that regulate mood and emotion (i.e., the hypothalamus and amygdala). Administration of SSRIs is known to dampen sex steroid–driven behaviors (specifically aggression) and may cause sexual dysfunction. Thus, SSRIs may also treat PMS and PMDD (where anger is a prominent symptom) through a primary increase in serotonin alone, in addition to allopregnanolone-mediated effects (Eriksson 2014).

Evidence supporting the serotonin hypothesis includes that serotonin-releasing agents, serotonin precursors (i.e., tryptophan), and serotonin receptor agonists (including buspirone) all improve premenstrual symptoms (Eriksson et al. 2008; Steinberg et

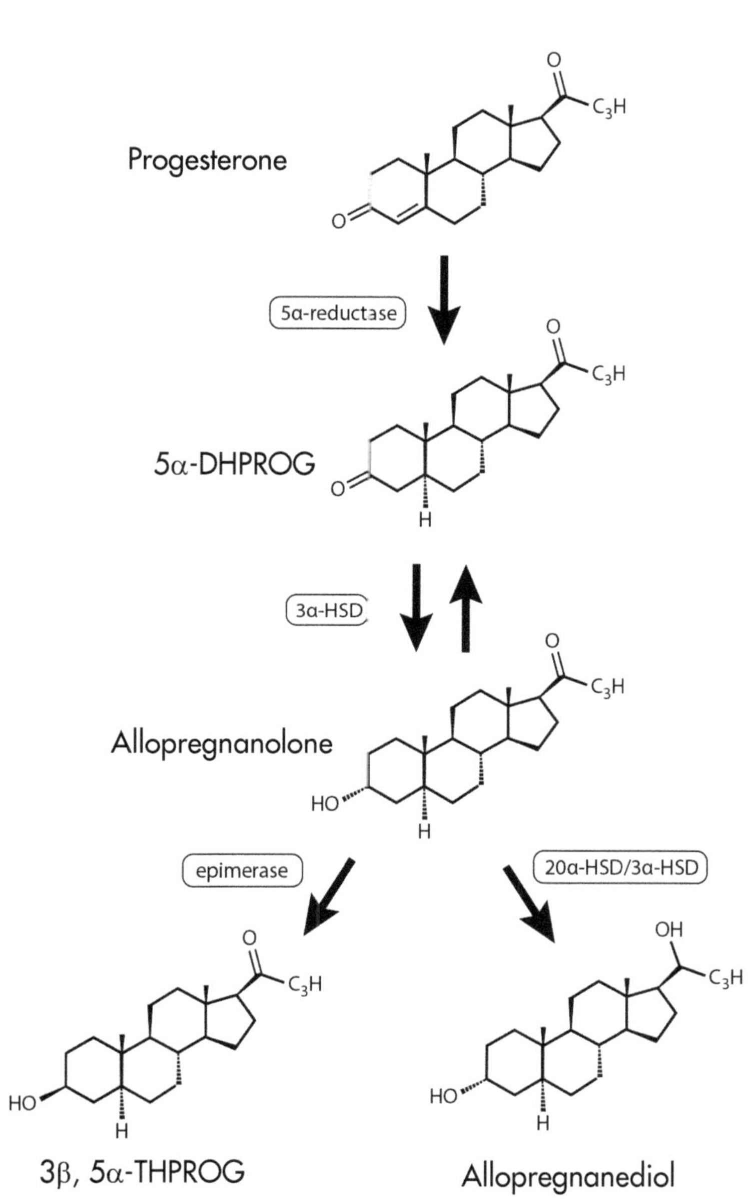


**FIGURE 6–1. The metabolic pathway of progesterone.**
DHPROG = dihydroprogesterone; HSD = hydroxysteroid dehydrogenase; THPROG = tetrahydroprogesterone.

al. 1999; Yonkers et al. 2008). Additionally, depleting serotonin via a tryptophan-free diet and blocking serotonin transmission via a serotonin receptor antagonist both have been shown to increase premenstrual symptoms (Li et al. 2013; Menkes et al. 1994). Furthermore, administering a serotonin receptor antagonist counteracts the symptom-reducing effects of fluoxetine in women with PMS (Roca et al. 2002), implying that its effect on the serotonin receptor mediates its premenstrual symptom–reducing effects. Decreased levels of serotonin have been found in the blood of women with PMS, and women with PMDD have exhibited lower serotonergic function in the luteal phase as compared with healthy control subjects (Inoue et al. 2007; Rapkin et al. 1987). Addi-

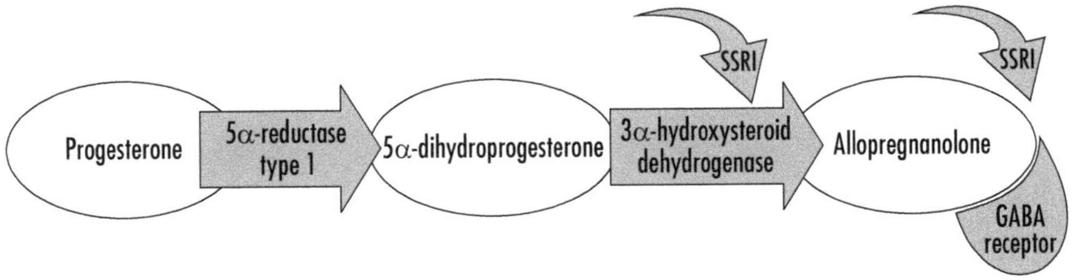


**FIGURE 6–2.** Influence of selective serotonin reuptake inhibitors (SSRIs) on allopregnanolone.

tional studies have shown that women with PMS or PMDD have dysregulated indexes of serotonin transmission, which may also contribute to the pathogenesis of the disorder (Yonkers et al. 2008).

Effective dosage of SSRIs for PMDD might point to a primary pathway for PMS or PMDD symptoms (i.e., allopregnanolone activity vs. serotonin activity), but the evidence is mixed. Some research indicates that treatment of PMS or PMDD requires doses comparable to antidepressant doses, at which point the serotonin reuptake receptor is inhibited (Eriksson 2014). Other studies, however, show that symptoms improve with lower doses of SSRIs (Kornstein et al. 2005; Steiner et al. 2003). Brain structure and functional changes have also been found in women with PMDD and PMS. Women with PMDD have been noted to have greater gray matter volume in the cerebellum, greater gray matter density in the left hippocampal cortex, and smaller volume in the parahippocampal cortex compared with healthy control subjects (Comasco and Sundström-Poromaa 2015; Hantsoo and Epperson 2015).

Women with PMS may have differences of the frontal cortex in areas that integrate emotional and physical input (i.e., the amygdala), due to hormonal influences. Evidence for this includes that women with PMDD demonstrate weakened frontocingulate cortex activation (Comasco et al. 2014) and greater anticipatory prefrontal cortex reactivity (both anterior medial and dorsal lateral) to negative emotional stimuli (Gingnell et al. 2013). Additionally, women with PMDD have been found to have greater abnormal dorsolateral prefrontal cortex activation during a cognitive task (Baller et al. 2013). In studies of depression, the dorsolateral prefrontal cortex demonstrates overactivity, which is believed to suggest a dysfunctional or inefficient response (Koenigs and Grafman 2009), and the same may be true in PMDD. This lack of top-down control (from overactive abnormal dorsolateral prefrontal cortex and underactive frontocingulate cortex) is in line with other studies that demonstrate increased amygdala activation to negative emotional stimuli during the luteal phase (Gingnell et al. 2013). This lack of top-down control and thus enhanced amygdala activation may lead to symptoms of impulsivity and impaired executive function and the expression of emotional symptoms (Baller et al. 2013; Yonkers and Simoni 2018), which are consistent with PMDD.

## Psychological Factors

Dysfunctional behavioral or cognitive responses to an emotion may predict a worsening of that emotion in a feedback-loop manner. Examples of maladaptive responses to emotion include difficulties with emotional awareness or regulation, rumination, and impulsive behavior (Dawson et al. 2018; Nolen-Hoeksema et al. 2008). Dysfunctional responses to emotion have been shown to influence the development or persistence of different psychiatric disorders, including PTSD, depression, and borderline personality disorder (Nolen-Hoeksema et al. 2008; Peters et al. 2015). Maladaptive emotional responses have also been found in patients with PMDD and seem to influence the severity and maintenance of symptoms (Dawson et al. 2018).

Responses to negative emotion documented in women with PMS or PMDD include difficulty with emotional regulation, behavioral impulsivity, impaired social connectedness, increased brooding rumination, greater self-focused attention (in response to negative affect), and elevated perceived stress (Dawson et al. 2018). Emotion-related impulsivity has been shown to predict premenstrual symptom severity and impairment, and depressive rumination has been associated with a greater increase in premenstrual depressive symptoms and a slower return to baseline. These maladaptive emotional responses serve as targets for cognitive-behavioral therapy (CBT) during PMDD treatment, as discussed later in the "Treatment Strategies" section.

In some studies, personality disorders have been found to be more common in women with PMDD (Sassoon et al. 2011), but other studies have not found this association (Critchlow et al. 2001). Several studies, however, have found that a wide range of personality traits, especially neuroticism, are more common in women with PMS and PMDD than in healthy control subjects (Fernández et al. 2019b); neuroticism traits have been found to be related to symptom severity and serotonin transporter polymorphisms in women with PMDD (Gingnell et al. 2010). Other commonly associated traits include obsessions (Critchlow et al. 2001), harm avoidance, novelty seeking, and reward dependence (Freeman et al. 1995). Higher levels of trait anger have been found in women with PMDD and PMS who attempted suicide (Ducasse et al. 2016).

### Social Considerations

Compared with control subjects, women with PMDD often report higher levels of psychosocial stress (Fontana and Palfai 1994), including work stress (Namavar Jahromi et al. 2011) or lack of work and lower socioeconomic status (de Carvalho et al. 2018). As previously mentioned (see "Epidemiology"), history of trauma has also been associated with risk for PMDD and is considered an important potential social factor in its etiology (Eisenlohr-Moul et al. 2016; Perkonigg et al. 2004). Social stresses may lead to greater vulnerability to stress responses, and studies of women with PMDD report alterations in hypothalamic-pituitary-adrenal axis function compared with control subjects (Hantsoo and Epperson 2015).

## Treatment Strategies

### Psychopharmacology

Once a diagnosis of PMDD has been made, the first steps in treatment should always be reassurance, support, and education. An understanding of the patient's unique values, racial or ethnic background, and sexuality, as well as gender identity, will influence the patient's experience of PMDD and should lead clinicians toward appropriate and educational discussions. Working with a patient in a sensitive manner unique to who that patient is can help reduce feelings of shame, guilt, and helplessness that people experiencing PMDD may feel.

## Antidepressant Medications

**Selective serotonin reuptake inhibitors.** SSRIs are considered the first-line treatment for PMDD. (When treating a woman of reproductive age, even if that patient is not planning a pregnancy, clinicians should always consider the safety of proposed medications for future pregnancies.) More than 30 well-designed double-blind randomized controlled trials (RCTs) have demonstrated the efficacy and safety of SSRIs for the treatment of PMDD (Marjoribanks et al. 2013). Therefore, much of the treatment of PMDD centers around the use of SSRIs. Within this class of medications, sertraline, fluoxetine, paroxetine, escitalopram, and citalopram have been specifically studied and deemed equally effective as treatment options; other SSRIs, however, should also be considered viable options as well.

Because of the decrease in serotonergic function during the luteal phase of the menstrual cycle, some patients diagnosed with PMDD are treated with SSRIs only during the 2 weeks prior to menses. Several studies have shown that this type of luteal-phase dosing is as effective as continuous dosing in reducing the symptoms of PMDD and PMS (Shah et al. 2008). Another treatment strategy for PMDD is to administer SSRIs only with symptom onset. Several small but well-designed RCTs have shown that symptom-onset dosing is an effective strategy in reducing PMDD symptoms, with minimal treatment days (Steiner and Li 2013; Yonkers et al. 2005b). Interestingly, in this research no symptom worsening was noted with discontinuation of treatment, and even with short-acting SSRIs such as paroxetine, withdrawal phenomena were not notable. Although there is more evidence, and therefore more support, for continuous-dosing strategies for SSRIs, both luteal-phase dosing and symptom-onset dosing represent reasonable strategies involving shorter treatment periods (with shorter exposure to side effects) for appropriate patients.

**Serotonin-norepinephrine reuptake inhibitors.** Much like SSRIs, the serotonin-norepinephrine reuptake inhibitors (SNRIs) are treatment options for PMDD due to their inhibitory effect on serotoninreuptake. Research has focused on two SNRIs, venlafaxine and duloxetine. A few studies have demonstrated that with continuous dosing, symptom remission rates for these two agents are superior to those of placebo (Freeman et al. 2001; Mazza et al. 2008; Ramos et al. 2009). Limited data exist on the intermittent use of SNRIs for PMDD. One study found intermittent dosing of venlafaxine to be efficacious in the treatment of PMDD, but some women experienced mild to moderate withdrawal-related symptoms (Cohen et al. 2004). Therefore, SNRIs represent an effective treatment strategy for PMDD but may be best used in patients who prefer continuous dosing.

**Tricyclic antidepressants.** Limited data exist to support the use of tricyclic antidepressants (TCAs) in the treatment of PMDD. In two studies with small numbers of subjects, clomipramine was shown to be superior to placebo in reducing premenstrual irritability and dysphoria; in one of those studies, both continuous and intermittent dosing appeared to be effective (Sundblad et al. 1992, 1993). Despite the limited data supporting its use, as well as the less desirable side effect profile for TCAs, clomipramine may be an effective treatment option for patients who cannot take first-line treatment. Some animal data support the effectiveness of amitriptyline and desipramine on some behaviors that may be related to PMDD (Li et al. 2012; Schneider and Popik 2007), and one trial for PMDD in humans could not distinguish between the effects of the SSRI sertraline and the TCA desipramine (Freeman et al. 1996). Other data indicate that antidepressants that work primarily through noradrenergic function are less effective than serotonergic antidepressants for PMDD (Eriksson et al. 1995).

## Anxiolytics

There has been some interest in benzodiazepines and the serotonin agonist buspirone in the treatment of PMDD. Although the benzodiazepine alprazolam did show improvement of symptoms compared with placebo, the response was not as robust as that from treatment with fluoxetine (Diegoli et al. 1998). Buspirone, however, did not show a statistically significant improvement in limited research (Landén et al. 2001). Both agents can increase sedation and somnolence, which is an undesired effect in a patient with PMDD who might be experiencing such symptoms as part of the underlying disorder.

## Hormonal Interventions

**Oral contraception.** Oral contraceptive pills (OCPs) have been explored as a treatment option based on the theory that cessation of ovulation would eliminate symptoms of PMS and PMDD. However, the evidence of any type of OCPs for treatment of PMDD is limited. In 2006, the FDA approved an OCP containing drospirenone for the treatment of PMDD. Drospirenone is a synthetic progestin derived from spironolactone rather than from the more commonly used 19-nortestosterone, which has been postulated to be associated with mood symptoms (Rapkin 2003). One multicenter, double-blind, placebo-controlled study evaluated the use of monophasic drospirenone 3 mg and ethinyl estradiol 20 μg administered for 24 days, followed by four inactive pills, in women with PMDD. They found that the treatment group's response rate to this formulation was similar to that of women taking SSRIs. Of note, premenstrual physical symptoms improved with drospirenone as well (Yonkers et al. 2005a). Although these results are encouraging, it should be noted that studies assessing drospirenone have had large placebo effects and have often lost large numbers of patients to follow-up (Lopez et al. 2012). Additional high-quality research is desired in this area.

In addition to the choice of agent, continuous versus cyclical dosing has also been studied. Some data have shown a benefit with continuous administration (without a hormone-free interval) of a formulation of the monophasic 19-nortestosterone derivative levonorgestrel and ethinyl estradiol in treating both physical and mental premenstrual symptoms, compared with placebo (Halbreich et al. 2012). Other reviews have shown inconsistencies in symptom reduction with this type of treatment (Freeman et al. 2012).

OCPs are not without risks. Side effects that may impair quality of life, such as decreased sexual interest, can occur (Sanders et al. 2001). In 2012, the FDA made a safety announcement warning that drospirenone may be associated with an increased risk of thromboembolism (U.S. Food and Drug Administration 2012). Vaginal bleeding has been reported in patients given continuous dosing of levonorgestrel. Therefore, decisions regarding treatment are best made on a case-by-case basis with careful attention to a patient's own unique mental and physical health factors. The higher risks associated with OCPs (vs. SSRIs) mean that they should be used as first-line treatment only in patients who are planning to use them for contraception anyway or those with existing medication regimens that preclude additional serotonin in the luteal phase (e.g., patients already taking the maximum dose of an SSRI or SNRI, those taking an monoamine oxidase inhibitor).

**Gonadotropin-releasing hormone agonists.** The GnRH agonist class of medications includes agents such as leuprolide and goserelin. GnRH agonists downregulate GnRH receptors, which leads to a decrease in both luteinizing and follicle-stimulating hormones and eventual decreases in production of ovarian estrogen and progesterone. That these hormonal changes result in anovulation, amenorrhea, and a menopause-type state is the basis of this type of treatment for PMS and PMDD. Studies evaluating GnRH agonists have shown them to be more effective than placebo in reducing PMDD symptoms (Wyatt et al. 2004).

Clearly, one issue with GnRH agonists is that by creating a menopausal state, they cause women to experience signs and symptoms of hypoestrogenism, such as hot flashes and night sweats, and present a risk for decreased bone mineral density (Dawood 1994). Therefore, some research has investigated the use of "add-back" estrogen and progesterone for women receiving GnRH agonists. Although research on this topic is limited, a small study demonstrated that when estrogen and progesterone were added back to the treatment, some symptoms of PMDD did occur. Addition of estrogen alone appeared to be most effective for prevention of menopausal symptoms without PMDD symptoms; however, this is not considered a safe option due to the risk for endometrial hyperplasia (Segebladh et al. 2009). Due to the complications associated with use of GnRH agonists and the unclear implications of long-term treatment with them, they are not considered a first-line treatment for PMDD and may come into play only as a temporary treatment for severe treatment-resistant cases.

**Danazol.** Danazol is a synthetic steroid with androgenic and antigonadotropic properties that suppresses ovulation. It has been shown to reduce premenstrual physical and mood symptoms in some cases (Hahn et al. 1995). However, this form of treatment is complicated by multiple side effects, such as decreased high-density lipoprotein cholesterol, weight gain, hirsutism, and acne. Consequently, as with GnRH agonists, danazol is not recommended as a first-line treatment for PMDD.

**Spironolactone.** Spironolactone is an aldosterone receptor antagonist and potassium-sparing diuretic. The best evidence for spironolactone appears to be in the treatment of premenstrual physical symptoms, such as swelling, breast tenderness, and food cravings. It has also been shown to reduce irritability and depression (Wang et al. 1995). Because this medication may increase potassium levels, careful monitoring for hyperkalemia is necessary.

**Bromocriptine and cabergoline.** Both bromocriptine and cabergoline are dopamine agonists that reduce prolactin levels. In doing so, they have been found to be effective in reducing premenstrual mastalgia. Additional symptom reduction has been inconsistent with bromocriptine. Cabergoline has been noted to have fewer side effects than bromocriptine, which has been associated with nausea, vomiting, and headaches

(Aydin et al. 2010). Additionally, these dopamine agonists must be carefully monitored for unwanted psychiatric side effects, such as worsening depression.

## Nonpharmacological Somatic Treatments

In all treatment efforts, a careful assessment with the patient about risk versus potential benefit is crucial. General health-oriented interventions with very low risk may include minimizing use of caffeine, salt, and alcohol, especially during the premenstrual week. Increasing other positive behaviors, such as sleep and exercise, is also recommended. Depending on symptom severity, interventions such as scheduling changes that reduce stress during the premenstrual week and other nonpharmacological approaches may be useful. A great amount of interest has been shown in dietary modifications for the treatment of PMDD. Areas that have been explored include intake of soy isoflavones, fat, protein, and carbohydrates. Some observational studies show associations between diet and PMS or PMDD, but the evidence is not consistent (Hashim et al. 2019; Houghton et al. 2017, 2018). Although some open-label studies have found improvements in symptoms with dietary modifications, others have not, and randomized evidence is lacking (Esmaeilpour et al. 2019; Houghton et al. 2019).

## Behavioral and Other Nonpharmacological Treatments

Support for psychotherapeutic treatments for PMDD remains inconclusive but promising. CBT has the most support, but many studies have had limitations in study design, including use of retrospective versus prospective PMDD diagnosis and existence of mainly open trials (Lustyk et al. 2009). In a randomized comparison study, women with prospectively confirmed PMDD were randomly assigned to 10 sessions of CBT alone, fluoxetine 20 mg/day alone, or combined CBT and fluoxetine. All groups demonstrated improvement in PMDD. Fluoxetine was associated with earlier improvement, and CBT was associated with greater maintenance of improvement at 1 year (Hunter et al. 2002). Recently, internet-based CBT was shown to be effective in addressing the functional and psychological impairments of PMDD (Weise et al. 2019). Although, to date, published studies on the use of mindfulness-based stress reduction therapies for PMDD are lacking, one small open study of women with menstrual-related mood symptoms found that participation in a mindfulness-based stress reduction class was associated with significant reduction in premenstrual symptoms, including decreased depressive symptoms, irritability, anxiety, and mood swings (Bluth et al. 2015). Thus, some data suggest efficacy of other low-risk interventions, such as mindfulness, to assist patients in stress reduction and coping during periods of illness.

Acupuncture has also been evaluated in the treatment of PMDD, and when compared with sham procedures, acupuncture and acupressure are associated with decreased PMS and PMDD symptoms in many trials. No studies have yet compared this modality with SSRIs, SNRIs, or OCPs (Armour et al. 2018).

## Supplements and Herbal Treatments

### Supplements

Calcium has been used as a generally low-risk supplement to reduce symptoms of PMS and PMDD. In a double-blind RCT of 466 women, calcium carbonate 1,200 mg/

day was found to significantly reduce PMS symptoms when compared with placebo (Thys-Jacobs et al. 2007). Compared with fluoxetine, calcium supplementation has a lower effect size (Yonkers et al. 2013); nevertheless, it is an important nutritional supplement that can be an important initial treatment approach in women reluctant to take antidepressants.

Vitamin E has been investigated in PMDD because it may have a role in prostaglandin synthesis and regulation of central neurotransmitters. In older small RCTs, vitamin E showed improvement in some specific symptoms reported by women, such as headache, crying, insomnia, forgetfulness, dizziness, and sweet craving (London et al. 1983, 1987). Although these results are promising, evidence to support vitamin E as an effective treatment for PMDD is still insufficient. Additionally, because vitamin E is a fat-soluble compound, there is a potential for toxicity at high doses and with prolonged use (Miller et al. 2005).

Other supplements, such as magnesium and vitamin $B_6$, have been studied, with inconsistent findings. Some research has indicated a benefit for women with premenstrual symptoms, and some has found no benefit (Whelan et al. 2009). Given the limited nature and inconsistencies in the results, it does not appear that these supplements represent a robust management approach at this time.

### Herbal Treatments

Historically, herbal treatment options have been used for the treatment of PMS and PMDD. Although some herbs such as St. John's wort (*Hypericum perforatum*) have been shown to be somewhat effective for PMS (Canning et al. 2010), they have not shown improvements in mood symptoms of PMDD. Chaste tree extract or chasteberry (*Vitex agnus-castus*) has shown some benefit in treating physical and mood-related PMS symptoms in multiple double-blind RCTs and in uncontrolled studies (Loch et al. 2000; Schellenberg 2001; Verkaik et al. 2017). The postulated mechanism of action for chaste tree extract is that it may bind to dopamine receptors and inhibit prolactin (Jarry et al. 1994) and also activate opioid receptors (Webster et al. 2011). Other promising herbal treatment strategies include saffron (Agha-Hosseini et al. 2008) and *Ginkgo biloba* (Ozgoli et al. 2009). Herbal remedies represent an interesting future direction for research, but additional research is needed before treatment recommendations can be made (Jang et al. 2014). As with any herbal treatments, which are not under the same governmental quality controls as pharmaceuticals, caution must be advised in the procurement and consumption of these products; actual formulations may differ widely even within the same brand due to the unregulated nature of the herbal treatment industry. Additionally, limited guidance is available about advising patients how best to administer and dose these supplements.

## Surgery

In patients with severe PMS and PMDD, for whom no other treatments have been effective and who do not desire future fertility, surgical oophorectomy has been performed as a last-line treatment. In small studies, oophorectomy with hysterectomy and estrogen replacement has been shown to be effective in patients with previously treatment-refractory disease (Cronje et al. 2004). Because this is an irreversible procedure, all other treatment options should be exhausted first. Proper discussion—including informed consent and a detailed understanding of the risks of hysterectomy and oophorectomy—is necessary. It is also crucial for patients considering this option to know that it is supported by only a limited amount of data at this time.

## Treatment Challenges: Partial Response, Treatment Resistance, and Comorbid Bipolar Disorder

No studies have been published on treatment-resistant PMDD, despite reports that 40% of women do not respond fully to SSRIs or OCPs (Halbreich 2008). For patients with poor treatment response to SSRIs and SNRIs, clinicians need to first reevaluate the diagnosis and rule out another mood or anxiety disorder with premenstrual exacerbation as the primary diagnosis, because many of the treatments for PMDD are either ineffective or potentially deleterious for primary mood or anxiety disorders. For instance, drospirenone-containing OCPs (Peters et al. 2017) and GnRH agonists (Freeman et al. 1997) are not effective for major depression with premenstrual exacerbation. Women with underlying bipolar disorder are at risk for antidepressant-induced hypomania or mixed episodes if they are not taking a mood stabilizer (Gitlin 2018; Viktorin et al. 2014).

To date, no RCTs are available to guide treatment of comorbid PMDD and bipolar disorder or of bipolar disorder with PME of mood symptoms. Current recommendations include first maximizing the mood stabilizer and then considering adding an OCP (Sepede et al. 2020). Support for this approach includes data from small studies of women with bipolar disorder who report improvement in cyclical mood fluctuations with OCPs (Frey and Minuzzi 2013) and with lamotrigine and OCPs compared with other mood stabilizers (Robakis et al. 2015).

Furthermore, to date no sequenced treatment trials for PMDD have been published. Only one small, open-label study has examined the effectiveness of switching from one SSRI, if not effective, to citalopram 20–40 mg/day for either the luteal phase or the full cycle (Freeman et al. 2002). Clinical improvement, defined as Daily Symptom Rating Scale decreases of >50% from baseline, were reported in 76% of the subjects, and no significant differences were found between the full- and half-cycle treatment groups. In a double-blind study, adjunctive quetiapine has been shown to reduce mood lability and depression in patients with PMDD who had only partial response to SSRIs (Jackson et al. 2015). Further studies are needed to guide treatment of partial response and treatment resistance.

# Conclusion

The treatment of PMDD remains an area in need of additional research for the best evidence-based treatment decisions. Currently, the recommended approach is for clinicians to involve patients in a multifaceted approach, including nutritional modifications, lifestyle choices, behavioral interventions and therapies, and, where appropriate, introduction of medical treatments. Working closely with patients to best understand their own unique values, risk assessment, and treatment choices is crucial to the most effective treatment strategy.

Premenstrual mood syndromes represent an area of reproductive psychiatry that truly welcomes a comprehensive assessment of each patient from a medical, psychological, and social standpoint. Millions of people worldwide are affected by PMDD, and the effects of the disorder are profound and debilitating for many. Even more women are affected by the less severe PMS, and women who have mood disorders commonly experience PME of their symptoms that does not meet criteria for PMDD. Although diseases that primarily affect women, including PMDD, have been understudied historically, changes are occurring, and additional emphasis is being placed on accurate diagnosis, treatment, and education. Additional research into PMDD will reveal future insight into and management strategies for this important disease.

## Key Points

- Premenstrual syndrome (PMS) affects most women worldwide, with physical or emotional symptoms or both, but it is not impairing.
- Premenstrual dysphoric disorder (PMDD) affects a much smaller number (up to 8% of women) and impairs function.
- PMDD only occurs in ovulatory menstrual cycles and can co-occur with other mood and anxiety disorders.
- PMDD must be differentiated from premenstrual exacerbation of underlying mood and anxiety disorders, such as bipolar disorder and major depression.
- Evidence-based treatments for PMDD include selective serotonin reuptake inhibitors (SSRIs), serotonin-norepinephrine reuptake inhibitors, and suppression of ovulation.
- Bipolar disorder and PMDD comorbidity is especially important to diagnose and requires treatment with mood stabilizers and contraceptives or a cautious trial of SSRIs.
- Nonpharmacological treatments are useful in the treatment of PMDD. These include calcium supplementation, cognitive-behavioral therapy, and acupuncture.

## References

Agha-Hosseini M, Kashani L, Aleyaseen A, et al: Crocus sativus L. (saffron) in the treatment of premenstrual syndrome: a double-blind, randomised and placebo-controlled trial. BJOG 115(4):515–519, 2008 18271889

Allen SS, McBride CM, Pirie PL: The shortened Premenstrual Assessment Form. J Reprod Med 36(11):769–772, 1991 1765953

American College of Obstetricians and Gynecologists: Guidelines for Women's Health Care: A Resource Manual, 4th Edition. Washington, DC, American College of Obstetricians and Gynecologists, 2014

American Psychiatric Association: Diagnostic and Statistical Manual of Mental Disorders, 4th Edition. Washington, DC, American Psychiatric Association, 1994

American Psychiatric Association: Diagnostic and Statistical Manual of Mental Disorders, 5th Edition. Arlington, VA, American Psychiatric Association, 2013

Armour M, Ee CC, Hao J, et al: Acupuncture and acupressure for premenstrual syndrome. Cochrane Database Syst Rev 8(8):CD005290, 2018 30105749

Aydin Y, Atis A, Kaleli S, et al: Cabergoline versus bromocriptine for symptomatic treatment of premenstrual mastalgia: a randomised, open-label study. Eur J Obstet Gynecol Reprod Biol 150(2):203–206, 2010 20206430
Bäckström T, Haage D, Löfgren M, et al: Paradoxical effects of GABA-A modulators may explain sex steroid induced negative mood symptoms in some persons. Neuroscience 191:46–54, 2011 21600269
Baker LJ, O'Brien PMS: Premenstrual syndrome (PMS): a peri-menopausal perspective. Maturitas 72(2):121–125, 2012 22534048
Baller EB, Wei SM, Kohn PD, et al: Abnormalities of dorsolateral prefrontal function in women with premenstrual dysphoric disorder: a multimodal neuroimaging study. Am J Psychiatry 170(3):305–314, 2013 23361612
Bertone-Johnson ER, Hankinson SE, Willett WC, et al: Adiposity and the development of premenstrual syndrome. J Womens Health (Larchmt) 19(11):1955–1962, 2010 20874240
Bertone-Johnson ER, Whitcomb BW, Missmer SA, et al: Early life emotional, physical, and sexual abuse and the development of premenstrual syndrome: a longitudinal study. J Womens Health (Larchmt) 23(9):729–739, 2014 25098348
Bicíková M, Dibbelt L, Hill M, et al: Allopregnanolone in women with premenstrual syndrome. Horm Metab Res 30(4):227–230, 1998 9623639
Bixo M, Ekberg K, Poromaa IS, et al: Treatment of premenstrual dysphoric disorder with the GABAA receptor modulating steroid antagonist sepranolone (UC1010): a randomized controlled trial. Psychoneuroendocrinology 80:46–55, 2017 28319848
Bluth K, Gaylord S, Nguyen K, et al: Mindfulness-based stress reduction as a promising intervention for amelioration of premenstrual dysphoric disorder symptoms. Mindfulness (NY) 6(6):1292–1302, 2015 26594254
Borenstein JE, Dean BB, Leifke E, et al: Differences in symptom scores and health outcomes in premenstrual syndrome. J Womens Health (Larchmt) 16(8):1139–1144, 2007 17937566
Bosman RC, Jung SE, Miloserdov K, et al: Daily symptom ratings for studying premenstrual dysphoric disorder: a review. J Affect Disord 189:43–53, 2016 26406968
Brockington IF: Menstrual psychosis: a bipolar disorder with a link to the hypothalamus. Curr Psychiatry Rep 13(3):193–197, 2011 21424263
Canning S, Waterman M, Orsi N, et al: The efficacy of Hypericum perforatum (St John's wort) for the treatment of premenstrual syndrome: a randomized, double-blind, placebo-controlled trial. CNS Drugs 24(3):207–225, 2010 20155996
Chocano-Bedoya PO, Manson JE, Hankinson SE, et al: Dietary B vitamin intake and incident premenstrual syndrome. Am J Clin Nutr 93(5):1080–1086, 2011 21346091
Chocano-Bedoya PO, Manson JE, Hankinson SE, et al: Intake of selected minerals and risk of premenstrual syndrome. Am J Epidemiol 177(10):1118–1127, 2013 23444100
Chung SH, Kim TH, Lee HH, et al: Premenstrual syndrome and premenstrual dysphoric disorder in perimenopausal women. J Menopausal Med 20(2):69–74, 2014 25371896
Cohen LS, Soares CN, Otto MW, et al: Prevalence and predictors of premenstrual dysphoric disorder (PMDD) in older premenopausal women. J Affect Disord 70(2):125–132, 2002 12117624
Cohen LS, Soares CN, Lyster A, et al: Efficacy and tolerability of premenstrual use of venlafaxine (flexible dose) in the treatment of premenstrual dysphoric disorder. J Clin Psychopharmacol 24(5):540–543, 2004 15349012
Comasco E, Sundström-Poromaa I: Neuroimaging the menstrual cycle and premenstrual dysphoric disorder. Curr Psychiatry Rep 17(10):77, 2015 26272540
Comasco E, Hahn A, Ganger S, et al: Emotional fronto-cingulate cortex activation and brain derived neurotrophic factor polymorphism in premenstrual dysphoric disorder. Hum Brain Mapp 35(9):4450–4458, 2014 24615932
Condon JT: The premenstrual syndrome: a twin study. Br J Psychiatry 162:481–486, 1993 8481739
Critchlow DG, Bond AJ, Wingrove J: Mood disorder history and personality assessment in premenstrual dysphoric disorder. J Clin Psychiatry 62(9):688–693, 2001 11681764
Cronje WH, Vashisht A, Studd JWW: Hysterectomy and bilateral oophorectomy for severe premenstrual syndrome. Hum Reprod 19(9):2152–2155, 2004 15229203

Dahlgren CL, Qvigstad E: Eating disorders in premenstrual dysphoric disorder: a neuroendocrinological pathway to the pathogenesis and treatment of binge eating. J Eat Disord 6:35, 2018 30386599
Dawood MY: Hormonal therapies for endometriosis: implications for bone metabolism. Acta Obstet Gynecol Scand Suppl 159:22–34, 1994 8209669
Dawson DN, Eisenlohr-Moul TA, Paulson JL, et al: Emotion-related impulsivity and rumination predict the perimenstrual severity and trajectory of symptoms in women with a menstrually related mood disorder. J Clin Psychol 74(4):579–593, 2018 28898408
de Carvalho AB, Cardoso TA, Mondin TC, et al: Prevalence and factors associated with premenstrual dysphoric disorder: a community sample of young adult women. Psychiatry Res 268:42–45, 2018 29986177
Devall AJ, Santos JM, Fry JP, et al: Elevation of brain allopregnanolone rather than 5-HT release by short term, low dose fluoxetine treatment prevents the estrous cycle-linked increase in stress sensitivity in female rats. Eur Neuropsychopharmacol 25(1):113–123, 2015 25498416
Dhingra V, Magnay JL, O'Brien PM, et al: Serotonin receptor 1A C(-1019)G polymorphism associated with premenstrual dysphoric disorder. Obstet Gynecol 110(4):788–792, 2007 17906010
Diegoli MS, da Fonseca AM, Diegoli CA, et al: A double-blind trial of four medications to treat severe premenstrual syndrome. Int J Gynaecol Obstet 62(1):63–67, 1998 9722128
Dubey N, Hoffman JF, Schuebel K, et al: The ESC/E(Z) complex, an effector of response to ovarian steroids, manifests an intrinsic difference in cells from women with premenstrual dysphoric disorder. Mol Psychiatry 22(8):1172–1184, 2017 28044059
Ducasse D, Jaussent I, Olié E, et al: Personality traits of suicidality are associated with premenstrual syndrome and premenstrual dysphoric disorder in a suicidal women sample. PLoS One 11(2):e0148653, 2016 26863007
Eisenlohr-Moul TA, Rubinow DR, Schiller CE, et al: Histories of abuse predict stronger within-person covariation of ovarian steroids and mood symptoms in women with menstrually related mood disorder. Psychoneuroendocrinology 67:142–152, 2016 26896670
Eisenlohr-Moul TA, Girdler SS, Schmalenberger KM, et al: Toward the reliable diagnosis of DSM-5 premenstrual dysphoric disorder: the Carolina Premenstrual Assessment Scoring System (C-PASS). Am J Psychiatry 174(1):51–59, 2017 27523500
Endicott J: The menstrual cycle and mood disorders. J Affect Disord 29(2–3):193–200, 1993 8300978
Endicott J, Nee J, Harrison W: Daily Record of Severity of Problems (DRSP): reliability and validity. Arch Women Ment Health 9(1):41–49, 2006 16172836
Eriksson E: SSRIs probably counteract premenstrual syndrome by inhibiting the serotonin transporter. J Psychopharmacol 28(2):173–174, 2014 24449218
Eriksson E, Hedberg MA, Andersch B, et al: The serotonin reuptake inhibitor paroxetin is superior to the noradrenaline reuptake inhibitor maprotiline in the treatment of premenstrual syndrome. Neuropsychopharmacology 12(2):167–176, 1995 7779245
Eriksson E, Ekman A, Sinclair S, et al: Escitalopram administered in the luteal phase exerts a marked and dose-dependent effect in premenstrual dysphoric disorder. J Clin Psychopharmacol 28(2):195–202, 2008 18344730
Esmaeilpour M, Ghasemian S, Alizadeh M: Diets enriched with whole grains reduce premenstrual syndrome scores in nurses: an open-label parallel randomised controlled trial. Br J Nutr 121(9):992–1001, 2019 30761961
Fernández MDM, Montes-Martínez A, Piñeiro-Lamas M, et al: Tobacco consumption and premenstrual syndrome: a case-control study. PLoS One 14:e0218794, 2019a
Fernández MDM, Regueira-Méndez C, Takkouche B: Psychological factors and premenstrual syndrome: a Spanish case-control study. PLoS One 14(3): 2019b 30840651
Fontana AM, Palfai TG: Psychosocial factors in premenstrual dysphoria: stressors, appraisal, and coping processes. J Psychosom Res 38(6):557–567, 1994 7990064
Freeman EW, Schweizer E, Rickels K: Personality factors in women with premenstrual syndrome. Psychosom Med 57(5):453–459, 1995 8552736
Freeman EW, Rickels K, Sondheimer SJ, et al: Sertraline versus desipramine in the treatment of premenstrual syndrome: an open-label trial. J Clin Psychiatry 57(1):7–11, 1996 8543554

Freeman EW, Sondheimer SJ, Rickels K: Gonadotropin-releasing hormone agonist in the treatment of premenstrual symptoms with and without ongoing dysphoria: a controlled study. Psychopharmacol Bull 33(2):303–309, 1997 9230648

Freeman EW, Rickels K, Yonkers KA, et al: Venlafaxine in the treatment of premenstrual dysphoric disorder. Obstet Gynecol 98(5 pt 1):737–744, 2001 11704162

Freeman EW, Jabara S, Sondheimer SJ, et al: Citalopram in PMS patients with prior SSRI treatment failure: a preliminary study. J Womens Health Gend Based Med 11(5):459–464, 2002 12165163

Freeman EW, Halbreich U, Grubb GS, et al: An overview of four studies of a continuous oral contraceptive (levonorgestrel 90 mcg/ethinyl estradiol 20 mcg) on premenstrual dysphoric disorder and premenstrual syndrome. Contraception 85(5):437–445, 2012 22152588

Freeman R, Lewis RM: The therapeutic role of estrogens in postmenopausal women. Endocrinol Metab Clin North Am 33(4):771–789, 2004 15501645

Frey BN, Minuzzi L: Comorbid bipolar disorder and premenstrual dysphoric disorder: real patients, unanswered questions. Arch Women Ment Health 16(1):79–81, 2013 23135309

Fry JP, Li KY, Devall AJ, et al: Fluoxetine elevates allopregnanolone in female rat brain but inhibits a steroid microsomal dehydrogenase rather than activating an aldo-keto reductase. Br J Pharmacol 171(24):5870–5880, 2014 25161074

Gehlert S, Song IH, Chang CH, et al: The prevalence of premenstrual dysphoric disorder in a randomly selected group of urban and rural women. Psychol Med 39(1):129–136, 2009 18366818

Gingnell M, Comasco E, Oreland L, et al: Neuroticism-related personality traits are related to symptom severity in patients with premenstrual dysphoric disorder and to the serotonin transporter gene-linked polymorphism 5-HTTPLPR. Arch Women Ment Health 13(5):417–423, 2010 20440524

Gingnell M, Bannbers E, Wikström J, et al: Premenstrual dysphoric disorder and prefrontal reactivity during anticipation of emotional stimuli. Eur Neuropsychopharmacol 23(11):1474–1483, 2013 24001875

Girdler SS, Straneva PA, Light KC, et al: Allopregnanolone levels and reactivity to mental stress in premenstrual dysphoric disorder. Biol Psychiatry 49(9):788–797, 2001 11331087

Gitlin MJ: Antidepressants in bipolar depression: an enduring controversy. Int J Bipolar Disord 6(1):25, 2018 30506151

Graze KK, Nee J, Endicott J: Premenstrual depression predicts future major depressive disorder. Acta Psychiatr Scand 81(2):201–205, 1990 2327284

Hahn PM, Van Vugt DA, Reid RL: A randomized, placebo-controlled, crossover trial of danazol for the treatment of premenstrual syndrome. Psychoneuroendocrinology 20(2):193–209, 1995 7899538

Halbreich U: Selective serotonin reuptake inhibitors and initial oral contraceptives for the treatment of PMDD: effective but not enough. CNS Spectr 13(7):566–572, 2008 18622361

Halbreich U, Endicott J, Schacht S, et al: The diversity of premenstrual changes as reflected in the Premenstrual Assessment Form. Acta Psychiatr Scand 65(1):46–65, 1982 6892280

Halbreich U, Borenstein J, Pearlstein T, et al: The prevalence, impairment, impact, and burden of premenstrual dysphoric disorder (PMS/PMDD). Psychoneuroendocrinology 28(suppl 3):1–23, 2003 12892987

Halbreich U, Freeman EW, Rapkin AJ, et al: Continuous oral levonorgestrel/ethinyl estradiol for treating premenstrual dysphoric disorder. Contraception 85(1):19–27, 2012 22067793

Haley CL, Sung SC, Rush AJ, et al: The clinical relevance of self-reported premenstrual worsening of depressive symptoms in the management of depressed outpatients: a STAR*D report. J Womens Health (Larchmt) 22(3):219–229, 2013 23480315

Hall E, Steiner M: Psychiatric symptoms and disorders associated with reproductive cyclicity in women: advances in screening tools. Womens Health (Lond) 11(3):397–415, 2015 26102476

Hantsoo L, Epperson CN: Premenstrual dysphoric disorder: epidemiology and treatment. Curr Psychiatry Rep 17(11):87, 2015 26377947

Hashemi S, Ramezani Tehrani F, Mohammadi N, et al: Comparison of metabolic and hormonal profiles of women with and without premenstrual syndrome: a community based cross-sectional study. Int J Endocrinol Metab 14(2):e28422, 2016 27679647

Hashim MS, Obaideen AA, Jahrami HA, et al: Premenstrual syndrome is associated with dietary and lifestyle behaviors among university students: a cross-sectional study from Sharjah, UAE. Nutrients 11(8):1939, 2019 31426498

Haywood A, Slade P, King H: Assessing the assessment measures for menstrual cycle symptoms: a guide for researchers and clinicians. J Psychosom Res 52(4):223–237, 2002 11943241

Hong JP, Park S, Wang HR, et al: Prevalence, correlates, comorbidities, and suicidal tendencies of premenstrual dysphoric disorder in a nationwide sample of Korean women. Soc Psychiatry Psychiatr Epidemiol 47(12):1937–1945, 2012 22538387

Houghton SC, Manson JE, Whitcomb BW, et al: Intake of dietary fat and fat subtypes and risk of premenstrual syndrome in the Nurses' Health Study II. Br J Nutr 118(10):849–857, 2017 29189192

Houghton SC, Manson JE, Whitcomb BW, et al: Carbohydrate and fiber intake and the risk of premenstrual syndrome. Eur J Clin Nutr 72(6):861–870, 2018 29379144

Houghton SC, Manson JE, Whitcomb BW, et al: Protein intake and the risk of premenstrual syndrome. Public Health Nutr 22(10):1762–1769, 2019 30774065

Hunter MS, Ussher JM, Browne SJ, et al: A randomized comparison of psychological (cognitive behavior therapy), medical (fluoxetine) and combined treatment for women with premenstrual dysphoric disorder. J Psychosom Obstet Gynaecol 23(3):193–199, 2002 12436805

Huo L, Straub RE, Roca C, et al: Risk for premenstrual dysphoric disorder is associated with genetic variation in ESR1, the estrogen receptor alpha gene. Biol Psychiatry 62(8):925–933, 2007 17599809

Hussein Shehadeh J, Hamdan-Mansour AM: Prevalence and association of premenstrual syndrome and premenstrual dysphoric disorder with academic performance among female university students. Perspect Psychiatr Care 54(2):176–184, 2018 28543046

Inoue Y, Terao T, Iwata N, et al: Fluctuating serotonergic function in premenstrual dysphoric disorder and premenstrual syndrome: findings from neuroendocrine challenge tests. Psychopharmacology (Berl) 190(2):213–219, 2007 17072588

Jackson C, Pearson B, Girdler S, et al: Double-blind, placebo-controlled pilot study of adjunctive quetiapine SR in the treatment of PMS/PMDD. Hum Psychopharmacol 30(6):425–434, 2015 26193781

Jahanfar S, Lye MS, Krishnarajah IS: The heritability of premenstrual syndrome. Twin Res Hum Genet 14(5):433–436, 2011 21962135

Jang SH, Kim DI, Choi MS: Effects and treatment methods of acupuncture and herbal medicine for premenstrual syndrome/premenstrual dysphoric disorder: systematic review. BMC Complement Altern Med 14:11, 2014 24410911

Jarry H, Leonhardt S, Gorkow C, et al: In vitro prolactin but not LH and FSH release is inhibited by compounds in extracts of Agnus castus: direct evidence for a dopaminergic principle by the dopamine receptor assay. Exp Clin Endocrinol 102(6):448–454, 1994 7890021

Kim DR, Gyulai L, Freeman EW, et al: Premenstrual dysphoric disorder and psychiatric comorbidity. Arch Women Ment Health 7(1):37–47, 2004 14963731

Koenigs M, Grafman J: The functional neuroanatomy of depression: distinct roles for ventromedial and dorsolateral prefrontal cortex. Behav Brain Res 201(2):239–243, 2009 19428640

Kornstein SG, Harvey AT, Rush AJ, et al: Self-reported premenstrual exacerbation of depressive symptoms in patients seeking treatment for major depression. Psychol Med 35(5):683–692, 2005 15918345

Landén M, Eriksson O, Sundblad C, et al: Compounds with affinity for serotonergic receptors in the treatment of premenstrual dysphoria: a comparison of buspirone, nefazodone and placebo. Psychopharmacology (Berl) 155(3):292–298, 2001 11432692

Li Y, Pehrson AL, Budac DP, et al: A rodent model of premenstrual dysphoria: progesterone withdrawal induces depression-like behavior that is differentially sensitive to classes of antidepressants. Behav Brain Res 234(2):238–247, 2012 22789402

Li Y, Raaby KF, Sánchez C, et al: Serotonergic receptor mechanisms underlying antidepressant-like action in the progesterone withdrawal model of hormonally induced depression in rats. Behav Brain Res 256:520–528, 2013 24016840

Loch EG, Selle H, Boblitz N: Treatment of premenstrual syndrome with a phytopharmaceutical formulation containing Vitex agnus castus. J Womens Health Gend Based Med 9(3):315–320, 2000 10787228
London RS, Sundaram GS, Murphy L, et al: The effect of alpha-tocopherol on premenstrual symptomatology: a double-blind study. J Am Coll Nutr 2(2):115–122, 1983 6350402
London RS, Murphy L, Kitlowski KE, et al: Efficacy of alpha-tocopherol in the treatment of the premenstrual syndrome. J Reprod Med 32(6):400–404, 1987 3302248
Lopez LM, Kaptein AA, Helmerhorst FM: Oral contraceptives containing drospirenone for premenstrual syndrome. Cochrane Database Syst Rev (2):CD006586, 2012 22336820
Lovick T: SSRIs and the female brain: potential for utilizing steroid-stimulating properties to treat menstrual cycle-linked dysphorias. J Psychopharmacol 27(12):1180–1185, 2013 23704364
Lustyk MK, Gerrish WG, Shaver S, et al: Cognitive-behavioral therapy for premenstrual syndrome and premenstrual dysphoric disorder: a systematic review. Arch Women Ment Health 12(2):85–96, 2009 19247573
Marjoribanks J, Brown J, O'Brien PM, et al: Selective serotonin reuptake inhibitors for premenstrual syndrome. Cochrane Database Syst Rev (6):CD001396, 2013 23744611
Marks JL, Hair CS, Klock SC, et al: Effects of menstrual phase on intake of nicotine, caffeine, and alcohol and nonprescribed drugs in women with late luteal phase dysphoric disorder. J Subst Abuse 6(2):235–243, 1994 7804022
Marrocco J, Einhorn NR, Petty GH, et al: Epigenetic intersection of BDNF Val66Met genotype with premenstrual dysphoric disorder transcriptome in a cross-species model of estradiol add-back. Mol Psychiatry 25(3):572–583, 2020 30356121
Martinez PE, Rubinow DR, Nieman LK, et al: 5′-reductase inhibition prevents the luteal phase increase in plasma allopregnanolone levels and mitigates symptoms in women with premenstrual dysphoric disorder. Neuropsychopharmacology 41(4):1093–1102, 2016 26272051
Mazza M, Harnic D, Catalano V, et al: Duloxetine for premenstrual dysphoric disorder: a pilot study. Expert Opin Pharmacother 9(4):517–521, 2008 18312154
Menkes DB, Coates DC, Fawcett JP: Acute tryptophan depletion aggravates premenstrual syndrome. J Affect Disord 32(1):37–44, 1994 7798465
Miller ER 3rd, Pastor-Barriuso R, Dalal D, et al: Meta-analysis: high-dosage vitamin E supplementation may increase all-cause mortality. Ann Intern Med 142(1):37–46, 2005 15537682
Mishell DR Jr: Premenstrual disorders: epidemiology and disease burden. Am J Manag Care 11(16 suppl):S473–S479, 2005 16336056
Monteleone P, Luisi S, Tonetti A, et al: Allopregnanolone concentrations and premenstrual syndrome. Eur J Endocrinol 142(3):269–273, 2000 10700721
Mortola JF, Girton L, Beck L, et al: Diagnosis of premenstrual syndrome by a simple, prospective, and reliable instrument: the calendar of premenstrual experiences. Obstet Gynecol 76(2):302–307, 1990 2371035
Namavar Jahromi B, Pakmehr S, Hagh-Shenas H: Work stress, premenstrual syndrome and dysphoric disorder: are there any associations? Iran Red Crescent Med J 13(3):199–202, 2011 22737463
National Health Service: Periods and fertility in the menstrual cycle. NHS.uk, August 5, 2019. Available at: https://www.nhs.uk/conditions/periods/fertility-in-the-menstrual-cycle. Accessed September 6, 2020.
Nobles CJ, Thomas JJ, Valentine SE, et al: Association of premenstrual syndrome and premenstrual dysphoric disorder with bulimia nervosa and binge-eating disorder in a nationally representative epidemiological sample. Int J Eat Disord 49(7):641–650, 2016 27206163
Nolen-Hoeksema S, Wisco BE, Lyubomirsky S: Rethinking rumination. Perspect Psychol Sci 3(5):400–424, 2008 26158958
O'Brien PM, Bäckström T, Brown C, et al: Towards a consensus on diagnostic criteria, measurement and trial design of the premenstrual disorders: the ISPMD Montreal consensus. Arch Women Ment Health 14(1):13–21, 2011 21225438
Osborne LM, Payne JL: Clinical updates in women's health care summary: mood and anxiety disorders: primary and preventive care review. Obstet Gynecol 130(3):674, 2017 28832483

Ozgoli G, Selselei EA, Mojab F, et al: A randomized, placebo-controlled trial of Ginkgo biloba L. in treatment of premenstrual syndrome. J Altern Complement Med 15(8):845–851, 2009 19678774
Padhy SK, Sarkar S, Beherre PB, et al: Relationship of premenstrual syndrome and premenstrual dysphoric disorder with major depression: relevance to clinical practice. Indian J Psychol Med 37(2):159–164, 2015 25969600
Parker MA, Sneddon AE, Arbon P: The menstrual disorder of teenagers (MDOT) study: determining typical menstrual patterns and menstrual disturbance in a large population-based study of Australian teenagers. BJOG 117(2):185–192, 2010 19874294
Perkonigg A, Yonkers KA, Pfister H, et al: Risk factors for premenstrual dysphoric disorder in a community sample of young women: the role of traumatic events and posttraumatic stress disorder. J Clin Psychiatry 65(10):1314–1322, 2004 15491233
Peters JR, Smart LM, Baer RA: Dysfunctional responses to emotion mediate the cross-sectional relationship between rejection sensitivity and borderline personality features. J Pers Disord 29(2):231–240, 2015 25102083
Peters W, Freeman MP, Kim S, et al: Treatment of premenstrual breakthrough of depression with adjunctive oral contraceptive pills compared with placebo. J Clin Psychopharmacol 37(5):609–614, 2017 28816924
Pilver CE, Kasl S, Desai R, et al: Health advantage for black women: patterns in pre-menstrual dysphoric disorder. Psychol Med 41(8):1741–1750, 2011a 21108869
Pilver CE, Levy BR, Libby DJ, et al: Posttraumatic stress disorder and trauma characteristics are correlates of premenstrual dysphoric disorder. Arch Women Ment Health 14(5):383–393, 2011b 21786081
Pinkerton JV, Guico-Pabia CJ, Taylor HS: Menstrual cycle-related exacerbation of disease. Am J Obstet Gynecol 202(3):221–231, 2010 20207238
Pradhan S, Gomez-Lobo V: Hormonal contraceptives, intrauterine devices, gonadotropin-releasing hormone analogues and testosterone: menstrual suppression in special adolescent populations. J Pediatr Adolesc Gynecol 32(5S suppl):S23–S29, 2019 30980941
Praschak-Rieder N, Willeit M, Winkler D, et al: Role of family history and 5-HTTLPR polymorphism in female seasonal affective disorder patients with and without premenstrual dysphoric disorder. Eur Neuropsychopharmacol 12(2):129–134, 2002 11872329
Qiao M, Zhang H, Liu H, et al: Prevalence of premenstrual syndrome and premenstrual dysphoric disorder in a population-based sample in China. Eur J Obstet Gynecol Reprod Biol 162(1):83–86, 2012 22377229
Raffi E, Freeman M: The etiology of premenstrual dysphoric disorder: 5 interwoven pieces. Curr Psychiatr 16(9):20–28, 2017
Ramos MG, Hara C, Rocha FL: Duloxetine treatment for women with premenstrual dysphoric disorder: a single-blind trial. Int J Neuropsychopharmacol 12(8):1081–1088, 2009 19250561
Rapkin A: A review of treatment of premenstrual syndrome and premenstrual dysphoric disorder. Psychoneuroendocrinology 28(3 suppl 3):39–53, 2003 12892989
Rapkin AJ, Edelmuth E, Chang LC, et al: Whole-blood serotonin in premenstrual syndrome. Obstet Gynecol 70(4):533–537, 1987 3627623
Rapkin AJ, Chang LC, Reading AE: Comparison of retrospective and prospective assessment of premenstrual symptoms. Psychol Rep 62(1):55–60, 1988 3363076
Rapkin AJ, Morgan M, Goldman L, et al: Progesterone metabolite allopregnanolone in women with premenstrual syndrome. Obstet Gynecol 90(5):709–714, 1997 9351749
Reed SC, Levin FR, Evans SM: Changes in mood, cognitive performance and appetite in the late luteal and follicular phases of the menstrual cycle in women with and without PMDD (premenstrual dysphoric disorder). Horm Behav 54(1):185–193, 2008 18413151
Reid RL: When should surgical treatment be considered for premenstrual dysphoric disorder? Menopause Int 18(2):77–81, 2012 22611227
Robakis TK, Holtzman J, Stemmle PG, et al: Lamotrigine and GABAA receptor modulators interact with menstrual cycle phase and oral contraceptives to regulate mood in women with bipolar disorder. J Affect Disord 175:108–115, 2015 25601310
Roca CA, Schmidt PJ, Smith MJ, et al: Effects of metergoline on symptoms in women with premenstrual dysphoric disorder. Am J Psychiatry 159(11):1876–1881, 2002 12411222

Rubinow DR, Roy-Byrne P: Premenstrual syndromes: overview from a methodologic perspective. Am J Psychiatry 141(2):163–172, 1984 6362441

Sanders SA, Graham CA, Bass JL, et al: A prospective study of the effects of oral contraceptives on sexuality and well-being and their relationship to discontinuation. Contraception 64(1):51–58, 2001 11535214

Sassoon SA, Colrain IM, Baker FC: Personality disorders in women with severe premenstrual syndrome. Arch Women Ment Health 14(3):257–264, 2011 21298551

Schellenberg R: Treatment for the premenstrual syndrome with agnus castus fruit extract: prospective, randomised, placebo controlled study. BMJ 322(7279):134–137, 2001 11159568

Schmidt PJ, Martinez PE, Nieman LK, et al: Premenstrual dysphoric disorder symptoms following ovarian suppression: triggered by change in ovarian steroid levels but not continuous stable levels. Am J Psychiatry 174(10):980–989, 2017 28427285

Schneider T, Popik P: Attenuation of estrous cycle-dependent marble burying in female rats by acute treatment with progesterone and antidepressants. Psychoneuroendocrinology 32(6):651–659, 2007 17561352

Segebladh B, Borgstrom A, Nyberg S, et al: Evaluation of different add back estradiol and progesterone treatments to gonadotropin-releasing agonist treatment in patients with premenstrual dysphoric disorder. Am J Obstet Gynecol 201(2):139.e1–139.e8, 2009 21501124

Segebladh B, Bannbers E, Kask K, et al: Prevalence of violence exposure in women with premenstrual dysphoric disorder in comparison with other gynecological patients and asymptomatic controls. Acta Obstet Gynecol Scand 90(7):746–752, 2011 21501124

Sepede G, Brunetti M, Di Giannantonio M: Comorbid premenstrual dysphoric disorder in women with bipolar disorder: management challenges. Neuropsychiatr Dis Treat 16:415–426, 2020 32103961

Shah NR, Jones JB, Aperi J, et al: Selective serotonin reuptake inhibitors for premenstrual syndrome and premenstrual dysphoric disorder: a meta-analysis. Obstet Gynecol 111(5):1175–1182, 2008 18448752

Shams-Alizadeh N, Maroufi A, Rashidi M, et al: Premenstrual dysphoric disorder and suicide attempts as a correlation among women in reproductive age. Asian J Psychiatr 31:63–66, 2018 29432986

Slyepchenko A, Frey BN, Lafer B, et al: Increased illness burden in women with comorbid bipolar and premenstrual dysphoric disorder: data from 1,099 women from STEP-BD study. Acta Psychiatr Scand 136(5):473–482, 2017 28846801

Steinberg S, Annable L, Young SN, et al: A placebo-controlled clinical trial of L-tryptophan in premenstrual dysphoria. Biol Psychiatry 45(3):313–320, 1999 10023508

Steiner M, Li T: Luteal phase and symptom-onset dosing of SSRIs/SNRIs in the treatment of premenstrual dysphoria: clinical evidence and rationale. CNS Drugs 27(8):583–589, 2013 23728922

Steiner M, Streiner DL: Validation of a revised visual analog scale for premenstrual mood symptoms: results from prospective and retrospective trials. Can J Psychiatry 50(6):327–332, 2005 15999948

Steiner M, Macdougall M, Brown E: The Premenstrual Symptoms Screening Tool (PSST) for clinicians. Arch Women Ment Health 6(3):203–209, 2003 12920618

Steiner M, Peer M, Macdougall M, et al: The Premenstrual Tension Syndrome Rating Scales: an updated version. J Affect Disord 135(1–3):82–88, 2011a 21802738

Steiner M, Peer M, Palova E, et al: The Premenstrual Symptoms Screening Tool revised for adolescents (PSST-A): prevalence of severe PMS and premenstrual dysphoric disorder in adolescents. Arch Women Ment Health 14(1):77–81, 2011b 21271266

Studd J: Hormone therapy for reproductive depression in women. Post Reprod Health 20(4):132–137, 2014 25398672

Sundblad C, Modigh K, Andersch B, et al: Clomipramine effectively reduces premenstrual irritability and dysphoria: a placebo-controlled trial. Acta Psychiatr Scand 85(1):39–47, 1992 1546547

Sundblad C, Hedberg MA, Eriksson E: Clomipramine administered during the luteal phase reduces the symptoms of premenstrual syndrome: a placebo-controlled trial. Neuropsychopharmacology 9(2):133–145, 1993 8216696

Takayama E, Tanaka H, Kamimoto Y, et al: Relationship between a high Edinburgh Postnatal Depression Scale score and premenstrual syndrome: a prospective, observational study. Taiwan J Obstet Gynecol 59(3):356–360, 2020 32416879
Takeo C, Negishi E, Nakajima A, et al: Association of cytosine-adenine repeat polymorphism of the estrogen receptor-beta gene with menopausal symptoms. Gend Med 2(2):96–105, 2005 16115604
Teatero ML, Mazmanian D, Sharma V: Effects of the menstrual cycle on bipolar disorder. Bipolar Disord 16(1):22–36, 2014 24467469
Thys-Jacobs S, McMahon D, Bilezikian JP: Cyclical changes in calcium metabolism across the menstrual cycle in women with premenstrual dysphoric disorder. J Clin Endocrinol Metab 92(8):2952–2959, 2007 17488795
U.S. Food and Drug Administration: FDA Drug Safety Communication: Updated information about the risk of blood clots in women taking birth control pills containing drospirenone. FDA.gov, April 10, 2012. Available at: https://www.fda.gov/drugs/drug-safety-and-availability/fda-drug-safety-communication-updated-information-about-risk-blood-clots-women-taking-birth-control. Accessed August 5, 2020.
Verkaik S, Kamperman AM, van Westrhenen R, et al: The treatment of premenstrual syndrome with preparations of Vitex agnus castus: a systematic review and meta-analysis. Am J Obstet Gynecol 217(2):150–166, 2017 28237870
Viktorin A, Lichtenstein P, Thase ME, et al: The risk of switch to mania in patients with bipolar disorder during treatment with an antidepressant alone and in combination with a mood stabilizer. Am J Psychiatry 171(10):1067–1073, 2014 24935197
Wang M, Hammarbäck S, Lindhe BA, et al: Treatment of premenstrual syndrome by spironolactone: a double-blind, placebo-controlled study. Acta Obstet Gynecol Scand 74(10):803–808, 1995 8533564
Webster DE, He Y, Chen SN, et al: Opioidergic mechanisms underlying the actions of Vitex agnus-castus L. Biochem Pharmacol 81(1):170–177, 2011 20854795
Weise C, Kaiser G, Janda C, et al: Internet-based cognitive-behavioural intervention for women with premenstrual dysphoric disorder: a randomized controlled trial. Psychother Psychosom 88(1):16–29, 2019 30783069
Whelan AM, Jurgens TM, Naylor H: Herbs, vitamins and minerals in the treatment of premenstrual syndrome: a systematic review. Can J Clin Pharmacol 16(3):e407–e429, 2009 19923637
Wittchen HU, Becker E, Lieb R, et al: Prevalence, incidence and stability of premenstrual dysphoric disorder in the community. Psychol Med 32(1):119–132, 2002 11883723
Wyatt KM, Dimmock PW, Ismail KM, et al: The effectiveness of GnRHa with and without 'add-back' therapy in treating premenstrual syndrome: a meta analysis. BJOG 111(6):585–593, 2004 15198787
Yen JY, Tu HP, Chen CS, et al: The effect of serotonin 1A receptor polymorphism on the cognitive function of premenstrual dysphoric disorder. Eur Arch Psychiatry Clin Neurosci 264(8):729–739, 2014 24158751
Yen JY, Liu TL, Chen IJ, et al: Premenstrual appetite and emotional responses to foods among women with premenstrual dysphoric disorder. Appetite 125:18–23, 2018 29407746
Yonkers KA, Simoni MK: Premenstrual disorders. Am J Obstet Gynecol 218(1):68–74, 2018 28571724
Yonkers KA, Brown C, Pearlstein TB, et al: Efficacy of a new low-dose oral contraceptive with drospirenone in premenstrual dysphoric disorder. Obstet Gynecol 106(3):492–501, 2005a 16135578
Yonkers KA, Pearlstein T, Fayyad R, et al: Luteal phase treatment of premenstrual dysphoric disorder improves symptoms that continue into the postmenstrual phase. J Affect Disord 85(3):317–321, 2005b 15780701
Yonkers KA, O'Brien PM, Eriksson E: Premenstrual syndrome. Lancet 371(9619):1200–1210, 2008 18395582
Yonkers KA, Pearlstein TB, Gotman N: A pilot study to compare fluoxetine, calcium, and placebo in the treatment of premenstrual syndrome. J Clin Psychopharmacol 33(5):614–620, 2013 23963058

CHAPTER 7

# Perimenopause

Nicole Leistikow, M.D.
Milena H. Smith, M.D., Ph.D.
Katherine E. Williams, M.D.
C. Neill Epperson, M.D.

Like other times of reproductive change in a woman's life, perimenopause increases the risk for the onset of symptoms affecting physical and mental health, as well as exacerbations of previously diagnosed mental illnesses. The greatest body of evidence exists for the recurrence of depression (Cohen et al. 2006; Freeman et al. 2014; Maki et al. 2018) and new-onset depression (Freeman et al. 2006). During perimenopause, hormones fluctuate significantly, and it is likely that these fluctuations, in addition to the overall waning amounts of estrogen and other hormones, are responsible for the increased risk of depression and the wide variety of symptoms that perimenopausal women may experience, including irritability, hot flashes, sleep disturbance, cognitive complaints, and sexual dysfunction. However, the role of these hormonal changes is complex and not yet fully understood, and additional factors, such as family history, adverse childhood experiences, changes with aging, and later life experiences, also have roles (Epperson et al. 2017; Woods et al. 2008).

In this chapter, we examine mental health at the end of the reproductive lifespan by focusing on the epidemiology, clinical features, presentation, pathophysiology, evaluation, and treatment of both perimenopausal depression and vasomotor symptoms (VMS) that are common and frequently complicate depression. We also review other prevalent and potentially related perimenopausal symptoms, such as sleep disturbance, sexual problems, and cognitive complaints. Much of the information we have about this time of life is informed by three large prospective cohort studies performed in the United States: the Study of Women's Health Across the Nation (SWAN), the Penn Ovarian Aging Study (POAS), and the Seattle Midlife Women's Health Study (SMWHS). These studies focus on women during the perimenopausal transition and offer significant evidence about the natural course and treatment of perimenopausal symptoms.

# Perimenopausal Depression

## Epidemiology

### Rates/Incidence

Cross-sectional studies suggest that perimenopausal women experience depressive symptoms at higher rates than premenopausal women: 45%–68% of women during the menopausal transition versus 28%–31% of women prior to this transition (Maki et al. 2018). Fewer studies measure actual rates of major depressive disorder (MDD) as women progress from premenopause to postmenopause. The large prospective SWAN reported increasing MDD rates across this transition: 5.8% in premenopausal, 9.1% in perimenopausal, and 9.8% in postmenopausal women (Bromberger et al. 2011). Similarly, POAS, which followed women over 8 years as many of them transitioned from premenopause to perimenopause, found that, after adjustments were made for risk factors such as smoking, BMI, history of premenstrual syndrome, estradiol levels, and VMS severity, perimenopausal women were more than five times as likely as premenopausal women to experience a first episode of depression (Freeman et al. 2006). The smaller Harvard Study of Moods and Cycles reported MDD in 9.5% of premenopausal women versus 16.6% of perimenopausal women (Cohen et al. 2006). Finally, a large cross-sectional survey of European women found a sevenfold increased risk of suicidal ideation in women during perimenopause compared with women in premenopause or postmenopause, independent of mood and anxiety disorders (Usall et al. 2009).

### Risk Factors

Women with a prior history of MDD are at increased risk of a recurrence during perimenopause (Maki et al. 2018). SWAN found that 58% of women with prior MDD experienced at least one major depressive episode over the study's 13-year follow-up period, compared with 28% of women with no prior history of depression, a twofold increase in risk (Bromberger et al. 2015). In addition, a greater degree of hormonal change, particularly as measured by blood levels of follicle-stimulating hormone (FSH) (Freeman et al. 2004) and estradiol (Freeman et al. 2006), is associated with increased depressive symptoms during perimenopause versus premenopause. Longer time spent in the menopausal transition may further increase the risk for a perimenopausal depression (Avis et al. 1994; Freeman et al. 2006), as does surgically induced menopause (Obermeyer et al. 2007). Other risk factors for perimenopausal depression include a history of anxiety, premenstrual syndrome, adverse experiences, a history of trauma during childhood, Black race or Hispanic ethnicity, financial stress, low social support, a history of violent or abusive relationships, VMS (hot flashes and night sweats) and other perimenopausal symptoms such as sleep problems, and health and lifestyle factors, including elevated BMI and smoking cigarettes (Bromberger et al. 2015; Cohen et al. 2006; Epperson et al. 2017; Freeman et al. 2004, 2006, 2014; Maki et al. 2018; Schmidt et al. 2004). Risk differences by race and ethnicity may be attenuated or explained by psychosocial differences. SWAN, for example, found that psychosocial and health factors accounted for higher odds of depressive symptoms among Black and Hispanic participants (Bromberger and Kravitz 2011). Table 7–1 summarizes the risk factors for menopausal depression.

TABLE 7–1. **Risk factors for perimenopausal depression**

| Demographic | Psychosocial | Menopause related | Medical |
|---|---|---|---|
| Younger age at menopause onset | Adverse childhood experiences | Vasomotor symptoms | History of anxiety or depression |
| Black race or Hispanic ethnicity | History of childhood trauma | Sleep disturbance | History of perimenstrual or perinatal mood symptoms |
| | Low social support | | High BMI |
| | Violent or abusive relationships | | Smoking |

## Other Mental Illnesses in Perimenopause

Although research is limited, existing evidence suggests that women are at an increased risk of new onset or exacerbation of other mental illnesses during perimenopause (Hu et al. 2016). A systematic review that included seven cross-sectional and two longitudinal studies found that women with bipolar I or II disorder were at increased risk of depressive episodes during perimenopause (Perich et al. 2017). In a small longitudinal study, women previously diagnosed with bipolar illness scored higher on scales measuring depressive and manic symptoms during late perimenopause and early postmenopause (Marsh et al. 2015). Findings from several studies suggest that perimenopause is a time of increased risk for schizophrenia, with a second wave being diagnosed between ages 45 and 54 (Crow et al. 2016; Gupta et al. 2012). Studies showing that estrogen and selective estrogen receptor modulators improve some symptoms of schizophrenia in women (Kulkarni et al. 2008; Searles et al. 2018) and that antipsychotics become less effective for women the more time elapses after menopause (González-Rodríguez et al. 2016) all suggest that the menopausal transition plays an important role in schizophrenia.

Anxiety disorders are less well studied during the menopausal transition, and current evidence is insufficient to establish an increased incidence during the menopausal transition. However, there is evidence of increased anxiety symptoms during perimenopause among women who previously had low baseline anxiety before beginning the menopausal transition, as well as a relationship between VMS and both anxiety and panic attacks (Bromberger et al. 2013; Bryant et al. 2012; Claudia et al. 2004; Freeman and Sammel 2016; Freeman et al. 2005; Hantsoo and Epperson 2017). Additionally, somatic anxiety preceding the menopausal transition is a risk factor for worse VMS during the transition, suggesting that treatment addressing anxiety may also improve hot flashes (Freeman and Sammel 2016).

The epidemiology of other disorders, such as substance misuse and eating disorders, requires further research. Perimenopause may be a time of increased vulnerability to a new onset or worsening of alcohol use disorder, and older women are more at risk from medical complications of alcohol use at lower levels of consumption than younger women or men (Milic et al. 2018). In addition, after controlling for other risk factors, a large study of women veterans with chronic pain found that having menopausal symptoms was associated with the potential iatrogenic risk of long-term and higher-dose opioid prescriptions (Gibson et al. 2019). Older women are also more likely than men to take prescribed sleep aids, which may lead to dependence and increased fall risk later in life (Pop et al. 2019). The transition to menopause, like puberty, may be a period of vulnerability to the development or recurrence of an eating disorder (Baker and Runfola 2016), although further research is needed to explore this association.

## Screening Methods for Perimenopausal Depression

There is currently no widespread agreement on the timing of or specific scales to use in screening for perimenopausal depression (Willi and Ehlert 2019) and no validated perimenopausal depression scale (Maki et al. 2018). Gynecologists wishing to screen at annual examinations may want to begin as early as late premenopause, or when one cycle has lengthened or shortened by at least 7 days in the past year, because studies show this to be when an increased risk of depressive symptoms begins (Freeman et al. 2006). The Center for Epidemiologic Studies Depression Scale (Radloff 1977) is used in numerous mood and menopause studies, but standard screening instruments used at other times of life, such as the Patient Health Questionnaire–9 (Spitzer et al. 1999), also can be used in the premenopausal population (Maki et al. 2018). The Patient Health Questionnaire–9 is a nine-item scale listing depressive symptoms based on DSM criteria, and a score ≥10 is considered a positive screen (Arroll et al. 2010). Before a patient starts taking antidepressants, the clinician should screen for bipolar disorder to prevent antidepressant-induced mania. The Mood Disorder Questionnaire is a brief screening tool that is frequently used for bipolar illness presenting in the postpartum period when sleep disturbance and somatic symptoms are higher; these characteristics are also found in the perimenopausal population (Clark and Wisner 2018).

## Clinical Features and Presentation

### Diagnostic Criteria

The diagnosis of perimenopausal depression is based on the same DSM-5 (American Psychiatric Association 2013) clinical criteria as the diagnosis of MDD at other times of life (see Chapter 13, "Depressive Disorders"). However, as discussed in sections that follow, other aspects of perimenopause, including VMS, sleep disturbances, sexual dysfunction, and cognitive symptoms, can complicate diagnosis and should be investigated and followed over the course of treatment.

### Clinical Presentation

The clinical presentation of perimenopausal depression has many of the features of depressive episodes outside the perimenopausal period: low mood, anhedonia, poor energy and low motivation, feelings of low self-worth, and sometimes suicidal ideation. Changes in sleep, appetite, concentration, and libido can also occur as part of MDD and can be challenging to distinguish from the symptoms of perimenopause. Sleep disruption is a common feature of depression in this period and can be mistaken for new-onset or previously undiagnosed bipolar disorder, which remains rare despite a possibly increased prevalence during perimenopause (see earlier subsection "Other Mental Illnesses in Perimenopause"). Perimenopause may trigger exacerbations of previously identified bipolar disorder, including manic episodes, although depressions are more common. The following case represents a typical constellation of symptoms that a provider may encounter and illustrates the challenge of distinguishing perimenopausal depression from both bipolar disorder and the somatic symptoms of perimenopause.

Ms. M is a 47-year-old woman referred to a psychiatrist by her gynecologist for symptoms of anxiety and low mood in the setting of irregular periods and hot flashes starting about 6 months prior. She presents with 12 weeks of difficulty sleeping, low energy, increased anxiety about her work, heightened irritability, poor concentration, and forgetfulness. She says she feels "moody" and is having trouble completing tasks at work. While talking with her gynecologist during a routine pap smear, Ms. M became tearful and said, "I feel like I'm failing everyone. Some days I wonder if I can go on."

Ms. M has a history of high anxiety that began during her senior year of high school and was treated successfully with psychotherapy. At age 20, after the birth of her first child, she experienced an episode of postpartum depression that resolved spontaneously after 6 months. During that episode, she had insomnia, frequent crying, and increased irritability and felt overwhelmed. She has no previous psychiatric hospitalizations. She has a history of episodes of increased irritability and anxiety, often occurring the week prior to menses. She does not smoke cigarettes or use any alcohol or drugs, including marijuana. She has no major medical conditions but has recently gained 5 lb and reports increased snacking at night before bed.

Social challenges are common in perimenopausal women and may trigger or exacerbate mood disturbances. Physical complaints or medical comorbidities may distract from or mask depressive etiologies in this population. Finally, alcohol and substance use often complicate the picture of depression at midlife. The following case illustrates the challenge of delineating social stressors, medical issues, and the use of medications, substances, or drugs in order to develop a differential diagnosis and appropriate treatment recommendations.

Ms. N is a 50-year-old woman who presents with difficulty sleeping and low mood that started about 3 months prior in the setting of her mother's death from breast cancer. She describes low energy, tearfulness, and trouble with both sleep initiation and maintenance. It takes up to an hour for her to fall asleep, and she then has several awakenings, each lasting about 30 minutes. Her sheets are sometimes damp when she wakes. She has had occasional, mild daytime hot flashes for several years without recent change in frequency or severity.

Ms. N has no prior history of mental illness. She has gained about 15 lb over the past 2 years and was diagnosed with type 2 diabetes 1 year ago; she has been taking metformin but has not seen her primary care doctor since. She has a family history of "thyroid problems." Ms. N smokes half a pack of cigarettes a day and does not use any drugs, including marijuana. She has been drinking one or two glasses of wine 4–5 nights a week for the past 2 months. She lives with her husband of 20 years and their two daughters, ages 15 and 18. Her aging father moved in with them recently after the death of her mother. She works as a trial attorney.

## Differential Diagnosis

The differential diagnosis of perimenopausal depression (Table 7–2) includes depression secondary to a general medical condition, subsyndromal depression, another mood disorder such as bipolar depression, adjustment disorder, bereavement or grief, substance misuse, and psychological distress that is elevated from baseline but does not meet criteria for an adjustment disorder. General screening laboratory tests are used as for any evaluation for symptoms of psychiatric illness at other times of a woman's life. These tests commonly include a complete blood count, comprehensive metabolic panel, thyroid-stimulating hormone, and vitamins D and $B_{12}$, as well as other tests as

**TABLE 7–2. Differential diagnosis for perimenopausal depression**

| |
|---|
| Adjustment disorder |
| Bereavement or grief |
| Depression secondary to a medical condition |
| Other mood disorder (especially bipolar affective disorder) |
| Psychological distress |
| Substance misuse |
| Subsyndromal depression |
| Thyroid disorder |

suggested by a particular woman's history and presentation. Women older than 40 are at increased risk of thyroid disorders, which can cause symptoms similar to depression, so it is particularly vital to assess thyroid function (Rossouw et al. 2002).

Levels of sex hormones are not typically assessed because levels of FSH, estradiol, progesterone, and luteinizing hormone can vary significantly day to day (Gordon et al. 2015). Although overall dysregulation and fluctuation of hormones have been linked to depressive symptom burden during perimenopause, clinicians are not able to identify when this occurs (Joffe et al. 2020). The exception to this guidance against checking sex hormone levels is when a woman is experiencing premature menopause; in this case, referring the patient to a gynecologist or a primary care provider for a comprehensive evaluation, typically including sex hormone levels and a pelvic examination, is indicated.

### Course and Prognosis

Perimenopausal depression has a similar course and prognosis as depression diagnosed at other times of life and responds similarly to treatments used at other times of life, with some caveats. Its diagnosis may be complicated or delayed due to symptoms related to perimenopause, such as VMS and sleep disturbance (resolution and treatment of these are discussed later). Additionally, other symptoms (e.g., migraines, which can worsen in perimenopause) may exacerbate depression or make its treatment more challenging (Pavlovic 2018). Some studies have suggested that perimenopausal women with depression may have lower rates of remission compared with premenopausal women or may respond better to combined treatment with antidepressants and hormone therapy (see "Treatment" subsection). However, other studies have yielded contradictory outcomes (Kornstein et al. 2013), and this is an area of ongoing research. Finally, women who experience recurrence of MDD in perimenopause are likely to continue to have a higher risk of depression after their final menstrual period, and some evidence indicates that women whose first episode of depression occurs during perimenopause are less likely to have further episodes after they stop menstruating (Freeman et al. 2014).

## Pathophysiology

### Biological Factors

During perimenopause, levels of reproductive steroids, including estradiol, progesterone, testosterone, and dehydroepiandrosterone sulfate, can vary widely. Because fluctuations in these hormones are known to affect mood, these changes likely play a role in the etiology of perimenopausal depression. Multiple studies indicate that the variability, not the absolute level, of peripherally measured hormones is central to the etiology of perimenopausal mood disturbances (Bromberger and Epperson 2018). In a study of women with no prior history of depression, fluctuations in estradiol, FSH, and luteinizing hormone relative to a woman's own mean level of these hormones when she was premenopausal were associated with greater depressive symptoms during perimenopause (Freeman et al. 2006). Furthermore, a subset of women with a history of either premenstrual dysphoric disorder or postpartum depression appears to be especially vulnerable to the dynamics of estrogen and progesterone withdrawal because these are associated with an increased risk of perimenopausal depression (Freeman et al. 2006; Woods and Mitchell 2005).

Strong evidence for the estrogen withdrawal hypothesis comes from a small randomized controlled trial (RCT) that included 56 asymptomatic postmenopausal women with a history of perimenopausal depression. The subjects were given 3 weeks of transdermal estradiol 100 μg/day and then randomized to either placebo or continued estradiol for another 3 weeks. When depressive symptomatology in the two groups was compared, the women who continued estradiol remained asymptomatic, but the women who were switched to placebo, and therefore were in estrogen withdrawal, had an increase in depressive symptoms (Schmidt et al. 2015). Polymorphisms in estrogen receptor genes may play a role in the etiology of perimenopausal depression (Bromberger and Epperson 2018). Studies such as SMWHS and SWAN have reported that polymorphisms in genes transcribing enzymes related to estrogen metabolism are associated with increased perimenopausal depression and hot flash risk in some women (Bromberger and Epperson 2018; Kravitz et al. 2006; Woods et al. 2018).

Fluctuating progesterone levels during perimenopause may also play an important role in the increased rates of anxiety symptoms during midlife. As women age, they experience more anovulatory cycles, and aging follicles lead to decreased progesterone concentrations even when ovulation occurs. As described in Chapter 6, "Premenstrual Mood Syndromes," progesterone is metabolized to allopregnanolone, and thus perimenopause is associated with fluctuating levels of allopregnanolone. Some women may not have $GABA_A$ receptors that adapt to this hormonal volatility; therefore, in perimenopause, as in premenstrual dysphoric disorder and postpartum depression, this dynamic change in allopregnanolone is associated with dysphoria and anxiety (Gordon et al. 2015; Hantsoo and Epperson 2020). Genetics may play a role in response to allopregnanolone alterations: $GABA_A$ receptor subunit polymorphisms have been found to be associated with an increased risk of depression, and it has been proposed that this be investigated in perimenopausal depression (Gordon et al. 2015).

## Psychological Factors

Psychological contributions to perimenopausal mood and anxiety disorders include attitudes toward menopause, personality traits, and cognitive styles, especially optimism and a self-critical cognitive style (Süss and Ehlert 2020). Most studies that include measures of attitudes toward menopause report that negative attitudes play a role in the etiology of menopausal depression and anxiety symptoms (Ayers et al. 2010). A bidirectional relationship likely exists, because women who have more depressive symptoms also have more negative attitudes (Ayers et al. 2010). Similarly, the psychological tendency toward self-criticism has been found to be an important moderator in the etiology of depressive symptoms: highly self-critical women with irritability are at higher risk for the development of depressive symptoms than women who are less self-critical (Mauas et al. 2014). Furthermore, women with depression during perimenopause have reported more unanticipated negative life events that were thought to be out of their control and decreased their self-esteem (Schmidt et al. 2004). Self-compassion, self-acceptance, and optimism are considered important resilience factors associated with more positive appraisal of the physical and emotional changes during perimenopause, and these are associated with fewer depressive symptoms and better quality of life (Süss and Ehlert 2020).

### Social and Cultural Considerations

In addition to biological and psychological factors, many social changes occur during the perimenopausal transition, and these may contribute to onset of depression and anxiety symptoms in vulnerable women. Role stress often escalates for women during this time as they attempt to juggle increased and varied responsibilities, which may include caring for aging family members, changing childcare needs, and new challenges at work and in their intimate relationships (Maki et al. 2018). To our knowledge, no large studies have attempted to quantify the contribution of these social and cultural differences to the etiology of perimenopausal depression. It is highly likely that differing cultural views of aging, and beliefs about the responsibilities associated with role changes, factor into the experience of stress and contribute to depressive symptoms experienced at this time of life. In their review of "empty nest psychosocial stress," Bougea et al. (2019) described the varying expectations that different families and cultures have regarding the care of elders, including whether living arrangements are independent or shared, and how these expectations shift in times of economic or social crisis (Bougea et al. 2019). Social stresses associated with increased depression at other times of life, such as interpersonal violence, racial discrimination, and poverty, likely also play a role in perimenopausal depressive symptoms. For instance, in a study of perimenopausal women in New York City, neighborhood characteristics of decreased safety and cohesiveness and increased racial discriminatory actions were associated with increased depressive symptoms (Gerber and Sievert 2018).

## Treatment

### Complete Evaluation That Identifies Contributing Factors

Treatment of a perimenopausal woman who has psychiatric symptoms begins with a comprehensive clinical interview that encompasses her current symptoms; prior history of psychiatric symptoms and treatment; medical history, including reproductive history; and social and family history (Stute et al. 2020). The interview should include a detailed review of current physical symptoms; list of current medications, including over-the-counter supplements; typical diet, sleep, and exercise habits; recent and ongoing stressors; and consumption of caffeine, alcohol, marijuana, and other substances. Information about recent menstrual cycle patterns, sexual function, and VMS should also be elicited (Canonico et al. 2007; Joffe et al. 2003; Krause and Nakajima 2015). A one-time hormone level is not terribly informative in the assessment and treatment of perimenopausal depression. Most often, the diagnosis is a clinical one based on VMS,

**TABLE 7–3. How to talk about perimenopausal depression**

| |
|---|
| How are you feeling about being near menopause? |
| Are you noticing any changes in your body that concern you? |
| Have you been having hot flashes or night sweats? |
| Have you had any problems with low mood, increased anxiety, or irritability? |
| Have you noticed any changes in your interest in or pleasure from sex? |
| Have you had any difficulty with urinating, with leaking urine, or with urinating more frequently or urgently? |
| Have you been having any problems with your memory or concentration? |
| Are you having any trouble sleeping? |
| How much pain are you in day to day? |
| Who are you caring for at this point in your life? |
| Have you found yourself turning to alcohol, drugs, or overeating to manage emotions? |
| How many alcoholic drinks per week are you having, and is this a change from your previous pattern? |
| Do you have anyone you can talk to whom you trust? |

vaginal dryness, and altered menstrual patterns. Although the FDA in 2018 approved a blood test for anti-Müllerian hormone, a measure of follicle reserve, as one of several indicators that a woman is in perimenopause (U.S. Food and Drug Administration 2018), the American College of Obstetricians and Gynecologists (2019) does not currently recommend its use as a predictor of estimated menopause onset in women who are currently premenopausal.

A recent study showed that most hot flashes occurring at night are associated with awakening (Thurston et al. 2019). Considering the impact of poor sleep on multiple psychiatric conditions, the clinician should ask about frequency of awakenings during the night and question whether bedding or clothing are damp or wet on awakening. Table 7–3 includes some questions that may assist providers in initiating these discussions. In addition, scales such as the Menopause Rating Scale (MRS; Heinemann et al. 2004), Greene Climacteric Scale (GCS; Greene 1976), Hot Flash Related Daily Interference Scale (HFRDIS; Carpenter 2001), Pittsburgh Sleep Quality Index (PSQI; Carpenter and Andrykowski 1998), and Montreal Cognitive Assessment (MoCA; Nasreddine et al. 2005) can be used to identify specific symptoms that may otherwise be missed.

## Psychopharmacology

**Antidepressants for perimenopausal depression.** A number of open trials in perimenopausal women provide evidence for the efficacy of antidepressants, including citalopram, duloxetine, escitalopram, mirtazapine, venlafaxine, and vortioxetine (Freeman et al. 2017; Joffe et al. 2001, 2007; Ladd et al. 2005; Soares et al. 2003, 2006). Use of desvenlafaxine is supported by two large RCTs, both of which show the medication's superiority to placebo (Clayton et al. 2013; Kornstein et al. 2010). Only one published trial compared particular agents directly, and the results did not demonstrate an efficacy difference between paroxetine and vortioxetine (Callegari et al. 2019). No evidence exists to contradict the conclusion that this efficacy is a class effect rather than specific to particular antidepressants; therefore, for a particular woman, preference should be given to any medication to which she has had a prior positive response.

When a woman has no prior history of depression or of a positive response to a specific drug, the choice of antidepressant is made based on data in women during perimenopause, as well as efficacy and tolerability in general. Given the high frequency of sexual dysfunction and weight gain with perimenopause, avoiding agents with a high risk of these side effects is sensible, and women should be closely monitored for their emergence. First-line agents include citalopram, desvenlafaxine, duloxetine, escitalopram, sertraline, venlafaxine, and vortioxetine, any of which may also confer improvement in sleep, anxiety, and pain (Maki et al. 2018). Dosage ranges are the same as those for other populations.

When depression occurs in the setting of VMS, an antidepressant that also has efficacy for VMS can be extremely helpful. Most of the first-line agents listed for the treatment of perimenopausal depression (e.g., citalopram, desvenlafaxine, duloxetine, escitalopram, venlafaxine, and vortioxetine), as well as fluoxetine and mirtazapine, have also shown some efficacy for treating VMS (Joffe et al. 2003, 2007; Maki et al. 2018; Soares et al. 2006). These medications are also used for VMS when menopausal hormone therapy (MHT) is contraindicated (see "Hormonal Treatment" section later in this chapter).

**Hormonal treatment for depression.** The extent to which MHT can have a direct positive effect on mood remains an open question. Multiple studies have attempted to determine whether estrogen therapy is effective as an antidepressant during and after the menopausal transition. Unfortunately, as discussed by Rubinow et al. (2015) in their assessment of 24 such studies (all RCTs) published between 1997 and 2014, drawing robust conclusions is made challenging by the studies' methodological differences; various studies used different definitions of the stages of menopause, as well as different forms of and timing of treatment with respect to the final menstrual period. Even more problematically, few of the studies assessed whether subjects had a prior history of depression or current VMS (both known to increase risk of MDD during the menopausal transition), only five studied women with depression, and only two were restricted to women in perimenopause (Rubinow et al. 2015). Therefore, although there is a theoretical basis and some evidence that estrogen therapy has direct positive effects on mood in women during perimenopause, perhaps particularly in women who experience VMS, this is not sufficiently established for it to be a standard treatment option (Chester et al. 2018). The only extant head-to-head trial comparing MHT (ethinyl estradiol/norethindrone acetate) with an antidepressant (escitalopram) for the treatment of low mood, VMS, and sleep disturbance in perimenopausal women showed improvement in sleep, VMS, and quality of life in both treatment groups, but escitalopram was more effective in the alleviation of symptoms of depression (Soares et al. 2006).

Another area in which knowledge is limited is whether MHT can prevent the occurrence of perimenopausal depression. The one extant study examining this in a prospective, placebo-controlled manner found that women who started MHT (transdermal estradiol plus sequential oral micronized progesterone) early, but not late, in the perimenopausal transition were less likely to experience depression during the 12-month study period than were those randomized to placebo. There was no obvious benefit of

MHT over placebo for women who started the study during the early postmenopause (Gordon et al. 2018). Widespread use of this strategy cannot be recommended until this result is replicated, but using MHT with the goal of preventing the recurrence of depression during the transition to menopause may be considered in the management of individual women with a history of severe depressive episodes, especially associated with other times of hormonal change.

In general, then, the paucity of data available to guide the use of estrogens for treatment of depression during perimenopause leaves antidepressants as the current standard of care. However, estradiol should be considered if perimenopausal symptoms of sleep disruption and VMS do not resolve with antidepressant treatment and if the patient has no contraindication to the use of MHT (see "Hormonal Treatment" section later). Among women with a uterus, the endometrial proliferative effects of estradiol must be managed with either concurrent or sequential use of progesterone. We recommend that any use of MHT by psychiatrists or psychiatric nurse practitioners be coordinated with the patient's gynecologist or primary care provider.

## Other Medical Interventions

Treatments such as electroconvulsive therapy or transcranial magnetic stimulation, for which there is sufficient evidence of efficacy in depression at other times of life, are reasonable options when indicated. (See Chapter 13 for further information about these treatments.)

## Behavioral and Somatic Treatments

**Psychotherapy.** Psychotherapy is the first-line treatment for mild to moderate depression in perimenopausal women, as it is in other populations. It is helpful to normalize the range of emotions that women experience about their changing bodies and social roles during perimenopause and to support healthy coping strategies, such as self-compassion and goal setting (Süss and Ehlert 2020). Cognitive-behavioral therapy (CBT) has Level I evidence for treatment of VMS and proven efficacy for depression and therefore is a particularly relevant therapeutic modality to consider for treatment of depression during perimenopause (Ayers et al. 2011; Mann et al. 2012).

**Alternative treatments for perimenopausal depression.** Currently, insufficient evidence exists to recommend alternative treatments for perimenopausal depression (Maki et al. 2018), although there are several promising areas of research, including soy isoflavones (Stute et al. 2020). A meta-analysis of 11 studies found that low- to moderate-intensity exercise might be helpful for depressive symptoms in midlife and older women (Pérez-López et al. 2017). Patients with depression should be encouraged to exercise to augment other evidence-based treatments; this is likely to have multiple benefits and confers low risk.

## Treatment Challenges

The largest challenge in treating perimenopausal depression often lies in distinguishing the symptoms of depression from the numerous symptoms of perimenopause, which overlap substantially. Perimenopausal symptoms can include VMS, sleep disturbances and fatigue, sexual problems and vaginal dryness, cognitive problems, urinary incontinence, muscle aches and joint pain, weight gain, and depressed or irritable mood

TABLE 7–4. **Overlapping symptoms of perimenopause and depression**

| Symptoms of perimenopause | Overlapping symptoms | Symptoms of depression |
|---|---|---|
| Breast tenderness | Decreased desire for sex | Anhedonia |
| Dyspareunia | Fatigue | Feeling worthless |
| Headache | Impaired concentration | Guilt |
| Hot flashes and night sweats (vasomotor symptoms) | Insomnia | Hopelessness |
| Menometrorrhagia | Irritability | Thoughts of death |
| Musculoskeletal pain | Low mood | |
| Palpitations | Memory complaints | |
| Restless legs | | |
| Vaginal dryness | | |

(Woods and Mitchell 2005). The remainder of this chapter addresses the most prevalent of these, focusing on aspects that will be helpful to psychiatric providers. Table 7–4 highlights the symptoms that are shared by or differentiate perimenopause and depression.

# Vasomotor Symptoms

## Epidemiology

### Rates

VMS are the most common physical complaints among menopausal women (Sussman et al. 2015; Woods and Mitchell 2005). They are experienced by up to 80% of women during perimenopause (Avis et al. 2018; Freeman and Sherif 2007; Williams et al. 2008); perimenopausal and surgically menopausal women are more likely to experience VMS than premenopausal or postmenopausal women (Obermeyer et al. 2007).

### Risk Factors and Screening

Risk factors for more frequent or more severe hot flashes include being Black or Hispanic, having a higher BMI, smoking, and having symptoms of anxiety or depression. Medical interventions such as a hysterectomy (even when the ovaries are conserved) or breast cancer treatment are also associated with more severe VMS (Avis et al. 2018) (Table 7–5).

Recommended screening tools are the MRS (Heinemann et al. 2004) and GCS (Greene 1976), which include VMS among a diverse list of additional symptoms. The HFRDIS (Carpenter 2001) measures the degree to which VMS specifically affect daily functioning.

## Clinical Features and Presentation

### Diagnostic Criteria

Perimenopausal VMS are experienced as a sudden onset of a feeling of heat, most often in the face, neck, and chest, followed by sweating and flushing and occasionally by chills (Mohyi et al. 1997). Symptoms may also include tachycardia and feelings of

TABLE 7–5. **Risk factors and screening tools for vasomotor symptoms**

| Risk factors | Screening tools |
|---|---|
| Black race | Greene Climacteric Scale |
| Hispanic ethnicity | Hot Flash Related Daily Interference Scale |
| Higher BMI | The Menopause Rating Scale |
| Smoking | |
| History of anxiety | |
| History of breast cancer treatment | |
| History of depression | |
| History of hysterectomy | |

anxiety and dread. Hot flashes typically last from 1 to 5 minutes and may occur multiple times a day and night (Bansal and Aggarwal 2019).

### Course and Differential Diagnosis

VMS vary greatly in severity, with studies suggesting that most women experience mild to moderate symptoms. VMS last a mean of 5 years but may last substantially longer for some women (Col et al. 2009; Freeman et al. 2011). In POAS, a 13-year longitudinal study involving assessment every 9–12 months of women from premenopause to postmenopause, the most common age at onset for moderate to severe VMS was 45–49 years, with an average duration of 10.2 years. Women with moderate to severe VMS onset at a later stage of menopause had a shorter duration of symptoms. The median durations were 11.6 years for women who experienced onset in the pre- and late premenopause stages, 7.4 years for those with onset in the early transition, and 3.8 years for those with onset in late perimenopause or early postmenopause. Moreover, Black women experienced a longer duration of VMS than white women in this study (Freeman et al. 2011) and in a study by Avis et al. (2015).

In general, VMS peak around the late perimenopausal or early postmenopausal period (Avis et al. 2015; Williams et al. 2008; Woods and Mitchell 2005). In one study, 24% of women ages 50–54 years had hot flashes, a percentage that decreased to 21% among women ages 55–59, to 10% among women ages 60–69, and to 5% among women ages 70–79 (Brunner et al. 2010). Perimenopausal VMS must be differentiated from other causes of flushing reactions (Table 7–6). The most common systemic causes include thyroid disorders, especially hyperthyroidism and medullary thyroid carcinoma, as well as pheochromocytoma and carcinoid syndrome. Medications commonly associated with hot flashes include tamoxifen, nicotinic acid, calcium channel blockers, and opiates (Mohyi et al. 1997).

## Pathophysiology

### Biological Factors

The pathophysiology of VMS is not yet fully understood. Hypotheses have included temperature dysregulation at the level of the hypothalamus, narrowing of the thermoneutral zone, and changes in local thermal control of skin blood flow. Women with VMS appear to have an extremely sensitive response to small rises in body temperature, leading to

TABLE 7–6. **Differential diagnosis for vasomotor symptoms**

| Biological conditions | Medications |
|---|---|
| Carcinoid syndrome | Calcium channel blockers |
| Pheochromocytoma | Nicotinic acid |
| Thyroid disorders, especially hyperthyroidism and medullary thyroid carcinoma | Opiates |
| | Tamoxifen |

rapid and excessive vasodilation of peripheral vasculature, which leads to a sense of heat and to sweating (Bansal and Aggarwal 2019). The hypothalamic thermoregulatory center appears to be affected by a range of hormonal and neurotransmitter inputs. Estrogen clearly affects the frequency and severity of hot flashes, with the precise biological mechanism of action still unknown (Bansal and Aggarwal 2019). The process of estrogen withdrawal, rather than the absolute level, appears to be a causative factor; women who are in a stable state of estrogen deficiency, such as prepubertal women and women with functional hypothalamic amenorrhea, do not report VMS (Ackerman et al. 2020).

Serotonin also plays an important role in VMS. In animal and human models, estrogen appears to modulate serotonin synthesis through multiple effects, including increased activity of tryptophan hydroxylase (the enzyme involved in serotonin biosynthesis), upregulation of serotonin 5-$HT_{2A}$ and 5-$HT_C$ receptors, and effects on the serotonin transporter (Krolick et al. 2018; Kugaya et al. 2003; Shanmugan and Epperson 2014). Hypothalamic neuronal systems involved in gonadotropin secretion, such as the kisspeptin, neurokinin B, and dynorphin (KND) signal system, have also been found in animal and human models to be associated with VMS (Bansal and Aggarwal 2019). The finding that injection of neurokinin B in postmenopausal women leads to hot flashes (Jayasena et al. 2015) triggered the development of neurokinin 3 receptor antagonists as a treatment strategy. Initial phase-2 double-blind RCTs have yielded promising results, and recent and ongoing studies include the investigation of optimal dosing and safety (Depypere et al. 2019; Prague et al. 2018).

## Psychological Factors

Psychosocial distress, including anxiety and depression, has been consistently associated with VMS (Avis et al. 2018). Cross-sectional studies do not allow the determination of whether VMS or psychological distress comes first, but longitudinal studies do allow this, and POAS found that anxiety and depression precede the onset of VMS (Freeman et al. 2005, 2009). In SWAN, the presence of symptoms of anxiety and depression along with VMS at subjects' first visit was associated with longer duration of VMS; furthermore, higher stress levels and higher sensitivity to symptoms are related to longer-lasting VMS (Avis et al. 2015). However, the directionality of causation is not completely understood, and it may indeed be bidirectional and complex. Not all women experience the same pattern of perimenopausal symptoms, and the relative roles of endocrinological and psychosocial factors may vary by subgroup (Avis et al. 2018).

## Social Considerations

Further complicating the understanding of how psychosocial factors influence perimenopausal symptoms, women in different cultures and countries report VMS at very different rates, which may be due to both biological factors that affect whether women develop VMS and nonbiological factors that affect the perception or reporting of VMS. Biological factors related to both VMS and culture include estrogen levels and varying genes involved in estrogen metabolism, lifestyle components (e.g., smoking, diet, body composition), and rates of gynecological surgeries (e.g., tubal ligation, hysterectomy, oophorectomy) (Avis et al. 2018). Nonbiological or social factors include education; attitudes toward menopause or VMS; sensitivity to VMS; language, which may affect the terminology used to describe or name VMS; and cultural norms around how the topic is regarded (Avis et al. 2018; Melby 2005; Melby et al. 2005, 2011; Pérez-Alcalá et al. 2013).

The effects that specific diets, alcohol consumption, and level of physical activity have on symptoms have been studied by several investigators, with conflicting results (Avis et al. 2018). High consumption of dietary phytoestrogens had been thought to be useful in limiting VMS, but SWAN was unable to show that phytoestrogen intake is inversely associated with VMS or to account for the lower levels of symptoms reported by Asian women (Gold et al. 2006). A survey of 745 women living primarily (91.6%) in the United States and undergoing the transition to menopause found a significant link between a vegan diet and less bothersome VMS and other physical symptoms of menopause and a trend toward less troublesome symptoms with lower consumption of meat and higher consumption of vegetables (Beezhold et al. 2018). However, this study's limitations are substantial, including self-report, recall bias, and the limited socioeconomic range of the participants, and replication with more rigorous methodology is needed.

## Treatment

### Psychopharmacology

The only antidepressant with FDA approval (in 2013) for the treatment of VMS related to menopause is paroxetine, based on two large RCTs. Both trials described significant improvement in VMS in women who received the active medication, which was also well tolerated (see Carroll et al. 2015). Of note, the dosing of paroxetine in these studies, using the formulation marketed as Brisdelle, was 7.5 mg/day, significantly lower than the dose typically required to treat mood and anxiety disorders (20–60 mg/day).

Similarly, as mentioned, many first-line agents used to treat perimenopausal depression, including citalopram, desvenlafaxine, duloxetine, escitalopram, fluoxetine, mirtazapine, venlafaxine, and vortioxetine, have also shown efficacy for treating VMS, often at lower doses than those used for clinical depression and anxiety, and are reasonable options (Joffe et al. 2003, 2007; Maki et al. 2018; Soares et al. 2006).

### Hormonal Treatment

The use of estrogen to treat symptoms of perimenopause has a complicated and at times controversial history; knowing highlights of this history can help clinicians address the hesitation many patients and providers have regarding estrogen therapy. Estrogen first became commercially available in the United States in 1933 and was used to treat a range of perimenopausal complaints. The popularity of estrogen products grew, and by 1975, estrogen was the fifth most commonly prescribed drug in the United States (Kohn et al. 2019). In the late 1970s, reports of an increased risk for endometrial cancer led to decreased use, but with the addition of progestogen or natural progesterone to decrease endometrial hypertrophy, use once again increased (Kohn et al. 2019).

Then, in the early 2000s, the results of one trial reshaped the history of MHT. The Women's Health Initiative (WHI), a large multicenter primary prevention RCT for coronary heart disease (CHD), was designed to assess the risks and benefits of MHT in healthy postmenopausal women. Because the prevention of CHD was the primary endpoint, the investigators intermittently examined the data to determine whether the benefits for CHD episodes outweighed the risks of MHT. The study had a planned duration of 8.5 years, with two active arms, both compared with placebo: 1) women with a uterus receiving oral conjugated equine estrogen (CEE) plus an oral progestogen (medroxyprogesterone acetate [MPA]) versus placebo, and 2) women with prior hysterectomy receiving CEE alone. In May 2002, however, the trial was stopped ahead of schedule because in the CEE+MPA group (after a mean of 5.2 years of follow-up), the test statistic for invasive breast cancer exceeded the stopping boundary, and the global index statistic suggested that risks were exceeding benefits. The absolute excess risks per 10,000 person-years were seven more CHD events, eight more strokes, eight more pulmonary emboli, and eight more invasive breast cancers. The absolute risk reductions per 10,000 person-years were six fewer colorectal cancers and five fewer hip fractures (Rossouw et al. 2002). After the publication of these initial results, which were widely covered in the press, prescriptions for MHT fell by as much as 80%, and provision of training in prescribing MHT dwindled rapidly (Chester et al. 2018).

Despite this initial panic, further consideration of the WHI results supports the provision of MHT to otherwise healthy women experiencing troublesome VMS. The average age of WHI participants at enrollment was 63 years, and many were not experiencing VMS. In fact, the presence of moderate VMS prevented women from enrolling in the study. The overall cohort thus differed significantly from the younger, symptomatic population of earlier observational studies and from the population that typically seeks treatment for symptoms of perimenopause. In fact, analysis of WHI data by age showed a *reduction* in myocardial infarction and all-cause mortality in women ages 50–59 treated with CEE alone; only women ages 70–79 had increased risks. For the group treated with CEE+MPA, the increased risk of myocardial infarction was minimal in women who were still within 10 years of their final menstrual period and younger than age 60. Risk of myocardial infarction increased with age and time since final menstrual period. Furthermore, *when* a particular woman develops VMS might provide information about her risk for cardiovascular disease: women in the WHI trial with VMS early in menopause had a lower risk of cardiovascular disease and all-cause mortality, whereas women still having hot flashes 14 years after menopause on average had a higher risk of CHD and all-cause mortality (Maclennan et al. 2004).

Research since the WHI has sought to reconcile its results with those of the many prior studies that encouraged the prescription of MHT. Recent studies have investigated younger women and lower doses of estrogen and have compared transdermal with oral estrogen preparations such as CEE or oral estradiol. The "timing hypothesis" posits that age and time since menopause are key; risks of MHT are lower when it is prescribed closer to the menopausal transition. Women who are <10 years from their final menstrual period at initiation of MHT, or age 50–59 years when MHT is started, have lower hazard ratios for CHD than women starting MHT at an older age. Furthermore, transdermal estrogen appears to convey a lower risk of thromboembolic events than oral estrogen and is as effective in treating VMS (Canonico et al. 2007).

Two well-designed trials support the conclusion that MHT does not increase risk of cardiovascular disease in younger women. The Kronos Early Estrogen and Prevention Study, a 4-year randomized double-blind prospective trial, studied 727 women ages 42–58 years (mean age 52) within three arms: oral estrogen (CEE, 0.45 mg/day) plus oral micronized progesterone (200 mg×12 days monthly); transdermal 17β-estradiol (50 μg/day) plus oral micronized progesterone (200 mg×12 days monthly); or placebo for both estrogen preparations and progesterone. Findings showed no significant effects on progression of atherosclerosis in either treatment arm compared with placebo (Miller et al. 2019) and no worsening in cognition (Gleason et al. 2015). The 7-year Early Versus Late Intervention Trial compared a total of 643 women taking oral 17β-estradiol (plus cyclical vaginal progesterone gel for those with a uterus) versus placebo in two groups: those <6 years past menopause and those ≥10 years past final menstrual period when started on MHT. For women closer to menopause, markers of cardiovascular disease progressed more slowly in the group given MHT. For women further from menopause, rate of progression of atherosclerosis was similar in the estradiol and placebo groups (Chester et al. 2018).

Thus, closer subanalyses of the WHI results, as well as studies conducted in its aftermath, yield adjusted recommendations for MHT in healthy women early in menopause. Multiple expert organizations, including the North American Menopause Society, the Endocrine Society, and the American Society for Reproductive Medicine, concur. Recommendations are no longer "the smallest dose possible for the shortest period of time" but rather the type, dose, and duration appropriate for each woman. The consensus of these multiple organizations is that for women younger than age 60 or within 10 years of the onset of menopause, and without contraindications, the benefit-risk ratio is favorable for treating moderate to severe VMS, as well as for the prevention of bone loss or fracture in those at elevated risk (Pinkerton et al. 2017; Stuenkel et al. 2015). Finally, nearly two decades after the abrupt cessation of the WHI study, analyses of all-cause mortality and mortality related to cancer or cardiovascular disease were not different for women in either of the hormone groups (CEE+MPA or CEE alone) compared with placebo (Manson et al. 2017).

Hormonal treatment of the VMS of perimenopause has positive effects on quality of life by improving sleep (through decreased awakenings due to night sweats), decreasing the discomfort and potential embarrassment of daytime VMS, and improving urogenital functioning, which can also reduce sexual dysfunction due to dyspareunia (Table 7–7) (American College of Obstetricians and Gynecologists 2014; Krause and Nakajima 2015). Estradiol is the most effective treatment for VMS and has FDA approval for the treatment of VMS and vulvovaginal atrophy. A 2004 Cochrane meta-analysis of 24 RCTs found a 75% reduction in weekly hot flash frequency with estradiol compared with placebo (Maclennan et al. 2004). Women with a uterus must use a progestogen (defined as having progesterone-like activity at progesterone receptors) or natural progesterone either continuously or sequentially with estrogen to prevent endometrial hyperplasia and to avoid increased risk of endometrial cancer. Although the progestogen or progesterone is often prescribed continuously and concurrently with estrogen because it reduces the frequency of bleeding, this practice is discouraged due to data suggesting an increased risk of breast cancer when the progestogen is prescribed continuously rather than sequentially (Brusselaers et al. 2018). The progestogen can be administered orally, through vaginal gel, or via an intrauterine device.

TABLE 7–7. **Effects of menopausal hormone therapy**

| Decreases | Increases* |
|---|---|
| Vaginal dryness | Risk of breast cancer |
| Vasomotor symptoms | Risk of coronary heart disease |
| Risk of colorectal cancer | Risk of stroke |
| Risk of hip and spine fracture | Risk of venous thromboembolic event |
| Risk of osteoporosis | |

*Risks vary related to age and time since menopause. Please see detailed explanations earlier in the chapter.

We recommend using natural progesterone (vs. synthetic progestins) whenever possible, because natural progesterone is metabolized to allopregnanolone, which has neuroprotective and anti-inflammatory effects (Yilmaz et al. 2019) and thus may counteract increases in proinflammatory cytokines associated with mood disorders and gonadal steroid fluctuations (Hantsoo and Epperson 2015). Due to allopregnanolone's benzodiazepine and barbiturate-like effects at the $GABA_A$ receptor, it is recommended that women take natural progesterone at bedtime (van Broekhoven et al. 2006). Interestingly, lower levels of allopregnanolone have been associated with depressive symptoms during late perimenopause and early postmenopause (Slopien et al. 2018), and allopregnanolone in the form of brexanolone has FDA approval for the treatment of postpartum depression (Kanes et al. 2017; Meltzer-Brody et al. 2018). In rodent models, allopregnanolone reverses chronic stress effects on hypothalamic-pituitary-adrenal axis function (Evans et al. 2012).

Psychiatric practitioners who choose hormonal strategies should consult with each patient's gynecologist or primary care provider to confirm that the patient is up to date on her annual examination and mammogram and has no contraindication to the use of MHT (Table 7–8). Specific training is available to psychiatric providers interested in becoming competent to prescribe MHT themselves, but conferring with the patient's gynecologist or primary physician is still recommended. These physicians are in a better position to surveille the endometrium and to manage any difficulties with bleeding patterns that might arise. If a patient's doctor is opposed to MHT and the psychiatrist is convinced of its effectiveness and safety for a particular patient, the psychiatrist and patient should request a second opinion from another gynecologist or primary care physician.

**Estrogen formulation and dosage.** Both oral and transdermal low-dose estrogen (<0.3 mg of conjugated estrogen, <0.5 mg of oral micronized estradiol, <2.5 μg of ethinyl estradiol, ≤25 μg of transdermal estradiol) effectively alleviate VMS in most women. Ultra-low-dose options, such as the 0.14-μg patch, have not been extensively studied but may reduce VMS. The dosage is increased if the initial dosage is not sufficient to treat symptoms and is decreased before discontinuation. Common side effects include vaginal bleeding, bloating, breast tenderness or enlargement, headaches, mood changes, and nausea.

**Estrogen delivery method.** Oral estrogen preparations are available, but transdermal preparations are generally preferred because they avoid first-pass liver metabolism and are less likely to adversely affect lipids, clotting factors, and inflammatory

**TABLE 7–8. Contraindications to menopausal hormone therapy**

| | |
|---|---|
| Relative | Smoking |
| Absolute | Breast cancer |
| | Other estrogen-sensitive malignancies |
| | Untreated endometrial hyperplasia |
| | Vaginal bleeding |
| | Liver disease |
| | Uncontrolled hypertension |
| | Thrombophilia |
| | History of venous thromboembolism (transdermal estrogen may be acceptable) |
| | Active or recent arterial thromboembolic event (e.g., myocardial infarction) |
| | Porphyria cutanea tarda |

*Source.* Adapted from Canonico et al. 2007; Pinkerton et al. 2017.

markers. FDA-approved products include transdermal estrogens available as patches, gels, an emulsion, and a spray. Estrogen patches are placed on a hairless area of the body other than the breasts, such as the abdomen or buttocks, and are changed once or twice a week. The gels (Divigel, Elestrin, EstroGel) and emulsion lotion (Estrasorb) are applied to the arms or legs as directed. The spray (Evamist) is applied to the inside of the forearm between the elbow and the wrist. Care must be taken not to expose other members of the household to these agents because the effects on pets and children in particular can be marked (North American Menopause Society 2021a).

Patients might ask about *bioidentical hormone therapy,* which refers to estrogen preparations prepared and dispensed by some compounding pharmacies. Claims that these preparations are "more natural" and "closer to the hormones produced by the body" and dispensed in formulations tailored to a particular woman are unfortunately unfounded. The FDA and Endocrine Society recognize *bioidentical* as a marketing term not based on scientific evidence. Some bioidentical hormones are made from components approved by the FDA, but other compounded hormones are not. Bioidentical hormone therapy is potentially inferior to FDA-approved treatments due to unknown pharmacokinetic properties and the risks of variability in purity and potency. No evidence base supports the efficacy or safety of individualizing hormone therapy doses based on salivary, serum, or urine testing of hormone levels. The current lack of data regarding the safety and efficacy of so-called bioidentical products means they should not be recommended or prescribed until such data become available (Committee on Gynecologic Practice and the American Society for Reproductive Medicine Practice Committee 2012; Maki et al. 2018).

Importantly, the 17β-estradiol found in FDA-approved oral and patch preparations is identical to the 17β-estradiol produced naturally by the human ovary. Likewise, oral micronized progesterone and vaginal progesterone creams are identical to natural progesterone produced by the corpus luteum at ovulation. A common practice for women who have significant side effects from oral progesterone is to utilize vaginal progesterone or a progesterone-emitting intrauterine device to protect the endometrium from hyperplasia while decreasing systemic exposure.

## Other Pharmacological Agents

Although MHT and antidepressants are the primary medications used in the management of VMS, data exist supporting the off-label use of a handful of other medications, including gabapentin, pregabalin, and clonidine, all of which are commonly used off-label by psychiatrists to treat symptoms such as pain, trouble falling asleep, and anxiety or impulsivity in the context of mood disorders. The most reliable evidence for using these agents during the perimenopausal transition is for the treatment of VMS. Gabapentin, which is FDA approved for peripheral neuropathy and postherpetic neuralgia, has Level I evidence for use in the treatment of VMS; RCTs using gabapentin 300 mg three times a day showed significantly decreased frequency of VMS. A 300-mg dose at bedtime has also demonstrated some efficacy for night sweats. However, the extent of improvement seen with gabapentin at dosages <2,400 mg/day is not comparable with that of MHT, and at this dosage gabapentin has poor tolerability. Because gabapentin is also used for the treatment of pain, restless legs syndrome, anxiety, and insomnia, it is an appealing option for some women during perimenopause, even though it does not have the same efficacy or tolerability as MHT (Guttuso et al. 2003; Hayes et al. 2011; Reddy et al. 2006). Pregabalin, a gabapentinoid, has Level II evidence for treatment of VMS, with one RCT showing significant improvement in symptoms and good tolerability at 7.5 mg twice daily (Loprinzi et al. 2010). Clonidine, an $\alpha_2$-adrenergic agonist, has Level II evidence for VMS, demonstrating moderate improvement in symptoms. Due to its limited efficacy and side effects, however, it is not commonly used (Nelson et al. 2006).

## Alternative Treatments

Up to 50%–80% of women turn to nonhormonal modalities for the treatment of VMS (Carpenter et al. 2015). Women elect nonhormonal treatments of symptoms of perimenopause for reasons that include medical contraindications and fear of the risks of taking prescription medications in general, or fear of hormones and antidepressants in particular. A smaller group of women turn to nonhormonal treatment due to an inability to tolerate the side effects of MHT. Due to the frequency of the use of alternative treatments, it is important that clinicians have a general understanding of the options available for the treatment of VMS beyond MHT and antidepressants, as well as the levels of existing evidence, to be prepared to discuss the risks and benefits of these strategies.

**Behavioral strategies.** Because VMS can be triggered by increases in ambient or body temperature, women often try cooling techniques with the goal of preventing and alleviating symptoms. They wear breathable clothing materials, dress in layers, and keep ice packs and fans nearby. Some women avoid doing activities that raise body temperature, eating spicy foods, or drinking alcohol. Although these strategies are not known to have medical risks, no evidence supports them as either preventing or alleviating symptoms.

Multiple RCTs have investigated the effects of exercise on VMS; none has shown a positive result. Given the known benefits of exercise for mood, anxiety, and general health, exercise should be encouraged in perimenopausal women, but not with any expectation that it will decrease VMS (Daley et al. 2014). Studies on yoga have been performed, but thus far RCTs have failed to show any significant difference in VMS between women randomized to yoga versus control subjects (Newton et al. 2014). Level II evidence is available to recommend weight loss as a strategy to reduce VMS; however, studies have varied in the baseline BMI of women and the amount of weight loss required to achieve benefit (Thurston et al. 2015).

Level I evidence is available from two large RCTs to recommend CBT as leading to a significant reduction of "problematic" hot flashes and night sweats. One of these trials was performed in women experiencing VMS following treatment for breast cancer (Mann et al. 2012) and the other in women undergoing natural menopause (Ayers et al. 2011). Interestingly, self-guided CBT was found to be as effective as group-based therapy. The therapeutic effect of this modality is thought to be due to developing a sense of control and increased understanding of and ability to tolerate symptoms. Along similar lines, there is Level II evidence for mindfulness-based stress reduction; one RCT showed a greater reduction in the intensity of VMS and the frequency of problematic symptoms in participants in a mindfulness-based stress reduction program compared with control subjects, but the result did not reach significance (Carmody et al. 2011).

Level I evidence is available to support the benefits of hypnosis (induction of a deep relaxation state and an altered state of awareness using imagery techniques) in the treatment of VMS (Elkins et al. 2013). However, multiple trials of relaxation strategies have been performed, both in women undergoing natural menopause and women undergoing treatment for cancer, with no significant benefits proven (Lindh-Åstrand and Nedstrand 2013; Saensak et al. 2014). Paced breathing (six to eight breaths per minute, inhaling through the nose and exhaling through the mouth) is sometimes taught as a means to manage VMS, but two RCTs showed no difference in symptoms with this technique (Carpenter et al. 2013; Sood et al. 2013).

**Procedures.** Acupuncture, among the most frequently used alternative therapies for VMS, has inconclusive evidence supporting its use. Although some studies show it reduces VMS compared with a waitlist control condition, others, in which acupuncture was compared with sham acupuncture (insertion of needles at nontherapeutic sites), found no significant difference in symptoms (Dodin et al. 2013; Ee et al. 2016). Four open-label studies have been performed to evaluate the efficacy of stellate ganglion block (using local anesthetic at the bilateral nerve group from vertebrae C6 to T2), with a reduction in VMS ranging from 34% to 90% (Walega et al. 2014). However, a randomized sham-controlled study showed no statistically significant overall change in VMS frequency between the two groups, although the group that received the actual procedure for moderate to severe VMS did have a statistically significant reduction in VMS frequency (Walega et al. 2014).

**Dietary supplements and herbal therapies.** The consumption of foods containing isoflavones (e.g., soybeans, soy products) and other phytoestrogens (e.g., seeds, whole grains, legumes) has been an appealing strategy for limiting VMS, based on the theory that eating foods containing compounds with estrogenic properties will lead to replenishment of waning levels of estrogen. However, multiple studies, including large RCTs, have failed to show significant benefits. Study designs and interpretations are limited by manufacturing variability, leading to inconsistent levels of isoflavones and phytoestrogens across products (Chen et al. 2015; Kronenberg and Fugh-Berman 2002; Lethaby et al. 2013).

**TABLE 7–9. Current recommendations for nonhormonal treatment of vasomotor symptoms**

| | |
|---|---|
| **Recommended** *(evidence to support efficacy and low risk)* | |
| Clonidine | Hypnosis |
| Cognitive-behavioral therapy | Pregabalin |
| Gabapentin | Selective serotonin reuptake inhibitors or serotonin-norepinephrine reuptake inhibitors |
| **Recommended with caution** *(some evidence to support efficacy)* | |
| Mindfulness | Stellate ganglion block |
| Soy derivatives | Weight loss |
| **Not enough evidence to recommend** *(no evidence to support efficacy in relieving or preventing vasomotor symptoms; may have other health benefits)* | |
| Acupuncture | Herbal supplements |
| Avoiding triggers | Paced breathing |
| Cooling techniques | Relaxation |
| Exercise | Yoga |

*Source.* Adapted from Carpenter et al. 2015.

Black cohosh (*Cimicifuga racemosa* or *Actaea racemosa*) is the most commonly purchased herbal supplement for the treatment of VMS. A Cochrane review of 16 RCTs, however, showed no significant difference in VMS in women taking black cohosh at an average dosage of 40 mg/day compared with control subjects. Several reports of hepatotoxicity with black cohosh products add to the standard concerns applicable to supplements, which lack federal oversight as to what is being sold and what production methods are used, leading to greater risk of contaminants (Leach and Moore 2012; Wuttke et al. 2008).

Dong quai (*Angelica sinensis*) is frequently used in traditional Chinese medicine to treat gynecological complaints. A Cochrane review of 22 RCTs showed no significant difference between the active ingredient and placebo. Furthermore, studies have raised concern for photosensitization, anticoagulation, and carcinogenicity, and side effects including taste changes, dyspepsia, diarrhea, and breast tenderness (Zhu et al. 2016). Multiple other supplements are marketed with claims for reducing symptoms of perimenopause. However, adequate data to support their use are not available.

In summary, nonhormonal treatments for VMS are an ongoing area of research. However, enough research currently exists to divide many of these treatments into one of three categories regarding their role in treating VMS: 1) those that current research supports as effective, 2) those that have some limited proof of effect, or 3) those that research has shown to lack effect. See Table 7–9. When deciding whether to recommend treating VMS with specific nonhormonal treatments or MHT, it is helpful to consider the larger picture, including whether the patient has a concurrent mood disorder or mood symptoms, whether the patient has contraindications to MHT, and whether the patient is interested in taking a prescription medication. See Figure 7–1 for an algorithm to assist in making these complex decisions.

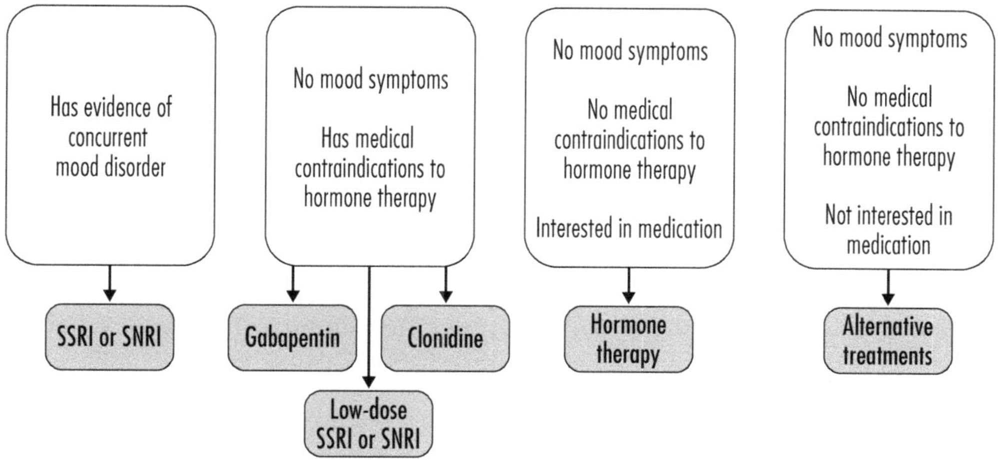


**FIGURE 7–1. Treatment options for vasomotor symptoms (VMS) affecting sleep and daily life.**
SNRI=serotonin-norepinephrine reuptake inhibitor; SSRI=selective serotonin reuptake inhibitor.

# Other Perimenopausal Symptoms

## Sleep Disturbance

### Rates and Risk Factors

Sleep disturbance, the second most common perimenopausal complaint after VMS, is often related to but not necessarily the direct result of VMS. Sleep disturbance typically consists of both trouble falling asleep and multiple awakenings (Kravitz et al. 2003). The percentage of women experiencing sleep disturbances increases from around 30% in premenopause (already a significant proportion of women) to 39%–60% in perimenopause and postmenopause, with the prevalence of sleep problems at its highest during the late perimenopausal transition (Kravitz et al. 2003, 2008; National Institutes of Health 2005). Sleep disturbance can be triggered or exacerbated by hot flashes, and hot flashes are not helped by sleep disturbance; research has shown that their relationship is complex (Baker et al. 2018; Kravitz et al. 2008). One study that objectively measured both hot flashes and night awakenings using skin conductance and actigraphy found that 78% of objectively measured hot flashes were associated with an awakening but that only 36% of awakenings were associated with a hot flash (Thurston et al. 2019).

Risk factors for sleep disturbance during perimenopause include VMS, surgical menopause (Kravitz et al. 2003), and breast cancer treatments, particularly chemotherapy but also radiotherapy and hormonal therapy in some studies (Costa et al. 2014). One study found that both surgical menopause and bilateral oophorectomy after natural menopause were associated with a higher risk of developing obstructive sleep apnea compared with natural menopause (Huang et al. 2018). Finally, one large study found an association between lower-quality sleep and white ethnicity, increased perceived stress, cigarette smoking, and lower self-reported quality of life (Kravitz et al. 2003).

### Further Screening

The PSQI, although not specific to perimenopause, can help identify the timing of sleep problems, their severity, and contributing factors (Carpenter and Andrykowski 1998). Given the greater risk for obstructive sleep apnea with aging and higher BMI (Perger et al. 2019), the increase in BMI commonly observed at midlife and with menopause (Montazeri et al. 2019), and the greater risk for obstructive sleep apnea among women with severe VMS (Gao et al. 2018), all midlife women with sleep complaints should be screened for symptoms of obstructive sleep apnea, with a low threshold for referring patients to sleep medicine specialists for full evaluation if indicated.

### Course

If due to perimenopause, symptoms such as sleep disturbance are generally most severe during the perimenopausal transition and tend to improve after menopause (Santoro 2016).

### Pharmacological Treatment

Sleep problems in perimenopause may be attributable to either VMS, perimenopausal depression, or both and may resolve with effective treatment of either. However, other sleep problems may not resolve, and other causes should be investigated. Evidence suggests that both sleep-disordered breathing (including obstructive sleep apnea) and restless legs syndrome may have an increased incidence in perimenopause and are important to diagnose and treat (Baker et al. 2018).

One small, industry-funded RCT of both perimenopausal and postmenopausal women with sleep disturbance but without clinical depression found that eszopiclone increased total sleep time and improved other measures of insomnia in this population (Joffe et al. 2010).

Given the evidence that endogenous melatonin decreases with age, particularly during perimenopause (Baker et al. 2018; Stute et al. 2020), an ongoing area of research is whether melatonin supplementation can help with perimenopausal symptoms. One small RCT found improvement in quality-of-life scores in the physical domain, including feeling worn out and tired, as well as in subjective reports of improved sleep in perimenopausal women randomized to melatonin 3 mg at bedtime (Kotlarczyk et al. 2012).

### Alternative Treatment

CBT for insomnia (CBT-I) has compelling evidence for efficacy in the population at large (see, e.g., Mitchell et al. 2012). In a study of 106 perimenopausal and postmenopausal women also experiencing VMS, CBT-I was found to reduce insomnia (but not VMS); improvement in symptoms was maintained at 6 months (McCurry et al. 2016).

## Sexual Problems

### Rates and Risk Factors

Sexual problems, including vaginal dryness and atrophy, which can lead to new-onset dyspareunia (pain with intercourse), are also commonly present in perimenopause.

There is evidence to suggest that overall sexual functioning declines around the time of the menopausal transition, with women experiencing increased pain and decreased sexual interest, arousal, ability to achieve orgasm, and emotional satisfaction. In one study, the steepest rate of decline in sexual functioning began around 20 months before the last menstrual period and continued for 1 year after the final menstrual period (Avis et al. 2017). Factors associated with the decline in sexual function in this study included VMS, vaginal dryness, and depression or anxiety. Women undergoing a hysterectomy before their final menstrual period also had a decline in sexual functioning after their surgery (Avis et al. 2017).

Vaginal dryness deserves particular attention because it is a highly prevalent symptom that women often fail to report to physicians. This symptom increases with advancing menopausal stages. In a large longitudinal study, 19% of women ages 42–53 reported vaginal dryness at baseline, and 34% of the same group reported the symptom at 17-year follow-up. Risk factors associated with vaginal dryness in this study included age since menopause, surgically induced menopause, anxiety, and being married (Waetjen et al. 2018). Vaginal dryness can be both the cause of dyspareunia and exacerbated by pain during intercourse. Among women who reported experiencing vaginal dryness in the prior 2 weeks in the study by Waetjen et al. (2018), 40% reported having pain sometimes or almost always with sexual intercourse, compared with 16% of women who reported no vaginal dryness in the prior 2 weeks. Both vaginal dryness and dyspareunia are underdiagnosed and therefore undertreated, although they can be improved by over-the-counter lubricants (Bygdeman and Swahn 1996), topical hormones, and MHT.

### Hormonal Treatment

If sexual problems are due to perimenopausal symptoms, vaginal estrogen cream or gel can be effective for dyspareunia and vaginal dryness (but not for hot flashes, which require systemic administration as described in the earlier section on treatment of VMS). Of note, evidence has shown that nonhormonal over-the-counter lubricants can be effective for the treatment of dyspareunia and vaginal dryness, and given their lower risk, they can be considered first-line treatment for women presenting with these symptoms alone or in women with contraindications to estrogen (Bygdeman and Swahn 1996). Women and their partners often have to try multiple lubricants to determine which is best for them. Water-based lubricants may require more frequent reapplication but are less irritating to sensitive skin.

## Cognitive Complaints

### Rates and Risk Factors

Complaints of cognitive symptoms during the menopausal transition are common, but symptoms that may be attributed to perimenopause are typically subtle, have gradual onset, and are challenging to distinguish from the normal symptoms of aging. Abrupt and serious cognitive decline should always be investigated to rule out other causes. Typical findings of cognitive changes due to perimenopause are of self-reported problems with verbal memory, such as remembering words or names (reported by 72% of women in SWAN), or with forgetting things (reported by 50%) (Greendale et al. 2010; Woods and Mitchell 2016).

When objective measures of cognitive performance are used, identifiable changes associated with perimenopause are typically subtle and may be transient. The first report that menopause stage—independent of age at the time of testing, baseline cognitive performance, race, and BMI—was associated with significant declines in immediate and delayed verbal recall came from POAS (Epperson et al. 2013). Although declines occurred across the transition, they became significant for immediate recall at the postmenopause stage ($P$=0.04) and for delayed recall in the early transition ($P$=0.002), when women reported having had one skipped period in the previous year.

One study examining processing speed, which is expected to improve over the course of repeated testing with the same instrument as subjects learn, found this expected improvement in women who were in premenopause, early perimenopause, or postmenopause but not in women at late perimenopause (Greendale et al. 2009). Another study, by Kuh et al. (2018), found that women who went through natural menopause at a later age had higher verbal memory scores but no changes in processing speed compared with women who completed menopause earlier. Although the authors hypothesized that hormone therapy could boost cognitive function in women going through the menopausal transition, they found no significant benefit for those taking MHT on either verbal memory or processing speed except for those who had menopause due to bilateral oophorectomy, who did show some benefit.

Not all cognitive domains are likely to be as negatively affected by the loss of estradiol. Given the impact of estradiol on neuronal morphology, receptors for various neurotransmitters, and neurochemistry in the prefrontal cortex, it is not surprising that many menopausal women complain of difficulties within the executive function domains of working memory, sustained attention, processing speed, and motivation for work (Epperson et al. 2015; Shanmugan and Epperson 2014; Shanmugan et al. 2020). Stimulant treatment may be beneficial for women with significant executive function complaints, but the potential adverse effects on blood pressure and heart rate should be considered, as well as the addictive potential of stimulant medications (Epperson et al. 2015).

Risk factors for self-reported memory problems during perimenopause included higher perceived levels of stress and depressed mood (Woods et al. 2000).

## Further Screening

The MoCA (Nasreddine et al. 2005) has high sensitivity and specificity for detecting mild cognitive impairment. If this is identified, causes other than perimenopause should be investigated. Women should be queried regarding undiagnosed ADHD if they present with significant symptoms of executive dysfunction. A recent study suggests that childhood adversity and current depression and anxiety can increase risk for executive function complaints among women who have undergone risk-reducing salpingo-oophorectomy due to having had breast or ovarian cancer or being at genetic risk for such cancers (Shanmugan et al. 2020). Tools such as the Brown Attention-Deficit Disorder Scale (Brown 1996; Sandra Kooij et al. 2008), Adult ADHD Self-Report Scale (Ustun et al. 2017), and Conners' Adult ADHD Rating Scale–Long Version (Conners et al. 1999; Sandra Kooij et al. 2008) can be used to assess severity of executive function difficulties both prior to and following stimulant treatment to assess the relative benefits and weigh these against the potential risks of long-term use.

## Additional Strategies for Changes in Sleep, Sexual Function, and Cognition

As discussed, successful treatment of mood disorders or VMS may result in improvements in sleep, sexual functioning, and cognition. However, for changes that do not improve with successful treatment of anxiety, depression, or VMS or with the specific treatments described earlier in this chapter, further investigation, education, and referral may be warranted. Further specialized treatment options are beyond the scope of this chapter and vary depending on the cause of the problem. Thus, the first step is to further characterize the problem using a scale, a diary, or other measurement system. Next, serious and treatable causes of the symptom should be explored and ruled out if possible so as to provide both reassurance and relief. Finally, the patient should be referred to specialists or additional sources of education. See Table 7–10 for specific steps to take in characterizing, investigating, and educating about these problems.

# Conclusion

Perimenopause is a time of reproductive change that confers increased risk of mental illness, as well as complex physical changes such as VMS, difficulty sleeping, sexual dysfunction, and cognitive complaints. Distinguishing between depression, the symptoms of perimenopause, and other psychological, behavioral, or medical causes of overlapping complaints can be challenging but will help guide decisions among the many treatment options, which include antidepressants, hormones, and alternative treatments. A growing evidence base is available to guide our understanding and treatment of patients at this time of life.

# Key Points

- Perimenopause is a time of increased risk for depression, especially for women with a prior history of depression.
- Typical symptoms of perimenopause can also include vasomotor symptoms (VMS), sleep disturbances, sexual dysfunction, and cognitive changes, among others. Executive function complaints should be assessed for severity and impact on daily functioning.
- The symptoms of depression and the symptoms of perimenopause can overlap, requiring a careful history and investigation to determine which treatments are recommended.
- Antidepressants can be effective for VMS as well as anxiety and depression.
- Menopausal hormone treatment is an effective treatment for VMS but has some contraindications.
- Evidence supports some alternative treatments as effective for VMS, but evidence also shows some alternative treatments to be ineffective or potentially harmful.

**TABLE 7–10. Additional strategies for changes in sleep, sexual functioning, and cognition**

| | Sleep | Sexual function | Cognition |
|---|---|---|---|
| **Characterize:** Describe and quantify problem using interview and scales | National Sleep Foundation Sleep Diary | Menopause Rating Scale | Mini-Mental State Examination[a] for more severe impairment |
| | Pittsburgh Sleep Quality Index | | Montreal Cognitive Assessment for more subtle impairment |
| | | | Various ADHD scales for executive function (see text for options) |
| **Rule out:** Consider serious and treatable causes | Caffeine or other stimulants | Dyspareunia | Dementia or neurocognitive disease |
| | Over-the-counter or illicit substances | History of trauma | Infectious, metabolic, or endocrine factors (complete blood count, comprehensive metabolic panel, thyroid stimulating hormone) |
| | Poor sleep hygiene | Intimate partner violence | |
| | Restless legs syndrome, obstructive sleep apnea, or other sleep disorders | Relationship stressors | Neurological disease (neurological examination if indicated) |
| | | Sexual side effects of antidepressants | |
| | | Urinary problems | Over-the-counter or illicit substances |
| | | Vaginal atrophy, dryness, or irritation | Polypharmacy |
| | | | Sleep disorders |
| **Educate:** Provide information and sources of further information | Cognitive-behavioral therapy for insomnia coaching application (Koffel et al. 2018) | National Institute on Aging[b] over-the-counter treatments for dyspareunia | National Institute on Aging[c] information on cognitive health |
| | National Institute on Aging[d] information on sleep hygiene and menopause | North American Menopause Society[e] information on sexual health | |

*Source.* [a]Folstein et al. 1975; [b]National Institute on Aging 2017a; [c]National Institute on Aging 2019a; [d]National Institute on Aging 2019b; [e]North American Menopause Society 2021b.

- Lingering changes in sleep, sexual function, or cognition should be characterized and investigated to rule out serious or treatable causes, and then patients should be educated and referred to specialists if indicated.

# References

Ackerman KE, Singhal V, Slattery M, et al: Effects of estrogen replacement on bone geometry and microarchitecture in adolescent and young adult oligoamenorrheic athletes: a randomized trial. J Bone Miner Res 35(2):248–260, 2020 31603998

American College of Obstetricians and Gynecologists: ACOG Practice Bulletin No. 141: management of menopausal symptoms. Obstet Gynecol 123(1):202–216, 2014 24463691

American College of Obstetricians and Gynecologists: ACOG Committee Opinion No. 773: the use of antimüllerian hormone in women not seeking fertility care. Obstet Gynecol 133(4):e274–e278, 2019 30913198

American Psychiatric Association: Diagnostic and Statistical Manual of Mental Disorders, 5th Edition. Arlington, VA, American Psychiatric Association, 2013

Arroll B, Goodyear-Smith F, Crengle S, et al: Validation of PHQ-2 and PHQ-9 to screen for major depression in the primary care population. Ann Fam Med 8(4):348–353, 2010 20644190

Avis NE, Brambilla D, McKinlay SM, et al: A longitudinal analysis of the association between menopause and depression: results from the Massachusetts Women's Health Study. Ann Epidemiol 4(3):214–220, 1994 8055122

Avis NE, Crawford SL, Greendale G, et al: Duration of menopausal vasomotor symptoms over the menopause transition. JAMA Intern Med 175(4):531–539, 2015 25686030

Avis NE, Colvin A, Karlamangla AS, et al: Change in sexual functioning over the menopausal transition: results from the Study of Women's Health Across the Nation. Menopause 24(4):379–390, 2017 27801705

Avis NE, Crawford SL, Green R: Vasomotor symptoms across the menopause transition: differences among women. Obstet Gynecol Clin North Am 45(4):629–640, 2018 30401547

Ayers B, Forshaw M, Hunter MS: The impact of attitudes towards the menopause on women's symptom experience: a systematic review. Maturitas 65(1):28–36, 2010 19954900

Ayers B, Mann E, Hunter MS: A randomised controlled trial of cognitive-behavioural therapy for women with problematic menopausal hot flushes: MENOS 2 trial protocol. BMJ Open 1(1):e000047, 2011 22021738

Baker FC, Lampio L, Saaresranta T, et al: Sleep and sleep disorders in the menopausal transition. Sleep Med Clin 13(3):443–456, 2018 30098758

Baker JH, Runfola CD: Eating disorders in midlife women: a perimenopausal eating disorder? Maturitas 85:112–116, 2016 26857889

Bansal R, Aggarwal N: Menopausal hot flashes: a concise review. J Midlife Health 10(1):6–13, 2019 31001050

Beezhold B, Radnitz C, McGrath RE, et al: Vegans report less bothersome vasomotor and physical menopausal symptoms than omnivores. Maturitas 112:12–17, 2018 29704911

Bougea A, Despoti A, Vasilopoulos E: Empty-nest-related psychosocial stress: conceptual issues, future directions in economic crisis. Psychiatriki 30(4):329–338, 2019 32283536

Bromberger JT, Epperson CN: Depression during and after the perimenopause: impact of hormones, genetics, and environmental determinants of disease. Obstet Gynecol Clin North Am 45(4):663–678, 2018 30401549

Bromberger JT, Kravitz HM: Mood and menopause: findings from the Study of Women's Health Across the Nation (SWAN) over 10 years. Obstet Gynecol Clin North Am 38(3):609–625, 2011 21961723

Bromberger JT, Kravitz HM, Chang YF, et al: Major depression during and after the menopausal transition: Study of Women's Health Across the Nation (SWAN). Psychol Med 41(9):1879–1888, 2011 21306662

Bromberger JT, Kravitz HM, Chang Y, et al: Does risk for anxiety increase during the menopausal transition? Study of Women's Health Across the Nation. Menopause 20(5):488–495, 2013 23615639

Bromberger JT, Schott L, Kravitz HM, et al: Risk factors for major depression during midlife among a community sample of women with and without prior major depression: are they the same or different? Psychol Med 45(8):1653–1664, 2015 25417760

Brown TE: Brown Attention-Deficit Disorder Scales. San Antonio, TX, Psychological Corporation, 1996

Brunner RL, Aragaki A, Barnabei V, et al: Menopausal symptom experience before and after stopping estrogen therapy in the Women's Health Initiative randomized, placebo-controlled trial. Menopause 17(5):946–954, 2010 20505547

Brusselaers N, Tamimi RM, Konings P, et al: Different menopausal hormone regimens and risk of breast cancer. Ann Oncol 29(8):1771–1776, 2018 29917061

Bryant C, Judd FK, Hickey M: Anxiety during the menopausal transition: a systematic review. J Affect Disord 139(2):141–148, 2012 21783260

Bygdeman M, Swahn ML: Replens versus dienoestrol cream in the symptomatic treatment of vaginal atrophy in postmenopausal women. Maturitas 23(3):259–263, 1996 8794418

Callegari C, Ielmini M, Caselli I, et al: Paroxetine versus vortioxetine for depressive symptoms in postmenopausal transition: a preliminary study. Psychopharmacol Bull 49(1):28–43, 2019 30858637

Canonico M, Oger E, Plu-Bureau G, et al: Hormone therapy and venous thromboembolism among postmenopausal women: impact of the route of estrogen administration and progestogens: the ESTHER study. Circulation 115(7):840–845, 2007 17309934

Carmody JF, Crawford S, Salmoirago-Blotcher E, et al: Mindfulness training for coping with hot flashes: results of a randomized trial. Menopause 18(6):611–620, 2011 21372745

Carpenter JS: The Hot Flash Related Daily Interference Scale: a tool for assessing the impact of hot flashes on quality of life following breast cancer. J Pain Symptom Manage 22(6):979–989, 2001 11738160

Carpenter JS, Andrykowski MA: Psychometric evaluation of the Pittsburgh Sleep Quality Index. J Psychosom Res 45(1):5–13, 1998 9720850

Carpenter JS, Burns DS, Wu J, et al: Paced respiration for vasomotor and other menopausal symptoms: a randomized, controlled trial. J Gen Intern Med 28(2):193–200, 2013 22936289

Carpenter JS, Gass MLS, Maki PM, et al: Nonhormonal management of menopause-associated vasomotor symptoms: 2015 position statement of The North American Menopause Society. Menopause 22(11):1155–1172, quiz 1173–1174, 2015 26382310

Carroll DG, Lisenby KM, Carter TL: Critical appraisal of paroxetine for the treatment of vasomotor symptoms. Int J Womens Health 7:615–624, 2015 26124682

Chen MN, Lin CC, Liu CF: Efficacy of phytoestrogens for menopausal symptoms: a meta-analysis and systematic review. Climacteric 18(2):260–269, 2015 25263312

Chester RC, Kling JM, Manson JE: What the Women's Health Initiative has taught us about menopausal hormone therapy. Clin Cardiol 41(2):247–252, 2018 29493798

Clark CT, Wisner KL: Treatment of peripartum bipolar disorder. Obstet Gynecol Clin North Am 45(3):403–417, 2018 30092918

Claudia P, Andrea C, Chiara C, et al: Panic disorder in menopause: a case control study. Maturitas 48(2):147–154, 2004 15172089

Clayton AH, Kornstein SG, Dunlop BW, et al: Efficacy and safety of desvenlafaxine 50 mg/d in a randomized, placebo-controlled study of perimenopausal and postmenopausal women with major depressive disorder. J Clin Psychiatry 74(10):1010–1017, 2013 24229754

Cohen LS, Soares CN, Vitonis AF, et al: Risk for new onset of depression during the menopausal transition: the Harvard Study of Moods and Cycles. Arch Gen Psychiatry 63(4):385–390, 2006 16585467

Col NF, Guthrie JR, Politi M, et al: Duration of vasomotor symptoms in middle-aged women: a longitudinal study. Menopause 16(3):453–457, 2009 19188852

Committee on Gynecologic Practice and the American Society for Reproductive Medicine Practice Committee: Committee opinion No. 532: compounded bioidentical menopausal hormone therapy. Obstet Gynecol 120(2 pt 1):411–415, 2012 22825109

Conners CK, Erhardt D, Sparrow EP: Conners' Adult ADHD Rating Scales (CAARS). Toronto, ON, Canada, Multi-Health Systems, 1999

Costa AR, Fontes F, Pereira S, et al: Impact of breast cancer treatments on sleep disturbances: a systematic review. Breast 23(6):697–709, 2014 25307946

Crow E, Jasberg S, Crow EA: Schizophrenia during menopausal transition. Ment Health Fam Med 12:190–195, 2016

Daley A, Stokes-Lampard H, Thomas A, et al: Exercise for vasomotor menopausal symptoms. Cochrane Database Syst Rev 11(11):CD006108, 2014 25431132

Depypere H, Timmerman D, Donders G, et al: Treatment of menopausal vasomotor symptoms with fezolinetant, a neurokinin 3 receptor antagonist: a phase 2a trial. J Clin Endocrinol Metab 104(12):5893–5905, 2019 31415087

Dodin S, Blanchet C, Marc I, et al: Acupuncture for menopausal hot flushes. Cochrane Database Syst Rev 20(7):CD007410, 2013 23897589

Ee C, Xue C, Chondros P, et al: Acupuncture for menopausal hot flashes: a randomized trial. Ann Intern Med 164(3):146–154, 2016 26784863

Elkins GR, Fisher WI, Johnson AK, et al: Clinical hypnosis in the treatment of postmenopausal hot flashes: a randomized controlled trial. Menopause 20(3):291–298, 2013 23435026

Epperson CN, Sammel MD, Freeman EW: Menopause effects on verbal memory: findings from a longitudinal community cohort. J Clin Endocrinol Metab 98(9):3829–3838, 2013 23836935

Epperson CN, Shanmugan S, Kim DR, et al: New onset executive function difficulties at menopause: a possible role for lisdexamfetamine. Psychopharmacology (Berl) 232(16):3091–3100, 2015 26063677

Epperson CN, Sammel MD, Bale TL, et al: Adverse childhood experiences and risk for first-episode major depression during the menopause transition. J Clin Psychiatry 78(3):e298–e307, 2017 28394509

Evans J, Sun Y, McGregor A, et al: Allopregnanolone regulates neurogenesis and depressive/anxiety-like behaviour in a social isolation rodent model of chronic stress. Neuropharmacology 63(8):1315–1326, 2012 22939998

Folstein MF, Folstein SE, McHugh PR: "Mini-mental state": a practical method for grading the cognitive state of patients for the clinician. J Psychiatr Res 12(3):189–198, 1975

Freeman EW, Sammel MD: Anxiety as a risk factor for menopausal hot flashes: evidence from the Penn Ovarian Aging cohort. Menopause 23(9):942–949, 2016 27433864

Freeman EW, Sherif K: Prevalence of hot flushes and night sweats around the world: a systematic review. Climacteric 10(3):197–214, 2007 17487647

Freeman EW, Sammel MD, Liu L, et al: Hormones and menopausal status as predictors of depression in women in transition to menopause Arch Gen Psychiatry 61(1):62–70, 2004 14706945

Freeman EW, Sammel MD, Lin H, et al: The role of anxiety and hormonal changes in menopausal hot flashes. Menopause 12(3):258–266, 2005 15879914

Freeman EW, Sammel MD, Lin H, et al: Associations of hormones and menopausal status with depressed mood in women with no history of depression. Arch Gen Psychiatry 63(4):375–382, 2006 16585466

Freeman EW, Sammel MD, Lin H: Temporal associations of hot flashes and depression in the transition to menopause. Menopause 16(4):728–734, 2009 19188849

Freeman EW, Sammel MD, Lin H, et al: Duration of menopausal hot flushes and associated risk factors. Obstet Gynecol 117(5):1095–1104, 2011 21508748

Freeman EW, Sammel MD, Boorman DW, et al: Longitudinal pattern of depressive symptoms around natural menopause. JAMA Psychiatry 71(1):36–43, 2014 24227182

Freeman MP, Cheng LJ, Moustafa D, et al: Vortioxetine for major depressive disorder, vasomotor, and cognitive symptoms associated with the menopausal transition. Ann Clin Psychiatry 29(4):249–257, 2017 29069110

Gao CC, Kapoor E, Lipford MC, et al: Association of vasomotor symptoms and sleep apnea risk in midlife women. Menopause 25(4):391–398, 2018 29088020
Gerber LM, Sievert LL: Neighborhood disorder, exposure to violence, and perceived discrimination in relation to symptoms in midlife women. Womens Midlife Health 4:14, 2018 30766724
Gibson CJ, Li Y, Huang AJ, et al: Menopausal symptoms and higher risk opioid prescribing in a national sample of women veterans with chronic pain. J Gen Intern Med 34(10):2159–2166, 2019 31414358
Gleason CE, Dowling NM, Wharton W, et al: Effects of hormone therapy on cognition and mood in recently postmenopausal women: findings from the randomized, controlled KEEPS–Cognitive and Affective Study. PLoS Med 12(6):e1001833, discussion e1001833, 2015 26035291
Gold EB, Colvin A, Avis N, et al: Longitudinal analysis of the association between vasomotor symptoms and race/ethnicity across the menopausal transition: study of women's health across the nation. Am J Public Health 96(7):1226–1235, 2006 16735636
González-Rodríguez A, Catalán R, Penadés R, et al: Antipsychotic response worsens with postmenopausal duration in women with schizophrenia. J Clin Psychopharmacol 36(6):580–587, 2016 27626286
Gordon JL, Girdler SS, Meltzer-Brody SE, et al: Ovarian hormone fluctuation, neurosteroids, and HPA axis dysregulation in perimenopausal depression: a novel heuristic model. Am J Psychiatry 172(3):227–236, 2015 25585035
Gordon JL, Rubinow DR, Eisenlohr-Moul TA, et al: Efficacy of transdermal estradiol and micronized progesterone in the prevention of depressive symptoms in the menopause transition: a randomized clinical trial. JAMA Psychiatry 75(2):149–157, 2018 29322164
Greendale GA, Huang MH, Wight RG, et al: Effects of the menopause transition and hormone use on cognitive performance in midlife women. Neurology 72(21):1850–1857, 2009 19470968
Greendale GA, Wight RG, Huang MH, et al: Menopause-associated symptoms and cognitive performance: results from the Study of Women's Health Across the Nation. Am J Epidemiol 171(11):1214–1224, 2010 20442205
Greene JG: A factor analytic study of climacteric symptoms. J Psychosom Res 20(5):425–430, 1976 1003364
Gupta R, Assalman I, Bottlender R: Menopause and schizophrenia. Menopause Int 18(1):10–14, 2012 22308532
Guttuso T Jr, Kurlan R, McDermott MP, et al: Gabapentin's effects on hot flashes in postmenopausal women: a randomized controlled trial. Obstet Gynecol 101(2):337–345, 2003 12576259
Hantsoo L, Epperson CN: Premenstrual dysphoric disorder: epidemiology and treatment. Curr Psychiatry Rep 17(11):87, 2015 26377947
Hantsoo L, Epperson CN: Anxiety disorders among women: a female lifespan approach. Focus 15(2):162–172, 2017 28966563
Hantsoo L, Epperson CN: Allopregnanolone in premenstrual dysphoric disorder (PMDD): evidence for dysregulated sensitivity to GABA-A receptor modulating neuroactive steroids across the menstrual cycle. Neurobiol Stress 12:100213, 2020 32435664
Hayes LP, Carroll DG, Kelley KW: Use of gabapentin for the management of natural or surgical menopausal hot flashes. Ann Pharmacother 45(3):388–394, 2011 21343402
Heinemann K, Ruebig A, Potthoff P, et al: The Menopause Rating Scale (MRS) scale: a methodological review. Health Qual Life Outcomes 2:45, 2004 15345062
Hu L-Y, Shen C-C, Hung J-H, et al: Risk of psychiatric disorders following symptomatic menopausal transition: a nationwide population-based retrospective cohort study. Medicine (Baltimore) 95(6):e2800, 2016 26871843
Huang T, Lin BM, Redline S, et al: Type of menopause, age at menopause, and risk of developing obstructive sleep apnea in postmenopausal women. Am J Epidemiol 187(7):1370–1379, 2018 29365014
Jayasena CN, Comninos AN, Stefanopoulou E, et al: Neurokinin B administration induces hot flushes in women. Sci Rep 5:8466, 2015 25683060

Joffe H, Groninger H, Soares CN, et al: An open trial of mirtazapine in menopausal women with depression unresponsive to estrogen replacement therapy. J Womens Health Gend Based Med 10(10):999–1004, 2001 11788110

Joffe H, Soares CN, Cohen LS: Assessment and treatment of hot flushes and menopausal mood disturbance. Psychiatr Clin North Am 26(3):563–580, 2003 14563098

Joffe H, Soares CN, Petrillo LF, et al: Treatment of depression and menopause-related symptoms with the serotonin-norepinephrine reuptake inhibitor duloxetine. J Clin Psychiatry 68(6):943–950, 2007 17592922

Joffe H, Petrillo L, Viguera A, et al: Eszopiclone improves insomnia and depressive and anxious symptoms in perimenopausal and postmenopausal women with hot flashes: a randomized, double-blinded, placebo-controlled crossover trial. Am J Obstet Gynecol 202(2):171.e1–171.e11, 2010 20035910

Joffe H, de Wit A, Coborn J, et al: Impact of estradiol variability and progesterone on mood in perimenopausal women with depressive symptoms. J Clin Endocrinol Metab 105(3):e642–e650, 2020 31693131

Kanes S, Colquhoun H, Gunduz-Bruce H, et al: Brexanolone (SAGE-547 injection) in post-partum depression: a randomised controlled trial. Lancet 390(10093):480–489, 2017 28619476

Koffel E, Kuhn E, Petsoulis N, et al: A randomized controlled pilot study of CBT-I Coach: feasibility, acceptability, and potential impact of a mobile phone application for patients in cognitive behavioral therapy for insomnia. Health Informatics J 24(1):3–13, 2018 27354394

Kohn GE, Rodriguez KM, Hotaling J, et al: The history of estrogen therapy. Sex Med Rev 7(3):416–421, 2019 31147294

Kornstein SG, Jiang Q, Reddy S, et al: Short-term efficacy and safety of desvenlafaxine in a randomized, placebo-controlled study of perimenopausal and postmenopausal women with major depressive disorder. J Clin Psychiatry 71(8):1088–1096, 2010 20797382

Kornstein SG, Toups M, Rush AJ, et al: Do menopausal status and use of hormone therapy affect antidepressant treatment response? Findings from the Sequenced Treatment Alternatives to Relieve Depression (STAR*D) study. J Womens Health (Larchmt) 22(2):121–131, 2013 23398127

Kotlarczyk MP, Lassila HC, O'Neil CK, et al: Melatonin Osteoporosis Prevention Study (MOPS): a randomized, double-blind, placebo-controlled study examining the effects of melatonin on bone health and quality of life in perimenopausal women. J Pineal Res 52(4):414–426, 2012 22220591

Krause MS, Nakajima ST: Hormonal and nonhormonal treatment of vasomotor symptoms. Obstet Gynecol Clin North Am 42(1):163–179, 2015 25681847

Kravitz HM, Ganz PA, Bromberger J, et al: Sleep difficulty in women at midlife: a community survey of sleep and the menopausal transition. Menopause 10(1):19–28, 2003 12544673

Kravitz HM, Janssen I, Lotrich FE, et al: Sex steroid hormone gene polymorphisms and depressive symptoms in women at midlife. Am J Med 119(9 suppl 1):S87–S93, 2006

Kravitz HM, Zhao X, Bromberger JT, et al: Sleep disturbance during the menopausal transition in a multi-ethnic community sample of women. Sleep 31(7):979–990, 2008 18652093

Krolick KN, Zhu Q, Shi H: Effects of estrogens on central nervous system neurotransmission: implications for sex differences in mental disorders. Prog Mol Biol Transl Sci 160:105–171, 2018 30470289

Kronenberg F, Fugh-Berman A: Complementary and alternative medicine for menopausal symptoms: a review of randomized, controlled trials. Ann Intern Med 137(10):805–813, 2002 12435217

Kugaya A, Epperson CN, Zoghbi S, et al: Increase in prefrontal cortex serotonin 2A receptors following estrogen treatment in postmenopausal women. Am J Psychiatry 160(8):1522–1524, 2003 12900319

Kuh D, Cooper R, Moore A, et al: Age at menopause and lifetime cognition: findings from a British birth cohort study. Neurology 90(19):e1673–e1681, 2018 29643079

Kulkarni J, de Castella A, Fitzgerald PB, et al: Estrogen in severe mental illness: a potential new treatment approach. Arch Gen Psychiatry 65(8):955–960, 2008 18678800

Ladd CO, Newport DJ, Ragan KA, et al: Venlafaxine in the treatment of depressive and vasomotor symptoms in women with perimenopausal depression. Depress Anxiety 22(2):94–97, 2005 16094663

Leach MJ, Moore V: Black cohosh (Cimicifuga spp.) for menopausal symptoms. Cochrane Database Syst Rev 2012(9):CD007244, 2012 22972105

Lethaby A, Marjoribanks J, Kronenberg F, et al: Phytoestrogens for menopausal vasomotor symptoms. Cochrane Database Syst Rev (12):CD001395, 2013 24323914

Lindh-Åstrand L, Nedstrand E: Effects of applied relaxation on vasomotor symptoms in postmenopausal women: a randomized controlled trial. Menopause 20(4):401–408, 2013 23149867

Loprinzi CL, Qin R, Balcueva EP, et al: Phase III, randomized, double-blind, placebo-controlled evaluation of pregabalin for alleviating hot flashes, N07C1. J Clin Oncol 28(4):641–647, 2010 19901102

Maclennan AH, Broadbent JL, Lester S, et al: Oral oestrogen and combined oestrogen/progestogen therapy versus placebo for hot flushes. Cochrane Database Syst Rev 2004(4):CD002978, 2004 15495039

Maki PM, Kornstein SG, Joffe H, et al: Guidelines for the evaluation and treatment of perimenopausal depression: summary and recommendations. Menopause 25(10):1069–1085, 2018 30179986

Mann E, Smith MJ, Hellier J, et al: Cognitive behavioural treatment for women who have menopausal symptoms after breast cancer treatment (MENOS 1): a randomised controlled trial. Lancet Oncol 13(3):309–318, 2012 22340966

Manson JE, Aragaki AK, Rossouw JE, et al: Menopausal hormone therapy and long-term all-cause and cause-specific mortality: the Women's Health Initiative randomized trials. JAMA 318(10):927–938, 2017 28898378

Marsh WK, Gershenson B, Rothschild AJ: Symptom severity of bipolar disorder during the menopausal transition. Int J Bipolar Disord 3(1):35, 2015 26296381

Mauas V, Kopala-Sibley DC, Zuroff DC: Depressive symptoms in the transition to menopause: the roles of irritability, personality vulnerability, and self-regulation. Arch Women Ment Health 17(4):279–289, 2014 24957780

McCurry SM, Guthrie KA, Morin CM, et al: Telephone-based cognitive behavioral therapy for insomnia in perimenopausal and postmenopausal women with vasomotor symptoms: a MsFLASH randomized clinical trial. JAMA Intern Med 176(7):913–920, 2016 27213646

Melby MK: Vasomotor symptom prevalence and language of menopause in Japan. Menopause 12(3):250–257, 2005 15879913

Melby MK, Lock M, Kaufert P: Culture and symptom reporting at menopause. Hum Reprod Update 11(5):495–512, 2005 15919681

Melby MK, Sievert LL, Anderson D, et al: Overview of methods used in cross-cultural comparisons of menopausal symptoms and their determinants: Guidelines for Strengthening the Reporting of Menopause and Aging (STROMA) studies. Maturitas 70(2):99–109, 2011 21840143

Meltzer-Brody S, Colquhoun H, Riesenberg R, et al: Brexanolone injection in post-partum depression: two multicentre, double-blind, randomised, placebo-controlled, phase 3 trials. Lancet 392(10152):1058–1070, 2018 30177236

Milic J, Glisic M, Voortman T, et al: Menopause, ageing, and alcohol use disorders in women. Maturitas 111:100–109, 2018 29673827

Miller VM, Naftolin F, Asthana S, et al: The Kronos Early Estrogen Prevention Study (KEEPS): what have we learned? Menopause 26(9):1071–1084, 2019 31453973

Mitchell MD, Gehrman P, Perlis M, Umscheid CA: Comparative effectiveness of cognitive behavioral therapy for insomnia: a systematic review. BMC Fam Pract 13:40, 2012 22631616

Mohyi D, Tabassi K, Simon J: Differential diagnosis of hot flashes. Maturitas 27(3):203–214, 1997 9288692

Montazeri SA, Ramezani Tehrani F, Bidhendi Yarandi R, et al: Effect of aging, menopause, and age at natural menopause on the trend in body mass index: a 15-year population-based cohort. Fertil Steril 111(4):780–786, 2019 30929733

Nasreddine ZS, Phillips NA, Bédirian V, et al: The Montreal Cognitive Assessment, MoCA: a brief screening tool for mild cognitive impairment. J Am Geriatr Soc 53(4):695–699, 2005 15817019
National Institute on Aging: Sex and Menopause: Treatment for Symptoms. Bethesda, MD, National Institute on Aging, 2017a. Available at: https://www.nia.nih.gov/health/sex-and-menopause-treatment-symptoms. Accessed November 18, 2019.
National Institute on Aging: Sleep Problems and Menopause: What Can I Do? Bethesda, MD, National Institute on Aging, 2017b. Available at: https://www.nia.nih.gov/health/sleep-problems-and-menopause-what-can-i-do. Accessed November 18, 2019.
National Institute on Aging: Cognitive Health and Older Adults. Bethesda, MD, National Institute on Aging, 2019a. Available at: https://www.nia.nih.gov/health/cognitive-health-and-older-adults. Accessed December 9, 2019.
National Institute on Aging: Memory, Forgetfulness, and Aging: What's Normal and What's Not? (online). Bethesda, MD, National Institute on Aging, 2019b. Available at: https://www.nia.nih.gov/health/memory-forgetfulness-and-aging-whats-normal-and-whats-not. Accessed December 9, 2019.
National Institutes of Health: National Institutes of Health State-of-the-Science Conference statement: management of menopause-related symptoms. Ann Intern Med 142(12 pt 1):1003–1013, 2005 15968015
Nelson HD, Vesco KK, Haney E, et al: Nonhormonal therapies for menopausal hot flashes: systematic review and meta-analysis. JAMA 295(17):2057–2071, 2006 16670414
Newton KM, Reed SD, Guthrie KA, et al: Efficacy of yoga for vasomotor symptoms: a randomized controlled trial. Menopause 21(4):339–346, 2014 24045673
North American Menopause Society: Dangers of Exposure to Topical Estrogen in Children and Pets: Menopause Education. Pepper Pike, OH, North American Menopause Society, 2021a. Available at: http://www.menopause.org/for-women/menopauseflashes/menopause-symptoms-and-treatments/dangers-of-exposure-to-topical-estrogen-in-children-pets. Accessed January 13, 2021.
North American Menopause Society: Sexual Health and Menopause Online. Pepper Pike, OH, North American Menopause Society, 2021b. Available at: http://www.menopause.org/for-women/sexual-health-menopause-online. Accessed January 13, 2021.
Obermeyer CM, Reher D, Saliba M: Symptoms, menopause status, and country differences: a comparative analysis from DAMES. Menopause 14(4):788–797, 2007 17507832
Pavlovic JM: Evaluation and management of migraine in midlife women. Menopause 25(8):927–929, 2018 29787480
Pérez-Alcalá I, Sievert LL, Obermeyer CM, et al: Cross-cultural analysis of determinants of hot flashes and night sweats: Latin-American immigrants to Madrid and their Spanish neighbors. Menopause 20(11):1111–1119, 2013 23571525
Pérez-López FR, Martínez-Domínguez SJ, Lajusticia H, et al: Effects of programmed exercise on depressive symptoms in midlife and older women: a meta-analysis of randomized controlled trials. Maturitas 106:38–47, 2017 29150165
Perger E, Mattaliano P, Lombardi C: Menopause and sleep apnea. Maturitas 124:35–38, 2019 31097176
Perich T, Ussher J, Meade T: Menopause and illness course in bipolar disorder: a systematic review. Bipolar Disord 19(6):434–443, 2017 28796389
Pinkerton JAV, Aguirre FS, Blake J, et al: The 2017 hormone therapy position statement of The North American Menopause Society. Menopause 24(7):728–753, 2017 28650869
Pop P, Bronskill SE, Piggott KL, et al: Management of sleep disorders in community-dwelling older women and men at the time of diagnosis. J Am Geriatr Soc 67(10):2094–2101, 2019 31225914
Prague JK, Roberts RE, Comninos AN, et al: Neurokinin 3 receptor antagonism rapidly improves vasomotor symptoms with sustained duration of action. Menopause 25(8):862–869, 2018 29533369
Radloff LS: The CES-D scale: a self-report depression scale for research in the general population. Appl Psychol Meas 1:385–401, 1977

Reddy SY, Warner H, Guttuso T Jr, et al: Gabapentin, estrogen, and placebo for treating hot flushes: a randomized controlled trial. Obstet Gynecol 108(1):41–48, 2006 16816054
Rossouw JE, Anderson GL, Prentice RL, et al: Risks and benefits of estrogen plus progestin in healthy postmenopausal women: principal results from the Women's Health Initiative randomized controlled trial. JAMA 288(3):321–333, 2002 12117397
Rubinow DR, Johnson SL, Schmidt PJ, et al: Efficacy of estradiol in perimenopausal depression: so much promise and so few answers. Depress Anxiety 32(8):539–549, 2015 26130315
Saensak S, Vutyavanich T, Somboonporn W, et al: Relaxation for perimenopausal and postmenopausal symptoms. Cochrane Database Syst Rev (7):CD008582, 2014 25039019
Sandra Kooij JJ, Marije Boonstra A, Swinkels SHN, et al: Reliability, validity, and utility of instruments for self-report and informant report concerning symptoms of ADHD in adult patients. J Atten Disord 11(4):445–458, 2008 18083961
Santoro N: Perimenopause: from research to practice. J Womens Health (Larchmt) 25(4):332–339, 2016 26653408
Schmidt PJ, Murphy JH, Haq N, et al: Stressful life events, personal losses, and perimenopause-related depression. Arch Women Ment Health 7(1):19–26, 2004 14963729
Schmidt PJ, Ben Dor R, Martinez PE, et al: Effects of estradiol withdrawal on mood in women with past perimenopausal depression: a randomized clinical trial. JAMA Psychiatry 72(7):714–726, 2015 26018333
Searles S, Makarewicz JA, Dumas JA: The role of estradiol in schizophrenia diagnosis and symptoms in postmenopausal women. Schizophr Res 196:35–38, 2018 28587815
Shanmugan S, Epperson CN: Estrogen and the prefrontal cortex: towards a new understanding of estrogen's effects on executive functions in the menopause transition. Hum Brain Mapp 35(3):847–865, 2014 23238908
Shanmugan S, Sammel MD, Loughead J, et al: Executive function after risk-reducing salpingo-oophorectomy in BRCA1 and BRCA2 mutation carriers: does current mood and early life adversity matter? Menopause 27(7):746–755, 2020 32187134
Slopien R, Pluchino N, Warenik-Szymankiewicz A, et al: Correlation between allopregnanolone levels and depressive symptoms during late menopausal transition and early postmenopause. Gynecol Endocrinol 34(2):144–147, 2018 28857628
Soares CN, Poitras JR, Prouty J, et al: Efficacy of citalopram as a monotherapy or as an adjunctive treatment to estrogen therapy for perimenopausal and postmenopausal women with depression and vasomotor symptoms. J Clin Psychiatry 64(4):473–479, 2003 12716252
Soares CN, Arsenio H, Joffe H, et al: Escitalopram versus ethinyl estradiol and norethindrone acetate for symptomatic peri- and postmenopausal women: impact on depression, vasomotor symptoms, sleep, and quality of life. Menopause 13(5):780–786, 2006 16894334
Sood R, Sood A, Wolf SL, et al: Paced breathing compared with usual breathing for hot flashes. Menopause 20(2):179–184, 2013 22990758
Spitzer RL, Kroenke K, Williams JBW: Validation and utility of a self-report version of PRIME-MD: the PHQ primary care study. Primary Care Evaluation of Mental Disorders. Patient Health Questionnaire. JAMA 282(18):1737–1744, 1999 10568646
Stuenkel CA, Davis SR, Gompel A, et al: Treatment of symptoms of the menopause: an Endocrine Society clinical practice guideline. J Clin Endocrinol Metab 100(11):3975–4011, 2015 26444994
Stute P, Spyropoulou A, Karageorgiou V, et al: Management of depressive symptoms in peri- and postmenopausal women: EMAS position statement. Maturitas 131:91–101, 2020 31740049
Süss H, Ehlert U: Psychological resilience during the perimenopause. Maturitas 131:48–56, 2020 31787147
Sussman M, Trocio J, Best C, et al: Prevalence of menopausal symptoms among mid-life women: findings from electronic medical records. BMC Womens Health 15:58, 2015 26271251
Thurston RC, Ewing LJ, Low CA, et al: Behavioral weight loss for the management of menopausal hot flashes: a pilot study. Menopause 22(1):59–65, 2015 24977456
Thurston RC, Chang Y, Buysse DJ, et al: Hot flashes and awakenings among midlife women. Sleep (Basel) 42(9):zsz131, 2019 31152182
U.S. Food and Drug Administration: FDA permits marketing of a diagnostic test to aid in the determination of menopausal status. FDA News Release, October 24, 2018

Usall J, Pinto-Meza A, Fernández A, et al: Suicide ideation across reproductive life cycle of women: results from a European epidemiological study. J Affect Disord 116(1–2):144–147, 2009 19155069

Ustun B, Adler LA, Rudin C, et al: The world health organization adult attention-deficit/hyperactivity disorder self-report screening scale for DSM-5. JAMA Psychiatry 74(5):520–527, 2017 28384801

van Broekhoven F, Bäckström T, Verkes RJ: Oral progesterone decreases saccadic eye velocity and increases sedation in women. Psychoneuroendocrinology 31(10):1190–1199, 2006 17034954

Waetjen LE, Crawford SL, Chang PY, et al: Factors associated with developing vaginal dryness symptoms in women transitioning through menopause: a longitudinal study. Menopause 25(10):1094–1104, 2018 29916947

Walega DR, Rubin LH, Banuvar S, et al: Effects of stellate ganglion block on vasomotor symptoms: findings from a randomized controlled clinical trial in postmenopausal women. Menopause 21(8):807–814, 2014 24496086

Willi J, Ehlert U: Assessment of perimenopausal depression: a review. J Affect Disord 249:216–222, 2019 30776662

Williams RE, Kalilani L, DiBenedetti DB, et al: Frequency and severity of vasomotor symptoms among peri- and postmenopausal women in the United States. Climacteric 11(1):32–43, 2008 18202963

Woods NF, Mitchell ES: Symptoms during the perimenopause: prevalence, severity, trajectory, and significance in women's lives. Am J Med 118(suppl 12B):14–24, 2005 16414323

Woods NF, Mitchell ES: The Seattle Midlife Women's Health Study: a longitudinal prospective study of women during the menopausal transition and early postmenopause. Womens Midlife Health 2:6, 2016 30766702

Woods NF, Mitchell ES, Adams C: Memory functioning among midlife women: observations from the Seattle Midlife Women's Health Study. Menopause 7(4):257–265, 2000 10914619

Woods NF, Smith-DiJulio K, Percival DB, et al: Depressed mood during the menopausal transition and early postmenopause: observations from the Seattle Midlife Women's Health Study. Menopause 15(2):223–232, 2008 18176355

Woods NF, Cray LA, Mitchell ES, et al: Polymorphisms in estrogen synthesis genes and symptom clusters during the menopausal transition and early postmenopause: observations from the Seattle Midlife Women's Health Study. Biol Res Nurs 20(2):153–160, 2018 29334760

Wuttke W, Jarry H, Becker T, et al: Phytoestrogens: endocrine disrupters or replacement for hormone replacement therapy? Maturitas 61(1–2):159–170, 2008 19434888

Yilmaz C, Karali K, Fodelianaki G, et al: Neurosteroids as regulators of neuroinflammation. Front Neuroendocrinol 55:100788, 2019 31513776

Zhu X, Liew Y, Liu ZL: Chinese herbal medicine for menopausal symptoms. Cochrane Database Syst Rev 3:CD009023, 2016 26976671

# PART II

## Pregnancy and the Postpartum Period

# CHAPTER 8

# A Clinical Approach to Psychiatric Diagnosis and Treatment During Pregnancy

Elizabeth M. Fitelson, M.D.
Lauren M. Osborne, M.D.
Jennifer L. Payne, M.D.

"Doctor, I just found out I'm pregnant! Is it safe to keep taking my antidepressant?" All clinicians who treat women of reproductive age are likely to hear this question at some point—most likely many times—over the course of their careers. Faced with the myriad sources of often contradictory information about treatment of perinatal psychiatric disorders, both patients and clinicians can feel overwhelmed or confused about how to balance keeping the mother well and protecting the future child. Many clinicians continue to recommend stopping all psychiatric medications during pregnancy out of concern for potential harm to the fetus. However, increasing evidence shows that untreated psychiatric illness during pregnancy poses significant risks to both the untreated mother and the developing child.

The importance of treating maternal mental illness is discussed elsewhere in this book and is not reiterated here in detail. Similarly, the safety and risks associated with specific psychiatric medications during pregnancy and recommendations for evaluating and treating specific syndromes are also covered elsewhere in this book. This chapter offers a general clinical approach to designing a treatment plan during pregnancy for women with psychiatric disorders. We should also note that although we frequently refer to our patients as women, we recognize and acknowledge that not everyone seeking care from a reproductive psychiatrist identifies as a woman. Anyone was assigned the female sex at birth—a group that includes cisgender women, transgender men, and nonbinary people—may have reproductive transitions associated with the female reproductive cycle and may therefore be subject to psychiatric illness at times of reproductive transition.

## Approach to Diagnosis

With any patient, a clinician cannot design a treatment plan without obtaining a proper understanding of the patient's symptoms and likely diagnosis. Arriving at the correct diagnosis is crucially important in the perinatal period. Because untreated psychiatric illness carries risks to both mother and child, and some psychiatric medications also carry risks, it is important to be sure that the illness is being treated appropriately. Pregnancy itself can induce physical symptoms, such as fatigue and appetite changes, that may be confused with mood symptoms. Also, the tendency of our society to equate motherhood with "glowing" and happiness may lead some women, and some clinicians, to downplay mood symptoms because they do not fit with deeply held expectations about pregnancy. Women living with considerable psychosocial stress may arrive in the perinatal period carrying prior diagnoses that may not be accurate but instead reflect inadequate evaluation or prejudice on the part of previous providers.

When a pregnant or postpartum woman presents for evaluation and treatment, it is important for the clinician to perform a thorough psychiatric interview to arrive at the correct diagnosis. The essential assessment components are listed in Table 8–1. Arriving at the correct diagnosis is the key first step in considering how to weigh the risks of medication versus those of untreated illness. One good example is the patient who presents with a long history of stimulant use and questions whether to continue her medication in pregnancy. An appropriate diagnostic interview will uncover the difference between the patient with severe ADHD, for whom this medication is essential to avoid car accidents and poor performance at work, and the patient without ADHD whose stimulant use was masking symptoms of anxiety and depression that might be better treated with an antidepressant.

## "Risk-Risk" Analysis

After arriving at a diagnosis, the clinician needs to help the patient arrive at a decision about risk. Clinicians are familiar with risk-benefit decision making when discussing treatment recommendations that balance the potential benefit of a treatment against the known risks and help patients make the most informed decision possible among a range of options. Because the risks of psychiatric illness in pregnancy have for so long been underestimated or misunderstood, a more helpful approach when discussing psychiatric treatment during pregnancy is a "risk-risk" analysis, which requires assessing the risks associated with psychiatric medication exposure to the fetus and pregnancy versus the risks of untreated psychiatric illness to the mother and the developing child.

Depression during pregnancy has been associated with preterm delivery, low birth weight, higher rates of preeclampsia and gestational diabetes, decreased infant motor

**TABLE 8–1. Components of assessment of mental disorders during pregnancy**

| |
|---|
| Thorough psychiatric interview to assess time course, quality, and severity of symptoms, with emphasis on review of any symptoms that might indicate previously undiagnosed bipolar disorder |
| Thorough review of the severity of past illness, including hospitalizations and suicidality |
| Gynecological history, including information about age at menarche, menstrual cycle–related mood symptoms, responses to hormonal contraception and/or hormonal interventions for infertility, and previous pregnancies (including terminations and miscarriages) |
| Gender and sexual history, including information about sexual orientation, gender identity, sexual partners, and sexually transmitted infections |
| Thorough family history, including information about antenatal or postpartum depression or psychosis in any female relatives and any family history of bipolar disorder |
| Use of standardized scales specifically designed for pregnancy |
| Edinburgh Postnatal Depression Scale (Cox et al. 1987) |
| Perinatal Anxiety Screening Scale (Somerville et al. 2014) |
| Laboratory tests for physical conditions common in pregnancy that may affect mood |
| Complete blood count for anemia |
| Thyroid-stimulating hormone for thyroid disease |
| Vitamins D and $B_{12}$ |
| Thorough review of past medication trials and the patient's response |
| Review of substance use |
| Social history, including any history of past traumas, intimate partner violence, chronic stress due to discrimination, and social supports available to the patient |
| Complete medical history, with special emphasis on any conditions that may affect the likelihood of psychiatric symptoms (e.g., autoimmune illness) |
| Assessment of the patient's ability to access and engage in nonpharmacological treatments |
| Assessment of the patient's feelings about pregnancy and impending motherhood (Was the pregnancy planned? Is it desired?) |

tone and activity, higher infant cortisol levels and poor reflexes, and overall worse infant health status (Ashman et al. 2002; Diego et al. 2004; Essex et al. 2002; Field et al. 2010; Halligan et al. 2004; Li et al. 2009; Orr et al. 2007). There is also a robust and replicated literature on the adverse effects of mothers' postpartum depression on infants and developing children, including lower IQ, slower language development, and higher rates of ADHD, behavior problems, and psychiatric illness (Grace et al. 2003). Similarly, maternal anxiety, psychosis, and mania are associated with poor pregnancy and infant outcomes and, in rare but tragic cases, infanticide (Jones et al. 2014; Vigod et al. 2014). Thus, exposure to maternal psychiatric illness during pregnancy or the postpartum period can lead to undesirable and negative outcomes for the exposed child.

Mental health conditions also are major contributors to all-cause maternal mortality (defined as the death of a woman in pregnancy or within a year after giving birth). With the rise of the opioid epidemic in the United States, maternal self-harm deaths, including both suicide and unintended overdose, are the leading cause of pregnancy-related death (Davis et al. 2019; Mangla et al. 2019; Shadigian and Bauer 2005). Systemic racial and ethnic disparities in many of the social determinants of health, such as housing stability, economic security, access to healthy food, environmental exposures, discrimination, and access to high quality health care, lead to higher levels of many maternal morbidities that are often comorbid with mental illness for Black women and other minoritized populations. Black women have higher rates of pregnancy hypertension and preterm births than do other ethnic groups, and Hispanic and Asian women have higher rates of gestational diabetes than other groups (U.S. Department of Health and Human Services, Health Resources and Services Administration, Maternal and Child Health Bureau 2013). Pregnancy-related death is three times as likely in Black women as in white women, regardless of education or income level, and is almost as high in American Indian and Alaskan Native populations (U.S. Department of Health and Human Services, Health Resources and Services Administration, Maternal and Child Health Bureau 2013).

Given all of these various dangers, clinicians from all disciplines who treat perinatal women with mental health conditions have a responsibility to partner with their patients to develop treatment plans that aim to mitigate *both* the risks of untreated or undertreated illness *and* the potential risks of treatment, including medication. Although most women would likely prefer not to take any medications during pregnancy, many face significant morbidity if psychiatric medications are discontinued, changed, or not initiated due to an imbalanced assessment of these risks. Also, many women may not have a real choice as to whether to continue or start medication if they are not presented with the full range of evidence-based treatment options available to treat their symptoms, including psychotherapy, lifestyle changes, and social supports.

The balance of risks will be different for every patient. Different risks will be faced by a patient with few psychosocial supports and few resources than by a financially comfortable woman with strong family support. Patients enduring ongoing challenges due to health care disparities for racial and sexual minorities will have different risk calculations than those in more privileged groups. The perinatal period represents a unique moment of opportunity for patients and families to engage in positive changes that can affect not only the course of a woman's psychiatric illness but also the well-being of her family. By engaging with a patient in a full risk-risk discussion that treats the risks of both illness and treatment seriously, clinicians prioritize the mother's well-being as essential to the health of the dyad rather than emphasizing the false dichotomy of sacrificing the mother's health for the benefit of the baby and respect patient autonomy and values as critical components of perinatal mental health care. Although such a discussion may appear daunting, the basic principles outlined in this chapter, applied along with the knowledge gleaned from the rest of this book, will enable clinicians to develop a rational psychiatric treatment plan for pregnancy.

## General Treatment Principles

### Expect the Unexpected Pregnancy and Prepare Ahead of Time

By age 44 years, 85% of U.S. women will be mothers (Livingston 2018). Unintended pregnancies, resulting from both failure to use contraception and failure of the contraceptive used, make up 50% of all pregnancies in the United States (Finer and Zolna 2014; Mosher and Bachrach 1996). The rate of unintended pregnancies has decreased slightly in recent years but remains highest among young women (ages 18–24 years), low-income women, cohabiting women, and women of color (Finer and Zolna 2016).

Every psychiatric provider who treats individuals with female reproductive organs who are between menarche and menopause will at some point (and possibly many times) manage a patient with a planned or unplanned pregnancy. Thus, it is imperative to consider the reproductive life cycle when initiating and continuing psychiatric treatment. This principle requires that the clinician make wise medication choices from the beginning of care and, for women of certain ages, begin with medications that have reassuring safety profiles in pregnancy. For example, although valproic acid can be extremely effective for bipolar mania, it should not be a first-line treatment for reproductive-age women with bipolar disorder because it is associated with a high rate of major organ malformations and intellectual disability in exposed children (Alsdorf and Wyszynski 2005; Kozma 2001; ten Berg et al. 2005). Women who have not tolerated or responded to other mood-stabilizing medications and may need to consider valproate should be advised of the significant teratogenic risk and counseled on effective birth control.

It is also important to discuss, when a medication is first prescribed, whether it can be safely used during pregnancy, even if the patient is not currently sexually active or planning pregnancy. Furthermore, clinicians must be careful of their own bias in considering whether patients with mental illness may become pregnant: although fertility rates among women with severe mental illness are lower than among the general population, most women with severe and persistent mental illness become mothers and describe motherhood as central to their existence (Jones et al. 2014). Asking women regularly about their plans to become pregnant, discussing contraceptive options, and questioning their plans in the event of an unplanned pregnancy help in rational treatment planning prior to conception, reduce the likelihood of a crisis, and may also reduce the likelihood of an unplanned pregnancy. It is vitally important to remember that this issue applies equally to transgender men and nonbinary people who may also plan future pregnancies.

### Revisit Diagnoses and Treatment Options: The Biopsychosocial Model

Most clinicians strive for diagnostic accuracy, but the course of psychiatric illness and responses to treatment are often complex and informed by a mix of biological factors (e.g., genetic vulnerability, medical illness, substance use), psychological factors (e.g., trauma, early attachments), and social determinants (e.g., partner or family support, education, financial resources, housing stability, bias or racism). Approaching treatment decisions for perinatal women necessitates careful consideration of these elements to properly understand the risks of the illness to the patient and her family and the most appropriate recommendations to mitigate these risks. In addition, psychiatric comorbidity is common, and response to treatment is often heterogeneous, complicating a simplistic algorithmic approach to treatment recommendations. However, to engage in a true risk-risk discussion and create a rational treatment plan, the clinician must understand as accurately as possible the nature of the psychiatric illness with which the perinatal patient presents, her response to past treatments, and the rationale for her current treatment (if she is already in treatment).

For example, a young woman with a history of childhood abuse who acts out and abuses substances may have been diagnosed in adolescence as "bipolar" and treated with mood stabilizers; however, a careful review of her history might reveal that she would be more appropriately diagnosed with PTSD and substance dependence. Another woman, diagnosed with depression and treated with antidepressants for years, might reveal in a careful review that she has had cycles of hypomania as well as depression. Many women who began treatment during an acute episode of depression might have been continued indefinitely on antidepressants by primary care providers without review of whether their depression is likely to recur or is comorbid with an anxiety disorder that may be amenable to other treatment options.

Each of these scenarios has profound implications for treatment recommendations. The young woman with trauma might benefit most from intensive trauma-focused psychotherapy and possibly an antidepressant medication and may not need to be maintained on mood stabilizers that confer more risk in pregnancy. The woman with mood cycling, in contrast, could be at higher risk for postpartum psychosis if her symptoms represent an undiagnosed bipolar disorder. A woman with a single past depressive episode could attempt to taper off medications safely prior to pregnancy but may benefit from cognitive-behavioral therapy (CBT) to address residual anxiety and to prevent relapse. Treatment planning in pregnancy necessitates this careful review of diagnosis so that patients and clinicians can consider the full range of appropriate treatment options that maximize safety and mental health.

## Consider Severity of Illness

It is important to consider the severity of illness when designing a treatment plan for pregnancy. Ultimately, the decision to continue or discontinue psychiatric medications for pregnancy will reside with the patient; however, the clinician can provide recommendations. For example, a woman with a history of mild illness that has been easily well controlled could be referred for psychotherapy while weaning off medication for pregnancy, whereas a woman with a more severe history might be encouraged to carefully consider the high rate of relapse and the risks of untreated psychiatric illness in pregnancy. All women should be monitored closely by their psychiatric providers during pregnancy and in the postpartum period, but women with a history of severe illness should be evaluated more often, particularly if they elect to discontinue medication.

## Maximize Behavioral and Somatic Treatments and Interventions

Accurate assessment of diagnosis and illness severity, as well as psychological factors, supports, and stressors, can help guide recommendations not only for psychiatric medications but also for evidence-based psychosocial interventions. Numerous studies support evidence-based psychotherapies such as interpersonal psychotherapy and CBT as effective interventions for mild to moderate depression in pregnancy and the postpartum period (Genovez et al. 2018). Although less studied in the perinatal population, evidence-based psychotherapies for diagnoses other than depression are likely to remain effective. For example, a patient with comorbid borderline personality disorder and anxiety who is engaging in self-injurious behaviors may benefit most from dialectical behavioral therapy. Psychotherapeutic interventions should be considered for every perinatal patient and included in a discussion of treatment options, not simply as alternatives to medications but as interventions that might help mitigate residual symptoms, reduce the need for adjunctive medications such as benzodiazepines, or allow for a trial reduction of medications.

In addition to traditional psychotherapy, some "complementary" treatments have evidence to suggest their benefit in mitigating the burden of psychiatric illness in perinatal women. Interventions such as exercise, yoga, acupuncture, or massage may have only modest evidence for benefit in clinical trials but, barring obstetric complications, are generally considered safe and may promote overall well-being (Reza et al. 2018). Bright light therapy is another example of an underutilized tool for depressive symptoms, with evidence of benefit when used alone or as augmentation in perinatal women (Deligiannidis and Freeman 2014). Given the clear connection between poor social or partner supports and perinatal depression, other interventions that shore up these supports might be appropriate, such as peer support, particularly for women with a history of childhood adversity (Racine et al. 2018). A comprehensive, individualized treatment plan for perinatal patients should include discussion of the breadth of nonpharmacological interventions that could offer benefit with minimal risk of harm. Unfortunately, given the wide health care disparities in our society, not all patients will have access to high-quality nonpharmacological interventions or to strong social supports, and this reality must also be factored into the treatment plan.

## Minimize the Number of Adverse Exposures

An important goal is to minimize potential adverse exposures to medication(s) and to maternal psychiatric illness. At one time, psychiatric providers often recommended discontinuing all psychiatric medications during the first trimester, when major organs are formed. However, the risk of psychiatric relapse is high with discontinuation of medications: up to 70% of women with major depression and 85% or more of women with bipolar disorder relapse when their psychiatric medications are discontinued for pregnancy (Cohen et al. 2006; Viguera et al. 2000, 2007). The developing infant is then potentially exposed to the adverse effects of psychiatric illness. In this situation, psychiatric medications are often restarted—and sometimes more are added in the case of a significant psychiatric relapse, resulting in the fetus being exposed to maternal psychiatric illness, the originally prescribed psychiatric medication(s), and potentially other psychiatric medications. Such risk of increased exposure to both illness and medications must be considered when discussing medication discontinuation, particularly for women with more severe illness pathology.

Nevertheless, simplifying a patient's regimen by eliminating medications that can be safely stopped is good practice when possible. At times, patients end up taking a complicated medication regimen when their doctors are trying several things at once to manage a severe illness or to reduce side effects, such as fatigue or sexual dysfunction. Patients and their physicians are often reluctant to change anything once stability is achieved because they are afraid of relapse. However, patients may be more willing to tolerate certain side effects in the context of pregnancy. Often, tapering of medications in a stable patient may reveal that one or more medications added as augmentation in an acute phase of illness is no longer needed. For example, sometimes sleep aids that were originally needed for an acute psychiatric illness can be eliminated or replaced with nonpharmacological interventions once the illness is under control. A carefully approached reduction of medications can effectively lower the exposure of the fetus to multiple medications. Ideally, such adjustment would be done prior to conception to avoid triggering relapse during pregnancy.

## Use Medications With Data When Possible

Although all new medications must undergo some animal testing to evaluate potential toxicity in gestation, pregnant and lactating women are generally excluded from clinical trials that test safety and efficacy of new drugs, so human data in pregnancy are collected after the drug is approved. Effectively, this means that the longer a medication has been available, the more data have been accumulated on the safety and risks of that medication in pregnancy. Medications new to the market generally do not have any human reproductive safety data; when possible, prescribers should consider the availability of such data when treating women of childbearing age and make recommendations accordingly, including considering a switch to an older medication that has more data if the patient is planning to conceive.

The FDA pregnancy categories A–D and X were misleading and caused confusion for many physicians when the FDA combined into Category B those medications that had 1) reassuring animal data but no human data and 2) demonstrated an adverse effect in animals but no risk in humans (U.S. Food and Drug Administration 2014). Thus, many providers concluded that if a medication was in Category B, it was safe to use during pregnancy or was preferable to a Category C or D medication. However, because medications new to the market usually had animal data but no human data in pregnancy, they were often placed in Category B. Switching to a Category B medication from a Category C or D medication is not always advisable because researchers may have much more data for and understand exactly what the risks are with those Category C or D medications than for the Category B medication. The FDA pregnancy categories have been phased out in favor of a new labeling plan that includes a summary of the known data in pregnancy for each medication and data for the illness(es) for which it is indicated. We have included this description of them here, however, because they continue to be available on the internet, and many patients still ask about them.

It is also important to understand that more data about a medication does not *necessarily* mean it is safer in pregnancy than a newer medication, particularly for a patient who did not do well in the past when taking an older medication. Clinicians must consider the person's past response to treatment as part of the "data" that help determine the safest medications in pregnancy. The safest medication is *usually* the one that is most effective and tolerated in treating a patient's illness. If an older medication with more reproductive safety data has been ineffective or not tolerated in the past, it is unlikely to be more effective or tolerated during pregnancy. Switching from a newer but effective medication to an older medication with more data may in fact be less "safe" in pregnancy if it increases the risk for relapse, noncompliance, or more medication changes.

## Plan Ahead: Make Medication Changes Prior to Pregnancy

In most cases, if medication changes are going to be made to decrease the risk to the fetus, they should be made prior to conception. Once a woman becomes pregnant while taking medication, the fetus has already been exposed to the medication. Switching at this point increases the number of medication exposures to the fetus and may increase the risk of relapse in the mother, in which case the fetus would be potentially exposed to the original medication and the new medication, as well as the mother's psychiatric illness. Unless a medication is a known teratogen, it makes more sense to continue the newer medication that is working well and thereby have one exposure for the fetus rather than two or more.

Two psychiatric medications—valproic acid and carbamazepine—should be avoided during pregnancy if at all possible due to their high risk of major organ malformations. Either of these medications should be switched to another mood stabilizer prior to pregnancy so as to prevent even brief exposure to a fetus. Their use in any females of reproductive age should be limited to severe cases that have failed other management strategies, and patients should be advised about the medications' risks in pregnancy and counseled on effective birth control.

## Consider Age and Other Risk Factors When Designing a Treatment Plan for Pregnancy

Other risk factors that can potentially impact pregnancy outcomes include, among others, maternal age, tobacco use, and substance use. When designing a treatment plan for pregnancy, these other risk factors should be taken into account. For example, a young woman who is taking a newer psychiatric medication with less safety data will have the luxury of time to attempt to switch to another medication with more data before becoming pregnant. In contrast, a woman in her early 40s might choose to proceed with attempting pregnancy sooner rather than wait for a medication change. Similarly, if a woman is using or abusing tobacco, marijuana, or other substances, these behaviors ideally should be addressed prior to attempting pregnancy so that the fetus is not exposed. In this case, smoking cessation and substance abuse treatment should take precedence over switching to a medication with more data. Likewise, if a woman with comorbid substance use disorder and psychiatric illness is more likely to relapse to using substances when psychiatrically ill, this risk is an important factor in any risk-risk discussion.

## Keep Mom Well—Do Not Err on the Side of Undertreating

In the setting of excitement about a pregnancy, both patients and providers may forget that the goal is to keep the mother well during pregnancy and to limit exposure of the fetus to both maternal psychiatric illness and medications. Often, women are given lower doses of medications to mitigate exposure in pregnancy. Although this can be a reasonable action—and using the lowest effective dose of medication is a solid principle in pregnancy—if the medication blood level drops below the therapeutic threshold, the woman is at higher risk of relapse and the fetus is at risk of exposure to both medication and illness. Because blood levels of most medications drop in later pregnancy due to increased blood volume, changes in glomerular filtration rate, and changes in liver metabolism (from about 20% for selective serotonin reuptake inhibitors to 50% for lamotrigine), the risk for relapse even in women who remain on medications is significant (Cohen et al. 2006). Although therapeutic drug monitoring is essential and helpful in a medication dosed by blood level, such as lithium, the primary determinant of medication dosing should be therapeutic effect. This means that dosing in pregnancy may sometimes exceed the FDA guidance on maximum dose. For example, a woman whose remission from OCD symptoms has required a dose of 200 mg/day of sertraline prior to pregnancy may experience breakthrough symptoms due to the metabolic and blood volume changes in late pregnancy, and increasing the dose of the medication above the FDA maximum to restabilize her symptoms is reasonable. In most cases, the dosage can be reduced again postpartum if the patient remains in remission.

Many women and their providers may be reluctant to increase psychiatric medications during pregnancy even in the setting of psychiatric relapse or worsening of symptoms. A better practice is to educate patients about these changes and risks in pregnancy proactively, monitor symptoms closely, and increase medications if needed, shortly after symptoms emerge, with the goal of a healthy mother who is more likely to have a healthy pregnancy and positive pregnancy and infant outcomes (DeVane et al. 2006; Tracy et al. 2005).

Stigma about psychiatric illness and the subtle idea that we, as humans, are in charge of our emotions and anxieties and that people with psychiatric conditions do not have real conditions—that their symptoms are "all in their heads"—lead to the idea that not treating or undertreating psychiatric illness during pregnancy is acceptable. Like other medical conditions regularly treated aggressively (albeit with some modifications) in pregnancy, such as asthma, hypertension, seizure disorders, and cancer, psychiatric illnesses are medical conditions with effects on many systems in the body. Psychiatrically ill mothers have worse personal, obstetrical, and infant outcomes (for details, see chapters on individual disorders). Therefore, psychiatric illness during pregnancy should be treated with the same goal as outside of pregnancy: to get the patient well. If the mother becomes psychiatrically ill during pregnancy, it is important to recognize that treatment is not working and to reengage in shared decision making; maximize current medications, accounting for the physiological changes of pregnancy (even at times above the FDA maximum if indicated); shore up the patient's support system; consider psychotherapy or other alternatives; evaluate for other medical complications that may be affecting symptoms; and not be afraid to add or switch medications if needed.

## Educate Everyone, Including Patients, Supports, and Other Providers

Education is one of the key elements to taking good care of a pregnant patient with psychiatric illness. Women receive conflicting messages about taking psychiatric medications during pregnancy—from the internet, their friends, their family, and their doctors. The psychiatric care provider should strive to make sure that everyone understands the rationale for the medication treatment plan during pregnancy. Scheduling a family meeting to discuss the plan and any concerns can be immensely helpful in preventing unneeded stress for both patient and family. It is also often helpful for the psychiatric care provider to reach out to the other members of the patient's medical team, including the obstetrician and the pediatrician. Early communication and understanding help to avoid mixed messages, confusion, and discontinuation of medications when discontinuation was not the plan.

### Be Calm: Approach to an Unplanned Pregnancy

In the case of an unplanned pregnancy, the first rule of thumb is not to panic. Ideally, the clinician and the patient will have already discussed the medication plan for pregnancy as described earlier (see "Expect the Unexpected Pregnancy and Prepare Ahead of Time"). Regardless, it is important not to immediately stop all psychiatric medications. Sudden discontinuation of psychiatric medications can cause great stress and anxiety for the patient, precipitate withdrawal, and may precipitate a relapse of mental illness (Einarson 2005). The best approach is to review the medication list based on the principles outlined previously for pre-pregnancy planning and, if the decision is to discontinue a medication, to taper its removal. The baby has been exposed already, and although stopping some medications may make sense to minimize the impact on the fetus, doing so in a controlled and logical fashion is generally ideal.

Also, in the setting of an unplanned pregnancy, it might not make sense to switch from a newer medication to an older one with more reproductive safety data. Such a switch might have made sense prior to pregnancy, but as mentioned, switching during pregnancy increases the number of exposures for the fetus, who has already been exposed to the newer medication. In addition, the likelihood that the patient would relapse while switching is high, and the exposure to the psychiatric illness would constitute a third exposure for the child. Unless a particular medication has been clearly associated with significant risk (i.e., valproic acid, carbamazepine), continuation of the current regimen may be most appropriate.

## Conclusion

In this chapter, we summarized a general treatment approach to designing a psychiatric treatment plan for pregnancy. General principles ideally include planning prior to pregnancy and minimizing the fetus's adverse exposures to medications and maternal psychiatric illness. Another major goal is to avoid erring on the side of undertreating a patient during pregnancy. Overall, the goal of psychiatric treatment during pregnancy is to keep the mother psychiatrically well in order to improve both maternal and infant outcomes.

## Key Points

- Ideally, the clinician and patient will make a treatment plan prior to pregnancy. Such treatment plans must be individualized and take into account not only the risks of illness versus the risks of medication but also the patient's psychosocial circumstances, access to health care, and health care disparities for racial and sexual minorities.
- The relapse rate of maternal psychiatric illness with discontinuation of medications is extremely high.
- An important treatment principle is to try to minimize the number of exposures for the fetus to both medications and the mother's psychiatric illness.
- It is also important to avoid undertreating the patient during pregnancy.

## References


Alsdorf R, Wyszynski DF: Teratogenicity of sodium valproate. Expert Opin Drug Saf 4(2):345–353, 2005 15794725

Ashman SB, Dawson G, Panagiotides H, et al: Stress hormone levels of children of depressed mothers. Dev Psychopathol 14(2):333–349, 2002 12030695

Cohen LS, Altshuler LL, Harlow BL, et al: Relapse of major depression during pregnancy in women who maintain or discontinue antidepressant treatment. JAMA 295(5):499–507, 2006 16449615

Cox JL, Holden JM, Sagovsky R: Detection of postnatal depression: development of the 10-item Edinburgh Postnatal Depression Scale. Br J Psychiatry 150:782–786, 1987 3651732

Davis NL, Smoots AN, Goodman DA: Pregnancy-related deaths: data from 14 U.S. Maternal Mortality Review Committees, 2008–2017. Centers for Disease Control and Prevention, U.S. Department of Health and Human Services, 2019. Available at: https://www.cdc.gov/reproductivehealth/maternal-mortality/erase-mm/MMR-Data-Brief_2019-h.pdf. Accessed January 14, 2021.

Deligiannidis KM, Freeman MP: Complementary and alternative medicine therapies for perinatal depression. Best Pract Res Clin Obstet Gynaecol 28(1):85–95, 2014 24041861

DeVane CL, Stowe ZN, Donovan JL, et al: Therapeutic drug monitoring of psychoactive drugs during pregnancy in the genomic era: challenges and opportunities. J Psychopharmacol 20(4 suppl):54–59, 2006 16785271

Diego MA, Field T, Hernandez-Reif M, et al: Prepartum, postpartum, and chronic depression effects on newborns. Psychiatry 67(1):63–80, 2004 15139586

Einarson A: Abrupt discontinuation of psychotropic drugs following confirmation of pregnancy: a risky practice. J Obstet Gynaecol Can 27(11):1019–1022, 2005 16529668

Essex MJ, Klein MH, Cho E, et al: Maternal stress beginning in infancy may sensitize children to later stress exposure: effects on cortisol and behavior. Biol Psychiatry 52(8):776–784, 2002 12372649

Field T, Diego M, Hernandez-Reif M: Prenatal depression effects and interventions: a review. Infant Behav Dev 33(4):409–418, 2010 20471091

Finer LB, Zolna MR: Shifts in intended and unintended pregnancies in the United States, 2001–2008. Am J Public Health 104(suppl 1):S43–S48, 2014 24354819

Finer LB, Zolna MR: Declines in unintended pregnancy in the United States. N Engl J Med 374(9):843–852, 2016 26962904

Genovez M, Vanderkruik R, Lemon E, et al: Psychotherapeutic treatments for depression during pregnancy. Clin Obstet Gynecol 61(3):562–572, 2018 29965823

Grace SL, Evindar A, Stewart DE: The effect of postpartum depression on child cognitive development and behavior: a review and critical analysis of the literature. Arch Women Ment Health 6(4):263–274, 2003 14628179

Halligan SL, Herbert J, Goodyer IM, et al: Exposure to postnatal depression predicts elevated cortisol in adolescent offspring. Biol Psychiatry 55(4):376–381, 2004 14960290

Jones I, Chandra PS, Dazzan P, et al: Bipolar disorder, affective psychosis, and schizophrenia in pregnancy and the post-partum period. Lancet 384(9956):1789–1799, 2014 25455249

Kozma C: Valproic acid embryopathy: report of two siblings with further expansion of the phenotypic abnormalities and a review of the literature. Am J Med Genet 98(2):168–175, 2001 11223853

Li D, Liu L, Odouli R: Presence of depressive symptoms during early pregnancy and the risk of preterm delivery: a prospective cohort study. Hum Reprod 24(1):146–153, 2009 18948314

Livingston G: They're waiting longer, but U.S. women today more likely to have children than a decade ago. Pew Research Center, January 18, 2018. Available at: https://www.pewsocialtrends.org/2018/01/18/theyre-waiting-longer-but-u-s-women-today-more-likely-to-have-children-than-a-decade-ago/. Accessed January 14, 2021.

Mangla K, Hoffman MC, Trumpff C, et al: Maternal self-harm deaths: an unrecognized and preventable outcome. Am J Obstet Gynecol 221(4):295–303, 2019 30849358

Mosher WD, Bachrach CA: Understanding U.S. fertility: continuity and change in the National Survey of Family Growth, 1988–1995. Fam Plann Perspect 28(1):4–12, 1996 8822409

Orr ST, Blazer DG, James SA, et al: Depressive symptoms and indicators of maternal health status during pregnancy. J Womens Health (Larchmt) 16(4):535–542, 2007 17521257

Racine N, Plamondon A, Madigan S, et al: Maternal adverse childhood experiences and infant development. Pediatrics 141(4):e20172495, 2018 29559588

Reza N, Deligiannidis KM, Eustis EH, et al: Complementary health practices for treating perinatal depression. Obstet Gynecol Clin North Am 45(3):441–454, 2018 30092920

Shadigian E, Bauer ST: Pregnancy-associated death: a qualitative systematic review of homicide and suicide. Obstet Gynecol Surv 60(3):183–190, 2005 16570396

Somerville S, Dedman K, Hagan R, et al: The Perinatal Anxiety Screening Scale: development and preliminary validation. Arch Womens Ment Health 17:443–454, 2014

ten Berg K, van Oppen ACC, Nikkels PGJ, et al: Complex cardiac defect with hypoplastic right ventricle in a fetus with valproate exposure. Prenat Diagn 25(2):156–158, 2005 15712340

Tracy TS, Venkataramanan R, Glover DD, et al: Temporal changes in drug metabolism (CYP1A2, CYP2D6 and CYP3A activity) during pregnancy. Am J Obstet Gynecol 192(2):633–639, 2005 15696014

U.S. Department of Health and Human Services, Health Resources and Services Administration, Maternal and Child Health Bureau: Child Health USA 2013. Rockville, MD, U.S. Department of Health and Human Services, 2013

U.S. Food and Drug Administration: Content and format of labeling for human prescription drug and biological products: requirements for pregnancy and lactation labeling. Final rule. Fed Regist 79(233):72063–72103, 2014 25509060

Vigod SN, Kurdyak PA, Dennis CL, et al: Maternal and newborn outcomes among women with schizophrenia: a retrospective population-based cohort study. BJOG 121(5):566–574, 2014 24443970

Viguera AC, Nonacs R, Cohen LS, et al: Risk of recurrence of bipolar disorder in pregnant and nonpregnant women after discontinuing lithium maintenance. Am J Psychiatry 157(2):179–184, 2000 10671384

Viguera AC, Whitfield T, Baldessarini RJ, et al: Risk of recurrence in women with bipolar disorder during pregnancy: prospective study of mood stabilizer discontinuation. Am J Psychiatry 164(12):1817–1824, 2007 18056236

CHAPTER 9

# A Clinical Approach to Psychiatric Diagnosis and Treatment in the Postpartum Period

Alyson Gorun, M.D.
Mira Zein, M.D.
Melisa Olgun, B.A.
Lisa A. Catapano, M.D., Ph.D.

The first postpartum months are often referred to as the "fourth trimester" to underscore the fact that the dependency of the newborn and the physical and emotional demands on the mother are no less—and in many ways more—than during pregnancy. This period is a time of drastic biological, emotional, and social change and, as a result, a time of psychiatric vulnerability. Great improvement in public awareness and understanding of postpartum depression (PPD) has occurred since the early 2000s, but providers are still generally inadequately trained to recognize and treat the full spectrum of mood and anxiety disorders that women can experience during this time, despite the prevalence of such disorders.

Two of the most critical considerations that must be at the center of good psychiatric care for postpartum women are 1) infant feeding and lactation and 2) sleep (or perhaps more accurately, sleep deprivation). The decision whether to breastfeed is difficult for many women, especially given the amount of social messaging around the topic. Women who do try to breastfeed have additional considerations: how to make it work, getting enough sleep, potential dietary restrictions, safety of medications in lactation, and involvement of the other parent or partner. In addition, regardless of whether the mother breastfeeds, sleep deprivation is near universal among new parents and has myriad consequences for cognitive, emotional, and physical well-being.

The previous chapter and this one are paired to discuss the clinical approach to psychiatric diagnosis and treatment of women during pregnancy (Chapter 8) and the postpartum period (this chapter). The first sections of the current chapter focus on optimizing care for the *individual*; we close this chapter by focusing on *systems and populations*, including systems of care for perinatal mental health, issues of access, and health care disparities. The significance of health care disparities is sorely overlooked in the literature and all too frequently in practice, but it has wide-ranging implications for women's reproductive mental health.

# General Treatment Principles

## Fourth Trimester

### Recognize the Enormity of the Transition

The postpartum period, defined as the 12 weeks after delivery, is an important time for a new mother and her family and can be considered a fourth trimester (Paladine et al. 2019). The weeks following birth are a critical period for a woman and her infant, setting the stage for long-term health and well-being (American College of Obstetricians and Gynecologists 2018a). The postpartum period is a time of significant challenge as the woman must adapt to hormonal and physical changes, recover from delivery, experience a change in family roles and responsibilities, and endure sleep deprivation—all while trying to care for and nourish a newborn (Spelke and Werner 2018).

In recognition of the importance of the postpartum period, in 2018 the American College of Obstetricians and Gynecologists (ACOG) issued updated recommendations for postpartum care, emphasizing the need to establish a postpartum care plan during pregnancy (American College of Obstetricians and Gynecologists 2018a). According to these recommendations, postpartum care should become an ongoing process rather than a single encounter, with services and support tailored to each woman's individual needs. The first postpartum visit should be within 3 weeks after birth, as opposed to the common practice of having the first follow-up visit at 6 weeks. The ACOG also recognizes the breadth and enormity of the transition into parenting and recommends that a comprehensive postpartum visit include a full assessment of physical, social, and psychological well-being, including the domains of mood and emotional well-being; infant care and feeding; sexuality, contraception, and birth spacing; sleep and fatigue; physical recovery from birth; chronic disease management; and health maintenance.

### Recognize That This Is a Time of Mental Health Vulnerability

The postpartum period can be a challenging time for many new mothers (and their loved ones) in terms of their mental health, including the development or exacerbation of psychiatric disorders. The etiology of postpartum psychiatric vulnerability is a complex interplay of psychological, biological, and social factors in addition to underlying genetic and environmental contributions (Meltzer-Brody et al. 2018). Postpartum disorders commonly include depression and anxiety but can, more rarely, include postpartum psychosis. In addition, they can include the new onset or exacerbation of OCD, PTSD, and eating disorders. These various disorders are described in detail throughout this textbook. The goal of treatment of postpartum mental health conditions is to reduce maternal symptoms and to support mother–child and family functioning; thus, in addition to treatment, women and their families should receive psychoeducation about mental health, including evidence-based discussions about the risks and benefits of treatment (Meltzer-Brody et al. 2018).

## Infant Feeding and Lactation

According to the Centers for Disease Control and Prevention (2018), in the United States, 83% of mothers have ever breastfed. More than half (57%) of mothers are breastfeeding at 6 months, and just over one-third of mothers (35.9%) are breastfeeding at 12 months. Mothers younger than age 30 are somewhat less likely to breastfeed (80.0%) than older mothers (86.3%). Further disparities in breastfeeding rates include fewer non-Hispanic Black infants ever having been breastfed (74.0%) compared with Hispanic infants (82.9%) and non-Hispanic white infants (86.6%). Moreover, infants born into families with low socioeconomic status are less likely to be breastfed, with infants who receive the Special Supplemental Nutrition Program for Women, Infants, and Children (WIC) less likely to be breastfed (75.5%) than children who are eligible but do not receive WIC (89.0%) or infants who are ineligible for WIC (92.7%).

Breastfeeding declined in the middle of the twentieth century, but by the 1970s there was renewed interest in high-income countries because of the natural foods movement and in low-income countries because of concerns about increased infant mortality from improper sterilization for formula (McIntyre et al. 2018). Despite substantial public relations campaigns since then (such as "breast is best" and the Baby-Friendly Hospital Initiative; McIntyre et al. 2018), only 37% of children younger than age 6 months are exclusively breastfed in low- and middle-income countries, with even shorter duration in high-income countries.

The mother's intention to breastfeed predicts both the initiation and the duration of breastfeeding. In addition to intrinsic motivations, extrinsic social factors such as breastfeeding encouragement from social networks and support from partners weigh into the decision (Lok et al. 2017). According to one study on infant feeding preferences, if the woman's husband and mother preferred exclusive breastfeeding, the mother was more likely to do so (Mueffelmann et al. 2015).

### Recognize That Decisions Around Infant Feeding Must Balance the Infant's Needs With the Mother's Well-Being

Decisions regarding infant feeding, particularly breastfeeding, highlight the complexities around optimizing the well-being of both the mother and the infant. Although breastfeeding is widely known to have clear health benefits, the medical, emotional, and logistical reasons that women may choose not to breastfeed are less commonly discussed. Several factors may affect the mental health and well-being (not to mention the preferences) of the mother and should also be taken into account. Breastfeeding does have demonstrated benefits in improving mental health for some women, but for other women it may contribute to the incidence and severity of anxiety or depressive symptoms; these women may choose not to breastfeed or terminate breastfeeding early

(McIntyre et al. 2018). As discussed later, women may choose not to breastfeed at all or to supplement with formula or may discontinue breastfeeding because of medical illness or medication, difficulty with nursing or lactation (and the stress associated with these difficulties), the need for sleep, the participation of the other parent or partner, anxiety or previous trauma, or reasons of lifestyle or personal choice.

Breastfeeding has been reported to be beneficial for both mother and baby. Studies have shown that breastfeeding has immediate benefits for the health and survival of the infant, particularly in low- and middle-income countries, where mortality rates for breastfed infants are lower; in meta-analyses of studies completed in these countries, three studies showed that infants younger than 6 months who were not breastfed had 3.5–4.1 times higher rates of mortality than those who received any breastmilk. In high-income countries, breastfeeding was associated with a 36% reduction in sudden infant deaths and a 58% decrease in necrotizing enterocolitis (Victora et al. 2016).

Breastfeeding also improves morbidity sequelae from infections; this benefit is due to the molecular composition of breast milk itself, which has both immunological and antibacterial properties (Allen and Hector 2005). Studies have shown that breastfed babies have lower rates of diarrhea, respiratory tract infections, otitis media, and other infections and a decreased risk of exposure to pathogens from formula preparation, all significant risks to infants in low- and middle-income countries (Shamir 2016; Victora et al. 2016). Studies have also demonstrated long-term benefits in children who are breastfed, with reductions in overweight and obesity (Shamir 2016; Victora et al. 2016). Some studies also show improved intellectual and motor development and increased intelligence in breastfed children (Shamir 2016; Victora et al. 2016), although demographic differences among families who choose to breastfeed may account for this.

Breastfeeding has also been shown to have both immediate and longer-term protective effects for the mother. The initiation of breastfeeding immediately after delivery stimulates the release of oxytocin, which helps contract the uterus, expel the placenta, and reduce postpartum bleeding (Victora et al. 2016). Furthermore, the combined effects of oxytocin, prolactin, and cortisol, which are released during lactation, are reported to have both antidepressant and anxiolytic effects and may help decrease rates of postpartum depression and anxiety (Godfrey and Lawrence 2010). Lastly, breastfeeding increases the period of amenorrhea, thus aiding in child spacing (Victora et al. 2016). Longer-term benefits include reduced risk of breast and ovarian cancers, type 2 diabetes, cardiovascular disease, rheumatoid arthritis, and osteoarthritis (Godfrey and Lawrence 2010). A dose-dependent preventive association of breastfeeding with premenopausal and postmenopausal breast cancer has been reported; according to one meta-analysis, breastfeeding for 12 months decreased the incidence of breast cancer between 3% and 4% (Victora et al. 2016). Table 9–1 lists excess risks of not breastfeeding for the health of both the child and the mother.

## Take Into Account the Mother's Mental Health and Need for Sleep

Women with psychiatric illness who plan to breastfeed may have significant challenges, including lactation and nursing difficulties, sleep deprivation, stress and uncertainty, history of physical or sexual trauma, and fears about medication exposure, among others. Certain mental health conditions pose particular challenges with breastfeeding. For example, women with bipolar disorder who are considering breastfeeding

**TABLE 9–1. Excess risks of not breastfeeding**

| Excess risk | Outcomes |
|---|---|
| For the child | |
| > 100% | Diarrhea and vomiting (gastrointestinal infection) |
| | Hospitalization for lower respiratory tract diseases in the first year |
| | Necrotizing enterocolitis (in preterm infants only) |
| > 50% | Acute ear infection (otitis media) |
| | Asthma, with family history |
| | Type 2 diabetes mellitus |
| | Sudden infant death syndrome |
| < 50% | Acute lymphocytic leukemia |
| | Acute myelogenous leukemia |
| | Asthma, no family history |
| | Childhood obesity |
| | Eczema (atopic dermatitis) |
| For the mother | |
| < 50% | Breast cancer |
| | Ovarian cancer |

*Source.* Adapted from Office of the Surgeon General et al. 2011.

will need to be counseled carefully by their clinician prior to delivery regarding specific risk factors associated with bipolar disorder, including the impact of sleep deprivation on mood relapse (Geddes and Miklowitz 2013) and the overall increased risk of mood relapse postpartum (Viguera et al. 2007). For women with bipolar disorder who are extremely sensitive to sleep deprivation, around-the-clock breastfeeding may be contraindicated. Frequent awakenings often needed during the night while exclusively breastfeeding may be a particularly significant risk factor that could be mitigated by using supplemental formula overnight or having a partner assist with overnight feedings. The additional risks of postpartum psychosis and other safety issues may shift the risk toward using medication prophylactically in the postpartum period (Jones et al. 2014).

Women with depression and anxiety during pregnancy are more likely to discontinue breastfeeding within 6 months of delivery and more likely to experience worsening of their mood and anxiety symptoms on cessation of breastfeeding (Ystrom 2012). PPD is associated with early breastfeeding cessation; however, the directionality of this association is unclear (Dias and Figueiredo 2015). The literature investigating the relationship between PPD and breastfeeding is often contradictory and has many methodological limitations. Some studies show that breastfeeding is not protective against PPD, whereas others show that it is (Pope and Mazmanian 2016). Those studies that show that breastfeeding is protective often do not control for confounders associated with depression, such as lack of social support or stressful life events (Pope et al. 2016). Higher levels of breastfeeding self-efficacy have been associated with fewer depressive symptoms and are also predictive of longer breastfeeding duration (Haga et al. 2012).

Lack of social support and insufficient emotion regulation strategies have also been associated with postpartum depressive symptoms and could be considered points for intervention by the clinician (Haga et al. 2012). Other factors associated with higher levels of depressive symptoms include breastfeeding difficulties, pain, worries, and negative attitudes (Dias and Figueiredo 2015). Most likely, many factors contribute to the relationship between breastfeeding and PPD. Sleep is a major consideration in postpartum well-being and in the choice to breastfeed. Women with psychiatric illness or sensitivity to sleep deprivation must factor in their need for sleep when making decisions about nocturnal infant care and feeding, as discussed in greater detail later in the section "Sleep."

### Support Choices Around Infant Feeding Nonjudgmentally

Mothers who cannot or choose not to breastfeed may experience both external shame and internal guilt about this decision (Lakshman et al. 2009; Lee 2007; Thomson et al. 2015). Women with depression, anxiety, and self-esteem issues, for example, may be more vulnerable to interpreting lactation and nursing difficulties as personal failures. Lack of breastfeeding can be experienced as not being a good mother or failing to live up to the ideals of womanhood (Taylor and Wallace 2012). Feelings of inadequacy and isolation may occur and can prevent a mother from seeking help, especially because many mothers, if they start to use formula, feel judged by health care professionals (Thomson et al. 2015; Schmied et al. 2011). Women who do not breastfeed, regardless of their reasons, are at higher risk of encountering shaming and stigma if their social network or their medical providers disagree with their decision (McIntyre et al. 2018).

Clinicians can support women's choices around lactation by taking a nonjudgmental approach that acknowledges these challenges while providing education about the risks and benefits, as well as helping to engage patients' support systems and access to professional intervention when available. It is important to support each mother in her decision-making process regardless of the decision made. The clinician's role is to enhance problem solving and flexibility around breastfeeding. Creating a space in which the mother can think about the risks and benefits of breastfeeding can help her come to her own decision. Often helpful are discussions around supplemental formula use instead of complete cessation of breastfeeding, or the role of the mother's partner in assisting with feedings. Directing a mother to obtain lactation support, whether through a group or a consultant, can be a helpful intervention as well. By directly addressing any negative feelings a mother has, clinicians can help mitigate the impact of these feelings. In addition, while discussing the benefits and potential disadvantages of breastfeeding with women, clinicians must be open to the psychosocial, cultural, and personal determinants affecting their decisions.

## Sleep

### Recognize That Postpartum Sleep Deprivation Is Common and Increases Risk of Psychiatric Illness

Sleep is often the most critical self-care issue a new parent faces and arguably the most important modifiable risk factor for postpartum psychiatric disorders. Postpartum sleep deficiency is common due to both postdelivery physiological changes and the mother's need to care for the newborn (Wilkerson and Uhde 2018). Preexisting sleep problems, such as apnea and restless legs syndrome, are often exacerbated during this time (Christian et al. 2019). Disrupted sleep may present as a cause or a consequence of psychiatric illness, or both.

Although it is universally recognized that postpartum women get poor sleep, the etiology, specific sleep parameters affected, and numerous physical and emotional sequelae of sleep deficiency in the postpartum period have only recently begun to be comprehensively studied. Women in the first several weeks postpartum have been shown to have poorer sleep on several different subjective and objective measures, including sleep quality, sleep latency, sleep efficiency, sleep medication usage, and daytime dysfunction (Christian et al. 2019; Wilkerson and Uhde 2018). Sleep deficiencies in the general population have broad consequences, including increasing the risk for chronic illness and all-cause mortality (Carroll et al. 2019). In the postpartum population in particular, sequelae include increased risk of PPD (McEvoy et al. 2019; Wilkerson and Uhde 2018), anxiety disorders (Okun et al. 2018), emotional dysregulation (Christian et al. 2019), interpersonal problems (Christian et al. 2019), and suicidal ideation (Sit et al. 2015), all of which present the possibility of much greater impairment and distress when they occur during the postpartum period.

### Do Anything You Can to Help New Mothers Sleep

To treat the postpartum population effectively, practitioners must be educated about the safety of sleep medicines (covered in Chapter 19, "Anxiety Disorders and Insomnia in the Perinatal Period"), as well as evidence-based nonpharmacological interventions such as massage, exercise, and other behavioral modifications (Owais et al. 2018; Wilkerson and Uhde 2018). On a psychosocial level, practitioners must be sensitive to the fact that during this time new mothers are learning to balance their own needs with the needs and demands of their infants. Sleep is often the first and primary ground for wrestling with this balance. Mothers who set poor boundaries with respect to their own sleep frequently do so out of a belief that self-sacrifice is a necessary part of being a good mother. Discussions about self-care and the necessity of "putting your own oxygen mask on first" are a critical part of helping new parents adjust to their new roles.

For patients with a partner, one useful strategy can be to ask the partner to attend a clinician visit late in the third trimester with the specific goal of creating a postpartum sleep plan. Even when women are breastfeeding, partners can take on other infant care tasks to help maximize the mother's sleep, and some couples choose a "tag-team" approach. For many families, obtaining a "sleep prescription" ahead of time can make it easier to divide tasks in ways that can help to preserve the mother's sleep, a particularly important goal for women with psychiatric illness.

## Systems of Perinatal Mental Health Care

The experiences of pregnancy, birth, and becoming a parent are transformational events in the lives of women and their families. Accompanying this set of enormous changes are physical and mental health challenges that have a clear impact on the mother and the infant; perinatal mental health and substance use disorders are associated with poor obstetrical, infant, and child outcomes (Britton et al. 2001; Deave et al. 2008; Forman et al. 2007; Grote et al. 2020; Paulson et al. 2009). The perinatal period represents an opportune time to identify and treat mental health disorders, in part because of frequent contact with health care providers (Smith et al. 2009).

A fragmented and deeply unequal system of physical and mental health care fails women at one of the most vulnerable times in their lives. When they are most in need of a robust safety net of support, the vast majority of pregnant women with mental health or substance abuse disorders go untreated (Carter et al. 2005; Marcus et al. 2003; Rowan et al. 2012). Moreover, health care disparities strongly affect perinatal mental health care. These disparities exist for a wide range of reasons, including lack of access to providers, geographical differences, differences in rates of private versus public insurance, differences in rates charged for people without insurance, communication differences, and cultural barriers (American College of Physicians 2010). In addition, racial and ethnic disparities in women's physical and mental health care serve as a barrier against quality and timely care.

Screening represents an important first step in the identification of perinatal mental health disorders. For example, the ACOG now recommends that screening for perinatal depression and anxiety take place at least once during the perinatal period (American College of Obstetricians and Gynecologists 2018b). Currently, more than 40 states have implemented guidelines and recommendations for screening for perinatal depression; however, it remains unclear if those steps have been successful in identifying—and treating—women with perinatal depression (Bauman et al. 2020). In a recent report, the Centers for Disease Control and Prevention noted that although screening captured a substantial prevalence of PPD, screening rates were highly variable across states, ranging from 50% to 90% (Bauman et al. 2020).

In addition, one of the most difficult dilemmas regarding access is how to pair identification and detection of perinatal mental health concerns with the resources needed to address positive screens. Several examples exist of innovative programs that aim to increase access and support for the mental health and well-being of mothers and their loved ones throughout pregnancy and the postpartum period. Examples include the integration of mental health care services into obstetrical (Goedde et al. 2020) and primary care settings (Lomonaco-Haycraft et al. 2018) and programs that increase access to specific populations, such as veterans (Katon et al. 2017). Another example is the Massachusetts Child Psychiatry Access Project for Moms, which aims to increase providers' capacity to address perinatal depression (Byatt et al. 2016). This cost-effective approach, now replicated in many other states, implements 1) trainings and toolkits on depression screening, assessment, and treatment; 2) telephonic access to perinatal psychiatric consultation for providers serving pregnant and postpartum women; and 3) care coordination to link women with individual psychotherapy and support groups (Byatt et al. 2016).

The timing of interventions is also important. There has been increasing recognition that the postpartum period is a particularly vulnerable time for women's mental health. In 2018, the ACOG issued updated recommendations regarding postpartum care, emphasizing the need for comprehensive postpartum assessments at 3 weeks postdelivery (American College of Obstetricians and Gynecologists 2018a). Services focused on the postpartum period have increased in number. One example is the Fourth Trimester Project, which is a woman-centered engagement program of postpartum support to meet the unmet needs of new mothers and their families in this vulnerable period (Tully et al. 2017).

Despite increasing attention on a systems level to maternal health and well-being, painfully obvious racial and ethnic disparities in women's health care remain. One needs only to look at the astonishingly high rates of maternal mortality among Black women in the United States to understand the breadth and depth of the problem (Holdt Somer et al. 2017). In addition, women of color in the United States, particularly in high-poverty neighborhoods, experience high rates of poor birth outcomes, including cesarean delivery, preterm birth, low birth weight, and infant mortality (Thomas et al. 2017). Although some of the disparities affecting new mothers begin preconception or in pregnancy (with higher rates of nearly all serious pregnancy morbidities affecting nonwhite women; Admon et al. 2018), in many cases they become apparent only during the postpartum period. Pregnancy-related deaths, most of which occur at or after delivery, are three times higher in Black women than white women (Creanga et al. 2017). Women of racial and ethnic minorities tend to deliver in lower-quality hospitals, with the 25% of hospitals that handle 75% of all Black women's deliveries performing lower on indicators of quality (Creanga et al. 2014; Howell et al. 2016).

Hospital quality, however, explains only part of the story; Black women who deliver in higher-quality hospitals still have disproportionate rates of mortality and morbidity (Howell et al. 2016). Women in racial and ethnic minority groups face additional challenges in the postpartum period. Children born to nonwhite and non-Asian women are far more likely to live in single-parent households (65% for Black, 53% for Native American, 41% for Hispanic, 24% for white, and 15% for Asian families) (Annie E. Casey Foundation 2020; O'Hare and Ritualo 2000). Although such rates do not factor in less formal partnership arrangements, they do likely reflect the fact that more Black women will enter the postpartum period as single parents, with no partner to help with nighttime care or the care of other children. This situation, in turn, may lead to greater sleep disruption, which can have both psychological and biological consequences. Poor sleep during pregnancy has been shown to be related to a more robust inflammatory response in African American women than in white women, for example, and to a higher risk for shortened gestation (Carroll et al. 2019). African Americans in general (and not only in the perinatal period) have notably higher rates of short sleep duration and poorer subjective sleep quality than do white Americans (Christian et al. 2019). Also, African American women are more likely to retain excess weight after pregnancy than are white women, and that excess weight can contribute to excess inflammation (Christian et al. 2019). Poor sleep and obesity are in turn related to rates of PPD, which are known to be higher among racial and ethnic minority populations (Bhati and Richards 2015; Cannon and Nasrallah 2019; Ertel et al. 2017).

Thus, it is crucial that programs exist that focus specifically on addressing perinatal health while simultaneously addressing racial and ethnic health care disparities. For example, doula care has been linked to improvements in many perinatal outcomes; however, women of color and low-income women often face barriers in accessing doula support (Thomas et al. 2017). Recent programs have implemented doula support for at-risk populations with the aim of reducing racial and income-based disparities in maternal and infant outcomes (Mottl-Santiago et al. 2020; Thomas et al. 2017).

Although addressing needs at the systems level is crucial, some of the aspects of improving systemic racism (Nature Medicine 2020; Obermeyer et al. 2019) and inequity within medical and mental health care start at the level of the doctor–patient relationship. Multiple studies of focus groups of Black women have examined their perceptions of the perinatal health care they received. One of the most salient themes was receiving substandard care based on implicit bias; participants expressed that racism and implicit bias must be addressed to start to decrease the disparities in perinatal health outcomes (Kalata et al. 2020; Roman et al. 2017; Salm Ward et al. 2013). Several studies have served to support this perception. For example, some systematic reviews found that implicit bias was common among health care providers, in terms of positive attitudes toward white patients and negative attitudes toward people of color (Dehon et al. 2017; Hall et al. 2015). In addition to the impact of bias on the care provided, the chronic stress of pervasive racism has a profound impact on health, and research is beginning to reveal both the psychosocial and biological effects of this chronic stress (Bichell 2017; Vines et al. 2006).

This textbook, with its focus on both biological and psychosocial aspects of mental health conditions related to reproductive transitions, is only one step in bringing attention—and, more importantly, badly needed change—to address widespread disparities in perinatal health care. In each chapter, we endeavor to present data about disparities where they are known, and we must acknowledge here the tremendous work yet to be done. Research studies are still overwhelmingly populated by white participants (with only 6% of participants being Black or Latinx) (Konkel 2015), so we are only in the beginning stages of understanding racial differences in etiology, pathophysiology, and treatment (separate from but compounded by the disparities mentioned here).

## Conclusion

The fourth trimester is a time of exquisite vulnerability for women due to the physical and emotional stress of delivering and caring for a newborn while establishing a new identity as a mother and managing a changing role in the family. Breastfeeding can be helpful or hurtful, depending on several factors, including how easily the process works, dietary problems, medical and medication issues, and managing sleep. Sleep deficiencies due to maternal hormonal changes and the baby's nocturnal needs significantly increase the possibility of depression and anxiety at a time when women are already at risk. The disparities that exist across health care systems are exacerbated during this time and further disadvantage minority women and their offspring, with long-lasting consequences for these individuals, their families, and their communities.

We must do better. Women's mental health presents clear examples of the need for a comprehensive health care system that optimizes quality, promotes access, and reduces the vast health care disparities of our society.

## Key Points

- The first postpartum months—the "fourth trimester"—are a time of significant psychiatric vulnerability.
- Decision-making around infant feeding must balance benefits to the infant with the mother's mental health and well-being.

- Sleep deprivation in new parents is nearly universal; has consequences for cognitive, physical and emotional well-being; and is arguably the most important modifiable risk factor for postpartum psychiatric disorders.
- Existing health care disparities are exacerbated during this vulnerable time and serve as a barrier to quality and timely care for minority women and their babies. Improved and more equitable screening and access to care for all is imperative to begin to address these disparities.

## References

Admon LK, Winkelman TNA, Zivin K, et al: Racial and ethnic disparities in the incidence of severe maternal morbidity in the United States, 2012–2015. Obstet Gynecol 132(5):1158–1166, 2018 30303912

Allen J, Hector D: Benefits of breastfeeding. NSW Public Health Bull 16(3–4):42–46, 2005 16106271

American College of Obstetricians and Gynecologists: ACOG Committee Opinion No. 736: optimizing postpartum care. Obstet Gynecol 131(5):e140–e150, 2018a 29683911

American College of Obstetricians and Gynecologists: ACOG Committee Opinion No. 757: screening for perinatal depression. Obstet Gynecol 132(5):e208–e212, 2018b 30629567

American College of Physicians: Racial and Ethnic Disparities in Healthcare. Philadelphia, PA, American College of Physicians, 2010

Annie E. Casey Foundation: 2020 KIDS COUNT Data Book: 2020 State Trends in Child Well-Being. Baltimore, MD, Annie E. Casey Foundation, 2020. Available at: https://www.aecf.org/resources/2020-kids-count-data-book. Accessed September 1, 2020.

Bauman BL, Ko JY, Cox S, et al: Vital signs: postpartum depressive symptoms and provider discussions about perinatal depression—United States, 2018. MMWR Morb Mortal Wkly Rep 69(19):575–581, 2020 32407302

Bhati S, Richards K: A systematic review of the relationship between postpartum sleep disturbance and postpartum depression. J Obstet Gynecol Neonatal Nurs 44(3):350–357, 2015 25819463

Bichell RE: Scientists are starting to tease out the subtler ways racism hurts health. National Public Radio Weekend Edition, November 11, 2017. Available at: https://www.npr.org/sections/health-shots/2017/11/11/562623815/scientists-start-to-tease-out-the-subtler-ways-racism-hurts-health. Accessed January 14, 2021.

Britton HL, Gronwaldt V, Britton JR: Maternal postpartum behaviors and mother-infant relationship during the first year of life. J Pediatr 138(6):905–909, 2001 11391337

Byatt N, Biebel K, Moore Simas TA, et al: Improving perinatal depression care: the Massachusetts Child Psychiatry Access Project for Moms. Gen Hosp Psychiatry 40:12–17, 2016 27079616

Cannon C, Nasrallah HA: A focus on postpartum depression among African American women: a literature review. Ann Clin Psychiatry 31(2):138–143, 2019 31046035

Carroll JE, Teti DM, Hall MH, et al: Maternal sleep in pregnancy and postpartum part II: biomechanisms and intervention strategies. Curr Psychiatry Rep 21(3):19, 2019 30826895

Carter FA, Carter JD, Luty SE, et al: Screening and treatment for depression during pregnancy: a cautionary note. Aust NZ J Psychiatry 39(4):255–261, 2005 15777362

Centers for Disease Control and Prevention: Breastfeeding Report Card: United States, 2018. Atlanta, GA, Centers for Disease Control and Prevention, 2018. Available at: https://www.cdc.gov/breastfeeding/pdf/2018breastfeedingreportcard.pdf. Accessed September 1, 2020.

Christian LM, Carroll JE, Teti DM, et al: Maternal sleep in pregnancy and postpartum part I: mental, physical, and interpersonal consequences. Curr Psychiatry Rep 21(3):20, 2019 30826881

Creanga AA, Bateman BT, Mhyre JM, et al: Performance of racial and ethnic minority-serving hospitals on delivery-related indicators. Am J Obstet Gynecol 211(6):647.e1–647.e16, 2014 24909341

Creanga AA, Syverson C, Seed K, Callaghan WM: Pregnancy-related mortality in the United States, 2011–2013. Obstet Gynecol 130(2):366–373, 2017 28697109
Deave T, Heron J, Evans J, et al: The impact of maternal depression in pregnancy on early child development. BJOG 115(8):1043–1051, 2008 18651886
Dehon E, Weiss N, Jones J, et al: A systematic review of the impact of physician implicit racial bias on clinical decision making. Acad Emerg Med 24(8):895–904, 2017 28472533
Dias CC, Figueiredo B: Breastfeeding and depression: a systematic review of the literature. J Affect Disord 171:142–154, 2015 25305429
Ertel KA, Huang T, Rifas-Shiman SL, et al: Perinatal weight and risk of prenatal and postpartum depressive symptoms. Ann Epidemiol 27(11):695–700, 2017 29110970
Forman DR, O'Hara MW, Stuart S, et al: Effective treatment for postpartum depression is not sufficient to improve the developing mother-child relationship. Dev Psychopathol 19(2):585–602, 2007 17459185
Geddes JR, Miklowitz DJ: Treatment of bipolar disorder. Lancet 381(9878):1672–1682, 2013 23663953
Godfrey JR, Lawrence RA: Toward optimal health: the maternal benefits of breastfeeding. J Womens Health (Larchmt) 19(9):1597–1602, 2010 20677994
Goedde D, Zidack A, Li YH, et al: Depression outcomes from a fully integrated obstetric mental health clinic: a 10-year examination. J Am Psychiatr Nurses Assoc January 3, 2020 31898913 Epub ahead of print
Grote NK, Bridge JA, Gavin AR, et al: A meta-analysis of depression during pregnancy and the risk of preterm birth, low birth weight, and intrauterine growth restriction. Arch Gen Psychiatry 67(10):1012–1024, 2020 31898913
Haga SM, Ulleberg P, Slinning K, et al: A longitudinal study of postpartum depressive symptoms: multilevel growth curve analyses of emotion regulation strategies, breastfeeding self-efficacy, and social support. Arch Women Ment Health 15(3):175–184, 2012 22451329
Hall WJ, Chapman MV, Lee KM, et al: Implicit racial/ethnic bias among health care professionals and its influence on health care outcomes: a systematic review. Am J Public Health 105(12):e60–e76, 2015 26469668
Holdt Somer SJ, Sinkey RG, Bryant AS: Epidemiology of racial/ethnic disparities in severe maternal morbidity and mortality. Semin Perinatol 41(5):258–265, 2017 28888263
Howell EA, Egorova N, Balbierz A, et al: Black-white differences in severe maternal morbidity and site of care. Am J Obstet Gynecol 214(1):122.e1–122.e7, 2016 26283457
Jones I, Chandra PS, Dazzan P, et al: Bipolar disorder, affective psychosis, and schizophrenia in pregnancy and the post-partum period. Lancet 384(9956):1789–1799, 2014 25455249
Kalata M, Kalata K, Yen H, et al: Community perspectives on the racial disparity in perinatal outcomes. J Mater Fetal Neonatal Med July 13, 2020 32654549 Epub ahead of print
Katon JG, Lewis L, Hercinovic S, et al: Improving perinatal mental health care for women veterans: description of a quality improvement program. Matern Child Health J 21(8):1598–1605, 2017 28168592
Konkel L: Racial and ethnic disparities in research studies: the challenge of creating more diverse cohorts. Environ Health Perspect 123(12):A297–A302, 2015 26625444
Lakshman R, Ogilvie D, Ong KK: Mothers' experiences of bottle-feeding: a systematic review of qualitative and quantitative studies. Arch Dis Child 94(8):596–601, 2009 19602520
Lee E: Health, morality, and infant feeding: British mothers' experiences of formula milk use in the early weeks. Sociol Health Illn 29(7):1075–1090, 2007 18092984
Lok KYW, Bai DL, Tarrant M: Family members' infant feeding preferences, maternal breastfeeding exposures and exclusive breastfeeding intentions. Midwifery 53:49–54, 2017 28755584
Lomonaco-Haycraft KC, Hyer J, Tibbits B, et al: Integrated perinatal mental health care: a national model of perinatal primary care in vulnerable populations. Prim Health Care Res Dev 20:1–8, 2018 29911521
Marcus SM, Flynn HA, Blow FC, et al: Depressive symptoms among pregnant women screened in obstetrics settings. J Womens Health (Larchmt) 12(4):373–380, 2003 12804344

McEvoy KM, Rayapati D, Washington Cole KO, et al: Poor postpartum sleep quality predicts subsequent postpartum depressive symptoms in a high-risk sample. Clin Sleep Med 15(9):1303–1310, 2019 31538601
McIntyre LM, Griffen AM, BrintzenhofeSzoc K: Breast is best…except when it's not. J Hum Lact 34(3):575–580, 2018 29787336
Meltzer-Brody S, Howard LM, Bergink V, et al: Postpartum psychiatric disorders. Nat Rev Dis Primers 4:18022, 2018 29695824
Mottl-Santiago J, Herr K, Rodrigues D, et al: The Birth Sisters Program: a model of hospital-based doula support to promote health equity. J Health Care Poor Underserved 31(1):43–55, 2020 32037316
Mueffelmann RE, Racine EF, Warren-Findlow J, et al: Perceived infant feeding preferences of significant family members and mothers' intentions to exclusively breastfeed. J Hum Lact 31(3):479–489, 2015 25311826
Nature Medicine: Ending systemic racism in medicine (editorial). Nat Med 26(7):985, 2020 32651578
Obermeyer Z, Powers B, Vogeli C, et al: Dissecting racial bias in an algorithm used to manage the health of populations. Science 366(6464):447–453, 2019 31649194
Office of the Surgeon General, Centers for Disease Control and Prevention, Office on Women's Health: The Surgeon General's Call to Action to Support Breastfeeding. Rockville, MD, Office of the Surgeon General, 2011
O'Hare WP, Ritualo AR: KIDS COUNT: identifying and helping America's most vulnerable. Stat Bull Metrop Life Insur Co 81(1):26–32, 2000 10666782
Okun ML, Mancuso RA, Hobel CJ, et al: Poor sleep quality increases symptoms of depression and anxiety in postpartum women. J Behav Med 41(5):703–710, 2018 30030650
Owais S, Chow CHT, Furtado M, et al: Non-pharmacological interventions for improving postpartum maternal sleep: a systematic review and meta-analysis. Sleep Med Rev 41:87–100, 2018 29449122
Paladine HL, Blenning CE, Strangas Y: Postpartum care: an approach to the fourth trimester. Am Fam Physician 100(8):485–491, 2019 31613576
Paulson JF, Keefe HA, Leiferman JA: Early parental depression and child language development. J Child Psychol Psychiatry 50(3):254–262, 2009 19175819
Pope CJ, Mazmanian D: Breastfeeding and postpartum depression: an overview and methodological recommendations for future research. Depress Res Treat 4765310:2016, 2016 27148457
Pope CJ, Mazmanian D, Bédard M, et al: Breastfeeding and postpartum depression: assessing the influence of breastfeeding intention and other risk factors. J Affect Disord 200:45–50, 2016 27126139
Roman LA, Raffo JE, Dertz K, et al: Understanding perspectives of African American Medicaid-insured women on the process of perinatal care: an opportunity for systems improvement. Matern Child Health J 21(suppl 1):81–92, 2017 28965183
Rowan P, Greisinger A, Brehm B, et al: Outcomes from implementing systematic antepartum depression screening in obstetrics. Arch Women Ment Health 15(2):115–120, 2012 22382279
Salm Ward TC, Mazul M, Ngui EM, et al: "You learn to go last": perceptions of prenatal care experiences among African-American women with limited incomes. Matern Child Health J 17(10):1753–1759, 2013 23180190
Schmied V, Beake S, Sheehan A, et al: Women's perceptions and experiences of breastfeeding support: a metasynthesis. Birth 38(1):49–60, 2011 21332775
Shamir R: The benefits of breast feeding. Nestle Nutr Inst Workshop Ser 86:67–76, 2016 27336781
Sit D, Luther J, Buysse D, et al: Suicidal ideation in depressed postpartum women: associations with childhood trauma, sleep disturbance and anxiety. J Psychiatr Res 66–67:95–104, 2015 26001587
Smith MV, Shao L, Howell H, et al: Success of mental health referral among pregnant and postpartum women with psychiatric distress. Gen Hosp Psychiatry 31(2):155–162, 2009 19269536
Spelke B, Werner E: The fourth trimester of pregnancy: committing to maternal health and well-being postpartum. RI Med J (2013) 101(8):30–33, 2018 30278599
Taylor E, Wallace L: For shame: feminism, breastfeeding advocacy, and maternal guilt. Hypatia 27:76–98, 2012

Thomas MP, Ammann G, Brazier E, et al: Doula services within a healthy start program: increasing access for an underserved population. Matern Child Health J 21(suppl 1):59–64, 2017 29198051
Thomson G, Ebisch-Burton K, Flacking R: Shame if you do—shame if you don't: women's experiences of infant feeding. Matern Child Nutr 11(1):33–46, 2015 25138617
Tully KP, Stuebe AM, Verbiest SB: The fourth trimester: a critical transition period with unmet maternal health needs. Am J Obstet Gynecol 217(1):37–41, 2017 28390671
Victora CG, Bahl R, Barros AJD, et al: Breastfeeding in the 21st century: epidemiology, mechanisms, and lifelong effect. Lancet 387(10017):475–490, 2016 26869575
Viguera AC, Whitfield T, Baldessarini RJ, et al: Risk of recurrence in women with bipolar disorder during pregnancy: prospective study of mood stabilizer discontinuation. Am J Psychiatry 164(12):1817–1824, quiz 1923, 2007 18056236
Vines AI, Baird DD, McNeilly M, et al: Social correlates of the chronic stress of perceived racism among Black women. Ethn Dis 16(1):101–107, 2006 16599356
Wilkerson AK, Uhde TW: Perinatal sleep problems: causes, complications, and management. Obstet Gynecol Clin North Am 45(3):483–494, 2018 30092923
Ystrom E: Breastfeeding cessation and symptoms of anxiety and depression: a longitudinal cohort study. BMC Pregnancy Childbirth 12(1):36, 2012 22621668

CHAPTER 10

# A Treatment Approach to Psychiatric Emergencies in the Perinatal Period

Jovana Martinovic, M.D.
Pooja Lakshmin, M.D.
Mira Zein, M.D.
Melisa Olgun, B.A.
Lucy A. Hutner, M.D.

The perinatal period is a particularly vulnerable time for the emergence or relapse of mental health disorders, some of which are associated with clinical emergencies. Health care providers, however, may be hesitant to treat emergencies in the perinatal population because of uncertainty about managing clinical issues, such as the use of psychotropic medications, in women who are pregnant or breastfeeding. In this chapter, we review some of the most common emergencies in reproductive psychiatry: suicidality, postpartum psychosis (PPP), acute agitation, substance intoxication and withdrawal, and catatonia. (For a fuller discussion of several of these syndromes, see Chapter 13, "Depressive Disorders"; Chapter 16, "Postpartum Psychosis"; and Chapter 21, "Substance Use Disorders.") We hope to help clinicians appreciate the clinical presentation, differential diagnosis, and treatment strategies for these emergencies and thereby gain confidence in identifying and treating these conditions in a rapid and safe manner.

## Suicide

Ms. O is a 27-year-old married woman who is 6 months postpartum with her first child. She had a difficult recovery after an emergency cesarean section and is having ongoing challenges with breastfeeding. She moved to a new city with her husband for his job. Their families live abroad, and she and her husband have not established strong social support in their new community. Her husband became worried and drove her to the emergency department after Ms. O told him she was having thoughts of suicide. She shares that she has been feeling sad and irritable since her baby was born. She is having trouble connecting with the baby and no longer gets pleasure out of anything. Although the baby is sleeping more now, Ms. O struggles with insomnia. She has had intermittent thoughts about suicide over the past month. Tonight, she was feeling more hopeless and, while her husband was caring for the baby, she began thinking about jumping off their balcony. The baby began to cry and interrupted her thoughts. Thinking about her baby and husband led Ms. O to share her thoughts with her husband and agree to seek help. She has a history of early childhood adversity and of recurrent depression dating back to adolescence, with a prior impulsive overdose with intent to die at age 16.

# Epidemiology

## Rates/Incidence

Ms. O, the patient in the case example, is affected by mental illness during the perinatal period. Psychiatric illness, most commonly depression, is a serious and treatable complication affecting up to 20% of women and has significant short- and long-term adverse effects on mother and child (O'Hara and Wisner 2014; Stuart-Parrigon and Stuart 2014). Although pregnancy and the postpartum period have historically been identified as protective time periods with respect to suicide risk, suicidality remains a significant public health issue. In fact, maternal suicide during pregnancy and the first year postpartum is a leading cause of death in developed countries (Austin et al. 2007; Lewis 2007; Oates 2003b; Palladino et al. 2011; Thornton et al. 2013). According to North American studies, the reported perinatal suicide rate is 3 per 100,000 live births in the United States (Palladino et al. 2011) and 2.58 per 100,000 live births in Ontario, Canada (Grigoriadis et al. 2017). The prevalence of suicidal ideation or thoughts of self-harm ranges from 5% to 14%, and completed suicide accounts for up to 20% of postpartum deaths (Lindahl et al. 2005). Although rates of attempted and completed suicide are lower in the peripartum period than at other times in a woman's life, certain subgroups of women may be at elevated risk—namely those with serious mental illness. Furthermore, women acting on suicidality during pregnancy and the postpartum period are more likely to use more lethal, violent means than do nonperipartum women, suggesting high intent and higher risk of completed suicide (Grigoriadis et al. 2017; Khalifeh et al. 2016; Lindahl et al. 2005; Oates 2003). In two studies that examined the timing of suicide, findings suggested that maternal suicides often occur later in the postpartum period, most frequently after the sixth month postpartum (Grigoriadis et al. 2017; Thornton et al. 2013).

Most women who have died by suicide in the perinatal period have been diagnosed with affective or anxiety disorders rather than psychotic illness (Gold et al. 2012; Grigoriadis et al. 2017). A large study in the United Kingdom found that almost half of those who died by suicide in the perinatal period had been diagnosed with depression. Unfortunately, this study also found that, compared with nonperipartum women, women who completed suicide in the peripartum period were less likely to be receiving active pharmacological or nonpharmacological treatment at the time of their deaths (Khalifeh et al. 2016).

## Risk Factors

Risk factors associated with suicide have been documented in various contexts, but literature on risk factors associated with maternal suicide in the perinatal period specifically is still emerging. As such, it may be helpful to keep in mind the World Health Organization (WHO) summary of key risk factors for suicide, which provides a useful framework for considering risks from the individual to health systems levels (World Health Organization 2014):

- Individual factors, such as previous suicide attempt, mental disorders, harmful use of alcohol, job or financial loss, hopelessness, chronic pain, family history of suicide, and genetic and biological factors
- Relationship factors, such as sense of isolation and lack of social support, conflict, discord, or loss
- Community factors, such as disaster, war and conflict, stresses of acculturation and dislocation, discrimination, and trauma or abuse
- Health systems factors, such as barriers to accessing health care, social factors such as access to means, inappropriate media reporting, and stigma associated with accessing care

Of these, the strongest risk factor is history of previous suicide attempt(s) (Yoshimasu et al. 2008). Findings from studies that reported on risk factors associated with peripartum suicide have some overlap with the risk factors identified in the WHO report but also indicate risk factors unique to this population and period of time. Table 10–1 lists the risk factors that have been associated with maternal suicide specifically, as synthesized from summaries in two review articles (Mangla et al. 2019; Orsolini et al. 2016).

Notably, women who are hospitalized for postpartum mental illness appear to be at higher risk of suicide, a fact consistent with the increased risk of suicide associated with inpatient admission and recent discharge seen in general psychiatric populations (Bolton et al. 2015). According to data from a Danish psychiatric registry, the risk of suicide among postpartum women following psychiatric admission was 70 times higher in the first year postpartum than the rate in the general population (Appleby et al. 1998). Some of this risk may be attributable to the type of inpatient care received. The United Kingdom Confidential Enquiries Into Maternal Deaths found that recently hospitalized postpartum women who completed suicide had been admitted to general psychiatry units and separated from their infants; they found no deaths among women admitted to specialized mother–baby units (Oates 2003b).

# Screening

Clinicians working in specialized mental health settings or in emergency departments are trained in careful risk assessment, but the reality is that opportunities for screening more often present in primary care settings (Bolton et al. 2015). Screening for maternal mental illness during pregnancy and the postpartum period has increased since universal screening guidelines for perinatal depression were endorsed by the U.S. Preventive Services Task Force (O'Connor et al. 2016), the American College of Obstetricians and Gynecologists (2018), and the American Academy of Pediatrics (Earls et al. 2010); however, screening is by no means universal. With each opportunity taken to screen

TABLE 10–1. **Risk factors for perinatal suicide**

| | |
|---|---|
| Individual factors | Prior psychiatric diagnoses (depression, anxiety, bipolar disorder, schizophrenia, borderline personality disorder, substance abuse disorder) |
| | History of self-harm or prior suicide attempt |
| | History of trauma |
| | Number of previous hospitalizations |
| | Medical comorbidity |
| | Recent illness onset and/or abrupt onset of symptoms |
| | No active treatment |
| | Family history of psychiatric disorder, suicidal ideation, or suicide attempt |
| Pregnancy-related factors | Nulliparity |
| | Interruption of medication |
| | Obstetrical or neonatal complication |
| | Unwanted/Unintended pregnancy |
| Interpersonal/Socioeconomic factors | Younger age |
| | Intimate partner violence and/or family conflict |
| | Lack of social support |
| | Unmarried/Unpartnered or partner who rejected paternity |
| | Social, racial, or gender discrimination or inequalities |
| | Low socioeconomic status and/or unemployment |
| | Crowded or inadequate housing or living in rural area |
| | Exposure to disaster, conflict, or war |
| Health system–related factors | Avoidance of health service due to fear of stigma or losing child custody |

*Source.* Adapted from Mangla et al. 2019; Orsolini et al. 2016.

for symptoms of perinatal depression, clinicians also have an opportunity to screen for suicidality; the Edinburgh Postnatal Depression Scale (Cox et al. 1987) and Patient Health Questionnaire–9 (Spitzer et al. 1999) have both been validated for peripartum use, and each includes a question about self-harm. Because suicide risk is elevated in patients with bipolar disorder, utilizing the Mood Disorder Questionnaire (Hirschfeld et al. 2000) to screen for bipolar disorder can also be helpful. These screening tools are briefly described in Table 10–2. The use of suicide-specific scales has been more controversial given repeated findings of low positive predictive value and specificity that limit the utility of these tools (Bolton et al. 2015).

## Differential Diagnosis

According to the WHO, *suicidal behavior* "refers to a range of behaviors that include thinking about suicide (or ideation), planning for suicide, attempting suicide and suicide itself" (World Health Organization 2014, p. 12); this cluster of suicidal thoughts and behaviors is also often referred to as *suicidality*. In assessing suicidality, clinicians should consider differential diagnosis of not only the thoughts about suicide or the

**TABLE 10–2. Screening tools for use during suicide assessment in maternal mental health settings**

| | |
|---|---|
| Edinburgh Postnatal Depression Scale (Stuart-Parrigon and Stuart 2014) | Self-report, 10 items<br>Screens for depression<br>Validated for peripartum use<br>Includes question about self-harm |
| Patient Health Questionnaire-9 (Spitzer et al. 1999) | Self-report, 9 items<br>Screens for depression<br>Validated for peripartum use<br>Includes question about self-harm |
| Mood Disorder Questionnaire (Hirschfeld et al. 2000) | Self-report, 17 items<br>Screens for bipolar disorder symptoms |

self-injurious behaviors themselves but also the underlying or comorbid psychiatric illness. This requires careful risk assessment, which will inform subsequent interventions. For example, thoughts about suicide may be symptoms of psychosis, such as command hallucinations, or may be ego-dystonic intrusive thoughts related to OCD. As discussed in the next part of this chapter, it is important to rule out PPP, which is an uncommon but high-risk psychiatric emergency. Suicidal behaviors are also distinct from nonsuicidal self-injury, in which the person has no intent to die (White Kress 2003).

## Assessment

If suicidal thoughts or behaviors are reported during screening, or if risk factors or psychiatric symptoms are identified, these should prompt more thorough exploration. A number of clinical practice guidelines exist regarding suicide risk assessment and intervention (Bolton et al. 2015), including from the American Psychiatric Association (Jacobs et al. 2003), and these guidelines can be used in the perinatal period. Guidelines for suicide risk assessment consistently recommend gathering information about the following (Bolton et al. 2015; Orsolini et al. 2016):

- Current stressors and psychosocial environment
- Presence of psychiatric symptoms and history of current illness
- Current substance use
- Current medications
- Current suicidal thoughts, including nature, timing, intent, and persistence
- Current suicidal plan, if applicable, including lethality, access to means, detail, and preparation
- Current or previous suicide attempt, if applicable, including timing, intent, method, and consequences
- Other risk factors
- Protective factors

Follow-up questions should include ones about preparation for death, such as the creation of a will, stockpiling pills, or securing childcare for children left behind after a suicide (Wisner et al. 2012). A complete maternal risk assessment should also include assessment of thoughts about harming the infant or infanticide (Orsolini et al. 2016). Barriers to completing a psychiatric risk assessment, especially in a primary care setting, are numerous, including reliance on a patient's subjective report; lack of practitioner training, comfort, and confidence; and time (Bolton et al. 2015; Orsolini et al. 2016). When available, information from other sources, including previous records, other health care providers, and family and friends, can be valuable in completing a psychiatric risk assessment (Jacobs et al. 2003).

## Management

If suicidality is elicited, then the assessing clinician should proceed to develop a safety plan and make a referral for specialized psychiatric assessment (Orsolini et al. 2016). Considerations around safety planning, treatment setting, and urgency of referral will depend on determination of level of risk; ideally, the treatment plan should be composed of the least restrictive interventions that are likely to be safe and efficacious (Jacobs et al. 2003). For patients who are at high risk and for whom acute safety concerns are present, hospitalization is likely to be required. Examples of patients who would be considered high risk include those who present immediately after a suicide attempt (especially with a history of prior attempts), have a suicide plan with immediate intent, are unable or unwilling to cooperate with assessment or treatment, or present with symptoms of psychosis (Jacobs et al. 2003; Orsolini et al. 2016). Treatment planning should proceed collaboratively as much as possible, with consideration and discussion of patient preferences, as well as of anticipated benefits and potential risks (Jacobs et al. 2003). Clinicians must be aware of local medical legislation and procedures regarding certification in high-risk cases for which involuntary admission may need to be considered.

Mental health care can reduce suicidality. Part of the risk assessment is to determine modifiable risk factors that can be mitigated and potential protective factors and strengths that can be optimized (Orsolini et al. 2016). Treatment of suicidality should also involve close attention to and evidence-based treatment of underlying or comorbid psychiatric illness. Evidence has shown that treatment of depression with antidepressants and of bipolar disorder with mood stabilizers reduces suicidal thoughts and behaviors (Bolton et al. 2015; Jacobs et al. 2003). Pharmacotherapy should also be considered for perinatal women with serious psychiatric disorders, with thoughtful risk-risk discussion around the developing fetus's and/or child's exposure to untreated maternal mental illness versus exposure to psychiatric medication during pregnancy, lactation, or both. (See Chapter 8, "A Clinical Approach to Psychiatric Diagnosis and Treatment During Pregnancy," for a discussion of risk-risk analysis.) Women taking selective serotonin reuptake inhibitors or other antidepressants should be carefully followed to monitor for the emergence of worsened suicidal thoughts, irritability, or agitation, which may indicate underlying bipolar symptomatology (Tondo et al. 2010). With respect to psychotherapeutic intervention, cognitive-behavioral therapy, dialectical behavioral therapy, and problem-solving therapy have shown promising results in reducing suicidality (Bolton et al. 2015). Various studies examining impacts of follow-up care for suicidal patients, ranging from low-cost interventions, such as

TABLE 10–3. **Principles of management of the suicidal perinatal patient**

| Low risk (suicidal thoughts but no plan or intent) | Medium risk (suicidal thoughts with plan but no intent, past attempt made) | High risk (suicidal thoughts with plan and immediate intent, attempts to avoid discovery) |
|---|---|---|
| Establish and maintain collaborative, therapeutic alliance | Establish and maintain collaborative, therapeutic alliance | Establish and maintain collaborative, therapeutic alliance |
| Regular follow-up with repeated assessment of risk | Close follow-up with repeated assessment of risk | Close follow-up once emergent management by psychiatry established |
| Referral to psychiatry | Urgent referral to psychiatry | |
| Treatment of underlying and comorbid mental health conditions; consider psychopharmacology | Treatment of underlying and comorbid mental health conditions, including psychopharmacology | Emergent assessment by psychiatry, possible hospitalization (on mother–baby unit where possible) |
| Psychotherapeutic intervention | Psychotherapeutic intervention | Treatment of underlying and comorbid mental health conditions, including psychopharmacology |
| Optimize social support | Optimize social support | |
| Psychoeducation for patient and supports | Psychoeducation for patient and supports | Psychotherapeutic intervention |
| | | Optimize social support |
| | | Psychoeducation for patient and supports |

sending letters by mail to follow up with suicidal patients, to more intensive case management interventions, have shown mixed results (Bolton et al. 2015).

In peripartum patients, preventive management, including antenatal psychiatric assessment and longer-term postpartum support, is strongly recommended to help lower the burden of maternal mental illness and to decrease the rates of perinatal suicide (Mangla et al. 2019; Orsolini et al. 2016). In addition, collaborative models of care, which integrate mental health services into primary care, pediatric, and obstetrical visits, are being increasingly implemented and are yielding positive results (Mangla et al. 2019). Table 10–3 summarizes the steps for suicidality assessment in patients in the perinatal period.

## Postpartum Psychosis

PPP is an important clinical emergency to recognize because it is associated with an elevated risk of both maternal suicide and harm to the infant, including infanticide (Oates 2003a; Spinelli 2004). Considerable controversy exists over what exactly PPP is; unfortunately, the name does not help. As the name might otherwise imply, *postpartum psychosis* is *not* the presentation of any and all psychosis in the postpartum period. Rather, it represents a distinct affective syndrome. In this section, we briefly describe the clinical presentation and then focus on the emergent management of PPP so that cases can be identified and treated in a rapid and safe manner. Chapter 16, "Postpartum Psychosis," covers the syndrome in greater detail.

> Ms. P is a 36-year-old woman, gravida 1 para 1, who is now 2 weeks postpartum with her first child. She has no known personal psychiatric history, but her father has a history of bipolar I disorder. She is brought to an emergency department by her worried wife, who reports that Ms. P seemed confused and "off." The patient states that immediately upon delivery, she had felt that "I just don't feel right in my body. Something is just wrong with me all over." She could not describe the feeling any further than that, and all medical workup was unremarkable. She had been discharged to home 36 hours after giving birth and had tried to reassure herself that her severe free-floating anxiety was normal. Ms. P was exclusively breastfeeding, and over the next week she was up during the night at least five to six times feeding the infant, with no more than 1–2 hours of sleep at a time. She began to notice that her thoughts were "racing"; she felt "on edge, wired"; and she did not need to sleep much at all. She felt that she had "so much energy that I was going to burst." She started to have intrusive thoughts that harm would come to the baby, although she denied homicidal ideation or command auditory hallucinations. Over the next couple of days, her symptoms progressed to the point that she believed she could not trust the intentions of other people and became convinced that they would harm her child. When a baby nurse came for her night shift and asked to hold the baby, Ms. P became convinced that the baby was going to be permanently harmed under the nurse's care, despite no evidence of any behavior that would have been of concern. Ms. P's wife noticed the patient starting to argue with the nurse and refusing to let her care for the baby, and she brought Ms. P to the emergency department for evaluation.

## Risk Factors

PPP is a rare but serious disorder affecting approximately 1–2 per 1,000 postpartum women (Osborne 2018; VanderKruik et al. 2017). Although the greatest risk factor is a prior history of PPP or bipolar disorder, most patients presenting with PPP have no previous mood episodes (Bergink et al. 2012; Blackmore et al. 2013; Munk-Olsen et al. 2009). A family history of bipolar disorder, particularly in first-degree relatives, also confers risk (Robertson et al. 2005). Other risk factors include primiparity, advanced maternal age, and the occurrence of a mood disorder during pregnancy (Bergink et al. 2012; Blackmore et al. 2006; Valdimarsdóttir et al. 2009).

## Clinical Features

### Diagnostic Criteria

PPP is not currently recognized as a distinct clinical disorder in DSM-5 (American Psychiatric Association 2013). The DSM-5 brief psychotic disorder diagnosis has a "with postpartum onset" specifier that is added if onset is during pregnancy or within 4 weeks postpartum. Because PPP is widely considered to be an affective disorder, this diagnosis often does not sufficiently describe the disorder.

### Clinical Presentation

Symptoms of PPP typically appear soon after birth, around 3–10 days postpartum. Symptom onset tends to be abrupt and follow a fulminant course (Bergink et al. 2012; Friedman et al. 2019; Valdimarsdóttir et al. 2009). Early warning signs can be difficult

TABLE 10–4. **Core clinical features of postpartum psychosis**

| | |
|---|---|
| Confusion | Irritability |
| Delusions/hallucinations | Mood state: mania, depression, mixed |
| Depersonalization | Thoughts of suicide and/or infanticide |
| Disorganization | Waxing and waning changes in consciousness |
| Insomnia | |

*Source.* Osborne 2018.

to differentiate from symptoms common to the postpartum period, such as difficulty sleeping, anxiety, and irritability (Osborne 2018). In addition, symptoms can often wax and wane, fluctuating significantly over time; therefore, assessing the patient at consecutive time points can lead to a more accurate clinical impression (Bergink et al. 2016; Osborne 2018).

Several distinct clinical features can help to distinguish PPP from other acute psychiatric disorders. These include a waxing and waning course, delirium-like alterations in consciousness, confusion, thought disorganization, and bizarre delusions (Bergink et al. 2016; Osborne 2018). Mood symptoms, such as mania, depression, or mixed states, are often present (Osborne 2018). Delusional content may be focused on childbirth or the newborn (e.g., "altruistic" delusions of suicide or infanticide) or on depressed psychotic thoughts, such as the baby being "better off" if the mother were dead (Bergink et al. 2016; Rodriguez-Cabezas and Clark 2018). Perceptual disturbances may occur, such as auditory or visual hallucinations with direct commands for suicide or infanticide (Bergink et al. 2016). Because of the waxing and waning nature of this syndrome, the clinician should question the patient directly about thoughts of suicide or infanticide at repeated intervals during the assessment (Bergink et al. 2016). A summary of key clinical features of PPP is found in Table 10–4.

## Assessment and Differential Diagnosis

The differential diagnosis of PPP is broad and includes medical conditions that may present during the postpartum period. Primary considerations regarding the psychiatric differential diagnoses include baby blues, postpartum depression, and postpartum OCD. A more thorough discussion of these differential diagnoses can be found in Chapter 16.

All patients should receive a physical examination, neurological examination, mental status examination, and cognitive assessment (e.g., the Montreal Cognitive Assessment [Nasreddine et al. 2005]). Laboratory workup should include complete blood count, complete metabolic profile, and urine toxicology screen. Depending on the clinical presentation, other laboratory tests should be ordered as indicated, such as complete thyroid function tests; serum calcium levels; vitamin $B_{12}$, thiamine, and folate levels; and markers of inflammation (Tinkelman et al. 2017). Patients presenting with neurological symptoms, such as altered mental status or seizure, should undergo head imaging, cerebrospinal fluid analysis, serum ammonia concentration, electroencephalogram, and screening for anti-NMDA receptor antibodies (Bergink et al. 2016). In first-episode cases or in patients with no known psychiatric history, more extensive workup may be warranted.

# Management

## Risk Assessment

Emergent management and treatment should begin with a risk assessment to ascertain the risks of suicide, child neglect or abuse, and infanticide because the risk of these outcomes are elevated in patients with PPP. Although the numbers of suicide attempts and deaths in pregnancy and in the postpartum period are lower than in the general population of women, suicide accounts for 20% of the deaths that occur in that time frame (Lindahl et al. 2005). In addition, a woman with PPP is at risk of child neglect or abuse because her confusion or delusions may get in the way of providing organized and responsive care to the infant (Friedman et al. 2019). Also, the risk of infanticide should be assessed because there is approximately a 4% risk of infanticide in PPP (Spinelli 2009). Altruistic or psychotic motives for infanticide are more likely to be linked to PPP than to fatal maltreatment, an unwanted child, or partner revenge (Friedman et al. 2019).

## Treatment Setting

Given the severity and high-risk nature of PPP, inpatient admission is warranted for rapid implementation of a safety plan, psychiatric stabilization, and treatment (Friedman et al. 2019). Ideally, hospitalization would occur in a dedicated mother–baby psychiatric unit that provides support for bonding, breastfeeding, and mother–infant dyadic treatment. This type of facility is considered best practice in most countries worldwide, although such units are scarce in the United States (Friedman et al. 2019).

## Treatment

Mood stabilizers and antipsychotics are the mainstay of the acute treatment of PPP. The choice of a medication regimen for a particular patient will depend on the clinical situation, symptom severity, previous response to medications, and adverse effects (Jones et al. 2014). Introduction of lithium early in the treatment course is recommended (Osborne 2018). One naturalistic study treated women with PPP with sequential use of benzodiazepines, antipsychotics, and lithium, achieving a 99% remission rate and 80% sustained remission rate after 9 months (Bergink et al. 2015). Electroconvulsive therapy (ECT) is also an effective treatment for PPP and can be a first-line treatment for high-risk patients in whom rapid improvement of symptoms is needed, including patients with catatonia, severe agitation, refusal to eat or drink with compromised nutritional status, severe suicidality, or treatment resistance (Focht and Kellner 2012).

# Acute Agitation

Acute agitation is a perinatal psychiatric emergency that might compromise the safety of the patient, the pregnancy, the patient's supports, and the treatment team. *Agitation* broadly refers to a behavior set that poses a risk to the safety of the patient or caregivers, impedes the implementation of care, or acutely impairs functioning (Yildiz et al. 2003). Patient agitation is also a leading cause of workplace injury for hospital staff and members of the treatment team (Gates et al. 2006; Lam 2002). Agitation can encompass a wide range of behaviors and underlying etiologies, including both psychiatric and medical conditions. Thus, the aim of treatment is to reduce agitation to reduce the risk of harm and to begin evaluation of the underlying cause. In this section, we summarize key steps in the identification, diagnosis, and management of the agitated perinatal patient, including the key steps of verbal deescalation and prevention of harm.

# Epidemiology

## Rates/Incidence

Relatively little comprehensive information has been written about the epidemiology of agitation, particularly in pregnancy. A systematic review estimated that in the United States, up to 1.7 million patient visits to emergency departments per year may involve episodes of agitation (Zeller and Rhoades 2010). A structured, retrospective multicenter chart review of patients presenting to an emergency department with psychiatric complaints revealed that 52% the patients had agitation as part of the clinical picture (Boudreaux et al. 2009).

## Risk Factors

Risk factors that predict agitation in the general adult population, the adult psychiatric population, or the perinatal population are scarcely described in the literature. One European expert consensus protocol described several categories of risk associated with agitation in the adult psychiatry population. These included demographic factors, such as male gender; psychosocial factors, such as a recent stressful life event; and clinical factors, such as active substance abuse (Vieta et al. 2017).

# Screening

To our knowledge, no screening tools are commonly used to detect agitation either in the general population or specifically in pregnant patients. One multicenter research collaboration (Lukens et al. 2006) measured agitation objectively using the Agitated Behavior Scale (Corrigan 1989), a well-validated, comprehensive scale to prospectively assess and quantify agitation.

# Clinical Features

## Diagnostic Criteria

DSM-5 does not have a formal set of diagnostic criteria for agitation. Agitation has been described as the physical manifestation of internal distress due to an underlying medical condition, such as delirium, or to a psychiatric condition, such as acute substance intoxication or withdrawal, mania, psychosis, or a personality disorder (Wilson et al. 2015).

## Clinical Presentation

Regarding the presentation of agitation, a clinician might say that "I know it when I see it"—an understandable response to behaviors that have broad presenting symptoms and a wide range of etiologies. Agitation typically refers to a state of increased arousal characterized by uncooperative or combative behavior, physical restlessness, increased verbal and motor activity, and extreme irritability (Nordstrom et al. 2012; Rodriguez-Cabezas and Clark 2018; Zeller and Rhoades 2010). Agitation symptoms can range from mild to severe, can fluctuate unpredictably, and can escalate sharply in a brief period of time (San et al. 2016). Agitation in the medical setting should be differentiated from *aggression*—behaviors that have the potential to harm another person (physically, sexually, verbally, or by other means), regardless of intent or whether harm actually occurs (Pekurinen et al. 2017; Zeller and Rhoades 2010). The following case example illustrates agitation in a pregnant patient.

> An unidentified, disheveled patient, appearing to be in her 30s, heavily gravid and in a highly agitated state, was brought to the emergency department by emergency medical technicians at 3 A.M. She refused to answer any questions, instead screaming loudly about how she had been invaded by aliens that resulted in her pregnancy, attracting concerned looks from other patients in the emergency department. She started to pace around the room, waving her arms around wildly and intermittently kicking the legs of a chair in the corner of the room with her bare foot. She refused any attempts by the nursing staff to evaluate her, including the taking of vital signs. When the attending physician entered the room, the patient became highly agitated and started waving her hands near the physician's face, shouting that angels were telling her that the emergency department doctors were there to harm her and her baby. A quick-thinking medical student retrieved a blanket, a bread roll, and some orange juice from outside the evaluation room. He offered it to the patient at arm's length, saying quietly, "Are you hungry or cold? I'm happy to get you more food if you want it." The patient noticeably calmed. A few minutes later, she was sitting in the chair, wrapped in the blanket and eating the roll. She remained highly suspicious but eventually accepted 0.5 mg of lorazepam and 2.5 mg of haloperidol orally. An hour later, she allowed the medical staff to take her vital signs and draw her blood.

## Course and Prognosis

Because the symptoms of agitation can range from mild to severe, fluctuate significantly, and arise from a number of different etiologies, the course and prognosis can be unpredictable. Clearly, however, uncontrolled agitation compromises the safety of the pregnant patient and the fetus and has been found to be associated with obstetrical complications such as preterm delivery, spontaneous abortion, postnatal death, and placental dysfunction (Aftab and Shah 2017).

## Pathophysiology

Although agitation is a common feature of many psychiatric conditions, such as schizophrenia, substance use disorders, bipolar disorder, and dementia, little is known about agitation itself as a unique entity (Sachs 2006). A unifying hypothesis for the etiology of agitation has not yet been described, but discrete factors have been linked to specific psychiatric disorders. For example, frontal lobe dysfunction, alterations in the catechol-*O*-methyltransferase gene involved in dopamine metabolism, and catecholamine inactivation have been implicated in the genesis of agitation in schizophrenia and bipolar disorder (Sachs 2006). A review of the pathophysiology of agitation suggests that various underlying etiologies are mediated by dysregulation of neurotransmitter systems to produce agitation symptoms, including the serotonergic, dopaminergic, noradrenergic, and GABAergic systems (Lindenmayer 2000).

## Differential Diagnosis

Agitation has many potential causes, including psychiatric illness, medical illness, and intoxication or withdrawal from prescribed medications or other substances. Many life-threatening medical etiologies can present with agitation, and they should be consid-

**TABLE 10–5. Examples of life-threatening medical etiologies of agitation in perinatal patients**

| | |
|---|---|
| Catatonia | Physical trauma |
| Coagulopathy/bleeding | Severe thyroid dysfunction |
| Eclampsia | Substance intoxication or withdrawal |
| Hypoxia or hypercapnia | Systemic infection |
| Immune-based disorders (e.g., NMDA encephalitis) | Venous or amniotic fluid thromboembolism |
| Intracranial hemorrhage | |

*Source.* Adapted from Niforatos et al. 2019; Nordstrom et al. 2012.

ered in every presentation. Particular attention should be given to signs and symptoms of *delirium,* which is an alteration in mental status that derives from a medical etiology. Core clinical features of delirium include altered arousal, impaired awareness and attention, disorientation, and confusion (European Delirium Association and American Delirium Society 2014). It is important to have a high index of suspicion for delirium in both general patients and pregnant patients, because the presentation tends to wax and wane and the symptoms and signs may be subtle (Nordstrom et al. 2012).

The most common psychiatric etiologies of agitation in the pregnant patient are substance intoxication and withdrawal, psychosis, mania, and extreme anxiety (Berkowitz and Mills 2019). Neuropsychiatric side effects of medications should be considered because symptoms such as akathisia can result in severe psychomotor restlessness (Pringsheim et al. 2018). Also, emotional distress due to pain or other stressors should be considered as a contributing factor to agitation (Berkowitz and Mills 2019).

## Assessment

The assessment of an agitated pregnant patient should begin with vital signs; assessment of the airway, breathing, and circulation; and measurement of oxygenation and blood glucose (Niforatos et al. 2019; Nordstrom et al. 2012). In the pregnant patient, vital signs might be outside the normal range yet physiologically appropriate. For example, a pregnant patient might have elevated resting heart rate due to decrease in systemic vascular resistance or have low blood pressure, which typically reaches its lowest point at about 24 weeks of gestation (Wilson et al. 2015). Temperature >100.4°F is typically consistent with a medical cause; temperatures this high are not usually seen with the mild physiological hyperthermia of pregnancy (Wilson et al. 2015). Examples of life-threatening medical etiologies of agitation in a pregnant patient are provided in Table 10–5.

Assessment of mental status can serve as a vital component of the initial screen of an agitated pregnant patient (Wilson et al. 2015). When possible, history gathering from the patient should follow. Collateral history and the description of inciting events by loved ones or observers, such as emergency medical technicians, can be useful, especially if the patient is unwilling or unable to cooperate with an interview (Niforatos et al. 2019; Stowell et al. 2012). Initial emergency assessment should include evaluation for delirium, trauma, intracranial hemorrhage, thrombocytopenia, coagulopathy, amniotic and venous thromboembolism, assessment of substance use or withdrawal, hypoxia or hypercapnia, and eclampsia (Berkowitz and Mills 2019; Niforatos et al. 2019).

# Management

## General Approach

In any intervention to address agitation, clinicians should actively monitor the physical status of the pregnant patient and the developing fetus, with frequent assessment of vital signs and clinical status and evaluation for adverse effects. Psychiatry and obstetrics teams should work together to monitor maternal and fetal health (including fetal heart monitoring and ultrasound) at all levels of agitation management. As with other clinical situations in reproductive psychiatry, performing a risk-risk analysis is important when considering the use of medications to treat agitation. Given the adverse consequences associated with untreated agitation in pregnancy, the benefits of using psychotropic medications generally outweigh risks (Aftab and Shah 2017). If the patient has a history of good response to a particular medication, every effort should be made to use the same medication to minimize exposing the fetus to an additional medication (Niforatos et al. 2019).

## Levels of Agitation Management

The approach to management of acute agitation should progress from least restrictive to more restrictive based on the level of agitation and response to each step of treatment. Deescalation techniques are prioritized as a first-line treatment for the pregnant patient given the desire to minimize extensive use of psychotropic medication and to avoid physical restraint when possible (Rodriguez-Cabezas and Clark 2018). Table 10–6 presents a stepwise approach to managing agitation in a pregnant patient.

In cases of mild agitation, the initial response should include moving the patient to a low-stimulus environment and utilizing both verbal and nonverbal deescalation techniques (Aftab and Shah 2017; Richmond et al. 2012; Rodriguez-Cabezas and Clark 2018). If a patient is moderately agitated or does not respond solely to deescalation, the clinician should progress to offering oral psychotropic medications. According to consensus guidelines, oral medications are clearly preferred over parenteral when possible (Allen et al. 2001).

If in the general adult population, a patient's severe agitation poses an acute danger to self or others, emergency interventions such as physical restraint, seclusion, or parenteral medication may be indicated. Expert consensus surveys have shown that most experts think emergency interventions are necessary in a minority of cases, from 1% to 20% of patients (Allen et al. 2001). Particular precautions need to be taken, however, in the case of a severely agitated pregnant patient. The use of four-point restraint with a patient in the supine position increases the risk of inferior vena cava syndrome and may affect fetal blood flow, particularly in the second and third trimesters (Niforatos et al. 2019; Rodriguez-Cabezas and Clark 2018). Therefore, especially later in pregnancy, physical restraint should be used only as an intervention of last resort. The patient who requires physical restraint should be placed in the left lateral decubitus position, 10–12 cm off the bed, with pillows and blankets for support. The patient should be monitored closely, with frequent assessment of vital signs and physical checks to minimize risk (Niforatos et al. 2019).

**TABLE 10–6. Stepwise approach to managing agitation in a pregnant patient**

| | |
|---|---|
| **Initial patient assessment** | Airway, breathing, circulation, disability, exposure, vital signs, pulse oximetry, blood glucose |
| **Emergency medical condition?** | Yes: Emergency medical management<br>No: Proceed to management steps for agitation |
| **Agitation severity** | |
| Mild | Verbal and nonverbal deescalation<br>Consider oral diphenhydramine<br>Reassess; if condition escalates, proceed to moderate/severe agitation management steps<br>Frequent assessment of vital signs and mental status<br>Obstetrical consultation for fetal monitoring and maternal health status |
| Moderate | Verbal and nonverbal deescalation<br>If known psychiatric history, offer patient's psychiatric medication<br>If unknown psychiatric history, offer oral antipsychotic ± benzodiazepine<br>Reassess; if condition escalates, proceed to severe agitation management step<br>Frequent assessment of vital signs and mental status<br>Obstetrical consultation for fetal monitoring and maternal health status |
| Severe | Verbal and nonverbal deescalation<br>Psychopharmacology: haloperidol + benzodiazepine ± diphenhydramine<br>Physical restraint only as last resort (left lateral decubitus, 10–12 cm off bed, with pillows and blankets for support)<br>Frequent assessment of vital signs and mental status<br>Obstetrical consultation for fetal monitoring and maternal health status |

*Source.* Niforatos et al. 2019.

## Psychopharmacology for Agitation in Pregnancy

The choice of medication to treat agitation should be based on a clinical assessment of the likely underlying cause, even if the diagnosis is provisional and subject to change when more data are available (Wilson et al. 2012). The best studied and most frequently used medications for agitation are the first-generation antipsychotics (FGAs), second-generation antipsychotics (SGAs), and benzodiazepines (Wilson et al. 2012). Antipsychotics have often been used for moderate to severe agitation both generally and in pregnancy. Extensive discussion of the pharmacology and clinical use of antipsychotic medication is found in Chapter 17, "Schizophrenia and Related Disorders." FGAs such as haloperidol have traditionally been used in emergency settings, although there has been increasing preference for SGAs such as quetiapine or olanzapine (Wilson et al. 2012) due to their lower risk of extrapyramidal symptoms.

Of the FGAs used to manage agitation, haloperidol is the most common, in part due to its long track record of efficacy and safety in the emergency setting (Ladavac et al. 2007; MacDonald et al. 2010; Wilson et al. 2012). Expert consensus guidelines support the use of haloperidol as the first-line treatment of acute agitation in pregnancy when the patient has no previous experience with neuroleptics, especially because medium- or high-potency FGAs are typically less sedating than low-potency ones, which may be important in the pregnant patient (Allen et al. 2005; Diav-Citrin et al. 2005). FGAs have the advantage of few adverse effects in terms of vital signs and anticholinergic side effects, and haloperidol has reassuring data about lack of teratogenicity from first-trimester exposure (Einarson 2005; Wilson et al. 2012). However, FGAs do carry the risks of extrapyramidal side effects, such as acute dystonia and neuroleptic malignant syndrome, and cardiac effects, such as QTc prolongation and torsades de pointes (Wilson et al. 2012). Exposure to high-potency antipsychotics may also be associated with neonatal extrapyramidal symptoms during and after delivery (Galbally et al. 2014).

SGAs such as quetiapine and olanzapine are increasingly used for the treatment of acute agitation (Allen et al. 2001). SGAs have several advantages over FGAs, including a reduced risk of acute extrapyramidal side effects and availability in a rapidly dissolving formulation, such as with olanzapine (Cohen et al. 2016). Early safety data on SGAs in pregnancy appear to be reassuring regarding risk of teratogenicity, with the possible exception of risperidone (Huybrechts et al. 2016). However, SGAs do carry side effects, including elevated risk of orthostatic hypotension, that may be of concern with acute use of these medications in pregnancy, particularly in a pregnant patient who may already have low resting blood pressure (Galbally et al. 2014; Wilson et al. 2012).

Benzodiazepines are also commonly used for management of acute agitation, and in cases of severe agitation in pregnancy, the benefit of using these medications may outweigh the risks. Early studies indicated an association between first-trimester benzodiazepine exposure and cleft lip and palate in the newborn, but further studies have not replicated this finding (Grigoriadis et al. 2019; Rodriguez-Cabezas and Clark 2018). Third-trimester exposure to benzodiazepines carries a concern for withdrawal or respiratory problems in the infant; however, these adverse effects are more common in women with chronic benzodiazepine use and less likely to arise from a one-time emergency dose (Enato et al. 2011).

Other medications to treat agitation may be useful in certain circumstances. For example, in a pregnant patient with mild agitation that is not related to delirium, oral medication such as diphenhydramine can be an appropriate first step. Although diphenhydramine is generally considered low risk for congenital malformations, anticholinergic medications can worsen symptoms of delirium, so this etiology is important to rule out (Li et al. 2013).

## Substance Intoxication and Withdrawal

The prevalence of substance use disorders, such as opioid use disorder, has been rising at an alarming pace in the United States, particularly among women of reproductive age (Saia et al. 2016). Pregnant women, however, face important barriers to substance use disorder treatment, including lack of access to care, fear of legal or custody consequences, and stigma (Saia et al. 2016). The use of substances during pregnancy can lead to significant adverse pregnancy outcomes (e.g., low birth weight, prematurity, placental dysfunction), and substance use disorders are often associated with psychiatric and medical comorbidities that may complicate the acute presentation of intoxication or withdrawal (DeVido et al. 2015). In this section, we focus on the management of the acute intoxication or withdrawal states that may require emergency assessment and intervention to avoid morbidity or mortality for the pregnant patient or the fetus. Chapter 21, "Substance Use Disorders," contains a full discussion of specific substances and their effects in the perinatal period.

## Alcohol

Alcohol intoxication is common in emergency settings. Key clinical features of intoxication include slurred speech, lack of coordination, impaired judgment, mood and personality changes, and somnolence (Pasha et al. 2020). These signs, familiar to most emergency physicians, are no different in pregnant women than in the general population. Acute alcohol withdrawal poses significant, life-threatening risks to pregnant women. Symptoms include tachycardia, hypertension, hyperthermia, restlessness, seizures, altered mental status, hallucinations, and agitation (DeVido et al. 2015). Potential consequences to the pregnancy from alcohol withdrawal include fetal distress, low birth weight, placental abruption, and preterm labor (DeVido et al. 2015; Rodriguez-Cabezas and Clark 2018). If alcohol withdrawal is suspected in a pregnant patient, all efforts should be made to treat the withdrawal in a setting that allows close medical monitoring.

Benzodiazepines are the mainstay of treatment for alcohol withdrawal in the general population (Aftab and Shah 2017). Data regarding their use for alcohol withdrawal in pregnant women are limited, but given the high risks associated with untreated withdrawal, benzodiazepines are the most recommendable option for alcohol withdrawal in pregnant patients (DeVido et al. 2015). Gabapentin may be an alternative, with some data indicating relative safety in pregnancy (Fujii et al. 2013). Anticonvulsants such as valproate and carbamazepine are associated with higher rates of congenital abnormalities and should be avoided (Heberlein et al. 2012).

## Cocaine and Methamphetamines

Stimulants, such as cocaine or methamphetamines, are the second most widely used and abused substance category in the United States after tobacco (Smid et al. 2019). According to the 2019 National Survey on Drug Use and Health, cocaine use remained stable in women of all age groups (>12 years), but methamphetamine use had a statistically significant increase in 2018–2019 as compared with 2016–2017 (Substance Abuse and Mental Health Services Administration 2020). Pregnant women with cocaine or methamphetamine toxicity can present with aggressive and irritable behavior, visual or other hallucinations, and grandiose and paranoid thought processes (Berkowitz and Mills 2019). Acute cocaine toxicity, which can lead to severe hypertension, hyperreflexia, proteinuria, edema, and seizures, may be mistaken for preeclampsia (Smid et al. 2019).

Maternal complications of cocaine or methamphetamine intoxication include myocardial infarction, renal failure, hepatic rupture, cerebral ischemia or infarction, and death (Kalaitzopoulos et al. 2018; Smid et al. 2019). Even small doses of cocaine may lead to cardiac morbidity and mortality in an otherwise healthy pregnant woman, potentially due to elevated progesterone concentrations, which increase cardiac muscle sensitivity to cocaine (Smid et al. 2019). β-adrenergic antagonists should not be used to treat cocaine-induced hypertension because they will create unopposed α-adrenergic stimulation; instead, hydralazine should be used for hypertension that is due to suspected maternal cocaine toxicity (Kuczkowski 2007).

### Opioids

Repeated opioid intoxication and withdrawal during pregnancy can result in complications that include fetal distress, intrauterine growth restriction, placental insufficiency, and preterm labor (Rodriguez-Cabezas and Clark 2018). Opioid withdrawal can cause permanent damage to fetal brain development and fetal demise (Rodriguez-Cabezas and Clark 2018). For pregnant women presenting with opioid withdrawal, the standard of care is acute agitation management and potential initiation of opioid maintenance therapy. Methadone and buprenorphine both have evidence of relative safety during pregnancy (Aftab and Shah 2017; Zedler et al. 2016). Medically assisted withdrawal ("detoxification") is not recommended for pregnant women because it is associated with high relapse rates and inherent overdose mortality risk (Saia et al. 2016).

## Catatonia

Catatonia is an important but easily missed perinatal psychiatric emergency. Significant life-threatening risks associated with its symptoms include agitation and prolonged immobility, both of which are common features of this condition.

### Epidemiology

#### Rates/Incidence

In the general population, catatonia is not uncommon. It has been reported to occur in 10%–18% of all acute psychiatric presentations (Llesuy et al. 2018; Rasmussen et al. 2016). However, catatonia in pregnancy has been described rarely. One retrospective chart review revealed only 3 case series (with 33, 15, and 13 patients in total) and 16 more individual case reports in the literature (Gonzales et al. 2014).

#### Risk Factors

Risk factors include underlying psychiatric illness (typically affective states, such as major depression and bipolar disorder), neurological illness, and medical illness.

### Screening

To our knowledge, screening for catatonia is not generally done in clinical practice. In terms of clinical assessment, the Bush-Francis Catatonia Rating Scale, among others, is widely used due to its validity, reliability, and ease of administration (Bush et al. 1996; Sienaert et al. 2011).

### Clinical Features

#### Diagnostic Criteria

The symptoms of catatonia can be divided into those that involve decreased, increased, or abnormal motor activities. Current research in catatonia links these varied abnormalities in the motor system to particular neural pathways, and it is clear that the many and varied features of this syndrome defy easy categorization (Walther et al. 2019). For clinicians, it can nevertheless be helpful to think of three broad subtypes of catatonia (Burrow et al. 2020): retarded, excited, and malignant. *Retarded catatonia* consists of hypoactive symptoms associated with a paucity of movement, including staring, mutism, prolonged immobility, withdrawal, and refusal to eat (Rasmussen et al. 2016). *Excited catatonia* refers to extreme psychomotor agitation with purposeless and excessive motor activity. *Malignant catatonia* is a severe version of excited catatonia that has potential complications such as hyperthermia, altered mental status, and autonomic dysfunction; it can be quickly fatal if not identified and effectively treated (Rasmussen et al. 2016). The symptoms of malignant catatonia can be nearly indistinguishable from neuroleptic malignant syndrome (Rodriguez et al. 2020). The term *catatonia* is described in multiple contexts across DSM-5, such as "catatonia due to a general medical condition" or "bipolar disorder with catatonia" (despite its somewhat awkward location in the "Schizophrenia Spectrum and Other Psychotic Disorders" section). Box 10–1 lists the diagnostic criteria for catatonia used as a specifier with another mental disorder.

### Box 10–1. Catatonia Associated With Another Mental Disorder (Catatonia Specifier)

A. The clinical picture is dominated by three (or more) of the following symptoms:

1. Stupor (i.e., no psychomotor activity; not actively relating to environment).
2. Catalepsy (i.e., passive induction of a posture held against gravity).
3. Waxy flexibility (i.e., slight, even resistance to positioning by examiner).
4. Mutism (i.e., no, or very little, verbal response [exclude if known aphasia]).
5. Negativism (i.e., opposition or no response to instructions or external stimuli).
6. Posturing (i.e., spontaneous and active maintenance of a posture against gravity).
7. Mannerism (i.e., odd, circumstantial caricature of normal actions).
8. Stereotypy (i.e., repetitive, abnormally frequent, non-goal-directed movements).
9. Agitation, not influenced by external stimuli.
10. Grimacing.
11. Echolalia (i.e., mimicking another's speech).
12. Echopraxia (i.e., mimicking another's movements).

**Coding note:** Indicate the name of the associated mental disorder when recording the name of the condition (i.e., 293.89 [F06.1] catatonia associated with major depressive disorder). Code first the associated mental disorder (e.g., neurodevelopmental disorder, brief psychotic disorder, schizophreniform disorder, schizophrenia, schizoaffective disorder, bipolar disorder, major depressive disorder, or other mental disorder) (e.g., 295.70 [F25.1] schizoaffective disorder, depressive type; 293.89 [F06.1] catatonia associated with schizoaffective disorder).

*Source.* Reprinted from American Psychiatric Association: *Diagnostic and Statistical Manual of Mental Disorders,* 5th Edition. Arlington, VA, 2013, pp. 119–120. 

## Clinical Presentation

Symptoms of catatonia can be highly variable; more than 60 clinical features have been described (Weder et al. 2008). Symptoms of retarded catatonia include withdrawal, prolonged immobility, and mutism (Espínola-Nadurille et al. 2007). Excited symptoms include restlessness, auditory and visual hallucinations, and disorganized speech and behavior, which can easily be misidentified as primarily psychotic in nature (Espínola-Nadurille et al. 2007). Malignant catatonia is characterized by severe agitation, autonomic instability, delirium, and a rapidly progressive course (Park et al. 2017).

### Course and Prognosis

The course of catatonia can be variable but can include serious, life-threatening complications. Symptoms that cause considerable safety risks to patients include agitation, negativism, mutism, prolonged immobility, and stupor (Gonzales et al. 2014). Immobility and withdrawal can lead to maternal malnutrition, dehydration, pressure ulcers, contractures, and aspiration pneumonia (Philbrick and Rummans 1994). Because pregnancy is a hypercoagulable state, immobility raises the potentially lethal risk of deep venous thrombosis and pulmonary embolism (Philbrick and Rummans 1994). Complications from malignant catatonia include rhabdomyolysis, renal failure, cardiac ischemia, metabolic acidosis, disseminated intravascular coagulation, and death (Philbrick and Rummans 1994). Notably, catatonia is a risk factor for neuroleptic malignant syndrome, which has a fatality rate of up to 10% (Rasmussen et al. 2016; Strawn et al. 2007).

### Differential Diagnosis and Assessment

It is important to distinguish catatonia from conditions with similar presentations, including extrapyramidal side effects, neuroleptic malignant syndrome, nonconvulsive status epilepticus, and akinetic mutism (Rasmussen et al. 2016). Gonzales et al. (2014), in their retrospective chart review of catatonia in pregnancy, noted a high incidence of medical etiologies in perinatal patients with catatonia. These included posterior reversible encephalopathy, neoplastic limbic encephalitis, cerebrovascular events, and eclampsia. The authors noted that catatonic patients in the perinatal period should be specifically ruled out for eclampsia because the seizures and posterior reversible encephalopathy can be both associated with and causative of catatonia. NMDA encephalitis is another condition diagnosed in a significant proportion of these cases; care should be taken to rule out this disorder in cases with similar presentations (Kumar et al. 2010).

### Pathophysiology

The pathophysiology of catatonia is not well understood. One hypothesis is that catatonia is a movement-based disorder similar to parkinsonism; another hypothesis is that catatonia is a form of extreme anxiety or an evolutionarily based fear response (Rasmussen et al. 2016). The GABA and glutamate neurotransmitter systems are thought to be implicated, particularly in the basal ganglia (Northoff 2002; Rasmussen et al. 2016). Other studies have examined structural (including the orbitofrontal, prefrontal, parietal, and motor cortical regions), genetic, and systemic contributors, such as the innate immune system, infection, and autoimmunity (Northoff 2002; Rogers et al. 2019; Walther et al. 2019).

## Management

The mainstay of treatment of catatonia in pregnant or postpartum patients is similar to the treatment of general adult patients with this condition—benzodiazepines as first-line treatment, followed by ECT if benzodiazepines alone are ineffective (Gonzales et al. 2014). Patients typically respond to benzodiazepines, such as lorazepam, which may be given in oral, intravenous, or intramuscular form. Patients may require elevated doses; doses as high as 20 mg/day orally have been reported in the general adult population (Gonzales et al. 2014). Doses of parenteral lorazepam as high as 6–8 mg/day have been administered safely to pregnant patients (Moeller 2013). At times ECT may be required; it is thought to be effective and can be administered safely in pregnancy with appropriate fetal monitoring (Pinna et al. 2015). (See Chapter 19, "Anxiety Disorders and Insomnia in the Perinatal Period," and Chapter 13, "Depressive Disorders," for more extensive discussion of benzodiazepines and ECT, respectively, in the perinatal period.)

## Conclusion

Patients in the perinatal period may be particularly vulnerable to the onset or exacerbation of mental health disorders. A number of important clinical emergencies need to be identified and treated rapidly and safely. This chapter highlighted several of these conditions, including acute suicidality, PPP, agitation, substance intoxication and withdrawal, and catatonia. By appreciating the clinical presentation, differential diagnosis, and treatment strategies for these emergencies, clinicians can rapidly identify and manage these conditions to minimize risk of maternal and fetal harm.

# Key Points

**Suicidality**

- Suicide is a leading cause of maternal death in developed countries, although rates of suicide are generally lower among perinatal than nonperinatal women.
- Risk of suicide is elevated for peripartum women with current or previous mental disorder.
- Awareness of risk factors for perinatal suicide, including historical and current experiences of trauma, is critical to understanding an individual patient's vulnerability and for guiding appropriate care.

**Postpartum Psychosis**

- Postpartum psychosis (PPP) is a psychiatric emergency. Although the condition is rare, it increases the risk of suicide and infanticide.
- PPP appears to be related to bipolar disorder; however, at times the syndrome is limited solely to the postpartum period.
- Risk factors include a history of bipolar disorder or prior PPP.
- Symptoms can wax and wane; therefore, repeated assessments over time can lead to a more accurate diagnostic picture.
- Treatment typically includes antipsychotics, benzodiazepines, and the early introduction of lithium.

### Acute Agitation

- Rapid and effective management of acute agitation is crucial for the safety of both the patient and the pregnancy.
- It is important to consider and rule out life-threatening medical and psychiatric causes of agitation in the pregnant patient.
- Deescalation using verbal and nonverbal techniques should be the first-line treatment.
- Treatment strategies include diphenhydramine for mild agitation, first- or second-generation neuroleptics, and judicious use of short-acting benzodiazepines.
- Physical restraint should be used only as a last resort due to the risk of inferior vena cava syndrome.

### Substance Intoxication and Withdrawal

- Alcohol withdrawal in pregnancy should be actively treated given the significant adverse obstetrical effects noted with untreated withdrawal.
- Benzodiazepines are the mainstay of alcohol withdrawal treatment in pregnancy; gabapentin may be a useful alternative.
- Maternal cocaine or methamphetamine intoxication can lead to serious adverse consequences, including hypertension, myocardial infarction, cerebrovascular accident, and death.
- In pregnancy, ingestion of even small amounts of cocaine may be cardiotoxic because elevated progesterone may increase the cardiac muscle's sensitivity to the effects of cocaine.
- Opioid intoxication and withdrawal may result in serious obstetrical adverse effects, including fetal demise.
- Maintenance is currently the standard of care in pregnancy for opioid use disorders, and medically assisted withdrawal is not recommended due to a high rate of relapse.

### Catatonia

- Catatonia is an important perinatal psychiatric emergency to recognize because it typically arises in concert with medical, neurological, or psychiatric conditions and can lead to life-threatening complications.
- Catatonia can be treated successfully with benzodiazepines; high doses may be required.
- Electroconvulsive therapy can also be a safe treatment in the pregnant patient if benzodiazepines are ineffective.

## References

Aftab A, Shah AA: Behavioral emergencies: special considerations in the pregnant patient. Psychiatr Clin North Am 40(3):435–448, 2017 28800800

Allen MH, Currier GW, Hughes DH, et al: The expert consensus guideline series. Treatment of behavioral emergencies. Postgrad Med (Spec No):1–88, quiz 89–90, 2001 11500996
Allen MH, Currier GW, Carpenter D, et al: The expert consensus guideline series. Treatment of behavioral emergencies 2005. J Psychiatr Pract 11(suppl 1):5–108, quiz 110–112, 2005 16319571
American College of Obstetricians and Gynecologists: ACOG Committee Opinion No. 757: screening for perinatal depression. Obstet Gynecol 132(5):e208–e212, 2018 30629567
American Psychiatric Association: Diagnostic and Statistical Manual of Mental Disorders, 5th Edition. Arlington, VA, American Psychiatric Association, 2013
Appleby L, Mortensen PB, Faragher EB: Suicide and other causes of mortality after post-partum psychiatric admission. Br J Psychiatry 173:209–211, 1998 9926095
Austin MP, Kildea S, Sullivan E: Maternal mortality and psychiatric morbidity in the perinatal period: challenges and opportunities for prevention in the Australian setting. Med J Aust 186(7):364–367, 2007 17407434
Bergink V, Bouvy PF, Vervoort JS, et al: Prevention of postpartum psychosis and mania in women at high risk. Am J Psychiatry 169(6):609–615, 2012 22407083
Bergink V, Burgerhout KM, Koorengevel KM, et al: Treatment of psychosis and mania in the postpartum period. Am J Psychiatry 172(2):115–123, 2015 25640930
Bergink V, Rasgon N, Wisner KL: Postpartum psychosis: madness, mania, and melancholia in motherhood. Am J Psychiatry 173(12):1179–1188, 2016 27609245
Berkowitz P, Mills M: Psychiatric emergencies in pregnancy, in Obstetric Intensive Care Manual, 5th Edition. Edited by Foley M, Strong T, Garite T. New York, McGraw Hill, 2019, pp 320–338
Blackmore ER, Jones I, Doshi M, et al: Obstetric variables associated with bipolar affective puerperal psychosis. Br J Psychiatry 188:32–36, 2006 16388067
Blackmore ER, Rubinow DR, O'Connor TG, et al: Reproductive outcomes and risk of subsequent illness in women diagnosed with postpartum psychosis. Bipolar Disord 15(4):394–404, 2013 23651079
Bolton JM, Gunnell D, Turecki G: Suicide risk assessment and intervention in people with mental illness. BMJ 351:h4978, 2015 26552947
Boudreaux ED, Allen MH, Claassen C, et al: The Psychiatric Emergency Research Collaboration-01: methods and results. Gen Hosp Psychiatry 31(6):515–522, 2009 19892209
Burrow JP, Spurling BC, Marwaha R: Catatonia, in StatPearls (internet). Treasure Island, FL, StatPearls Publishing, 2020
Bush G, Fink M, Petrides G, et al: Catatonia. I. Rating scale and standardized examination. Acta Psychiatr Scand 93(2):129–136, 1996 8686483
Cohen LS, Viguera AC, McInerney KA, et al: Reproductive safety of second-generation antipsychotics: current data from the Massachusetts General Hospital National Pregnancy Registry for Atypical Antipsychotics. Am J Psychiatry 173(3):263–270, 2016 26441156
Corrigan JD: Development of a scale for assessment of agitation following traumatic brain injury. J Clin Exp Neuropsychol 11(2):261–277, 1989 2925835
Cox JL, Holden JM, Sagovsky R: Detection of postnatal depression: development of the 10-item Edinburgh Postnatal Depression Scale. Br J Psychiatry 150:782–786, 1987 3651732
DeVido J, Bogunovic O, Weiss RD: Alcohol use disorders in pregnancy. Harv Rev Psychiatry 23(2):112–121, 2015 25747924
Diav-Citrin O, Shechtman S, Ornoy S, et al: Safety of haloperidol and penfluridol in pregnancy: a multicenter, prospective, controlled study. J Clin Psychiatry 66(3):317–322, 2005 15766297
Earls MF, Siegel BS, Dobbins MI, et al: Incorporating recognition and management of perinatal and postpartum depression into pediatric practice. Pediatrics 126(5):1032–1039, 2010 20974776
Einarson A: The safety of psychotropic drug use during pregnancy: a review. MedGenMed 7(4):3, 2005 16614625
Enato E, Moretti M, Koren G: The fetal safety of benzodiazepines: an updated meta-analysis. J Obstet Gynaecol Can 33(1):46–48, 2011 21272436
Espínola-Nadurille M, Ramírez-Bermúdez J, Fricchione GL: Pregnancy and malignant catatonia. Gen Hosp Psychiatry 29(1):69–71, 2007 17189750
European Delirium Association; American Delirium Society: The DSM-5 criteria, level of arousal and delirium diagnosis: inclusiveness is safer. BMC Med 12:141, 2014 25300023

Focht A, Kellner CH: Electroconvulsive therapy (ECT) in the treatment of postpartum psychosis. J ECT 28(1):31–33, 2012 22330704
Friedman S, Prakash C, Nagle-Yang S: Postpartum psychosis: protecting mother and infant. Curr Psychiatr 18(4):13–21, 2019
Fujii H, Goel A, Bernard N, et al: Pregnancy outcomes following gabapentin use: results of a prospective comparative cohort study. Neurology 80(17):1565–1570, 2013 23553472
Galbally M, Snellen M, Power J: Antipsychotic drugs in pregnancy: a review of their maternal and fetal effects. Ther Adv Drug Saf 5(2):100–109, 2014 25083265
Gates DM, Ross CS, McQueen L: Violence against emergency department workers. J Emerg Med 31(3):331–337, 2006 16982376
Gold KJ, Singh V, Marcus SM, et al: Mental health, substance use and intimate partner problems among pregnant and postpartum suicide victims in the National Violent Death Reporting System. Gen Hosp Psychiatry 34(2):139–145, 2012 22055329
Gonzales N, Quinn DK, Rayburn W: Perinatal catatonia: a case report and literature review. Psychosomatics 55(6):708–714, 2014 25262045
Grigoriadis S, Wilton AS, Kurdyak PA, et al: Perinatal suicide in Ontario, Canada: a 15-year population-based study. CMAJ 189(34):E1085–E1092, 2017 28847780
Grigoriadis S, Graves L, Peer M, et al: Benzodiazepine use during pregnancy alone or in combination with an antidepressant and congenital malformations: systematic review and meta-analysis. J Clin Psychiatry 80(4):18r12412, 2019 31294935
Heberlein A, Leggio L, Stichtenoth D, et al: The treatment of alcohol and opioid dependence in pregnant women. Curr Opin Psychiatry 25(6):559–564, 2012 23037965
Hirschfeld RM, Williams JB, Spitzer RL, et al: Development and validation of a screening instrument for bipolar spectrum disorder: the Mood Disorder Questionnaire. Am J Psychiatry 157(11):1873–1875, 2000 11058490
Huybrechts KF, Hernández-Díaz S, Patorno E, et al: Antipsychotic use in pregnancy and the risk for congenital malformations. JAMA Psychiatry 73(9):938–946, 2016 27540849
Jacobs DG, Baldessarini RJ, Conwell Y, et al: Practice guideline for the assessment and treatment of patients with suicidal behaviors. APA Practice Guidelines, 2003. Available at: https://www.psychiatryonline.org/pb/assets/raw/sitewide/practice_guidelines/guidelines/suicide.pdf. Accessed January 15, 2021.
Jones I, Chandra PS, Dazzan P, et al: Bipolar disorder, affective psychosis, and schizophrenia in pregnancy and the post-partum period. Lancet 384(9956):1789–1799, 2014 25455249
Kalaitzopoulos DR, Chatzistergiou K, Amylidi AL, et al: Effect of methamphetamine hydrochloride on pregnancy outcome: a systematic review and meta-analysis. J Addict Med 12(3):220–226, 2018 29509557
Khalifeh H, Hunt IM, Appleby L, et al: Suicide in perinatal and non-perinatal women in contact with psychiatric services: 15 year findings from a U.K. national inquiry. Lancet Psychiatry 3(3):233–242, 2016 26781366
Kuczkowski KM: The effects of drug abuse on pregnancy. Curr Opin Obstet Gynecol 19(6):578–585, 2007 18007137
Kumar MA, Jain A, Dechant VE, et al: Anti-N-methyl-D-aspartate receptor encephalitis during pregnancy. Arch Neurol 67(7):884–887, 2010 20625099
Ladavac AS, Dubin WR, Ning A, Stuckeman PA: Emergency management of agitation in pregnancy. Gen Hosp Psychiatry 29(1):39–41, 2007 17189743
Lam LT: Aggression exposure and mental health among nurses. Australian e-Journal for the Advancement of Mental Health 1(2):89–100, 2002
Lewis G (ed): Saving Mothers' Lives: Reviewing Maternal Deaths to Make Motherhood Safer—2003–2005. Seventh Report on Confidential Enquiries into Maternal Deaths in the United Kingdom. London, The Confidential Enquiry into Maternal and Child Health, 2007
Li Q, Mitchell AA, Werler MM, et al: Assessment of antihistamine use in early pregnancy and birth defects. J Allergy Clin Immunol Pract 1(6):666–74.e1, 2013 24565715
Lindahl V, Pearson JL, Colpe L: Prevalence of suicidality during pregnancy and the postpartum. Arch Women Ment Health 8(2):77–87, 2005 15883651

Lindenmayer JP: The pathophysiology of agitation. J Clin Psychiatry 61(suppl 14):5–10, 2000 11154018

Llesuy JR, Medina M, Jacobson KC, et al: Catatonia under-diagnosis in the general hospital. J Neuropsychiatry Clin Neurosci 30(2):145–151, 2018 29325478

Lukens TW, Wolf SJ, Edlow JA, et al: Clinical policy: critical issues in the diagnosis and management of the adult psychiatric patient in the emergency department. Ann Emerg Med 47(1):79–99, 2006 16387222

MacDonald K, Wilson MP, Minassian A, et al: A retrospective analysis of intramuscular haloperidol and intramuscular olanzapine in the treatment of agitation in drug- and alcohol-using patients. Gen Hosp Psychiatry 32(4):443–445, 2010 20633750

Mangla K, Hoffman MC, Trumpff C, et al: Maternal self-harm deaths: an unrecognized and preventable outcome. Am J Obstet Gynecol 221(4):295–303, 2019 30849358

Moeller K: Favorable pregnancy outcomes following continual intramuscular lorazepam use in late pregnancy. Ment Health Clin 3(2):96–98, 2013

Munk-Olsen T, Laursen TM, Mendelson T, et al: Risks and predictors of readmission for a mental disorder during the postpartum period. Arch Gen Psychiatry 66(2):189–195, 2009 19188541

Nasreddine ZS, Phillips NA, Bédirian V, et al: The Montreal Cognitive Assessment, MoCA: a brief screening tool for mild cognitive impairment. J Am Geriatr Soc 53(4):695–699, 2005 15817019

Niforatos JD, Wanta JW, Shapiro AP, et al: How should I treat acute agitation in pregnancy? Cleve Clin J Med 86(4):243–247, 2019 30951449

Nordstrom K, Zun LS, Wilson MP, et al: Medical evaluation and triage of the agitated patient: consensus statement of the American Association for Emergency Psychiatry Project BETA Medical Evaluation Workgroup. West J Emerg Med 13(1):3–10, 2012 22461915

Northoff G: Catatonia and neuroleptic malignant syndrome: psychopathology and pathophysiology. J Neural Transm (Vienna) 109(12):1453–1467, 2002 12486486

Oates M: Perinatal psychiatric disorders: a leading cause of maternal morbidity and mortality. Br Med Bull 67:219–229, 2003a 14711766

Oates M: Suicide: the leading cause of maternal death. Br J Psychiatry 183:279–281, 2003b 14519602

O'Connor E, Rossom RC, Henninger M, et al: Primary care screening for and treatment of depression in pregnant and postpartum women: evidence report and systematic review for the U.S. Preventive Services Task Force. JAMA 315(4):388–406, 2016 26813212

O'Hara MW, Wisner KL: Perinatal mental illness: definition, description and aetiology. Best Pract Res Clin Obstet Gynaecol 28(1):3–12, 2014 24140480

Orsolini L, Valchera A, Vecchiotti R, et al: Suicide during perinatal period: epidemiology, risk factors, and clinical correlates. Front Psychiatry 7:138, 2016 27570512

Osborne LM: Recognizing and managing postpartum psychosis: a clinical guide for obstetric providers. Obstet Gynecol Clin North Am 45(3):455–468, 2018 30092921

Palladino CL, Singh V, Campbell J, et al: Homicide and suicide during the perinatal period: findings from the National Violent Death Reporting System. Obstet Gynecol 118(5):1056–1063, 2011 22015873

Park J, Tan J, Krzeminski S, et al: Malignant catatonia warrants early psychiatric-critical care collaborative management: two cases and literature review. Case Rep Crit Care 2017:1951965, 2017 28250995

Pasha AK, Chowdhury A, Sadiq S, et al: Substance use disorders: diagnosis and management for hospitalists. J Community Hosp Intern Med Perspect 10(2):117–126, 2020 32850046

Pekurinen V, Willman L, Virtanen M, et al: Patient aggression and the wellbeing of nurses: a cross-sectional survey study in psychiatric and non-psychiatric settings. Int J Environ Res Public Health 14(10):1245, 2017 29057802

Philbrick KL, Rummans TA: Malignant catatonia. J Neuropsychiatry Clin Neurosci 6(1):1–13, 1994 7908547

Pinna M, Manchia M, Pillai G, et al: Efficacy and safety of electroconvulsive therapy in the first trimester of pregnancy: a case of severe manic catatonia. Bipolar Disord 17(5):567–571, 2015 25854818

Pringsheim T, Gardner D, Addington D, et al: Assessment and treatment of antipsychotic-induced akathisia. Can J Psychiatry 63(11):719–729, 2018 29685069
Rasmussen SA, Mazurek MF, Rosebush PI: Catatonia: our current understanding of its diagnosis, treatment and pathophysiology. World J Psychiatry 6(4):391–398, 2016 28078203
Richmond JS, Berlin JS, Fishkind AB, et al: Verbal de-escalation of the agitated patient: consensus statement of the American Association for Emergency Psychiatry Project BETA De-escalation Workgroup. West J Emerg Med 13(1):17–25, 2012 22461917
Robertson E, Jones I, Haque S, et al: Risk of puerperal and non-puerperal recurrence of illness following bipolar affective puerperal (post-partum) psychosis. Br J Psychiatry 186:258–259, 2005 15738508
Rodriguez S, Dufendach KA, Weinreib RM: Neuroleptic malignant syndrome or catatonia? A case report. J Crit Care Med (Targu Mures) 6(3):190–193, 2020 32864466
Rodriguez-Cabezas L, Clark C: Psychiatric emergencies in pregnancy and postpartum. Clin Obstet Gynecol 61(3):615–627, 2018 29794819
Rogers JP, Pollak TA, Blackman G, David AS: Catatonia and the immune system: a review. Lancet Psychiatry 6(7):620–630, 2019 31196793
Sachs GS: A review of agitation in mental illness: burden of illness and underlying pathology. J Clin Psychiatry 67(suppl 10):5–12, 2006 16965190
Saia KA, Schiff D, Wachman EM, et al: Caring for pregnant women with opioid use disorder in the USA: expanding and improving treatment. Curr Obstet Gynecol Rep 5(3):257–263, 2016 27563497
San L, Marksteiner J, Zwanzger P, et al: State of acute agitation at psychiatric emergencies in Europe: the STAGE Study. Clin Pract Epidemiol Ment Health 12:75–86, 2016 27857778
Sienaert P, Rooseleer J, De Fruyt J: Measuring catatonia: a systematic review of rating scales. J Affect Disord 135(1–3):1–9, 2011 21420736
Smid MC, Metz TD, Gordon AJ: Stimulant use in pregnancy: an under-recognized epidemic among pregnant women. Clin Obstet Gynecol 62(1):168–184, 2019 30601144
Spinelli MG: Maternal infanticide associated with mental illness: prevention and the promise of saved lives. Am J Psychiatry 161(9):1548–1557, 2004 15337641
Spinelli MG: Postpartum psychosis: detection of risk and management. Am J Psychiatry 166(4):405–408, 2009 19339365
Spitzer RL, Kroenke K, Williams JB: Validation and utility of a self-report version of PRIME-MD: the PHQ primary care study. Primary Care Evaluation of Mental Disorders. Patient Health Questionnaire. JAMA 282(18):1737–1744, 1999 10568646
Strawn JR, Keck PE Jr, Caroff SN: Neuroleptic malignant syndrome. Am J Psychiatry 164(6):870–876, 2007 17541044
Stowell KR, Florence P, Harman HJ, et al: Psychiatric evaluation of the agitated patient: consensus statement of the American Association for Emergency Psychiatry Project Beta Psychiatric Evaluation Workgroup. West J Emerg Med 13(1):11–16, 2012 22461916
Stuart-Parrigon K, Stuart S: Perinatal depression: an update and overview. Curr Psychiatry Rep 16(9):468, 2014 25034859
Substance Abuse and Mental Health Services Administration: 2019 National Survey on Drug Use and Health: Women. Washington, DC, Substance Abuse and Mental Health Services Administration, U.S. Department of Health and Human Services, September 2020
Thornton C, Schmied V, Dennis CL, et al: Maternal deaths in NSW (2000–2006) from nonmedical causes (suicide and trauma) in the first year following birth. BioMed Res Int 2013:623743, 2013 24024205
Tinkelman A, Hill EA, Deligiannidis KM: Management of new onset psychosis in the postpartum period. J Clin Psychiatry 78(9):1423–1424, 2017 29125722
Tondo L, Vázquez G, Baldessarini RJ: Mania associated with antidepressant treatment: comprehensive meta-analytic review. Acta Psychiatr Scand 121(6):404–414, 2010 19958306
Valdimarsdóttir U, Hultman CM, Harlow B, et al: Psychotic illness in first-time mothers with no previous psychiatric hospitalizations: a population-based study. PLoS Med 6(2):e13, 2009 19209952

VanderKruik R, Barreix M, Chou D, et al: The global prevalence of postpartum psychosis: a systematic review. BMC Psychiatry 17(1):272, 2017 28754094
Vieta E, Garriga M, Cardete L, et al: Protocol for the management of psychiatric patients with psychomotor agitation. BMC Psychiatry 17(1):328, 2017 28886752
Walther S, Stegmayer K, Wilson JE, et al: Structure and neural mechanisms of catatonia. Lancet Psychiatry 6(7):610–619, 2019 31196794
Weder ND, Muralee S, Penland H, et al: Catatonia: a review. Ann Clin Psychiatry 20(2):97–107, 2008 18568581
White Kress VE: Self-injurious behaviors: assessment and diagnosis. Journal of Counseling and Development 81:490–496, 2003
Wilson MP, Pepper D, Currier GW, et al: The psychopharmacology of agitation: consensus statement of the American Association for Emergency Psychiatry Project Beta Psychopharmacology Workgroup. West J Emerg Med 13(1):26–34, 2012 22461918
Wilson MP, Nordstrom K, Shah AA, et al: Psychiatric emergencies in pregnant women. Emerg Med Clin North Am 33(4):841–851, 2015 26493527
Wisner K, Sit D, Reynolds S, et al: Mental health and behavioral disorders in pregnancy, in Obstetrics: Normal and Problem Pregnancies, 6th Edition. Edited by Gabbe S, Niebyl J, Galan H, et al. Philadelphia, PA, Elsevier Saunders, 2012, pp 1156–1188
World Health Organization: Preventing Suicide: A Global Imperative. Geneva, Switzerland, World Health Organization, 2014
Yildiz A, Sachs GS, Turgay A: Pharmacological management of agitation in emergency settings. Emerg Med J 20(4):339–346, 2003 12835344
Yoshimasu K, Kiyohara C, Miyashita K: Suicidal risk factors and completed suicide: meta-analyses based on psychological autopsy studies. Environ Health Prev Med 13(5):243–256, 2008 19568911
Zedler BK, Mann AL, Kim MM, et al: Buprenorphine compared with methadone to treat pregnant women with opioid use disorder: a systematic review and meta-analysis of safety in the mother, fetus and child. Addiction 111(12):2115–2128, 2016 27223595
Zeller SL, Rhoades RW: Systematic reviews of assessment measures and pharmacologic treatments for agitation. Clin Ther 32(3):403–425, 2010 20399981

# CHAPTER 11

# Stress in Pregnancy

## Impacts on Mother and Child

Lea Takács, Ph.D.
Vanessa Babineau, Ph.D.
Catherine Monk, Ph.D.

Research conducted over the past 30 years has demonstrated that maternal emotional stress in pregnancy is associated with somatic diseases for children in later life (Painter et al. 2012; Tamashiro and Moran 2010). Although less studied than risks related to physical health, convincing evidence exists regarding detrimental effects of prenatal stress on child neurodevelopment, behavior, and mental health (Glover 2011; Graignic-Philippe et al. 2014; Van den Bergh et al. 2017). Such effects have been found not only for maternal distress related to a psychiatric disorder but also for various types of stress that do not fall within any definable category of mental illness. More specifically, there is a distinction between prenatal stress and distress, whereby *prenatal stress* includes daily hassles, perceived stress, pregnancy-related worries, and major life events, and *prenatal distress* includes psychological symptoms and disorders such as anxiety and depression, both of which have been associated with adverse fetal and child outcomes.

The effects of prenatal stress have usually been studied under the fetal programming hypothesis, which postulates that environmental risk factors to which a fetus is exposed in utero (e.g., malnutrition) alter fetal development, exerting sustained effects on child health (Barker 1995a, 1995b). This hypothesis, also known as the Barker hypothesis or the developmental origins of health and disease (DOHaD) model (Fleming et al. 2015), suggests that the fetus adapts in reaction to environmental cues on physiological, neuroendocrine, and metabolic levels by programming or reprogramming its biological systems while they are still immature and therefore extremely malleable. Gestation is a particularly vulnerable period for brain development, and even subtle alterations in brain structure and function resulting from environmental conditions can have long-term consequences. Most studies report negative effects of prenatal exposure to maternal stress on brain–behavior development, indicating greater child susceptibility to mental health problems and disorders later in life.

Surprisingly, some studies report positive effects of prenatal stress (DiPietro et al. 2006, 2010; Kantonen et al. 2015; Lin et al. 2014; Rothenberger et al. 2011) and elevated maternal cortisol in pregnancy (Glynn and Sandman 2012) on child outcomes, suggesting that prenatal stress is not necessarily pathogenic. Several hypotheses have been proposed to explain such findings, diverging from the traditional diathesis–stress model (Zuckerman 1999) that links stress with increased vulnerability to disease. According to some authors, prenatal stress may provide more stimulation for the fetus, enhancing fetal sensitivity (and physiological and behavioral reactivity) to environmental cues and, thereby, postnatal developmental plasticity. This may be a risk factor but also an opportunity, depending on the child's postnatal environment (Hartman et al. 2018, 2019). More sensitive and reactive children may be at a higher risk of mental health problems if exposed to postnatal adversity (e.g., low parenting quality); conversely, they may benefit more from postnatal supportive environments compared with children without prenatal stress exposure (Hartman et al. 2018). Another explanation may be that the exposure to prenatal stress leads to fetal adaptations or "programmed" changes (e.g., heightened vigilance, alertness, aggressiveness, or impulsivity) that may improve children's chance for survival, preparing them for the demands of the extrauterine world. As some authors put it (Sandman et al. 2012b), it is not the stress, per se, but rather the incongruity between the pre- and postnatal environments that leads to less favorable outcomes in children who are exposed prenatally to conditions that differ from those into which they are born.

What seems to be of pivotal importance is the magnitude of prenatal stress. While reporting positive effects for moderate levels of stress, DiPietro et al. (2006) and Laplante et al. (2008) also found detrimental outcomes for high levels of stress. In addition, Hartman et al. (2020) observed that children who were exposed to the least prenatal stress were the most affected by maternal postnatal stress. It seems, therefore, that both too little and too much stress may be pathogenic, whereas moderate levels of stress might be beneficial (DiPietro 2004, 2012). Yet these results must be interpreted with caution because they may apply to specific samples only. The studies showing positive effects of prenatal stress are mostly based on data from families of higher socioeconomic and educational status (DiPietro 2012; Laplante et al. 2008). Although there may be a positive association between moderate prenatal stress and specific child outcomes, little is known about the factors modulating such association (e.g., timing and type of stress) or the direction of the effects in different developmental domains (e.g., such that better performance in one domain is accompanied by worse performance in another domain).

Despite some inconsistencies, the bulk of existing research shows a higher risk of detrimental neurodevelopmental outcomes and mental health disorders following exposure to stress in utero. As such, maternal stress in pregnancy may function as a "third pathway" of familial transmission of risk for psychiatric disorder, apart from shared genes and quality of parental care. It should, however, be emphasized that most children exposed to prenatal stress remain unaffected, and as such, the nature of this association consists in *increasing the risk* rather than causing inevitable mental health problems and disorders. Figure 11–1 summarizes the relationships between maternal stress and child outcomes.

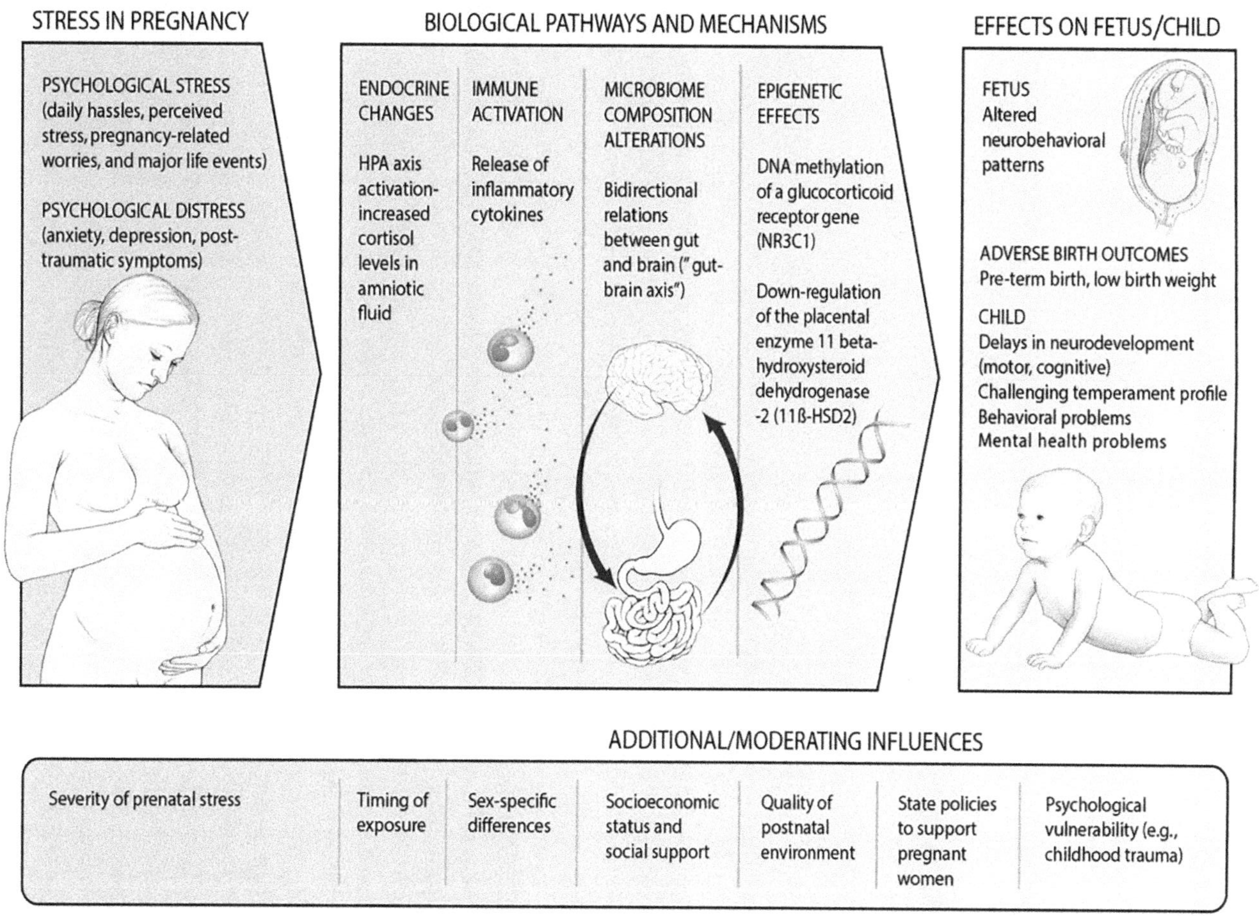


**FIGURE 11–1. The effects of stress in pregnancy on child outcomes: biological mechanisms and moderating factors.**
*Source.* Image by David Rini.

## Types of Prenatal Stress and Distress

The term *prenatal stress* refers to a wide range of different types of stress that can occur during pregnancy. These include daily hassles, such as job strain; perceived stress, such as feeling overwhelmed or out of control; pregnancy-related anxieties, such as worrying about the baby's health or fear of giving birth; and major life events, such as the death of a loved one (Class et al. 2011) or natural and manmade disasters. *Prenatal distress,* on the other hand, includes a range of psychological symptoms and disorders, such as depression and anxiety, which can be either preexisting to the pregnancy or onset during pregnancy (Table 11–1). These stresses and distresses can occur in the form of a single event, a series of events, or on a daily chronic basis in women with or without definable psychiatric illnesses (Mulder et al. 2002). Although we can make distinctions among different types of prenatal stress and distress, it remains unclear whether these distinctions coincide with differential effects on fetal and child outcomes (Monk et al. 2018). Nevertheless, they provide meaningful insights for treatment, and potential differences in outcomes continue to be investigated.

Distinctions among different types of prenatal stress and distress can be made based on prevalence, because their estimated prevalence varies depending on the type of stress or distress being considered (Monk et al. 2019b; Van den Bergh et al. 2017; Ward et al. 2017). During pregnancy, 8%–12% of women are estimated to meet diagnostic criteria for major depressive disorder (Melville et al. 2010), a rate that doubles in low-income and socioeconomically disadvantaged samples (Fisher et al. 2012). Similarly, 13% of pregnant women are estimated to meet criteria for an anxiety disorder (Vesga-López et al. 2008). These estimates increase when symptoms are self-reported. For instance, Loomans et al. (2013) found that 30% of women self-report high levels of concurrent depression and state anxiety during pregnancy. Loomans et al. (2013) additionally found that up to 52% of pregnant women experience daily stress, such as job strain, during pregnancy and 9% experience pregnancy-related anxiety, although neither of these identified groups report high levels of depression or state anxiety. Depression and anxiety are the most common mental health disorders during pregnancy, and other common nonpsychotic disorders include PTSD and personality disorders, with estimated prevalence rates of 6%–8% and 6%, respectively (Howard et al. 2014).

Although distinct, the different types of stress and distress are often correlated. For example, depression and anxiety are often comorbid during the prenatal period, and women who are depressed during pregnancy are more likely to meet criteria for an anxiety disorder than those who are not (Dindo et al. 2017). Additionally, women who have experienced a trauma prior to being pregnant are nearly five times more likely to be depressed in pregnancy than women without a trauma history (Seng et al. 2010). Even trauma that occurs as far back as childhood is associated with increased symptoms of both depression and anxiety during pregnancy (Letourneau et al. 2019). Comorbid prenatal stresses can thus be considered not only in terms of additive but also interactive effects, whereby one type of preexisting stress can enhance the likelihood of risk for another type of stress. The proper identification of different prenatal stresses and their comorbidities has the potential to lead toward more precise treatment, as opposed to treatment that fails to recognize comorbidities and thus alleviates distress only partially (Dindo et al. 2017).

TABLE 11–1. **Types of prenatal stress and distress and their estimated prevalence**

| Prenatal stress (estimated prevalence) | Prenatal distress (estimated prevalence) |
|---|---|
| Stressful life events (63%) | Prenatal anxiety (13%) |
| Daily hassles (52%) | Prenatal depression (8%–12%) |
| Pregnancy-related anxieties (9%) | PTSD (6%–8%) |
| Perceived stress (8%–11%) | Personality disorders (6%) |
| Severe life events (1%) | |

# Fetal and Child Outcomes

## Prenatal Stress and Fetal Neurobehavior

Research focusing on the effects of prenatal stress on fetal neurobehavior most frequently examines two indicators of fetal response to stress: motor activity and heart rate/heart rate variability (HRV) or reactivity. In general, studies investigate either the effects of maternal chronic stress (sometimes depression or anxiety) or the effects of stress that was induced experimentally.

Maternal chronic stress in pregnancy has been linked to a higher fetal activity and heart rate. For example, DiPietro et al. (2002) found that the fetuses of stressed mothers were more active across gestation compared with those whose mothers showed more positive emotionality. In line with this finding, Dieter et al. (2001) reported increased fetal activity in depressed mothers. In another study, DiPietro et al. (2010) observed no association between maternal trait anxiety and fetal motor activity or heart rate, but they did find a link between higher maternal pregnancy-specific stress and marginally higher motor activity, increased coupling of fetal motor activity and heart rate, and higher fetal HRV. Higher HRV is typically considered a mark of better emotion regulation (Sloan et al. 2017) and may be regarded as an index of more advanced CNS maturation. A recent study (Walsh et al. 2019) reported lower coupling of fetal motor activity and heart rate in physically stressed pregnant women (i.e., women with physical indicators of stress, such as higher average blood pressure), but not in those with psychological stress. However, Monk et al. (2016) found an indirect effect of high perceived stress in pregnancy on lower fetal coupling through placental DNA methylation.

Because the literature on fetal responses to maternal stress is variable, researchers have focused on the effects of experimentally induced stress to measure these effects more directly. Using the Stroop color-word task in a series of studies, Monk et al. (2000, 2003, 2004, 2011) found significant increases in fetal heart rate in response to the stressor in a group of mothers with psychological vulnerability (anxiety and depression) but not in those without such vulnerability. DiPietro et al. (2003) reported no changes in fetal heart rate using the same method to induce mild stress in pregnant women, but their results were based on a general sample of mothers regardless of psychological vulnerability. Other studies employed direct stimulation of the fetus. For example, Makino et al. (2009) observed that fetuses showed a different heart rate pattern in response to vibroacoustic stimulation depending on maternal trait anxiety scores. Fetuses of mothers from a high trait anxiety scores group displayed a biphasic response pattern characterized by acceleration followed by deceleration, whereas the response of fetuses from mothers with low trait anxiety scores consisted of a single long period of acceleration, one acceleration lasting >1 minute, or at least two accelerations lasting >15 seconds. Maternal psychological status thus seems to be of crucial importance, modulating fetal reactivity to stress possibly as a consequence of shaping fetal development over gestation. Moreover, different types of psychological vulnerability may elicit differential fetal response. Reissland et al. (2018) reported that anxiety was associated with an increased fetal response (eye-blink reactions), whereas depression was associated with a decreased fetal response to sound and light stimulation.

Taken together, maternal psychological status—chronic mood or distress—in pregnancy affects fetal neurobehavior and reactivity to stressful stimuli. Both chronic and acute stress elicit fetal response characterized mostly by higher intensity of motor activity and heart rate. Some authors suggest that this is not necessarily a developmental disadvantage; higher fetal motor activity has been linked with more optimal motor maturation and development (DiPietro et al. 2010). It is, however, too early to draw final conclusions in this regard because the results of previous studies are ambiguous—prenatal stress has also been associated with delayed fetal maturation (Sandman et al. 2012a).

## Prenatal Stress and Birth Outcomes

According to the fetal programming hypothesis, the prenatal environment is of crucial importance to health throughout the lifespan (Barker 1995b). Originally, birth weight was considered a proxy for the quality of environment in utero (Barker 1990). Indeed, low birth weight and other unfavorable birth outcomes, such as preterm birth, have been linked with various prenatal factors, including maternal stress, as exemplified in several studies (Copper et al. 1996; Lima et al. 2018; Wadhwa et al. 1993).

However, the assertion that prenatal stress results in unfavorable birth outcomes is not without controversy. In his seminal work, Istvan (1986) suggested that although there is sound evidence of the negative effects of stress on birth outcomes in animal research, the results for humans remain inconsistent and unconvincing due to methodological study limitations. Those limitations include retrospective assessment of stress in pregnancy or failure to account for important confounders, such as biomedical factors that increase obstetrical risks (e.g., hypertension in pregnancy, preeclampsia). A later meta-analysis supported this line of reasoning by concluding that there is no evidence for the association between general or pregnancy-specific anxiety and detrimental birth outcomes and that the significant associations that have been found were primarily in studies with lower-quality methodology (Littleton et al. 2007). A meta-analysis conducted by the same research team several years later reported that the association between prenatal psychosocial stress and low birth weight was in fact significant but very small (Littleton et al. 2010). Finally, a meta-analysis that was limited to prospective studies published from 1970 to 2012 (Bussières et al. 2015) substantiated the association between prenatal stress and low birth weight and preterm birth, with findings specific to different types of stress: pregnancy-related anxiety and stress yielded a stronger association than general stress, life events, or natural disasters. Nevertheless, the results of the studies remain conflicting. For example, a recent study distinguishing different prenatal stress phenotypes (i.e., mental health or mood symptoms and physical indicators of stress) found that women showing physical but not psychological indicators of stress had increased risk of preterm birth compared with the healthy group (Walsh et al. 2019).

# Prenatal Stress and Child Neurodevelopment and Psychopathology

## State Regulation, Stress Reactivity, and Temperament

Several studies have shown that infants of mothers who had depressive symptoms in pregnancy have poorer regulation of behavioral states, autonomic stability, and neurobehavioral maturity in the first days of the postpartum period (Figueiredo et al. 2017; Gerardin et al. 2011; Pacheco and Figueiredo 2012). The child's stress reactivity is another frequently studied outcome in the context of prenatal stress, exposure to which has been linked with altered child's hypothalamic-pituitary-adrenal (HPA) axis functioning. However, the direction of this effect is inconsistent and has been shown to vary depending on the type of stress, with different types eliciting blunted or increased HPA axis reactivity. For example, Romero-Gonzalez et al. (2018) found that maternal perceived stress in pregnancy predicted lower cortisol but that pregnancy-specific stress predicted higher cortisol in neonates. Measuring cortisol and cortisone in the first morning urine of 45-month-old children, Send et al. (2019) found a lower nocturnal rate of cortisol and cortisone in children who had been exposed to prenatal stress. In a similar study, children age 6 years had higher hair cortisone, but not cortisol, levels detected in association with prenatal stress (Molenaar et al. 2019). Cortisone is a metabolite of cortisol, with the enzyme 11β hydroxysteroid dehydrogenase type 2 (11β-HSD2) converting cortisol to cortisone in the peripheral tissues. Measuring cortisone in addition to cortisol may thus provide a more complete picture of the cumulative amount of active and inactive corticosteroids (Molenaar et al. 2019).

Prenatal stress has been linked with more difficult child temperament and negative emotionality, but this association appears to be modulated by child sex and by the type and timing of stress. For example, Simcock et al. (2017a) found that higher levels of objective hardship related to a flood disaster (Queensland Flood in 2011) during pregnancy were associated with more irritable temperament in boys but not in girls at age 6 months; moreover, the mothers with higher emotional response to the flood reported more active-reactive infants. Laplante et al. (2016), too, assessed the effects of disaster-related prenatal stress on infant temperament 6 months postpartum and observed poorer temperament in children exposed to higher maternal stress in utero.

Examining the differential effects of various types of prenatal stress on infant temperament at 3 months of age, Chong et al. (2016) demonstrated evidence for the effects of anxiety (both state and trait) on infants' negative emotionality and poor attention regulation but found no effects of prenatal depression. Similarly, Nolvi et al. (2016) attempted to disentangle the effects of prenatal depression, anxiety, and pregnancy-specific anxiety on infant emotional reactivity at 6 months postpartum and concluded that only pregnancy-specific anxiety predicted infant reactivity (more specifically, overall negative emotional reactivity and its aspects fearfulness and falling reactivity). In a study by Austin et al. (2005b), only trait anxiety—not depression or perceived stress in pregnancy—predicted "difficult" infant temperament.

Overall, it appears that maternal anxiety is a much stronger predictor of infants' traits associated with temperament than is maternal depression, although depressive symptoms in pregnancy were found to be associated with higher activity/impulsivity and sleep problems in young children (Gerardin et al. 2011). Nevertheless, most studies on the effects of prenatal distress on child temperament used parent-report questionnaires, which makes it impossible to disentangle child behavior from maternal perceptions of it that may be biased by maternal psychological status. As for the timing of stress, Sandman et al. (2012a) observed the strongest association between stress and impaired emotion regulation in infants if the stress occurred early in gestation, but research to date is insufficient to draw final conclusions about the effects of timing of prenatal stress on child reactivity and regulation.

## Motor Development

Studies about the effects of prenatal stress focus frequently on motor development in infancy because it is strongly predictive of later outcomes across different developmental domains. Substantial evidence shows that prenatal stress, such as depressive symptoms or stressful life events, predicts poorer motor skills and delayed motor development in young children (Cao et al. 2014; Gerardin et al. 2011; Lin et al. 2017; Moss et al. 2017) despite several positive or null findings. For example, Simcock et al. (2016) found better motor development outcomes in 2-month-old infants whose mothers were exposed to a flood during pregnancy, but this effect changed with increasing child age, such that prenatal exposure to a flood predicted delayed motor development in the children at 6 and 16 months of age. Sandman et al. (2012b) found positive effects of prenatal depressive symptoms on motor development in the first postpartum year, but only in infants whose mothers had experienced congruent levels of depressive symptoms in pregnancy and postpartum. This was true even for children of mothers with relatively high levels of pre- and postpartum depression. Nevertheless, Koutra et al. (2013) found no association between prenatal stress and motor development in young children.

The effect of prenatal stress on motor development appears to be stronger if the exposure occurs in late pregnancy (Cao et al. 2014; Grace et al. 2016; Moss et al. 2017; Simcock et al. 2016). Additionally, differential effects according to the type of stress have also been found. For example, Simcock et al. (2016) observed that delayed motor development was associated with exposure to a flood in utero but not with maternal traumatic stress symptoms related to the flood. In contrast, Moss et al. (2017) found a negative effect of disaster-related stress on motor development in 16-month-old children, but only for negative maternal appraisal of the overall flood consequences and not due to the flood exposure per se. Effects on motor development are documented beyond the period of early childhood. Grace et al. (2016), following children until adolescence, evidenced suboptimal neuromuscular development at ages 10, 14, and 17 years in children whose mothers experienced a higher number of stressful life events in late pregnancy. However, stressful events occurring earlier in pregnancy were not associated with child's later motor outcomes in this study.

## Cognitive Development

Prenatal maternal stress is also associated with adverse outcomes in cognitive development domains, including word comprehension, nonverbal cognitive tasks (Henrichs et al. 2011), language development (King et al. 2012), problem solving (Simcock et al. 2017b), IQ, working memory (Evans et al. 2012), and performance in math tasks (Pearson et al. 2016). A meta-analysis by Tarabulsy et al. (2014) detected a significant association, albeit with a small effect size, between prenatal stress and cognitive development, with a larger effect documented in studies assessing prenatal stress retrospectively. Moreover, they found that studies with objective indicators of prenatal stress (e.g., objective severity of a natural disaster or a number of stressful events) reported greater effect sizes as compared with those examining subjective indicators (e.g., perceived stress, pregnancy-related stress or anxiety). This conclusion is also supported by other research groups (Moss et al. 2017; Simcock et al. 2017b).

Differential effects were found for depressive symptoms, anxiety, and pregnancy-related anxiety. For example, Koutra et al. (2013) found detrimental effects of depressive symptoms, but not of anxiety, on child cognitive performance. Depression was associated with lower IQ score in children 8 years of age (Evans et al. 2012), whereas anxiety was associated with impaired working memory in children of the same age in another study (Pearson et al. 2016). Buss et al. (2011) observed that lower visuospatial working memory in children ages 6–9 years was related to pregnancy-related anxiety; neither state anxiety nor depression explained any additional variance.

The effects of prenatal stress on child cognition appear to be more severe for girls than for boys. Investigating the association between perceived stress during pregnancy and infant cognition at the age of 4.5 months, Merced-Nieves et al. (2020) observed that maternal stress is associated with delayed development of physical reasoning, but this effect was only true for girls and not for boys. Li et al. (2013) also observed sex-specific effects at 10 years of age in association with maternal life stress events (e.g., job loss, residential move) in pregnancy, finding that prenatal exposure to stress was associated with lower reading scores in girls but with higher reading and math scores in boys. Simcock et al. (2017b) reported that at high levels of maternal subjective flood-related stress in pregnancy, girls had lower scores on the problem-solving domain than boys at 6 months of age. In addition, Buss et al. (2011) found that pregnancy-specific anxiety was associated with lower inhibitory control in girls only at ages 6–9 years. However, King et al. (2012) found adverse effects of a natural disaster (Quebec Ice Storm of 1998) during pregnancy on boys but not girls in terms of their IQ scores at 11 years of age.

Similar to the motor development domain, the timing of the stress exposure may be decisive for the severity of outcomes in the cognitive domain. However, although late pregnancy has been found to be a critical period for motor development, the effects on cognitive performance appear to be stronger if stress occurs early in gestation (Sandman et al. 2012a). Moreover, the intensity of prenatal stress appears to alter cognitive outcomes. Laplante et al. (2008) found a curvilinear and not a linear relation between prenatal stress and cognitive and language abilities in preschoolers, indicating that high levels of prenatal stress are related to less optimal performance in children, whereas moderate levels of stress may enhance it.

Although evidence links prenatal stress with less optimal cognitive development, study results have been mixed, with some authors reporting no association (Karam et al. 2016) and others reporting positive effects (Li et al. 2013). Importantly, studies that accounted for maternal IQ observed that the significant association between prenatal stress and child cognitive outcomes does not persist after taking this additional factor into consideration (Van den Bergh et al. 2017). Thus, despite evidence for this association, further research is needed to draw firm conclusions. Table 11–2 summarizes the relationship between stress and several neurodevelopmental outcomes.

TABLE 11–2. **Effects of prenatal stress on fetal and child behavior and neurodevelopment**

| Domain | Specific outcomes | Type of distress and timing |
|---|---|---|
| Fetal neurobehavior | ↑ Motor activity | Chronic stress, depression |
| | ↑ Heart rate reactivity | Experimentally induced stress in psychologically vulnerable women |
| | ↑ Heart rate variability | Pregnancy-specific stress |
| | ↑ ↓ Coupling of fetal motor activity and heart rate | Pregnancy-specific stress, perceived stress |
| Child temperament | ↑ Negative emotionality | Maternal anxiety appears to have greater effect than depression |
| | ↓ Emotion/attention regulation | No conclusive evidence regarding timing |
| | ↑ Emotional reactivity | |
| | ↑ Temperamental "difficulty" | |
| Child neurodevelopment | ↓ Motor development | Exerts stronger effects if occurs in late pregnancy |
| | | Findings about effects of different types are conflicting |
| | ↓ Cognitive development | Objective indicators (e.g., objective severity of a natural disaster) have greater effect than subjective indicators |
| | | Stronger effects if occurs in early pregnancy |

## Mental Health

Accumulating evidence shows an association between maternal distress in pregnancy and offspring mental health problems (Table 11–3), particularly internalizing (emotional) and externalizing (behavioral) symptoms (Cents et al. 2013; Hentges et al. 2019; Lahti et al. 2017; Leis et al. 2014; Loomans et al. 2011; O'Donnell et al. 2014; Pickles et al. 2017; Robinson et al. 2008, 2011; Tearne et al. 2015). Internalizing and externalizing behaviors have been found to be predicted by different types of stressful events, both those beyond mother's control (e.g., death of a relative) and those at least partly within her control (e.g., marital problems) (Robinson et al. 2011) and have been linked to prenatal depressive symptoms, anxiety (Cents et al. 2013; Lahti et al. 2017; Leis et al. 2014; Loomans et al. 2011; O'Donnell et al. 2014), and pregnancy-specific anxiety (Pickles et al. 2017).

There are, however, some discrepancies in the current research on the effects of maternal prenatal distress on externalizing and internalizing behaviors in offspring. For example, Korhonen et al. (2014) observed that prenatal depression was associated with externalizing but not internalizing problems in adolescents, whereas Betts et al. (2014) found the opposite. In addition, a study assessing the effects of natural disaster–related stress found that internalizing problems in young children were linked to maternal objective flood-related hardship (e.g., financial loss related to the disaster) rather than to stress experienced in response to the flood (McLean et al. 2019). How-

**TABLE 11–3. Effects of prenatal stress on offspring mental health**

| Mental health domain | Types of maternal prenatal distress associated with offspring mental health outcomes |
|---|---|
| ADHD | Stressful life events; major life events (bereavement); anxiety |
| Anxiety | Perceived stress, depressive symptoms, anxiety, pregnancy-related anxiety, exposure to a natural disaster |
| Autism | Stressful life events; major life events (bereavement) |
| Borderline personality disorder | Anxiety, depression |
| Conduct disorder | Anxiety; stressful life events |
| Depressive symptoms | Perceived stress, stressful life events, depression, anxiety |
| Eating disorders | Exposure to a natural disaster |
| Internalizing and externalizing problems | Stressful events, depression, anxiety, pregnancy-specific anxiety, exposure to a natural disaster |
| Schizophrenia | Daily life stress, but results of studies are mixed |

ever, in a similar study, maternal subjective distress in response to the storm exposure, rather than the exposure itself, predicted both internalizing and externalizing problems in children (King et al. 2012). Nevertheless, it can be difficult to distinguish prenatal from postnatal effects; Velders et al. (2011) found that parental postnatal psychological functioning, rather than prenatal depressive symptoms, was associated with child emotional and behavioral problems.

Interestingly, no differences in the effects of prenatal stress with respect to the time of exposure were observed in the study by Robinson et al. (2011); effects on child behavioral problems due to exposure to stressful life events in the first 18 weeks of pregnancy were similar to those of exposure at 34 weeks of gestation. Similarly, Lahti et al. (2017) found no effect of timing of maternal depression across pregnancy on child behavioral problems. However, they did find an effect of depression severity, whereby the most detrimental outcomes were detected in children whose mothers had shown clinically significant levels of depressive symptoms during pregnancy.

The effects of prenatal stress on emotional and behavioral problems may persist from infancy to adolescence and into adulthood. These childhood outcomes have been reported in children ages 3–5 years (Cents et al. 2013; King et al. 2012; Loomans et al. 2011; O'Donnell et al. 2014; Pickles et al. 2017), 6–9 years (King et al. 2012; O'Donnell et al. 2014), 10–11 years (King et al. 2012; Leis et al. 2014; O'Donnell et al. 2014), 12–13 years (O'Donnell et al. 2014), 14 years (Betts et al. 2014), 16 years (Korhonen et al. 2014), and 21 years (Betts et al. 2014).

Prenatal stress has also been linked with childhood anxiety. In one study, prenatal depression was associated with higher scores on a generalized anxiety scale in 1-year-old infants (Gerardin et al. 2011). Similar results were found in another study where maternal exposure to flood in pregnancy predicted anxiety in 4-year-old children; however, objective flood-related hardship, rather than subjective distress, predicted childhood anxiety (McLean et al. 2019). Evidence suggests that the effects of prenatal distress (e.g., perceived stress, depressive symptoms, anxiety, pregnancy-related anxiety) on anxiety symptoms in offspring may extend to preadolescence (Davis and Sandman 2012) and even into adulthood (Capron et al. 2015).

Children exposed to prenatal stress also appear to be at an increased risk for symptoms of depression, which were observed at different ages throughout childhood. For example, prenatal stress has been associated with depressive symptoms at 12 years of age (Davis et al. 2020), and stressful life events in early pregnancy have been linked with high levels of depressive symptoms in children 10–19 years of age (Kingsbury et al. 2016). Maternal prenatal anxiety and depression have been found to be associated with an increased risk of depression in the offspring up to 18 years of age (Capron et al. 2015; Pearson et al. 2013).

Evidence also suggests that prenatal stress might play a role in the development of autism (Class et al. 2014; Rijlaarsdam et al. 2017; Ronald et al. 2011), particularly in boys. For instance, Ronald et al. (2011) found that stressful events in pregnancy, such as divorce or a residential move, predicted autistic traits in boys but not girls at the age of 2 years. The timing of prenatal stress may modulate the effects on autism, as evidenced in one study that showed a higher risk of autism following maternal bereavement specifically in the third trimester of pregnancy (Class et al. 2014). Nevertheless, the association between prenatal stress and autism is ambiguously supported; for example, a study by Rai et al. (2012), based on data from two large population studies, found no link between major life events in pregnancy and autism.

Similarly, the risk for ADHD related to prenatal stress exposure has also been reported to be higher in males than in females (Li et al. 2010; Loomans et al. 2011). However, not all studies documenting the association between prenatal stress and ADHD have found sex-specific results (Class et al. 2014; Ronald et al. 2011). Additionally, Class et al. (2014) reported a greater risk for ADHD in children who were exposed to stress specifically in late pregnancy.

Prenatal distress has also been found to enhance the risk of conduct disorder (Glasheen et al. 2013; MacKinnon et al. 2018), an association that has also been shown to be particularly pronounced in boys (Glasheen et al. 2013). Other mental health outcomes linked with prenatal distress exposure include eating disorders (St-Hilaire et al. 2015), borderline personality disorder (Winsper et al. 2015), and psychosis (Fineberg et al. 2016). Moreover, the risk for schizophrenia related to prenatal stress exposure also appears to be higher in male offspring (Fineberg et al. 2016). Nevertheless, in a review of prenatal stress effects on a risk of schizophrenia (Lipner et al. 2019), the authors concluded that the results of studies are mixed and that the question of whether specific types of prenatal stress or timing of exposure have differential effects remains unresolved.

## Biological Mechanisms

The DOHaD hypothesis contends that maternal stress in pregnancy can affect the developing fetus through stress-based alterations in maternal biology, with potentially long-lasting implications for the offspring's health. However, some doubts have been expressed regarding the causality of such associations. For example, women who experience stress during pregnancy are more likely to be living in poverty, which represents an environmental factor that is directly linked with child outcomes (Lefmann and Combs-Orme 2014). They might also smoke or drink alcohol more frequently and lack an appropriate diet and adequate physical activity (Goodwin et al. 2017; Hurley et al. 2005; Schetter and Glynn 2011). Moreover, pregnant women who are stressed are more likely to also be stressed in the postpartum period (Field 2011; Lin et al. 2017), which might, in turn, lead to less favorable parenting practices (Huizink et al. 2017; Schechter et al. 2017) and difficulties in bonding (Figueiredo and Costa 2009). In fact, maternal stress in pregnancy is related to several factors that are linked with child outcomes; thus, the effects of stress are difficult to disentangle from those of other related factors. In addition, it is reasonable to expect that mothers who appraise their pregnancy period as being more stressful have specific genetic predispositions that may be passed onto their children.

It can thus be difficult to determine whether direct biological mechanisms connect maternal prenatal stress and child psychopathology in addition to indirect pathways, such as behavioral, and shared genetic factors (Glover 2019). Is it indeed biological fetal programming that mediates, at least partially, the association between prenatal stress and offspring psychopathology? Based on results from animal studies, this question can be answered affirmatively. Animal research provides strong evidence that offspring exposed prenatally to maternal stress are affected in several ways, including changes in HPA axis activity (Maccari et al. 1995), functional and structural alterations of the brain (Adrover et al. 2015; Charil et al. 2010; Coe et al. 2003), epigenetic changes (Jensen Peña et al. 2012; Weaver et al. 2004), and alterations in gut microbiota (Bailey et al. 2004), all of which also relate to variations in behavioral outcomes, such as increased fear behavior and distractibility or reduced sociability (Austin et al. 2005a).

Moreover, studies with human subjects have shown that stress experienced by mothers during pregnancy holds a stronger association with child outcomes than stress experienced by fathers during the same period, which implies that the effects of prenatal stress cannot be attributed solely to shared genes (Capron et al. 2015). Although the biological pathways suggested in animal research may also apply to humans, there are considerable differences between humans and animals on physiological and neuroendocrine levels (Glover et al. 2010). Overall, the mechanisms by which prenatal stress may affect human offspring are emerging, and research has explored several systems that could be involved.

One frequently studied domain is HPA axis functioning. The end product of the HPA axis—that is, the stress hormone cortisol—has been hypothesized as a leading agent in the association between prenatal stress exposure and child outcomes. It has been assumed that maternal stress results in increased cortisol levels that, in turn, lead to a higher fetal exposure to cortisol, affecting the development of the fetal and child nervous system (Davis et al. 2017; Graham et al. 2019). Indeed, higher cortisol levels in amniotic fluid have been found to predict lower scores in cognitive development in 17-month-old infants (Bergman et al. 2010). Higher maternal cortisol levels have also been associated with decrements in child cognitive performance at 7 years of age (LeWinn et al. 2009).

However, the results of the studies are conflicting, reporting both positive and negative effects of fetal exposure to higher cortisol levels. For instance, higher levels of maternal cortisol in late pregnancy have been shown to enhance fetal neurodevelopment (Glynn and Sandman 2012) and cognitive development in infancy and middle childhood (Davis and Sandman 2010; Davis et al. 2017). Making matters even more complex, maternal cortisol levels do not always correspond to maternal levels of perceived distress, which is especially true later in pregnancy, where there is often a weak or no association between perceived stress and cortisol levels (Davis et al. 2011; Voegtline et al. 2013; Werner et al. 2013).

Given the lack of association between maternal perceived stress and cortisol levels in late pregnancy, it is unlikely that the effects of maternal stress in pregnancy on child outcomes can be explained primarily by an increase in maternal cortisol levels. Therefore, other pathways have been investigated, including downregulation of the placental enzyme 11β-HSD2 (Bowers and Yehuda 2016; Monk et al. 2016; O'Donnell et al. 2012; Togher et al. 2017). 11β-HSD2 converts cortisol to an inactive form (i.e., cortisone), thus regulating the degree of maternal cortisol passing through the placenta to the fetal compartment. When this enzyme is downregulated, possibly through epigenetic changes on gene regulation (Seth et al. 2015), the fetus may become exposed to higher levels of cortisol without increases in maternal levels. Indeed, Glover et al. (2009) observed that the association between maternal and amniotic fluid cortisol varies based on maternal anxiety status, with a stronger association occurring among more anxious pregnant women. For all women, levels of 11β-HSD2 decrease during the third trimester to enable a higher proportion of maternal cortisol to circulate in the placenta, a process that is necessary for fetal lung maturation and preparation for birth; however, if maternal cortisol levels have been high for a longer period, the fetus becomes exposed to atypical cortisol levels, with a potential programming effect on its development and health (DeSocio 2018). Monk et al. (2016) observed the association between greater maternal stress and higher placental DNA methylation of *HSD11B2*, which, in turn, was linked with lower coupling of fetal movements and heart rate, an indicator of less mature CNS development.

Prenatal stress has been associated with other epigenetic changes. The most frequently studied epigenetic mechanism is DNA methylation, consisting of the addition of methyl groups to the promoter region of genes. Since the HPA axis is considered the main regulator of the stress response, research in this area has focused on the association between prenatal stress and methylation of a glucocorticoid receptor gene (*NR3C1*). Methylation of this gene prevents the expression of the glucocorticoid receptors in the hippocampus, resulting in suppression of negative feedback that turns down HPA axis activity when cortisol levels are too high for an extended period (DeSocio 2018). Variation in *NR3C1* regulation has been studied in the placenta as an indicator of variation in cortisol that may reach the fetus; it has also been studied in other samples thought to be representative of children's biology.

Conradt et al. (2013) reported that maternal depression was related to greater placental DNA methylation of *NR3C1*, which in turn predicted lower self-regulation and higher hypotonia and lethargy in infants. Also, maternal emotional distress during pregnancy was linked with methylation of *NR3C1* in cord blood (Harris and Seckl 2011; Hompes et al. 2013), and changes in *NR3C1* methylation have been associated with a higher risk of psychopathology (Dadds et al. 2015; Tyrka et al. 2016). Investigating the effects of intimate partner violence during pregnancy on *NR3C1* methylation, Radtke et al. (2011) found no effect on methylation in the mothers but did find an effect in their adolescent children. The link between maternal distress and offspring methylation of *NR3C1* is further supported by a meta-analytic study by Palma-Gudiel et al. (2015), which reported a significant correlation between stress in pregnancy and methylation levels at a CpG site located at the *NR3C1* promoter. Regulation of other genes also seems to be involved in the association between maternal prenatal distress and child behavior (Cao-Lei et al. 2017).

Maternal immune response might also be a pathway by which maternal prenatal stress exerts its effects on the fetus. Research has indicated that not only infection but also maternal psychosocial stress elicits a release of the proinflammatory cytokines. More specifically, depressive symptoms in pregnant women have been found to be associated with higher levels of circulating proinflammatory cytokines interleukin (IL)-6 and IL-15, tumor necrosis factor (TNF)-α, and C-C motif chemokine 3 (CCL3) (Christian et al. 2009; Osborne et al. 2019). Another study reported higher levels of IL-1β and IL-6 in association with stress in pregnant women (Coussons-Read et al. 2007). Maternal infections during pregnancy have been linked with neuropsychiatric disease in offspring later in life (Brown 2011), yet the evidence for the mediating role of maternal cytokines is still emerging. Existing studies are mostly based on animal models, and those conducted in humans have shown no effect of most of the proinflammatory maternal cytokines on the offspring's psychopathology; positive associations have been found between specific maternal cytokines (e.g., TNF-α or IL-8) and neuropsychiatric disease in the offspring, but they have not always been successfully replicated in other studies (Rakers et al. 2017).

Nevertheless, recent research has suggested an association between maternal cytokines (IL-6) and infant brain changes and cognitive development. Spann et al. (2018) observed an association between maternal IL-6 levels in pregnancy and resting state functional connectivity in newborn brain and toddler cognitive outcomes, suggesting that maternal immune activation in pregnancy influences the human nervous system in both the short and long term (Spann et al. 2018). In addition, Graham et al. (2018) found that above-average concentrations of maternal proinflammatory cytokine IL-6 during pregnancy is associated with larger newborn right amygdala volume and stronger left amygdala connectivity in the newborn, which are in turn associated with lower impulse control at 2 years of age.

A promising area of research is the role of the microbiome in prenatal stress programming. Altered gut microbiota composition has been linked with metabolic and immune disorders and with brain development and behavior (O'Mahony et al. 2017). Recognizing this association has led to establishing the so-called gut-brain axis (Bercik et al. 2012). Communication between gut microbiota and the brain appears to be bidirectional, such that the brain exerts influence on gut microbiota, and the gut microbiota affects neurodevelopment (de Weerth 2017).

Distress and anxiety experienced in pregnancy have been associated with changes in the composition of the maternal intestinal and vaginal microbiome (Gur et al. 2017; Hechler et al. 2019; Jašarevic et al. 2015), suggesting that the microbiome might be a link between prenatal stress and neurodevelopment (Gur et al. 2015). Although offspring gut colonization has long been thought to commence during birth by passage through the birth canal and to develop with subsequent breastfeeding, the "sterility of the uterus" dogma has been challenged by several studies, indicating that offspring gut microbiome colonization may occur in utero. Nevertheless, studies are only beginning to investigate the intrauterine transmission of microbes from mother to fetus resulting in fetal colonization (Chong et al. 2018).

## Additional/Moderating Influences

The inconsistency in research findings indicates that exploration of moderating factors that buffer or exacerbate the effects of prenatal stress on fetal and child outcomes is paramount. As previously mentioned, the intensity of prenatal stress may modulate its effects on offspring, with some authors suggesting that moderate levels of stress might even be beneficial and others showing that the opposite is true for high levels of prenatal stress (DiPietro et al. 2006; Laplante et al. 2008). Nevertheless, researchers have indicated that these positive effects, such as advanced maturation and resilience to stress in later life, do not come without cost, because prenatal stress is associated with alterations in brain development (Van den Bergh et al. 2017). Moreover, it may be the case that the potential benefits of prenatal stress only manifest under specific circumstances, such as a supportive postnatal environment and high-quality parental care (Hartman et al. 2018).

Although the timing of prenatal stress may also play a role, to date research has not identified a particular period more vulnerable to stress. It is more likely that the effects of stress differ depending on the gestational period in which the exposure occurs, concurring with sensitive windows for the development of specific brain regions (Van den Bergh et al. 2017). For example, first- and second-trimester exposure has been associated with effects on cognitive development, and the first trimester of pregnancy has been linked with behavioral problems (Van den Bergh et al. 2017). Further research is needed to corroborate these initial findings about specific effects of stress at specific gestational ages.

The term *prenatal distress* covers various types of stress whose effects need to be disentangled despite their intercorrelation. For example, depression and anxiety are often comorbid, but they may have differential effects on the developing child. As indicated, several authors have reported that anxiety, not prenatal depression, is associated with temperamental features in infants (Austin et al. 2005b; Chong et al. 2016). Nolvi et al. (2016) identified only pregnancy-related anxiety (and not general anxiety or depression) as being related to infant temperament. On the other hand, suboptimal cognitive functioning has been associated with prenatal depression but not anxiety (Koutra et al. 2013). Research has also shown the differences between the effects of natural disasters (i.e., objective hardship due to exposure to the event) and their subjective appraisal, demonstrating that their effects often diverge and that they may exert differential effects for specific child outcomes. For example, McLean et al. (2019) observed that internalizing problems were associated with objective disaster-related hardship, whereas Moss et al. (2017) found that only maternal subjective distress, and not objective hardship related to the flood, was directly associated with delays in child motor development.

Moreover, sex-specific differences in the effects of prenatal stress imply that child sex may modify prenatal programming. In their review, Sutherland and Brunwasser (2018) reported that sex-dependent results were found primarily in studies evaluating the impact of prenatal stress on nervous system development and temperament. Girls were found to be at a higher risk of elevated negative emotionality and reactivity, anxiety, and internalizing symptoms and displayed delayed motor and cognitive development more frequently if exposed to stress in utero. Boys, on the other hand, showed reduced reactivity and emotionality and had a higher risk of externalizing problems and schizophrenia.

These findings can be interpreted within an evolutionary framework. Male fetuses are more vulnerable to stress in terms of viability, which manifests in a diminished secondary sex ratio (males to females born) in the context of prenatal stress (Walsh et al. 2019). Although it threatens viability in males (where the fittest are more likely to survive), prenatal stress leads to a higher vulnerability in later development in females, who are disposed to develop strategies for surviving in an adverse prenatal environment but pay the price of being more susceptible to delayed neurodevelopment, increased reactivity, and mood-related problems (Sandman et al. 2013). In fact, higher reactivity and greater vigilance in a stressful environment could have been an evolutionary advantage for females, who looked after the children, whereas males may have benefited more from lower stress reactivity so as to better explore the environment and face potential dangers (Glover and Hill 2012). Thus, both males and females are likely affected by prenatal stress, but the consequences and developmental domains concerned appear to differ (Van den Bergh et al. 2017). It is of note that sex-specific differences in the effects of prenatal stress may contribute to the well-known sex differences in psychopathology, particularly an increased risk for internalizing problems in females (Hicks et al. 2019).

Family socioeconomic status is another factor to consider as a moderator of the effects of prenatal stress on child outcomes. As indicated, positive effects of moderate levels of stress are found in higher-income populations, where families have more economic, social, and cultural resources that are expected to buffer the potential detrimental effects of stress (DiPietro 2012; Laplante et al. 2008). Given the adverse effects of low socioeconomic status on child development (Bradley and Corwyn 2002), we can expect that the positive effects of moderate doses of stress do not apply to disadvantaged populations, who are also more prone to experience extreme stress. For example, Robinson et al. (2016) reported that women from ethnic minority groups are more likely to experience depression and anxiety during pregnancy than are women who identify themselves as white.

The effects of prenatal stress may also be modulated by state policies to support women during pregnancy. Comparing the levels of depression and anxiety symptoms in pregnant women in the United States and the Netherlands, Gartstein et al. (2020) found higher levels of depression and anxiety in the U.S. population. The authors hypothesized that different workplace and health care policies (e.g., access to health care and paid maternity leave) in those countries may have contributed to different levels of stress in pregnancy. Thus, the strength of the effects of prenatal stress might be modulated not only by the difference between low- and high-income countries but also by disparities in the support provided to pregnant women and new mothers in Western cultures that are economically similar.

Currently, research has indicated that maternal stress in pregnancy is associated with a prior maternal history of childhood trauma (e.g., abuse, neglect) and may thus function as a pathway underlying the intergenerational transmission of maternal trauma to offspring. Maternal childhood trauma has been found to be associated with several adverse outcomes in the offspring, including altered autonomic nervous system regulation (Gustafsson et al. 2017), altered brain structure (Moog et al. 2018), and behavioral problems (Plant et al. 2017). There is evidence that women with a trauma history are more likely to experience distress in pregnancy, especially symptoms of depression or anxiety (Ghosn et al. 2019; Plant et al. 2017). Interestingly, Plant et al. (2013) found that maternal childhood maltreatment and prenatal depression combined (but neither separately) predicted a higher risk of adolescent antisocial behavior in the offspring. Moreover, women with childhood trauma show raised placental cortisol-releasing hormone (Moog et al. 2016) and elevated levels of the proinflammatory cytokine TNF-α in pregnancy (Blackmore et al. 2011), which may suggest that intergenerational transmission of trauma involves placental-fetal stress physiology and immune system activation.

Social support is another factor to be considered in the context of prenatal stress, but it is seldom measured. A positive effect of partner support in pregnancy on maternal emotional well-being and infant temperament was reported by Stapleton et al. (2012). Zhu et al. (2015) observed an interaction between prenatal stressful life events and social support in an analysis stratified by child sex, such that boys whose mothers experienced severe stressful events accompanied by lower social support were at a higher risk of developing ADHD symptoms. Walsh et al. (2019) reported that controlling for social support largely mitigated the effects of prenatal stress on birth outcomes.

Women who experience prenatal stress are more likely to experience stress in the postnatal period as well (Field 2011; Lin et al. 2017). To avoid confounding by postnatal stress, most recent studies focusing on the effects of prenatal stress have controlled carefully for this variable. Postnatal stress may nevertheless moderate the association between prenatal stress and child neurodevelopmental outcomes. As previously described, there are conflicting findings regarding the nature of such moderation: on the one hand, postnatal stress has been found to exacerbate detrimental effects of prenatal stress (Hartman et al. 2020); on the other hand, some authors have observed more optimal outcomes for children whose mothers experienced congruent levels of both pre- and postpartum stress, regardless of its intensity, suggesting that postnatal stress may actually result in favorable outcomes if combined with comparable levels of prenatal stress (Sandman et al. 2012b).

## Screening, Treatment, and Prevention

There are bidirectional psychological and biological influences between the mother and her fetus or child, which underscores the need for a dyadic approach to treatment that takes into consideration both the mother's and the child's well-being (Monk et al. 2019a). For example, in addition to the woman's own experience of distress during pregnancy, that distress can lead to adverse fetal and child neurobehavioral outcomes, which can also in turn produce increased distress for the mother in a dyadic back-and-forth relationship between mother and child. Although the precise mechanisms of transmission from mother to child (i.e., the mechanisms by which maternal prenatal distress can transcend to the fetus) are not yet fully understood, a complete understanding of these pathways is not necessary to provide treatment, especially when considering how distress or symptoms of depression and anxiety are modifiable with access to adequate health services (Monk et al. 2018).

When maternal distress during pregnancy goes unidentified by health care professionals, most women will not seek treatment for themselves (MacLennan et al. 1996). To ensure that distressed pregnant women do receive treatment, the first step is to perform routine screening for prenatal mental health issues as recommended by leading professional and government organizations. As of 2015, the American College of Obstetricians and Gynecologists (ACOG) issued a formal recommendation that all obstetrical care providers screen women for depression and anxiety at least once during pregnancy, in addition to screening in the postpartum period (American College of Obstetricians and Gynecologists 2018). The U.S. Preventive Services Task Force (USPSTF) also recommends screening for maternal depression during and after pregnancy (Siu et al. 2016). These recommendations by ACOG and USPSTF are supported by conclusions in a systematic review that demonstrated that screening for depression during both pregnancy and postpartum can lead to 1) reduced prevalence of depression, and 2) increased remission (O'Connor et al. 2016). (For specific recommendations on screening and measures to use, please consult Chapter 13, "Depressive Disorders," Chapter 19, "Anxiety Disorders and Insomnia in the Perinatal Period," and chapters on individual disorders.)

However, in addition to screening for prenatal depression and anxiety, screening for adverse childhood experiences may also be warranted, given that women who have a history of early life trauma are more likely to experience depression and anxiety during pregnancy (Letourneau et al. 2019). The standard measure of assessing a history of trauma is the Adverse Childhood Experiences questionnaire (Felitti et al. 1998), a 10-item self-report scale that has been validated in both research and clinical settings (Glowa et al. 2016) and is suitable for use during pregnancy (Monk et al. 2018). Given that obstetrical care providers and other women's health providers play a key role in the evaluation and management of women who survive sexual assault, ACOG recommends routine screening for a history of sexual assault, including screening during pregnancy (American College of Obstetricians and Gynecologists 2019).

Interventions that focus on treating prenatal distress can improve women's experience during pregnancy and prevent postpartum depression (Monk et al. 2018). Full recommendations for treatment modalities are given in the chapters on anxiety (Chapter 19) and depression (Chapter 13) and include specific psychotherapies (e.g., rational-emotive behavior therapy; Anton and David 2015) and mindfulness-based cognitive therapy adapted for women with perinatal depression (Dimidjian et al. 2015), as well as pharmacotherapy where indicated. In addition, interventions aimed at reducing distress among women who may not be identified as having clinically significant illness can be helpful. Practical Resources for Effective Postpartum Parenting, a dyadic treatment that begins in pregnancy and is designed to teach women about infant cues and sleep patterns, has been associated with reduced symptoms of maternal depression and anxiety and with less infant fussiness and crying behavior at 6 weeks postpartum (Werner et al. 2016).

When prevention is focused on improving mood during pregnancy, this offers an opportunity to foster more positive representations of the child in utero. These approaches, in turn, can carry over into the quality of the mother–child attachment and promote the healthy development of the child (Glover and Capron 2017). Screening, prevention, and treatment of maternal pre- and postnatal stress are intended to improve the mental health and well-being of both the mother and her child, and evidence supports the positive effects they bring to both.

## Special Considerations

Regardless of whether one engages in research or clinical practice, there are considerations to be made when working with women who are experiencing distress during pregnancy. When designing a study, interpreting results, or considering potential clinical applications, confounding factors must be taken into account both in the pre- and postnatal environment. For example, a common factor to consider when investigating the influence of maternal prenatal mood on child outcomes is maternal *postnatal* mood. Other examples, among many possible confounds or factors, include maternal social support, socioeconomic status, maternal age, child sex, child gestational age at birth and birth weight, birth complications, maternal history of trauma, race, ethnicity, and cultural background.

The generalizability of findings should also be considered, especially given the lack of diversity in trial samples, which do not match the U.S. population. For example, Latinx and Black Americans represent nearly one-third of the U.S. population, yet comprise only 6% of participants in federally funded clinical trials (Coakley et al. 2012). Lack of diversity in research is both an ethical and a scientific problem because race and ethnicity can lead to increased risk for disease and decreased likelihood of responding to treatment (Monk et al. 2019a). In prenatal stress research, the communities and minority groups who are underrepresented are often those at greater risk of prenatal stress. Thus, greater diversity in sampling is needed to better reflect the reality of women who are disproportionately exposed to adversity throughout pregnancy and the postpartum period.

A final and fundamental consideration in research and clinical practice that supports women with prenatal stress is how to not blame the mother. Researchers and clinicians who work with women during pregnancy can engage in thoughtful, deliberate, and dynamic practices such that women and mothers are not blamed for ways in which their fetus or child's development can be affected. Research and clinical practice in this domain have the purpose of supporting women's health and experience during pregnancy, as well as supporting the health of their fetuses and children. Pressure can be relieved by reinforcing how prenatal stress is only one of a multitude of factors that can influence fetal and child development and by emphasizing that support is being provided for both the mother and the child's health and well-being, as individuals and as a dyad.

## Conclusion

Several decades ago, David Barker formulated his hypothesis that adult disease might be programmed in utero. This hypothesis was extended from physical to mental health outcomes, including the hypothesis that environmental factors occurring early in life—including maternal stress—can alter neurodevelopment and increase risk of later psychiatric disorder. Evidence has been provided to support the association between prenatal stress and child developmental outcomes, including psychopathology, yet further identification of mechanisms and the role of moderating factors remain to be discovered. Although clinical, translational, and basic researchers continue to make new discoveries in DOHaD research as it relates to maternal stress and child outcomes, clinicians can rely on evidenced-based interventions to provide women and their future children with support.

## Key Points

- Prenatal (di)stress includes daily hassles, perceived stress, and major life events and a range of mental health problems, such as depression and anxiety.
- Prenatal (di)stress is associated with adverse neurobehavioral outcomes throughout fetal, infant, and child development.
- Traumatic events prior to pregnancy can influence prenatal (di)stress.
- The influence of prenatal (dis)tress can be moderated by factors such as socioeconomic status and social support.
- Evidence-based screening tools are available to identify prenatal (di)stress.
- Evidence-based interventions are available for the treatment of prenatal depression and other mood disturbances.
- Careful considerations must be made to avoid blaming mothers and women for the influence of prenatal (di)stress on child outcomes.

## References

Adrover E, Pallarés ME, Baier CJ, et al: Glutamate neurotransmission is affected in prenatally stressed offspring. Neurochem Int 88:73–87, 2015 26026592

American College of Obstetricians and Gynecologists: ACOG Committee Opinion No. 757: screening for perinatal depression. Obstet Gynecol 132(5):e208–e212, 2018 30629567

American College of Obstetricians and Gynecologists: ACOG Committee Opinion No. 777: sexual assault. Obstet Gynecol 133(4):e296–e302, 2019 30913202

Anton R, David D: A randomized clinical trial of a new preventive rational emotive and behavioral therapeutical program of prepartum and postpartum emotional distress. J Evid Based Psychother 15:3–15, 2015

Austin MP, Hadzi-Pavlovic D, Leader L, et al: Maternal trait anxiety, depression and life event stress in pregnancy: relationships with infant temperament. Early Hum Dev 81(2):183–190, 2005a 15748973

Austin MP, Leader LR, Reilly N: Prenatal stress, the hypothalamic-pituitary-adrenal axis, and fetal and infant neurobehaviour. Early Hum Dev 81(11):917–926, 2005b 16169164

Bailey MT, Lubach GR, Coe CL: Prenatal stress alters bacterial colonization of the gut in infant monkeys. J Pediatr Gastroenterol Nutr 38(4):414–421, 2004 15085020

Barker DJ: The fetal and infant origins of adult disease. BMJ 301(6761):1111, 1990 2252919

Barker DJ: Fetal origins of coronary heart disease. BMJ 311(6998):171–174, 1995a 7613432

Barker DJ: Intrauterine programming of adult disease. Mol Med Today 1(9):418–423, 1995b 9415190

Bercik P, Collins SM, Verdu EF: Microbes and the gut-brain axis. Neurogastroenterol Motil 24(5):405–413, 2012 22404222

Bergman K, Sarkar P, Glover V, et al: Maternal prenatal cortisol and infant cognitive development: moderation by infant-mother attachment. Biol Psychiatry 67(11):1026–1032, 2010 20188350

Betts KS, Williams GM, Najman JM, et al: Maternal depressive, anxious, and stress symptoms during pregnancy predict internalizing problems in adolescence. Depress Anxiety 31(1):9–18, 2014 24395339

Blackmore ER, Moynihan JA, Rubinow DR, et al: Psychiatric symptoms and proinflammatory cytokines in pregnancy. Psychosom Med 73(8):656–663, 2011 21949424

Bowers ME, Yehuda R: Intergenerational transmission of stress in humans. Neuropsychopharmacology 41(1):232–244, 2016 26279078

Bradley RH, Corwyn RF: Socioeconomic status and child development. Annu Rev Psychol 53:371–399, 2002 11752490
Brown AS: Exposure to prenatal infection and risk of schizophrenia. Front Psychiatry 2:63, 2011 22131978
Buss C, Davis EP, Hobel CJ, et al: Maternal pregnancy-specific anxiety is associated with child executive function at 6–9 years age. Stress 14(6):665–676, 2011 21995526
Bussières EL, Tarabulsy GM, Pearson J, et al: Maternal prenatal stress and infant birth weight and gestational age: a meta-analysis of prospective studies. Dev Rev 36:179–199, 2015
Cao X, Laplante DP, Brunet A, et al: Prenatal maternal stress affects motor function in 5½-year-old children: project ice storm. Dev Psychobiol 56(1):117–125, 2014 23143986
Cao-Lei L, De Rooij SR, King S, et al: Prenatal stress and epigenetics. Neurosci Biobehav Rev 117:198–210, 2017 28528960
Capron LE, Glover V, Pearson RM, et al: Associations of maternal and paternal antenatal mood with offspring anxiety disorder at age 18 years. J Affect Disord 187:20–26, 2015 26301478
Cents RA, Diamantopoulou S, Hudziak JJ, et al: Trajectories of maternal depressive symptoms predict child problem behaviour: the Generation R study. Psychol Med 43(1):13–25, 2013 22490169
Charil A, Laplante DP, Vaillancourt C, et al: Prenatal stress and brain development. Brain Res Brain Res Rev 65(1):56–79, 2010 20550950
Chong CYL, Bloomfield FH, O'Sullivan JM: Factors affecting gastrointestinal microbiome development in neonates. Nutrients 10(3):274, 2018 29495552
Chong SC, Broekman BF, Qiu A, et al: Anxiety and depression during pregnancy and temperament in early infancy: findings from a multi-ethnic, Asian, prospective birth cohort study. Infant Ment Health J 37(5):584–598, 2016 27548536
Christian LM, Franco A, Glaser R, et al: Depressive symptoms are associated with elevated serum proinflammatory cytokines among pregnant women. Brain Behav Immun 23(6):750–754, 2009 19258033
Class QA, Lichtenstein P, Langstrom N, D'Onofrio BM: Timing of prenatal maternal exposure to severe life events and adverse pregnancy outcomes: a population study of 2.6 million pregnancies. Psychosom Med 73:234–241, 2011
Class QA, Abel KM, Khashan AS, et al: Offspring psychopathology following preconception, prenatal and postnatal maternal bereavement stress. Psychol Med 44(1):71–84, 2014 23591021
Coakley M, Fadiran EO, Parrish LJ, et al: Dialogues on diversifying clinical trials: successful strategies for engaging women and minorities in clinical trials. J Womens Health (Larchmt) 21(7):713–716, 2012 22747427
Coe CL, Kramer M, Czéh B, et al: Prenatal stress diminishes neurogenesis in the dentate gyrus of juvenile rhesus monkeys. Biol Psychiatry 54(10):1025–1034, 2003 14625144
Conradt E, Lester BM, Appleton AA, et al: The roles of DNA methylation of NR3C1 and 11beta-HSD2 and exposure to maternal mood disorder in utero on newborn neurobehavior. Epigenetics 8(12):1321–1329, 2013 24135662
Copper RL, Goldenberg RL, Das A, et al: The preterm prediction study: maternal stress is associated with spontaneous preterm birth at less than thirty-five weeks' gestation. Am J Obstet Gynecol 175(5):1286–1292, 1996 8942502
Coussons-Read ME, Okun ML, et al: Psychosocial stress increases inflammatory markers and alters cytokine production across pregnancy. Brain Behav Immun 21(3):343–350, 2007 17029703
Dadds MR, Moul C, Hawes DJ, et al: Individual differences in childhood behavior disorders associated with epigenetic modulation of the cortisol receptor gene. Child Dev 86(5):1311–1320, 2015 26152664
Davis EP, Sandman CA: The timing of prenatal exposure to maternal cortisol and psychosocial stress is associated with human infant cognitive development. Child Dev 81(1):131–148, 2010 20331658
Davis EP, Sandman CA: Prenatal psychobiological predictors of anxiety risk in preadolescent children. Psychoneuroendocrinology 37(8):1224–1233, 2012 22265195
Davis EP, Glynn LM, Waffarn F, et al: Prenatal maternal stress programs infant stress regulation. J Child Psychol Psychiatry 52(2):119–129, 2011 20854366

Davis EP, Head K, Buss C, et al: Prenatal maternal cortisol concentrations predict neurodevelopment in middle childhood. Psychoneuroendocrinology 75:56–63, 2017 27771566
Davis EP, Hankin BL, Glynn LM, et al: Prenatal maternal stress, child cortical thickness, and adolescent depressive symptoms. Child Dev 91(2):e432–e450, 2020 31073997
DeSocio JE: Epigenetics, maternal prenatal psychosocial stress, and infant mental health. Arch Psychiatr Nurs 32(6):901–906, 2018 30454636
de Weerth C: Do bacteria shape our development? Crosstalk between intestinal microbiota and HPA axis. Neurosci Biobehav Rev 83:458–471, 2017 28918360
Dieter JNI, Field T, Hernandez-Reif M, et al: Maternal depression and increased fetal activity. J Obstet Gynaecol 21(5):468–473, 2001 12521799
Dimidjian S, Goodman SH, Felder JN, et al: An open trial of mindfulness-based cognitive therapy for the prevention of perinatal depressive relapse/recurrence. Arch Women Ment Health 18(1):85–94, 2015 25298253
Dindo L, Elmore A, O'Hara M, et al: The comorbidity of Axis I disorders in depressed pregnant women. Arch Women Ment Health 20(6):757–764, 2017 28842756
DiPietro JA: The role of prenatal maternal stress in child development. Curr Dir Psychol Sci 13(2):71–74, 2004
DiPietro JA: Maternal stress in pregnancy: considerations for fetal development. J Adolesc Health 51(2 suppl):S3–S8, 2012 22794531
DiPietro JA, Hilton SC, Hawkins M, et al: Maternal stress and affect influence fetal neurobehavioral development. Dev Psychol 38(5):659–668, 2002 12220045
DiPietro JA, Costigan KA, Gurewitsch ED: Fetal response to induced maternal stress. Early Hum Dev 74:125–138, 2003 14580752
DiPietro JA, Novak MF, Costigan KA, et al: Maternal psychological distress during pregnancy in relation to child development at age two. Child Dev 77(3):573–587, 2006 16686789
DiPietro JA, Kivlighan KT, Costigan KA, et al: Prenatal antecedents of newborn neurological maturation. Child Dev 81(1):115–130, 2010 20331657
Evans J, Melotti R, Heron J, et al: The timing of maternal depressive symptoms and child cognitive development: a longitudinal study. J Child Psychol Psychiatry 53(6):632–640, 2012 22211468
Felitti VJ, Anda RF, Nordenberg D, et al: Relationship of childhood abuse and household dysfunction to many of the leading causes of death in adults: the Adverse Childhood Experiences (ACE) study. Am J Prev Med 14(4):245–258, 1998 9635069
Field T: Prenatal depression effects on early development: a review. Infant Behav Dev 34(1):1–14, 2011 20970195
Figueiredo B, Costa R: Mother's stress, mood and emotional involvement with the infant: 3 months before and 3 months after childbirth. Arch Women Ment Health 12(3):143–153, 2009 19259772
Figueiredo B, Pinto TM, Pacheco A, et al: Fetal heart rate variability mediates prenatal depression effects on neonatal neurobehavioral maturity. Biol Psychol 123:294–301, 2017 27984086
Fineberg AM, Ellman LM, Schaefer CA, et al: Fetal exposure to maternal stress and risk for schizophrenia spectrum disorders among offspring: differential influences of fetal sex. Psychiatry Res 236:91–97, 2016 26753951
Fisher J, Cabral de Mello M, Patel V, et al: Prevalence and determinants of common perinatal mental disorders in women in low- and lower-middle-income countries: a systematic review. Bull World Health Organ 90(2):139G–149G, 2012 22423165
Fleming TP, Velazquez MA, Eckert JJ: Embryos, DOHaD and David Barker. J Dev Orig Health Dis 6(5):377–383, 2015 25952250
Gartstein MA, Erickson NL, Cooijmans KHM, et al: Is prenatal maternal distress context-dependent? Comparing United States and the Netherlands. J Affect Disord 260:710–715, 2020 31561114
Gerardin P, Wendland J, Bodeau N, et al: Depression during pregnancy: is the developmental impact earlier in boys? A prospective case-control study. J Clin Psychiatry 72(3):378–387, 2011 21208585
Ghosn F, Almansa B, Moreno-Giménez A, et al: Trajectories of stress biomarkers and anxious-depressive symptoms from pregnancy to postpartum period in women with a trauma history. Eur J Psychotraumatol 10(1):1601990, 2019 31069025

Glasheen C, Richardson GA, Kim KH, et al: Exposure to maternal pre- and postnatal depression and anxiety symptoms: risk for major depression, anxiety disorders, and conduct disorder in adolescent offspring. Dev Psychopathol 25(4 Pt 1):1045–1063, 2013 24229548

Glover V: Annual Research Review: Prenatal stress and the origins of psychopathology: an evolutionary perspective. J Child Psychol Psychiatry 52(4):356–367, 2011 21250994

Glover V: Is the association between maternal stress during pregnancy and the child's depression partly causal, and what should we do about it? Acta Psychiatr Scand 139(4):301–303, 2019 30891746

Glover V, Capron L: Prenatal parenting. Curr Opin Psychol 15:66–70, 2017 28813271

Glover V, Hill J: Sex differences in the programming effects of prenatal stress on psychopathology and stress responses: an evolutionary perspective. Physiol Behav 106(5):736–740, 2012 22353310

Glover V, Bergman K, Sarkar P, et al: Association between maternal and amniotic fluid cortisol is moderated by maternal anxiety. Psychoneuroendocrinology 34(3):430–435, 2009 19019559

Glover V, O'Connor TG, O'Donnell K: Prenatal stress and the programming of the HPA axis. Neurosci Biobehav Rev 35(1):17–22, 2010 19914282

Glowa PT, Olson AL, Johnson DJ: Screening for adverse childhood experiences in a family medicine setting: a feasibility study. J Am Board Fam Med 29(3):303–307, 2016 27170787

Glynn LM, Sandman CA: Sex moderates associations between prenatal glucocorticoid exposure and human fetal neurological development. Dev Sci 15(5):601–610, 2012 22925508

Goodwin RD, Cheslack-Postava K, Nelson DB, et al: Serious psychological distress and smoking during pregnancy in the United States: 2008–2014. Nicotine Tob Res 19(5):605–614, 2017 28403468

Grace T, Bulsara M, Robinson M, et al: The impact of maternal gestational stress on motor development in late childhood and adolescence: a longitudinal study. Child Dev 87(1):211–220, 2016 26462448

Graham AM, Rasmussen JM, Rudolph MD, et al: Maternal systemic interleukin-6 during pregnancy is associated with newborn amygdala phenotypes and subsequent behavior at 2 years of age. Biol Psychiatry 83(2):109–119, 2018 28754515

Graham AM, Rasmussen JM, Entringer S, et al: Maternal cortisol concentrations during pregnancy and sex-specific associations with neonatal amygdala connectivity and emerging internalizing behaviors. Biol Psychiatry 85(2):172–181, 2019 30122286

Graignic-Philippe R, Dayan J, Chokron S, et al: Effects of prenatal stress on fetal and child development: a critical literature review. Neurosci Biobehav Rev 43:137–162, 2014 24747487

Gur TL, Worly BL, Bailey MT: Stress and the commensal microbiota: importance in parturition and infant neurodevelopment. Front Psychiatry 6:5, 2015 25698977

Gur TL, Shay L, Palkar AV, et al: Prenatal stress affects placental cytokines and neurotrophins, commensal microbes, and anxiety-like behavior in adult female offspring. Brain Behav Immun 64:50–58, 2017 28027927

Gustafsson H, Doyle C, Gilchrist M, et al: Maternal abuse history and reduced fetal heart rate variability: abuse-related sleep disturbance is a mediator. Dev Psychopathol 29(3):1023–1034, 2017 27760572

Harris A, Seckl J: Glucocorticoids, prenatal stress and the programming of disease. Horm Behav 59(3):279–289, 2011 20591431

Hartman S, Freeman SM, Bales KL, et al: Prenatal stress as a risk—and an opportunity—factor. Psychol Sci 29(4):572–580, 2018 29412055

Hartman S, Sayler K, Belsky J: Prenatal stress enhances postnatal plasticity: the role of microbiota. Dev Psychobiol 61(5):729–738, 2019 30575950

Hartman S, Eilertsen EM, Ystrom E, et al: Does prenatal stress amplify effects of postnatal maternal depressive and anxiety symptoms on child problem behavior? Dev Psychol 56(1):128–137, 2020 31682144

Hechler C, Borewicz K, Beijers R, et al: Association between psychosocial stress and fecal microbiota in pregnant women. Sci Rep 9(1):4463, 2019 30872645

Henrichs J, Schenk JJ, Kok R, et al: Parental family stress during pregnancy and cognitive functioning in early childhood: the Generation R Study. Early Child Res Q 26:332–343, 2011

Hentges RF, Graham SA, Plamondon A, et al: A developmental cascade from prenatal stress to child internalizing and externalizing problems. J Pediatr Psychol 44(9):1057–1067, 2019 31166597

Hicks LM, Swales DA, Garcia SE, et al: Does prenatal maternal distress contribute to sex differences in child psychopathology? Curr Psychiatry Rep 21(2):7, 2019 30729361

Hompes T, Izzi B, Gellens E, et al: Investigating the influence of maternal cortisol and emotional state during pregnancy on the DNA methylation status of the glucocorticoid receptor gene (NR3C1) promoter region in cord blood. J Psychiatr Res 47(7):880–891, 2013 23566423

Howard LM, Molyneaux E, Dennis CL, et al: Non-psychotic mental disorders in the perinatal period. Lancet 384(9956):1775–1788, 2014 25455248

Huizink AC, Menting B, De Moor MHM, et al: From prenatal anxiety to parenting stress: a longitudinal study. Arch Women Ment Health 20(5):663–672, 2017 28634716

Hurley KM, Caulfield LE, Sacco LM, et al: Psychosocial influences in dietary patterns during pregnancy. J Am Diet Assoc 105(6):963–966, 2005 15942549

Istvan J: Stress, anxiety, and birth outcomes: a critical review of the evidence. Psychol Bull 100(3):331–348, 1986 3797559

Jašarevic E, Howerton CL, Howard CD, et al: Alterations in the vaginal microbiome by maternal stress are associated with metabolic reprogramming of the offspring gut and brain. Endocrinology 156(9):3265–3276, 2015 26079804

Jensen Peña C, Monk C, Champagne FA: Epigenetic effects of prenatal stress on 11beta-hydroxysteroid dehydrogenase-2 in the placenta and fetal brain. PLoS One 7(6):e39791, 2012 22761903

Kantonen T, Karlsson L, Nolvi S, et al: Maternal alexithymic traits, prenatal stress, and infant temperament. Infant Behav Dev 41:12–16, 2015 26263082

Karam F, Sheehy O, Huneau MC, et al: Impact of maternal prenatal and parental postnatal stress on 1-year-old child development: results from the OTIS antidepressants in pregnancy study. Arch Women Ment Health 19(5):835–843, 2016 26957509

King S, Dancause K, Turcotte-Tremblay AM, et al: Using natural disasters to study the effects of prenatal maternal stress on child health and development. Birth Defects Res C Embryo Today 96(4):273–288, 2012 24203917

Kingsbury M, Weeks M, MacKinnon N, et al: Stressful life events during pregnancy and offspring depression: evidence from a prospective cohort study. J Am Acad Child Adolesc Psychiatry 55(8):709.e2–716.e2, 2016 27453085

Korhonen M, Luoma I, Salmelin R, et al: Maternal depressive symptoms: associations with adolescents' internalizing and externalizing problems and social competence. Nord J Psychiatry 68(5):323–332, 2014 24070429

Koutra K, Chatzi L, Bagkeris M, et al: Antenatal and postnatal maternal mental health as determinants of infant neurodevelopment at 18 months of age in a mother-child cohort (Rhea Study) in Crete, Greece. Soc Psychiatry Psychiatr Epidemiol 48(8):1335–1345, 2013 23248031

Lahti M, Savolainen K, Tuovinen S, et al: Maternal depressive symptoms during and after pregnancy and psychiatric problems in children. J Am Acad Child Adolesc Psychiatry 56(1):30.e7–39.e7, 2017 27993226

Laplante DP, Brunet A, Schmitz N, et al: Project Ice Storm: prenatal maternal stress affects cognitive and linguistic functioning in 5½-year-old children. J Am Acad Child Adolesc Psychiatry 47(9):1063–1072, 2008 18665002

Laplante DP, Brunet A, King S: The effects of maternal stress and illness during pregnancy on infant temperament: Project Ice Storm. Pediatr Res 79(1–1):107–113, 2016 26375472

Lefmann T, Combs-Orme T: Prenatal stress, poverty, and child outcomes. Child and Adolescent Social Work Journal 31(6):577–590, 2014

Leis JA, Heron J, Stuart EA, et al: Associations between maternal mental health and child emotional and behavioral problems: does prenatal mental health matter? J Abnorm Child Psychol 42(1):161–171, 2014 23748337

Letourneau N, Dewey D, Kaplan BJ, et al: Intergenerational transmission of adverse childhood experiences via maternal depression and anxiety and moderation by child sex. J Dev Orig Health Dis 10(1):88–99, 2019 30175696

LeWinn KZ, Stroud LR, Molnar BE, et al: Elevated maternal cortisol levels during pregnancy are associated with reduced childhood IQ. Int J Epidemiol 38(6):1700–1710, 2009 19423658
Li J, Olsen J, Vestergaard M, et al: Attention-deficit/hyperactivity disorder in the offspring following prenatal maternal bereavement: a nationwide follow-up study in Denmark. Eur Child Adolesc Psychiatry 19(10):747–753, 2010 20495989
Li J, Robinson M, Malacova E, et al: Maternal life stress events in pregnancy link to children's school achievement at age 10 years. J Pediatr 162(3):483–489, 2013 23084705
Lima SAM, El Dib RP, Rodrigues MRK, et al: Is the risk of low birth weight or preterm labor greater when maternal stress is experienced during pregnancy? A systematic review and meta-analysis of cohort studies. PLoS One 13(7):e0200594, 2018 30048456
Lin B, Crnic KA, Luecken LJ, et al: Maternal prenatal stress and infant regulatory capacity in Mexican Americans. Infant Behav Dev 37(4):571–582, 2014 25113917
Lin Y, Xu J, Huang J, et al: Effects of prenatal and postnatal maternal emotional stress on toddlers' cognitive and temperamental development. J Affect Disord 207:9–17, 2017 27665073
Lipner E, Murphy SK, Ellman LM: Prenatal maternal stress and the cascade of risk to schizophrenia spectrum disorders in offspring. Curr Psychiatry Rep 21(10):99, 2019 31522269
Littleton HL, Breitkopf CR, Berenson AB: Correlates of anxiety symptoms during pregnancy and association with perinatal outcomes: a meta-analysis. Am J Obstet Gynecol 196(5):424–432, 2007 17466693
Littleton HL, Bye K, Buck K, et al: Psychosocial stress during pregnancy and perinatal outcomes: a meta-analytic review. J Psychosom Obstet Gynaecol 31(4):219–228, 2010 21039328
Loomans EM, van der Stelt O, van Eijsden M, et al: Antenatal maternal anxiety is associated with problem behaviour at age five. Early Hum Dev 87(8):565–570, 2011 21576004
Loomans EM, van Dijk AE, Vrijkotte TG, et al: Psychosocial stress during pregnancy is related to adverse birth outcomes: results from a large multi-ethnic community-based birth cohort. Eur J Public Health 23(3):485–491, 2013 22850187
Maccari S, Piazza PV, Kabbaj M, et al: Adoption reverses the long-term impairment in glucocorticoid feedback induced by prenatal stress. J Neurosci 15(1 Pt 1):110–116, 1995 7823121
MacKinnon N, Kingsbury M, Mahedy L, et al: The association between prenatal stress and externalizing symptoms in childhood: evidence from the Avon Longitudinal Study of Parents and Children. Biol Psychiatry 83(2):100–108, 2018 28893381
MacLennan A, Wilson D, Taylor A: The self-reported prevalence of postnatal depression. Aust N Z J Obstet Gynaecol 36(3):313, 1996 8883758
Makino I, Matsuda Y, Yoneyama M, et al: Effect of maternal stress on fetal heart rate assessed by vibroacoustic stimulation. J Int Med Res 37(6):1780–1788, 2009 20146876
McLean MA, Cobham VE, Simcock G, et al: Toddler temperament mediates the effect of prenatal maternal stress on childhood anxiety symptomatology: the QF2011 Queensland Flood Study. Int J Environ Res Public Health 16(11):1998, 2019 31195616
Melville JL, Gavin A, Guo Y, et al: Depressive disorders during pregnancy: prevalence and risk factors in a large urban sample. Obstet Gynecol 116(5):1064–1070, 2010 20966690
Merced-Nieves FM, Aguiar A, Dzwilewski KLC, et al: Association of prenatal maternal perceived stress with a sexually dimorphic measure of cognition in 4.5-month-old infants. Neurotoxicol Teratol 77:106850, 2020 31812786
Molenaar NM, Tiemeier H, van Rossum EFC, et al: Prenatal maternal psychopathology and stress and offspring HPA axis function at 6 years. Psychoneuroendocrinology 99:120–127, 2019 30223193
Monk C, Fifer WP, Myers MM, et al: Maternal stress responses and anxiety during pregnancy: effects on fetal heart rate. Dev Psychobiol 36(1):67–77, 2000 10607362
Monk C, Myers MM, Sloan RP, et al: Effects of women's stress-elicited physiological activity and chronic anxiety on fetal heart rate. J Dev Behav Pediatr 24(1):32–38, 2003 12584483
Monk C, Sloan RP, Myers MM, et al: Fetal heart rate reactivity differs by women's psychiatric status: an early marker for developmental risk? J Am Acad Child Adolesc Psychiatry 43(3):283–290, 2004 15076261
Monk C, Fifer WP, Myers MM, et al: Effects of maternal breathing rate, psychiatric status, and cortisol on fetal heart rate. Dev Psychobiol 53(3):221–233, 2011 21400485

Monk C, Feng T, Lee S, et al: Distress during pregnancy: epigenetic regulation of placenta glucocorticoid-related genes and fetal neurobehavior. Am J Psychiatry 173(7):705–713, 2016 27013342
Monk C, Foss S, Desai P, Glover V: L'esposizicne del feto ai disturbi psicologici della madre, in Psicologia Clinica Perinatale: Dalla Teoria Alla Pratica. Edited by Grussu P, Quatraro RM. Trento, Italy, Erickson, 2018, pp 71–104
Monk C, Lugo-Candelas C, Trumpff C: Prenatal developmental origins of future psychopathology: mechanisms and pathways. Annu Rev Clin Psychol 15:317–344, 2019a 30795695
Monk C, Webster RS, McNeil RB, et al: Associations of perceived prenatal stress and adverse pregnancy outcomes with perceived stress years after delivery. Arch Womens Ment Health 23:361–369, 2019b 31256258
Moog NK, Buss C, Entringer S, et al: Maternal exposure to childhood trauma is associated during pregnancy with placental-fetal stress physiology. Biol Psychiatry 79(10):831–839, 2016 26444076
Moog NK, Entringer S, Rasmussen JM, et al: Intergenerational effect of maternal exposure to childhood maltreatment on newborn brain anatomy. Biol Psychiatry 83(2):120–127, 2018 28842114
Moss KM, Simcock G, Cobham V, et al: A potential psychological mechanism linking disaster-related prenatal maternal stress with child cognitive and motor development at 16 months: the QF2011 Queensland Flood Study. Dev Psychol 53(4):629–641, 2017 28333525
Mulder EJH, Robles de Medina PG, Huizink AC, et al: Prenatal maternal stress: effects on pregnancy and the (unborn) child. Early Hum Dev 70(1–2):3–14, 2002 12441200
Nolvi S, Karlsson L, Bridgett DJ, et al: Maternal prenatal stress and infant emotional reactivity six months postpartum. J Affect Disord 199:163–170, 2016 27107891
O'Connor E, Rossom RC, Henninger M, et al: Primary care screening for and treatment of depression in pregnant and postpartum women: evidence report and systematic review for the US Preventive Services Task Force. JAMA 315(4):388–406, 2016 26813212
O'Donnell KJ, Bugge Jensen A, Freeman L, et al: Maternal prenatal anxiety and downregulation of placental 11beta-HSD2. Psychoneuroendocrinology 37(6):818–826, 2012 22001010
O'Donnell KJ, Glover V, Barker ED, et al: The persisting effect of maternal mood in pregnancy on childhood psychopathology. Dev Psychopathol 26(2):393–403, 2014 24621564
O'Mahony SM, Clarke G, Dinan TG, et al: Early life adversity and brain development: is the microbiome a missing piece of the puzzle? Neuroscience 342:37–54, 2017 26432952
Osborne LM, Yenokyan G, Fei K, et al: Innate immune activation and depressive and anxious symptoms across the peripartum: an exploratory study. Psychoneuroendocrinology 99:80–86, 2019 30195110
Pacheco A, Figueiredo B: Mother's depression at childbirth does not contribute to the effects of antenatal depression on neonate's behavioral development. Infant Behav Dev 35(3):513–522, 2012 22717759
Painter RC, Roseboom TJ, de Rooij SR: Long-term effects of prenatal stress and glucocorticoid exposure. Birth Defects Res C Embryo Today 96(4):315–324, 2012 24203920
Palma-Gudiel H, Córdova-Palomera A, Eixarch E, et al: Maternal psychosocial stress during pregnancy alters the epigenetic signature of the glucocorticoid receptor gene promoter in their offspring: a meta-analysis. Epigenetics 10(10):893–902, 2015 26327302
Pearson RM, Evans J, Kounali D, et al: Maternal depression during pregnancy and the postnatal period: risks and possible mechanisms for offspring depression at age 18 years. JAMA Psychiatry 70(12):1312–1319, 2013 24108418
Pearson RM, Bornstein MH, Cordero M, et al: Maternal perinatal mental health and offspring academic achievement at age 16: the mediating role of childhood executive function. J Child Psychol Psychiatry 57(4):491–501, 2016 26616637
Pickles A, Sharp H, Hellier J, et al: Prenatal anxiety, maternal stroking in infancy, and symptoms of emotional and behavioral disorders at 3.5 years. Eur Child Adolesc Psychiatry 26(3):325–334, 2017 27464490
Plant DT, Barker ED, Waters CS, et al: Intergenerational transmission of maltreatment and psychopathology: the role of antenatal depression. Psychol Med 43(3):519–528, 2013

Plant DT, Jones FW, Pariante CM, et al: Association between maternal childhood trauma and offspring childhood psychopathology: mediation analysis from the ALSPAC cohort. Br J Psychiatry 211(3):144–150, 2017 28729357
Radtke KM, Ruf M, Gunter HM, et al: Transgenerational impact of intimate partner violence on methylation in the promoter of the glucocorticoid receptor. Transl Psychiatry 1:e21, 2011 22832523
Rai D, Golding J, Magnusson C, et al: Prenatal and early life exposure to stressful life events and risk of autism spectrum disorders: population-based studies in Sweden and England. PLoS One 7(6):e38893, 2012 22719977
Rakers F, Rupprecht S, Dreiling M, et al: Transfer of maternal psychosocial stress to the fetus. Neurosci Biobehav Rev S0149–7634(16):30719–9, 2017 28237726
Reissland N, Froggatt S, Reames E, et al: Effects of maternal anxiety and depression on fetal neuro-development. J Affect Disord 241:469–474, 2018 30149334
Rijlaarsdam J, van IJzendoorn MH, Verhulst FC, et al: Prenatal stress exposure, oxytocin receptor gene (OXTR) methylation, and child autistic traits: the moderating role of OXTR rs53576 genotype. Autism Res 10(3):430–438, 2017 27520745
Robinson AM, Benzies KM, Cairns SL, et al: Who is distressed? A comparison of psychosocial stress in pregnancy across seven ethnicities. BMC Pregnancy Childbirth 16(1):215, 2016 27514674
Robinson M, Oddy WH, Li J, et al: Pre- and postnatal influences on preschool mental health: a large-scale cohort study. J Child Psychol Psychiatry 49(10):1118–1128, 2008 19017026
Robinson M, Mattes E, Oddy WH, et al: Prenatal stress and risk of behavioral morbidity from age 2 to 14 years: the influence of the number, type, and timing of stressful life events. Dev Psychopathol 23(2):507–520, 2011 23786692
Romero-Gonzalez B, Caparros-Gonzalez RA, Gonzalez-Perez R, et al: Newborn infants' hair cortisol levels reflect chronic maternal stress during pregnancy. PLoS One 13(7):e0200279, 2018 29979751
Ronald A, Pennell CE, Whitehouse AJ: Prenatal maternal stress associated with ADHD and autistic traits in early childhood. Front Psychol 1:223, 2011 21833278
Rothenberger SE, Resch F, Doszpod N, et al: Prenatal stress and infant affective reactivity at five months of age. Early Hum Dev 87(2):129–136, 2011 21194854
Sandman CA, Davis EP, Buss C, et al: Exposure to prenatal psychobiological stress exerts programming influences on the mother and her fetus. Neuroendocrinology 95(1):7–21, 2012a 21494029
Sandman CA, Davis EP, Glynn LM: Prescient human fetuses thrive. Psychol Sci 23(1):93–100, 2012b 22173740
Sandman CA, Glynn LM, Davis EP: Is there a viability-vulnerability tradeoff? Sex differences in fetal programming. J Psychosom Res 75(4):327–335, 2013 24119938
Schechter JC, Brennan PA, Smith AK, et al: Maternal prenatal psychological distress and preschool cognitive functioning: the protective role of positive parental engagement. J Abnorm Child Psychol 45(2):249–260, 2017 27150387
Schetter CD, Glynn LM: Stress in pregnancy: empirical evidence and theoretical issues to guide interdisciplinary researchers, in Handbook of Stress Science Biology, Psychology, and Health. Edited by Contrada R, Baum A. New York, Springer, 2011, pp 321–343
Send TS, Bardtke S, Gilles M, et al: Prenatal maternal stress is associated with lower cortisol and cortisone levels in the first morning urine of 45-month-old children. Psychoneuroendocrinology 103:219–224, 2019 30711899
Seng JS, Rauch SA, Resnick H, et al: Exploring posttraumatic stress disorder symptom profile among pregnant women. J Psychosom Obstet Gynaecol 31(3):176–187, 2010 20482290
Seth S, Lewis AJ, Saffery R, et al: Maternal prenatal mental health and placental 11beta-HSD2 gene expression: initial findings from the Mercy Pregnancy and Emotional Wellbeing Study. Int J Mol Sci 16(11):27482–27496, 2015 26593902
Simcock G, Kildea S, Elgbeili G, et al: Age-related changes in the effects of stress in pregnancy on infant motor development by maternal report: the Queensland Flood Study. Dev Psychobiol 58(5):640–659, 2016 27004939

Simcock G, Elgbeili G, Laplante DP, et al: The effects of prenatal maternal stress on early temperament: the 2011 Queensland Flood Study. J Dev Behav Pediatr 38(5):310–321, 2017a 28448308

Simcock G, Laplante DP, Elgbeili G, et al: Infant neurodevelopment is affected by prenatal maternal stress: the QF2011 Queensland Flood Study. Infancy 22(3):282–302, 2017b 33158359

Siu AL, Bibbins-Domingo K, Grossman DC, et al: Screening for depression in adults: US Preventive Services Task Force recommendation statement. JAMA 315(4):380–387, 2016 26813211

Sloan RP, Schwarz E, McKinley PS, et al: Vagally mediated heart rate variability and indices of well-being: results of a nationally representative study. Health Psychol 36(1):73–81, 2017 27570892

Spann MN, Monk C, Scheinost D, et al: Maternal immune activation during the third trimester is associated with neonatal functional connectivity of the salience network and fetal to toddler behavior. J Neurosci 38(11):2877–2886, 2018 29487127

St-Hilaire A, Steiger H, Liu A, et al: A prospective study of effects of prenatal maternal stress on later eating-disorder manifestations in affected offspring: preliminary indications based on the Project Ice Storm cohort. Int J Eat Disord 48(5):512–516, 2015 25808647

Stapleton LR, Schetter CD, Westling E, et al: Perceived partner support in pregnancy predicts lower maternal and infant distress. J Fam Psychol 26(3):453–463, 2012 22662772

Sutherland S, Brunwasser SM: Sex differences in vulnerability to prenatal stress: a review of the recent literature. Curr Psychiatry Rep 20(11):102, 2018 30229468

Tamashiro KL, Moran TH: Perinatal environment and its influences on metabolic programming of offspring. Physiol Behav 100(5):560–566, 2010 20394764

Tarabulsy GM, Pearson J, Vaillancourt-Morel MP, et al: Meta-analytic findings of the relation between maternal prenatal stress and anxiety and child cognitive outcome. J Dev Behav Pediatr 35(1):38–43, 2014 24345757

Tearne JE, Allen KL, Herbison CE, et al: The association between prenatal environment and children's mental health trajectories from 2 to 14 years. Eur Child Adolesc Psychiatry 24(9):1015–1024, 2015 25431038

Togher KL, Treacy E, O'Keeffe GW, et al: Maternal distress in late pregnancy alters obstetric outcomes and the expression of genes important for placental glucocorticoid signalling. Psychiatry Res 255:17–26, 2017 28511050

Tyrka AR, Parade SH, Welch ES, et al: Methylation of the leukocyte glucocorticoid receptor gene promoter in adults: associations with early adversity and depressive, anxiety and substance-use disorders. Transl Psychiatry 6(7):e848, 2016 27378548

Van den Bergh BRH, Van den Heuvel MI, Lahti M, et al: Prenatal developmental origins of behavior and mental health: the influence of maternal stress in pregnancy. Neurosci Biobehav Rev 117:26–64, 2017 28757456

Velders FP, Dieleman G, Henrichs J, et al: Prenatal and postnatal psychological symptoms of parents and family functioning: the impact on child emotional and behavioural problems. Eur Child Adolesc Psychiatry 20(7):341–350, 2011 21523465

Vesga-López O, Blanco C, Keyes K, et al: Psychiatric disorders in pregnant and postpartum women in the United States. Arch Gen Psychiatry 65(7):805–815, 2008 18606953

Voegtline KM, Costigan KA, Kivlighan KT, et al: Concurrent levels of maternal salivary cortisol are unrelated to self-reported psychological measures in low-risk pregnant women. Arch Women Ment Health 16(2):101–108, 2013 23269500

Wadhwa PD, Sandman CA, Porto M, et al: The association between prenatal stress and infant birth weight and gestational age at birth: a prospective investigation. Am J Obstet Gynecol 169(4):858–865, 1993 8238139

Walsh K, McCormack CA, Webster R, et al: Maternal prenatal stress phenotypes associate with fetal neurodevelopment and birth outcomes. Proc Natl Acad Sci USA 116(48):23996–24005, 2019 31611411

Ward TS, Kanu FA, Robb SW: Prevalence of stressful life events during pregnancy and its association with postpartum depressive symptoms. Arch Womens Ment Health 20:161–171, 2017

Weaver IC, Cervoni N, Champagne FA, et al: Epigenetic programming by maternal behavior. Nat Neurosci 7(8):847–854, 2004 15220929

Werner E, Zhao Y, Evans L, et al: Higher maternal prenatal cortisol and younger age predict greater infant reactivity to novelty at 4 months: an observation-based study. Dev Psychobiol 55(7):707–718, 2013 22778036

Werner EA, Gustafsson HC, Lee S, et al: PREPP: postpartum depression prevention through the mother-infant dyad. Arch Women Ment Health 19(2):229–242, 2016 26231973

Winsper C, Wolke D, Lereya T: Prospective associations between prenatal adversities and borderline personality disorder at 11–12 years. Psychol Med 45(5):1025–1037, 2015 25171495

Zhu P, Hao JH, Tao RX, et al: Sex-specific and time-dependent effects of prenatal stress on the early behavioral symptoms of ADHD: a longitudinal study in China. Eur Child Adolesc Psychiatry 24(9):1139–1147, 2015 25791080

Zuckerman M: Diathesis-stress models, in Vulnerability to Psychopathology: A Biosocial Model. Washington, DC, American Psychological Association, 1999, pp 3–23

# CHAPTER 12

# Infant Mental Health and the Parent–Infant Relationship

## Essentials, Assessment, and Treatment

Soudabeh Givrad, M.D.
Jennifer J. Paul, Ph.D.
Christine Wittmann, M.D.
Mireya Nadal-Vicens, M.D., Ph.D.
Celeste St. John-Larkin, M.D.

Psychiatrists and other mental health clinicians treating women during the perinatal period have a unique opportunity to assess infant mental health and to provide early intervention during a sensitive developmental period. In the prenatal and immediate postpartum periods, a complex interplay between biological and environmental factors sets the stage for the offspring's lifelong physical, neurocognitive, and social-emotional development. The quality of the main caregiving relationships is among the most influential environmental factors in infancy and early childhood. Infants grow in an interpersonal context, and they start to learn about themselves and the world they live in via their daily interactions with their primary caregivers. Of note, throughout this chapter we use the terms *primary caregivers* and *parents* interchangeably, although we realize that parents are not always the primary or the only primary caregivers for infants and young children.

We begin with an overview of infant mental health and its lifelong impact on health and well-being. We then review key components of the parent–infant relationship as they affect infant mental health, including attachment, biological pathways that influence infant neurodevelopment, and elements of the parent–infant dyad. We close by describing specific conditions that influence infant mental health, such as the neonatal intensive care setting, and touching on important issues in parenting and infant mental health for fathers, nonbirth parents, adoptive parents, and LGBTQ+ families. We hope that by understanding the importance of infant mental health, clinicians will gain an appreciation of the importance of the early life environment, both pre- and postnatally, in affecting the trajectory of mental and physical health throughout the lifespan.

Ms. Q is a 32-year-old gravida 1, para 1 woman who comes to see you for assessment and treatment of postpartum anxiety. She brings her 3-week-old baby boy, R, with her. During the visit, she appears both highly anxious and very tired, stating that she has been getting an average of 2–3 hours of sleep per night since R was born. She frequently turns to R and adjusts the way she is holding him, rarely keeping him in one position for more than a few seconds. As the minutes go by, she takes the pacifier in and then out of his mouth, puts a blanket on him and then takes it off, and alternates between standing up and sitting down, stating she just does not know what to do to soothe him. Baby R is making vocalizations that show he is neither settled nor content. Ms. Q reports feeling very flustered about this, and she apologizes to you about her baby's fussing. She then attempts to nurse him, and R appears to calm down temporarily, but you observe that he does not appear to be held in a comfortable position. Ms. Q is focused on his latching on and states that she often feels pain with nursing but believes she just has to put up with it. She seems irritated and says she feels guilty about complaining about the pain. She states that being a mother seems to come so naturally to other people she knows, and she wonders why it is not the same way with her: "I just don't know what he wants and how to calm him down, and it makes me feel like I am a terrible mother." You notice that she barely makes eye contact with R during the session. At one point she looks at R while he is nursing. He is looking intently into her eyes. She turns to you and, with a tone of sadness, says, "See? I can't tell what he wants from me when he looks at me like this."

## Infant Mental Health

*Infant mental health* has been defined as "the developing capacity of the child from birth to age three to experience, regulate, and express emotions; form close and secure interpersonal relationships; and explore the environment and learn—all in the context of family, community and cultural expectations for young children" (Zero to Three Infant Mental Health Task Force Steering Committee 2001). An understanding of infant mental health is important even for clinicians who focus on adult mental health, because one of its founding principles is that early life experiences—whether positive or adverse—shape the brain and have a lifelong impact on health, behavior, and cognition into adulthood (Clinton et al. 2016).

The Adverse Childhood Experiences study is one example that highlights the importance of the early environment in affecting health and well-being into adulthood. This study showed that adverse childhood experiences (ACEs) such as abuse, neglect, and trauma had a dose-response, lifelong effect on the incidence of conditions linked to the risk of mortality, such as depression, suicide attempts, alcoholism, substance abuse, cigarette smoking, cardiovascular events, and cancer (Felitti et al. 1998). A subsequent systematic review and meta-analysis showed that the number of ACEs that co-occur (e.g., four or more) was strongly associated with poor mental, physical, and sexual health in adulthood and was linked with outcomes that affect families across generations, such as substance abuse, mental illness, and violence (Hughes et al. 2017). Researchers have calculated that six or more ACEs results in a ≥20-year reduction in life expectancy (Price et al. 2013). Research is now beginning to focus on factors that promote positive health outcomes in the setting of adverse events—that is, resilience—especially in the setting of chronic external stressors, such as resource inequity (Kinner and Borschmann 2017).

Additionally, there is greater understanding about the influence of the parent–infant relationship on the neurodevelopment of the infant. Evidence has consistently demonstrated that a secure attachment relationship leads to development of neural structures that lay the foundation for child mental health and well-being and positively influences the hypothalamic-pituitary axis, which regulates the response to external stress (Clinton et al. 2016). When these early relationships are highly stressful (e.g., with absence, neglect, or violence), the neural pathways attuned toward reactivity are accentuated, setting children up for ongoing challenges throughout life (Clinton et al. 2016). In contrast, a sound social and emotional base through secure attachment creates a foundation for robust physical, cognitive, and motor development (Clinton et al. 2016).

## The Parent–Infant Relationship

### Attachment

Human infants, through repeated interactions with caregivers, learn to seek comfort and protection from a selective number of reliable caregivers (Finelli et al. 2019). *Attachment* describes this bond with a main caregiver, from whom the infant seeks safety and nurturance. Attachment between infants and caregivers is crucial for their development because it increases the likelihood of infant survival and serves as the bedrock of cognitive, social, and emotional development (Insel and Young 2001). Attachment, in terms of behaviors that govern connections between infant and caregiver, can be observed throughout mammalian development (Insel and Young 2001). The concept of *attachment* was first named by John Bowlby, who defined it as "a lasting psychological connectedness between human beings" (Bowlby 1969, p. 194) and concluded that "what is believed to be essential for mental health is that the infant and young child should experience a warm, intimate, and continuous relationship with his mother (or permanent mother substitute) in which both find satisfaction and enjoyment" (Bowlby 1951, p. 11).

Caregivers promote development of secure attachment in their infant by meeting the infant's needs with reasonable reliability and warmth. Similarly, following the infant's lead in terms of engagement, with the appropriate amount of eye contact, expressivity of the face, and tolerance of the infant's negative emotions, is a critical component of the caregiver's role in this process (Sroufe 1985). Many parents have an expectation, reinforced by social myths, that bonding happens the instant the infant is placed on the mother's chest after delivery or makes eye contact. In reality, the process of attachment and bonding is much more nuanced and can change over time. This is important because it allows for interventions that can address any difficulty that may be present initially or develop over time.

Several concepts related to attachment and development of an optimal relationship between parents and infants are important in understanding the parent–infant relationship. The first concept is infant *self-regulation*. When caregivers respond promptly to an infant's distress, the infants adjust without needing to escalate their demands. In turn, this makes it easier for infants to self-soothe and self-regulate because their level of distress experienced is not severe. Thus, the ability to self-soothe and self-regulate is the result of a healthy attachment with a responsive caregiver, through a process of coregulation. Through repeated interactions with emotionally available caregivers, infants not only begin to learn how to manage basic biological rhythms (e.g., sleeping, waking, eating) but also develop early self-control through emotional regulation and negotiation. Sameroff and Fiese (2000) proposed that, at birth, infants are primarily dependent on the "other" or primary caregiver for maintaining self-regulation. As the infants mature, they become increasingly capable and responsible for their own self-regulation, but they continue to function within the context of coregulation with significant others into adulthood and throughout life (Sameroff and Fiese 2000).

The second concept is infant temperament. Broadly speaking, *temperament* refers to individual differences in emotional and motor reactivity that are mostly stable across situations and over time (Rothbart and Derryberry 1981). Processes that serve to modulate reactivity include attentional control, attention shifting, and inhibitory control; these processes serve as the basis for self-regulation (Gartstein and Skinner 2018). In the past, temperament was described as a fixed, "constitutional" set of traits and was thought to be a highly heritable platform for social and emotional development (Lewis et al. 2015). However, recent research has highlighted the dynamic processes involved in infant temperament formation, including such factors as the epigenetic effects of stress and the impact of maternal mental health disorders (Gartstein and Skinner 2018; Lewis et al. 2015). Variations in infant temperament highlight the importance of noting what infants bring to the relationship and the effects of that on the parents. This also leads to the concept of *goodness of fit* between a parent and an infant; a parent might be able to more easily establish an optimal coregulatory process and bond with one child but find another child more challenging, in part due to differences in their temperament (Chess and Thomas 1991).

Our understanding of attachment as it relates to the parent–infant relationship has developed throughout the past several decades. Some early pioneers of this work were Mary Ainsworth and colleagues, who created a research method called the Strange Situation Protocol (SSP) to provide a standardized way of assessing toddlers' attachment to a given caretaker (Ainsworth and Bell 1970). The SSP involves observing toddlers' behavior in several different laboratory settings: with the caregiver, with the caregiver and a stranger, with the stranger alone, entirely alone, and upon reunion with the caregiver. Based on the toddlers' behavior in these settings—their reaction to separation and reunion with their primary caregiver—their attachment style to that caregiver can be described. Ainsworth and colleagues categorized attachment into two overarching styles: secure and insecure, with two branches of insecure or anxious attachment (avoidant and ambivalent/resistant) (Ainsworth and Bell 1970; Ainsworth et al. 1978). Table 12–1 summarizes the attachment styles of infancy and the anticipated responses to the SSP. Main and Solomon (1986, 1990) later proposed an additional type of insecure attachment, *disorganized*, suggesting that these infants experienced fear of the parent that resulted in an inconsistent response to that parent's return. Infants with a disorga-

**TABLE 12–1. Attachment categorizations and associated examples of infant/young child behavior**

| Attachment style | Secure (type B)* | Insecure | | |
|---|---|---|---|---|
| | | Avoidant (type A)* | Ambivalent/Resistant (type C)* | Disorganized/Disoriented (type D)** |
| Infant/Young child behavioral examples | Happily interacts with caregiver<br>Explores environment freely while occasionally checking in with caregiver<br>Friendly toward stranger when caregiver is present<br>Exhibits distress upon separation from caregiver<br>Avoids stranger and limits exploration while separated from caregiver<br>Enthusiastically greets caregiver upon return<br>Seeks caregiver when distressed and is easily soothed by caregiver<br>Trusts that caregiver will be available to meet needs | Explores environment without acknowledging caregiver<br>Limits emotional expression across range of emotions despite physiological arousal<br>No outward indication of distress upon separation from caregiver<br>Plays as usual when stranger is present and caregiver is absent<br>Shows little interest in interaction with caregiver upon return by not moving toward caregiver or seeking contact<br>May avoid or ignore caregiver generally, as well as when distressed | Shows unwillingness to explore environment and exhibits fear of stranger<br>Displays clingy behavior and may cry and seek out caregiver even prior to separation<br>Exhibits intense distress upon separation from caregiver<br>Demonstrates ambivalence toward caregiver upon return by vacillating between contact-seeking and contact-rejecting behavior<br>Expresses anger or anxiety when caregiver attempts to soothe<br>Struggles to regulate intense emotions and may exaggerate emotional response in effort to elicit attention from caregiver<br>Difficult to soothe and responds poorly to caregiver's attempts to comfort | Displays inconsistent, unpredictable, and directionless behavior<br>Expresses fear and confusion when interacting with caregiver<br>Demonstrates unusual and sometimes contradictory behavior in response to caregiver, such as freezing, posturing, or engaging in self-stimulatory behavior (e.g., head-banging)<br>Struggles to cope or be comforted when distressed |

*Source.* *Adapted from Ainsworth et al. 1978. **Adapted from Main and Solomon 1990.

nized attachment style have an increased likelihood of having a history of maltreatment or having a primary caregiver with unresolved trauma or loss (Granqvist et al. 2017). Attachment is specific to the infant and a particular caregiver. Infants can form different attachment styles to individual caretakers; they may have a secure attachment with one caregiver and an insecure attachment with another (Dagan and Sagi-Schwartz 2018).

Many studies have looked at characteristics of children who were observed to have insecure attachment early in life. These children appear to be at increased risk for greater negativity in early childhood, slower cognitive development, and externalizing behaviors in adolescence (Boldt et al. 2017; Ding et al. 2014). In addition to its effect on interpersonal relationships, attachment also predicts ability to self-regulate (Davis et al. 2011). Infants with disorganized attachment demonstrate greater increases in cortisol in response to a stressful situation than infants with organized attachment (Bernard and Dozier 2010).

Attachment provides the earliest model for human relationships. Thus, children with insecure attachment may grow up to be adults who struggle to form stable, loving, and trusting relationships with others. This research has led to efforts to characterize attachment patterns in adults, and the Adult Attachment Interview (AAI) was created to address this need (George et al. 1985). This instrument asks adults to recount aspects of their childhood and childhood relationships with each parent, then scores their responses. Their ability to form a coherent and nuanced narrative, independent of the actual events experienced, is analyzed to gain insight into adult individuals' conceptualization of relationship with their own attachment figures and family environment as a child and the degree to which an organized pattern of experience has been developed. AAI categorizes adults into four categories of secure-autonomous (F), dismissing (D), preoccupied (E), and disoriented/disorganized (U/D). For example, an adult whose AAI reveals patchy or broken narratives without much substance may be categorized as being in the dismissive category.

The dynamic nature of attachment offers hope for the potential benefits of clinical intervention. Parents and caregivers who have psychiatric illnesses that impede their ability to respond warmly and consistently to the needs of infants and toddlers will benefit from standard treatment of those illnesses, as well as parent–child dyad therapies or coaching about the types of parental behaviors necessary for healthy child development. When infants have developed a disorganized attachment, interventions to address this are associated with improvements in the security and organization of attachment (Cicchetti et al. 2006; Facompré et al. 2018).

One criticism of studies of attachment has been that early studies looked only at mothers and their infants and primarily at white, middle-class families (Van IJzendoorn and Kroonenberg 1988). Through the framework of infant mental health, the Irving Harris Professional Development Network established Diversity Informed Tenets for Work with Infants, Children and Families to address the impact of institutional and cultural barriers that lead to class, race, and other inequities (St. John and Thomas 2012). There are 10 tenets based on the following core concepts: diversity-informed practice, equity, intersectionality, privilege, reflective capacity, and social justice (Irving Harris Foundation 2018). Dr. Ghosh Ippen explained this further: "Diversity-informed practice is dynamic, focusing not just on values, beliefs or experiences of a group or individual but on interactions among people with different views.…Perspectives are shaped not only by their own experience but also by the larger sociopolitical and historical context" (Ghosh Ippen et al. 2012, p. 33). This framework is especially helpful, given the increased recognition of the social determinants of health and related health disparities, to ensure that all women, infants, and families receive the best care possible.

## Neurobiology of Attachment

The parent–infant relationship serves to set the neurobiological tone for the infant brain, which in turn affects how that infant deals with stress. Critical to infant neurodevelopment—and foundational to the development of attachment—are the opposing concepts of the promotion of self-regulation and the transmission of stress. Interestingly, there is some evidence for genomic intergenerational transmission of trauma. Women who survived the Tutsi genocide while pregnant had children with alterations in the hippocampus-pituitary-adrenal axis (HPA), including lower cortisol and higher mineralocorticoid receptor signaling together with genomic changes in glucocorticoid receptors (Perroud et al. 2014).

Surprisingly, there is also evidence of paternal transmission of a trauma history, presumably through genomic modifications of spermal chromatin. Children of male Holocaust survivors show a modification in a glucocorticoid receptor that is associated with an increase in stress reactivity (Yehuda et al. 2014). These findings have been validated in animal studies showing that male rodents exposed to an olfactory fear paradigm transmit odor-specific fear to their progeny. These progeny then, in turn, transmit that fear to their own progeny, meaning that the biological underpinnings (through epigenetic changes transmitted via spermal chromatin) exist for the transmission of trauma through multiple generations (Dias and Ressler 2014). Although stress is clearly transmitted along both parental lines to infants who may show evidence of that stress later in life, those markings can be offset by postnatal experiences such as parent–infant relationships that promote self-regulation and thus enhance resiliency.

Biologically, behaviorally, and psychologically, the parent–infant relationship begins in the prenatal period for both the parent and the developing fetus. The maternal environment is transmitted to the infant in various ways. Proposed mechanisms include the maternal HPA axis resulting in fetal stress hormone exposure, placental epigenetics, placental mitochondrial dysfunction, maternal immune system activation, and the maternal microbiome. The first two pathways, HPA axis and epigenetics, are discussed here; please see Chapter 11, "Stress in Pregnancy," for a detailed discussion of the mechanisms through which parental stress gets transmitted to the offspring.

It has long been appreciated that maternal stress is associated with adverse infant outcomes. We now know that maternal stress is associated with changes in fetal brain development in ways that may alter the stress response of infants throughout their lifespan. For example, stress during pregnancy is associated with long-lasting changes in infants' HPA axis; in humans, these alterations are detectable at 6 months, 5 years, and even 10 years after birth (Lupien et al. 2009). Perinatal stress tends to affect the HPA axis and how sensitive it is to stress in the child's environment. One mechanism is by having the perinatal environment modify the chromatin around the genes relevant to the stress response, known as *epigenetic modification*, which can lead to multigenerational transfer of altered stress response. In addition, prenatal exposure to maternal stress is also associated with modifications of at least two brain areas critical for emotional regulation: the size of the hippocampus and the reactivity of the amygdala (Qiu et al. 2015; Rifkin-Graboi et al. 2015). Exposure to significant prenatal stress may even affect infants' later cognitive functioning (Davis and Sandman 2010). This effect may be mediated simply through exposure to stress hormones (glucocorticoids); glucocorticoid administration in the absence of external stress is associated with smaller hippocampal size in both infants and monkeys (Lupien et al. 2009).

As discussed in detail in Chapter 11 and Chapter 19 ("Anxiety Disorders and Insomnia in the Perinatal Period"), delineating the differential impact of different types of perinatal distress can be challenging, given the overlap of—and comorbidity among—distress, perceived stress, anxiety disorders, pregnancy-related anxiety, depressive disorders, and other disorders, such as PTSD. That said, specific maternal mental health conditions, such as anxiety and depressive disorders, have been associated with many of the same infant neurobiological changes produced by chronic stress in pregnancy, such as HPA stress axis alterations, decreased hippocampal size, and increased amygdalar reactivity (Qiu et al. 2015; Rifkin-Graboi et al. 2013, 2015). In humans, infants exposed to maternal depression and anxiety show altered stress responses detectable even in later childhood, for example, at age 10 (Lupien et al. 2009). Interestingly, in rodent models, selective serotonin reuptake inhibitors (SSRIs) reverse the effects of prenatal stress exposure on hippocampal volume (Rayen et al. 2011).

After birth, the parent–infant relationship continues to be a highly dynamic combination of nature and nurture. Two main neurobiological pathways are thought to be involved in the parent–infant attachment bond: 1) the dopaminergic "reward" pathway and 2) the oxytocinergic system (Scatliffe et al. 2019; Strathearn et al. 2009). Oxytocin is a neuromodulatory hormone produced in the hypothalamus that plays a key role in physiological processes, such as labor and lactation. Oxytocin is also believed to be critical to the emergence and maintenance of the behavior that forms the basis of the parent–infant bond (Kim et al. 2014). Oxytocin is released in response to stimuli such as infant suckling or the sight or sound of a nursing mother's infant (McNeilly et al. 1983). Evidence suggests a relationship between oxytocin and prosocial effects, such as enhanced social memory, improved eye gaze when looking at faces, increased recognition of faces and facial expressions, and increased manifestations of trust (Baumgartner et al. 2008; Domes et al. 2007; Guastella et al. 2008a, 2008b; Kosfeld et al. 2005; Savaskan et al. 2008). Likewise, oxytocin is thought to mediate multiple behavioral components of the parent–infant relationship, including physical contact, synchrony, and responsiveness. These effects are notably seen in both mother–infant and father–infant pairs (Kim et al. 2014; Scatliffe et al. 2019; Vittner et al. 2018). Oxytocin receptors are located in the ventral striatum, an important dopaminergic brain region, and animal models have demonstrated that oxytocin receptor binding is associated with maternal prosocial behaviors (Olazábal and Young 2006). Thus, it is thought that oxytocin may link social cues to dopamine-associated reinforcement pathways (Strathearn et al. 2009).

Of the multiple ways that the early parent–infant relationship affects infant neurodevelopment, most is known about the role of physical contact. One of the benefits of being held close to a parent's chest is that the infant regulates breathing and heart rate to more closely match those of the adult, which in turn lowers overall stress tone. For example, Meaney and Szyf (2005) have shown in animal rodent models that increased frequency of being licked as an infant (a form of maternal nurturing behavior) lowered anxiety levels in adulthood by modifying the HPA axis and that decreased licking and grooming in infancy resulted in higher stress levels in adult rodents (Meaney and Szyf 2005; Weaver et al. 2004). They found that exposure to licking produced epi-

**TABLE 12–2. Benefits of skin-to-skin contact after birth**

| Maternal benefits | Infant benefits |
|---|---|
| Earlier expulsion of placenta | Decrease in the "stress of being born" |
| Reduced postpartum bleeding | Improved thermoregulation |
| Increased breastfeeding self-efficacy | Less crying |
| Lowered maternal stress levels | Increased breastfeeding initiation |
| Promotion of mother–infant bonding (perhaps mediated through elevated postbirth oxytocin levels) | Heart rate variability regulation |
| | Decreased pain and distress |
| | Improved breathing patterns and oxygen saturation levels |
| | Improved sleep |
| | Improved digestion and weight gain |
| | Improved survival and shorter neonatal intensive care unit admission for premature infants |
| | Accelerated pace of oral microbial repertoire maturity |

*Source.* Cleveland et al. 2017; Hendricks-Muñoz et al. 2015; Mitchell et al. 2013; Moore et al. 2016; Rojas et al. 2003; Samra et al. 2013; Widström et al. 2019.

genetic changes in one of the stress response receptors that were adopted for the life of the animal (Francis et al. 1999; Weaver et al. 2004). The same epigenetic DNA changes have been found in humans; for example, the DNA structure that encodes the stress response molecules in rodents is similar to the DNA structure in humans with a history of child abuse who later committed suicide (McGowan et al. 2009).

Physical contact between mother and infant has important clinical benefits. For example, skin-to-skin contact (SSC)—also referred to as Kangaroo Care—has clear evidence of benefit for mother and newborn after birth, such as helping the newborn transition to extrauterine life, increasing rates of breastfeeding, and promoting early parent–infant bonding (United Nations Children's Fund and World Health Organization 2009). These benefits have led to the implementation of SSC as part of the requirements for the World Health Organization (WHO)'s Baby-Friendly Hospital Initiative (United Nations Children's Fund and World Health Organization 2009). See Table 12–2 for a summary of the benefits of SSC. Given its efficacy, cost-effectiveness, and feasibility, SSC has been recommended as the standard of high-quality care for all newborn infants, no matter what the gestational age, geographical location, or socioeconomic environment (Campbell-Yeo et al. 2015).

Physical contact is also very important in its absence. Physical separation from a caring adult increases stress and, if prolonged, results in long-term increases in stress reactivity. In rodents, even separations of 3 hours per day, if repeated, are associated with long-lasting changes in stress tone and in the neurobiology of the hippocampus, a brain area critical to learning and emotional response (Lupien et al. 2009). Humans deprived of physical contact in early infancy have myriad neurobiological changes that go well beyond the hippocampus and amygdala to include global brain size, attention, IQ, verbal functioning, executive functioning, working memory, and more

(Nelson et al. 2007). The clinical implications of this issue were highlighted recently in the setting of the COVID-19 pandemic. In the early days of the pandemic, there was discussion of physically separating mothers with suspected or proven COVID-19 infection from their newborns (Stuebe 2020). However, the initial policies enacted were mixed, reflecting the tension between the desire to reduce the risk of transmission between mother and infant and the known clinical benefits of physical contact. The WHO recommended against separation, stating that infants with mothers with suspected or confirmed COVID-19 should be "enabled to stay together, practicing skin to skin contact," whereas the Centers for Disease Control and Prevention initially advised that facilities "consider separating the mother from her infant" until the mother was considered no longer contagious (Centers for Disease Control and Prevention 2020; Stuebe 2020; World Health Organization 2020).

## The Parent–Infant Dyad

The parent–infant relationship comprises the *observable aspects* of the interaction and the *unobservable aspects* (i.e., mental, emotional, representational) of the relationship.

### Observable Interactions

The observable aspects of the parent–infant relationship consist of the nuances of their interactions with each other. Infants are born with unique capabilities at birth, including having a preference for maternal smell (Macfarlane 1975; Sullivan and Toubas 1998) and voice (DeCasper and Fifer 1980) and preferring the mother's face over other shapes and objects or even a stranger's face (Bushnell et al. 1989; Field et al. 1984; Pascalis et al. 1995). From the beginning, they are active participants in their environment and their interactions with their caregivers. The relationship between the parent and infant is very intimate and made up of physical closeness through touch, nonverbal interactions (e.g., gaze), mutual communication through vocalizations and protoconversations, and coregulation, such as the level of reciprocity between mother and infant. Many facets of the parent–infant dyad influence the quality of the interaction, including parental responsiveness, handling of disruption and repair, and the pleasure experienced by both parent and infant. The microanalytic research, which looks at early mother–infant interactions, shows that infants and mothers engage in a rich and detailed back-and-forth exchange, which, if studied at 4 months of age, can predict the development of secure versus avoidant attachment patterns at 1 year (Koulomzin et al. 2002).

### Unobservable Interactions

Parents often evolve a rich set of imaginations and expectations regarding their infants and regarding themselves as parents, which are referred to as *parental representational mind*. These thoughts and fantasies are affected by the parents' history with their own caregivers, culture, life events, hopes, dreams, fears, and history of trauma, among other factors (Stern 1985, 1995). Another important concept is *parental reflective functioning*. Parental reflective functioning has been described as parents' capacity to understand their own and their child's mental states, and the effects these have on behaviors and interactions between them (De Roo et al. 2019). Parental reflective functioning is associated with better parent–child coregulation and is linked to the quality of the parent–child attachment (Moser et al. 2019).

In turn, through interactions with their primary caregivers, infants begin forming mental patterns of how they are perceived in each interaction, how they are expected to respond, and what they can expect from the other person. Over time, they might start internalizing these images and identifying with them. These internalized images, or *mental representations*, of themselves and the world around them are also called *internal working models* (Crittenden 1990). Galinsky (1987) theorized that parent and child development are intertwined, such that the child's and parent's developmental processes shape each other; the parental stages of development correspond with the baby's own age and developmental trajectory. Just as children advance through several developmental stages, adults also continue to move through developmental stages within the context of the transition to parenthood.

The infant's psychological life begins in the parents' mind (Gilmore and Meersand 2013). Galinsky (1987) proposed six progressive psychological stages of parenthood: Image-Making, Nurturing, Authority, Interpretive, Interdependent, and Departure. In Galinsky's model, Stage 1 (Image-Making)—when parents form images about their infants and begin to imagine who and how they will be as parents—begins at conception and continues through delivery. Parental mental representations have been hypothesized to become more elaborate as the pregnancy progresses and to continue into the postnatal period, when parents encounter the real infant. These mental representations can translate into feelings about the pregnancy, infant, and their evolving family and might be associated with parents projecting or attributing characteristics to the infant pre- or postnatally. These attributions might have a positive or negative valence. Even when positive, they may not be accurate and therefore not match the real infant. In effect, the imagined infant may or may not reflect the real infant.

Of note, adults' own experiences of being parented may affect how they parent their own children. Negative experiences of being parented as a child and their influence on how these adults parent their own children have been described as "ghosts in the nursery" (Fraiberg et al. 1975). These "ghosts" can be transmitted from one generation to the next and seem to influence parent–child interaction, silently and negatively, in the present moment, potentially leading to an intergenerational cycle of abuse and trauma. More recently, "angels in the nursery" have been proposed as a positive counterpart, representing benevolent parenting experiences (Lieberman et al. 2005b). Early positive experiences of parenting in childhood lead to security and self-confidence in adulthood. This, in turn, affects adults' experience of and responses to their own children. It can also serve to interrupt negative patterns of interaction or abuse.

## Assessment

Assessment of parent–infant relationships can start during pregnancy, before the infant is born. During the prenatal period, the clinician can get a sense of parental mental representations by noticing how the parents talk about their infant and about themselves as parents. The clinician can also ask the parents what they think their baby will be like, how they imagine their relationship with their baby will be, if they have any worries about being a parent, and how the transition to parenthood has been affecting their understanding and feelings about each other. Later, when the infant is born, the clinician can explore whether the experience of having this infant and the transition to parenthood have been similar to what they imagined and, if not, how they have been different. Within the psychotherapy context, there is space to evaluate and understand attributions to the infant that might be related to the parent's history of relational experiences, traumas, and other societal and cultural beliefs. Research has shown that early alteration of unbalanced or disrupted parental attachment representations can decrease the rates of internalizing and externalizing disorders in childhood (Tooten et al. 2014).

The assessment phase continues after the child's birth in terms of analyzing various components of the interactions between parents and their infant. Several formal methods of assessment and observation of parent–infant interactions have been developed. Some of the main factors identified and evaluated in these interactions consist of maternal sensitivity, responsiveness, contingency, dyadic reciprocity, disruption and repair, level of intrusiveness or control, and the pleasure experienced by the parent and the infant. Several of the formalized assessment measures include the Crowell Parent–Child Interaction Procedure (Crowell et al. 1988); the Face-to-Face Still-Face Procedure (Tronick et al. 1978); the Marschak Interaction Method (Marschak 1960); and the Early Relational Assessment (Clark 1999).

The perinatal mental health clinician who is seeing the mother or both parents in the postpartum period can also obtain rich information from clinically observing the interactions between parents and their infant, including the quality of the gaze, the touch, the vocalization between the parents and the infant, and the affective tone between them. Moreover, the clinician should assess the level of reciprocity within the dyad—how the infant responds to various verbal and nonverbal communications and contact from the parents, and vice versa. Does the dyad seem to reciprocate, engage, be soothed by, and enjoy the interactions?

Parents and infants go through various cycles and can experience mismatches or disruptions regularly, even when all is going well between them. Mismatches are often followed by repair and eventually get to a point of harmony (Tronick and Gianino 1986). Therefore, when observing parent–infant interactions, the goal is not to draw conclusions based on each and every observable interaction but, rather, to consider them as a cumulative set of data that, when considered with the information the clinician has about the parent's psychology, psychopathology, relationships, history of trauma, and representational mind, can help with better assessment of any relational problems between parents and infants.

## Touch

Touch is one of the main ways in which parents and infants connect and communicate. The extensive research on the importance and necessity of physical closeness, touch, and SSC from the first moments after birth has translated into policies and practices that aim at supporting mothers, and increasingly fathers, in providing this experience for infants, including those born prematurely (Cleveland et al. 2017; Field et al. 2010). When assessing touch and the ways in which the infant is physically handled in the perinatal setting, one can pay attention to things such as

- Is the parent able to be physically close to the infant and hold him or her?
- How does the parent touch and handle the infant?
- Do the parent and infant appear comfortable, and is the parent attuned to what the infant is expressing?
- Is the quality of touch affectionate and gentle, or intrusive and rough?
- Does the parent enjoy physical closeness to the infant?

- How does the infant respond to being physically close to the parent? Is the infant able to nestle against the parent's body? Is the infant able to be soothed when held or rocked, or is his or her body rigid and uncomfortable?

## Gaze

So much of the communication between parents and infants is nonverbal, and gaze is one of the main ways that infants communicate with others (Negri 2007). In fact, gaze aversion in infants is thought to be one of their main ways of disengaging or signaling dislike, distress, or disconnect and at times a way to self-regulate before being able to reengage in more direct interactions. Parents can also have difficulty engaging in face-to-face interaction, which includes periods of mutual gaze with the infant. When assessing gaze in the dyad, some things to notice are

- Is the parent able to engage in face-to-face interaction with the infant?
- What is the quality of gaze (e.g., soft and affectionate vs. cold and distant)?
- Are the parent and the infant able to engage in mutual gaze?
- What happens when an infant averts his or her gaze? Is the parent able to wait for the infant to self-regulate and reengage, or is this too distressing for the parent, who must find a way to make eye contact with the infant again?
- Is the infant able to look at the clinician and make eye contact?

Of course, these interactions vary based on the infant's age and developmental stage and the infant's arousal state at the time of observation, such as whether the infant is interactive and playful or sleepy and restful.

## Vocalizations

Parents and infants also communicate verbally and through vocalization. Infants and their caregivers engage in vocal turn-taking prior to the development of speech, called *protoconversations*. These protoconversations set the stage for bonding, language, and social development of the infant (Yoo et al. 2018). From a very early age, infants start vocalizing different sounds, to which parents respond in various ways (Bornstein et al. 2015). This sets the stage for contingent interactions within the pair. The rate of conversation turn-taking may vary within different communities and cultures; however, to date, our knowledge indicates that mothers universally respond to their infant's vocalizations and that infant vocalization is also contingent on maternal verbal communication. Within these interactions, and more so in the beginning, mothers are more responsive to their infants than vice versa (Bornstein et al. 2015). By 6 months of age, infants have learned that their vocalizations have social value and that parental engagement can be altered by the level and type of vocalization (Franklin et al. 2014). In perinatal mental health settings, the clinician can pay attention to the presence or absence of any conversational turn-taking, the affective tone of the vocalizations in both the parent and the infant, the match or mismatch in the tone and rhythmicity of this interaction, and the content (in the parent with a preverbal infant).

## Treatment

When parents and infants face problems and challenges in their relationship, whether due to parental psychopathology, medical traumas, attachment problems, or other reasons, it is important to address these issues because both parents and infants can be significantly affected by them. Parents seen in perinatal mental health settings receive treatment for their mental health issues, such as depression or anxiety. However, studies have shown that treatment of maternal psychopathology alone does not always translate into better connection and relationship with the infant (Forman et al. 2007). When there are concerns about the parent–infant relationship,the psychopathology and relational issues ideally should be addressed simultaneously whenever possible.

Parent–infant psychotherapy focuses on the relationship between the parent and the infant as the main target of treatment and intervention. It is a strength-based, culturally informed model of care in which the therapist identifies and draws on the existing strengths in the relationship and family system. The treatment consists of a range of interventions, some practical (e.g., making sure the parent and infant have the basic necessities of a safe living environment), some behavioral (e.g., focusing on the observable interactions between the parent and the infant), and some geared toward the mental representations and emotional dynamics between the parent and the infant. Additionally, educating and informing parents about normal development and realistic expectations can be a significant part of treatment. This is especially true for first-time parents and those who have a child with medical or developmental problems.

Ms. S is a 28-year-old woman, gravida 1 para 0, at 34 weeks+3 days who is referred to you by her obstetrician for concerns about mood and anxiety. In your intake session, she reveals a past psychiatric history of generalized anxiety disorder and tells you she had been on a stable dose of escitalopram for the past 5 years. Recently her anxiety has been worse, and she thinks her mood is becoming more depressed. Ms. S is a graduate student in chemistry at a laboratory in an academic center nearby, and she reports that it is highly stressful work. You explore the circumstances around her pregnancy and how she feels about the pregnancy and her baby. She reports that this was a planned pregnancy, but she is now feeling more anxious because she is realizing that this is not an ideal time to pause her experiments. She is worried about how this will affect her project and the paper she wants to write and if competing laboratories will use this opportunity to publish ahead of her. She is hoping the baby does not come soon, so that she can have more time to wrap up some of her experiments. She feels guilty about these thoughts and feelings and is anxious about whether she is able to be a good and dedicated mother because she believes she should be more focused on her pregnancy and on becoming a mother. Her own mother stopped working when she had a child and later was always resentful about not being able to have the career she had wanted. Ms. S believes that part of her identity is deeply tied to her career and education, and she finds her work a great source of joy. When exploring her mental representations of her baby, she tells you that she imagines her daughter will be a strong, curious, and independent baby.

At the end of the session, you suggest an increase in the dose of escitalopram to optimize her treatment and explore whether she is open to psychotherapy. She reports that, due to time constraints, she cannot participate in weekly psychotherapy at this point. As part of her treatment, when you see her every 2–3 weeks, you start exploring her mental representations of her child and herself as a mother. You discuss her ambivalence about changes in her identity and career trajectory, her fear of her baby being needy or fussy, and how this all is affecting her connection with her baby. You also start to speak more about her own childhood and her relationship with her parents, particularly her mother. Her mother always appeared envious of her friends who continued working and were more financially independent. Despite her mother not pursuing her career, Ms. S always experienced her mother as distant and preoccupied. She is worried about being able to respond to her baby's needs.

> Over time, Ms. S is able to build a much more elaborate and nuanced narrative of her relationship with her mother and to imagine her mother's experiences and challenges and her own experiences and feelings during childhood and as an adult. She is also gradually able to voice a wider range of feelings about her transition to motherhood and the joys and challenges she might face. In your last prenatal appointment at 39 weeks+4 days, she talks with excitement about meeting her baby girl soon and tells you: "I am so excited to meet my baby and get to know her."

There are several evidence-based models of care for infants and their caregivers (Njoroge and Yang 2012). These are listed in Table 12–3. Additionally, some other interventions with a focus on the mother–infant dyad address maternal mental health. Two with promising results are Mother-Infant Therapy Group (M-ITG) and Mom Power. M-ITG is a 12-week manualized program of individualized support in the context of a psychotherapeutic group setting for mothers with PMADs and their infants (Clark et al. 2003, 2008). Mom Power is an attachment-based, trauma-informed multifamily parenting and mental health intervention for high-risk mothers and their young children (Muzik et al. 2015; Rosenblum et al. 2017, 2018).

Even though different treatment models use different frames, the therapist working with parents and their young children needs to maintain a certain level of flexibility. For instance, the therapist needs to be able to shift between sessions in which the infant is present to individual sessions or to sessions focusing on issues within the parental couple that may be affecting the infant, based on the needs for each dyad and family. At times, the focus of a session might be on figuring out how the mother can access more support, whereas at other times the focus might be on exploring how past traumas and experiences are shaping parental perception of the infant or on how the parent makes meaning of the infant's behavior.

## Special Considerations

### Premature/Medically Ill Infants

Each year, about 8%–10% of infants born in the United States need admission to a neonatal intensive care unit (NICU) due to prematurity or medical complications (Harrison and Goodman 2015). NICU admission brings on many challenges for infants and their parents and possibly within their relationship. NICU infants experience early separation, unnatural environments, painful and intrusive procedures, problems with physiological regulation, and long periods of isolation (Maroney 2003). They have been hypothesized to be neurologically more susceptible to both positive and negative environmental factors (Krugers et al. 2016).

In turn, NICU parents have a significantly higher rate of depression, anxiety, and PTSD, as well as generally higher levels of psychological stress (Roque et al. 2017). The transition to parenthood often happens in an abrupt, unexpected, and traumatic manner for these parents. They may struggle with parental self-efficacy because they are often dependent on NICU staff to care for their infant. They must adjust to caring for a medically vulnerable infant and communicate with multiple medical providers (Vance et al. 2020), and they may have fears of possibly hurting their infant themselves. NICU parents may experience a process of grief and of feeling robbed of the experiences that

**TABLE 12–3. Evidence-based models of care and promising practices for parent–child relationship treatment**

| Dyadic intervention tools | Brief description | Intended age of child, *years* | Key references |
|---|---|---|---|
| Attachment and Biobehavioral Catch-up[a] | Dyadic intervention designed to increase parental nurturance and parent–child reciprocity through parent coaching for children who have experienced neglect or other types of interpersonal trauma | 0–2 | Bernard et al. 2012; Dozier and Bernard 2019a, 2019b; Dozier et al. 2018 |
| Child-Parent Psychotherapy[a,b] | Relationship-based, manualized intervention to treat trauma sequelae in young children and their caregivers | 0–5 | Ghosh Ippen et al. 2012; Lieberman et al. 2005a, 2006, 2015, 2019 |
| Circle of Security Intervention[b] | Relationship-based, attachment-informed group treatment targeting caregiver sensitivity and responsiveness to promote child attachment security | 0–5 | Coyne et al. 2019; Powell et al. 2014; Ramsauer et al. 2014; Yaholkoski et al. 2016 |
| Incredible Years (basic parent training and child training intervention [Dinosaur School])[a,b] | Two components of three-pronged developmentally centered group-based curriculum to promote positive parenting practices and child prosocial behaviors, as well as treat children's disruptive behaviors | 0–12 (basic); 3–8 (child training) | Menting et al. 2013; Reid and Webster-Stratton 2011; Seabra-Santos et al. 2016; Webster-Stratton 2011; Webster-Stratton and Reid 2003 |
| Parent-Child Interaction Therapy[a,b] | Dyadic, manualized treatment for children with disruptive behavior disorders and their caregivers | 2–7 | Carpenter et al. 2014; Eyberg 1988; Eyberg et al. 2001; Stevens and N'zi 2019; Thomas and Herschell 2013; Thomas and Zimmer-Gembeck 2012 |
| Promoting First Relationships[a,c] | Home visiting prevention/intervention program utilizing parent training strategies to promote secure and healthy relationships between caregivers and young children | 0–3 | Kelly et al. 2008; Oxford et al. 2016; Spieker et al. 2012 |

**TABLE 12–3. Evidence-based models of care and promising practices for parent–child relationship treatment *(continued)***

| Dyadic intervention tools | Brief description | Intended age of child, *years* | Key references |
|---|---|---|---|
| Theraplay[a,c] | Structured play therapy intervention intended to enhance attachment, self-esteem, trust, and joyful engagement for children who exhibit behavioral problems and their caregivers; frequently used with foster and adoptive parents | 0–18 | Booth and Jernberg 2009; Tucker et al. 2017; Wettig et al. 2011 |
| Trauma-focused cognitive-behavioral therapy[a,b] | Treatment for PTSD and other trauma-related symptoms in children, with primary caregivers typically observing sessions and participating in several sessions | 3–18 | Cohen et al. 2006; Scheeringa 2015; Scheeringa et al. 2011 |
| Watch, Wait, and Wonder | Dyadic intervention utilizing infant-led play sessions to strengthen the attachment relationship between caregiver and child experiencing relational or developmental difficulties | 0–4 | Cohen et al. 1999, 2002; Muir et al. 1999 |

[a]Evidence-based model per the California Evidence-Based Clearinghouse for Child Welfare (www.cebc4cw.org).
[b]Evidence-based model per Njoroge and Yang 2012.
[c]Categorized as promising research evidence.

they had imagined they would have, such as holding and nursing their infant and taking their infant home. Many NICU families also face complicated psychosocial difficulties, such as financial issues if parents do not return to work, problems with childcare for siblings, and housing and commuting issues (Lewis et al. 2019). There are also disparities in the quality of care that infants of color, especially Black and Hispanic infants, receive at structural, procedural, and outcome levels (Sigurdson et al. 2019).

NICU parent–infant pairs are a vulnerable population and, as a result of all these challenges, may have more challenges in forming an optimal parent–infant relationship, particularly earlier on (Scala et al. 2021). They may therefore need additional layers of assessment and treatment or support. Psychological interventions in the NICU can be broadly divided into developmental care practices, interventions targeting parental mental health, and interventions targeting infant mental health and parent–infant attachment (Scala et al. 2021). Developmental care practices are interventions that aim at decreasing infant pain and stress, providing appropriate sensory stimulation, improving parental presence and self-efficacy, and familiarizing parents with premature infant communication and needs (Scala et al. 2021). As an example, promoting and facilitating SSC between parent and infant is part of developmental care practices. SSC has proved to be highly beneficial, with significant health benefits specifically for premature infants (Campbell-Yeo et al. 2015). Benefits of SSC for premature infants include reduced mortality, improved physiology (thermoregulation and cardiovascular stability), improved behaviors (breastfeeding initiation, sleep), less procedural discomfort, and improved neurodevelopment (Campbell-Yeo et al. 2015).

A number of formal programs are available, each of which utilizes a different combination of interventions to improve infant and parental outcomes for NICU families. The Newborn Individualized Developmental Care and Assessment Program, Family Nurture Intervention, Mother-Infant Transaction Program, Creating Opportunities for Parent Empowerment, Auditory Tactile Visual Vestibular Interventions, NICU Family Support Core Curriculum, and Close Collaboration With Parents are among the more established and studied formal NICU programs (Scala et al. 2021). Despite advances in addressing infant and parental distress in the NICU, a significant challenge remains for identifying interventions that can support parental involvement in the NICU, support infant development, and optimize preterm neurodevelopmental outcomes (Aucott et al. 2002).

## Parent–Infant Relationship and Mental Health in Fathers/Nonbirth Parents, LGBTQ+ Parents, and Adoptive Parents

### Fathers

Fathers and partners play a crucial—yet less well understood—role in infants' psychosocial and neurobiological development. At the same time, there is increasing recognition that the perinatal period is a vulnerable time for fathers' mental health. Two meta-analyses found an 8%–10% prevalence rate of paternal depression (with the highest incidence between 3 and 6 months postpartum) compared with the 4% prevalence rate of depression in men in the general population (Cameron et al. 2016; Paulson and Bazemore 2010). A meta-analysis of studies from 12 countries underscored the higher risk fathers experience during the perinatal period and showed high levels of paternal anxiety during this time (Lieferman et al. 2021). The rate of paternal anxiety during perinatal period was estimated to be 10.7%, which is a significant increase from the baseline prevalence of anxiety in men of about 2%–4% (Lieferman et al. 2021). Studies have found that depressive symptoms may begin during pregnancy and continue in the transition to parenthood, and there may be a correlation between paternal and maternal depression (de Magistris et al. 2013; Paulson and Bazemore 2010).

Fathers can be key attachment figures, and a positive perception of the parenting role is consistently associated with paternal caregiving activities and interpersonal warmth (Lucassen et al. 2011). As with maternal involvement, paternal involvement begins prior to birth; for example, internal parental representations during the mother's pregnancy are positively associated with later child development (Maas et al. 2012; Vreeswijk et al. 2014). After birth, paternal caregiving is particularly important in infancy, in part due to alleviating maternal stress (Kim et al. 2016). However, there is still much to learn about the father–infant relationship, particularly in early infancy (Ramchandani et al. 2013; Tamis-LeMonda et al. 2004).

## LGBTQ+ Parents

A similar need for further study is in the role of other nonbirth parents, such as for LGBTQ+ families. A steadily increasing number of same-gender and nonbinary couples are building families and raising children, and this number is likely to continue to grow (American Academy of Pediatrics Committee on Psychosocial Aspects of Child and Family Health 2013). According to the U.S. Census, between 2 million and 3.7 million children under age 18 have an LGBTQ+ parent, and approximately 200,000 of these children are being raised by a same-sex couple (Family Equality Council 2017).

Extensive evidence supports the lack of relationship between parents' sexual orientation and children's emotional, psychosocial, and behavioral development (Farr et al. 2010; Golombok and Badger 2010; Stacey and Biblarz 2001; Tasker 2005; Wainright et al. 2004). In contrast, many studies have attested to the normal development of children in same-gender families when the child is wanted, the parents have a commitment to shared parenting, and the parents have strong economic and social support. This has led current researchers to conclude that the same set of factors determine healthy child development no matter what the sex or gender of their parents:

> In all, it is now well-established that the adjustment of children and adolescents is best accounted for by variations in the quality of the relationships with their parents, the quality of the relationship between the parents or significant adults in the children's and adolescents' lives, and the availability of economic and socio-economic resources. (Lamb 2012, p. 106)

The American Academy of Pediatrics (AAP) has clear policy statements supporting these facts:

> To promote optimal health and well-being of all children, the [AAP] supports access for all children to (1) civil marriage rights for their parents and (2) willing and capable foster and adoptive parents, regardless of the parents' sexual orientation…the AAP has supported families in all their diversity, because the family has always been the basic social unit in which children develop the supporting and nurturing relationships with adults

that they need to thrive. (American Academy of Pediatrics Committee on Psychosocial Aspects of Child and Family Health 2013, p. 827)

These families nevertheless have a particular need for advocacy and support from mental health professionals and health care providers, because families headed by sexual minority groups encounter significant barriers to care and health equity, including lack of provider knowledge, external societal stigma, and homophobia, despite greater visibility and wider cultural acceptance (Mayer et al. 2008; Webster and Telingator 2016). Additionally, there are aspects specific to each subpopulation in this group, such as pregnancy, birth, and parenting in LGBTQ+ families.

There remains a wide knowledge gap in the study of LGBTQ+ families and their experiences through pregnancy, the transition to parenthood, the experiences of early parenting, and parent–infant interactions; this is in part because pregnancy and parenting research is still centered on a heteronormative framework (Charter et al. 2018; Darwin and Greenfield 2019). Some research has focused on lesbian experiences of reproductive and maternity care but very little on the experience of pregnancy and parenting; research focusing on the experiences of gay male parents and transgender parents remains scarce (Darwin and Greenfield 2019; Hafford-Letchfield et al. 2019; Tornello and Bos 2017; Van Rijn-van Gelderen et al. 2018). In addition, although there has been increasing focus on paternal mental health, a heteronormative approach to these data risks conflating gender (manhood/fatherhood) with the role of coparenting or co-caretaking (Darwin and Greenfield 2019).

Much remains to be understood in terms of the complexity of family structures, such as a lesbian couple with a child who is biologically connected to a nonbirth parent or the existence of more than one birth parent within a particular family (Darwin and Greenfield 2019; Goldberg 2006). Despite these limitations, important concepts are emerging. For example, recent research has started to examine the experiences of preconception, pregnancy, and new motherhood from the perspective of lesbian nonbiological mothers (McKelvey 2014; Wojnar and Katzenmeyer 2014). One descriptive phenomenology study concluded that nonbirth lesbian parents experience an overall theme of "feeling different" (e.g., legal and biological concerns, losing relationships, feeling incomplete, and the need to carve out a unique role) that permeate their preconception, pregnancy, birth, and early parenting experiences (Wojnar and Katzenmeyer 2014).

## Adoptive Parents

Adoption is an important area of overlap with the discussion of LGBTQ+ parents and a topic of extensive study unto itself. There are approximately 1.5 million adopted children living in the United States, or about 2% of all U.S. children (Kreider and Lofquist 2014). Recent trends in adoption include changes in the demographics of infants and children over the past two decades. International adoptions into the United States peaked with nearly 23,000 per year in both 2004 and 2005. Due to various legal and political changes, by 2019, just under 3,000 children were adopted into the United States (U.S. Department of State Bureau of Consular Affairs 2020). Increasingly, these children tend to be older and may have had more placements in foster care or orphanages prior to adoption. The number of children in foster care in the United States has increased slightly over the past decade, although it was decreasing from 2009 to 2012. In 2019, there were a record high 66,000 adoptions out of foster care. In 2018, of the

63,000 adoptions from foster care, 51% were adopted by their foster parent(s) and 35% by a relative (Congressional Coalition on Adoption Institute 2018; U.S. Department of Health and Human Services 2020).

Racial disparities also may affect the health and well-being of adoptive children. Approximately 15,000 infants per year are adopted directly from birth, and these are more likely to be white infants, most often through "open adoptions." Most domestic adoptions in the United States are from foster care following abuse or neglect in the child's original home. "Most of these children have suffered traumatic losses, are no longer infants, are of color, are in sibling groups that should be placed together, and/or have special physical, learning, or behavioral health needs that have been identified or are yet to emerge" (Siegel 2015, p. 19). Lack of "secure and enduring relationships with committed and nurturing adults" (American Academy of Pediatrics Committee on Psychosocial Aspects of Child and Family Health 2013, p. 827) in early life, deemed necessary by the AAP, can have long lasting impacts for adopted children and their families.

Like the many constellations of parents, adopted children comprise a heterogenous group. Preadoption experiences and degree of maltreatment or neglect, age at adoption, length of time exposed to adversities prior to adoption, and in-utero exposures to substances all have a direct impact on child outcome (Harwood et al. 2013). Adoption type could be associated with some of these factors; for instance, children adopted through international or foster care pathways show poorer school outcomes and increased health care needs that are at least partially related to differences in preadoption placement settings (Harwood et al. 2013). However, most adopted children form secure attachments with their adoptive parents and do well developmentally (van Londen et al. 2007). As with the general infant and young child population, the quality of parent–child relationships can at least partially mediate the effects of adverse pre- and postnatal adversities and lead to better social and cognitive development (Stams et al. 2002). A study by Niemann and Weiss (2012) evaluated factors affecting attachment 6 months after international adoption for children who were adopted late in the first or second year of life. Children with fewer placements prior to adoption and lower stress levels after adoption (as measured by basal salivary cortisol) were more likely to have attachment security with their adoptive mothers (Niemann and Weiss 2012). It is hypothesized that a lower infant stress level may be a protective factor in promoting bonding with the adoptive mother, and, alternatively, responsive care from the mother may buffer HPA axis dysregulation, leading to a lower stress level in the infant who is developing an attachment bond with the adoptive mother.

As with all parent–infant dyads, the adoptee's temperament can play a role in the dynamics of the relationship with the parent. Adopted children with a more difficult temperament have lower social and cognitive development and higher level of internalizing and externalizing behavior problems at age 7 (Stams et al. 2002). Multiple studies have evaluated short- and long-term predictors of development in adoptive infants and children. Maternal sensitivity appears to be the strongest factor in promoting secure attachment and positive social-emotional development, although responsive and flexible parenting in general and adult attachment style are also factors (Roberson 2006). Maternal sensitivity is important both during early childhood and as children grow into adolescence and can help maintain a secure attachment. A large, longitudinal study of early infant international adoptees in the Netherlands also found that an increase in maternal sensitive support from early childhood into adolescence can lead to changing of attachment patterns from insecure to secure by early adolescence (Beijersbergen et al. 2012).

A randomized controlled trial was recently published of an intervention focused on increasing maternal sensitivity in 83 families with internationally adopted children in Italy. Video-Feedback Intervention to Promote Positive Parenting in Adoption and Foster Care is a home visiting program developed in the Netherlands to promote positive parenting over 4–6 months and uses emotional availability as a measure of maternal sensitivity (Barone et al. 2019). Children showed improvement in emotional availability and externalizing behaviors at 6-month follow up, mediated by maternal improvements in emotional availability during the intervention. The highest benefit was noted in children with the most temperamental negative affect whose mother's emotional availability score increased over the course of the study (Barone et al. 2019). This highlights one possible intervention for supporting adoptive parents in improving sensitive and responsive caregiving and thereby improving outcomes for their adopted children even beyond early childhood.

Adoptive parents may also face unique challenges that increase their risk of depressive symptoms, including infertility, financial stressors, and undergoing evaluation by adoption agencies (Fields et al. 2010). For example, rates of depression in 39 adoptive mothers were 25.6% before adoption and 15.4% 6 weeks after adoption (Senecky et al. 2009). A longer-term study of 86 families also found decreasing rates of depression over the first-year following adoption, as measured by a modified version of the Edinburgh Postnatal Depression Scale. The rates were 27.9% at 0–4 weeks, 25.6% at 5–12 weeks, and 12.8% at 13–52 weeks postadoption. Stress and adjustment difficulties predicted depression in this study (Fields et al. 2010). A larger study of rates of depression and anxiety symptoms in adoptive mothers compared with postpartum mothers found similar rates of depression between the two groups but less anxiety in adoptive mothers. Higher levels of reported sleep deprivation, history of infertility, past psychological disorder, and lower marital satisfaction predicted higher rates of depression (Mott et al. 2011). Foli et al. (2012) evaluated predictors and proposed a theory of postadoption depression, suggesting the assessment of factors including parents' expectations of themselves as parents and of family and friends, their expectations for the child, feelings of rest, history of depression and low self-esteem, and interpersonal variables such as parent–child bonding, marital satisfaction, and perceived support. Further research is needed on optimal times to screen for postadoption depression and other parental mental health concerns, given the increased stressors these families often face.

## Conclusion

As discussed, pregnancy and the postpartum period are critical times for both infant and parental development. Although this is a time of increased risk for the onset or exacerbation of mental illness, it is also an important period for the developing fetus and infant in terms of stress response, emotional regulation, and developing a sense of security in relationships, setting the stage for subsequent emotional and neurocognitive development. By observing and addressing parent–infant relationship disturbances and challenges, medical and mental health providers caring for women during this vulnerable time can have a long-term positive impact for the families in their care and potentially for future generations.

Neurobiological evidence exists for alterations of HPA axis activity, decreased hippocampal size, increased amygdala reactivity, and stress response in infants exposed to stress in utero. Although genetics and stress exposure are important factors, research in both animal models and humans has shown that physical contact and proximity and parental nurturing behaviors can lead to epigenetic changes that can override these heritable traits. Mental health conditions may interfere with these nurturing behaviors, but early detection of any parent–infant relational difficulties and appropriate intervention can lead to better self-regulation in the infant, encourage healthy attachment relationships, and result in improved psychoemotional well-being in infants as they grow and develop.

Mental health clinicians can help parents by observing and understanding the nuances of parent–infant interactions and by exploring parent perceptions of the infant and of themselves as parents. This process is especially salient in the setting of pregnancy and postpartum mood or anxiety disorders. Important areas to notice include the quality of physical contact, gaze, and vocalizations between the parent and infant, as well as the affective tone, mutual coregulation, and any mismatches and repairs within the back and forth of interactions.

Several other populations may also require additional support. Parents who are members of racial minority groups are subject to health care disparities that are pronounced in terms of perinatal care and peripartum outcomes and are raising children within the context of the additional stressors associated with racist political and cultural structures. Parents of infants who require care in the NICU are faced with additional pressures and anxieties associated with worries about the health of their child, as well as the logistical and emotional difficulties of having a child with a prolonged hospital stay and potentially continued medical complexities. Parents who have a history of trauma and poor attachment with their own primary caregivers are more likely to struggle. Parents may need support around having realistic expectations for themselves and their infants at different developmental stages.

Other parental groups that may have unique needs require additional study. We know that fathers are at increased risk for depression after the birth of a child, yet little is known regarding the best way to screen for these difficulties and to provide services successfully. LGBTQ+ couples who become parents have rarely been the focus of studies looking at attachment and early adaptation to the role of parent, although research has demonstrated that children raised in same-sex households are at no increased risk for emotional and psychiatric difficulties. There is little research on attachment in families with transgender or nonbinary parents. Adopted infants and children and their parents are another important population to keep in mind when screening for parental mental health concerns and addressing infant mental health and attachment in new parents. Ongoing research into the needs of these parents will enable us to ensure that the care we provide to families is data informed and culturally responsive.

Attachment and other aspects of the parent–infant relationship are rich fields with many nuances beyond what we have been able to cover in this chapter. Although the nature of clinical work focuses on identifying parents and families at increased need for support, we can be encouraged and hopeful about the opportunities to collaborate with families to remediate these difficulties and set infants on a healthier developmental path. Intervening with culturally sensitive, diversity-informed, strength-based approaches can provide lasting benefits for parents, infants, and the family relationships.

## Key Points

- Early interactions between the infant and caregiver set a template for long-standing effects on the well-being of the infant.
- Parental mental illness can have adverse effects on parent–infant interactions.
- Neurobiological mechanisms of stress transmission during pregnancy, and of responsive parenting behavior during infancy, can affect the child's stress response, self-regulation, and attachment into adulthood.
- Negative patterns of interactions between parent and infant can be identified in the clinical setting and are amenable to intervention. Intervening during pregnancy and infancy offers an opportunity to achieve long-standing benefits for both the child and parents.
- Evidence-based models of care are available that incorporate treatment for the mother, the infant, and their relationship with culturally informed and strength-based approaches.
- Parents of infants who require care in the neonatal intensive care unit (NICU) face particular stressors and may need additional supports specific to their experience; racial and ethnic disparities in NICU care augment these stressors for families of color.
- Fathers, LGBTQ+ parents, and adoptive parents are also at increased risk of depression in the period after the birth or adoption of an infant and also benefit from screening and treatment.

## References

Ainsworth MD, Bell SM: Attachment, exploration, and separation: illustrated by the behavior of one-year-olds in a strange situation. Child Dev 41(1):49–67, 1970 5490680

Ainsworth MDS, Blehar MC, Waters E, et al: Patterns of Attachment: A Study of the Strange Situation. Hillsdale, NJ, Erlbaum, 1978

American Academy of Pediatrics Committee on Psychosocial Aspects of Child and Family Health: Promoting the well-being of children whose parents are gay or lesbian. Pediatrics 131(4):827–830, 2013 23519941

Aucott S, Donohue PK, Atkins E, et al: Neurodevelopmental care in the NICU. Ment Retard Dev Disabil Res Rev 8(4):298–308, 2002 12454906

Barone L, Ozturk Y, Lionetti F: The key role of positive parenting and children's temperament in post-institutionalized children's socio-emotional adjustment after adoption placement: a RCT study. Social Development 28(1):136–151, 2019

Baumgartner T, Heinrichs M, Vonlanthen A, et al: Oxytocin shapes the neural circuitry of trust and trust adaptation in humans. Neuron 58(4):639–650, 2008 18498743

Beijersbergen MD, Juffer F, Bakermans-Kranenburg MJ, et al: Remaining or becoming secure: parental sensitive support predicts attachment continuity from infancy to adolescence in a longitudinal adoption study. Dev Psychol 48(5):1277–1282, 2012 22369333

Bernard K, Dozier M: Examining infants' cortisol responses to laboratory tasks among children varying in attachment disorganization: stress reactivity or return to baseline? Dev Psychol 46(6):1771–1778, 2010 20873923
Bernard K, Dozier M, Bick J, et al: Enhancing attachment organization among maltreated children: results of a randomized clinical trial. Child Dev 83(2):623–636, 2012 22239483
Boldt LJ, Kochanska G, Jonas K: Infant attachment moderates paths from early negativity to preadolescent outcomes for children and parents. Child Dev 88(2):584–596, 2017 27569427
Booth PB, Jernberg AM: Theraplay: Helping Parents and Children Build Better Relationships Through Attachment-Based Play, 3rd Edition. San Francisco, CA, Jossey-Bass, 2009
Bornstein MH, Putnick DL, Cote LR, et al: Mother-infant contingent vocalizations in 11 countries. Psychol Sci 26(8):1272–1284, 2015 26133571
Bowlby J: Maternal care and mental health. Bull World Health Organ 3(3):355–533, 1951 14821768
Bowlby J: Attachment and Loss, Vol 1: Loss. New York, Basic Books, 1969, p 194
Bowlby J: Attachment theory and its therapeutic implications. Adolesc Psychiatry 6:5–33, 1978 742687
Bushnell IWR, Sai F, Mullin JT: Neonatal recognition of the mother's face. Br J Dev Psychol 7(1):3–15, 1989
Cameron EE, Sedov ID, Tomfohr-Madsen LM: Prevalence of paternal depression in pregnancy and the postpartum: an updated meta-analysis. J Affect Disord 206:189–203, 2016 27475890
Campbell-Yeo ML, Disher TC, Benoit BL, et al: Understanding kangaroo care and its benefits to preterm infants. Pediatric Health Med Ther 6:15–32, 2015 29388613
Carpenter AL, Puliafico AC, Kurtz SM, et al: Extending parent-child interaction therapy for early childhood internalizing problems: new advances for an overlooked population. Clin Child Fam Psychol Rev 17(4):340–356, 2014 25212716
Centers for Disease Control and Prevention: Interim considerations for infection prevention and control of coronavirus disease 2019 (COVID-19) in inpatient obstetric healthcare settings. CDC.gov, February 18, 2020. Available at: https://stacks.cdc.gov/view/cdc/85196. Accessed January 21, 2021.
Charter R, Ussher JM, Perz J, et al: The transgender parent: experiences and constructions of pregnancy and parenthood for transgender men in Australia. Int J Transgenderism 19(1):64–77, 2018
Chess S, Thomas A: Temperament and the concept of goodness of fit, in Explorations in Temperament: Perspectives on Individual Differences. Edited by Strelau J, Angleitner A. Boston, MA, Springer, 1991, pp 15–28
Cicchetti D, Rogosch FA, Toth SL: Fostering secure attachment in infants in maltreating families through preventive interventions. Dev Psychopathol 18(3):623–649, 2006 17152394
Clark R: The Parent–Child Early Relational Assessment: a factorial validity study. Educational and Psychological Measurement 59(5):821–846, 1999
Clark R, Tluczek A, Wenzel A: Psychotherapy for postpartum depression: a preliminary report. Am J Orthopsychiatry 73(4):441–454, 2003 14609406
Clark R, Tluczek A, Brown R: A mother-infant therapy group model for postpartum depression. Infant Ment Health J 29(5):514–536, 2008 28636219
Cleveland L, Hill CM, Pulse WS, et al: Systematic review of skin-to-skin care for full-term, healthy newborns. J Obstet Gynecol Neonatal Nurs 46(6):857–869, 2017 28950108
Clinton J, Feller AF, Williams RC: The importance of infant mental health. Paediatr Child Health 21(5):239–241, 2016 27441014
Cohen JA, Mannarino AP, Deblinger E: Treating Trauma and Traumatic Grief in Children and Adolescents. New York, Guilford, 2006
Cohen NJ, Muir E, Lojkasek M, et al: Watch, wait, and wonder: testing the effectiveness of a new approach to mother-infant psychotherapy. Infant Ment Health J 20(4):429–451, 1999
Cohen NJ, Lojkasek M, Muir E, et al: Six-month follow-up of two mother-infant psychotherapies: convergence of therapeutic outcomes. Infant Mental Health J 23(4):361–380, 2002
Congressional Coalition on Adoption Institute: Fact Sheet: U.S. adoption and foster care statistics. The AFCARS Report: preliminary FY 2017 estimates as of September 24, 2018. Available at: https://www.ccainstitute.org/resources/fact-sheets. Accessed August 23, 2020.

Coyne J, Powell B, Hoffman K, et al: The circle of security, in Handbook of Infant Mental Health, 4th Edition. Edited by Zeanah C. New York, Guilford, 2019, pp 500–513
Crittenden PM: Internal representational models of attachment relationships. Infant Mental Health Journal 11(3):259–277, 1990
Crowell JA, Feldman SS, Ginsberg N: Assessment of mother-child interaction in preschoolers with behavior problems. J Am Acad Child Adolesc Psychiatry 27(3):303–311, 1988 2454223
Dagan O, Sagi-Schwartz A: Early attachment network with mother and father: an unsettled issue. Child Dev Perspect 12(2):115–121, 2018
Darwin Z, Greenfield M: Mothers and others: the invisibility of LGBTQ people in reproductive and infant psychology. J Reprod Infant Psychol 37(4):341–343, 2019 31387370
Davis EP, Sandman CA: The timing of prenatal exposure to maternal cortisol and psychosocial stress is associated with human infant cognitive development. Child Dev 81(1):131–148, 2010
Davis EP, Glynn LM, Waffarn F, et al: Prenatal maternal stress programs infant stress regulation. J Child Psychol Psychiatry 52(2):119–129, 2011 20854366
DeCasper AJ, Fifer WP: Of human bonding: newborns prefer their mothers' voices. Science 208(4448):1174–1176, 1980 7375928
de Magistris A, Carta M, Fanos V: Postpartum depression and the male partner. Journal of Pediatric and Neonatal Individualized Medicine 2(1):15–27, 2013
De Roo M, Wong G, Rempel GR, et al: Advancing optimal development in children: examining the construct validity of a parent reflective functioning questionnaire. JMIR Pediatr Parent 2(1):e11561, 2019 31518301
Dias BG, Ressler KJ: Parental olfactory experience influences behavior and neural structure in subsequent generations. Nat Neurosci 17(1):89–96, 2014 24292232
Ding YH, Xu X, Wang ZY, et al: The relation of infant attachment to attachment and cognitive and behavioural outcomes in early childhood. Early Hum Dev 90(9):459–464, 2014 25000392
Domes G, Heinrichs M, Michel A, et al: Oxytocin improves "mind-reading" in humans. Biol Psychiatry 61(6):731–733, 2007 17137561
Dozier M, Bernard K: Attachment and biobehavioral catch-up, in Handbook of Infant Mental Health, 4th Edition. Edited by Zeanah C. New York, Guilford, 2019a, pp 514–526
Dozier M, Bernard K: Development of the ABC intervention, in Coaching Parents of Vulnerable Infants: The Attachment and Biobehavioral Catch-Up Approach. Edited by Dozier M, Bernard K. New York, Guilford, 2019b, pp 41–59
Dozier M, Bernard K, Roben CKP: Attachment and biobehavioral catch-up, in Handbook of Attachment-Based Interventions. Edited by Steele H, Steele M. New York, NY, Guilford, 2018, pp 27–49
Eyberg S: PCIT: integration of traditional and behavioral concern. Child and Family Behavioral Therapy 10(1):33–46, 1988
Eyberg SM, Funderburk BW, Hembree-Kigin T, et al: Parent-child interaction therapy with behavior problem children: one- and two-year maintenance of treatment effects in the family. Child and Family Behavioral Therapy 23(4):1–20, 2001
Facompré CR, Bernard K, Waters TEA: Effectiveness of interventions in preventing disorganized attachment: a meta-analysis. Dev Psychopathol 30(1):1–11, 2018 28397637
Family Equality Council: LGBTQ Family Factsheet: In Support of August 2017 Presentation to NAC Undercount of Young Children Working Group. Washington, DC, U.S. Census Bureau, 2017. Available at: https://www2.census.gov/cac/nac/meetings/2017-11/LGBTQ-families-factsheet.pdf. Accessed August 24, 2020
Farr RH, Forsell SL, Patterson CJ: Parenting and child development in adoptive families: does parental sexual orientation matter? Applied Developmental Science 14(3):164–178, 2010
Felitti VJ, Anda RF, Nordenberg D, et al: Relationship of childhood abuse and household dysfunction to many of the leading causes of death in adults: the Adverse Childhood Experiences (ACE) study. Am J Prev Med 14(4):245–258, 1998 9635069
Field TM, Cohen D, Garcia R, et al: Mother-stranger face discrimination by the newborn. Infant Behav Dev 7(1):19–25, 1984
Field T, Diego M, Hernandez-Reif M: Preterm infant massage therapy research: a review. Infant Behav Dev 33(2):115–124, 2010 20137814

Fields ES, Meuchel JM, Jaffe CJ, et al: Post adoption depression. Arch Women Ment Health 13(2):147–151, 2010 20119862

Finelli J, Zeanah CH Jr, Smyke AT: Attachment disorders in early childhood, in Handbook of Infant Mental Health, 4th Edition. Edited by Zeanah CH. New York, Guilford, 2019, pp 452–456

Foli KJ, South SC, Lim E: Rates and predictors of depression in adoptive mothers: moving toward theory. ANS Adv Nurs Sci 35(1):51–63, 2012 22293610

Forman DR, O'Hara MW, Stuart S, et al: Effective treatment for postpartum depression is not sufficient to improve the developing mother-child relationship. Dev Psychopathol 19(2):585–602, 2007 17459185

Fraiberg S, Adelson E, Shapiro V: Ghosts in the nursery: a psychoanalytic approach to the problems of impaired infant-mother relationships. J Am Acad Child Psychiatry 14(3):387–421, 1975

Francis D, Diorio J, Liu D, et al: Nongenomic transmission across generations of maternal behavior and stress responses in the rat. Science 286(5442):1155–1158, 1999 10550053

Franklin B, Warlaumont AS, Messinger D, et al: Effects of parental interaction on infant vocalization rate, variability and vocal type. Lang Learn Dev 10(3):279–2996, 2014 25383061

Galinsky E: Six Stages of Parenthood. Reading, MA, Perseus Books, 1987

Gartstein MA, Skinner MK: Prenatal influences on temperament development: the role of environmental epigenetics. Dev Psychopathol 30(4):1269–1303, 2018 29229018

George C, Kaplan N, Main M: The Adult Attachment Interview (unpublished manuscript). University of California at Berkeley, 1985

Ghosh Ippen C: Integrating a diversity-informed approach into evidence-based practice, in Trauma Therapy in Context: The Science and Craft of Evidence-Based Practice, 1st Edition. Edited by McMackin A, Newman E, Fogler J, Keane T. Washington, DC, American Psychological Association, 2012, pp 29–50

Gilmore K, Meersand P: Normal Child and Adolescent Development: A Psychodynamic Primer. Washington, DC, American Psychiatric Publishing, 2013

Goldberg A: The transition to parenthood for lesbian couples. J GLBT Fam Stud 2(1):13–42, 2006

Golombok S, Badger S: Children raised in mother-headed families from infancy: a follow-up of children of lesbian and single heterosexual mothers, at early adulthood. Hum Reprod 25(1):150–157, 2010 19840989

Granqvist P, Sroufe LA, Dozier M, et al: Disorganized attachment in infancy: a review of the phenomenon and its implications for clinicians and policy-makers. Attach Hum Dev 19(6):534–558, 2017 28745146

Guastella AJ, Mitchell PB, Dadds MR: Oxytocin increases gaze to the eye region of human faces. Biol Psychiatry 63(1):3–5, 2008a 17888410

Guastella AJ, Mitchell PB, Mathews F: Oxytocin enhances the encoding of positive social memories in humans. Biol Psychiatry 64(3):256–258, 2008b 18343353

Hafford-Letchfield T, Cocker C, Rutter D, et al: What do we know about transgender parenting? Findings from a systematic review. Health Soc Care Community 27(5):1111–1125, 2019 30983067

Harrison W, Goodman D: Epidemiologic trends in neonatal intensive care, 2007–2012. JAMA Pediatr 169(9):855–862, 2015 26214387

Harwood R, Feng X, Yu S: Preadoption adversities and postadoption mediators of mental health and school outcomes among international, foster, and private adoptees in the United States. J Fam Psychol 27(3):409–420, 2013 23750523

Hendricks-Muñoz KD, Xu J, Parikh HI, et al: Skin-to-skin care and the development of the preterm infant oral microbiome. Am J Perinatol 32(13):1205–1216, 2015 26007311

Hughes K, Bellis MA, Hardcastle KA, et al: The effect of multiple adverse childhood experiences on health: a systematic review and meta-analysis. Lancet Public Health 2(8):e356–e366, 2017

Insel TR, Young LJ: The neurobiology of attachment. Nat Rev Neurosci 2(2):129–136, 2001 11252992

Irving Harris Foundation: The Tenets: Diversity Informed Tenets for Work With Infants, Children and Families, 2018. Available at: https://diversityinformedtenets.org. Accessed July 5, 2020.

Kelly JF, Zuckerman T, Rosenblatt S: Promoting first relationships: a relationship-focused early intervention approach. Infants and Young Children 21(4):285–295, 2008

Kim M, Kang SK, Yee B, et al: Paternal involvement and early infant neurodevelopment: the mediation role of maternal parenting stress. BMC Pediatr 16(1):212, 2016 27955632

Kim S, Fonagy P, Koos O, et al: Maternal oxytocin response predicts mother-to-infant gaze. Brain Res 1580:133–142, 2014 24184574
Kinner SA, Borschmann R: Inequality and intergenerational transmission of complex adversity. Lancet Public Health 2(8):e342–e343, 2017 29253468
Kosfeld M, Heinrichs M, Zak PJ, et al: Oxytocin increases trust in humans. Nature 435(7042):673–676, 2005 15931222
Koulomzin M, Beebe B, Anderson S, et al: Infant gaze, head, face and self-touch at 4 months differentiate secure vs. avoidant attachment at 1 year: a microanalytic approach. Attach Hum Dev 4(1):3–24, 2002 12065027
Kreider RM, Lofquist DM: Adopted Children and Stepchildren: 2010. Washington, DC, U.S. Census Bureau, April 23, 2014. Available at: https://www.census.gov/library/publications/2014/demo/p20-572.html. Accessed January 21, 2021.
Krugers HJ, Arp JM, Xiong H, et al: Early life adversity: lasting consequences for emotional learning. Neurobiol Stress 6:14–21, 2016 28229105
Lamb ME: Mothers, fathers, families, and circumstances: factors affecting children's adjustment. Appl Dev Sci 16(2):98–111, 2012
Leiferman JA, Farewell CV, Jewell J, et al: Anxiety among fathers during the prenatal and postpartum period: a meta-analysis. J Psychosom Obstet Gynaecol 42(2):152–161, 2021
Lewis AJ, Austin E, Knapp R, et al: Perinatal maternal mental health, fetal programming and child development. Healthcare (Basel) 3(4):1212–1227, 2015 27417821
Lewis TP, Andrews KG, Shenberger E, et al: Caregiving can be costly: a qualitative study of barriers and facilitators to conducting kangaroo mother care in a US tertiary hospital neonatal intensive care unit. BMC Pregnancy Childbirth 19(1):227, 2019 31272398
Lieberman AF, Padrón E, Van Horn P, et al: Angels in the nursery: the intergenerational transmission of benevolent parental influences. Infant Ment Health J 26(6):504–520, 2005a 28682485
Lieberman AF, Van Horn P, Ippen CG: Toward evidence-based treatment: child-parent psychotherapy with preschoolers exposed to marital violence. J Am Acad Child Adolesc Psychiatry 44(12):1241–1248, 2005b 16292115
Lieberman AF, Ghosh Ippen C, Van Horn P: Child-parent psychotherapy: 6-month follow-up of a randomized controlled trial. J Am Acad Child Adolesc Psychiatry 45(8):913–918, 2006 16865033
Lieberman AF, Ghosh Ippen C, Van Horn P: Don't Hit My Mommy! A Manual for Child-Parent Psychotherapy With Young Children Exposed to Violence and Other Trauma, 2nd Edition. Washington, DC, Zero to Three Press, 2015
Lieberman AF, Hernandez Dimmler M, Ghosh Ippen CM: Child-parent psychotherapy: a trauma-informed treatment for young children and their caregivers, in Handbook of Infant Mental Health, 4th Edition. Edited by Zeanah C. New York, Guilford, 2019, pp 485–499
Lucassen N, Tharner A, Van Ijzendoorn MH, et al: The association between paternal sensitivity and infant-father attachment security: a meta-analysis of three decades of research. J Fam Psychol 25(6):986–992, 2011 22004434
Lupien SJ, McEwen BS, Gunnar MR, et al: Effects of stress throughout the lifespan on the brain, behaviour and cognition. Nat Rev Neurosci 10(6):434–445, 2009 19401723
Maas AJ, Vreeswijk CM, de Cock ES, et al: "Expectant parents": study protocol of a longitudinal study concerning prenatal (risk) factors and postnatal infant development, parenting, and parent-infant relationships. BMC Pregnancy Childbirth 12:46, 2012 22686874
Macfarlane A: Olfaction in the development of social preferences in the human neonate. Ciba Found Symp 33(33):103–117, 1975 1045976
Main M, Solomon J: Discovery of an insecure-disorganized/disoriented attachment pattern, in Affective Development in Infancy. Edited by Brazelton TB, Yogman MW. Westport, CT, Ablex Publishing, 1986, pp 95–124
Main M, Solomon J: Procedures for identifying infants as disorganized/disoriented during the Ainsworth strange situation, in Attachment in the Preschool Years: Theory, Research, and Intervention. Edited by Greenberg MT, Cicchetti D, Cummings EM. Chicago, IL, University of Chicago Press, 1990, pp 121–160
Maroney DI: Recognizing the potential effect of stress and trauma on premature infants in the NICU: how are outcomes affected? J Perinatol 23(8):679–683, 2003 14647168

Marschak M: A method for evaluating child-parent inter-action under controlled conditions. J Genet Psychol 97:3–22, 1960 14421486
Mayer KH, Bradford JB, Makadon HJ, et al: Sexual and gender minority health: what we know and what needs to be done. Am J Public Health 98(6):989–995, 2008 18445789
McGowan PO, Sasaki A, D'Alessio AC, et al: Epigenetic regulation of the glucocorticoid receptor in human brain associates with childhood abuse. Nat Neurosci 12(3):342–348, 2009 19234457
McKelvey MM: The other mother: a narrative analysis of the postpartum experiences of nonbirth lesbian mothers. ANS Adv Nurs Sci 37(2):101–116, 2014 24786200
McNeilly AS, Robinson IC, Houston MJ, et al: Release of oxytocin and prolactin in response to suckling. Br Med J (Clin Res Ed) 286(6361):257–259, 1983 6402061
Meaney MJ, Szyf M: Maternal care as a model for experience-dependent chromatin plasticity? Trends Neurosci 28(9):456–463, 2005 16054244
Menting ATA, Orobio de Castro B, Matthys W: Effectiveness of the Incredible Years parent training to modify disruptive and prosocial child behavior: a meta-analytic review. Clin Psychol Rev 33(8):901–913, 2013 23994367
Mitchell AJ, Yates C, Williams K, et al: Effects of daily kangaroo care on cardiorespiratory parameters in preterm infants. J Neonatal Perinatal Med 6(3):243–249, 2013 24246597
Moore ER, Bergman N, Anderson GC, et al: Early skin-to-skin contact for mothers and their healthy newborn infants. Cochrane Database Syst Rev 11(11):CD003519, 2016 27885658
Moser DA, Suardi F, Rossignol AS, et al: Parental reflective functioning correlates to brain activation in response to video-stimuli of mother-child dyads: links to maternal trauma history and PTSD. Psychiatry Res Neuroimaging 293(3):110985, 2019 31627112
Mott SL, Schiller CE, Richards JG, et al: Depression and anxiety among postpartum and adoptive mothers. Arch Women Ment Health 14(4):335–343, 2011 21725836
Muir E, Lojkasek M, Cohen NJ: Watch, Wait and Wonder: A Manual Describing a Dyadic Infant-Led Approach to Problems in Infancy and Early Childhood. Toronto, ON, Hincks-Dellcrest Institute, 1999
Muzik M, Rosenblum KL, Alfafara EA, et al: Mom Power: preliminary outcomes of a group intervention to improve mental health and parenting among high-risk mothers. Arch Womens Ment Health18:507–21, 2015
Negri R: Therapeutic consultation, early detection of alarm symptoms in infants and treatment with parent-infant psychotherapy, in Innovations in Parent-Infant Psychotherapy. Edited by Monzo MP, Tydeman B. London, Routledge, 2007, pp 95–116
Nelson CA3rd, Zeanah CH, Fox NA, et al: Cognitive recovery in socially deprived young children: the Bucharest Early Intervention Project. Science 318(5858):1937–1940, 2007 18096809
Niemann S, Weiss S: Factors affecting attachment in international adoptees at 6 months post adoption. Child Youth Serv Rev 34(1):205–212, 2012 22267885
Njoroge WF, Yang D: Evidence-based psychotherapies for preschool children with psychiatric disorders. Curr Psychiatry Rep 14(2):121–128, 2012 22258435
Olazábal DE, Young LJ: Oxytocin receptors in the nucleus accumbens facilitate "spontaneous" maternal behavior in adult female prairie voles. Neuroscience 141(2):559–568, 2006 16725274
Oxford ML, Marcenko M, Fleming CB, et al: Promoting birth parents' relationships with their toddlers upon reunification: results from Promoting First Relationships® home visiting program. Child Youth Serv Rev 61:109–116, 2016 26869740
Pascalis O, de Schonen S, Morton J, et al: Mother's face recognition in neonates: a replication and an extension. Infant Behavior and Development 18(1):79–85, 1995
Paulson JF, Bazemore SD: Prenatal and postpartum depression in fathers and its association with maternal depression: a meta-analysis. JAMA 303(19):1961–1969, 2010 20483973
Perroud N, Rutembesa E, Paoloni-Giacobino A, et al: The Tutsi genocide and transgenerational transmission of maternal stress: epigenetics and biology of the HPA axis. World J Biol Psychiatry 15(4):334–345, 2014 24690014
Powell B, Cooper G, Hoffman K, et al: The Circle of Security Intervention: Enhancing Attachment in Early Parent-Child Relationships. New York, Guilford, 2014
Price LH, Kao HT, Burgers DE, et al: Telomeres and early life stress: an overview. Biol Psychiatry 73(1):15–23, 2013 22831981

Qiu A, Anh TT, Li Y, et al: Prenatal maternal depression alters amygdala functional connectivity in 6-month-old infants. Transl Psychiatry 5:e508, 2015 25689569

Ramchandani PG, Domoney J, Sethna V, et al: Do early father-infant interactions predict the onset of externalising behaviours in young children? Findings from a longitudinal cohort study. J Child Psychol Psychiatry 54(1):56–64, 2013 22808985

Ramsauer B, Lotzin A, Mühlhan C, et al: A randomized controlled trial comparing Circle of Security Intervention and treatment as usual as interventions to increase attachment security in infants of mentally ill mothers: study protocol. BMC Psychiatry 14(1):24, 2014 24476106

Rayen I, van den Hove DL, Prickaerts J, et al: Fluoxetine during development reverses the effects of prenatal stress on depressive-like behavior and hippocampal neurogenesis in adolescence. PLoS One 6(9):e24003, 2011 21912658

Reid MJ, Webster-Stratton C: The Incredible Years parent, teacher, and child intervention: targeting multiple areas of risk for a young child with pervasive conduct problems using a flexible, manualized, treatment program. Cognitive and Behavioral Practice 8(4):377–386, 2011

Rifkin-Graboi A, Bai J, Chen H, et al: Prenatal maternal depression associates with microstructure of right amygdala in neonates at birth. Biol Psychiatry 74(11):837–844, 2013 23968960

Rifkin-Graboi A, Meaney MJ, Chen H, et al: Antenatal maternal anxiety predicts variations in neural structures implicated in anxiety disorders in newborns. J Am Acad Child Adolesc Psychiatry 54(4):313–321, 2015 25791148

Roberson KC: Attachment and caregiving behavioral systems in intercountry adoption: a literature review. Children and Youth Services Review 28(7):727–740, 2006

Rojas MA, Kaplan M, Quevedo M, et al: Somatic growth of preterm infants during skin-to-skin care versus traditional holding: a randomized, controlled trial. J Dev Behav Pediatr 24(3):163–168, 2003 12806228

Roque ATF, Lasiuk GC, Radünz V, et al: Scoping review of the mental health of parents of infants in the NICU. J Obstet Gynecol Neonatal Nurs 46(4):576–587, 2017 28506679

Rosenblum KL, Muzik M, Morelen DM, et al: A community-based randomized controlled trial of mom power parenting intervention for mothers with interpersonal trauma histories and their young children. Arch Womens Ment Health 20:673–86, 2017

Rosenblum KL, Lawler J, Alfafara E, et al: Improving maternal representations in high-risk mothers: a randomized, controlled trial of the mom power parenting intervention. Child Psychiatry Hum Dev 49:372–84, 2018

Rothbart MK, Derryberry D: Development of individual differences in temperament, in Advances in Developmental Psychology. Edited by Lamb ME, Brown AL. Hillsdale, NJ, Lawrence Erlbaum Associates, 1981, pp 37–86

Sameroff AJ, Fiese BH: Models of development and developmental risk, in Handbook of Infant Mental Health, 2nd Edition. Edited by Zeanah JR. New York, Guilford, 2000, pp 3–19

Samra NM, Taweel AE, Cadwell K: Effect of intermittent kangaroo mother care on weight gain of low birth weight neonates with delayed weight gain. J Perinat Educ 22(4):194–200, 2013

Savaskan E, Ehrhardt R, Schulz A, et al: Post-learning intranasal oxytocin modulates human memory for facial identity. Psychoneuroendocrinology 33(3):368–374, 2008 18221838

Scala M, Givrad S, Shaw RJ: Psychological interventions in the NICU, in The Treatment of Psychological Distress in Parents of Premature Infants: PTSD in the NICU. Edited by Shaw RJ, Horwitz SM. Washington, DC, American Psychiatric Association Publishing, 2021, pp 127–182

Scatliffe N, Casavant S, Vittner D, et al: Oxytocin and early parent-infant interactions: a systematic review. Int J Nurs Sci 6(4):445–453, 2019 31728399

Scheeringa MS: Treating PTSD in Preschoolers: A Clinical Guide. New York, Guilford, 2015

Scheeringa MS, Weems CF, Cohen JA, et al: Trauma-focused cognitive-behavioral therapy for posttraumatic stress disorder in three-through six year-old children: a randomized clinical trial. J Child Psychol Psychiatry 52(8):853–860, 2011 21155776

Seabra-Santos MJ, Gaspar MF, Azevedo AF, et al: Incredible Years parent training: what changes, for whom, how, for how long? J Appl Dev Psychol 6(44):93–104, 2016

Senecky Y, Agassi H, Inbar D, et al: Post-adoption depression among adoptive mothers. J Affect Disord 115(1–2):62–68, 2009 18950870

Siegel DH: Adoption trends today. Social Work Today 15(6):18, 2015

Sigurdson K, Mitchell B, Liu J, et al: Racial/ethnic disparities in neonatal intensive care: a systematic review. Pediatrics 144(2):e20183114, 2019 31358664
Spieker SJ, Oxford ML, Kelly JF, et al: Promoting first relationships: randomized trial of a relationship-based intervention for toddlers in child welfare. Child Maltreat 17(4):271–286, 2012 22949743
Sroufe LA: Attachment classification from the perspective of infant-caregiver relationships and infant temperament. Child Dev 56(1):1–14, 1985 3987395
Stacey J, Biblarz TJ: (How) does the sexual orientation of parents matter? Am Sociol Rev 66(2):159–183, 2001
Stams GJJM, Juffer F, van IJzendoorn MH: Maternal sensitivity, infant attachment, and temperament in early childhood predict adjustment in middle childhood: the case of adopted children and their biologically unrelated parents. Dev Psychol 38(5):806–821, 2002 12220057
Stern DN: The Interpersonal World of the Infant: A View from Psychoanalysis and Developmental Psychology. New York, Basic Books, 1985
Stern DN: The Motherhood Constellation: A Unified View of Parent-Infant Psychotherapy. New York, Basic Books, 1995
Stevens M, N'zi A: Parent-child interaction therapy, in Handbook of Infant Mental Health, 4th Edition. Edited by Zeanah C. New York, Guilford, 2019, pp 542–552
St. John MS, Thomas K: Infant mental health professional development: together in the struggle for social justice. Zero to Three 33(1):13–22, 2012
Strathearn L, Fonagy P, Amico J, et al: Adult attachment predicts maternal brain and oxytocin response to infant cues. Neuropsychopharmacology 34(13):2655–2666, 2009 19710635
Stuebe A: Should infants be separated from mothers with COVID-19? First, do no harm. Breastfeed Med 15(5):351–352, 2020 32271625
Sullivan RM, Toubas P: Clinical usefulness of maternal odor in newborns: soothing and feeding preparatory responses. Biol Neonate 74(6):402–408, 1998 9784631
Tamis-LeMonda CS, Shannon JD, Cabrera NJ, et al: Fathers and mothers at play with their 2- and 3-year-olds: contributions to language and cognitive development. Child Dev 75(6):1806–1820, 2004 15566381
Tasker F: Lesbian mothers, gay fathers, and their children: a review. J Dev Behav Pediatr 26(3):224–240, 2005 15956875
Thomas R, Herschell AD: Parent-child interaction therapy: a manualized intervention for the therapeutic child welfare sector. Child Abuse Negl 37(8):578–584, 2013 23561022
Thomas R, Zimmer-Gembeck MJ: Parent-child interaction therapy: an evidence-based treatment for child maltreatment. Child Maltreat 17(3):253–266, 2012 22942167
Tooten A, Hall RA, Hoffenkamp HN, et al: Maternal and paternal infant representations: a comparison between parents of term and preterm infants. Infant Behav Dev 37(3):366–379, 2014
Tornello SL, Bos H: Parenting intentions among transgender individuals. LGBT Health 4(2):115–120, 2017 28212056
Tronick EZ, Gianino A: Interactive mismatch and repair: challenges to the coping infant. Zero to Three 6(3):1–6, 1986
Tronick E, Als H, Adamson L, et al: The infant's response to entrapment between contradictory messages in face-to-face interaction. J Am Acad Child Psychiatry 17(1):1–13, 1978 632477
Tucker C, Schieffer K, Willis T, et al: Enhancing social-emotional skills in at-risk preschool students through Theraplay based groups: the Sunshine Circle Model. International Journal of Play Therapy 26(4):185–195, 2017
United Nations Children's Fund, World Health Organization: Baby-Friendly Hospital Initiative: Revised, Updated and Expanded for Integrated Care. New York, United Nations Children's Fund, 2009. Available at: https://www.unicef.org/nutrition/files/BFHI_2009_s1.pdf. Accessed August 6, 2020.
U.S. Department of Health and Human Services: Trends in Foster Care and Adoption: FY 2010–2019. Washington, DC, Administration for Children and Families, August 2020. Available at: https://www.acf.hhs.gov/cb/resource/trends-in-foster-care-and-adoption. Accessed August 24, 2020.

U.S. Department of State Bureau of Consular Affairs: Annual Report on Intercountry Adoption. Washington, DC, U.S. Department of State, March 2020. Available at: https://travel.state.gov/content/dam/NEWadoptionassets/pdfs/FY%202019%20Annual%20Report%20.pdf. Accessed January 19, 2021.

Van IJzendoorn MH, Kroonenberg PM: Cross-cultural patterns of attachment: a meta-analysis of the strange situation. Child Dev 59(1):147–156, 1988

van Londen WM, Juffer F, van Ijzendoorn MH: Attachment, cognitive, and motor development in adopted children: short-term outcomes after international adoption. J Pediatr Psychol 32(10):1249–1258, 2007 17709336

Van Rijn-van Gelderen L, Bos HWM, Jorgensen TD, et al: Wellbeing of gay fathers with children born through surrogacy: a comparison with lesbian-mother families and heterosexual IVF parent families. Hum Reprod 33(1):101–108, 2018 29145594

Vance AJ, Pan W, Malcolm WH, et al: Development of parenting self-efficacy in mothers of high-risk infants. Early Hum Dev 141:104946, 2020 31901656

Vittner D, McGrath J, Robinson J, et al: Increase in oxytocin from skin-to-skin contact enhances development of parent-infant relationship. Biol Res Nurs 20(1):54–62, 2018 29017336

Vreeswijk CM, Maas AJ, Rijk CH, et al: Stability of fathers' representations of their infants during the transition to parenthood. Attach Hum Dev 16(3):292–306, 2014 24684586

Wainright JL, Russell ST, Patterson CJ: Psychosocial adjustment, school outcomes, and romantic relationships of adolescents with same-sex parents. Child Dev 75(6):1886–1898, 2004 15566386

Weaver ICG, Cervoni N, Champagne FA, et al: Epigenetic programming by maternal behavior. Nat Neurosci 7(8):847–854, 2004 15220929

Webster CR Jr, Telingator CJ: Lesbian, gay, bisexual, and transgender families. Pediatr Clin North Am 63(6):1107–1119, 2016 27865336

Webster-Stratton C: The Incredible Years Parents, Teachers, and Children's Training Series: Program Content, Methods, Research and Dissemination, 1980–2011. Seattle, WA, Incredible Years, 2011

Webster-Stratton C, Reid MJ: Treating conduct problems and strengthening social and emotional competence in young children: The Dina Dinosaur treatment program. J Emot Behav Disord 1(3):130–143, 2003

Wettig HHG, Coleman AR, Geider FJ: Evaluating the effectiveness of Theraplay in treating shy, socially withdrawn children. International Journal of Play Therapy 20(1):26–37, 2011

Widström AM, Brimdyr K, Svensson K, et al: Skin-to-skin contact the first hour after birth, underlying implications and clinical practice. Acta Paediatr 108(7):1192–1204, 2019 30762247

Wojnar DM, Katzenmeyer A: Experiences of preconception, pregnancy, and new motherhood for lesbian nonbiological mothers. J Obstet Gynecol Neonatal Nurs 43(1):50–60, 2014 24354595

World Health Organization: Clinical Management of Severe Acute Respiratory Infection (SARI) When COVID-19 Disease Is Suspected: Interim Guidance (No. WHO/2019-nCoV/clinical/2020.4). Geneva, World Health Organization, 2020

Yaholkoski A, Hurl K, Theule J: Efficacy of the Circle of Security intervention: a meta-analysis. J Infant Child Adolesc Psychother 15(1):95–103, 2016

Yehuda R, Daskalakis NP, Lehrner A, et al: Influences of maternal and paternal PTSD on epigenetic regulation of the glucocorticoid receptor gene in Holocaust survivor offspring. Am J Psychiatry 171(8):872–880, 2014 24832930

Yoo H, Bowman DA, Oller DK: The origin of protoconversation: an examination of caregiver responses to cry and speech-like vocalizations. Front Psychol 9:1510, 2018 30197615

Zero to Three Infant Mental Health Task Force Steering Committee: Definition of Infant Mental Health. National Center for Clinical Infant Programs. Washington, DC, Zero to Three, 2001

# CHAPTER 13

# Depressive Disorders

Lauren M. Osborne, M.D.
Catherine Birndorf, M.D.

The reproductive years represent a period of heightened risk in women for major depressive disorder (MDD), with some women particularly vulnerable to mood symptoms that arise at moments of reproductive transition, such as menarche (Patton et al. 1996; Shen et al. 2019), the premenstruum (Miller and Miller 2001), pregnancy and the postpartum period, and perimenopause (Bromberger and Epperson 2018). For example, prior to puberty, MDD presents in equal rates in boys and girls. However, in the reproductive years, it is twice as common in women as in men. Postmenopause, the opposite is true: the rate of MDD in women dips below that of men. The focus of this chapter is on depressive disorders in pregnancy and postpartum. (See Chapter 6, "Premenstrual Mood Syndromes," and Chapter 7, "Perimenopause," for discussion of other reproductive transition periods.)

*Perinatal depression*—an umbrella term that includes both antenatal depression (AD) and postpartum depression (PPD)—is a serious mental health disorder affecting at least 15% of women in the developed world and 20%–40% of women worldwide (Bennett et al. 2004; Gaynes et al. 2005; Le Strat et al. 2011; Wisner et al. 2002). With more than 4 million live births in the United States each year, at least 600,000 families will be affected, making depression the most common complication of childbirth (Grace et al. 2003)—far outstripping such common complications as gestational diabetes (Dabelea et al. 2005), preterm birth (Saigal and Doyle 2008), and preeclampsia (Umesawa and Kobashi 2017). Perinatal depression affects the entire family, increasing partner conflict, disrupting mother–infant bonding, leading to poor occupational and social functioning, and affecting the cognitive, emotional, and social development of the child (Conroy et al. 2012; Grace et al. 2003). The societal costs of untreated perinatal depression are severe, with a recent estimate of $14.2 billion for all births in the United States in 2017 (or $32,000 per mother–child pair) (Luca et al. 2019).

At one time, pregnancy was thought to be "protective" against depression, but we now know that pregnancy itself confers neither protection nor risk—a woman is no more or less likely to develop depression during pregnancy than at any other time in her life (Vesga-López et al. 2008). Yet many women with preexisting depression stop treatment during pregnancy, leading to relapse rates perhaps as high as 65% (Cohen et al. 2006). Moreover, the postpartum period poses a time of elevated risk (O'Hara and McCabe 2013), and many women with PPD—perhaps as much as 80% (Whitton et al. 1996)—are never diagnosed or treated (Pearlstein 2008). Underdiagnosis is likely due to a combination of stigma against mental illness, struggles with access to care, attribution of neurovegetative symptoms to normal pregnancy changes, and lack of coordination between obstetrical and psychiatric care providers.

Although awareness of perinatal depression, and especially PPD, has increased in recent years, with both the American College of Obstetricians and Gynecologists (ACOG; 2015, 2018) and the U.S. Preventive Services Task Force (USPSTF) (O'Connor et al. 2016) recommending screening in both pregnancy and postpartum, scientists' knowledge of the pathophysiology still has major gaps. Moreover, the knowledge of both physicians and the public about how to balance the potential risks of treatment with the potential risks of *lack of* treatment lags behind the evidence, leading to often unnecessary suffering on the part of mothers and children.

## Epidemiology

### Rates/Incidence

Estimates of the rates of both AD and PPD vary widely. In the United States, most studies and current data from the Centers for Disease Control and Prevention show rates of 10%–15% during pregnancy (Centers for Disease Control and Prevention 2015; Gaynes et al. 2005), although some recent studies show rates as low as 6% in previously healthy women (Ashley et al. 2016). One factor that complicates the calculations of the incidence and prevalence of perinatal depression is prior history of depression, because perinatal depression can represent either a new onset of a mood disorder or an exacerbation of a prior disorder.

Rates around the world are similar to those of the United States and even higher, with higher rates more common in low- and middle-income countries (Al-Azri et al. 2016; Castro e Couto et al. 2016; George et al. 2016; Ogbo et al. 2018), with one recent study in Saudi Arabia finding a rate as high as 58% (Bawahab et al. 2017). In the postpartum period, a recent worldwide meta-analysis found an incidence of 12% and a prevalence of 17%, with rates being highest in the Middle East and lowest in Europe (Shorey et al. 2018), whereas another meta-analysis focused on perinatal depression found a worldwide prevalence of 11.9%, with rates highest in low- and middle-income countries (Woody et al. 2017). Recent country-specific studies find rates ranging from 14% to 25% in low- and middle-income countries (Doe et al. 2017; Hartmann et al. 2017; Özcan et al. 2017; Upadhyay et al. 2017). In higher-income countries, rates are overall lower, but women in immigrant and minority groups have higher rates than women in other groups (Doe et al. 2017; Falah-Hassani et al. 2015). One recent meta-analysis found that Black women, overall, are more likely to report symptoms but are less likely to seek care due to cultural stigma about mental illness (Cannon and Nasrallah 2019).

**TABLE 13–1. Psychosocial risk factors for perinatal depression**

| Antenatal | Postpartum |
|---|---|
| Anxiety | Breastfeeding problems |
| History of depression | Depression or anxiety during the index pregnancy |
| Intimate partner violence | Family history of postpartum depression |
| Lack of social support/Poor relationship quality | Fetal or newborn loss |
| Low income and/or education | Infant in neonatal intensive care unit |
| Single mothers | Low social support |
| Smoking | Preterm birth |
| Stress | Prior history of depression |
| Teen pregnancy | Traumatic birth experience or stressful events during the perinatal period |
| Unintended pregnancy | |

## Risk Factors

The biological risk factors for perinatal depression, about which we have limited knowledge, are still evolving and are discussed later (see "Pathophysiology"). Although any woman can develop depression during pregnancy or postpartum, and the commonly cited "one in seven" figure for perinatal mood and anxiety disorders refers to the general population, identified risk factors increase a woman's likelihood of becoming ill (Table 13–1). The strongest psychosocial risk factors for PPD are anxiety and depression in pregnancy, history of prior psychiatric illness, stressful life events during the perinatal period, and poor social support (Robertson et al. 2004). For women with prior affective illness, particularly prior MDD, studies show rates as high as 40% for PPD and 75% for the combined antenatal and postpartum periods (Guintivano et al. 2018; Kimmel et al. 2015). Family history also plays a strong role: in the same study, 53% of those with a family history of PPD developed the illness, compared with only 11% of those without a family history.

Other well-established risk factors include low socioeconomic status, single motherhood, adolescent pregnancy, low education status, unwanted pregnancy, childhood trauma, intimate partner violence, and obstetrical and delivery complications (Gelaye et al. 2016; Kimmel et al. 2015; Lancaster et al. 2010; Stuart-Parrigon and Stuart 2014). Some risk factors vary according to cultural context; for example, stressful life events in one large meta-analysis were an important risk factor only in non-Asian samples, and the sex of the child may be a risk factor in some cultures (Robertson et al. 2004). Although many studies indicate higher rates in Black and Latinx populations, a lack of social support, lack of access, and lack of trust in the medical establishment may explain some of this discrepancy (Cannon and Nasrallah 2019). In addition, some studies find that ethnicity and race are no longer predictive once marital status, poverty, education, and subjective socioeconomic status are taken into account (Dolbier et al. 2013). Other studies have indicated that social support can buffer symptom severity and that those buffering effects do not differ according to race or ethnicity (Pao et al. 2019).

## Screening Methods

The most important aspect of screening for perinatal depression as a routine component of obstetrical care is that it be done. Implementing some method of screening is vastly preferable to not implementing it, so clinicians should not hesitate to put screening procedures into practice even if the ideal cannot be achieved. Screening can and should be carried out by any clinician who treats a perinatal woman, including not only obstetrical clinicians but also primary care and mental health clinicians. By far, the most commonly used tool is the Edinburgh Postnatal Depression Scale (EPDS; Figure 13–1), which was created by a perinatal psychiatrist and has been validated in both pregnancy and the postpartum period and translated into more than 50 languages (Cox et al. 1987).

Several aspects of this 10-item self-report scale make it particularly advantageous during pregnancy and postpartum. First, it includes a mini-anxiety screener (three questions), which can be used both to assess the anxious symptoms that are often part of perinatal depression and to evaluate for anxiety itself. Second, it excludes neurovegetative and other physical symptoms of depression, such as changes in sleep patterns, appetite, and weight, that can be confused with symptoms of pregnancy and thus lead patients at times to dismiss them and clinicians to discount them even if endorsed. Finally, the EPDS is long enough to be relatively comprehensive while also being short enough to not be a burden; many patients can complete it in 5 minutes or less. (See Table 13–2 for more information.) The EPDS has been validated in many different racial and ethnic groups. Although the factor structure of the scale appears to differ slightly among ethnic and racial groups (Chiu et al. 2017; Hartley et al. 2014; King 2012), no data have suggested that it is not valid as a screening tool in any of these populations.

Although other screening tools lack the advantages described for perinatal patients, they can nonetheless be useful and are worth administering if the EPDS is not feasible (as in electronic medical records that have just one screening tool built in). Both the Beck Depression Inventory and the Zung Self-Rating Depression Scale are comprehensive rating scales for depression, but at more than 20 questions each—including constitutional symptoms—they may be burdensome to complete and have not been validated in this population (Schaefer et al. 1985; Wang and Gorenstein 2013).

Screening in and of itself is not enough. A positive screening result on the EPDS or any other scale is not a diagnosis of depression; it must be followed by a clinical evaluation. Misuse of screening measures as diagnostic tools can lead to potential harm by leading the clinician either to undervalue a patient's report of depressive symptoms or to misdiagnose a patient who does not meet criteria for a major depressive episode. In fact, studies on the EPDS show that nearly all patients with false-positive screening results, or patients who screened positive but did not have a diagnosis of depression on further evaluation, did indeed have a diagnosable mental health condition (Milgrom and Gemmill 2014).

Although universal screening using the EPDS or other measures during and after pregnancy can increase the detection of perinatal depression, it is also important to acknowledge that detection alone is not the goal. If detection does not lead to treatment and reduction of suffering, it is of limited value. Clinicians must go beyond screening

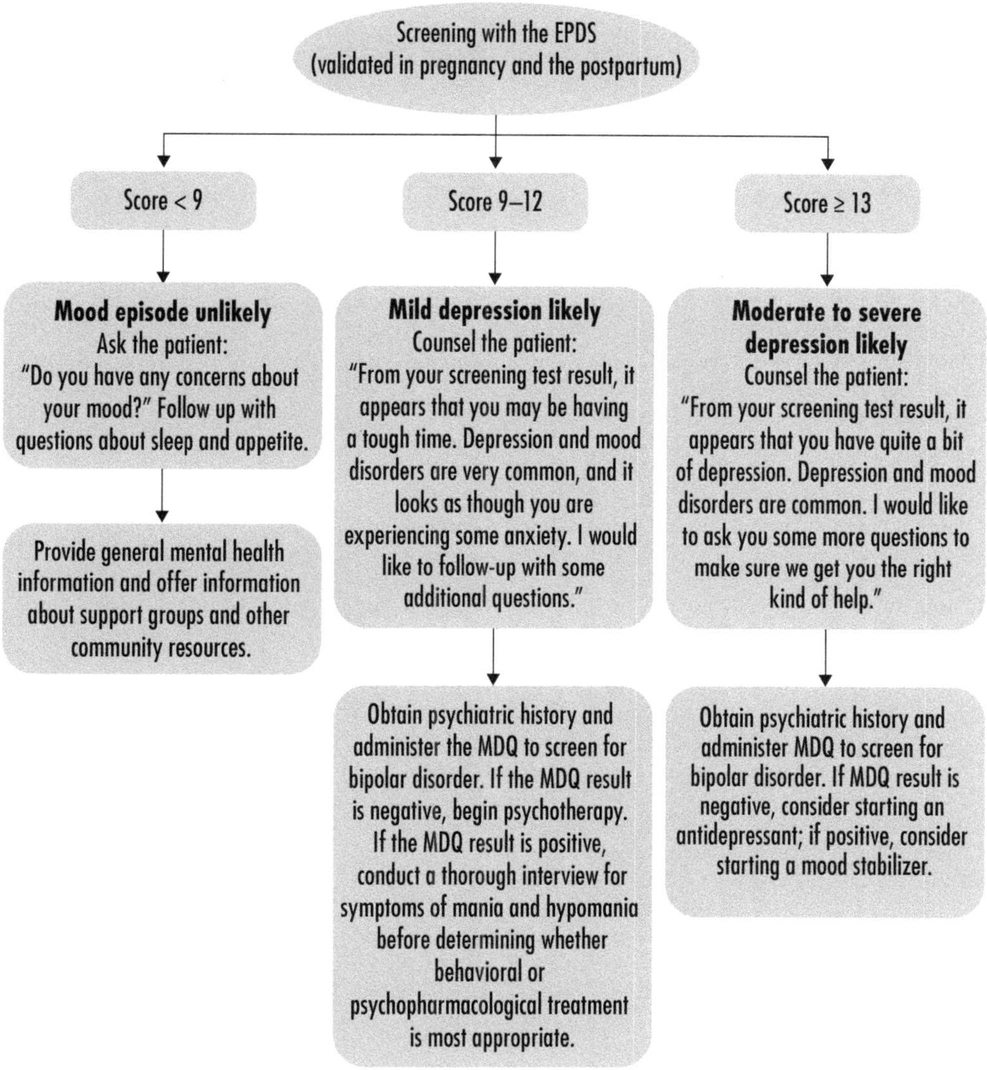


**FIGURE 13–1.** Using the Edinburgh Postnatal Depression Scale (EPDS).
MDQ=Mood Disorder Questionnaire.

to developing evaluation and targeted referral processes for women who screen positive. Even when this is provided, we must consider the barriers to treatment that many perinatal women face, from logistical issues (e.g., transportation and childcare) to the stigma associated with mental health treatment. Models that integrate mental health care into an obstetrical or primary care setting can address many of these barriers and improve both engagement in mental health care and the depression treatment effect for perinatal women. The recent transition to telehealth in many mental health settings, prompted by the COVID-19 pandemic, may in fact prove to be a boon to perinatal women because it will eliminate some of these barriers.

**TABLE 13–2. Screening tools for perinatal depression**

| Tool | Purpose | Items, *N* | Scoring | Advantages | Disadvantages | Comments |
|---|---|---|---|---|---|---|
| Beck Depression Inventory | Depression | 21 | 11–16 = mild<br>17–20 = borderline<br>21–30 = moderate<br>31–40 = severe<br>>40 = extremely severe | Comprehensive | Has many questions on appetite, sex, weight, and sleep; copyrighted and must pay for use | |
| Edinburgh Postnatal Depression Scale | Peripartum depression | 10 | 0–8 = limited or no symptoms<br>9–12 = mild symptoms<br>13–18 = moderate symptoms<br>≥19 = severe symptoms | Validated for antepartum and postpartum; eliminates constitutional symptoms; has anxiety | | Available in >50 languages; most widely used |
| Patient Health Questionnaire | Depression | 2 or 9 | 5–9 = mild<br>10–14 = moderate<br>15–19 = moderately severe<br>20–27 = severe | Incorporated into many primary care work flows; two-item version very quick | Has constitutional questions | Very widely used in general population |
| Quick Inventory of Depressive Symptomatology (Self-Report) | Depression | 16 | 8–12 = mild<br>13–16 = moderate<br>17–20 = moderate-severe<br>≥21 = severe | Comprehensive but a little shorter than Beck and Zung | Has constitutional questions | |
| Zung Self-Rating Depression Scale | Depression | 20 | 50–59 = mild<br>60–69 = moderate<br>≥70 = severe | Has both positive and negatively worded questions | No direct suicide question | |

# Clinical Features

## Diagnostic Criteria and Evaluation

Ms. T is a 28-year-old first-time mother with no prior psychiatric history and a desired pregnancy. She is no longer involved with the baby's father, but she lives with her sister, who is strongly supportive, and has other family members close by. She works as a teacher's aide and is highly conscientious, with very firm ideas prior to birth of what an "ideal birth experience" will be. At 37 weeks, she presents for a routine check and is found to have elevated blood pressure and protein in her urine. She is hospitalized for induction, and eventually has a cesarean section delivery after failing to progress. Her baby is small for gestational age and has to spend 24 hours in intensive care for low blood sugar.

In the initial days after the birth, Ms. T feels somewhat "giddy," both laughing and crying easily. She experiences some difficulty with latching and poor milk supply, and within 3 weeks she is frequently tearful and confides to her sister that she is "a terrible mom." She constantly reviews the events of the birth, convinced that she should and could have done something to prevent the cesarean section: "I should have known I had high blood pressure"; "I should have tried harder in labor." She ruminates about these events and about her breastfeeding difficulties and begins to have thoughts that her child might be better off without her.

The diagnosis of perinatal depression is at once simple and complex: simple because the core diagnostic features of MDD can also be used in the perinatal period, complex because unique clusters and emphases of symptoms occur in this period and because not all clinicians and governing bodies agree on the definition. The current definition, according to DSM-5 (American Psychiatric Association 2013), is the onset of a major depressive episode during pregnancy or within 4 weeks of childbirth (see Box 13–1). This definition conflates AD and PPD, which may be two biologically distinct entities, and although onset within 4 weeks postpartum likely captures those women for whom parturition is a biological trigger for symptoms, it fails to capture the significant population who may have onset later as a result of psychosocial triggers or hormonal disruption due to weaning (Burke et al. 2019).

### Box 13–1. DSM-5 Criteria for Major Depressive Disorder

A. Five (or more) of the following symptoms have been present during the same 2-week period and represent a change from previous functioning; at least one of the symptoms is either (1) depressed mood or (2) loss of interest or pleasure.

**Note:** Do not include symptoms that are clearly attributable to another medical condition.

1. Depressed mood most of the day, nearly every day, as indicated by either subjective report (e.g., feels sad, empty, hopeless) or observation made by others (e.g., appears tearful). (**Note:** In children and adolescents, can be irritable mood.)
2. Markedly diminished interest or pleasure in all, or almost all, activities most of the day, nearly every day (as indicated by either subjective account or observation).
3. Significant weight loss when not dieting or weight gain (e.g., a change of more than 5% of body weight in a month), or decrease or increase in appetite nearly every day. (**Note:** In children, consider failure to make expected weight gain.)
4. Insomnia or hypersomnia nearly every day.

5. Psychomotor agitation or retardation nearly every day (observable by others, not merely subjective feelings of restlessness or being slowed down).
6. Fatigue or loss of energy nearly every day.
7. Feelings of worthlessness or excessive or inappropriate guilt (which may be delusional) nearly every day (not merely self-reproach or guilt about being sick).
8. Diminished ability to think or concentrate, or indecisiveness, nearly every day (either by subjective account or as observed by others).
9. Recurrent thoughts of death (not just fear of dying), recurrent suicidal ideation without a specific plan, or a suicide attempt or a specific plan for committing suicide.

B. The symptoms cause clinically significant distress or impairment in social, occupational, or other important areas of functioning.

C. The episode is not attributable to the physiological effects of a substance or another medical condition.

**Note:** Criteria A–C represent a major depressive episode.

**Note:** Responses to a significant loss (e.g., bereavement, financial ruin, losses from a natural disaster, a serious medical illness or disability) may include the feelings of intense sadness, rumination about the loss, insomnia, poor appetite, and weight loss noted in Criterion A, which may resemble a depressive episode. Although such symptoms may be understandable or considered appropriate to the loss, the presence of a major depressive episode in addition to the normal response to a significant loss should also be carefully considered. This decision inevitably requires the exercise of clinical judgment based on the individual's history and the cultural norms for the expression of distress in the context of loss.

D. The occurrence of the major depressive episode is not better explained by schizoaffective disorder, schizophrenia, schizophreniform disorder, delusional disorder, or other specified and unspecified schizophrenia spectrum and other psychotic disorders.

E. There has never been a manic episode or a hypomanic episode.

**Note:** This exclusion does not apply if all of the manic-like or hypomanic-like episodes are substance-induced or are attributable to the physiological effects of another medical condition.

In recording the name of a diagnosis, terms should be listed in the following order: major depressive disorder, single or recurrent episode, severity/psychotic/remission specifiers, followed by as many of the following specifiers without codes that apply to the current episode.

*Specify*:

**With anxious distress**
**With mixed features**
**With melancholic features**
**With atypical features**
**With mood-congruent psychotic features**
**With mood-incongruent psychotic features**
**With catatonia**. **Coding note:** Use additional code 293.89 (F06.1).
**With peripartum onset**
**With seasonal pattern** (recurrent episode only)

**With peripartum onset:** This specifier can be applied to the current or, if full criteria are not currently met for a major depressive episode, most recent episode of major depression if onset of mood symptoms occurs during pregnancy or in the 4 weeks following delivery.

---

*Source.* Reprinted from American Psychiatric Association: *Diagnostic and Statistical Manual of Mental Disorders,* 5th Edition. Arlington, VA, 2013, p. 160–161, 186. 

**Table 13–3. How to talk about perinatal depression with moms**

| |
|---|
| How are you feeling about being pregnant/a mother? |
| Was this a desired pregnancy? |
| What things are you most happy about? |
| What things are you most concerned about? |
| Do you have anyone you can talk to that you trust? |
| How is your partner doing? |
| Are you able to enjoy your baby? |

*Source.* Adapted from materials made available by HealthTeamWorks and the Colorado Department of Public Health and Environment (CDPHE) and from MCPAP for Moms (www.healthteamworks.org/guidelines/depression.htm).

**Table 13–4. Assessing suicidal ideation in perinatal women**

| Lower risk | Higher risk |
|---|---|
| No prior attempts | History of suicide attempt |
| No plan | High lethality of prior attempt(s) |
| No intent | Current plan |
| No substance use | Current intent |
| Protective factors (what prevents you from acting?) | Substance use |
| | Lack of protective factors (including social support) |

*Source.* Adapted from materials made available by HealthTeamWorks and the Colorado Department of Public Health and Environment (CDPHE) and from MCPAP for Moms (www.healthteamworks.org/guidelines/depression.htm).

When evaluating a woman for depression, it is important to understand not only whether she meets criteria for the disorder but also how to talk with her about difficult and painful feelings and about risk. Some women may feel ashamed or unwilling to admit thoughts that are scary to them, and they must be approached in an open, nonjudgmental fashion. Some women may also be concerned about adverse consequences (e.g., referral to child protective services) that may result from being open about such thoughts. See Tables 13–3 and 13–4 for tips.

## Clinical Presentation

The clinical presentation of perinatal depression has many of the features of depressive episodes outside the postpartum period, with low mood, anhedonia, poor energy and concentration, low motivation, feelings of low self-worth, and sometimes suicidal ideation. Changes in sleep, appetite, and libido can also occur but are at times difficult to discern due to the effects of pregnancy (or to the patient's or physician's assumption of what pregnancy does). Anxious distress is a common feature of depression in this period, with high rates of rumination and worry—often about the mother's or baby's health—and intrusive thoughts (Collardeau et al. 2019; DeJong et al. 2016; Moulds et al. 2018). Recent research has begun to identify different clinical phenotypes within perinatal depression. The international consortium Postpartum Depression: Action Towards Causes and Treatment (PACT) assembled data from 19 international sites and used principal component and factor analysis to identify symptom dimensions, identifying five clinical phenotypes with different clusters of symptoms and timing of onset: severe anxious depression, moderate anxious depression, anxious anhedonia, pure anhedonia, and resolved depression, with anxiety and anhedonia especially prominent in women who had postpartum onset (Putnam et al. 2017). Few data indicate whether those in different racial and ethnic groups present differently in the perinatal period. Outside the perinatal period, evidence indicates that Black, Latinx, and Asian groups may be more likely than white patients to present with somatic complaints (Das et al. 2006), and clinicians may display greater uncertainty in diagnosing depression in minority populations (Adams et al. 2014).

> Ms. U is a 35-year-old married woman in a stable relationship. She has a 3-year-old son and a prior history of one episode of depression in college (treated to remission with citalopram and psychotherapy), mild premenstrual mood lability, and an episode of PPD following the birth of her son. That episode was severe and resulted in a brief hospitalization followed by 4 weeks in a day hospital program. In the hospital, Ms. U was treated with escitalopram and lorazepam; on discharge, the lorazepam was discontinued, and she eventually stabilized on 20 mg of escitalopram. Ms. U is now 21 weeks pregnant with her second child, and prior to the conception she elected to discontinue the escitalopram because "I was doing so well, and I didn't want to hurt my baby."
>
> For several months prior to conceiving and during her first trimester, Ms. U did well, maintaining a stable mood and prioritizing self-care with occasional sessions with her therapist and a daily exercise routine. At 15 weeks' gestation, however, she began to feel the return of her depressive symptoms, characterized by low self-worth, low motivation, and significant anxious distress. She feared for the safety of her husband and son and began following the husband when he left in the morning to ensure that he dropped their son off at day care. She has been calling the daycare multiple times each day to check up on her son, and she calls her husband frequently at work to make sure he is all right. She knows rationally that this is not necessary, but she cannot help it.

## Differential Diagnosis

Although diagnosis can be straightforward when classic depressive symptoms alone are present, several other disorders can be confused with depression in the perinatal period (Table 13–5). "Baby blues," which affects up to 75% of women (Nonacs and Cohen 1998), refers to mild mood lability in the immediate postpartum period. Some women with perinatal mood and anxiety symptoms may mistakenly believe that their symptoms are consistent with the blues, but both patients and clinicians should know that this resolves by 2 weeks postpartum and is never associated with severe symptoms, such as suicidality. Symptoms of anxiety disorders may overlap with those of depressive disorders, with a high rate of comorbidity between the two (Jordan and Minikel 2019). Medical disorders, such as hypothyroidism, anemia, or the rare Sheehan's disorder, may present with symptoms such as lethargy and fatigue, which may be confused with symptoms of depression (Kang et al. 2020; Wilson et al. 2019). Either intoxication or withdrawal from substances can be confused with symptoms of depression, so substance use disorders must always be included in the differential diagnosis. Finally, any woman presenting with depressive symptoms in the perinatal period may in fact have bipolar disorder—in fact, some research indicates that a high proportion of women with first-time depressive episodes in the postpartum later go on to be diagnosed with

**TABLE 13–5. Differential diagnosis**

| |
|---|
| Anemia |
| Anxiety disorder |
| Baby blues (if postpartum) |
| Endocrine disorders (e.g., hypothyroidism, Sheehan's syndrome) |
| Organic brain disorder (e.g., encephalitis, multiple sclerosis) |
| Other mood disorder (especially bipolar affective disorder) |
| Postpartum psychosis |
| Substance use disorder |

bipolar disorder (Sharma et al. 2018). Screening with the Mood Disorders Questionnaire and a careful clinical interview for symptoms of mania, hypomania, and rapid cycling may help clarify diagnosis in these cases (Sharma and Baczynski 2019). Women with psychotic or mixed symptoms should be suspected of having postpartum psychosis, which is often part of bipolar disorder (see Chapter 15, "Bipolar Disorder and Related Disorders," and Chapter 16, "Postpartum Psychosis," for further discussion.)

## Course/Prognosis

Left untreated, perinatal depression can have a devastating impact on mother, child, and the entire family (Beck 1998; Conroy et al. 2012; Goodman et al. 2011; Grote et al. 2010; Murray and Cooper 1997). AD is associated with higher rates of obstetrical complications, such as preeclampsia, preterm birth, low birth weight, and operative delivery (Hu et al. 2015; Jarde et al. 2016) and, independent of PPD, with negative sequelae for the child, including increased rates of internalizing disorders and altered cognitive development (Conroy et al. 2012; Zhu et al. 2014). In addition, AD is the biggest risk factor for PPD, which has the potential to lead to poor mother–infant bonding and to emotional and cognitive dysregulation for the child (Hoffman et al. 2017).

In addition to its effects on the pregnancy and child, perinatal depression can have long-lasting effects on the woman herself. The natural course of the illness is not entirely clear because most studies have focused exclusively on the postpartum period, and few have followed women beyond 6 months postpartum. A strong majority of women (70%–75%) will have persistent depressive symptoms at 6 months postpartum (Paulson et al. 2016; Torres et al. 2019), and some evidence shows that, although more than half of women will experience gradual remission, more than one-third will still have clinically significant depressive symptoms at 12 months postpartum (Fisher et al. 2019).

A 2014 review of longitudinal studies found decreasing levels of depression over time (with follow-up between 1 and 3.5 years) but great variability; at any time point between 4 months and 3 years, about 30% of mothers diagnosed with PPD in community samples and about 50% in clinical samples remained symptomatic (Vliegen et al. 2014). An examination of subgroups showed that, in most studies, there was a persistently depressed group and that women who remitted prior to 6 months often then relapsed later, although sometimes only with subthreshold symptoms. Demographic factors such as age, socioeconomic status, ethnicity, and education have at times been linked to chronicity, but that evidence has been mixed, and no clear consensus has been found (Vliegen et al. 2014). However, some risk factors for PPD have been shown to be related to the chronicity of course, including poor partner/social support, prior history of mental health problems, contextual factors (e.g., stress or financial worries), and personality factors (e.g., maladaptive coping styles and excessive self-criticism) (Vliegen et al. 2014). Another small study followed women with a prior history of MDD from an index pregnancy for an average of 12.9 years and found that only one-third of subjects reported sustained remission, with one-fifth endorsing depression at least 50% of the time (Freeman et al. 2018).

Some studies have looked at differences in course and symptoms according to time of symptom onset. Women with onset during pregnancy have been found to have higher rates of prior depressive episodes and higher rates of psychosocial stressors than women with onset in the postpartum, who are more likely to have obsessive-compulsive and psychotic symptoms (Altemus et al. 2012). Another group recently examined the trajectory of depressive symptoms across time in the perinatal period and identified four groups: two that were stable over time, with persistent symptoms of either low or moderate severity; one group with more severe symptoms during pregnancy that decreased in the postpartum; and another group that had few or moderate symptoms during pregnancy but developed severe symptoms in the postpartum (Ahmed et al. 2018). Certain characteristics predicted which women would belong to which group. Those women who reported more stress were more likely to belong to the higher-severity groups. Women with a prior history of depression were most likely to belong to the antepartum or moderate-stable groups. Being nonwhite and having poor partner support were also associated with the antepartum group, and only young maternal age was associated with the postpartum group. Another group that looked at symptoms in pregnancy only found three classes—increasing, decreasing, and stable—and similarly found that poor partner support was the key distinguishing factor for women whose symptoms worsened (Boekhorst et al. 2019).

Although perinatal depression is not known to have a different natural course than that of depression outside the perinatal period (although research is sparse), this illness may have lasting effects on a woman's health long after the acute symptoms have passed. Women with perinatal depression may have a "reproductive subtype" of depression and may have symptoms at other times of hormonal transition, including the premenstrual period and perimenopause (Payne et al. 2009). In addition, perinatal depression is associated with other morbidities of pregnancy (e.g., gestational diabetes, preeclampsia, preterm birth) that have lasting effects on the woman's or child's health. Gestational diabetes is associated with an increased risk of subsequent Type II diabetes and preeclampsia with a subsequent increased risk of cardiovascular disease (Chasan-Taber 2016; Perry et al. 2018).

# Pathophysiology

## Biological Factors

Considerable research is available on the genetics and epigenetics of PPD (McEvoy et al. 2017). (This work has, by and large, not extended yet to include AD, so this section focuses on PPD only.) Family and twin studies from the 1990s forward have indicated a genetic basis for PPD when it is defined as a mood episode beginning within 4 weeks of parturition; some of these studies have also found familiality to PPD in families with MDD or bipolar affective disorder (Forty et al. 2006; Murphy-Eberenz et al. 2006; Payne et al. 2008; Treloar et al. 1999). Genome-wide linkage and association studies have found variations on areas of chromosomes 1 and 9, and a single nucleotide polymorphism study identified the potential involvement of two estrogen-responsive genes (Carroll et al. 2006; Green and Galea 2008; Mahon et al. 2009; Mehta et al. 2014). In addition, candidate gene studies have implicated polymorphisms in several promising genes, including the serotonin transporter gene (Hu et al. 2019; Pinheiro et al. 2013; Zhang et al. 2015), the catechol-*O*-methyltransferase (*COMT*) gene (Alvim-Soares et al. 2013; Comasco et al. 2011; Doornbos et al. 2009; Klein et al. 2016), and the estrogen receptor alpha (*ESR1*) gene (Costas et al. 2010; Pinsonneault et al. 2013). Data are mixed on the involvement of several other genes, including brain-derived neurotrophic factor (*BDNF*) (Comasco et al. 2011; Figueira et al. 2010), the oxytocin receptor (*OXTR*) (Bell et al. 2015; Jonas et al. 2013; Mileva-Seitz et al. 2013), hemicentin 1 (*HMCN1*) (Alvim-Soares et al. 2014; Mahon et al. 2009), and monoamine oxidase A (*MAOA*) (Comasco et al. 2011; Doornbos et al. 2009; Ivorra et al. 2010). The one commonality across all of these genetic studies is the issue of timing, with results often positive when symptoms are measured close to delivery but negative for depressions that begin later. This may indicate that there is a genetic basis to PPD only when the timing is clearly linked to the hormonal trigger of childbirth.

Genetics is only a part of the landscape of heritable risk factors for PPD, and recent work has also identified and replicated epigenetic biomarkers that consistently predict the development of PPD with an accuracy of more than 80%. Two loci have been identified at the *HP1BP3* and *TTC9B* genes—identified originally by linking estrogen-responsive loci in the mouse hippocampus to DNA methylation differences in blood samples from pregnant and postpartum women with mood disorders—and replicated subsequently in diverse populations both with and without preexisting mood disorders (Guintivano et al. 2014; Osborne et al. 2016). Although the function of these two genes is not entirely clear, both are known to be responsive to gonadal hormones (Cao et al. 2006; Nassa et al. 2011).

In addition to the genetic and epigenetic risk factors mentioned, we can also point to substantial evidence of biological risk factors that may not be driven by heritability. The most obviously involved biological system is the endocrine system, because all women undergo massive shifts in reproductive hormones across pregnancy, leading to a dramatic drop shortly after delivery, and perhaps related to the high rate of the baby blues. However, only some women develop perinatal depression, meaning that individual women's vulnerability is far more important than absolute levels of hormones. This was elegantly demonstrated two decades ago when women with prior PPD and healthy control subjects were subjected to an identical, pregnancy-mimicking hormone regimen, and only women with prior PPD became ill (Bloch et al. 2000).

Initial research on estrogen and progesterone as risk factors for PPD was unilluminating. Animal studies have suggested that estradiol withdrawal induces depressive symptoms (Bethea et al. 2002; Galea et al. 2001), and early studies indicated that estradiol affects levels of serotonin and that its administration could improve symptoms of PPD (Ahokas et al. 2001; Gregoire et al. 1996). However, numerous studies have also found no differences in either estradiol levels or rate of estradiol withdrawal in women with PPD compared with healthy women (Chatzicharalampous et al. 2011; Okun et al. 2011). More recent work has begun to pinpoint both metabolites of and receptors for these hormones. For progesterone, considerable evidence indicates that dysregulation of allopregnanolone (one of the 3α-5α reduced metabolites of progesterone) is related to risk for perinatal depression. Lower allopregnanolone levels in pregnancy and poor allopregnanolone response to stress during pregnancy have been associated with both AD and PPD (Crowley et al. 2016; Hellgren et al. 2014, 2017; Osborne et al. 2017); other GABAergic neurosteroids may also play a role but have been less studied. The FDA's 2019 decision to declare brexanolone (a synthetic version of allopregnanolone) the first approved drug for PPD was informed by considerable basic science research into GABAergic dysregulation.

Other hormonal systems may also be involved in the pathophysiology of perinatal depression. The neurosteroid system works in close concert with the hypothalamic-pituitary-adrenal axis, and a number of studies have examined dysregulation of the cortisol response in perinatal mood symptoms. Corticotropin-releasing hormone is produced by the placenta, and elevated levels have been tied to later PPD (Yim et al. 2009). PPD has also been connected with altered cortisol responsiveness and altered levels of adrenocorticotropic hormone (Cox et al. 2015; Groër et al. 2005; Iliadis et al. 2015; Jolley et al. 2007; Scheyer and Urizar 2016), although data are mixed, and the directionality is not always consistent. Some studies have implicated dysregulation of the thyroid system (Kuijpens et al. 2001; Lambrinoudaki et al. 2010), but systematic reviews have failed to find consistent associations (Szpunar and Parry 2018; Yim et al. 2009). Finally, oxytocin has been an area of interest, with studies showing that lower pregnancy oxytocin is associated with higher levels of both AD and PPD symptoms (Skrundz et al. 2011), that women who went on to develop PPD have a drop in oxytocin prior to parturition (whereas healthy women have an increase) (Jobst et al. 2016), and that oxytocin levels in the third trimester can predict the development of PPD only for women with a history of prior MDD (Massey et al. 2016). Prolactin has also been investigated and is thought to mediate normal maternal behavior but with little evidence thus far for a specifically different role in depression (Payne and Maguire 2019).

Another system that may be implicated in perinatal depression is the immune system. A connection between immune dysregulation and MDD is well established (Dowlati et al. 2010; Howren et al. 2009; Miller et al. 2009), but the directionality of this connection—and whether it applies only to certain subsets of depressed people (Raison et al. 2013)—is still in question. It is logical to wonder whether women in the perinatal period comprise one of those subsets because there is substantial immune dysregulation in healthy pregnancy, allowing the body to adjust to the presence of a "foreign pathogen" (i.e., a fetus whose genetic material is at least half foreign). Early work in this area looked primarily at levels of proinflammatory cytokines, and both methods and outcomes were mixed (Osborne and Monk 2013). Numerous studies since then have found both elevations (Liu et al. 2016; Osborne et al. 2019; Simpson et al. 2016) and decreases (Bränn et al. 2017, 2020; Edvinsson et al. 2017) in proinflammatory cytokines associated with perinatal depression, with the bulk of the evidence concerning increases in interleukin-6, a cytokine with both pro- and anti-inflammatory properties that is integral to the acute phase response and to B- and T-cell activation. More recently, some groups have begun to look at summative inflammatory scores (Bränn et al. 2017) and at antibodies (Wesseloo et al. 2018) and immune cell populations (Krause et al. 2014; Osborne et al. 2020), directions that may prove fruitful to solidify a connection

**Table 13–6. Potential pathophysiological factors**

| | |
|---|---|
| **Inherent biological** | |
| | Altered activity in amygdala, prefrontal cortex, cingulate cortex, and insula (cause or consequence?) |
| | Epigenetic factors (*HP1BP3* and *TTC9B*) |
| | Genetic factors (especially *SERT* and *ESR1*) |
| | Hypothalamic-pituitary-adrenal axis |
| | Immune system |
| | Neurosteroids (especially allopregnanolone) |
| | Oxytocin |
| **Obstetrical** | |
| | Preterm birth |

that remains tenuous despite its theoretical plausibility. The immune system may also in part be responsible for the connection between preterm birth, which is associated with local inflammation, and PPD (Fransson et al. 2012).

Much current research into biological factors comes from neuroimaging studies of altered network activity and altered white matter connectivity. In the resting state, attenuated activity has been observed in numerous brain regions, including the anterior cingulate cortex, amygdala, hippocampus, and dorsolateral prefrontal cortex (Deligiannidis et al. 2013). Decreased corticocortical, corticolimbic (Deligiannidis et al. 2013), and posterior cingulate cortex–right amygdala (Chase et al. 2014) connectivity has also been observed, along with changes in homogeneity across numerous brain regions. Task-based functional MRI studies have also identified altered activity in response to an infant's cry or images of an infant, with the greatest evidence for the amygdala, prefrontal cortex, cingulate cortex, and insula (as summarized in Payne and Maguire 2019). Limited studies using PET and magnetic resonance spectroscopy confirm alterations in these same regions. To date, few studies have examined changes in white matter connectivity, although one has found lower fractional anisotropy in the anterior limb of the internal capsule, the retrolenticular internal capsule, and corpus callosum (Silver et al. 2018). Future areas of research that hold the potential for discovery in perinatal depression include neuronal oscillations (particularly with respect to GABAergic signaling) and circuit changes in the maternal care network, for which there is already significant animal research regarding healthy maternal behavior but few data specific to depression. Table 13–6 summarizes potential biological factors.

## Psychosocial Factors

As covered earlier (see "Risk Factors" and Table 13–1), prior psychiatric history is the strongest predictor of the development of PPD, with significant evidence not only for MDD but also for anxiety disorders, prior reproductive mood disorders (PPD or premenstrual dysphoric disorder), personality disorders, and any psychiatric disorders (as reviewed in Guintivano et al. 2018). This applies both to psychiatric illness that preceded the pregnancy and to antenatal illness. Stressful life events or past or current physical, sexual, or psychological abuse (including intimate partner violence) is also significantly predictive (Agrawal et al. 2014; Cerulli et al. 2011; Robertson-Blackmore et al. 2013; Woolhouse et al. 2012). Some studies have found evidence for maternal age as a risk factor (with both the youngest and oldest mothers at greater risk than those in the middle). Although race and ethnicity are not consistently identified with risk, Black women who develop perinatal depression are less likely to be identified and treated (Guintivano et al. 2018).

Another important etiological factor that is both biological and psychosocial is sleep. Considerable evidence supports a role for impaired sleep in concurrent symptoms of both AD and PPD, with some evidence also showing that impaired sleep may predict the development of future symptoms (McEvoy et al. 2019; Okun et al. 2011). (See Chapter 9, "A Clinical Approach to Psychiatric Diagnosis and Treatment in the Postpartum Period," for further details on sleep.)

## Treatment

Before deciding on a particular mode of treatment for depression during the perinatal period, it is important to consider the severity of a woman's illness. The great fear that many clinicians have about prescribing in pregnancy can often override considerations about the most appropriate treatment for the patient's illness. As discussed in Chapter 8, "A Clinical Approach to Psychiatric Diagnosis and Treatment in Pregnancy," there is no completely risk-free decision when a woman with depression is pregnant. Sometimes the best way to balance her risks will be to prescribe medication, but sometimes it will not. A woman's ability to access care is also an important part of this equation. In many communities, low-income women have little access to quality psychotherapy, for example, which may affect the decision of what treatment to use. One recent study showed that Black women have higher rates of hospital treatment for PPD, which likely reflects the fact that Black women may have less access to the outpatient care that might prevent hospitalization (Chan et al. 2020).

In cases in which issues of access do not force the clinician's hand, the primary consideration about whether to use medication has to do with the severity of illness and prior response. Table 13–7 offers clinical tips for how to determine whether medication is warranted.

### Psychopharmacology

As discussed in Chapters 8 and 9, considerable controversy remains about treating depression in pregnancy and during breastfeeding. We have no randomized controlled trials about medication risks and very few studies about medication efficacy, alternative treatments, or dosage alterations that may be required due to metabolic changes in pregnancy. Decisions about treatment must therefore rely on observational evidence only. Although there is some evidence of risks associated with antidepressant usage, those risks appear to be few now that studies (primarily of selective serotonin reuptake inhibitors [SSRIs]) are being conducted with appropriate control groups and controlling for appropriate confounders. The substantial body of evidence we have concerning the risks of untreated psychiatric illness to both mother and child (Field et al. 2006, 2010; Li et al. 2009; Orr et al. 2007; Zuckerman et al. 1989) must be weighed against any known risks of medication.

**TABLE 13–7. Indications for medication use for perinatal depression**

| Suggests medication may not be indicated | Suggests medication treatment should be considered |
|---|---|
| Mild depression based on clinical assessment | Moderate/severe depression based on clinical assessment |
| No suicidal ideation | Suicidal ideation |
| Able to care for self/baby | Difficulty functioning or caring for self/baby |
| Depression has improved with psychotherapy in past | Psychotic symptoms present |
| Engaged in psychotherapy or other nonmedication treatment | History of severe depression or suicidal ideation/attempts |
| Strong preference for and access to psychotherapy | Comorbid anxiety disorders or symptoms |

*Source.* Adapted from materials made available by HealthTeamWorks and the Colorado Department of Public Health and Environment (CDPHE) and from MCPAP for Moms (www.healthteamworks.org/guidelines/depression.htm).

To understand the risks of antidepressant usage in pregnancy, it is important to understand the differences between women who use antidepressants and those who do not. Women with depression have higher rates of diabetes mellitus, obesity, smoking, substance use, and cesarean section than women who do not have depression (De Hert et al. 2011). Therefore, studies that fail to account for risks conferred either directly by the illness or symptoms themselves (e.g., by elevated cortisol or inflammation) or indirectly through health behaviors may find apparent associations between antidepressants and risks that may not be caused by the medication itself but rather by characteristics associated with the women taking the medication. This means that any association found when comparing women taking antidepressants with healthy women (the control group used in the vast majority of studies) is spurious.

With these caveats in mind, current evidence shows few consistent and sustained risks associated with antidepressant usage. We review here current knowledge about several areas that have been investigated for risk.

## Risk Considerations During Early Pregnancy

**Congenital malformations.** Some studies have found statistically significant but clinically negligible associations (i.e., with odds ratios just above 1) between overall congenital malformations and the use of antidepressants (Einarson 2012; Grigoriadis et al. 2013). Some but not all early studies found potential associations between use of antidepressants in pregnancy and heart defects (Chisolm and Payne 2016). In 2005, the FDA issued a warning concerning heart defects with paroxetine. These studies generally compared psychiatric with nonpsychiatric populations, an error of inaccurate control group that unfortunately continues, as shown in a recent large population study (Wemakor et al. 2015). Better-designed studies have not upheld these associations. Large studies (with populations approaching or exceeding 1 million women) and meta-analyses that compare women with depression who took antidepressants with those who did not take antidepressants have found no association between SSRI use in the first trimester and overall congenital or heart defects (Huybrechts et al. 2014a; Wang et al. 2015). Of course, a large study or meta-analysis depends upon the choice of studies included, and some meta-analyses continue to find increased rates of cardiac defects with paroxetine. Such analyses still do not account for the risk of the underlying illness and continue to use comparator groups that are not comparable (Bérard et al. 2016). The best available evidence therefore indicates that antidepressant usage does not increase the risk of congenital malformations.

**Spontaneous abortion (miscarriage).** Several studies have found increased rates of spontaneous abortion in women using antidepressants (Einarson et al. 2009; Santone et al. 2009). Spontaneous abortion has also been associated with depression itself (Nakano et al. 2004). Large database studies and meta-analyses of the highest-quality studies indicate that antidepressants likely confer no added risk of spontaneous abortion beyond the risk conferred by the illness itself (Kjaersgaard et al. 2013; Ross et al. 2013).

## Other Pregnancy Risks

**Persistent pulmonary hypertension.** In 2006, the FDA issued an alert for a potential, and seemingly alarming, association between SSRI usage and persistent pulmonary hypertension of the newborn (Chambers et al. 2006). Subsequent studies were mixed, with about half confirming this association (albeit with considerably lower odds ratios) and the other half failing to find it (Andrade et al. 2009; Källén and Olausson 2008; Kieler et al. 2012; Wichman et al. 2009; Wilson et al. 2011). A recent study in almost 4,000,000 women found an unadjusted OR of 1.51 (95% CI, 1.35–1.69) for an association between SSRI use and persistent pulmonary hypertension of the newborn, but when the analysis was adjusted for potential confounders, the relationship vanished (with the exception of remaining statistically significant when cases were limited to full-term infants only [OR 1.28; 95% CI 1.01–1.64]) (Huybrechts et al. 2015).

**Infant growth.** Most studies that do not control for depression show a small, statistically significant relationship between antidepressant exposure and a reduction in birth weight, with very small effect size (<100 g) (Huang et al. 2014; Ross et al. 2013). Those studies that have directly compared the effects on infant growth of antidepressant exposure with those of depression have found no differences; in one case, both groups were associated with slower growth (El Marroun et al. 2012), and in another, neither was associated (Wisner et al. 2013). It therefore seems likely that there is no significant effect of antidepressants directly on infant growth—and if there is any effect, it is very small and not clinically meaningful.

**Fetal behavior and neurodevelopment.** Several studies have indicated that depression or stress in pregnancy can alter fetal heart rate, fetal heart rate variability, and the coupling of heart rate to movement (Field et al. 2006; Monk et al. 2004) and can be associated in particular with male vulnerability (Walsh et al. 2019). (See Chapter 11, "Stress in Pregnancy," for additional information.) It is unclear what the long-term consequences are of this altered fetal behavior. Some studies also show differences in fetal neurodevelopment with SSRI use, including alterations in the development of neural circuitry in the somatosensory cortex in animals (Xu et al. 2004) and an increase in connectivity between the right amygdala and insula (Lugo-Candelas et al. 2018) and widespread changes in white matter microstructure (Jha et al. 2016) in humans. Other studies have shown that the administration of SSRIs actually reversed changes in fetal brain structure associated with maternal stress (Velasquez et al. 2019), whereas still others have shown that both depression and antidepressants may affect fetal brain structure, but in different ways (Rotem-Kohavi et al. 2019). Many of the existing studies have not been able to control for confounders, including severity of illness, and it is not yet clear what these changes mean for long-term consequences in children.

**Preterm birth.** Several studies have found an association between antidepressant usage and preterm birth (i.e., birth prior to 37 weeks' gestation). Recent research, including large database studies and high-quality meta-analyses, has upheld this association, finding a small but significant risk of preterm birth with antidepressant usage (Huybrechts et al. 2014b; Ross et al. 2013) even when controlling for depression. One study that directly compared the effects on labor of depression with those of antidepressant exposure found them to be about equal (Wisner et al. 2009). In most studies, the average reduction in gestational age is about 3–4 days (Yonkers et al. 2012). In this case, then, there does appear to be a statistical association with risk, but when making treatment decisions, we must consider whether this is a *clinically* important association and how it compares with the risks of no medication. Another recent study confirmed that untreated depression is associated with significantly increased risks of preterm birth and low birth weight (Jarde et al. 2016), meaning that women with depression, regardless of whether they take medications, may be at risk for preterm birth, thus indicating that this is a risk we cannot change. Thus, the decision about medication use should be made using other bases.

## Neonatal Outcomes

**Hypothalamic-pituitary-adrenal axis reactivity.** Several studies have shown that babies born to mothers depressed in pregnancy have elevated cortisol and possibly other biochemical changes reflective of their mothers' depression (Fernandes et al. 2015; Field et al. 2006; Oberlander et al. 2008; Osborne et al. 2018; Talge et al. 2007). In some cases, studies have shown altered infant reactivity to stress associated with these changes. The elevations in cortisol have been shown to persist at least until adolescence (O'Donnell et al. 2013). Although some evidence indicates that SSRI exposure may alter this biochemical balance (Pawluski et al. 2012), it is unclear whether antidepressant exposure in depressed women would alter this balance for better or worse, and considerable additional research is needed before drawing conclusions.

**Neonatal adaptation.** One newborn outcome thought to be associated with antidepressant use in pregnancy is poor neonatal adaptation syndrome. The first observation of "withdrawal" from antidepressants in infants was published in 1973 (Webster 1973), but it is now uncertain whether the behavioral syndrome observed in about 30% of babies whose mothers have taken SSRIs in the third trimester is actually withdrawal (rather than toxicity), leading to the current descriptive term, "poor neonatal adaptation syndrome." There is no consistent definition of this syndrome nor any specific measurement tool or blinded rating scale, but repeated observations led the FDA in 2004 to require that labels for both SSRI and serotonin-norepinephrine reuptake inhibitor (SNRI) antidepressants contain a warning that third-trimester exposure to these drugs may be associated with "respiratory distress, cyanosis, apnea, seizures, temperature instability, feeding difficulty, vomiting, hypoglycemia, hypotonia, hypertonia, hyperreflexia, tremor, jitteriness, irritability, and constant crying" (O'Connor et al. 2016). Most cases of the poor neonatal adaptation syndrome appear to be mild and self-limited (although increased with polypharmacy) (Oberlander et al. 2004) and are not associated with lasting repercussions (Moses-Kolko et al. 2005), but these data are quite limited (Salisbury et al. 2016). The common clinical practice of tapering antidepressants in the third trimester to avoid this syndrome has no scientific basis and can lead to other negative sequelae because plasma levels drop 40%–50% (Deligiannidis et al. 2014) across the course of pregnancy, and tapering—or even maintaining a steady pre-pregnancy dose—may lead to relapse in vulnerable women.

**Long-term effects.** Cognitive and behavioral effects of antidepressant exposure on children have been well studied, and there is no evidence of associated IQ deficits or long-term behavioral problems (Nulman et al. 1997, 2002, 2012). Depression in pregnancy and the postpartum period is associated with both cognitive and behavioral problems in children, including both internalizing and externalizing disorders, that are both acute and long lasting (Capron et al. 2015; O'Connor et al. 2007; O'Donnell et al. 2013; Smith-Nielsen et al. 2016). Alarming newspaper headlines have linked the use of antidepressants in pregnancy to autism based on initial studies that found an increase in risk (Croen et al. 2011; Rai et al. 2013). Subsequent studies that considered confounds more carefully have found no increased risk. Women with depression have a higher risk of giving birth to a child with autism, but the medication itself does not appear to confer additional risk (Andrade 2017a, 2017b; Hviid et al. 2013; Sørensen et al. 2013).

When making treatment decisions, clinicians must always weigh the risks discussed here against the risks to both mother and child of untreated illness in pregnancy (Table 13–8). For the mother, relapse into a mood episode (including possible suicidality) is substantial, and a considerable body of evidence points to increased risks for the child from AD (Field et al. 2006; Grace et al. 2003). Moreover, untreated depression in pregnancy is the biggest risk factor for PPD, which has known and devastating effects on children and families (Grace et al. 2003). Impaired bonding can lead to insecure attachment (Hipwell et al. 2000), and PPD has also been associated with increased colic, impaired parenting behavior, increases in harsh discipline, impaired emotional and language development, impaired attention and cognition, and long-term behavioral problems (Akman et al. 2006; Flynn et al. 2004; McLearn et al. 2006).

## Management During Pregnancy

As discussed in Chapters 8 and 9, any decision about medication use in pregnancy and lactation must be individual; for each woman, the balance of risk of medications versus risks of untreated illness will be different. The FDA's new pregnancy and lactation labeling rule offers extremely useful—although lengthy—information about the risks of individual drugs. The defunct FDA categories (A, B, C, D, X) are not useful for understanding the risks of antidepressants; clinicians tend to assume that this is a graded scale, with B being better than C, but in reality drugs are assigned to category B when there is insufficient information about risk to determine whether they belong in group A (no risk to humans) or group C (evidence of risk to humans). Because so much about medication use in pregnancy is unknown, it is wiser to choose an older drug about which we have more data (which might be category C rather than B), because then the

**TABLE 13–8. Risks of psychiatric disorder versus risks of selective serotonin reuptake inhibitor (SSRI) use in pregnancy**

| Reproductive domain | Risks associated with psychiatric disorder | Risks associated with SSRI treatment |
|---|---|---|
| Congenital malformations | Unlikely | Early studies: cardiac defects |
| | | More recent studies: no or very low association after corrections |
| Spontaneous abortion | Unlikely | Equivocal studies; low odds ratios and same for women who stop SSRI prior to pregnancy |
| Length of pregnancy | Preterm delivery | Preterm delivery |
| Size effects | Infant small for gestational age | Infant small for gestational age |
| Short-term risks (withdrawal) | Impaired bonding with baby in postpartum period | Serotonergic withdrawal in newborn: |
| | Increased risk of postpartum depression | Gastrointestinal |
| | | Neuromuscular |
| | | Pulmonary |
| | | Psychiatric/Behavioral |
| | | Transient (24–48 hours); no treatment needed |
| Long-term risks (development) | Associated with poor bonding to baby/parent | Developmental studies show promise: |
| | Maternal depression leads to increased risk of child developing depression | Prospective trials show catching up of any initial delays |
| | Fetal neurodevelopment studies show changes in brain structure, but significance is unclear | Behavioral problems also occur in children of mothers with depression |
| | | Autism studies poorly constructed; no associations when sibling analyses and paternal factors are included |
| | | Fetal neurodevelopment studies show changes in brain structure, but significance is unclear |
| Other (e.g., obstetrical risks) | Poor prenatal care | None known |
| | Increased risk of suicide | |
| | Increased smoking, substance use, poor diet | |

*Note.* Table compares risks of both psychiatric illness and medication use to pregnancy, child, and mother. It is organized by reproductive domains, so risks discussed by pregnancy timing in the text are regrouped here into sections that are easily classified together for ease in patient communication.

risks are known rather than unknown. Although these categories have been phased out, they may still appear on labels of older drugs, so all clinicians must be aware of the pitfalls of relying on them.

In general, all SSRIs and SNRIs can be used in pregnancy and lactation, as can tricyclic antidepressants. (Please see the Appendix for a detailed chart of dosage suggestions and pregnancy and lactation considerations.) We have fewer data on bupropion and mirtazapine, although the growing amount of evidence on these two drugs is reassuring. (Mirtazapine has the added benefits of being helpful for both sleep and nausea.) Newer SSRIs, such as vortioxetine and vilazodone, have no evidence for their use in pregnancy, so they should not be considered first-line in a patient with no prior drug trials. They may, however, be the best choice for patients who have failed trials with other SSRIs and for whom these medications are known to provide stability, or for patients who present already stable on one of these medications postconception.

Because we have little evidence about polypharmacy and no evidence of increased risk with increased doses, it is wise to try to maximize the dose of a single medication rather than use low doses of several medications. In addition, because the risks are comparable, it is wisest to use a drug to which the woman has responded in the past rather than choosing a drug that may appear to have lower risk (Payne 2019). *There is no "one safe drug" for pregnancy; the choice depends on the woman's history.* Although we have more evidence of safety for sertraline and fluoxetine than for many others, the risk for all older SSRIs is low. There is slightly more evidence of risk with paroxetine (although, as described earlier, recent studies do not support this risk). It therefore makes sense, if starting a drug in a patient with no prior antidepressant exposure, to avoid paroxetine as the first choice—but again, it makes little sense to switch a patient away from paroxetine if that is the drug that has kept her stable in the past.

Dosage considerations in pregnancy are also important. Many clinicians will be inclined to decrease doses in the third trimester to lower the risk for neonatal adaptation syndrome, but there is no evidence supporting this approach. In fact, because pharmacokinetic changes and volume of distribution in pregnancy mean that serum concentrations of most drugs will drop by 40%–50% by the end of the third trimester, many women will need *increased* rather than decreased doses. There are currently no clinical guidelines on how to manage this, but many experienced clinicians will raise doses prophylactically or closely monitor symptoms in late pregnancy so that dosage adjustments may be made expediently if necessary.

## Lactation

For all women with mood disorders, the decision about whether to breastfeed must take into account both the significant benefits of breastfeeding to both mother and child and the risks of sleep disruption to the mother's mood. (For further discussion of this issue, see Chapter 9.) The postpartum period is a time for heightened risk for depression, both for women with previously diagnosed illness and for those with new-onset PPD. Many women are fearful of the possible risks of medication exposure through breastmilk; this can be particularly true for those with new-onset illness who have never had to consider medication risk in the past.

Fortunately, the necessary considerations around the use of antidepressant medication in lactation are few. The American Academy of Pediatrics considers a relative infant dose of <10% to be acceptable in lactation (see Chapter 9 for a full discussion of relative infant dose). All SSRI antidepressants fall below this level and can be used safely in lactation. Sertraline has the lowest passage into breast milk, at around 0.5%. Fluoxetine was initially thought to pose greater risk due to its long half-life and early case reports of sedated infants, but no additional data have supported higher risk. Tricyclic antidepressants also have evidence of safety in lactation and can be used. Fewer data are available concerning newer antidepressants, such as bupropion and mirtazapine, but the available evidence is reassuring. (See Chapter 23, "Attention-Deficit/Hyperactivity Disorder," for further discussion of bupropion in pregnancy.) As with pregnancy, the very newest drugs have no data regarding use in lactation and should therefore be used with caution and only when a patient has failed trials of drugs with more data.

### Other Medication Treatment

Because PPD arises at a time of vast changes in reproductive hormones, hormonal remedies have seemed an obvious route to try and have been cited as perhaps more appealing to women who are reluctant to try psychotropic drugs (Moses-Kolko et al. 2009). Some early case reports and open-label trials showed promise for the use of estrogen (usually transdermal estradiol) to treat PPD (Gregoire et al. 1996), particularly in women with a deficiency of estradiol (Ahokas et al. 1999, 2001) or those who also had premenstrual mood symptoms (Studd 2014). A randomized trial in 2015 was designed to compare transdermal estradiol with placebo but was unable to evaluate this question fully because serum concentrations of estradiol on a variety of doses were not higher than those of women given placebo (Wisner et al. 2015). A similar randomized trial in 2020 showed promising differences in response between placebo and estradiol groups, but the numbers were too small to determine whether these differences were due to chance (Li et al. 2020), leaving unanswered the question of whether transdermal estradiol might be effective as a treatment for PPD.

While the field was failing to find an answer as to whether estradiol could be used as treatment, other researchers chose to investigate the progesterone system, focusing on the metabolite allopregnanolone. Allopregnanolone is an allosteric modulator of the $GABA_A$ receptor, and the link between this system and PPD made it an attractive treatment target. Brexanolone, a synthetic version of allopregnanolone for injection, was recently developed and tested in three double-blind, randomized, placebo-controlled trials, each of which showed a reduction in depressive symptoms compared with placebo (Kanes et al. 2017; Meltzer-Brody et al. 2018). Integrated data from all three trials showed a separation from placebo both at 60 hours (primary endpoint) and 30 days (secondary endpoint) (Meltzer-Brody and Kanes 2020), and on the strength of these studies brexanolone became in 2019 the first drug to be FDA approved for the treatment of PPD. Although the excitement of having a "first-ever" drug has been substantial, critics have pointed out the large placebo effects in each trial. In addition, the difficulties of administration (a 3-day infusion requiring an inpatient stay, with few data yet about breastfeeding safety, and a price tag of $34,000) mean that this drug at the moment is usable by only a tiny minority of women. An oral compound is currently in testing.

## Nonpharmacological Somatic Treatments

Electroconvulsive therapy (ECT) is an effective option for the treatment of severe mood symptoms, especially in the context of associated catatonia, psychotic agitation, suicidality, or severe physical decline (e.g., malnutrition or dehydration) (Ward et al. 2018).

ECT offers a rapid treatment response and serves as an alternative to pharmacological treatment or when pharmacotherapy fails. The safety and efficacy of ECT during pregnancy have been established over decades and support its role as a treatment option for pregnant women when clinically indicated (Ward et al. 2018). ECT also has evidence to support its efficacy in the treatment of postpartum affective disorders, and some suggest it should be considered a first-line treatment in women with severe symptoms in this setting (Forray and Ostroff 2007). As with pharmacotherapy, any risks of ECT in pregnancy must be weighed against the risks of untreated mental illness. The risks and adverse reactions in pregnancy are similar to those in nonpregnant patients and include memory loss, prolonged seizure, and risks related to anesthesia (Ward et al. 2018). ECT is not associated with increased risk of congenital malformations, miscarriage, preterm delivery, or infant neurodevelopmental concerns. The most common reported maternal risk is premature contractions, which have been found to occur in up to 24% of patients and is seen most frequently in the latter half of pregnancy (Ward et al. 2018). The most reported fetal risk is transient fetal bradyarrhythmias, likely due to hypoxia (Anderson and Reti 2009).

Although ECT is a safe and efficacious treatment option for the treatment of depression during pregnancy, its accessibility to pregnant women is often limited by logistical considerations and by the comfort level of community ECT providers in treating pregnant patients. ECT during pregnancy should be done in a setting that allows for obstetrical monitoring and support and for access to neonatal care if necessary. Further specific and practical protocol recommendations regarding ECT during pregnancy can be found in a recent comprehensive review (Ward et al. 2018). Modification of medications (e.g., tapering off anticonvulsants) may be required for patients considering ECT.

Repetitive transcranial magnetic stimulation (rTMS), although a much newer technique than ECT, is also building a body of evidence for both safety and efficacy in pregnancy and the postpartum. rTMS is approved by the FDA for use in patients who have failed at least one antidepressant. It has the potential to be widely useful in the perinatal period because it avoids questions of fetal risk posed by some medications and is also less invasive than ECT. It nevertheless represents a significant patient burden because treatment is generally carried out 5 days a week. Randomized controlled trials are lacking, but the open-label pilot studies and case series that have been conducted have been associated with an improvement in symptoms, with no indication of adverse effects for the fetus (Felipe and Ferrão 2016; Johansen et al. 2019). rTMS has also been studied for PPD, with promising initial results (Garcia et al. 2010).

## Behavioral Treatments

### Psychotherapy

For many women with perinatal depression, particularly those with mild to moderate symptoms, psychotherapy will be the first-choice treatment. There is considerable evidence of the effectiveness of manualized, evidence-based psychotherapies for both prevention and treatment of perinatal depression, with the best evidence for cognitive-behavioral therapy (CBT) and interpersonal therapy. Two systematic reviews have addressed psychotherapy in both antenatal and postpartum populations (Loughnan et al. 2019; Sockol et al. 2011) and found good overall effect sizes, with some evidence that effect sizes may be greater for postpartum than for antenatal women. For postpartum women only, there have been moderate to good effect sizes in several trials; those with the most rigorous methodology showed substantial reductions in symptoms for any type of psychotherapy but little difference between different active treatment arms, which have included interpersonal therapy, CBT, psychodynamic therapy, directive and nondirective cognitive counseling, and both group and individual deliveries (Cooper et al. 2003; Milgrom et al. 2005, 2011; O'Hara et al. 2000). Many of the existing studies suffer from small sample sizes, limited follow-up, and inadequate control groups. For summaries of the existing evidence for prevention and treatment, see Stuart and Koleva (2014) and Werner et al. (2015).

#### Sleep Interventions

Both education about sleep hygiene and CBT for insomnia have some evidence of efficacy in the perinatal population, but research in this area is still young. Studies have focused largely on infant sleep regulation, and those that have examined maternal depressive symptoms have found a positive effect (Hiscock et al. 2014; Johansen et al. 2019; Phillips et al. 2010; Smart and Hiscock 2007). Two preliminary open pilot studies of CBT for insomnia in perinatal women have promising results (Swanson et al. 2013; Tomfohr-Madsen et al. 2017).

### Alternative and Complementary Treatments

Psychotherapy and psychopharmacological agents at this point hold the greatest body of evidence for safety and efficacy in pregnancy and lactation, but evidence is building for some alternative and complementary therapies. Because patients often see these modalities as desirable, clinicians must understand the evidence base and know which modalities have evidence of safety and which may be helpful. Although many patients believe such approaches will be safe "because they are natural," the reality is that such agents are outside of the FDA approval process and thus unregulated, so there is little control over them. Most vitamins, minerals, and nutraceuticals have little evidence of either safety or efficacy and should thus be avoided in pregnancy, with the possible exception of omega-3 fatty acids (Reza et al. 2018). Bright light therapy has been found to be both safe and acceptable and superior to a dim-light placebo for AD, but a randomized controlled trial in PPD failed to show a difference, and more research is clearly needed (Johansen et al. 2019). Physical activity in general has evidence of safety and acceptability in AD and PPD, although research is lacking on whether it is effective for either treating or preventing perinatal depression (Reza et al. 2018). More evidence exists for yoga, which is also safe and acceptable and shows greater reduction of depressive symptoms when compared with waitlist, treatment as usual, massage, social support, and parenting education (Davis et al. 2015; Field et al. 2012, 2013a, 2013b). For further details on the evidence base for integrative approaches to the treatment of perinatal depression, please see Chapter 14, "Integrative Approaches to Perinatal Depression."

## Conclusion

Depression during pregnancy and the postpartum period affects 15%–20% of women (with higher rates in developing countries) and can have devastating consequences for the woman, her child, and her entire family. It is associated with adverse health behaviors in women, including increased rates of substance use and less adherence to prenatal care. In its severest manifestations it can lead to suicide, a major cause of maternal deaths in the first year postpartum (Goldman-Mellor and Margerison 2019). Maternal depression is also associated with poor behavioral, emotional, and cognitive outcomes for children. It is important to screen pregnant and postpartum women for depressive illness and to treat that illness when found. Because psychiatrists are not typically educated about the risks of untreated perinatal depression, many physicians overestimate the relative risks of using antidepressant drugs, with the result that many women with depression in pregnancy and postpartum are untreated. Mild symptoms can respond to nonpharmacological treatments, and most antidepressants can be used safely in pregnancy and the postpartum.

## Key Points

- Depression is common both in pregnancy and postpartum, with an elevated biological risk in the early postpartum period.
- A personal or family history of depression is the strongest single risk factor of perinatal depression.
- Suicide is a leading cause of peripartum mortality, and all decisions about treatment in this period must bear that in mind.
- Although changes in reproductive hormones may be involved in triggering postpartum depressive symptoms, little evidence shows that levels of estrogen and progesterone differ between women with depression and healthy women; rather, some women appear to be vulnerable to shifting hormones.
- Good screening tools, including the Edinburgh Postnatal Depression Scale, are important but cannot take the place of a clinical diagnosis.
- Women with mild or moderate symptoms can often be treated successfully with psychotherapy and other nonpharmacological approaches, but differences in access to care may affect women's ability to engage in such treatment.
- Women with moderate to severe symptoms usually require pharmacological treatment.
- Although very few randomized controlled trials have been published, increasingly sophisticated statistical techniques have resulted in rigorous data from observational trials over the past few years.
- Most data indicate that the risks of untreated illness often outweigh the risks of medication, so clinicians should not hesitate to prescribe medication for women who are ill, if indicated.

# References


Adams A, Vail L, Buckingham CD, et al: Investigating the influence of African American and African Caribbean race on primary care doctors' decision making about depression. Soc Sci Med 116:161–168, 2014 25014268

Agrawal A, Ickovics J, Lewis JB, et al: Postpartum intimate partner violence and health risks among young mothers in the United States: a prospective study. Matern Child Health J 18(8):1985–1992, 2014 24562504

Ahmed A, Feng C, Bowen A, et al: Latent trajectory groups of perinatal depressive and anxiety symptoms from pregnancy to early postpartum and their antenatal risk factors. Arch Women Ment Health 21(6):689–698, 2018 29654413

Ahokas A, Kaukoranta J, Aito M: Effect of oestradiol on postpartum depression. Psychopharmacology (Berl) 146(1):108–110, 1999 10485972

Ahokas A, Kaukoranta J, Wahlbeck K, et al: Estrogen deficiency in severe postpartum depression: successful treatment with sublingual physiologic 17beta-estradiol: a preliminary study. J Clin Psychiatry 62(5):332–336, 2001 11411813

Akman I, Kusçu K, Özdemir N, et al: Mothers' postpartum psychological adjustment and infantile colic. Arch Dis Child 91(5):417–419, 2006 16452109

Al-Azri M, Al-Lawati I, Al-Kamyani R, et al: Prevalence and risk factors of antenatal depression among Omani women in a primary care setting: cross-sectional study. Sultan Qaboos Univ Med J 16(1):e35–e41, 2016 26909211

Altemus M, Neeb CC, Davis A, et al: Phenotypic differences between pregnancy-onset and postpartum-onset major depressive disorder. J Clin Psychiatry 73(12):e1485–e1491, 2012 23290332

Alvim-Soares A, Miranda D, Campos SB, et al: Postpartum depression symptoms associated with Val158Met COMT polymorphism. Arch Women Ment Health 16(4):339–340, 2013 23636476

Alvim-Soares AM, Miranda DM, Campos SB, et al: HMNC1 gene polymorphism associated with postpartum depression. Br J Psychiatry 36(1):96–97, 2014 24604465

American College of Obstetricians and Gynecologists: ACOG Committee Opinion No. 630: screening for perinatal depression. Obstet Gynecol 125(5):1268–1271, 2015 25932866

American College of Obstetricians and Gynecologists: ACOG Committee Opinion No. 757: screening for perinatal depression. Obstet Gynecol 132(5):e208–e212, 2018 30629567

American Psychiatric Association: Diagnostic and Statistical Manual of Mental Disorders, 5th Edition. Arlington, VA, American Psychiatric Association, 2013

Anderson EL, Reti IM: ECT in pregnancy: a review of the literature from 1941 to 2007. Psychosom Med 71(2):235–242, 2009 19073751

Andrade C: Antidepressant exposure during pregnancy and risk of autism in the offspring, 1: meta-review of meta-analyses. J Clin Psychiatry 78(8):e1047–e1051, 2017a 28994903

Andrade C: Antidepressant exposure during pregnancy and risk of autism in the offspring, 2: do the new studies add anything new? J Clin Psychiatry 78(8):e1052–e1056, 2017b 29099558

Andrade SE, McPhillips H, Loren D, et al: Antidepressant medication use and risk of persistent pulmonary hypertension of the newborn. Pharmacoepidemiol Drug Saf 18(3):246–252, 2009 19148882

Ashley JM, Harper BD, Arms-Chavez CJ, et al: Estimated prevalence of antenatal depression in the US population. Arch Women Ment Health 19(2):395–400, 2016 26687691

Bawahab JA, Alahmadi JR, Ibrahim AM: Prevalence and determinants of antenatal depression among women attending primary health care centers in Western Saudi Arabia. Saudi Med J 38(12):1237–1242, 2017 29209674

Beck CT: The effects of postpartum depression on child development: a meta-analysis. Arch Psychiatr Nurs 12(1):12–20, 1998 9489170

Bell AF, Carter CS, Steer CD, et al: Interaction between oxytocin receptor DNA methylation and genotype is associated with risk of postpartum depression in women without depression in pregnancy. Front Genet 6:243, 2015 26257770

Bennett HA, Einarson A, Taddio A, et al: Prevalence of depression during pregnancy: systematic review. Obstet Gynecol 103(4):698–709, 2004 15051562
Bérard A, Iessa N, Chaabane S, et al: The risk of major cardiac malformations associated with paroxetine use during the first trimester of pregnancy: a systematic review and meta-analysis. Br J Clin Pharmacol 81(4):589–604, 2016 26613360
Bethea CL, Lu NZ, Gundlah C, et al: Diverse actions of ovarian steroids in the serotonin neural system. Front Neuroendocrinol 23(1):41–100, 2002 11906203
Bloch M, Schmidt PJ, Danaceau M, et al: Effects of gonadal steroids in women with a history of postpartum depression. Am J Psychiatry 157(6):924–930, 2000 10831472
Boekhorst MGBM, Beerthuizen A, Endendijk JJ, et al: Different trajectories of depressive symptoms during pregnancy. J Affect Disord 248:139–146, 2019 30731281
Bränn E, Papadopoulos F, Fransson E, et al: Inflammatory markers in late pregnancy in association with postpartum depression—a nested case-control study. Psychoneuroendocrinology 79:146–159, 2017 28285186
Bränn E, Fransson E, White RA, et al: Inflammatory markers in women with postpartum depressive symptoms. J Neurosci Res 98(7):1309–1321, 2020 30252150
Bromberger JT, Epperson CN: Depression during and after the perimenopause: impact of hormones, genetics, and environmental determinants of disease. Obstet Gynecol Clin North Am 45(4):663–678, 2018 30401549
Burke CS, Susser LC, Hermann AD: GABAA dysregulation as an explanatory model for late-onset postpartum depression associated with weaning and resumption of menstruation. Arch Women Ment Health 22(1):55–63, 2019 29968131
Cannon C, Nasrallah HA: A focus on postpartum depression among African American women: a literature review. Ann Clin Psychiatry 31(2):138–143, 2019 31046035
Cao S, Iyer JK, Lin V: Identification of tetratricopeptide repeat domain 9, a hormonally regulated protein. Biochem Biophys Res Commun 345(1):310–317, 2006 16678794
Capron LE, Glover V, Pearson RM, et al: Associations of maternal and paternal antenatal mood with offspring anxiety disorder at age 18 years. J Affect Disord 187:20–26, 2015 26301478
Carroll JS, Meyer CA, Song J, et al: Genome-wide analysis of estrogen receptor binding sites. Nat Genet 38(11):1289–1297, 2006 17013392
Castro e Couto T, Cardoso MN, Brancaglion MY, et al: Antenatal depression: prevalence and risk factor patterns across the gestational period. J Affect Disord 192:70–75, 2016 26707350
Centers for Disease Control and Prevention: Selected 2012 Through 2015 Maternal and Child Health Indicators Aggregate by State. Atlanta, GA, Centers for Disease Control and Prevention, 2015. Available at: https://www.cdc.gov/prams/prams-data/2015-mch-indicators.html. Accessed July 31, 2019.
Cerulli C, Talbot NL, Tang W, et al: Co-occurring intimate partner violence and mental health diagnoses in perinatal women. J Womens Health (Larchmt) 20(12):1797–1803, 2011 21923282
Chambers CD, Hernandez-Diaz S, Van Marter LJ, et al: Selective serotonin-reuptake inhibitors and risk of persistent pulmonary hypertension of the newborn. N Engl J Med 354(6):579–587, 2006 16467545
Chan AL, Guo N, Popat R, et al: Racial and ethnic disparities in hospital-based care associated with postpartum depression. J Racial Ethn Health Disparities 8(1):220–229, 2020 32474833
Chasan-Taber L: It is time to view pregnancy as a stress test. J Womens Health (Larchmt) 25(1):2–3, 2016 26667129
Chase HW, Moses-Kolko EL, Zevallos C, et al: Disrupted posterior cingulate-amygdala connectivity in postpartum depressed women as measured with resting BOLD fMRI. Soc Cogn Affect Neurosci 9(8):1069–1075, 2014 23709351
Chatzicharalampous C, Rizos D, Pliatsika P, et al: Reproductive hormones and postpartum mood disturbances in Greek women. Gynecol Endocrinol 27(8):543–550, 2011 20653338
Chisolm MS, Payne JL: Management of psychotropic drugs during pregnancy. BMJ 532:h5918, 2016 26791406
Chiu YM, Sheffield PE, Hsu HL, et al: Subconstructs of the Edinburgh Postnatal Depression Scale in a multi-ethnic inner-city population in the U.S. Arch Women Ment Health 20(6):803–810, 2017 28770342

Cohen LS, Altshuler LL, Harlow BL, et al: Relapse of major depression during pregnancy in women who maintain or discontinue antidepressant treatment. JAMA 295(5):499–507, 2006 16449615

Collardeau F, Corbyn B, Abramowitz J, et al: Maternal unwanted and intrusive thoughts of infant-related harm, obsessive-compulsive disorder and depression in the perinatal period: study protocol. BMC Psychiatry 19(1):94, 2019 30898103

Comasco E, Sylvén SM, Papadopoulos FC, et al: Postpartum depression symptoms: a case-control study on monoaminergic functional polymorphisms and environmental stressors. Psychiatr Genet 21(1):19–28, 2011 21099450

Conroy S, Pariante CM, Marks MN, et al: Maternal psychopathology and infant development at 18 months: the impact of maternal personality disorder and depression. J Am Acad Child Adolesc Psychiatry 51(1):51–61, 2012 22176939

Cooper PJ, Murray L, Wilson A, et al: Controlled trial of the short- and long-term effect of psychological treatment of post-partum depression. I. Impact on maternal mood. Br J Psychiatry 182:412–419, 2003 12724244

Costas J, Gratacòs M, Escaramís G, et al: Association study of 44 candidate genes with depressive and anxiety symptoms in post-partum women. J Psychiatr Res 44(11):717–724, 2010 20092830

Cox EQ, Stuebe A, Pearson B, et al: Oxytocin and HPA stress axis reactivity in postpartum women. Psychoneuroendocrinology 55:164–172, 2015 25768266

Cox JL, Holden JM, Sagovsky R: Detection of postnatal depression: development of the 10-item Edinburgh Postnatal Depression Scale. Br J Psychiatry 150(6):782–786, 1987 3651732

Croen LA, Grether JK, Yoshida CK, et al: Antidepressant use during pregnancy and childhood autism spectrum disorders. Arch Gen Psychiatry 68(11):1104–1112, 2011 21727247

Crowley SK, O'Buckley TK, Schiller CE, et al: Blunted neuroactive steroid and HPA axis responses to stress are associated with reduced sleep quality and negative affect in pregnancy: a pilot study. Psychopharmacology (Berl) 233(7):1299–1310, 2016 26856852

Dabelea D, Snell-Bergeon JK, Hartsfield CL, et al: Increasing prevalence of gestational diabetes mellitus (GDM) over time and by birth cohort: Kaiser Permanente of Colorado GDM Screening Program. Diabetes Care 28(3):579–584, 2005 15735191

Das AK, Olfson M, McCurtis HL, et al: Depression in African Americans: breaking barriers to detection and treatment. J Fam Pract 55(1):30–39, 2006 16388764

Davis K, Goodman SH, Leiferman J, et al: A randomized controlled trial of yoga for pregnant women with symptoms of depression and anxiety. Complement Ther Clin Pract 21(3):166–172, 2015 26256135

De Hert M, Correll CU, Bobes J, et al: Physical illness in patients with severe mental disorders. I. Prevalence, impact of medications and disparities in health care. World Psychiatry 10(1):52–77, 2011 21379357

DeJong H, Fox E, Stein A: Rumination and postnatal depression: a systematic review and a cognitive model. Behav Res Ther 82:38–49, 2016 27203622

Deligiannidis KM, Sikoglu EM, Shaffer SA, et al: GABAergic neuroactive steroids and resting-state functional connectivity in postpartum depression: a preliminary study. J Psychiatr Res 47(6):816–828, 2013 23499388

Deligiannidis KM, Byatt N, Freeman MP: Pharmacotherapy for mood disorders in pregnancy: a review of pharmacokinetic changes and clinical recommendations for therapeutic drug monitoring. J Clin Psychopharmacol 34(2):244–255, 2014 24525634

Doe S, LoBue S, Hamaoui A, et al: Prevalence and predictors of positive screening for postpartum depression in minority parturients in the South Bronx. Arch Women Ment Health 20(2):291–295, 2017 28025705

Dolbier CL, Rush TE, Sahadeo LS, et al: Relationships of race and socioeconomic status to postpartum depressive symptoms in rural African American and non-Hispanic white women. Matern Child Health J 17(7):1277–1287, 2013 22961387

Doornbos B, Dijck-Brouwer DA, Kema IP, et al: The development of peripartum depressive symptoms is associated with gene polymorphisms of MAOA, 5-HTT and COMT. Prog Neuropsychopharmacol Biol Psychiatry 33(7):1250–1254, 2009 19625011

Dowlati Y, Herrmann N, Swardfager W, et al: A meta-analysis of cytokines in major depression. Biol Psychiatry 67(5):446–457, 2010 20015486

Edvinsson Å, Bränn E, Hellgren C, et al: Lower inflammatory markers in women with antenatal depression brings the M1/M2 balance into focus from a new direction. Psychoneuroendocrinology 80:15–25, 2017 28292683

Einarson A: Challenges for healthcare providers in treating women with psychiatric disorders during pregnancy. J Popul Ther Clin Pharmacol 19(3):e371–e375, 2012 23075467

Einarson A, Choi J, Einarson TR, et al: Rates of spontaneous and therapeutic abortions following use of antidepressants in pregnancy: results from a large prospective database. J Obstet Gynaecol Can 31(5):452–456, 2009 19604427

El Marroun H, Jaddoe VW, Hudziak JJ, et al: Maternal use of selective serotonin reuptake inhibitors, fetal growth, and risk of adverse birth outcomes. Arch Gen Psychiatry 69(7):706–714, 2012 22393202

Falah-Hassani K, Shiri R, Vigod S, et al: Prevalence of postpartum depression among immigrant women: a systematic review and meta-analysis. J Psychiatr Res 70:67–82, 2015 26424425

Felipe RM, Ferrão YA: Transcranial magnetic stimulation for treatment of major depression during pregnancy: a review. Trends Psychiatry Psychother 38(4):190–197, 2016 28076639

Fernandes M, Stein A, Srinivasan K, et al: Foetal exposure to maternal depression predicts cortisol responses in infants: findings from rural South India. Child Care Health Dev 41(5):677–686, 2015 25131942

Field T, Diego M, Hernandez-Reif M: Prenatal depression effects on the fetus and newborn: a review. Infant Behav Dev 29(3):445–455, 2006 17138297

Field T, Diego M, Hernandez-Reif M: Prenatal depression effects and interventions: a review. Infant Behav Dev 33(4):409–418, 2010 20471091

Field T, Diego M, Hernandez-Reif M, et al: Yoga and massage therapy reduce prenatal depression and prematurity. J Bodyw Mov Ther 16(2):204–209, 2012 22464118

Field T, Diego M, Delgado J, et al: Tai chi/yoga reduces prenatal depression, anxiety and sleep disturbances. Complement Ther Clin Pract 19(1):6–10, 2013a 23337557

Field T, Diego M, Delgado J, et al: Yoga and social support reduce prenatal depression, anxiety and cortisol. J Bodyw Mov Ther 17(4):397–403, 2013b 24138994

Figueira P, Malloy-Diniz L, Campos SB, et al: An association study between the Val66Met polymorphism of the BDNF gene and postpartum depression. Arch Women Ment Health 13(3):285–289, 2010 20169377

Fisher SD, Sit DK, Yang A, et al: Four maternal characteristics determine the 12-month course of chronic severe postpartum depressive symptoms. Depress Anxiety 36(4):375–383, 2019 30645006

Flynn HA, Davis M, Marcus SM, et al: Rates of maternal depression in pediatric emergency department and relationship to child service utilization. Gen Hosp Psychiatry 26(4):316–322, 2004 15234828

Forray A, Ostroff RB: The use of electroconvulsive therapy in postpartum affective disorders. J ECT 23(3):188–193, 2007 17804998

Forty L, Jones L, Macgregor S, et al: Familiality of postpartum depression in unipolar disorder: results of a family study. Am J Psychiatry 163(9):1549–1553, 2006 16946179

Fransson E, Dubicke A, Byström B, et al: Negative emotions and cytokines in maternal and cord serum at preterm birth. Am J Reprod Immunol 67(6):506–514, 2012 22017458

Freeman MP, Claypoole LD, Burt VK, et al: Course of major depressive disorder after pregnancy and the postpartum period. Depress Anxiety 35(12):1130–1136, 2018 30192044

Galea LA, Wide JK, Barr AM: Estradiol alleviates depressive-like symptoms in a novel animal model of post-partum depression. Behav Brain Res 122(1):1–9, 2001 11287071

Garcia KS, Flynn P, Pierce KJ, et al: Repetitive transcranial magnetic stimulation treats postpartum depression. Brain Stimul 3(1):36–41, 2010 20633429

Gaynes BN, Gavin N, Meltzer-Brody S, et al: Perinatal depression: prevalence, screening accuracy, and screening outcomes. Evid Rep Technol Assess (Summ) (119):1–8, 2005 15760246

Gelaye B, Rondon MB, Araya R, et al: Epidemiology of maternal depression, risk factors, and child outcomes in low-income and middle-income countries. Lancet Psychiatry 3(10):973–982, 2016 27650773
George C, Lalitha AR, Antony A, et al: Antenatal depression in coastal South India: prevalence and risk factors in the community. Int J Soc Psychiatry 62(2):141–147, 2016 26443716
Goldman-Mellor S, Margerison CE: Maternal drug-related death and suicide are leading causes of postpartum death in California. Am J Obstet Gynecol 221(5):489.e1–489.e9, 2019 31173749
Goodman SH, Rouse MH, Connell AM, et al: Maternal depression and child psychopathology: a meta-analytic review. Clin Child Fam Psychol Rev 14(1):1–27, 2011 21052833
Grace SL, Evindar A, Stewart DE: The effect of postpartum depression on child cognitive development and behavior: a review and critical analysis of the literature. Arch Women Ment Health 6(4):263–274, 2003 14628179
Green AD, Galea LA: Adult hippocampal cell proliferation is suppressed with estrogen withdrawal after a hormone-simulated pregnancy. Horm Behav 54(1):203–211, 2008 18423635
Gregoire AJ, Kumar R, Everitt B, et al: Transdermal oestrogen for treatment of severe postnatal depression. Lancet 347(9006):930–933, 1996 8598756
Grigoriadis S, VonderPorten EH, Mamisashvili L, et al: The effect of prenatal antidepressant exposure on neonatal adaptation: a systematic review and meta-analysis. J Clin Psychiatry 74(4):e309–e320, 2013 23656856
Groër M, Davis M, Casey K, et al: Neuroendocrine and immune relationships in postpartum fatigue. MCN Am J Matern Child Nurs 30(2):133–138, 2005 15775810
Grote NK, Bridge JA, Gavin AR, et al: A meta-analysis of depression during pregnancy and the risk of preterm birth, low birth weight, and intrauterine growth restriction. Arch Gen Psychiatry 67(10):1012–1024, 2010 20921117
Guintivano J, Arad M, Gould TD, et al: Antenatal prediction of postpartum depression with blood DNA methylation biomarkers. Mol Psychiatry 19(5):560–567, 2014 23689534
Guintivano J, Manuck T, Meltzer-Brody S: Predictors of postpartum depression: a comprehensive review of the last decade of evidence. Clin Obstet Gynecol 61(3):591–603, 2018 29596076
Hartley CM, Barroso N, Rey Y, et al: Factor structure and psychometric properties of English and Spanish versions of the Edinburgh Postnatal Depression Scale among Hispanic women in a primary care setting. J Clin Psychol 70(12):1240–1250, 2014 24807217
Hartmann JM, Mendoza-Sassi RA, Cesar JA: [Postpartum depression: prevalence and associated factors] [in Portuguese]. Cad Saude Publica 33(9):e00094016, 2017 29019521
Hellgren C, Åkerud H, Skalkidou A, et al: Low serum allopregnanolone is associated with symptoms of depression in late pregnancy. Neuropsychobiology 69(3):147–153, 2014 24776841
Hellgren C, Comasco E, Skalkidou A, et al: Allopregnanolone levels and depressive symptoms during pregnancy in relation to single nucleotide polymorphisms in the allopregnanolone synthesis pathway. Horm Behav 94:106–113, 2017 28666923
Hipwell AE, Goossens FA, Melhuish EC, et al: Severe maternal psychopathology and infant-mother attachment. Dev Psychopathol 12(2):157–175, 2000 10847622
Hiscock H, Cook F, Bayer J, et al: Preventing early infant sleep and crying problems and postnatal depression: a randomized trial. Pediatrics 133(2):e346–e354, 2014 24394682
Hoffman C, Dunn DM, Njoroge WFM: Impact of postpartum mental illness upon infant development. Curr Psychiatry Rep 19(12):100, 2017 29105008
Howren MB, Lamkin DM, Suls J: Associations of depression with C-reactive protein, IL-1, and IL-6: a meta-analysis. Psychosom Med 71(2):171–186, 2009 19188531
Hu J, Zhou B, Li Y, et al: The interaction between estradiol change and the serotonin transporter gene (5-HTTLPR) polymorphism is associated with postpartum depressive symptoms. Psychiatr Genet 29(4):97–102, 2019 31246736
Hu R, Li Y, Zhang Z, Yan W: Antenatal depressive symptoms and the risk of preeclampsia or operative deliveries: a meta-analysis. PLoS One 10(3):e0119018, 2015 25789626
Huang H, Coleman S, Bridge JA, et al: A meta-analysis of the relationship between antidepressant use in pregnancy and the risk of preterm birth and low birth weight. Gen Hosp Psychiatry 36(1):13–18, 2014 24094568

Huybrechts KF, Palmsten K, Avorn J, et al: Antidepressant use in pregnancy and the risk of cardiac defects. N Engl J Med 370(25):2397–2407, 2014a 24941178
Huybrechts KF, Sanghani RS, Avorn J, et al: Preterm birth and antidepressant medication use during pregnancy: a systematic review and meta-analysis. PLoS One 9(3):e92778, 2014b 24671232
Huybrechts KF, Bateman BT, Palmsten K, et al: Antidepressant use late in pregnancy and risk of persistent pulmonary hypertension of the newborn. JAMA 313(21):2142–2151, 2015 26034955
Hviid A, Melbye M, Pasternak B: Use of selective serotonin reuptake inhibitors during pregnancy and risk of autism. N Engl J Med 369(25):2406–2415, 2013 24350950
Iliadis SI, Comasco E, Sylvén S, et al: Prenatal and postpartum evening salivary cortisol levels in association with peripartum depressive symptoms. PLoS One 10(8):e0135471, 2015 26322643
Ivorra JL, Sanjuan J, Jover M, et al: Gene-environment interaction of child temperament. J Dev Behav Pediatr 31(7):545–554, 2010 20729761
Jarde A, Morais M, Kingston D, et al: Neonatal outcomes in women with untreated antenatal depression compared with women without depression: a systematic review and meta-analysis. JAMA Psychiatry 73(8):826–837, 2016 27276520
Jha SC, Meltzer-Brody S, Steiner RJ, et al: Antenatal depression, treatment with selective serotonin reuptake inhibitors, and neonatal brain structure: a propensity-matched cohort study. Psychiatry Res Neuroimaging 253:43–53, 2016 27254086
Jobst A, Krause D, Maiwald C, et al: Oxytocin course over pregnancy and postpartum period and the association with postpartum depressive symptoms. Arch Women Ment Health 19(4):571–579, 2016 27320943
Johansen SL, Robakis TK, Williams KE, et al: Management of perinatal depression with non-drug interventions. BMJ 364:l322, 2019 30803997
Jolley SN, Elmore S, Barnard KE, et al: Dysregulation of the hypothalamic-pituitary-adrenal axis in postpartum depression. Biol Res Nurs 8(3):210–222, 2007 17172320
Jonas W, Mileva-Seitz V, Girard AW, et al: Genetic variation in oxytocin rs2740210 and early adversity associated with postpartum depression and breastfeeding duration. Genes Brain Behav 12(7):681–694, 2013 23941164
Jordan V, Minikel M: Postpartum anxiety: more common than you think. J Fam Pract 68(3):165, 168, 170, 174, 2019 31039214
Källén B, Olausson PO: Maternal use of selective serotonin re-uptake inhibitors and persistent pulmonary hypertension of the newborn. Pharmacoepidemiol Drug Saf 17(8):801–806, 2008 18314924
Kanes S, Colquhoun H, Gunduz-Bruce H, et al: Brexanolone (SAGE-547 injection) in post-partum depression: a randomised controlled trial. Lancet 390(10093):480–489, 2017 28619476
Kang SY, Kim HB, Sunwoo S: Association between anemia and maternal depression: a systematic review and meta-analysis. J Psychiatr Res 122:88–96, 2020 31945502
Kieler H, Artama M, Engeland A, et al: Selective serotonin reuptake inhibitors during pregnancy and risk of persistent pulmonary hypertension in the newborn: population based cohort study from the five Nordic countries. BMJ 344:d8012, 2012 22240235
Kimmel M, Hess E, Roy PS, et al: Family history, not lack of medication use, is associated with the development of postpartum depression in a high-risk sample. Arch Women Ment Health 18(1):113–121, 2015 24980575
King PA: Replicability of structural models of the Edinburgh Postnatal Depression Scale (EPDS) in a community sample of postpartum African American women with low socioeconomic status. Arch Women Ment Health 15(2):77–86, 2012 22297555
Kjaersgaard MI, Parner ET, Vestergaard M, et al: Prenatal antidepressant exposure and risk of spontaneous abortion: a population-based study. PLoS One 8(8):e72095, 2013 24015208
Klein M, Schmoeger M, Kasper S, et al: Meta-analysis of the COMT Val158Met polymorphism in major depressive disorder: the role of gender. World J Biol Psychiatry 17(2):147–158, 2016 26813412
Krause D, Jobst A, Kirchberg F, et al: Prenatal immunologic predictors of postpartum depressive symptoms: a prospective study for potential diagnostic markers. Eur Arch Psychiatry Clin Neurosci 264(7):615–624, 2014 24595743

Kuijpens JL, Vader HL, Drexhage HA, et al: Thyroid peroxidase antibodies during gestation are a marker for subsequent depression postpartum. Eur J Endocrinol 145(5):579–584, 2001 11720875
Lambrinoudaki I, Rizos D, Armeni E, et al: Thyroid function and postpartum mood disturbances in Greek women. J Affect Disord 121(3):278–282, 2010 19632726
Lancaster CA, Gold KJ, Flynn HA, et al: Risk factors for depressive symptoms during pregnancy: a systematic review. Am J Obstet Gynecol 202(1):5–14, 2010 20096252
Le Strat Y, Dubertret C, Le Foll B: Prevalence and correlates of major depressive episode in pregnant and postpartum women in the United States. J Affect Disord 135(1–3):128–138, 2011 21802737
Li D, Liu L, Odouli R: Presence of depressive symptoms during early pregnancy and the risk of preterm delivery: a prospective cohort study. Hum Reprod 24(1):146–153, 2009 18948314
Li HJ, Martinez PE, Li X, et al: Transdermal estradiol for postpartum depression: results from a pilot randomized, double-blind, placebo-controlled study. Arch Women Ment Health 23(3):401–412, 2020 31372757
Liu H, Zhang Y, Gao Y, Zhang Z: Elevated levels of Hs-CRP and IL-6 after delivery are associated with depression during the 6 months post partum. Psychiatry Res 243:43–48, 2016 27359302
Loughnan SA, Joubert AE, Grierson A, et al: Internet-delivered psychological interventions for clinical anxiety and depression in perinatal women: a systematic review and meta-analysis. Arch Women Ment Health 22(6):737–750, 2019 31101993
Luca DL, Garlow N, Staatz C, et al: Society Costs of Untreated Perinatal Mood and Anxiety Disorders in the United States. Issue Brief. Princeton, NJ, Mathematica Policy Research, 2019
Lugo-Candelas C, Cha J, Hong S, et al: Associations between brain structure and connectivity in infants and exposure to selective serotonin reuptake inhibitors during pregnancy. JAMA Pediatr 172(6):525–533, 2018 29630692
Mahon PB, Payne JL, MacKinnon DF, et al: Genome-wide linkage and follow-up association study of postpartum mood symptoms. Am J Psychiatry 166(11):1229–1237, 2009 19755578
Massey SH, Schuette SA, Pournajafi-Nazarloo H, et al: Interaction of oxytocin level and past depression may predict postpartum depressive symptom severity. Arch Women Ment Health 19(5):799–808, 2016 26957508
McEvoy K, Osborne LM, Nanavati J, et al: Reproductive affective disorders: a review of the genetic evidence for premenstrual dysphoric disorder and postpartum depression. Curr Psychiatry Rep 19(12):94, 2017 29082433
McEvoy KM, Rayapati D, Washington Cole KO, et al: Poor postpartum sleep quality predicts subsequent postpartum depressive symptoms in a high-risk sample. J Clin Sleep Med 15(9):1303–1310, 2019 31538601
McLearn KT, Minkovitz CS, Strobino DM, et al: The timing of maternal depressive symptoms and mothers' parenting practices with young children: implications for pediatric practice. Pediatrics 118(1):e174–e182, 2006 16818531
Mehta D, Newport DJ, Frishman G, et al: Early predictive biomarkers for postpartum depression point to a role for estrogen receptor signaling. Psychol Med 44(11):2309–2322, 2014 24495551
Meltzer-Brody S, Kanes SJ: Allopregnanolone in postpartum depression: role in pathophysiology and treatment. Neurobiol Stress 12:100212, 2020 32435663
Meltzer-Brody S, Colquhoun H, Riesenberg R, et al: Brexanolone injection in post-partum depression: two multicentre, double-blind, randomised, placebo-controlled, phase 3 trials. Lancet 392(10152):1058–1070, 2018 30177236
Mileva-Seitz V, Steiner M, Atkinson L, et al: Interaction between oxytocin genotypes and early experience predicts quality of mothering and postpartum mood. PLoS One 8(4):e61443, 2013 23637833
Milgrom J, Gemmill AW: Screening for perinatal depression. Best Pract Res Clin Obstet Gynaecol 28(1):13–23, 2014 24095728
Milgrom J, Negri LM, Gemmill AW, et al: A randomized controlled trial of psychological interventions for postnatal depression. Br J Clin Psychol 44(Pt 4):529–542, 2005 16368032
Milgrom J, Holt CJ, Gemmill AW, et al: Treating postnatal depressive symptoms in primary care: a randomised controlled trial of GP management, with and without adjunctive counselling. BMC Psychiatry 11:95, 2011

Miller AH, Maletic V, Raison CL: Inflammation and its discontents: the role of cytokines in the pathophysiology of major depression. Biol Psychiatry 65(9):732–741, 2009 19150053

Miller MN, Miller BE: Premenstrual exacerbations of mood disorders. Psychopharmacol Bull 35(3):135–149, 2001 12397883

Monk C, Sloan RP, Myers MM, et al: Fetal heart rate reactivity differs by women's psychiatric status: an early marker for developmental risk? J Am Acad Child Adolesc Psychiatry 43(3):283–290, 2004 15076261

Moses-Kolko EL, Bogen D, Perel J, et al: Neonatal signs after late in utero exposure to serotonin reuptake inhibitors: literature review and implications for clinical applications. JAMA 293(19):2372–2383, 2005 15900008

Moses-Kolko EL, Berga SL, Kalro B, et al: Transdermal estradiol for postpartum depression: a promising treatment option. Clin Obstet Gynecol 52(3):516–529, 2009 19661765

Moulds ML, Black MJ, Newby JM, et al: Repetitive negative thinking and its role in perinatal mental health. Psychopathology 51(3):161–166, 2018 29694970

Murphy-Eberenz K, Zandi PP, March D, et al: Is perinatal depression familial? J Affect Disord 90(1):49–55, 2006 16337009

Murray L, Cooper P: Effects of postnatal depression on infant development. Arch Dis Child 77(2):99–101, 1997 9301345

Nakano Y, Oshima M, Sugiura-Ogasawara M, et al: Psychosocial predictors of successful delivery after unexplained recurrent spontaneous abortions: a cohort study. Acta Psychiatr Scand 109(6):440–446, 2004 15117289

Nassa G, Tarallo R, Ambrosino C, et al: A large set of estrogen receptor β-interacting proteins identified by tandem affinity purification in hormone-responsive human breast cancer cell nuclei. Proteomics 11(1):159–165, 2011 21182203

Nonacs R, Cohen LS: Postpartum mood disorders: diagnosis and treatment guidelines. J Clin Psychiatry 59(suppl 2):34–40, 1998 9559758

Nulman I, Rovet J, Stewart DE, et al: Neurodevelopment of children exposed in utero to antidepressant drugs. N Engl J Med 336(4):258–262, 1997 8995088

Nulman I, Rovet J, Stewart DE, et al: Child development following exposure to tricyclic antidepressants or fluoxetine throughout fetal life: a prospective, controlled study. Am J Psychiatry 159(11):1889–1895, 2002 12411224

Nulman I, Koren G, Rovet J, et al: Neurodevelopment of children following prenatal exposure to venlafaxine, selective serotonin reuptake inhibitors, or untreated maternal depression. Am J Psychiatry 169(11):1165–1174, 2012 23128923

O'Connor E, Rossom RC, Henninger M, et al: Primary care screening for and treatment of depression in pregnant and postpartum women: evidence report and systematic review for the US Preventive Services Task Force. JAMA 315(4):388–406, 2016 26813212

O'Connor TG, Caprariello P, Blackmore ER, et al: Prenatal mood disturbance predicts sleep problems in infancy and toddlerhood. Early Hum Dev 83(7):451–458, 2007 17008033

O'Donnell KJ, Glover V, Jenkins J, et al: Prenatal maternal mood is associated with altered diurnal cortisol in adolescence. Psychoneuroendocrinology 38(9):1630–1638, 2013 23433748

O'Hara MW, McCabe JE: Postpartum depression: current status and future directions. Annu Rev Clin Psychol 9:379–407, 2013 23394227

O'Hara MW, Stuart S, Gorman LL, et al: Efficacy of interpersonal psychotherapy for postpartum depression. Arch Gen Psychiatry 57(11):1039–1045, 2000 11074869

Oberlander TF, Misri S, Fitzgerald CE, et al: Pharmacologic factors associated with transient neonatal symptoms following prenatal psychotropic medication exposure. J Clin Psychiatry 65(2):230–237, 2004 15003078

Oberlander TF, Weinberg J, Papsdorf M, et al: Prenatal exposure to maternal depression, neonatal methylation of human glucocorticoid receptor gene (NR3C1) and infant cortisol stress responses. Epigenetics 3(2):97–106, 2008 18536531

Ogbo FA, Eastwood J, Hendry A, et al: Determinants of antenatal depression and postnatal depression in Australia. BMC Psychiatry 18(1):49, 2018 29463221

Okun ML, Luther J, Prather AA, et al: Changes in sleep quality, but not hormones predict time to postpartum depression recurrence. J Affect Disord 130(3):378–384, 2011 20708275

Orr ST, Blazer DG, James SA, Reiter JP: Depressive symptoms and indicators of maternal health status during pregnancy. J Womens Health (Larchmt) 16(4):535–542, 2007 17521257
Osborne LM, Monk C: Perinatal depression: the fourth inflammatory morbidity of pregnancy? Theory and literature review. Psychoneuroendocrinology 38(10):1929–1952, 2013 23608136
Osborne L, Clive M, Kimmel M, et al: Replication of epigenetic postpartum depression biomarkers and variation with hormone levels. Neuropsychopharmacology 41(6):1648–1658, 2016 26503311
Osborne LM, Gispen F, Sanyal A, et al: Lower allopregnanolone during pregnancy predicts postpartum depression: an exploratory study. Psychoneuroendocrinology 79:116–121, 2017 28278440
Osborne LM, Yenokyan G, Fei K, et al: Innate immune activation and depressive and anxious symptoms across the peripartum: an exploratory study. Psychoneuroendocrinology 99:80–86, 2019 30195110
Osborne LM, Gilden J, Kamperman AM, et al: T-cell defects and postpartum depression. Brain Behav Immun 87:397–403, 2020 31926288
Osborne S, Biaggi A, Chua TE, et al: Antenatal depression programs cortisol stress reactivity in offspring through increased maternal inflammation and cortisol in pregnancy: The Psychiatry Research and Motherhood—Depression (PRAM-D) Study. Psychoneuroendocrinology 98:211–221, 2018 30033161
Özcan NK, Boyacioglu NE, Dinç H: Postpartum depression prevalence and risk factors in Turkey: a systematic review and meta-analysis. Arch Psychiatr Nurs 31(4):420–428, 2017 28693880
Pao C, Guintivano J, Santos H, et al: Postpartum depression and social support in a racially and ethnically diverse population of women. Arch Women Ment Health 22(1):105–114, 2019 29968129
Patton GC, Hibbert ME, Carlin J, et al: Menarche and the onset of depression and anxiety in Victoria, Australia. J Epidemiol Community Health 50(6):661–666, 1996 9039386
Paulson JF, Bazemore SD, Goodman JH, et al: The course and interrelationship of maternal and paternal perinatal depression. Arch Women Ment Health 19(4):655–663, 2016 26790687
Pawluski JL, Brain UM, Underhill CM, et al: Prenatal SSRI exposure alters neonatal corticosteroid binding globulin, infant cortisol levels, and emerging HPA function. Psychoneuroendocrinology 37(7):1019–1028, 2012 22177580
Payne JL: Psychopharmacology in pregnancy and breastfeeding. Med Clin North Am 103(4):629–650, 2019 31078197
Payne JL, Maguire J: Pathophysiological mechanisms implicated in postpartum depression. Front Neuroendocrinol 52:165–180, 2019 30552910
Payne JL, MacKinnon DF, Mondimore FM, et al: Familial aggregation of postpartum mood symptoms in bipolar disorder pedigrees. Bipolar Disord 10(1):38–44, 2008 18199240
Payne JL, Palmer JT, Joffe H: A reproductive subtype of depression: conceptualizing models and moving toward etiology. Harv Rev Psychiatry 17(2):72–86, 2009 19373617
Pearlstein T: Perinatal depression: treatment options and dilemmas. J Psychiatry Neurosci 33(4):302–318, 2008 18592032
Perry H, Khalil A, Thilaganathan B: Preeclampsia and the cardiovascular system: an update. Trends Cardiovasc Med 28(8):505–513, 2018 29884568
Phillips J, Sharpe L, Nemeth D: Maternal psychopathology and outcomes of a residential mother-infant intervention for unsettled infant behaviour. Aust N Z J Psychiatry 44(3):280–289, 2010 20180728
Pinheiro RT, Coelho FM, Silva RA, et al: Association of a serotonin transporter gene polymorphism (5-HTTLPR) and stressful life events with postpartum depressive symptoms: a population-based study. J Psychosom Obstet Gynaecol 34(1):29–33, 2013 23394411
Pinsonneault JK, Sullivan D, Sadee W, et al: Association study of the estrogen receptor gene ESR1 with postpartum depression—a pilot study. Arch Women Ment Health 16(6):499–509, 2013 23917948
Putnam KT, Wilcox M, Robertson-Blackmore E, et al: Clinical phenotypes of perinatal depression and time of symptom onset: analysis of data from an international consortium. Lancet Psychiatry 4(6):477–485, 2017 28476427

Rai D, Lee BK, Dalman C, et al: Parental depression, maternal antidepressant use during pregnancy, and risk of autism spectrum disorders: population based case-control study. BMJ 346:f2059, 2013 23604083

Raison CL, Rutherford RE, Woolwine BJ, et al: A randomized controlled trial of the tumor necrosis factor antagonist infliximab for treatment-resistant depression: the role of baseline inflammatory biomarkers. JAMA Psychiatry 70(1):31–41, 2013 22945416

Reza N, Deligiannidis KM, Eustis EH, Battle CL: Complementary health practices for treating perinatal depression. Obstet Gynecol Clin North Am 45(3):441–454, 2018 30092920

Robertson E, Grace S, Wallington T, et al: Antenatal risk factors for postpartum depression: a synthesis of recent literature. Gen Hosp Psychiatry 26(4):289–295, 2004 15234824

Robertson-Blackmore E, Putnam FW, Rubinow DR, et al: Antecedent trauma exposure and risk of depression in the perinatal period. J Clin Psychiatry 74(10):e942–e948, 2013 24229763

Ross LE, Grigoriadis S, Mamisashvili L, et al: Selected pregnancy and delivery outcomes after exposure to antidepressant medication: a systematic review and meta-analysis. JAMA Psychiatry 70(4):436–443, 2013 23446732

Rotem-Kohavi N, Williams LJ, Muller AM, et al: Hub distribution of the brain functional networks of newborns prenatally exposed to maternal depression and SSRI antidepressants. Depress Anxiety 36(8):753–765, 2019 31066992

Saigal S, Doyle LW: An overview of mortality and sequelae of preterm birth from infancy to adulthood. Lancet 371(9608):261–269, 2008 18207020

Salisbury AL, O'Grady KE, Battle CL, et al: The roles of maternal depression, serotonin reuptake inhibitor treatment, and concomitant benzodiazepine use on infant neurobehavioral functioning over the first postnatal month. Am J Psychiatry 173(2):147–157, 2016 26514656

Santone G, Ricchi G, Rocchetti D, et al: Is the exposure to antidepressant drugs in early pregnancy a risk factor for spontaneous abortion? A review of available evidences. Epidemiol Psichiatr Soc 18(3):240–247, 2009 20034202

Schaefer A, Brown J, Watson CG, et al: Comparison of the validities of the Beck, Zung, and MMPI Depression Scales. J Consult Clin Psychol 53(3):415–418, 1985 4008725

Scheyer K, Urizar GG Jr: Altered stress patterns and increased risk for postpartum depression among low-income pregnant women. Arch Women Ment Health 19(2):317–328, 2016 26275372

Sharma V, Baczynski C: Is bipolar post-partum depression overlooked? Lancet Psychiatry 6(11):891–892, 2019 31631869

Sharma V, Al-Farayedhi M, Doobay M, et al: Should all women with postpartum depression be screened for bipolar disorder? Med Hypotheses 118:26–28, 2018 30037609

Shen Y, Varma DS, Zheng Y, et al: Age at menarche and depression: results from the NHANES 2005–2016. PeerJ 7:e7150, 2019 31223544

Shorey S, Chee CYI, Ng ED, et al: Prevalence and incidence of postpartum depression among healthy mothers: a systematic review and meta-analysis. J Psychiatr Res 104:235–248, 2018 30114665

Silver M, Moore CM, Villamarin V, et al: White matter integrity in medication-free women with peripartum depression: a tract-based spatial statistics study. Neuropsychopharmacology 43(7):1573–1580, 2018 29453442

Simpson W, Steiner M, Coote M, et al: Relationship between inflammatory biomarkers and depressive symptoms during late pregnancy and the early postpartum period: a longitudinal study. Br J Psychiatry 38(3):190–196, 2016 27579595

Skrundz M, Bolten M, Nast I, et al: Plasma oxytocin concentration during pregnancy is associated with development of postpartum depression. Neuropsychopharmacology 36(9):1886–1893, 2011 21562482

Smart J, Hiscock H: Early infant crying and sleeping problems: a pilot study of impact on parental well-being and parent-endorsed strategies for management. J Paediatr Child Health 43(4):284–290, 2007 17444831

Smith-Nielsen J, Tharner A, Krogh MT, et al: Effects of maternal postpartum depression in a well-resourced sample: early concurrent and long-term effects on infant cognitive, language, and motor development. Scand J Psychol 57(6):571–583, 2016 27611177

Sockol LE, Epperson CN, Barber JP: A meta-analysis of treatments for perinatal depression. Clin Psychol Rev 31(5):839–849, 2011 21545782
Sørensen MJ, Grønborg TK, Christensen J, et al: Antidepressant exposure in pregnancy and risk of autism spectrum disorders. Clin Epidemiol 5:449–459, 2013 24255601
Stuart S, Koleva H: Psychological treatments for perinatal depression. Best Pract Res Clin Obstet Gynaecol 28(1):61–70, 2014 24269903
Stuart-Parrigon K, Stuart S: Perinatal depression: an update and overview. Curr Psychiatry Rep 16(9):468, 2014 25034859
Studd J: Hormone therapy for reproductive depression in women. Post Reprod Health 20(4):132–137, 2014 25398672
Swanson LM, Flynn H, Adams-Mundy JD, et al: An open pilot of cognitive-behavioral therapy for insomnia in women with postpartum depression. Behav Sleep Med 11(4):297–307, 2013 23216373
Szpunar MJ, Parry BL: A systematic review of cortisol, thyroid-stimulating hormone, and prolactin in peripartum women with major depression. Arch Women Ment Health 21(2):149–161, 2018 29022126
Talge NM, Neal C, Glover V: Antenatal maternal stress and long-term effects on child neurodevelopment: how and why? J Child Psychol Psychiatry 48(3–4):245–261, 2007 17355398
Tomfohr-Madsen LM, Clayborne ZM, Rouleau CR, et al: Sleeping for two: an open-pilot study of cognitive behavioral therapy for insomnia in pregnancy. Behav Sleep Med 15(5):377–393, 2017 27124405
Torres A, Gelabert E, Roca A, et al: Course of a major postpartum depressive episode: a prospective 2 years naturalistic follow-up study. J Affect Disord 245:965–970, 2019 30699882
Treloar SA, Martin NG, Bucholz KK, et al: Genetic influences on post-natal depressive symptoms: findings from an Australian twin sample. Psychol Med 29(3):645–654, 1999 10405086
Umesawa M, Kobashi G: Epidemiology of hypertensive disorders in pregnancy: prevalence, risk factors, predictors and prognosis. Hypertens Res 40(3):213–220, 2017 27682655
Upadhyay RP, Chowdhury R, Aslyeh Salehi, et al: Postpartum depression in India: a systematic review and meta-analysis. Bull World Health Organ 95(10):706–717C, 2017 29147043
Velasquez JC, Zhao Q, Chan Y, et al: In utero exposure to citalopram mitigates maternal stress effects on fetal brain development. ACS Chem Neurosci 10(7):3307–3317, 2019 31184110
Vesga-López O, Blanco C, Keyes K, et al: Psychiatric disorders in pregnant and postpartum women in the United States. Arch Gen Psychiatry 65(7):805–815, 2008 18606953
Vliegen N, Casalin S, Luyten P: The course of postpartum depression: a review of longitudinal studies. Harv Rev Psychiatry 22(1):1–22, 2014 24394219
Walsh K, McCormack CA, Webster R, et al: Maternal prenatal stress phenotypes associate with fetal neurodevelopment and birth outcomes. Proc Natl Acad Sci USA 116(48):23996–24005, 2019 31611411
Wang S, Yang L, Wang L, et al: Selective serotonin reuptake inhibitors (SSRIs) and the risk of congenital heart defects: a meta-analysis of prospective cohort studies. J Am Heart Assoc 4(5):e001681, 2015 25991012
Wang YP, Gorenstein C: Psychometric properties of the Beck Depression Inventory–II: a comprehensive review. Br J Psychiatry 35(4):416–431, 2013 24402217
Ward HB, Fromson JA, Cooper JJ, et al: Recommendations for the use of ECT in pregnancy: literature review and proposed clinical protocol. Arch Women Ment Health 21(6):715–722, 2018 29796968
Webster PA: Withdrawal symptoms in neonates associated with maternal antidepressant therapy. Lancet 2(7824):318–319, 1973 4124794
Wemakor A, Casson K, Garne E, et al: Selective serotonin reuptake inhibitor antidepressant use in first trimester pregnancy and risk of specific congenital anomalies: a European register-based study. Eur J Epidemiol 30(11):1187–1198, 2015 26148560
Werner E, Miller M, Osborne LM, et al: Preventing postpartum depression: review and recommendations. Arch Women Ment Health 18(1):41–60, 2015 25422150

Wesseloo R, Kamperman AM, Bergink V, et al: Thyroid peroxidase antibodies during early gestation and the subsequent risk of first-onset postpartum depression: a prospective cohort study. J Affect Disord 225:399–403, 2018 28850854

Whitton A, Warner R, Appleby L: The pathway to care in post-natal depression: women's attitudes to post-natal depression and its treatment. Br J Gen Pract 46(408):427–428, 1996 8776916

Wichman CL, Moore KM, Lang TR, et al: Congenital heart disease associated with selective serotonin reuptake inhibitor use during pregnancy. Mayo Clin Proc 84(1):23–27, 2009 19121250

Wilson KL, Zelig CM, Harvey JP, et al: Persistent pulmonary hypertension of the newborn is associated with mode of delivery and not with maternal use of selective serotonin reuptake inhibitors. Am J Perinatol 28(1):19–24, 2011 20607643

Wilson N, Lee JJ, Bei B: Postpartum fatigue and depression: a systematic review and meta-analysis. J Affect Disord 246:224–233, 2019 30584956

Wisner KL, Parry BL, Piontek CM: Clinical practice. Postpartum depression. N Engl J Med 347(3):194–199, 2002 12124409

Wisner KL, Sit DK, Hanusa BH, et al: Major depression and antidepressant treatment: impact on pregnancy and neonatal outcomes. Am J Psychiatry 166(5):557–566, 2009 19289451

Wisner KL, Sit DK, McShea MC, et al: Onset timing, thoughts of self-harm, and diagnoses in postpartum women with screen-positive depression findings. JAMA Psychiatry 70(5):490–498, 2013 23487258

Wisner KL, Sit DK, Moses-Kolko EL, et al: Transdermal estradiol treatment for postpartum depression: a pilot, randomized trial. J Clin Psychopharmacol 35(4):389–395, 2015 26061609

Woody CA, Ferrari AJ, Siskind DJ, et al: A systematic review and meta-regression of the prevalence and incidence of perinatal depression. J Affect Disord 219:86–92, 2017 28531848

Woolhouse H, Gartland D, Hegarty K, et al: Depressive symptoms and intimate partner violence in the 12 months after childbirth: a prospective pregnancy cohort study. BJOG 119(3):315–323, 2012 22145631

Xu Y, Sari Y, Zhou FC: Selective serotonin reuptake inhibitor disrupts organization of thalamocortical somatosensory barrels during development. Brain Res Dev Brain Res 150(2):151–161, 2004 15158078

Yim IS, Glynn LM, Dunkel-Schetter C, et al: Risk of postpartum depressive symptoms with elevated corticotropin-releasing hormone in human pregnancy. Arch Gen Psychiatry 66(2):162–169, 2009 19188538

Yonkers KA, Norwitz ER, Smith MV, et al: Depression and serotonin reuptake inhibitor treatment as risk factors for preterm birth. Epidemiology 23(5):677–685, 2012 22627901

Zhang X, Wang L, Huang F, et al: Evaluation of the promoter region polymorphism (5-HTTLPR) in the serotonin transporter gene in females with postpartum depression. Exp Ther Med 9(1):245–249, 2015 25452810

Zhu P, Sun MS, Hao JH, et al: Does prenatal maternal stress impair cognitive development and alter temperament characteristics in toddlers with healthy birth outcomes? Dev Med Child Neurol 56(3):283–289, 2014 24512346

Zuckerman B, Amaro H, Bauchner H, et al: Depressive symptoms during pregnancy: relationship to poor health behaviors. Am J Obstet Gynecol 160(5 pt 1):1107–1111, 1989 2729387

# CHAPTER 14

# Integrative Approaches to Perinatal Depression

Madeleine A. Becker, M.D., M.A.
M. Camille Hoffman, M.D., M.Sc.
Nina T. Ballone, M.D.
Ripal Shah, M.D., M.P.H.

Integrative medicine is a medical subspecialty recognized by the American Board of Physician Subspecialties. It combines conventional medicine with evidence-based complementary medicine, which includes but is not limited to lifestyle approaches, nutrition, supplements, and mind-body approaches. This subspecialty recognizes the integration between ancient and conventional medicine in the approach to the treatment of disease. Additionally, integrative medicine has a holistic health approach and emphasizes wellness and prevention of illness. Many integrative medicine interventions have been studied for the treatment of women and are often used along with conventional treatments (Clarke et al. 2015).

Approximately one-third of American adults reported using at least one integrative health approach in the past year (Clarke et al. 2015). Data show that women use integrative treatments more often than men, and use is common throughout the reproductive years (Adams et al. 2009; Steel et al. 2020). Although data exist on integrative treatments for depression in pregnancy, they are less robust than the literature on psychopharmacology and psychotherapy for the treatment and prevention of perinatal depression. Nonetheless, women are highly likely to use integrative strategies, and 37% of pregnant women and 28% of postpartum women report use in the past 12 months, compared with 40% of nonpregnant/nonpostpartum women. Mind-body practices were the most common modality reported (25% of pregnant women). Diets and dietary supplements (excluding vitamins and minerals) were used during the postpartum period by 8% of women (Birdee et al. 2014).

This chapter focuses on widely used supplements that include botanicals (herbs), vitamins, and minerals; mind-body therapies including yoga and meditation; and other treatments such as bright light therapy and their evidence and effects on perinatal depression. Except where indicated, we focus on those interventions that have robust data to support their use. This chapter is designed to augment Chapter 13, "Depressive Disorders"; please consult that chapter for a thorough description of perinatal depression and a discussion of its pathophysiology.

# Nutrition

The foods that we eat—and the nutrients that are derived from them—play a critical role in both our survival and our overall state of health, wellness, and disease. Pregnant and lactating women have elevated nutrient needs, and these needs may be difficult to meet through normal diet or maternal stores (Bodnar and Wisner 2005). Because pregnancy and lactation are major nutritional stressors, childbearing-age women may be particularly vulnerable to the impact of nutritional deficiencies on mood, specifically depression (Bodnar and Wisner 2005). This section addresses dietary patterns, nutrients, and specific foods that are thought to play important roles in healthy pregnancy outcomes and also have an impact on perinatal mood.

## Diet

Evidence consistently suggests that certain overall dietary patterns during pregnancy may be protective for healthy outcomes. Specifically, diets that are higher in vegetables, fruits, fiber, nuts and seeds, legumes, and seafood—and lower in processed meats and fried foods—appear to be the most protective (Raghavan et al. 2019) and may reduce the risk of preterm birth (Chia et al. 2019). A systematic review of dietary patterns in association with perinatal depression and anxiety found an inverse relationship between diets consisting of whole foods, fruits, vegetables, fish, and seafood and perinatal depression and anxiety (Silva et al. 2019; Sparling et al. 2017). Conversely, poor dietary quality is being studied as a modifiable risk factor in depression (Bodnar and Wisner 2005).

## Nutrients and Dietary Supplements

In addition to a generally healthy diet, specific nutrients are recommended for healthy pregnancy outcomes, and some of them may have an impact on perinatal mood. Table 14–1 summarizes the current recommendations by the American College of Obstetricians and Gynecologists (ACOG) for daily nutrient intake during pregnancy.

### Folic Acid

Folate, also known as vitamin $B_9$, is a micronutrient found in foods such as green leafy vegetables. Its name is derived from the Latin word for leaf (*folium*). Folate is an essential micronutrient—that is, humans and most other mammals cannot synthesize it *de novo* and instead must obtain it from their diet (Naninck et al. 2019). Folate is a cofactor and regulatory molecule in many crucial biological processes, such as the synthesis and metabolism of neurotransmitters and the regulation of homocysteine levels in the vasculature (Bottiglieri 1996). It is also crucial in supporting healthy fetal growth and development in pregnancy (Bottiglieri 1996). An adequate maternal folate supply is

**TABLE 14–1. Recommendations for nutrient intake in pregnancy**

| Nutrient (daily amount) | Role in fetal development | Example sources |
|---|---|---|
| Calcium (1,000 mg) | Bones, teeth | Milk, yogurt, dark leafy greens |
| Iron (27 mg) | Oxygen delivery | Lean red meat, poultry, beans/peas |
| Iodine (220 μg) | Brain, thyroid | Iodized table salt, meat, eggs |
| Choline (450 mg) | Brain, spinal cord | Meat, beef liver, eggs |
| Vitamin A (770 μg) | Skin, eyesight, bones | Carrots, leafy greens, sweet potatoes |
| Vitamin C (85 mg) | Teeth, gums, bones | Citrus, broccoli, strawberries |
| Vitamin D (600 IU) | Bones, teeth, eyesight, skin | Sunlight, fatty fish (e.g., salmon) |
| Vitamin $B_6$ (1.9 mg) | Red blood cells, nutrition | Beef, whole-grain cereals, bananas |
| Vitamin $B_{12}$ (2.6 μg) | CNS, red blood cells | Beef, milk, poultry, fish |
| Folic acid (600 μg) | CNS, overall development | Dark leafy greens, citrus, beans |

*Source.* Adapted from American College of Obstetricians and Gynecologists 2020.

important because the developing fetus receives folate through the placenta through polarized folate transporters (Naninck et al. 2019).

The U.S. Preventive Services Task Force recommends that all women who are either planning or capable of pregnancy take a daily supplement containing 400–800 μg of folic acid daily. This dose of daily folate—started prior to conception and continued throughout pregnancy—has been associated with decreased risk of neural tube defects (Freedman et al. 2018). It is difficult to obtain the recommended amount of folate consistently by diet, and in 1998, the FDA mandated fortification of foods. Since then, prevalence rates of infants born with neural tube defects have decreased significantly (Bibbins-Domingo et al. 2017). Maternal folate status also has other important effects on the fetus. A study found that low folate levels in early pregnancy may affect later cognitive functioning in children, even in the absence of neural tube defects. Low maternal folate levels have been associated with a smaller total brain volume and predicted poorer performance on language and visuospatial assessments in the children. Thus, folate insufficiency in early pregnancy may have long-lasting effects on fetal brain development (Ars et al. 2019).

In terms of perinatal depression, folate deficiency has been associated with increased antenatal depression scores, and prolonged folate supplementation (>6 months) during pregnancy has been associated with a decreased risk of postpartum depression (PPD) in Chinese women (Chong et al. 2014; Yan et al. 2017). A small, open-label trial of a prenatal supplement in depressed versus healthy women with a history of depression found that folate supplementation may have some efficacy in both prevention and treatment of perinatal depression (Freedman et al. 2018). In addition, evidence supports the use of folate as an antidepressant augmentation strategy for depression during pregnancy (Deligiannidis and Freeman 2010).

Of note, folate is typically ingested in its natural form (dihydrofolate) in foods or in its synthetic form in vitamin supplements, which is then converted to the active form (L-methylfolate) by the enzyme methylene tetrahydrofolate reductase (*MTHFR*). The *MTHFR* gene has polymorphisms (seen in up to 50% of individuals in the United States) that affect the conversion of ingested folate (Naninck et al. 2019). Individuals with these polymorphisms may be more prone to folate deficiency; thus, it has been hypothesized that carriers of these polymorphisms in genes might benefit from methylated folate supplementation instead of folate. Methylated folate and folic acid have comparable physiological activity, bioavailability, and absorption at equimolar doses; because methylated folate does not need to be converted to its active form, it may offer some advantages, but little is known about its efficacy (Obeid et al. 2013; Pietrzik et al. 2010). High-dose folate supplementation (4–5 g) is recommended when antiepileptic medications are used in pregnancy due to the higher rates of neural tube defects with these medications (Wilson et al. 2007).

## Vitamin D

Vitamin D receptors are widespread throughout the human body, and it has many functions beyond its role in calcium homeostasis (Agarwal et al. 2018). Low vitamin D intake, or low 25(OH)D-levels, have been associated with preeclampsia, gestational diabetes, bacterial vaginosis, shorter length of gestation, and PPD (Christesen et al. 2012). Conversely, vitamin D supplementation during pregnancy may be associated with reduced risk of preeclampsia and gestational diabetes. It also may reduce the risks of low birth weight and postpartum hemorrhage (Palacios et al. 2019). Vitamin D supplementation has also been associated with positive fetal/infant outcomes, such as decreased risk of infant wheezing and of schizophrenia (Freedman et al. 2018).

Low vitamin D levels have also been associated with both antenatal and postnatal depression and depressive symptoms (Aghajafari et al. 2018; Wang et al. 2018; Williams et al. 2016). There appears to be an inverse relationship between low serum vitamin D levels and both pre- and postnatal depression (Trujillo et al. 2018). In one of the most robust meta-analyses (in nonpregnant women), an improvement was seen in depression with supplementation of vitamin D ≥800 IU/day (and concomitant change in serum vitamin D levels) compared with antidepressant medication (Spedding 2014). Vitamin D supplementation during pregnancy is low risk (at recommended doses, typically around 800–1000 IU daily), has benefits for general health, and may serve an adjunctive role in treatment of perinatal depression.

## *S*-Adenosyl Methionine

*S*-adenosyl methionine (SAM-e) is a methyl donor in the brain. It is involved in the synthesis of hormones, neurotransmitters, nucleic acids, proteins, and phospholipids, and it acts as an intermediate in the synthesis of norepinephrine, dopamine, and serotonin (Mischoulon 2009). SAM-e has been found to be efficacious in the treatment of major depressive disorder and superior to placebo and equivalent to tricyclic antidepressants, with fewer side effects (Deligiannidis and Freeman 2010; Sarris et al. 2016). To our knowledge, no studies have examined the efficacy or safety of SAM-e for depression specifically during pregnancy. One placebo-controlled study of SAM-e for postnatal depressive symptoms found a significant decrease in depressive symptoms with SAM-e compared with placebo (Cerutti et al. 1993; Deligiannidis and Freeman 2014). Supplementation with SAM-e has been used to treat intrahepatic cholestasis during pregnancy, and it has generally been well tolerated with no adverse effects noted when used for this purpose. When used for depression in nonpregnant patients, side effects may include increased anxiety, mania, or hypomania in patients with bipolar depression. Therefore, care must be taken with patients who have a history of bipolar disorder (Mischoulon 2009). We do not recommend SAM-e as an antidepressant during pregnancy because more data are needed to determine efficacy, dosing, and safety in this population.

## Omega-3 Fatty Acids

Omega-3 fatty acids (n-3s) are found primarily in oily, cold-water fish and certain nuts and seeds. The three main forms of n-3s are docosahexaenoic acid (DHA), eicosapentaenoic acid (EPA), and alpha linolenic acid (ALA). Both DHA and EPA are biologically active n-3 fatty acids and are critical to fetal growth and development. They are also important in visual and cognitive function in newborns, children, and adults. ALA can be obtained from plant sources such as flax seeds, walnuts, kale, and spinach. However, because only ~10% of ALA is converted to DHA, those who consume only these plant sources of n-3s (ALA) need to eat significantly larger quantities to obtain adequate daily amounts.

Evidence of the effect of n-3s and their benefits in pregnancy are mixed. A Cochrane review of studies found a modest reduction in preterm birth (<37 weeks), early preterm birth (<34 weeks), and low birth weight babies in women consuming n-3s and a small increase in birth weight and length of gestation (Middleton et al. 2018; Newberry et al. 2016). On the other hand, in a meta-analysis assessing the association of n-3s with multiple perinatal factors, supplementation was not associated with prevention of preterm birth, preeclampsia risk reduction, decreased fetal growth restriction/small for gestational age infants, decreased rates of PPD, or improved child neurodevelopment (Saccone et al. 2016). In terms of fetal development, n-3s have been correlated with benefits, such as enhanced neonatal visual development, improved CNS functioning, and improved childhood intelligence scores. DHA and EPA also appear to reduce the risk of childhood allergic diseases, such as asthma, autoimmune diseases, atopic dermatitis, and allergic rhinitis (Freedman et al. 2018).

A review of n-3 supplementation and its effects on depression in nonpregnant populations found that n-3s have been associated with a reduction in depressive symptoms (Qureshi and Al-Bedah 2013). In a review that examined studies looking at timing of intervention, type and dose of n-3 used, and existing maternal depressive symptoms, EPA supplementation was associated with reduced depressive symptoms both during pregnancy and postpartum (Hsu et al. 2018). A randomized trial of higher-dose n-3 supplementation in overweight and obese pregnant women using a combined dose of 2 g/day of DHA+EPA found that the subjects had comparatively lower C-reactive protein levels (CRP) and decreased adipose and placental proinflammatory cytokines than control subjects (Haghiac et al. 2015). Maternal inflammation in the form of elevated CRP and proinflammatory cytokines has been associated with both depressive symptoms and adverse fetal/infant brain development (Hunter et al. 2019).

In summary, n-3s may improve obstetrical outcomes and perinatal depressive symptoms and may reduce inflammatory cytokines. Variations in dose and methods across studies have made interpretation of the data complicated. However, based on tolerability and possible benefits during pregnancy, low risk of use, and benefits for general health, n-3s may serve an adjunctive role for supplementation during pregnancy (Deligiannidis and Freeman 2010). Most experts in perinatal mental health recommend that perinatal women with depression consume 1 g/day of EPA+DHA in addition to receiving psychotherapy or pharmacotherapy (Reza et al. 2018).

## Probiotics

Probiotics are living microorganisms that may play a beneficial role in health, and the use of probiotics during pregnancy to reduce rates of multiple adverse pregnancy outcomes has become a common study interest. The proposed mechanisms of action of probiotics in the mental health literature focus on a bidirectional relationship between the brain and gastrointestinal tract (i.e., the "gut-brain axis"). Clear mechanisms of action, however, remain the topic of research and are primarily theoretical at this time (Noonan et al. 2020). Probiotics are theorized to affect the genitourinary-gastrointestinal tract relationship and to interfere with pathogens and inflammatory cytokines associated with preterm labor (Reid and Bocking 2003).

Unfortunately, recent studies have been lackluster regarding probiotics and reduced risks of preterm birth, gestational diabetes, small or large for gestational age infants, or premature rupture of membranes. Study variables are considerably heterogeneous, including timing of intervention, type of probiotic supplemented, stated versus actual content of probiotic, and duration of the intervention, which makes it difficult to interpret the evidence (Jarde et al. 2018). The Probiotics in Pregnancy study sought to evaluate the impact of the probiotic *Lactobacillus rhamnosus* HN001 on pregnancy and postpartum outcomes through a large randomized controlled trial. Women who received the probiotic had significantly lower Edinburgh Postnatal Depression Scale scores and lower rates of anxiety screening scores than those who received placebo (Slykerman et al. 2017). Although effects were modest, *L. rhamnosus* may be a reasonable recommendation as an adjunct for mild depression and anxiety, along with standard-of-care screening and treatment recommendations during pregnancy.

## Melatonin

Melatonin is a hormone secreted by the pineal gland (and the placenta during pregnancy) and is involved in regulating normal sleep-wake cycles by influencing circadian rhythm timing. It has also been shown to have antioxidant, anti-inflammatory, and antiapoptotic effects (Yang et al. 2018). Melatonin supplements are typically created synthetically (although they can be derived from animals or microorganisms) and are sold over the counter as a supplement for insomnia and circadian rhythm problems, such as jet lag.

From existing human and animal data, we understand that the interaction between normal circadian rhythms and melatonin production is important across human reproduction. During human pregnancies, melatonin serum concentrations increase markedly, and this is thought to stimulate luteal progesterone production and to decrease prostaglandin production (Brzezinski et al. 1992). Melatonin both crosses the placenta and is produced by the placenta in normal pregnancies (Reiter et al. 2014). Melatonin also plays several roles in normal pregnancy, including fetal maturation and the onset of labor, in association with oxytocin. Researchers are currently examining the use of exogenous melatonin in reducing adverse neurodevelopmental outcomes in "at-risk" fetuses due to either growth restriction or the risk of prematurity (Palmer et al. 2019; Wilkinson et al. 2016). In addition, there is currently research on melatonin's capacity to mitigate placental oxidative stress during pregnancy; placental oxidative stress has been associated with recurrent miscarriages, preeclampsia, intrauterine growth restriction, and stillbirth (Rodrigues Helmo et al. 2018).

However, despite widespread use of melatonin during pregnancy, there remains a dearth of literature on its safety and effectiveness. For example, there is scarce understanding of what constitutes adequate dosing in pregnancy, as well as theoretical concerns regarding how exogenous prenatal melatonin exposure might interfere with circadian rhythms during prenatal-to-postnatal development (Davis 1997).

### Tryptophan

L-Tryptophan, an essential amino acid, serves as a precursor to the monoamine neurotransmitter serotonin and the hormone melatonin. During the perinatal period, levels of total tryptophan are lower starting in the second trimester until delivery (van Lee et al. 2018). This decreased level of tryptophan may result in a decreased serotonin level producing symptoms of depression or anxiety, as well as a decreased melatonin level that may disrupt the sleep-wake cycle (Bell et al. 2001). Limited trials have suggested that in healthy, nonpregnant adults, supplementation of L-tryptophan and 5-hydroxytryptophan (5-HTP, a metabolite of L-tryptophan) may improve symptoms of depression and anxiety (Birdsall 1998; Kikuchi et al. 2021). However, due to limited data evaluating efficacy and safety and to concerns about contamination, the routine use of L-tryptophan or 5-HTP supplements as antidepressants is not recommended during pregnancy (Shaw et al. 2002).

## Specific Foods

Delineating which parts of the diet are the most beneficial—the individual foods, the nutrients contained in them, or perhaps the entire diet itself—is complex. However, certain foods as described here may be particularly beneficial to perinatal outcomes, particularly in regard to perinatal depression and anxiety.

### Fish and Seafood

A cohort study was conducted in 1966 in Finland based on the finding that n-3s—found in smaller cold-water fish—were related to mood. In this study, higher frequency of fish consumption was associated with a lower risk of depression, and lower frequency of fish consumption was associated with increased risk of depression in women but not in men (Timonen et al. 2004). Although these data do not appear to translate directly to pregnant women in many studies, the Pregnancy Diet and Associated Outcomes in the Avon Longitudinal Study of Parents and Children study data suggest that consumption of fish and shellfish high in n-3s and iodine was independently associated with lower frequency of maternal depressive and anxiety symptoms. Furthermore, there was a lower frequency of fetal growth restriction and improved measures of neurocognitive development in the children of these women. These findings support the recommendation by multiple organizations that pregnant women eat at least two servings of low/no-mercury fish or shellfish weekly as part of a healthy pregnancy diet (Emmett et al. 2015). See the previous section, "Omega-3 Fatty Acids," for detailed information on these nutrients as they relate to fish and seafood intake.

### Dark Chocolate

Cocoa and chocolate products are rich in flavonoids, a group of polyphenols that are potent antioxidants and have anti-inflammatory effects. A recent large cross-sectional survey in nonpregnant subjects found that dark chocolate was associated with significantly lower odds of depressive symptoms (Deligiannidis and Freeman 2010; Jackson et al. 2019). In a systematic review of the effects of chocolate consumption in pregnancy, chocolate intake was found to be beneficial, with both acute stimulatory effects on fetal reactivity and antihypertensive effects in mothers (Latif 2019). Other recent studies found that chocolate consumption of 30 g (~1 oz) of 70% cocoa daily reduced blood pressure without increasing weight gain or total cholesterol level in pregnant women (Di Renzo et al. 2012). Among pregnant Japanese women, those with the highest chocolate consumption (87.5 g/week) had a significantly lower risk of developing gestational diabetes than those with the lowest consumption (Dong et al. 2019). Dark chocolate consumption in pregnancy seems to reduce the negative effects of prenatal maternal stress on infant temperament and may be associated with a greater positive reactivity and activity in infants at 6 months (Brillo and Di Renzo 2015). Dark chocolate should be consumed in moderation, especially during pregnancy, due to both the caffeine content (which should be limited during pregnancy) and the caloric intake.

## Botanicals

The use of supplements and herbal products (botanicals) is popular among pregnant women (Dante et al. 2014). However, knowledge about both the efficacy and safety of these products in pregnancy and lactation is lacking (Dugoua et al. 2006). These products are not subject to the same stringent regulation by the FDA as pharmacological agents. Thus, there may be more variation in content and dosing compared with an FDA-approved medication. This section reviews a sample of commonly used supplements and botanicals in pregnancy, with a focus on perinatal mood effects.

### St. John's Wort (*Hypericum Perforatum*)

*Hypericum perforatum* is derived from a naturally occurring plant, St. John's wort (SJW). SJW has been used since ancient times for its medicinal properties (Deligiannidis and Freeman 2014). Several of its bioactive components, such as hypericin, hyperforin, and flavonoids, have affinity for neurotransmitter systems important in the pathophysiology (and pharmacotherapy) of major depression, including activity at GABA, NMDA, and serotonin receptors (Deligiannidis and Freeman 2014). It may also inhibit interleukin-6 and increase cortisol production, resulting in both anti-inflammatory and antidepressant effects (Butterweck 2003). One Cochrane review suggested that it is as effective as conventional antidepressants (and superior to placebo) for mild to moderate depression, with fewer adverse side effects (Linde et al. 2008). A major safety concern about SJW is its ability to alter the pharmacokinetics or clinical response of a variety of clinically important drugs because it is a strong inducer of the cytochrome P450 3A4 enzyme. For example, SJW can lower the levels of hormonal contraceptives, increasing the risk of an unplanned pregnancy (Soleymani et al. 2017).

The data on the effects of SJW on human pregnancy are very limited. In a series of 58 pregnancies exposed to SJW (49 of which included first-trimester exposure) compared with two control groups, no increase was reported in the rate of major malformations, preterm birth, or live birth (Moretti et al. 2009). Most experts do not recommend the use of SJW during pregnancy due to the concerns regarding drug-drug interactions and its limited safety data (Mischoulon 2009). There is little evidence of adverse effects on the infant when using SJW in breastfeeding; possible associations with colic and lethargy have been reported in a few cases (Lee et al. 2003).

### Cannabis

With the legalization of cannabis (marijuana) for either medical or recreational use in several states in the United States (and all of Canada), reports of use during pregnancy have increased markedly. Morning sickness, depression, stress, and anxiety are all commonly cited reasons for patients to choose to use cannabis during pregnancy (Brown et al. 2017; Roberson et al. 2014). As with other supplements, cannabis is often favored by women who want something "natural" to treat their symptoms, despite recommendations by the ACOG to avoid cannabis in pregnancy. Current data suggest a negative impact on fetal brain development that has been associated with problems with behavioral self-regulation, a precursor to later and more serious problems in adulthood. Children of mothers who used marijuana beyond 10 weeks' gestation were found to be at increased risk for regulation problems at 3 months of age compared with infants who were not exposed to cannabis (or those whose mothers stopped using cannabis prior to 10 weeks' gestation) (Hoffman et al. 2020). For these reasons, avoidance of all forms of cannabis is recommended during pregnancy.

## Mind-Body Practices

Mind-body interventions are a broad category of integrative practices that focus on the connections between the brain, mind, body, and behavior. A broad range of interventions can be included under the category of mind-body, ranging from a focus on exercise and sleep to formal mind-body interventions such as yoga and meditation. According to the 2012 National Health Interview Survey, the most common mind and body practices used by adults include yoga and meditation practices, including programs that incorporate mindfulness-based interventions (Clarke et al. 2018; National Center for Complementary and Integrative Health 2018). An analysis of data from the 2007 National Health Interview Survey looking at the use of integrative medicine approaches found that mind-body practices were the most common modality used by women during pregnancy and postpartum (Birdee et al. 2014).

Mind-body treatments have demonstrated effectiveness in helping lower anxiety and depression in pregnancy (Sheffield and Woods-Giscombé 2016). These practices may affect mood states by inducing relaxation and improving neuroplasticity, as measured by serum biomarkers including brain-derived neurotrophic factor, sirtuin 1, cortisol, interleukin-6, dehydroepiandrosterone sulfate, and markers of oxidative stress (Tolahunase et al. 2018). A systematic review of nonpharmacological interventions for managing anxiety in pregnancy showed that women who participated in mind-body practices rated them to be enjoyable, positive, and beneficial (Evans et al. 2020).

## Mindfulness Practice

As mindfulness-based interventions (MBIs) have gained popularity over the past decade, more focus has been dedicated to the potential benefits that these interventions may provide for alleviating symptoms of depression and anxiety for women during the perinatal period. Reviews evaluating MBIs, such as mindfulness-based stress reduction and mindfulness-based cognitive therapy, have shown efficacy in reducing the severity of perinatal depression and anxiety and in alleviating perinatal anxiety and depression symptoms (Shi and MacBeth 2017) and stress symptoms (Lever Taylor et al. 2016). They have also been found beneficial in improving other aspects of maternal well-being, including negative affect and stress (Lever Taylor et al. 2016; Matvienko-Sikar et al. 2016). One randomized controlled trial evaluating the effectiveness of MBIs for preventing a relapse of depression in pregnant women found that MBIs were superior to treatment as usual (Dimidjian et al. 2016).

## Yoga

The practice of yoga usually refers to its three main components: postures, breathing, and meditation. Yoga practices have been associated with reducing sympathetic activity, improving vagal tone, balancing heart rate variability, normalizing hypothalamic-pituitary-adrenal axis activity, and influencing monoamine changes. These effects likely explain how yoga affects mood (Brown and Gerbarg 2005; Streeter et al. 2012).

A systematic review and meta-analysis of randomized controlled trials to determine the effectiveness of yoga practice for prenatal depression found that women both with and without depression rated decreased depressive symptoms with yoga compared with standard prenatal care, antenatal exercises, or social support. Furthermore, this review found that an integrated yoga intervention (including breathing and meditation as well as movement) significantly reduced the level of prenatal depression, whereas exercise-based yoga alone did not show this same effect (Gong et al. 2015). However, another large systematic review found that depression and anxiety during the perinatal period were significantly reduced regardless of yoga intervention style.

Yoga interventions were also found to have a beneficial effect on outcomes such as stress, pain, biomarkers (cortisol, progesterone, and estriol), anger, mindfulness, birth weight, gestational age, maternal–fetal attachment, heart rate variability, optimism and power, and well-being (Jiang et al. 2015; Sheffield and Woods-Giscombé 2016). In another review of yoga interventions during pregnancy, women participating in yoga intervention groups had significantly improved relationships and reduced anxiety, depression, anger, and stress. Even a one-time 20-minute yoga session led to significant improvements in anxiety and depression. Longer-term interventions showed significant improvements in anxiety, depression, and stress; reduced anger; and lower cortisol levels (Jiang et al. 2015; Sheffield and Woods-Giscombé 2016).

Yoga modified for pregnancy is an activity recommended as safe by the ACOG for women engaging in regular physical activity during pregnancy. Guidelines note that exposure to excess heat, as with "hot yoga," should be avoided, as well as postures that may result in decreased venous return or hypotension (American College of Obstetricians and Gynecologists 2020).

## Exercise

Regular physical activity is one of the most beneficial therapies available for numerous physical and mental health conditions. Exercise is beneficial in the perinatal period in nearly all pregnancies for the health of both the mother and the baby. Physical activity and exercise can also have a positive effect on mood. Exercise leads to an increase in body and brain temperature, which leads to a feeling of general relaxation and tranquility. Exercise can have effects on depression that are comparable with those of antidepressant medications. It is hypothesized that this is due at least in part to the secretion of endogenous opioid peptides in the brain that accompany exercise of sufficient intensity and duration (Dinas et al. 2011). Exercise may improve autonomic nervous system functioning by increasing heart rate variability and reducing symptoms of anxiety (Stubbs et al. 2017).

Exercise has been studied in relation to both the prevention and the treatment of perinatal depression. When exercise was systematically reviewed for the prevention of antenatal depression, significant reductions were noted in all six of the included randomized controlled trials, with no difference in efficacy between aerobic and non-aerobic exercise (Daley et al. 2015). In addition, exercise has a positive impact on both anxiety and stress reduction, and it improves the overall quality of life (Kołomanska et al. 2019). When an exercise program was initiated in previously inactive pregnant women, significant reductions in depression, anger, tension, fatigue, and anxiety were noted after only 4 weeks of recorded episodes of moderate-to-vigorous exercise for 30 minutes, four times per week (Gaston and Prapavessis 2013). Regular exercise (three times per week) has been shown to decrease the symptoms and incidence of depression in pregnant women (Perales et al. 2015). Even light-to-moderate physical activity has been associated with reduced PPD symptoms and, in cases of preexisting PPD, has also been shown to increase the odds of resolving depression by 54% (McCurdy et al. 2017).

Physical exercise during pregnancy and the postpartum period is a safe strategy for achieving better psychological well-being and reducing depressive symptoms in women (Poyatos-León et al. 2017). Healthy women should try to get at least 150 minutes of moderate-intensity aerobic activity over the course of each week. Women who regularly engage in vigorous-intensity aerobic activity may continue at this level provided that their condition and health remain unchanged or as recommended by their obstetrical care provider (American College of Obstetricians and Gynecologists 2020). In addition to mood benefits, regular physical activity has other benefits for pregnancy, including reducing the risk of excessive gestational weight gain, low back pain, gestational diabetes, and cesarean delivery (Bauer et al. 2020; Domenjoz et al. 2014; Nascimento et al. 2012).

## Acupuncture

Although acupuncture is a common complementary intervention used by women for both physical and mental health symptoms, there remain few studies and inconsistent findings regarding its utility for treatment of depression during pregnancy (van Ravesteyn et al. 2017). A large review found that acupuncture may be an effective complementary approach for depression in pregnancy (Smith et al. 2019). This is largely based on one study in which antenatal depression outcomes were improved with treatment with acupuncture for 8 weeks perinatally as compared with control subjects

(Manber et al. 2004). Another study found no difference in the use of acupuncture versus sham intervention for treatment of postnatal depression (Chung et al. 2012). At this time, not enough evidence supports the use of acupuncture as treatment for perinatal major depressive disorder.

## Other Approaches

### Bright Light Therapy

As mentioned, women with depression during pregnancy may be hesitant to use medications due to the fear of exposure to the fetus. Bright light therapy is a reasonable treatment for perinatal depression because it is low cost, home-based, and has a much lower side effect profile than medications. Fatigue and sleep disturbances are some of the most commonly reported symptoms in women with perinatal depression, and bright light therapy may alleviate these comorbidities (Crowley and Youngstedt 2012).

Studies have suggested that disturbances in the regulation of melatonin and circadian rhythms are associated with depression during pregnancy and postpartum. Timed bright light treatment can synchronize circadian rhythms and has been used in the treatment of mood disorders (Parry et al. 2008). Small studies have found bright light therapy to be effective for perinatal depression. Significant decreases in depressive symptoms scored by depression rating scales were found with 5 weeks of treatment (Epperson et al. 2004). Larger randomized controlled studies are needed. Recommendations are an initial dosing of 15–30 minutes of exposure within the first 10 minutes of awakening with a 10,000–15,000 lux commercial ultraviolet-blocked light box, and the light should be <12 inches from the face. Side effects are uncommon and usually mild; they may include nausea, sleep disturbance, or, in some cases, emergent symptoms of hypomania (Deligiannidis and Freeman 2014). Light therapy can be used alone or to augment pharmacotherapy (Lam et al. 2016). It can also be used in combination with "critically timed wake therapy" (Parry et al. 2019), which is discussed in the section that follows.

### Sleep

Poor sleep, either in duration, continuity, or quality, is linked with increased risk for negative health outcomes such as cardiovascular disease, diabetes, depression, and anxiety (Khan and Aouad 2017; McHill and Wright 2017). Pregnant women have demonstrated changes in sleep patterns, such as longer sleep-onset latency, more nighttime awakenings, less total sleep time, less slow wave sleep, lower sleep efficiency, and a lower percentage of rapid eye movement (REM) sleep (Bei et al. 2015; Hedman et al. 2002). It has been hypothesized that these changes in sleep patterns may explain some of the reasons why the perinatal period may increase the risk of a mood disorder. Poor sleep quality in the perinatal period is associated with PPD and anxiety (Okun et al. 2018), increased pain perception, increased rates of cesarean delivery, and increased risk of preterm birth and low birth weight infants (Okun et al. 2018; Reichner 2015). Please see Chapter 9, "A Clinical Approach to Psychiatric Diagnosis and Treatment in the Postpartum Period," and Chapter 19, "Anxiety Disorders and Insomnia in the Perinatal Period," for detailed discussion of insomnia in these perinatal periods.

Some intervention studies have demonstrated efficacy in improving perinatal sleep. A yoga program that included poses, breathing practices, and meditation led to less sleep disturbance and decreased anxiety, depression, stress, and low back pain (Babbar and Shyken 2016). In addition, regular physical activity, massage, and acupuncture have been associated with improved sleep quality and reduced insomnia during pregnancy (Hollenbach et al. 2013). Cognitive-behavioral therapy for insomnia (CBT-i) is a nonpharmacological insomnia-focused psychotherapy that is recommended as the first-line treatment for insomnia by American and European guidelines (Riemann et al. 2017; Schutte-Rodin et al. 2008). CBT-i has also been identified by pregnant women as their treatment of choice, compared with pharmacotherapy and acupuncture (Sedov et al. 2017).

Another promising area of research is "critically timed wake therapy" to improve both antenatal and postpartum depressive symptoms. For prenatal depression, "early wake therapy," in which women are kept awake late into the night and then permitted to sleep between 3 A.M. and 7 A.M. (for 1 night only) led to delayed melatonin onset and advanced sleep onset the following night. For postpartum women, "late wake therapy," in which sleep was permitted between 9 P.M. and 1 A.M. and then the patient was awakened (for 1 night only), led to increased total sleep time the following night. These improvements, when they were further augmented by bright light therapy, expedited symptom improvement such that 1 week of combined critically timed wake therapy plus bright light therapy was equivalent to 6 weeks of bright light therapy alone (Parry et al. 2011, 2019).

General sleep hygiene recommendations that can safely be recommended to pregnant women include keeping the sleeping area dark and cool (60°–68°F), avoiding blue-wavelength light from screens for 1–3 hours before bedtime, being exposed to natural sunlight before noon daily, avoiding caffeine and nicotine in the afternoon or evening, getting regular physical activity (after reviewing with their obstetrician), and limiting daytime naps to 20–30 minutes (Burkhart and Phelps 2009; Harding et al. 2019; Walker 2017).

## Special Considerations

Nausea and vomiting are commonly experienced in early pregnancy (Einarson et al. 2013). For mild cases, ginger, pyridoxine (vitamin $B_6$, 25 mg every 8 hours), antihistamines, and metoclopramide have all been associated with greater benefit than placebo (Firouzbakht et al. 2014). For moderate cases, pyridoxine-doxylamine, promethazine, and metoclopramide have been associated with greater benefit than placebo (McParlin et al. 2016). Ginger, chamomile, pyridoxine, and acupuncture are all recommended for the relief of nausea in early pregnancy, based on a woman's preferences and available options, per the World Health Organization (2016) first-line recommendations for treating nausea and vomiting during pregnancy. Taking a multivitamin early in pregnancy, and even prior to conception, has been associated with decreased nausea and vomiting (Emelianova et al. 1999). Hypnosis can be helpful for nausea and vomiting generally as well, although it has not been studied specifically during the perinatal period. Many studies on self-hypnosis have been related to mitigating chemotherapy-induced nausea and vomiting. A meta-analysis showed conflicting data on the use of self-hypnosis and its use for hyperemesis gravidarum (McCormack 2010).

## Conclusion

An integrative approach addresses the physiological, psychiatric, and emotional/spiritual aspects of human functioning and wellness. The use of integrative interventions is high among women, including during pregnancy and the postpartum period, in part due to relative limitations and concerns regarding pharmacotherapy options during these periods. Although pharmacological treatment is effective and often necessary for treating perinatal depression and anxiety, many pregnant women may be concerned about exposure and potential adverse effects on the fetus. Although far less studied in the perinatal population, integrative approaches potentially offer women and their providers adjunctive or alternative options for treatment of perinatal depression and anxiety. Many women, even after discontinuing breastfeeding, elect to continue these integrative modalities when they are effective.

Despite the high prevalence of integrative treatment use during pregnancy and breastfeeding periods, there remains a paucity of research focused on evaluating its efficacy and effectiveness. Therefore, empirical evidence is limited regarding the safety and benefit of integrative medicine to treat mental health symptoms during pregnancy and lactation, particularly approaches that use herbal supplements. Many encouraging studies examining the use of integrative medicine as both a preventive strategy and an adjunct to treatment during the perinatal period were discussed in this chapter, with recommendations made where adequate data to support efficacy and safety exist.

## Key Points

- Diets consisting of whole foods, fruits, vegetables, fish, and seafood have been associated with decreased perinatal depression and anxiety.
- Folate has multiple important effects on fetal growth and neurodevelopment. Deficiencies have been associated with neural tube defects, cleft lip, poor cognitive functioning, and emotional problems in children and may also be associated with maternal depression.
- Omega-3 fatty acids may improve obstetrical outcomes, reduce inflammatory cytokines, and improve perinatal depressive symptoms.
- There is limited evidence on the effectiveness of melatonin for insomnia during pregnancy.
- Mind-body treatments have demonstrated effectiveness in helping lower anxiety and depression in pregnancy.
- Exercise, even light-to-moderate physical activity, has been associated with reduced depression, stress, and anxiety in pregnancy; reduced postpartum depressive symptoms; and other health benefits in pregnancy.
- Insomnia increases the risk of a mood disorder, and poor sleep quality is strongly associated with postpartum depression and anxiety.
- Bright light therapy is a low-cost and home-based treatment that may alleviate sleep disturbance and depression.

# References

Adams J, Lui CW, Sibbritt D, et al: Women's use of complementary and alternative medicine during pregnancy: a critical review of the literature. Birth 36(3):237–245, 2009 19747271

Agarwal S, Kovilam O, Agrawal DK: Vitamin D and its impact on maternal-fetal outcomes in pregnancy: a critical review. Crit Rev Food Sci Nutr 58(5):755–769, 2018 27558700

Aghajafari F, Field CJ, Weinberg AR, et al: Both mother and infant require a vitamin D supplement to ensure that infants' vitamin D status meets current guidelines. Nutrients 10(4):429, 2018 29596362

American College of Obstetricians and Gynecologists: Physical activity and exercise during pregnancy and the postpartum period: ACOG Committee opinion summary, Number 804. Obstet Gynecol 135(4):991–993, 2020 32217974

Ars CL, Nijs IM, Marroun HE, et al: Prenatal folate, homocysteine and vitamin B12 levels and child brain volumes, cognitive development and psychological functioning: the Generation R Study. Br J Nutr 122(s1):S1–S9, 2019 31638501

Babbar S, Shyken J: Yoga in Pregnancy. Clin Obstet Gynecol 59(3):600–612, 2016 27152528

Bauer I, Hartkopf J, Kullmann S, et al: Spotlight on the fetus: how physical activity during pregnancy influences fetal health: a narrative review. BMJ Open Sport Exerc Med 6(1):e000658, 2020 32206341

Bei B, Coo S, Trinder J: Sleep and mood during pregnancy and the postpartum period. Sleep Med Clin 10(1):25–33, 2015 26055670

Bell C, Abrams J, Nutt D: Tryptophan depletion and its implications for psychiatry. Br J Psychiatry 178:399–405, 2001 11331552

Bibbins-Domingo K, Grossman DC, Curry SJ, et al: Folic acid supplementation for the prevention of neural tube defects: US preventive services task force recommendation statement. JAMA 317(2):183–189, 2017 28097362

Birdee GS, Kemper KJ, Rothman R, et al: Use of complementary and alternative medicine during pregnancy and the postpartum period: an analysis of the National Health Interview Survey. J Womens Health (Larchmt) 23(10):824–829, 2014 25268759

Birdsall TC: 5-Hydroxytryptophan: a clinically-effective serotonin precursor. Altern Med Rev 3(4):271–280, 1998 9727088

Bodnar LM, Wisner KL: Nutrition and depression: implications for improving mental health among childbearing-aged women. Biol Psychiatry 58(9):679–685, 2005 16040007

Bottiglieri T: Folate, vitamin B12, and neuropsychiatric disorders. Nutr Rev 54(12):382–390, 1996 9155210

Brillo E, Di Renzo GC: Chocolate and other cocoa products: effects on human reproduction and pregnancy. J Agric Food Chem 63(45):9927–9935, 2015 26218965

Brown QL, Sarvet AL, Shmulewitz D, et al: Trends in marijuana use among pregnant and nonpregnant reproductive-aged women, 2002–2014. JAMA 317(2):207–209, 2017 27992619

Brown RP, Gerbarg PL: Sudarshan Kriya yogic breathing in the treatment of stress, anxiety, and depression, part I: neurophysiologic model. J Altern Complement Med 11(1):189–201, 2005 15750381

Brzezinski A, Fibich T, Cohen M, et al: Effects of melatonin on progesterone production by human granulosa lutein cells in culture. Fertil Steril 58(3):526–529, 1992 1521647

Burkhart K, Phelps JR: Amber lenses to block blue light and improve sleep: a randomized trial. Chronobiol Int 26(8):1602–1612, 2009 20030543

Butterweck V: Mechanism of action of St John's wort in depression: what is known? CNS Drugs 17(8):539–562, 2003 12775192

Cerutti R, Sichel MP, Perin M, et al: Psychological distress during puerperium: a novel therapeutic approach using S-adenosylmethionine. Current Therapeutic Research 53(6):707–716, 1993

Chia AR, Chen LW, Lai JS, et al: Maternal dietary patterns and birth outcomes: a systematic review and meta-analysis. Adv Nutr 10(4):685–695, 2019 31041446

Chong MFF, Wong JXY, Colega M, et al: Relationships of maternal folate and vitamin B12 status during pregnancy with perinatal depression: the GUSTO study. J Psychiatr Res 55:110–116, 2014 24774647
Christesen HT, Falkenberg T, Lamont RF, et al: The impact of vitamin D on pregnancy: a systematic review. Acta Obstet Gynecol Scand 91(12):1357–1367, 2012 22974137
Chung KF, Yeung WF, Zhang ZJ, et al: Randomized non-invasive sham-controlled pilot trial of electroacupuncture for postpartum depression. J Affect Disord 142(1–3):115–121, 2012 22840621
Clarke TC, Black LI, Stussman BJ, et al: Trends in the use of complementary health approaches among adults: United States, 2002–2012. Natl Health Stat Rep (79):1–16, 2015 25671660
Clarke TC, Barnes PM, Black LI, et al: Use of yoga, meditation, and chiropractors among U.S. adults aged 18 and over. NCHS Data Brief (325):1–8, 2018 30475686
Crowley SK, Youngstedt SD: Efficacy of light therapy for perinatal depression: a review. J Physiol Anthropol 31:15, 2012 22738716
Daley AJ, Foster L, Long G, et al: The effectiveness of exercise for the prevention and treatment of antenatal depression: systematic review with meta-analysis. BJOG 122(1):57–62, 2015 24935560
Dante G, Bellei G, Neri I, Facchinetti F: Herbal therapies in pregnancy: what works? Curr Opin Obstet Gynecol 26(2):83–91, 2014 24535321
Davis FC: Melatonin: role in development. J Biol Rhythms 12(6):498–508, 1997 9406023
Deligiannidis KM, Freeman MP: Complementary and alternative medicine for the treatment of depressive disorders in women. Psychiatr Clin North Am 33(2):441–463, 2010 20385346
Deligiannidis KM, Freeman MP: Complementary and alternative medicine therapies for perinatal depression. Best Pract Res Clin Obstet Gynaecol 28(1):85–95, 2014 24041861
Dimidjian S, Goodman SH, Felder JN, et al: Staying well during pregnancy and the postpartum: a pilot randomized trial of mindfulness-based cognitive therapy for the prevention of depressive relapse/recurrence. J Consult Clin Psychol 84(2):134–145, 2016 26654212
Dinas PC, Koutedakis Y, Flouris AD: Effects of exercise and physical activity on depression. Ir J Med Sci 180(2):319–325, 2011 21076975
Di Renzo GC, Brillo E, Romanelli M, et al: Potential effects of chocolate on human pregnancy: a randomized controlled trial. J Matern Fetal Neonatal Med 25(10):1860–1867, 2012 22537244
Domenjoz I, Kayser B, Boulvain M: Effect of physical activity during pregnancy on mode of delivery. Am J Obstet Gynecol 211(4):401.e1–401.e11, 2014 24631706
Dong J-Y, Kimura T, Ikehara S, et al: Chocolate consumption and risk of gestational diabetes mellitus: the Japan Environment and Children's Study. Br J Nutr 122(8):936–941, 2019 31337446
Dugoua JJ, Mills E, Perri D, et al: Safety and efficacy of St. John's wort (Hypericum) during pregnancy and lactation. Can J Clin Pharmacol 13(3):e268–e276, 2006 17085775
Einarson TR, Piwko C, Koren G: Quantifying the global rates of nausea and vomiting of pregnancy: a meta analysis. J Popul Ther Clin Pharmacol 20(2):e171–e183, 2013 23863575
Emelianova S, Mazzotta P, Einarson A, et al: Prevalence and severity of nausea and vomiting of pregnancy and effect of vitamin supplementation. Clin Invest Med 22(3):106–110, 1999 10410832
Emmett PM, Jones LR, Golding J: Pregnancy diet and associated outcomes in the Avon Longitudinal Study of Parents and Children. Nutr Rev 73(suppl 3):154–174, 2015 26395341
Epperson CN, Terman M, Terman JS, et al: Randomized clinical trial of bright light therapy for antepartum depression: preliminary findings. J Clin Psychiatry 65(3):421–425, 2004 15096083
Evans K, Spiby H, Morrell JC: Non-pharmacological interventions to reduce the symptoms of mild to moderate anxiety in pregnant women: a systematic review and narrative synthesis of women's views on the acceptability of and satisfaction with interventions. Arch Women Ment Health 23(1):11–28, 2020 30613846
Firouzbakht M, Nikpour M, Jamali B, et al: Comparison of ginger with vitamin B6 in relieving nausea and vomiting during pregnancy. Ayu 35(3):289–293, 2014 26664238
Freedman R, Hunter SK, Hoffman MC: Prenatal primary prevention of mental illness by micronutrient supplements in pregnancy. Am J Psychiatry 175(7):607–619, 2018 29558816
Gaston A, Prapavessis H: Tired, moody and pregnant? Exercise may be the answer. Psychol Health 28(12):1353–1369, 2013 23837826

Gong H, Ni C, Shen X, et al: Yoga for prenatal depression: a systematic review and meta-analysis. BMC Psychiatry 15:14, 2015 25652267

Haghiac M, Yang XH, Presley L, et al: Dietary omega-3 fatty acid supplementation reduces inflammation in obese pregnant women: a randomized double-blind controlled clinical trial. PLoS One 10(9):e0137309, 2015 26340264

Harding EC, Franks NP, Wisden W: The temperature dependence of sleep. Front Neurosci 13:336, 2019 31105512

Hedman C, Pohjasvaara T, Tolonen U, et al: Effects of pregnancy on mothers' sleep. Sleep Med 3(1):37–42, 2002 14592252

Hoffman MC, Hunter SK, D'Alessandro A, et al: Interaction of maternal choline levels and prenatal marijuana's effects on the offspring. Psychol Med 50(10):1716–1726, 2020 31364525

Hollenbach D, Broker R, Herlehy S, et al: Non-pharmacological interventions for sleep quality and insomnia during pregnancy: a systematic review. J Can Chiropr Assoc 57(3):260–270, 2013 23997252

Hsu MC, Tung CY, Chen HE: Omega-3 polyunsaturated fatty acid supplementation in prevention and treatment of maternal depression: putative mechanism and recommendation. J Affect Disord 238:47–61, 2018 29860183

Hunter SK, Hoffman MC, D'Alessandro A, et al: Male fetus susceptibility to maternal inflammation: C-reactive protein and brain development. Psychol Med December 2, 2019 31787129 Epub ahead of print

Jackson SE, Smith L, Firth J, et al: Is there a relationship between chocolate consumption and symptoms of depression? A cross-sectional survey of 13,626 US adults. Depress Anxiety 36(10):987–995, 2019 31356717

Jarde A, Lewis-Mikhael A-M, Moayyedi P, et al: Pregnancy outcomes in women taking probiotics or prebiotics: a systematic review and meta-analysis. BMC Pregnancy Childbirth 18(1):14, 2018 29310610

Jiang Q, Wu Z, Zhou L, et al: Effects of yoga intervention during pregnancy: a review for current status. Am J Perinatol 32(6):503–514, 2015 25535930

Khan MS, Aouad R: The effects of insomnia and sleep loss on cardiovascular disease. Sleep Med Clin 12(2):167–177, 2017 28477772

Kikuchi AM, Tanabe A, Iwahori Y: A systematic review of the effect of L-tryptophan supplementation on mood and emotional functioning. J Diet Suppl 18(3):316–333, 2021 32272859

Kołomanska D, Zarawski M, Mazur-Bialy A: Physical activity and depressive disorders in pregnant women—a systematic review. Medicina (Kaunas) 55(5):212, 2019 31130705

Lam RW, Levitt AJ, Levitan RD, et al: Efficacy of bright light treatment, fluoxetine, and the combination in patients with nonseasonal major depressive disorder: a randomized clinical trial. JAMA Psychiatry 73(1):56–63, 2016 26580307

Latif R: Maternal and fetal effects of chocolate consumption during pregnancy: a systematic review. J Matern Fetal Neonatal Med 32(17):2915–2927, 2019 29534636

Lee A, Minhas R, Matsuda N, et al: The safety of St. John's wort (Hypericum perforatum) during breastfeeding. J Clin Psychiatry 64(8):966–968, 2003 12927015

Lever Taylor B, Cavanagh K, Strauss C: The effectiveness of mindfulness-based interventions in the perinatal period: a systematic review and meta-analysis. PLoS One 11(5):e0155720, 2016 27182732

Linde K, Berner MM, Kriston L: St John's wort for major depression. Cochrane Database Syst Rev (4):CD000448, 2008 18843608

Manber R, Schnyer RN, Allen JJB, et al: Acupuncture: a promising treatment for depression during pregnancy. J Affect Disord 83(1):89–95, 2004 15546651

Matvienko-Sikar K, Lee L, Murphy G, et al: The effects of mindfulness interventions on prenatal well-being: a systematic review. Psychol Health 31(12):1415–1434, 2016 27539908

McCormack D: Hypnosis for hyperemesis gravidarum. J Obstet Gynaecol 30(7):647–653, 2010 20925602

McCurdy AP, Boulé NG, Sivak A, et al: Effects of exercise on mild-to-moderate depressive symptoms in the postpartum period: a meta-analysis. Obstet Gynecol 129(6):1087–1097, 2017 28486363

McHill AW, Wright KP Jr: Role of sleep and circadian disruption on energy expenditure and in metabolic predisposition to human obesity and metabolic disease. Obes Rev 18(suppl 1):15–24, 2017 28164449

McParlin C, O'Donnell A, Robson SC, et al: Treatments for hyperemesis gravidarum and nausea and vomiting in pregnancy: a systematic review. JAMA 316(13):1392–1401, 2016 27701665

Middleton P, Gomersall JC, Gould JF, et al: Omega-3 fatty acid addition during pregnancy. Cochrane Database Syst Rev 11:CD003402, 2018 30480773

Mischoulon D: Update and critique of natural remedies as antidepressant treatments. Obstet Gynecol Clin North Am 36(4):789–807, x, 2009 19944301

Moretti ME, Maxson A, Hanna F, et al: Evaluating the safety of St. John's Wort in human pregnancy. Reprod Toxicol 28(1):96–99, 2009 19491000

Naninck EFG, Stijger PC, Brouwer-Brolsma EM: The importance of maternal folate status for brain development and function of offspring. Adv Nutr 10(3):502–519, 2019 31093652

Nascimento SL, Surita FG, Cecatti JG: Physical exercise during pregnancy: a systematic review. Curr Opin Obstet Gynecol 24(6):387–394, 2012 23014142

National Center for Complementary and Integrative Health: Complementary, Alternative, or Integrative Health: What's In a Name? Bethesda, MD, National Institutes of Health, 2018. Available at: https://www.nccih.nih.gov/health/complementary-alternative-or-integrative-health-whats-in-a-name. Accessed April 27, 2020.

Newberry SJ, Chung M, Booth M, et al: Omega-3 fatty acids and maternal and child health: an updated systematic review. Evid Rep Technol Assess (Full Rep) (224):1–826, 2016 30307735

Noonan S, Zaveri M, Macaninch E, et al: Food and mood: a review of supplementary prebiotic and probiotic interventions in the treatment of anxiety and depression in adults. BMJ Nutrition, Prevention, and Health 3:351–362, 2020

Obeid R, Holzgreve W, Pietrzik K: Is 5-methyltetrahydrofolate an alternative to folic acid for the prevention of neural tube defects? J Perinat Med 41(5):469–483, 2013 23482308

Okun ML, Mancuso RA, Hobel CJ, et al: Poor sleep quality increases symptoms of depression and anxiety in postpartum women. J Behav Med 41(5):703–710, 2018 30030650

Palacios C, Kostiuk LK, Peña-Rosas JP: Vitamin D supplementation for women during pregnancy. Cochrane Database Syst Rev 7:CD008873, 2019 31348529

Palmer KR, Mockler JC, Davies-Tuck ML, et al: Protect-me: a parallel-group, triple blinded, placebo-controlled randomised clinical trial protocol assessing antenatal maternal melatonin supplementation for fetal neuroprotection in early onset fetal growth restriction. BMJ Open 9(6):e028243, 2019 31230020

Parry BL, Meliska CJ, Sorenson DL, et al: Plasma melatonin circadian rhythm disturbances during pregnancy and postpartum in depressed women and women with personal or family histories of depression. Am J Psychiatry 165(12):1551–1558, 2008 18829869

Parry BL, Meliska CJ, Sorenson DL, et al: Reduced phase-advance of plasma melatonin after bright morning light in the luteal, but not follicular, menstrual cycle phase in premenstrual dysphoric disorder: an extended study. Chronobiol Int 28(5):415–424, 2011 21721857

Parry BL, Meliska CJ, Lopez AM, et al: Early versus late wake therapy improves mood more in antepartum versus postpartum depression by differentially altering melatonin-sleep timing disturbances. J Affect Disord 245:608–616, 2019 30445386

Perales M, Refoyo I, Coteron J, et al: Exercise during pregnancy attenuates prenatal depression: a randomized controlled trial. Eval Health Prof 38(1):59–72, 2015 24872442

Pietrzik K, Bailey L, Shane B: Folic acid and L-5-methyltetrahydrofolate: comparison of clinical pharmacokinetics and pharmacodynamics. Clin Pharmacokinet 49(8):535–548, 2010 20608755

Poyatos-León R, García-Hermoso A, Sanabria-Martínez G, et al: Effects of exercise-based interventions on postpartum depression: a meta-analysis of randomized controlled trials. Birth 44(3):200–208, 2017 28589648

Qureshi NA, Al-Bedah AM: Mood disorders and complementary and alternative medicine: a literature review. Neuropsychiatr Dis Treat 9:639–658, 2013 23700366

Raghavan R, Dreibelbis C, Kingshipp BL, et al: Dietary patterns before and during pregnancy and birth outcomes: a systematic review. Am J Clin Nutr 109(suppl 7):729S–756S, 2019 30982873

Reichner CA: Insomnia and sleep deficiency in pregnancy. Obstet Med 8(4):168–171, 2015 27512475
Reid G, Bocking A: The potential for probiotics to prevent bacterial vaginosis and preterm labor. Am J Obstet Gynecol 189(4):1202–1208, 2003 14586379
Reiter RJ, Tan DX, Korkmaz A, et al: Melatonin and stable circadian rhythms optimize maternal, placental and fetal physiology. Hum Reprod Update 20(2):293–307, 2014 24132226
Reza N, Deligiannidis KM, Eustis EH, et al: Complementary health practices for treating perinatal depression. Obstet Gynecol Clin North Am 45(3):441–454, 2018 30092920
Riemann D, Baglioni C, Bassetti C, et al: European guideline for the diagnosis and treatment of insomnia. J Sleep Res 26(6):675–700, 2017 28875581
Roberson EK, Patrick WK, Hurwitz EL: Marijuana use and maternal experiences of severe nausea during pregnancy in Hawai'i. Hawaii J Med Public Health 73(9):283–287, 2014 25285255
Rodrigues Helmo F, Etchebehere RM, Bernardes N, et al: Melatonin treatment in fetal and neonatal diseases. Pathol Res Pract 214(12):1940–1951, 2018 30377024
Saccone G, Saccone I, Berghella V: Omega-3 long-chain polyunsaturated fatty acids and fish oil supplementation during pregnancy: which evidence? J Matern Fetal Neonatal Med 29(15):2389–2397, 2016 26382010
Sarris J, Murphy J, Mischoulon D, et al: Adjunctive nutraceuticals for depression: a systematic review and meta-analyses. Am J Psychiatry 173(6):575–587, 2016 27113121
Schutte-Rodin S, Broch L, Buysse D, et al: Clinical guideline for the evaluation and management of chronic insomnia in adults. J Clin Sleep Med 4(5):487–504, 2008 18853708
Sedov ID, Goodman SH, Tomfohr-Madsen LM: Insomnia treatment preferences during pregnancy. J Obstet Gynecol Neonatal Nurs 46(3):e95–e104, 2017 28343943
Shaw K, Turner J, Del Mar C: Tryptophan and 5-hydroxytryptophan for depression. Cochrane Database Syst Rev (1):CD003198 2002 11869656
Sheffield KM, Woods-Giscombé CL: Efficacy, feasibility, and acceptability of perinatal yoga on women's mental health and well-being: a systematic literature review. J Holist Nurs 34(1):64–79, 2016 25896571
Shi Z, MacBeth A: The effectiveness of mindfulness-based interventions on maternal perinatal mental health outcomes: a systematic review. Mindfulness (NY) 8(4):823–847, 2017 28757900
Silva DFO, Cobucci RN, Gonçalves AK, et al: Systematic review of the association between dietary patterns and perinatal anxiety and depression. BMC Pregnancy Childbirth 19(1):212, 2019 31234821
Slykerman RF, Hood F, Wickens K, et al: Effect of Lactobacillus rhamnosus HN001 in pregnancy on postpartum symptoms of depression and anxiety: a randomised double-blind placebo-controlled Trial. EBioMedicine 24:159–165, 2017 28943228
Smith CA, Shewamene Z, Galbally M, et al: The effect of complementary medicines and therapies on maternal anxiety and depression in pregnancy: a systematic review and meta-analysis. J Affect Disord 245:428–439, 2019 30423471
Soleymani S, Bahramsoltani R, Rahimi R, et al: Clinical risks of St John's wort (Hypericum perforatum) co-administration. Expert Opin Drug Metab Toxicol 13(10):1047–1062, 2017 28885074
Sparling TM, Henschke N, Nesbitt RC, et al: The role of diet and nutritional supplementation in perinatal depression: a systematic review. Matern Child Nutr 13(1), 2017 26840379
Spedding S: Vitamin D and depression: a systematic review and meta-analysis comparing studies with and without biological flaws. Nutrients 6(4):1501–1518, 2014 24732019
Steel A, Goldenberg JZ, Hawrelak JA, et al: Integrative physiology and traditional naturopathic practice: results of an international observational study. Integr Med Res 9(4):100424, 2020 32509521
Streeter CC, Gerbarg PL, Saper RB, et al: Effects of yoga on the autonomic nervous system, gamma-aminobutyric-acid, and allostasis in epilepsy, depression, and post-traumatic stress disorder. Med Hypotheses 78(5):571–579, 2012 22365651
Stubbs B, Vancampfort D, Rosenbaum S, et al: An examination of the anxiolytic effects of exercise for people with anxiety and stress-related disorders: a meta-analysis. Psychiatry Res 249:102–108, 2017 28088704

Timonen M, Horrobin D, Jokelainen J, et al: Fish consumption and depression: the Northern Finland 1966 birth cohort study. J Affect Disord 82(3):447–452, 2004 15555697

Tolahunase MR, Sagar R, Faiq M, et al: Yoga- and meditation-based lifestyle intervention increases neuroplasticity and reduces severity of major depressive disorder: a randomized controlled trial. Restor Neurol Neurosci 36(3):423–442, 2018 29614706

Trujillo J, Vieira MC, Lepsch J, et al: A systematic review of the associations between maternal nutritional biomarkers and depression and/or anxiety during pregnancy and postpartum. J Affect Disord 232:185–203, 2018 29494902

van Lee L, Cai S, Loy SL, et al: Relation of plasma tryptophan concentrations during pregnancy to maternal sleep and mental well-being: the GUSTO cohort. J Affect Disord 225:523–529, 2018 5667743

van Ravesteyn LM, Lambregtse-van den Berg MP, Hoogendijk WJG, et al: Interventions to treat mental disorders during pregnancy: a systematic review and multiple treatment meta-analysis. PLoS One 12(3):e0173397, 2017 28358808

Walker M: Why We Sleep: Unlocking the Power of Sleep and Dreams. New York, Scribner, 2017

Wang J, Liu N, Sun W, et al: Association between vitamin D deficiency and antepartum and postpartum depression: a systematic review and meta-analysis of longitudinal studies. Arch Gynecol Obstet 298(6):1045–1059, 2018 30264203

Weinert LS, Silveiro SP: Maternal-fetal impact of vitamin D deficiency: a critical review. Matern Child Health J 19(1):94–101, 2015 24748216

Wilkinson D, Shepherd E, Wallace EM: Melatonin for women in pregnancy for neuroprotection of the fetus. Cochrane Database Syst Rev 3:CD010527, 2016 27022888

Williams JA, Romero VC, Clinton CM, et al: Vitamin D levels and perinatal depressive symptoms in women at risk: a secondary analysis of the mothers, omega-3, and mental health study. BMC Pregnancy Childbirth 16(1):203, 2016 27485050

Wilson RD, Genetics Committee, Motherisk: Pre-conceptional vitamin/folic acid supplementation 2007: the use of folic acid in combination with a multivitamin supplement for the prevention of neural tube defects and other congenital anomalies. J Obstet Gynaecol Can 29(12):1003–1013, 2007 18053387

World Health Organization: WHO Recommendations on Antenatal Care for a Positive Pregnancy Experience. Geneva, World Health Organization, 2016

Yan J, Liu Y, Cao L, et al: Association between duration of folic acid supplementation during pregnancy and risk of postpartum depression. Nutrients 9(11):1206, 2017 29099069

Yang HL, Zhou WJ, Gu CJ, et al: Pleiotropic roles of melatonin in endometriosis, recurrent spontaneous abortion, and polycystic ovary syndrome. Am J Reprod Immunol 80(1):e12839, 2018 29493042

CHAPTER 15

# Bipolar Disorder and Related Disorders

Sarah M. Nagle-Yang, M.D.
Sarah A. DeBrunner, M.D.
Andrea Favini, M.D.
Andrew M. Novick, M.D., Ph.D.
Caitlin Hasser, M.D.
Chandni Prakash, M.D.
Margo Nathan, M.D.

Bipolar disorder (BD) is a common psychiatric illness often associated with significant impairments in quality of life and psychosocial functioning (Yatham et al. 2018). BD frequently presents in adolescence or early adulthood, coinciding with peak reproductive years. Although the sex ratio of BD is roughly equal, there are distinctions in the phenomenology of the illness between women and men. The typical age of onset is later in women than in men, and women with BD may experience symptom exacerbation in accordance with menstrual cycle hormonal fluctuations, in the perinatal period, and in the menopausal transition (Freeman and Gelenberg 2005). BD is a chronic illness that typically requires ongoing management during both acute episodes and periods of maintenance.

This chapter provides an overview of BD in the context of the female reproductive lifespan, with a detailed review of treatment considerations for women with BD in the perinatal period. For a more detailed review of the clinical approach in reproductive

---

We wish to acknowledge Ran Zhao and Crystal Clark for their contribution to the curriculum.

**TABLE 15–1. Risk factors for postpartum mood episodes for women with bipolar disorder**

| | |
|---|---|
| Discontinuation of maintenance medication | Primiparity |
| Family history of perinatal mood episode | Unplanned pregnancy |
| Mood symptoms during pregnancy | Younger age |
| Previous perinatal mood episode | |

psychiatry or the underlying physiology and pharmacological considerations across the reproductive life cycle, please see the corresponding chapters in this text.

# Epidemiology

## Rates/Incidence

Prevalence estimates suggest a cumulative 12-month prevalence of 2.4% for bipolar spectrum disorders and lower rates for individual subtypes such as BD type I (BDI; 0.6%) and BD type II (BDII; 0.4%) (Yatham et al. 2018). Age of onset is typically between 12 and 30 years of age, coinciding with the peak reproductive years (Epstein et al. 2014).

## Risk Factors

General risk factors for BD include a family history of mood disorder, traumatic life events, and substance use (Roberts 2019). A previous perinatal mood episode is the strongest predictor for a perinatal recurrence of illness for women with BD (Di Florio et al. 2018). Primiparity has also been associated with a higher risk of a postpartum manic or psychotic episode in women with BD. In a study that included 934 women with BDI, 35% reported an episode of mania or psychotic depression after their first pregnancy, compared with 20.5% after their second pregnancy and 14.6% after their third pregnancy (Di Florio et al. 2014). Other important risk factors for a postpartum mood episode in BDI include mood symptoms during pregnancy, younger age, unplanned pregnancy, and a family history of a perinatal mood episode (Table 15–1) (Doyle et al. 2012).

## Screening Methods

Identifying women with BD during pregnancy and postpartum may be aided by the use of screening tools. Although screening for depression during these periods is recommended by the American College of Obstetricians and Gynecologists (ACOG), the U.S. Preventive Services Task Force, and the American Academy of Pediatrics, no formal recommendations for BD screening as a part of routine obstetrical care have been established (American College of Obstetricians and Gynecologists 2018; Earls et al. 2019; Siu et al. 2016). Postpartum depression is more common among women with BD than among women with major depressive disorder, and most postpartum mood episodes experienced by women with BD are depressive, so screening for depression without also screening for BD risks misclassifying bipolar depression as unipolar de-

**TABLE 15–2. Validated screening instruments for detection of bipolar disorders**

| |
|---|
| Bipolar Spectrum Diagnostic Scale |
| Hypomania Checklist |
| Mood Disorders Questionnaire |
| Mood Swings Questionnaire |

pression (Wisner et al. 2013). Thus, many experts recommend simultaneous screening using the Edinburgh Postnatal Depression Scale (EPDS) and the Mood Disorder Questionnaire (MDQ) at initial presentation during pregnancy and at the first postpartum visit to aid in further diagnostic evaluation (Clark and Wisner 2018). The EPDS is a brief, 10-item scale designed to identify depression that is easy to score and has been translated into many languages (Cox et al. 1987). The MDQ is a 13-item scale used to identify a lifetime history of mania or hypomania (Hirschfeld et al. 2000). Merrill et al. (2015) screened women during their initial prenatal visit and found that 21.4% of participants with a positive EPDS (score ≥10) also had a positive MDQ. Similarly, Wisner et al. (2013) found that 22.6% of postpartum women who screened positive on the EPDS (score ≥10) were diagnosed with BD by further evaluation using the Structured Clinical Interview for DSM-IV. Other validated screening instruments for BD include the Hypomania Checklist (increased accuracy for detecting BDII), the Bipolar Spectrum Diagnostic Scale, and the Mood Swings Questionnaire (Table 15–2) (Carvalho et al. 2015; Parker et al. 2012).

# Diagnostic Criteria

BDs comprise a spectrum of diagnostic subtypes distinguished primarily by the symptoms and symptom severity experienced during the acute phases of the illness. The subtypes included in DSM-5's (American Psychiatric Association 2013) "Bipolar and Related Disorders" section are BDI, BDII, cyclothymic disorder, other specified bipolar and related disorder, unspecified bipolar and related disorder, substance/medication-induced bipolar and related disorder, and bipolar and related disorder due to another medical condition. DSM-5 also contains a range of specifiers that may further clarify a patient's clinical features, course, or severity. The "with peripartum onset" specifier can be applied to the current or most recent manic, hypomanic, or depressive episode if onset occurs either during pregnancy or in the first 4 weeks postpartum.

The essential feature of BDI is the occurrence of a manic episode (Box 15–1). Although depressive episodes are not necessary to meet the diagnostic criteria for BDI, manic episodes are often preceded or followed by hypomanic or major depressive episodes. In contrast, the diagnosis of BDII disorder requires at least one major depressive episode and at least one hypomanic episode over the disease course. Cyclothymic disorder is characterized by subthreshold presentation of depressive and hypomanic episodes (American Psychiatric Association 2013). Patients with BD often have one or more comorbid psychiatric diagnoses. Anxiety disorders, substance use disorders, impulse control disorders, and personality disorders are the most common comorbidities (Yatham et al. 2018).

### Box 15–1. DSM-5 Criteria for Bipolar I Disorder

For a diagnosis of bipolar I disorder, it is necessary to meet the following criteria for a manic episode. The manic episode may have been preceded by and may be followed by hypomanic or major depressive episodes.

**Manic Episode**

A. A distinct period of abnormally and persistently elevated, expansive, or irritable mood and abnormally and persistently increased activity or energy, lasting at least 1 week and present most of the day, nearly every day (or any duration if hospitalization is necessary).

B. During the period of mood disturbance and increased energy or activity, three (or more) of the following symptoms (four if the mood is only irritable) are present to a significant degree and represent a noticeable change from usual behavior:

   1. Inflated self-esteem or grandiosity.
   2. Decreased need for sleep (e.g., feels rested after only 3 hours of sleep).
   3. More talkative than usual or pressure to keep talking.
   4. Flight of ideas or subjective experience that thoughts are racing.
   5. Distractibility (i.e., attention too easily drawn to unimportant or irrelevant external stimuli), as reported or observed.
   6. Increase in goal-directed activity (either socially, at work or school, or sexually) or psychomotor agitation (i.e., purposeless non-goal-directed activity).
   7. Excessive involvement in activities that have a high potential for painful consequences (e.g., engaging in unrestrained buying sprees, sexual indiscretions, or foolish business investments).

C. The mood disturbance is sufficiently severe to cause marked impairment in social or occupational functioning or to necessitate hospitalization to prevent harm to self or others, or there are psychotic features.

D. The episode is not attributable to the physiological effects of a substance (e.g., a drug of abuse, a medication, other treatment) or another medical condition.

   **Note:** A full manic episode that emerges during antidepressant treatment (e.g., medication, electroconvulsive therapy) but persists at a fully syndromal level beyond the physiological effect of that treatment is sufficient evidence for a manic episode and, therefore, a bipolar I diagnosis.

**Note:** Criteria A–D constitute a manic episode. At least one lifetime manic episode is required for the diagnosis of bipolar I disorder.

*Source.* Reprinted from American Psychiatric Association: *Diagnostic and Statistical Manual of Mental Disorders,* 5th Edition. Arlington, VA, 2013, p. 124. 

# Clinical Features

## Clinical Presentation

Ms. V is a 26-year-old woman with a history of BDI who presents for a preconception visit to discuss a treatment plan in the context of trying to conceive. She has no previous pregnancies. Ms. V was diagnosed with BDI at age 20 while admitted to an inpatient psychiatric unit during an acute manic episode. Symptoms during that episode included decreased need for sleep, pressured speech, flight of ideas, elevated and expansive mood, hypersexuality, and erotomanic delusions. She was treated effectively during that inpatient admission with mood-stabilizing medications but since that time has experienced two other similar episodes, each in the context of nonadherence to pharmacotherapy.

At presentation, Ms. V reports that her mood has been stable and euthymic for the past 2 years on her current medication regimen, which includes lithium 900 mg/day and lurasidone 40 mg/day. Previous medication trials (e.g., quetiapine, risperidone, lamotrigine, and olanzapine) have been limited due to tolerability. She remembers that when she was started on lithium, her previous psychiatrist told her that if she were to ever become pregnant, she would need to stop taking the medication immediately because it "causes birth defects." She inquires how she should safely discontinue this medication and which medications for BD are "safe in pregnancy."

Although the sex ratio of BDI is approximately 1:1, there are sex differences in the clinical presentation. Compared with men, women are more likely to experience hypomanic episodes, and the prevalence rate of BDII is higher among women (Baldassano et al. 2005; Moses-Kolko et al. 2019). Women may be slightly older than men on initial presentation and are more likely to experience comorbid thyroid disease (Baldassano et al. 2005), anxiety disorders (Saunders et al. 2012), and eating disorders (McElroy et al. 2016). Alternatively, men are more likely than women to present with comorbid substance use disorders (Grover et al. 2019). Although some studies have indicated that women are more likely than men to experience predominant depressive episodes (Altshuler et al. 2010; Grover et al. 2019) and rapid cycling subtype (Di Florio and Jones 2010; Erol et al. 2015), this literature is mixed, and other studies have not found such associations (Baldassano et al. 2005).

## Course/Prognosis

BD is a chronic illness that typically requires ongoing management throughout all stages of the disease course. On average, people living with BD experience symptoms of the disease for approximately half of their lives (Yatham et al. 2018). Although the psychosocial functioning of people with BD varies greatly among individuals, overall, BD is associated with significant morbidity and is one of the leading causes of years lost to disability worldwide. Factors associated with more significant functional impairments include higher frequency of acute episodes, prominent depressive symptoms, and lower cognitive status (Yatham et al. 2018). Patients with BD have an elevated risk of suicide relative to the general population, and approximately 6%–7% of patients with BD die by suicide (Schaffer et al. 2015).

### Influence of Reproductive Transitions

**Menses.** Research suggests that most women with BD experience an exacerbation of mood symptoms in the premenstrual period and that this exacerbation is a predictor of more severe disease course for women with BD (Dias et al. 2011; Payne et al. 2007; Teatero et al. 2014). Women with premenstrual exacerbation have been found to have greater symptom severity and greater frequency of mood episodes over the course of the disease (Dias et al. 2011). Women with comorbid premenstrual dysphoric disorder (PMDD) have an earlier age of onset of BD, higher rates of rapid cycling, more frequent mood episodes, and higher rates of psychiatric comorbidity and are more likely to report mood symptoms related to contraceptive use (Slyepchenko et al. 2017). To diagnose PMDD in women with BD, assessment should occur during a period of euthymia, utilizing the standard of 2 months of prospective mood charting (Yatham et al. 2018).

The effect of BD and associated treatments on the menstrual cycle is also a developing area of research (Reynolds-May et al. 2014; Teatero et al. 2014). Women with BD are more likely than healthy control subjects to retrospectively report menstrual abnormalities early in the reproductive years that predate the onset of BD (Joffe et al. 2006; Rasgon et al. 2000). Medications used to treat BD also may adversely affect the hypothalamic-pituitary-gonadal (HPG) axis, resulting in menstrual and other hormonal abnormalities (Kenna et al. 2009). Valproate has been the mood stabilizer most strongly linked to HPG dysfunction. A study by Joffe et al. (2006) showed that 10% of women with BD treated with valproate developed oligomenorrhea with hyperandrogenism. It is important therefore to monitor women with BD for menstrual and hormonal abnormalities. Encourage patients to record monthly onset of their cycles (particularly in the first several months after starting a new pharmacological agent), which will help them detect more subtle abnormalities or changes. Women with BD should also be educated about signs of hormonal dysfunction, such as virilization and changes in the menstrual cycle (Kenna et al. 2009). All women of reproductive age who are treated with valproate must be counseled about the risks of valproate exposure in pregnancy (as detailed later) and the need for adequate contraception.

To date, there are few studies of the treatment of exacerbation of mood symptoms in the premenstruum in patients with BD. For women who do not have contraindications to oral contraception (see Chapter 4, "Contraception"), suppression of the HPG axis with an oral contraceptive may be considered. To date, limited existing studies suggest that oral contraceptives are not associated with destabilization of mood in BD (Pagano et al. 2016). Case studies and small observational studies have also reported that lamotrigine may be an especially useful mood stabilizer to consider in this subpopulation of women with BD. Women receiving lamotrigine therapy are reported to have fewer menstrual cycle mood fluctuations than women receiving other mood stabilizers, and lamotrigine and oral contraceptives appear to be an especially useful combination (Robakis et al. 2015). When using this combination, be aware that lamotrigine levels are likely to decrease during the active oral contraceptive pill weeks because estradiol increases the clearance of lamotrigine via induction of hepatic glucuronidation (Reddy 2010). Changes in the pharmacokinetics of mood stabilizers across the menstrual cycle should also be considered in the differential diagnosis of women with BD with premenstrual mood exacerbations, although to date studies regarding the influence of the menstrual cycle on lithium and valproate metabolism are limited (Carmassi et al. 2019).

**Menopause.** Most women with BD will experience menopause, yet the clinical disease course during this transition remains understudied. In the general population, mood symptoms are common but not universal during perimenopause and can include irritability, anxiety, depression, lability, and difficulty with concentration and sleep (Minuzzi et al. 2012). Marsh et al. (2008) monitored mood symptoms of women with BD ages 45–55 and found that the frequency of depressive episodes increased during perimenopause relative to the patients' report of their disease course in reproductive years. In a prospective study of women with BD at various stages of menopause, greater depression and mood elevation symptoms were reported during late menopause and early postmenopause relative to reproductive age or early menopause, supporting the theory that a subset of women likely has a sensitivity to fluctuations in reproductive hormones rather than to the absolute reproductive hormone levels (Marsh et al. 2015). Importantly, women with major depressive disorder who experience illness exacerbation during the menopausal transition have an increased risk of diagnostic conversion to BD compared with women with a history of depression who remain stable during perimenopause (Chen et al. 2017). To date, no studies have been published of specific treatment recommendations for women with BD during the menopausal transition. Sleep disturbance is a well-known potential precipitant for mood destabilization, and many perimenopausal women experience sleep disturbances, so early intervention for sleep disturbances (and contributing factors, such as hot flashes) is recommended.

**Preconception.** The potential for pregnancy introduces an additional level of complexity in the psychiatric management of women with BD. Approximately 50% of pregnancies in the United States are unplanned, and women with BD are even more likely to have unplanned pregnancy than women in the general population (Finer and Zolna 2016; Marengo et al. 2015). Many commonly used mood stabilizers carry a risk of teratogenicity at the earliest stages of fetal development; thus, it is critical that discussions about family planning occur early in the treatment of any woman of reproductive age as part of routine care. Psychiatrists should inquire about all women's obstetrical history, plans for pregnancy, and contraceptive practices and preferences. Women with BD should be counseled about the risk of hypersexuality or high-risk sexual behaviors as a component of mania, as well as about the availability of long-acting reversible contraceptive options and methods to protect against sexually transmitted infections.

When prescribing medication treatment, potential teratogenic effects should be included in any discussion with women of reproductive age. Patients should be encouraged to engage proactively in preconception planning in collaboration with the treating psychiatrist. Preconception planning is more fully discussed in Chapter 8, "A Clinical Approach to Psychiatric Diagnosis and Treatment During Pregnancy," but should include consideration of risks related to the underlying disease and the risks of clinically indicated pharmacological treatments. Comorbid substance use disorders or medical conditions should also be discussed. A desire for pregnancy may provide an important opportunity to encourage healthy behaviors and adherence to treatment.

**Pregnancy and Postpartum.** The onset of mood episodes in women with BD has been strongly associated with reproductive events. In one study of 887 mothers with BD, 28% experienced their first lifetime episode of BD in relation to childbirth (Di Florio et al. 2018). Current evidence suggests that pregnancy is not protective against mood episodes for women with BD, and the postpartum period has been identified as particularly high risk. Women with BD are seven times as likely to experience a first-time psychiatric admission and twice as likely to experience a psychiatric readmission in the first postpartum month as women in the general population (Terp and Mortensen 1998). Viguera et al. (2000) found that, among women with BD who discontinued lithium maintenance, pregnant women had a rate of recurrence similar to that of nonpregnant women over a 9-month period (52% and 58%), and postpartum women had an increased risk of recurrence nearly three times that of nonpregnant women (70% vs. 24%). Findings from Di Florio et al. (2014) indicate that mood episodes were more likely to occur during the postpartum period for BDI (91.4%) and BDII (81.6%) as com-

TABLE 15–3. **Risks of untreated bipolar disorder during pregnancy**

| Risks to maternal health | Obstetrical complications | Risks to neonatal health |
|---|---|---|
| Decreased compliance with prenatal care | Antepartum hemorrhage | Adverse neurodevelopmental outcomes |
| Increased rates of obesity or overweight | Higher rate of cesarean sections | Low birth weight |
| Increased rates of substance abuse | Intrauterine growth restriction | Neonatal hypoglycemia |
| Increased risk of postpartum psychosis | Placental abnormalities | Preterm birth (<37 weeks) |
| Increased risk of suicide* | Poor prenatal follow-up | Small for gestational age infant |
| Risky or impulsive behaviors | Preeclampsia | Smaller head circumference |

*Suicide is one of the leading causes of maternal death in the peripartum and accounts for approximately 20% of postpartum deaths.

pared with during pregnancy. During the postpartum period, most episodes among women with BDI and BDII occurred within the first 4 weeks (80% and 53% respectively), and women with BDI experienced a shorter latency for manic and psychotic episodes than for episodes of nonpsychotic depression.

Postpartum psychosis (PPP) is a rare but serious condition typically considered to be a psychiatric emergency. Although PPP may occur outside of the setting of BD, there is a close link between BD and this distinct clinical syndrome. For a large percentage of women who experience PPP, the episode can be understood as either a first episode or a recurrence of an underlying BD (Wesseloo et al. 2016). A personal or family history of BD is one of the greatest risk factors for PPP (Bergink et al. 2016; Jones and Craddock 2001). For a thorough discussion of PPP, including its clinical presentation, epidemiology, and treatment, please see Chapter 16,"Postpartum Psychosis."

Decisions regarding maintenance medications in pregnant women with BD strongly influence the risk of recurrence. One prospective cohort study examined the risk of mood episode recurrence in pregnancy among women with BD who were euthymic at conception. Women who discontinued mood stabilizer treatment experienced twice as many episodes of recurrence as those who continued maintenance treatment. Women who discontinued medication quickly (over a period of <2 weeks), experienced a more rapid relapse as opposed to those who tapered mood stabilizer medication more gradually. Most mood episodes were characterized as major depression, followed by mixed state, hypomania, and mania (Viguera et al. 2007).

## Risk of Untreated Bipolar Disorder During Pregnancy

Maternal, obstetrical, and fetal risks related to BD are many and are summarized in Table 15–3. Careful consideration of these factors prior to conception and during periods of mood stability allow for the patient and her psychiatrist to form a collaborative treatment plan that optimizes the health of both the patient and the fetus. Although it is always the patient's decision when or whether to try to conceive, sensitive inquiry into reproductive planning by the psychiatrist may encourage the pa-

**TABLE 15–4. Differential diagnosis of manic episodes**

| | |
|---|---|
| Anatomical lesions (e.g., carcinoid) | Neurological conditions (e.g., multiple sclerosis, Huntington's disease) |
| Delirium | Other psychiatric conditions |
| Epilepsy (e.g., complex partial seizures) | ADHD |
| Frontotemporal dementia | Borderline personality disorder |
| Infectious disease (e.g., viral encephalitis) | PTSD |
| Medication induced (e.g., L-dopa, thyroxine, corticosteroids) | Substance use disorder (e.g., cocaine, hallucinogens) |
| Metabolic or endocrine disorders (e.g., hyperthyroidism, Wilson's disease, Cushing's disease) | Traumatic brain injury |

tient to share her plans in an ongoing way and to work with her provider to develop a plan that best balances associated risks.

### Differential Diagnosis

Even when presenting during times of reproductive events, BD is diagnosed based on a thorough psychiatric history. The differential diagnosis includes unipolar depression, especially anxious phenotype, as well as other illnesses with some overlapping mood symptoms, including PTSD and borderline personality disorder. Additionally, intoxication or withdrawal from substances such as cocaine or alcohol can mimic affective episodes, and therefore substance use disorders should also be considered. Aside from psychiatric illness, many medical illnesses (e.g., thyroid disorders) and medications (e.g., steroids) may also cause mood symptoms and therefore should be included in the differential diagnosis (Roberts 2019). See Table 15–4 for additional differential diagnostic considerations in the setting of acute mania (Freudenreich et al. 2019).

## Pathophysiology

Clinical and epidemiological research has demonstrated that times of hormonal fluctuation place women with BD at greater risk for relapse (Frey and Dias 2014; Gogos et al. 2019). This suggests that reproductive hormones such as estradiol and progesterone play significant roles in the pathophysiology of BD, and perinatal BD in particular. Unfortunately, there is a paucity of direct research on specific mechanisms underlying BD in the perinatal period. The reason for this might be the difficulty in understanding the pathophysiology of BD in general. Although many psychiatric disorders likely have multiple biological pathways that lead to similar symptomatic manifestations, this might be particularly true for BD (Maletic and Raison 2014). As such, current research suggests a diverse set of neurobiological aberrations in BD, including genetic and epigenetic factors, inflammation and oxidative stress, circadian rhythm abnormalities, differences in brain networks regulating emotion, and impairments in neuronal signaling and plasticity (Maletic and Raison 2014; Muneer 2016; Newberg et al. 2008). In this section, we provide a brief review of research on the pathophysiology of BD, focusing on potential interactions with reproductive hormones.

BD is known to have one of the largest genetic components of all psychiatric disorders, with heritability as high as 90% (Craddock and Sklar 2013). Despite this, genetic studies, including genome-wide association studies, have failed to find reliably specific genes that are definitively linked to the disorder, suggesting that it is a polygenic condition (Craddock and Sklar 2013; McMahon et al. 2010). Repeated identification of polymorphisms in L-type calcium channel genes has garnered significant attention, and this is particularly relevant given that some calcium channel blockers (including lamotrigine) can be effective mood stabilizers. Furthermore, at higher levels, estradiol can block L-type calcium channels (Vega-Vela et al. 2017), suggesting a mechanism by which low levels might lead to mood instability.

A number of studies have found increased levels of inflammatory cytokines in patients with BD, both in the periphery and postmortem in areas of the prefrontal cortex (Maletic and Raison 2014; Rosenblat and McIntyre 2016; Thomas et al. 2004). Such inflammatory changes are associated with suppressed neuroplasticity and with changes in monoaminergic transmission (Raison et al. 2006). Both estradiol and progesterone are known to have anti-inflammatory effects, decreasing cytokines in the CNS; however, this has yet to be studied directly in BD (Frey and Dias 2014; De Nicola et al. 2018).

Like many psychiatric disorders, uncontrolled BD can have neurodegenerative effects that are likely mediated by increases in oxidative stress, excitotoxicity, and suppression of neurotrophic factors (Maletic and Raison 2014; Muneer 2016; Newberg et al. 2008). This can be seen anatomically, with increases in lateral ventricle size that correspond with the number of manic episodes (Strakowski et al. 2002). Estrogens and progestins have well-known neuroprotective effects, such as increasing brain-derived neurotrophic factor (Heberden 2017; Singh and Su 2013) and protecting against oxidative stress and excitotoxicity (Frey and Dias 2014; Irwin et al. 2008; Numakawa et al. 2011), which emphasizes a potential modulating role of these steroids in bipolar pathophysiology.

Overall, current research has yet to elucidate a definitive or unique pathophysiology of BD during the perinatal period. For BD as a whole, various interrelated mechanisms likely contribute to the episodic disturbances in mood that characterize this illness. Furthermore, estrogens and progestins appear to have an overall protective effect on pathophysiological processes associated with BD, such as inflammation, oxidative stress, and suppression of neuroplasticity. Thus, when these hormones are in flux during the perinatal period (and during other reproductive transitions), a pathophysiological disinhibition may occur, placing women at greater risk for bipolar episodes.

## Treatment

### Pharmacology in Pregnancy

Pharmacological intervention is a critical component in the management of acute bipolar illness and in the prevention of recurrent mood episodes. Treatment of BD in the perinatal period requires balancing risks associated with untreated illness against risks of medication exposure. In this section, we review risk profiles of available treatments for BD in pregnancy, highlighting risk of congenital malformations, obstetrical outcomes, and neonatal and neurodevelopmental outcomes, as well as key elements

**TABLE 15–5. Agents with favorable balance between efficacy and reassuring safety data for treatment of acute episodes of bipolar disorder during pregnancy**

| Acute manic episode | Acute depressive episode |
|---|---|
| Aripiprazole | Lamotrigine |
| Haloperidol | Lithium |
| Lithium | Quetiapine |
| Quetiapine | |

*Note.* Decisions should always be focused on minimizing risk after considering an individual patient's presentation and treatment history.

of management during pregnancy. Because no risk-free option exists in this treatment setting, the focus is necessarily on minimizing risks after consideration of the patient's unique presentation, illness course, previous treatment responses, and social supports.

Lithium is one of the most established treatments in BD, with efficacy in all phases of the disease and recent evidence supporting its efficacy in prophylaxis of postpartum mood episodes (Bergink et al. 2012; Yatham et al. 2018). Although early research emphasized the potential for teratogenicity with lithium, growing evidence regarding its safety profile (reviewed in detail later) supports its use in women who are unlikely to achieve or maintain euthymia with lamotrigine or antipsychotic medication monotherapy. Although valproate is a foundation of treatment in general for BD, especially for mixed states, it is rarely considered a treatment option prior to or during pregnancy due to its high teratogenic risk and considerable concern about neurodevelopmental outcomes in exposed infants (Yatham et al. 2018).

In the setting of acute mania in pregnancy, the treating psychiatrist might also consider quetiapine or aripiprazole, given the efficacy of each of these medications in treating acute manic episodes and its reassuring (although limited) safety information during pregnancy (Huybrechts et al. 2016). Other experts favor haloperidol due to its more developed reproductive safety data (see Chapter 17, "Schizophrenia and Related Disorders,") (Epstein et al. 2014). For acute bipolar depression during pregnancy, lamotrigine is often considered a preferred agent due to its reassuring safety profile and evidence for efficacy in bipolar depression in the general population (Epstein et al. 2014). Quetiapine has efficacy to support its use in acute bipolar depression, as well as a limited but reassuring safety profile in pregnancy (Huybrechts et al. 2016). Although lurasidone has evidence to support its use in bipolar depression in the general population, data regarding its safety in pregnancy are limited relative to many second-generation antipsychotics. Table 15–5 provides a summary of agents that generally show a favorable balance between efficacy and reassuring safety data for treatment of acute episodes of BD during pregnancy. Clinical treatment plans should aim to minimize risk after considering an individual patient's presentation and treatment history.

In the setting of maintenance treatment for patients who are not acutely symptomatic, the severity of the patient's disease course prior to presentation should be a primary consideration. A history of inpatient hospitalization, frequent or recent mood episodes, psychotic symptoms associated with mood episodes, suicidal ideation or attempts, medication failures, and previous attempts to taper medications should be considered in the analysis of disease severity and the necessity of medication during pregnancy. If the patient has a history limited to mild or remote symptoms, a gradual medication taper with close monitoring may be considered. In this case, a recurrence of symptoms should prompt the patient and physician to reevaluate her need for medication. Women with moderate or severe symptoms should be considered for ongoing maintenance pharmacotherapy with the agent that best balances efficacy with risk (Yonkers et al. 2004). Some women might elect to switch to a medication with a more favorable reproductive risk profile before or during pregnancy, but any plan to change a medication regimen should take into account the anticipated effectiveness of the treatment options, the inherent risk of relapse in the setting of medication changes, and, in the setting of switching during pregnancy, the risk of multiple medication exposures across fetal development. Figure 15–1 provides a useful algorithm to guide decision making around maintenance treatment prior to and during pregnancy.

Once the decision is made to use a medication during pregnancy, awareness of pregnancy-related pharmacokinetic changes and the potential need for dosage adjustments is an important component of care that may further reduce risk of relapse and avoid unintentional supratherapeutic dosing. Therapeutic drug monitoring can complement close clinical monitoring. For medications without a standardized therapeutic range, a woman's individual level at a point of euthymia will allow the physician to establish a target medication level throughout and after pregnancy (Deligiannidis et al. 2014). General tenets of prescribing during pregnancy are described further in Chapter 8.

Ms. W is a 32-year-old woman with a history of BDII who was referred by her obstetrician for a consultation at a reproductive psychiatry practice. She is currently pregnant, at 34 weeks' gestation. Her current medications include a prenatal vitamin and lamotrigine 200 mg daily. Although her pregnancy has been medically uncomplicated, she reports increasing depressive symptoms over the past month. She describes feeling depressed most of each day, takes hours to fall asleep at night, and is not feeling motivated to do her normal activities (i.e., cooking, nightly walks with her partner, preparing the baby's room). Ms. W states that although she is not having suicidal thoughts, she does notice that her worldview has become more negative in recent weeks, and she spends a lot of her time doubting her ability to be a "good mom" to her baby.

Ms. W reports that previous trials of antidepressants (i.e., selective serotonin reuptake inhibitors and serotonin-norepinephrine reuptake inhibitors) have not been effective and in many cases "made things worse." Prior to pregnancy, she was treated effectively with lamotrigine 150 mg/day for 3 years. Her treating psychiatrist increased her lamotrigine dose to 200 mg/day after onset of these symptoms 3 weeks ago. However, because she is now on the maximum dose of lamotrigine, he has informed her that there is no more he can do pharmacologically to treat her depression. Ms.W tells the reproductive psychiatrist, "I am so worried that this will get worse. I don't want to have postpartum depression, have trouble bonding with my baby, or do something to hurt myself or my baby. I'm really freaked out and feel like I need help!"

## Lithium

Lithium is a first-line medication for BD, with an evidence base for acute and maintenance treatment of manic and depressive symptoms (Munk-Olsen et al. 2018). It also has established antisuicidal properties and emerging evidence to support its use in the treatment and prevention of PPP in women at elevated risk (Bergink et al. 2012; Poels et al. 2018).

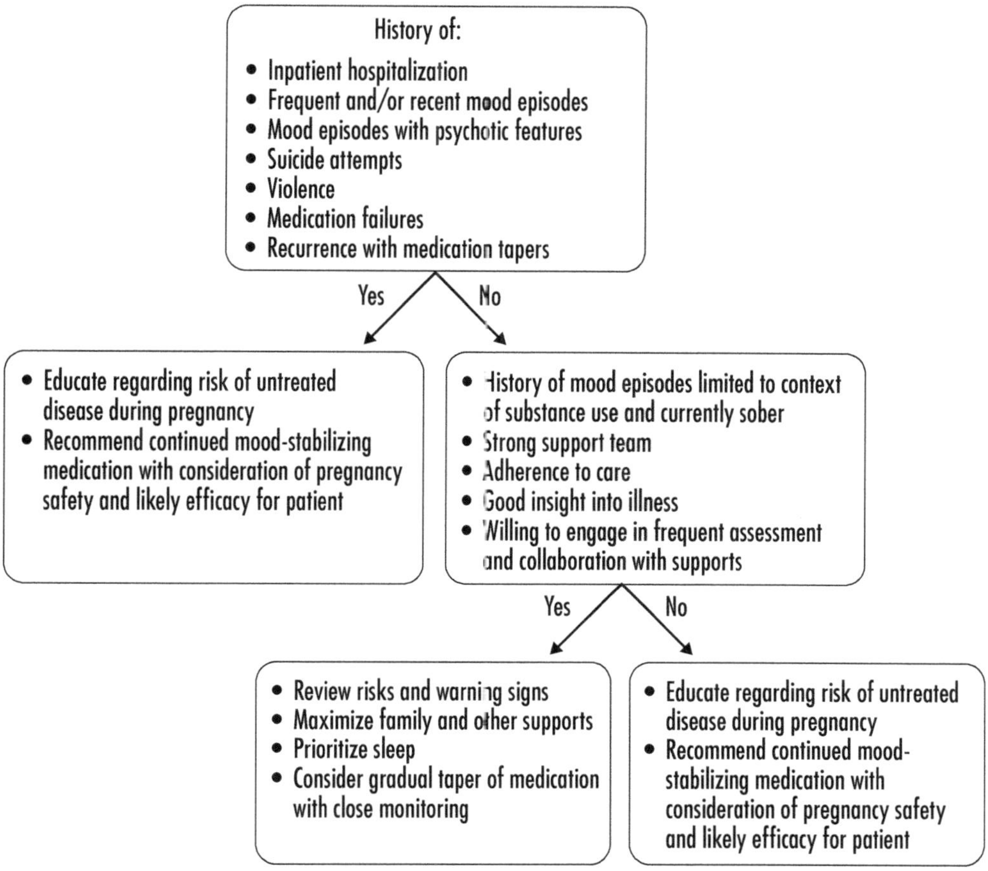


**FIGURE 15–1. Maintenance medication treatment algorithm.**
In this setting, the severity of the patient's disease course prior to presentation is a primary consideration.

**Early pregnancy.** A strong association between in utero lithium exposure and congenital heart defects was first proposed in the 1970s based on reports from The International Register of Lithium Babies, an international registry of infants born to women treated with lithium in the first trimester of pregnancy (Cohen et al. 1994). Publications from this registry suggested that Ebstein's anomaly, a rare right ventricular outflow defect involving downward displacement of the tricuspid valve, was 400 times more common in infants with first-trimester lithium exposure than in the general population (occurring in 6 of the 225 reported births), thus establishing lithium as a human teratogen (Epstein et al. 2014). Not until 20 years later was the strength of this association critically questioned by Cohen et al. (1994), who suggested an overestimation of risk due to the registry's retrospective enrollment of voluntarily submitted cases and lack of a control group.

Several more recent large-scale studies have provided further clarity on the risk of malformations with first-trimester lithium exposure. In 2017, Patorno and colleagues published a U.S. cohort study that included 1,325,563 pregnancies, of which 663 were exposed to lithium and 1,945 were exposed to lamotrigine. They found an adjusted risk ratio for cardiac malformations among infants with first-trimester lithium exposure of

1.65 (95% CI 1.02–2.68). This risk was dose dependent, with those who were receiving more than 900 mg/day at the highest risk (RR 3.22; 95% CI 1.47–7.02) (Patorno et al. 2017). The following year, Munk-Olsen et al. (2018) completed a large meta-analysis that compared 727 lithium-exposed pregnancies with 21,397 reference pregnancies in mothers with a mood disorder. Although this study found an overall increase in malformation of any kind (adjusted OR 1.71; 95% CI 1.07–2.72), it did not find a statistically significant difference in the rate of cardiac malformations between the two groups (Munk-Olsen et al. 2018).

In 2019, another large-scale meta-analysis ($N$=1,349,563 pregnancies) had similar findings (Fornaro et al. 2020). This study also found an increased risk of overall malformations for lithium-exposed infants (OR 1.81; 95% CI 1.35–2.41). Although the risk of cardiac malformations was increased in lithium-exposed infants when compared with unexposed control subjects (OR 1.86; 95% CI 1.16–2.96), when the comparison group was women with affective disorders, the difference was not statistically significant (OR 1.59; 95% CI 0.91–2.77). Cumulatively, these data suggest that although lithium may indeed have an association with cardiac or overall malformations, this risk occurs at a much lower magnitude than previously postulated. Although the overestimation of risk in previous decades was likely largely due to methodological research challenges, it is likely that the underlying illness is also a confounding factor.

Although less is known about the risk of spontaneous abortion associated with lithium use in pregnancy, recent data raise the possibility of increased risk. A 2014 study reported an increased rate of spontaneous abortion among women with BD who were taking lithium during pregnancy compared with a random selection of women who called a teratology information service regarding exposures not known to be teratogenic (adjusted OR 1.94; 95% CI 1.08–3.48). This was investigated as a secondary endpoint in a study for which malformations were the primary outcome of interest (Diav-Citrin et al. 2014). In 2020, Poels and colleagues examined pregnancy outcomes among women with BDI for whom data about medication use were available. In this sample of 443 women, spontaneous abortion occurred more often in lithium-exposed pregnancies compared with pregnancies not exposed to lithium; both groups comprised women with verified BDI. Although the authors noted that the study and control groups did not differ in age of illness onset (one indicator of disease severity in patients with BD), the medications utilized in the control group during pregnancy, acute mood episodes during pregnancy, and additional measures of disease severity were not reported. Thus, underlying illness remains a potential confounder (Poels et al. 2020).

**Obstetrical outcomes.** Lithium has not been found to increase the risk of preeclampsia, gestational diabetes, rates of cesarean delivery, preterm birth, low birth weight, or postpartum hemorrhage when women taking it have been compared with disease-matched control subjects (Fornaro et al. 2020; Munk-Olsen et al. 2018). Two case reports describe polyhydramnios in women taking lithium during pregnancy (Poels et al. 2018).

**Neonatal outcomes.** Neonatal effects associated with lithium use in the second and third trimester of pregnancy include reversible neonatal hypothyroidism, goiter, nephrogenic diabetes insipidus, and cardiac arrhythmias (Kozma 2005). In addition, high infant lithium concentrations at birth can be associated with respiratory difficulties, hypotonicity, poor suck and grasp, lethargy, and tremor (Epstein et al. 2014). Typically, these symptoms resolve in 1–2 weeks without intervention, but infants with signs of toxicity may require intensive monitoring. Lithium exposure during pregnancy has been associated with higher rates of neonatal hospital admission (Munk-Olsen et al. 2018).

**Long-term effects.** Limited data show that in-utero exposure to lithium does not adversely affect IQ scores (Forsberg et al. 2018).

**Management during pregnancy.** Lithium freely crosses the placental barrier and thus maternal lithium therapy does result in fetal exposure (Poels et al. 2018). Excretion of lithium occurs almost exclusively via the kidneys; thus, its pharmacokinetics are influenced considerably by intravascular volume and glomerular filtration rate (GFR). Lithium has an established therapeutic drug level of 0.6–1.2 mEq/L, representing a narrow therapeutic index. During pregnancy, as renal blood flow, GFR, and plasma volume increase, the clearance of lithium increases by 30%–50%, causing plasma levels to decrease substantially. The decline in lithium serum level presents a risk for illness recurrence. After delivery, lithium clearance quickly returns to pre-pregnancy levels (Deligiannidis et al. 2014). No consensus has been reached on how frequently to monitor lithium levels in pregnancy, but levels should be checked regularly throughout pregnancy and anytime the patient is at risk for dehydration (e.g., hyperemesis gravidarum) or has impaired renal function (e.g., preeclampsia). For routine monitoring, one common strategy is to check the patient's lithium level monthly starting early in pregnancy, then weekly starting 4 weeks prior to expected delivery. Split daily dosing of lithium can serve to minimize peak serum levels and thus theoretically reduce teratogenic risk (Wesseloo et al. 2017).

Close monitoring of maternal serum lithium levels proximal to delivery is critical, and adequate hydration should be provided if labor is prolonged. Although some experts recommend cessation of lithium 24–48 hours prior to a scheduled cesarean delivery or at onset of labor as a strategy to mitigate the risk of neonatal toxicity, no current evidence supports that this strategy decreases the risk of complication in the infant, and thus any management plan should also include consideration of risk of relapse postpartum (Molenaar et al. 2020; Poels et al. 2018). It is prudent to measure a postpartum lithium level approximately 24 hours after delivery and to consider restarting the patient on the pre-pregnancy lithium dosage after delivery if the dosage has been increased incrementally during pregnancy (Deligiannidis et al. 2014) because a quick return to baseline GFR and rapid decrease in plasma volume in the postpartum period can place the patient at risk of toxicity.

Women who are maintained on lithium during pregnancy should have periodic monitoring of their thyroid and renal function. Nephrotoxic medication and nonsteroidal anti-inflammatory medications should be avoided (Khan et al. 2016). Although the recent evidence summarized here has questioned the association between lithium and cardiac malformations, it is recommended that women maintained on lithium in the first trimester have a high-resolution ultrasound and fetal echocardiography at 16–20 weeks' gestation to evaluate for cardiac malformations (Poels et al. 2018). Due to the risk of neonatal symptoms, some experts recommend that women maintained on lithium in late pregnancy deliver in a hospital setting with access to high-level neonatology services. An umbilical cord blood sample should be obtained for measurement of infant lithium level and thyroid function (Poels et al. 2018). See Figure 15–2 for a visual representation of management considerations of lithium throughout the perinatal period.

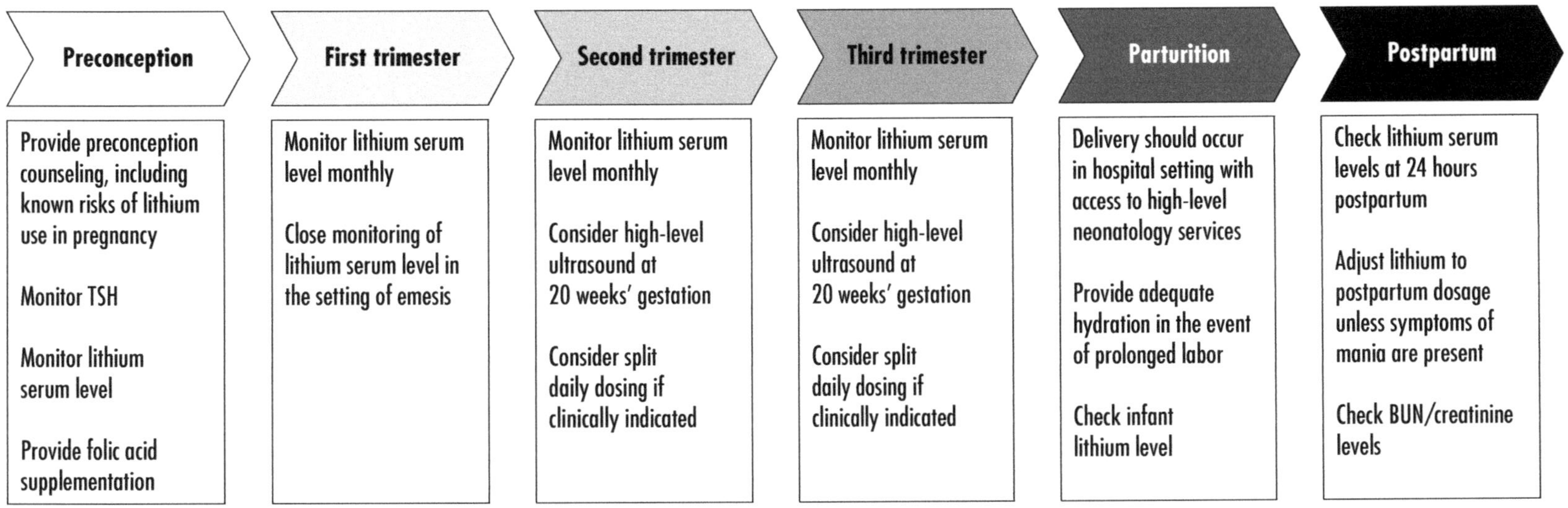


**FIGURE 15–2.** Lithium in pregnancy.
BUN=blood urea nitrogen; TSH=thyroid-stimulating hormone.

## Lamotrigine

Lamotrigine is an antiepileptic drug approved by the FDA for treatment of bipolar depression and maintenance treatment of BD. Lamotrigine does not have evidence to support its use in acute mania (Yatham et al. 2018). Lamotrigine's relative reproductive safety and emerging evidence base in the perinatal period make it an emerging first-line option for treatment of BD during pregnancy, particularly in women with a preponderance of depressive episodes. A small naturalistic study showed that lamotrigine was effective in preventing symptom relapse during pregnancy and the postpartum period when women with BD were continued on the drug during pregnancy (Prakash et al. 2016). A population-based cohort study found that lamotrigine was as effective as lithium in preventing postpartum relapse in women with BD; this study, however, was limited by its small number of participants and observational design (Wesseloo et al. 2017). Because participants in this study with a history of acute mania were more likely to be taking lithium, whereas participants with a vulnerability toward depressive episodes were more likely to be taking lamotrigine, the results should be understood in the context of potential confounding by indication.

**Early pregnancy.** Although an initial publication from the North American Antiepileptic Pregnancy Registry reported a small increased risk for oral clefts in 684 infants exposed to lamotrigine in the first trimester (Holmes et al. 2008), more recently, a population-based case-control study of 10.1 million births did not observe an association between lamotrigine in pregnancy and overall malformation, including no increased risk of cleft palate (Dolk et al. 2016). This large study is consistent with several international registries that reported no elevated risk of malformations with lamotrigine use in the first trimester (Campbell et al. 2014; Cunnington et al. 2005; Tomson et al. 2018).

**Obstetrical outcomes.** A recent systematic review and meta-analysis did not find an increase in rates of spontaneous abortions, stillbirths, preterm deliveries, or small for gestational age infants with exposure to lamotrigine in pregnancy (Pariente et al. 2017).

**Neonatal outcomes.** Lamotrigine exposure during pregnancy has not been associated with adverse neonatal effects (Epstein et al. 2014).

**Long-term effects.** Available data on infant neurodevelopmental outcomes demonstrate no significant concerns on cognitive scores (Baker et al. 2015; Epstein et al. 2014; Meador et al. 2013).

**Management during pregnancy.** Lamotrigine is metabolized almost completely via glucuronic acid conjugation to its inactive metabolite in the liver. Estradiol upregulates hepatic glucuronidation; thus, rising estradiol levels across pregnancy result in increased clearance of lamotrigine and decreased serum lamotrigine concentrations (Clark et al. 2013). The metabolism of lamotrigine increases as early as 8 weeks' gestation, continues progressively into the third trimester, then declines precipitously over the first 2 weeks postpartum. Although individual variability exists, lamotrigine clearance potentially increases more than 300% throughout pregnancy (Deligiannidis et al. 2014). Because the therapeutic serum concentration range for lamotrigine maintenance treatment of BD is not defined, a preconception trough serum lamotrigine level can help guide dosage in pregnancy. Once a baseline level is obtained, some recommend monitoring the level monthly and increasing the dose by 20%–25% to maintain the patient's baseline serum level or in conjunction with clinical symptoms (Clark et al. 2013).

In the absence of a reference preconception lamotrigine level, dosage adjustments should be guided by clinical presentation. If the lamotrigine dosage is increased in pregnancy, it should be decreased in the postpartum period, with close monitoring to avoid toxicity (Deligiannidis et al. 2014). Some experts recommend an immediate postpartum decrease of 25%, with further decreases every 3–4 days until pre-pregnancy dosing is reached (Clark and Wisner 2018). Symptoms of toxicity include dizziness, ataxia, and blurred vision. There is preliminary evidence in favor of split daily dosing in pregnancy (Clark et al. 2016). See Figure 15–3 for a visual representation of management considerations of lamotrigine throughout the perinatal period.

## Valproate

Valproate is an antiepileptic drug with a wide spectrum of efficacy in BD. Although it has the strongest evidence to support its use in acute mania, efficacy has been established for its use in acute bipolar depression and in maintenance treatment of BD. Due to valproate's substantial teratogenic and neurodevelopmental risks, the FDA and European Medicine Agency recommend that it be avoided in women of reproductive age if alternative therapies are available and effective. If valproate must be used in women of reproductive age, contraception is advised, and adequate documentation of its clinical justification and discussion of risks is recommended (Khan et al. 2016).

**Early pregnancy.** Valproate is considered a human teratogen. Exposure to valproate in pregnancy is associated with a significant increase in the risk of congenital malformations and adverse neurodevelopmental effects, a risk that exceeds that of other antiepileptics and mood stabilizers. The risk of major malformations has been reported to be 5%–11% with first-trimester valproate monotherapy (Campbell et al. 2014; Diav-Citrin et al. 2008; Epstein et al. 2014; Tomson et al. 2018; Weston et al. 2016) and includes neural tube defects, craniofacial defects, cardiovascular anomalies, skeletal and limb malformations, and genitourinary defects. The risk has been found to be dose dependent, rising significantly (up to 20-fold) with daily doses over 1,000 mg (Diav-Citrin et al. 2008; Epstein et al. 2014; Morrow et al. 2006).

**Obstetrical outcomes.** Literature on the reproductive risk of valproate has focused heavily on congenital malformations and neurodevelopmental outcomes. There are no consistent reports of increased risk of obstetrical adverse outcomes, such as spontaneous abortion or preterm delivery. Although intrauterine growth restriction has been associated with valproate, this is typically associated with the "valproate syndrome," which also includes skeletal and limb malformations (Epstein et al. 2014).

**Neonatal outcomes.** Antenatal valproate exposure has been associated with increased risk of neonatal heart rate decelerations, hypoglycemia, hepatotoxicity, low fibrinogen levels, abnormal tone, and feeding difficulties (Yonkers et al. 2004).

**Long-term effects.** Higher rates of developmental delay, reduced IQ scores, learning difficulties, impaired verbal abilities, and autistic spectrum disorder (ASD) have been consistently associated with valproate exposure and appear to be dose dependent (Baker et al. 2015; Bromley et al. 2013; Meador et al. 2013).

| Preconception | First trimester | Second trimester | Third trimester | Postpartum |
|---|---|---|---|---|
| Provide preconception counseling, including known risks of lamotrigine use in pregnancy<br><br>Note lamotrigine level to establish therapeutic range for patient<br><br>Provide folic acid supplementation | Monitor clinical symptoms closely<br><br>Check lamotrigine level if clinically indicated<br><br>Increase lamotrigine as needed | Monitor clinical symptoms closely<br><br>Check lamotrigine level if clinically indicated<br><br>Increase lamotrigine as needed | Monitor clinical symptoms closely<br><br>Check lamotrigine level if clinically indicated<br><br>Increase lamotrigine as needed | If lamotrigine level has increased during pregnancy, decrease dosage by 25% every 3–4 days until pre-pregnancy dosage is reached |

**FIGURE 15–3.** Lamotrigine in pregnancy.

**Management during pregnancy.** Preconception valproate levels can help guide dosage adjustments in pregnancy, and the lowest effective dosage should be used. The metabolism of valproate is complex because it is metabolized by glucuronidation and oxidation. Valproate is also highly protein bound; its pharmacological activity is, however, dependent on the free or unbound drug, which is able to cross the blood-brain barrier. Importantly, although an increase in the clearance of valproate and an overall decrease in plasma concentration of the medication have been observed in late pregnancy, no significant changes have been found in the unbound (active) concentration of the medication. To monitor valproate levels accurately during pregnancy, both free and total plasma levels should be measured (Deligiannidis et al. 2014).

## Carbamazepine

Carbamazepine is an antiepileptic drug that has traditionally been considered an alternative agent in the treatment of BD rather than as a first-line mood stabilizer. Efficacy has been established in acute mania, with some evidence to support its use in maintenance treatment. Carbamazepine has limited evidence to support its efficacy in acute depression (Yatham et al. 2018). Most experts agree that carbamazepine should be used in pregnancy only when clearly clinically indicated above other alternatives, given its teratogenicity, less established efficacy profile, significant drug-drug interactions, and associated risk of neonatal hemorrhage (Yonkers et al. 2004).

**Early pregnancy.** Carbamazepine exposure prenatally has been associated with 5%–8% risk for major malformation, which is higher than the baseline risk of 3%–5% (Campbell et al. 2014; Tomson et al. 2018; Vajda et al. 2016). A recent report from an international antiepileptic drug registry showed that major malformation risk with carbamazepine exposure appears to be dose dependent, with more substantial risk at doses >700 mg/day (4.5% vs. 7.2%) (Tomson et al. 2018). Although overall malformation rates with first-trimester carbamazepine exposure are lower than corresponding rates with valproate, it is also considered a human teratogen (Yonkers et al. 2004). The most common malformations associated with exposure are neural tube defects, craniofacial abnormalities, and cardiac and urinary tract defects. Combination of carbamazepine with another antiepileptic drug further increases the risk of malformations (Margulis et al. 2019; Yonkers et al. 2004).

**Obstetrical outcomes.** Carbamazepine has been associated with small but significant reductions in birth weight and head circumference (Yonkers et al. 2004).

**Neonatal outcomes.** Carbamazepine use in late pregnancy has been associated with transient hepatic toxicity, coagulopathy, vitamin K deficiency, and low birth weight (Epstein et al. 2014; Yonkers et al. 2004).

**Long-term effects.** Studies examining neurodevelopmental outcomes in infants exposed to carbamazepine in utero have yielded mixed results and have not consistently shown a pattern of associated cognitive dysfunction (Epstein et al. 2014).

**Management during pregnancy.** Carbamazepine is metabolized hepatically via glucuronidation, conjugation, and hydroxylation. It induces the cytochrome P450 system and can affect the metabolism of coadministered agents. Some studies have reported a decline in total carbamazepine concentrations across pregnancy, but the concentration of free carbamazepine generally either shows a slight decline or remains at baseline (Deligiannidis et al. 2014). Because the measurement of total carbamazepine concentration may be misleading, both free and total concentrations should be monitored (Epstein et al. 2014). As with other mood stabilizers, dosage adjustments should be guided by clinical presentation, and the lowest effective dose should be used in pregnancy, with rapid reduction after delivery to pre-pregnancy levels. Vitamin K supplementation is recommended during pregnancy and should be administered intramuscularly to the newborn (Yonkers et al. 2004).

### Second-Generation Antipsychotics

Second-generation antipsychotics are prescribed for the management of BD at increasing rates, likely secondary to their FDA approval for the acute treatment of manic and depressive episodes, as well as for the maintenance treatment of BD (Yatham et al. 2018). For a comprehensive review of prescribing considerations of these agents in the perinatal period, see Chapter 17.

## Pharmacology in Lactation

The postpartum period is a time of substantially elevated risk for women with BD. Childbirth can also be a trigger for new onset of mood or psychotic symptoms in previously healthy women (Yonkers et al. 2004). When acute symptoms present in the postpartum period, a thorough assessment of safety should be the priority; if needed, inpatient admission should be recommended. For women with known BD or a personal history of PPP, prophylactic treatment in the immediate postpartum period is considered the standard of care (Bergink et al. 2012).

Because breastfeeding is associated with multiple well-established benefits for both mother and infant, many women with BD prefer to breastfeed their infants. Treating psychiatrists should discuss infant feeding preferences with a patient early in her pregnancy and regularly as the pregnancy progresses. Assuming the patient has capacity to make decisions about breastfeeding, the psychiatrist should provide available evidence about the risks and benefits of breastfeeding for the patient's specific situation and the associated risks of formula feeding versus indicated medications. If the patient has been treated with an efficacious medication during pregnancy, consideration should be given to continuing the effective medication, because switching medication during a high-risk period will not only introduce the infant to multiple exposures but also increase risk for symptom relapse for the patient.

When a woman with BD does aim to breastfeed her infant, the treating psychiatrist should proactively discuss a plan for maternal and infant monitoring that includes collaboration with the treating pediatrician and use of the lowest effective maternal medication dose. Information about available lactation services should be provided. Strategies to maximize sleep while breastfeeding should be discussed. These might include family members bringing the infant to feed at the breast at night and then assuming all other night care of the infant (i.e., changing diapers, burping, soothing back to sleep). For single mothers who live alone, such conversations should include strategizing about friends or family who might be able to come for extended visits. Once breastfeeding is established, the family member might bottle-feed the infant expressed breastmilk at night, allowing the patient uninterrupted sleep. Women with acute mania, psychosis, suicidality, or homicidality may not be capable of safely breastfeeding their infants. Inpatient hospitalization for any indication may also interrupt a patient's access to her infant and thus establishment of breastfeeding. In these cases, patients can be supported in pumping breastmilk if desired and clinically appropriate to preserve breastmilk production.

In some cases, women with BD might choose to formula-feed their infants, either due to personal preference or after a risk/benefit discussion with their psychiatrist, obstetrician, or pediatric physician. Mothers of infants with prematurity or other medical problems or women in need of polypharmacy treatment for BD may determine that the risks of medication exposure outweigh the benefits of breastfeeding. Women with a known sensitivity to sleep deprivation may determine that formula-feeding by a support person overnight to allow prolonged uninterrupted sleep is a critical need in achieving or maintaining euthymia. Psychiatrists and other providers should be supportive patients who choose to formula-feed because this decision often induces feelings of shame and guilt that can be inadvertently reinforced by medical providers or family members. Validating the patient's decision to make an informed decision and, when appropriate, to prioritize her own health in order to care for her baby can be a powerful intervention for a new mother during a vulnerable time.

Regardless of how the patient chooses to feed her infant, use of sedating medications (i.e., quetiapine, benzodiazepines) may present a safety concern. When such medications are prescribed, the patient should be instructed to exercise caution during feedings and to follow established safe sleep recommendations. Although the American Academy of Pediatrics universally recommends against parent–infant bed sharing due to the associated increased risk of sudden infant death syndrome, sedating medications are specifically noted to further increase this risk (Task Force on Sudden Infant Death Syndrome 2016).

Although the lactation profile of specific medications relevant to the treatment of BD is discussed later, further discussion of general tenets of prescribing during lactation are described in Chapter 1, "The Reproductive Life Cycle." Of note, the relative infant dose (RID) is an important consideration in the safety profile of medications during pregnancy, and the RID of relevant medications is provided in Table 15–6. An RID of <10% is generally considered acceptable in breastfeeding (Newton and Hale 2015).

## Lithium

Although historically, experts have recommended against breastfeeding while taking lithium, current data suggest that breastfeeding can be a safe option for women receiving lithium therapy who have a full-term infant, can readily adhere to frequent blood draws, and are capable of close monitoring of their infant's behaviors and alertness in collaboration with a pediatrician. Exposure to lithium through breastmilk is substantially less than via placental transfer. Reports of the RID are variable, ranging from 10% to 30%, but are generally higher than the accepted 10% value considered to be low risk (Newmark et al. 2019; Poels et al. 2018). Although numerous reports are available of infants breastfed by women receiving lithium therapy without signs of toxicity or adverse effects (Bogen et al. 2012; Moretti et al. 2003), data do suggest that lithium exposure through breastfeeding can cause adverse effects in cases of dehydration, prematurity, or impaired renal function. When lithium is prescribed to a breastfeeding woman, collaboration with and close monitoring by the pediatrician is recommended. If the mother's lithium dosage has been increased during pregnancy, maternal serum

**TABLE 15–6. Relative infant doses**

| Medication | Relative infant dose (RID)* |
|---|---|
| Aripiprazole | 1% |
| Carbamazepine | 3.8%–5.9% |
| Lamotrigine | 9.2%–18.27% |
| Lithium | 12%–30.1% |
| Lurasidone | No data |
| Olanzapine | 0.3%–2.2% |
| Quetiapine | 0.07%–0.1% |
| Risperidone | 2.8%–9.1% |
| Valproate | 0.99%–5.6% |
| Ziprasidone | 0.07%–1.2% |

*RID=infant dose via breastmilk (mg/kg/day) divided by maternal dose (mg/kg/day). An RID of <10% is generally considered acceptable in breastfeeding.

levels should be closely monitored postpartum to avoid toxicity. Monitoring of infant serum levels, blood urea nitrogen, creatinine, and thyroid-stimulating hormone is recommended when clinically indicated by sedation, feeding difficulties, restlessness, abnormal growth, or signs of dehydration.

## Lamotrigine

Breastfeeding with lamotrigine is associated with an estimated RID of 9.2%–18.3%, and lamotrigine is not a contraindication to breastfeeding in full-term healthy infants. Wide ranges of lamotrigine concentrations in infants are reported, likely due to interindividual variation in lamotrigine metabolism by mother and infant (Clark et al. 2013). Although most infants have not exhibited adverse reactions, adverse reactions in infants exposed to lamotrigine via breastfeeding have occasionally been reported. When lamotrigine is prescribed to a breastfeeding woman, maternal serum lamotrigine concentration should be monitored after delivery, and infants should be monitored for apnea, rash, drowsiness, or poor sucking. If clinically indicated, infant serum lamotrigine levels, platelet count, and liver function may be monitored (Clark and Wisner 2018). If an infant exposed to lamotrigine via breastmilk develops a rash, the mother should cease breastfeeding until the infant has been clinically evaluated and the source has been determined (Lactmed 2020). Limited data suggest no adverse effects on growth or development due to lamotrigine exposure through breastmilk (Meador et al. 2013).

## Valproate

Valproate has very low passage into breastmilk and is considered compatible with breastfeeding. Although no definite adverse reactions have been reported in infants exposed to valproate via breastmilk, one questionable case of thrombocytopenia has been reported, and there is a theoretical risk of hepatotoxicity. When valproate is prescribed to a breastfeeding woman, her infant should be monitored for jaundice, abnormal bleeding, and abnormal bruising. Monitoring of infant valproate levels, platelets, and liver enzymes may be performed if clinically indicated (Lactmed 2020).

## Carbamazepine

Carbamazepine has relatively high levels in breastmilk, but carbamazepine therapy is considered compatible with breastfeeding because few associated adverse effects have been reported. Although most infants exposed to carbamazepine have not had adverse reactions, sedation and problems with feeding have been reported. Hepatic dysfunction has been reported in three cases in the setting of additional intrauterine exposure and concurrent drug therapy, When carbamazepine is prescribed to a breastfeeding woman, her infant should be monitored for sedation, jaundice, and weight gain. If clinically indicated, infant carbamazepine level, liver enzymes, and complete blood count may be monitored (Lactmed 2020).

## Other Medication Treatment: Folic Acid

Since the 1970s, low plasma levels of folate have been linked with increased risk of neural tube defects (Smithells et al. 1976). To prevent this, the United States has required mandatory folic acid fortification of cereal grain since 1998, and the U.S. Preventive Services Task Force recommends that "all women planning for or capable of pregnancy" take 400–800 μg of folic acid daily (Bibbins-Domingo et al. 2017; Huhta and Linask 2015). Because neural tube formation begins early in pregnancy, preconception folate supplementation is critical, ideally beginning 1 month prior to conception and continuing through the first 3 months of pregnancy (Bibbins-Domingo et al. 2017).

Folic acid supplementation with 4 mg/day is strongly recommended for women of reproductive age who are maintained on valproate given its high teratogenic potential, although this strategy does not completely alleviate risk (Tomson et al. 2018). Rationale for higher-dosage folic acid supplementation with other antiepileptic medications remains uncertain. Because lamotrigine therapy does not affect the folate pathway or increase risk of neural tube or other congenital anomalies, folic acid supplementation beyond the standard 400–800 μg daily may not be necessary, particularly because some data show that folic acid can decrease lamotrigine effectiveness (Geddes et al. 2016).

In addition to reducing risk of neural tube defects, there is increasing evidence that folic acid supplementation reduces risk and severity of fetal cardiac malformations induced by environmental exposures, such as lithium, alcohol, and elevated homocysteine (Huhta and Linask 2015). Folate works to suppress lithium-induced upregulation of a Wnt/β-catenin signaling pathway critical in embryonic cardiogenesis, thus potentially exerting a protective effect (Huhta and Linask 2015). Although folic acid supplementation beyond standard requirements has been recommended by some experts for women maintained on lithium in pregnancy, no current consensus has been found on this recommendation or on specifics such as formulation (folic acid vs. L-methylfolate), dosing (recommendations range from 1 mg/day to 5 mg/day or higher), or duration of treatment (Huhta and Linask 2015). More research is needed on the effects of high-dose folic acid supplementation on fetal neurocognitive development; although some studies show a reduced risk of ASD with folate supplementation, others have reported detrimental effects on fetal neural development and an increased risk of ASD with excess folic acid supplementation (Wiens and DeSoto 2017).

# Nonpharmacological Somatic Treatments

## Electroconvulsive Therapy

Electroconvulsive therapy (ECT) is an effective option for the treatment of severe mood symptoms, especially in the context of associated catatonia, psychotic agitation, suicidality, or severe physical decline (e.g., malnutrition or dehydration) (Ward et al. 2018). ECT offers a rapid treatment response and serves as an alternative to pharmacological treatment or as a second-line agent when pharmacotherapy fails. The safety and efficacy of ECT during pregnancy and postpartum have been established over decades and support its role as a treatment option for perinatal women when clinically indicated (Ward et al. 2018). For a detailed discussion of ECT in pregnancy and postpartum, please see Chapter 13, "Depressive Disorders."

## Bright Light Therapy

Bright light therapy is an effective and safe treatment option for bipolar depression when prescribed as augmentation with a mood-stabilizing medication. Sit et al. (2018) performed a randomized, double-blind, placebo-controlled trial in adults with BDI and BDII and found that midday 7,000-lux bright light therapy in conjunction with a mood-stabilizing medication led to a robust antidepressant response (68.2% remission rate of depression vs. 22.2% with placebo) after 4–6 weeks. Midday timing of light therapy (between 12 P.M. and 2:30 P.M.) was not associated with switching to mania, hypomania, or mixed states. Advantages of bright light therapy in the perinatal period include the absence of drug transfer in utero or via breastfeeding and a minimal side effect profile. The bright light box should be a broad-spectrum, bright white light that provides ultraviolet filtration and emits 7,000 to 10,000 lux. It should be placed at an optimal distance of 12 inches from the eyes (Sit et al. 2018). Light dosing starts with 15 minutes a day at midday for the first week, then increases by 15 minutes per day each week until the target dose of 45–60 minutes a day by week 4 is reached or until symptoms have fully remitted (Sit et al. 2018).

# Behavioral Treatments

## Psychoeducation and Psychotherapy

Although pharmacotherapy is the mainstay of treatment for BD, both psychoeducation and select psychotherapy modalities are useful adjunctive tools for the treatment of acute depressive episodes and prevention of relapse. Use of these modalities in the setting of acute mania is not supported by current evidence (Yatham et al. 2018).

Models of evidence-based psychoeducation for individuals with BD may be delivered individually or in a group setting over numerous sessions and focus on developing skills to identify warning signs of depression and mania, manage stress, minimize denial of chronic illness, improve medication adherence, and develop healthy lifestyles (Yatham et al. 2018). Evidence-based psychotherapy modalities for BD include cognitive-behavioral therapy, family-focused therapy, and interpersonal and social rhythms therapy. Peer support is an evidence-based modality in the maintenance phase of the illness only (Yatham et al. 2018). Although data regarding the use of these treatments in pregnant or postpartum women with BD are extremely limited, it is reasonable to assume they may be beneficial, particularly for women experiencing adversity, relationship stress, disruption of sleep and wake cycles, or other stress (Epstein et al. 2014).

### Lifestyle Considerations

In addition to the dramatic fluctuations in female sex hormones across the perinatal period, multiple biological, psychological, and social changes can contribute to a relapse in BD. Treatment discussions with the perinatal woman and family should include these factors in a manner that is mindful of the patient's social and financial resources. The patient may consider planning to limit predictable stressors during pregnancy and the postpartum period by reducing work hours, deferring the start of new projects at home or work, or other means to simplify her schedule. Bolstering psychosocial supports helps to provide emotional and physical support. A family member or friend may be identified to watch for early warning signs of relapse, monitor medication compliance, or contribute to infant care postpartum. When financially feasible, instrumental support in newborn care, such as a postpartum doula or night nanny, can be recommended.

The perinatal period is associated with normative alterations in sleep physiology and sleep disruptions. Nighttime infant feedings further contribute to poor sleep quality in the postpartum period and may contribute to postpartum depressive symptoms (Park et al. 2013). Sleep disruption is a commonly reported precursor to mania in patients with BD, and women with BD who have a personal history of mania precipitated by sleep loss have an increased risk for PPP (Lewis et al. 2018). Several practical strategies can be considered to minimize maternal sleep disruption. In the hospital setting, approaches for women at elevated risk for postpartum mood disorders may include rooming them away from noise and traffic, assessing vital signs during waking hours only, clustering medication administration with lab draws to minimize room traffic, encouraging visitors to adhere to specific visiting hours, opening blinds during the day to increase exposure to natural light, and the option of rooming-out the infant at night. At home, patients and families may be given a "prescription" for prioritizing sleep and family, and trusted supports can be asked to provide overnight bottle feeding of expressed breastmilk or supplementation with formula. When clinically indicated, conventional sedative hypnotic medications may be considered, with the goal of reestablishing a normal sleep-wake rhythm (Ross et al. 2005).

## Conclusion

Competent psychiatric care of women with BD across the reproductive lifespan requires the psychiatrist to appreciate the potential influence of fluctuations in female reproductive hormones. In women of reproductive age, the potential for pregnancy adds a layer of complexity to treatment planning. Preconception planning should be a routine component of psychiatric care for reproductive-age women with BD and should include inquiry about plans for pregnancy and contraceptive practices. When prescribing medications with teratogenic or other obstetrical risk, these risks should be part of a balanced risk-risk discussion with the patient or her proxy. When treating BD during pregnancy or the postpartum period, it is critical to take a comprehensive approach to treatment that includes psychological and pharmacological options and to prioritize the need for adequate sleep and social supports. Pharmacological decisions should be made with consideration of the risk of the underlying disease to both the mother and infant, as well as risk of clinically indicated medications.

## Key Points

- Women with bipolar disorder (BD) may experience exacerbation of illness during times of reproductive hormone fluctuation, such as the premenstrual, postpartum, and perimenopausal periods.
- The potential for pregnancy introduces added complexity in the treatment of women with BD, and family planning is a critical component of psychiatric care.
- Treatment planning for women with BD during and after pregnancy should necessarily include psychological and pharmacological options. Adequate sleep should be a priority.
- Decisions around maintenance medications in the perinatal period strongly influence the risk of recurrence for women with BD.
- Lithium is one of the most established treatments for BD, and growing evidence regarding its safety profile supports its use in women who are unlikely to maintain euthymia with lamotrigine or antipsychotic monotherapy.
- Lamotrigine's relative reproductive safety and emerging evidence base in the perinatal period make it an emerging first-line option for treatment of BD in pregnancy, particularly for women with a preponderance of depressive episodes.

## References

Altshuler LL, Kupka RW, Hellemann G, et al: Gender and depressive symptoms in 711 patients with bipolar disorder evaluated prospectively in the Stanley Foundation bipolar treatment outcome network. Am J Psychiatry 167(6):708–715, 2010 20231325

American College of Obstetricians and Gynecologists: ACOG committee opinion no. 757: screening for perinatal depression. Obstet Gynecol 132(5):e208–e212, 2018 30629567

American Psychiatric Association: Diagnostic and Statistical Manual of Mental Disorders, 5th Edition. Arlington, VA, American Psychiatric Association, 2013

Baker GA, Bromley RL, Briggs M, et al: IQ at 6 years after in utero exposure to antiepileptic drugs: a controlled cohort study. Neurology 84(4):382–390, 2015 25540307

Baldassano CF, Marangell LB, Gyulai L, et al: Gender differences in bipolar disorder: retrospective data from the first 500 STEP-BD participants. Bipolar Disord 7(5):465–470, 2005 16176440

Bergink V, Bouvy PF, Vervoort JS, et al: Prevention of postpartum psychosis and mania in women at high risk. Am J Psychiatry 169(6):609–615, 2012 22407083

Bergink V, Rasgon N, Wisner KL: Postpartum psychosis: madness, mania, and melancholia in motherhood. Am J Psychiatry 173(12):1179–1188, 2016 27609245

Bibbins-Domingo K, Grossman DC, Curry SJ, et al: Folic acid supplementation for the prevention of neural tube defects: US Preventive Services Task Force recommendation statement. JAMA 317(2):183–189, 2017 28097362

Bogen DL, Sit D, Genovese A, et al: Three cases of lithium exposure and exclusive breastfeeding. Arch Women Ment Health 15(1):69–72, 2012 22277970

Bromley RL, Mawer GE, Briggs M, et al: The prevalence of neurodevelopmental disorders in children prenatally exposed to antiepileptic drugs. J Neurol Neurosurg Psychiatry 84(6):637–643, 2013 23370617
Campbell E, Kennedy F, Russell A, et al: Malformation risks of antiepileptic drug monotherapies in pregnancy: updated results from the UK and Ireland Epilepsy and Pregnancy Registers. J Neurol Neurosurg Psychiatry 85(9):1029–1034, 2014 24444855
Carvalho AF, Takwoingi Y, Sales PM, et al: Screening for bipolar spectrum disorders: a comprehensive meta-analysis of accuracy studies. J Affect Disord 172:337–346, 2015 25451435
Carmassi C, Del Grande C, Masci I, et al: Lithium and valproate serum level fluctuations within the menstrual cycle: a systematic review. Int Clin Psychopharmacol 34(3):143–150, 2019 30907774
Chen LC, Yang AC, Su TP, et al: Symptomatic menopausal transition and subsequent bipolar disorder among midlife women with major depression: a nationwide longitudinal study. Arch Women Ment Health 20(3):463–468, 2017 28429098
Clark CT, Wisner KL: Treatment of peripartum bipolar disorder. Obstet Gynecol Clin North Am 45(3):403–417, 2018 30092918
Clark CT, Klein AM, Perel JM, et al: Lamotrigine dosing for pregnant patients with bipolar disorder. Am J Psychiatry 170(11):1240–1247, 2013 24185239
Clark CT, Wisner KL, Stika C, et al: Lamotrigine pharmacokinetics across pregnancy: implications for treatment of bipolar disorder in pregnancy. Clin Pharmacol Ther 99(suppl 1):S93–S94, 2016
Cohen LS, Friedman JM, Jefferson JW, et al: A reevaluation of risk of in utero exposure to lithium. JAMA 271(2):146–150, 1994 8031346
Cox JL, Holden JM, Sagovsky R: Detection of postnatal depression: development of the 10-item Edinburgh Postnatal Depression Scale. Br J Psychiatry 150(6):782–786, 1987 3651732
Craddock N, Sklar P: Genetics of bipolar disorder. Lancet 381(9878):1654–1662, 2013 23663951
Cunnington M, Tennis P, International Lamotrigine Pregnancy Registry Scientific Advisory Committee: Lamotrigine and the risk of malformations in pregnancy. Neurology 64(6):955–960, 2005 15781807
De Nicola AF, Garay LI, Meyer M, et al: Neurosteroidogenesis and progesterone anti-inflammatory/neuroprotective effects. J Neuroendocrinol 30(2):e12502, 2018 28675779
Deligiannidis KM, Byatt N, Freeman MP: Pharmacotherapy for mood disorders in pregnancy: a review of pharmacokinetic changes and clinical recommendations for therapeutic drug monitoring. J Clin Psychopharmacol 34(2):244–255, 2014 24525634
Diav-Citrin O, Shechtman S, Bar-Oz B, et al: Pregnancy outcome after in utero exposure to valproate: evidence of dose relationship in teratogenic effect. CNS Drugs 22(4):325–334, 2008 18336060
Diav-Citrin O, Shechtman S, Tahover E, et al: Pregnancy outcome following in utero exposure to lithium: a prospective, comparative, observational study. Am J Psychiatry 171(7):785–794, 2014 24781368
Di Florio A, Jones I: Is sex important? Gender differences in bipolar disorder. Int Rev Psychiatry 22(5):437–452, 2010 21047158
Di Florio A, Jones L, Forty L, et al: Mood disorders and parity: a clue to the aetiology of the postpartum trigger. J Affect Disord 152–154:334–339, 2014 24446553
Di Florio A, Gordon-Smith K, Forty L, et al: Stratification of the risk of bipolar disorder recurrences in pregnancy and postpartum. Br J Psychiatry 213(3):542–547, 2018 30113284
Dias RS, Lafer B, Russo C, et al: Longitudinal follow-up of bipolar disorder in women with premenstrual exacerbation: findings from STEP-BD. Am J Psychiatry 168(4):386–394, 2011 21324951
Dolk H, Wang H, Loane M, et al: Lamotrigine use in pregnancy and risk of orofacial cleft and other congenital anomalies. Neurology 86(18):1716–1725, 2016 27053714
Doyle K, Heron J, Berrisford G, et al: The management of bipolar disorder in the perinatal period and risk factors for postpartum relapse. Eur Psychiatry 27(8):563–569, 2012 21924587
Earls MF, Yogman MW, Mattson G, et al: Incorporating recognition and management of perinatal depression into pediatric practice. Pediatrics 143(1):e20183259, 2019 30559120
Epstein RA, Moore KM, Bobo WV: Treatment of bipolar disorders during pregnancy: maternal and fetal safety and challenges. Drug Healthc Patient Saf 7:7–29, 2014 25565896

Erol A, Winham SJ, McElroy SL, et al: Sex differences in the risk of rapid cycling and other indicators of adverse illness course in patients with bipolar I and II disorder. Bipolar Disord 17(6):670–676, 2015 26529373

Finer LB, Zolna MR: Declines in unintended pregnancy in the United States, 2008–2011. N Engl J Med 374(9):843–852, 2016 26962904

Fornaro M, Maritan E, Ferranti R, et al: Lithium exposure during pregnancy and the postpartum period: a systematic review and meta-analysis of safety and efficacy outcomes. Am J Psychiatry 177(1):76–92, 2020 31623458

Forsberg L, Adler M, Römer Ek I, et al: Maternal mood disorders and lithium exposure in utero were not associated with poor cognitive development during childhood. Acta Paediatr 107(8):1379–1388, 2018 29150869

Freeman MP, Gelenberg AJ: Bipolar disorder in women: reproductive events and treatment considerations. Acta Psychiatr Scand 112(2):88–96, 2005 15992389

Freudenreich O, Francis A, Fricchione G: Psychosis, mania, and catatonia, in The American Psychiatric Association Publishing Textbook of Psychosomatic Medicine and Consultation-Liaison Psychiatry, 3rd Edition. Edited by Levenson JL. Washington, DC, American Psychiatric Association Publishing, 2019, pp 249–279

Frey BN, Dias RS: Sex hormones and biomarkers of neuroprotection and neurodegeneration: implications for female reproductive events in bipolar disorder. Bipolar Disord 16(1):48–57, 2014 24206266

Geddes JR, Gardiner A, Rendell J, et al: Comparative evaluation of quetiapine plus lamotrigine combination versus quetiapine monotherapy (and folic acid versus placebo) in bipolar depression (CEQUEL): a 2 × 2 factorial randomised trial. Lancet Psychiatry 3(1):31–39, 2016 26687300

Gogos A, Ney LJ, Seymour N, et al: Sex differences in schizophrenia, bipolar disorder, and post-traumatic stress disorder: are gonadal hormones the link? Br J Pharmacol 176(21):4119–4135, 2019 30658014

Grover S, Sahoo S, Chaudhary S, et al: Gender differences, family size and fertility rate among patients with bipolar disorder: a study from India. Psychiatry Res 272:562–568, 2019 30616124

Heberden C: Sex steroids and neurogenesis. Biochem Pharmacol 141:56–62, 2017 28571999

Hirschfeld RM, Williams JB, Spitzer RL, et al: Development and validation of a screening instrument for bipolar spectrum disorder: the Mood Disorder Questionnaire. Am J Psychiatry 157(11):1873–1875, 2000 11058490

Holmes LB, Baldwin EJ, Smith CR, et al: Increased frequency of isolated cleft palate in infants exposed to lamotrigine during pregnancy. Neurology 70(22 Pt 2):2152–2158, 2008 18448870

Huhta JC, Linask K: When should we prescribe high-dose folic acid to prevent congenital heart defects? Curr Opin Cardiol 30(1):125–131, 2015 25389654

Huybrechts KF, Hernández-Díaz S, Patorno E, et al: Antipsychotic use in pregnancy and the risk for congenital malformations. JAMA Psychiatry 73(9):938–946, 2016 27540849

Irwin RW, Yao J, Hamilton RT, et al: Progesterone and estrogen regulate oxidative metabolism in brain mitochondria. Endocrinology 149(6):3167–3175, 2008 18292191

Joffe H, Cohen LS, Suppes T, et al: Valproate is associated with new-onset oligoamenorrhea with hyperandrogenism in women with bipolar disorder. Biol Psychiatry 59(11):1078–1086, 2006 16448626

Jones I, Craddock N: Familiality of the puerperal trigger in bipolar disorder: results of a family study. Am J Psychiatry 158(6):913–917, 2001 11384899

Kenna HA, Jiang B, Rasgon NL: Reproductive and metabolic abnormalities associated with bipolar disorder and its treatment. Harv Rev Psychiatry 17(2):138–146, 2009 19373621

Khan SJ, Fersh ME, Ernst C, et al: Bipolar disorder in pregnancy and postpartum: principles of management. Curr Psychiatry Rep 18(2):13, 2016 26781551

Kozma C: Neonatal toxicity and transient neurodevelopmental deficits following prenatal exposure to lithium: another clinical report and a review of the literature. Am J Med Genet A 132A(4):441–444, 2005 15633173

Lactmed: Drugs and Lactation Database. National Institutes of Health, 2020. Available at: https://www.ncbi.nlm.nih.gov/books/NBK501268. Accessed June 2021.

Lewis KJS, Di Florio A, Forty L, et al: Mania triggered by sleep loss and risk of postpartum psychosis in women with bipolar disorder. J Affect Disord 225:624–629, 2018 28889048

Maletic V, Raison C: Integrated neurobiology of bipolar disorder. Front Psychiatry 5:98, 2014 25202283

Marengo E, Martino DJ, Igoa A, et al: Unplanned pregnancies and reproductive health among women with bipolar disorder. J Affect Disord 178:201–205, 2015 25827504

Margulis AV, Hernandez-Diaz S, McElrath T, et al: Relation of in-utero exposure to antiepileptic drugs to pregnancy duration and size at birth. PLoS One 14(8):e0214180, 2019 31381574

Marsh WK, Templeton A, Ketter TA, et al: Increased frequency of depressive episodes during the menopausal transition in women with bipolar disorder: preliminary report. J Psychiatr Res 42(3):247–251, 2008 17266987

Marsh WK, Gershenson B, Rothschild AJ: Symptom severity of bipolar disorder during the menopausal transition. Int J Bipolar Disord 3(1):35, 2015 26296381

McElroy SL, Crow S, Blom TJ, et al: Prevalence and correlates of DSM-5 eating disorders in patients with bipolar disorder. J Affect Disord 191:216–221, 2016 26682490

McMahon FJ, Akula N, Schulze TG, et al: Meta-analysis of genome-wide association data identifies a risk locus for major mood disorders on 3p21.1. Nat Genet 42(2):128–131, 2010 20081856

Meador KJ, Baker GA, Browning N, et al: Fetal antiepileptic drug exposure and cognitive outcomes at age 6 years (NEAD study): a prospective observational study. Lancet Neurol 12(3):244–252, 2013 23352199

Merrill L, Mittal L, Nicoloro J, et al: Screening for bipolar disorder during pregnancy. Arch Women Ment Health 18(4):579–583, 2015 25968603

Minuzzi L, Frey BN, Soares CN: Depression during the menopausal transition: an update on epidemiology and biological treatments. Focus 10(1):22–27, 2012

Molenaar NM, Poels EMP, Robakis T, et al: Management of lithium dosing around delivery: an observational study. Bipolar Disord June 11, 2020 32526071 Epub ahead of print

Moretti ME, Koren G, Verjee Z, et al: Monitoring lithium in breast milk: an individualized approach for breastfeeding mothers. Clin Pharmacol Ther 73(2):9–9, 2003

Morrow J, Russell A, Guthrie E, et al: Malformation risks of antiepileptic drugs in pregnancy: a prospective study from the UK Epilepsy and Pregnancy Register. J Neurol Neurosurg Psychiatry 77(2):193–198, 2006 16157661

Moses-Kolko EL, Clark CT, DeBrunner S, et al: Reproductive-age women with bipolar II disorder, in Bipolar II Disorder: Recognition, Understanding, and Treatment. Edited by Swartz HA, Suppes T. Washington, DC, American Psychiatric Association Publishing, 2019, pp 263–286

Muneer A: The neurobiology of bipolar disorder: an integrated approach. Chonnam Med J 52(1):18–37, 2016 26865997

Munk-Olsen T, Liu X, Viktorin A, et al: Maternal and infant outcomes associated with lithium use in pregnancy: an international collaborative meta-analysis of six cohort studies. Lancet Psychiatry 5(8):644–652, 2018 29929874

Newberg AR, Catapano LA, Zarate CA, et al: Neurobiology of bipolar disorder. Expert Rev Neurother 8(1):93–110, 2008 18088203

Newmark RL, Bogen DL, Wisner KL, et al: Risk-benefit assessment of infant exposure to lithium through breast milk: a systematic review of the literature. Int Rev Psychiatry 31(3):295–304, 2019 31180257

Newton ER, Hale TW: Drugs in breast milk. Clin Obstet Gynecol 58(4):868–884, 2015 26457856

Numakawa T, Matsumoto T, Numakawa Y, et al: Protective action of neurotrophic factors and estrogen against oxidative stress-mediated neurodegeneration. J Toxicol 2011:405194, 2011 21776259

Pagano HP, Zapata LB, Berry-Bibee EN, et al: Safety of hormonal contraception and intrauterine devices among women with depressive and bipolar disorders: a systematic review. Contraception 94(6):641–649, 2016 27364100

Pariente G, Leibson T, Shulman T, et al: Pregnancy outcomes following in utero exposure to lamotrigine: a systematic review and meta-analysis. CNS Drugs 31(6):439–450, 2017 28434134

Park EM, Meltzer-Brody S, Stickgold R: Poor sleep maintenance and subjective sleep quality are associated with postpartum maternal depression symptom severity. Arch Women Ment Health 16(6):539–547, 2013 23733081

Parker G, Graham R, Hadzi-Pavlovic D, et al: Further examination of the utility and comparative properties of the MSQ and MDQ bipolar screening measures. J Affect Disord 138(1–2):104–109, 2012 22285793

Patorno E, Huybrechts KF, Bateman BT, et al: Lithium use in pregnancy and the risk of cardiac malformations. N Engl J Med 376(23):2245–2254, 2017 28591541

Payne JL, Roy PS, Murphy-Eberenz K, et al: Reproductive cycle-associated mood symptoms in women with major depression and bipolar disorder. J Affect Disord 99(1–3):221–229, 2007 17011632

Poels EMP, Bijma HH, Galbally M, et al: Lithium during pregnancy and after delivery: a review. Int J Bipolar Disord 6(1):26, 2018 30506447

Poels EMP, Kamperman AM, Vreeker A, et al: Lithium use during pregnancy and the risk of miscarriage. J Clin Med 9(6):1819, 2020 32545238

Prakash C, Hatters-Friedman S, Moller-Olsen C, et al: Maternal and fetal outcomes after lamotrigine use in pregnancy: a retrospective analysis from an urban maternal mental health centre in New Zealand. Psychopharmacol Bull 46(2):63–69, 2016 27738382

Raison CL, Capuron L, Miller AH: Cytokines sing the blues: inflammation and the pathogenesis of depression. Trends Immunol 27(1):24–31, 2006 16316783

Rasgon NL, Altshuler LL, Gudeman D, et al: Medication status and polycystic ovary syndrome in women with bipolar disorder: a preliminary report. J Clin Psychiatry 61(3):173–178, 2000 10817101

Reddy DS: Clinical pharmacokinetic interactions between antiepileptic drugs and hormonal contraceptives. Expert Rev Clin Pharmacol 3(2):183–192, 2010 20369030

Reynolds-May MF, Kenna HA, Marsh W, et al: Evaluation of reproductive function in women treated for bipolar disorder compared to healthy controls. Bipolar Disord 16(1):37–47, 2014 24262071

Robakis TK, Holtzman J, Stemmle PG, et al: Lamotrigine and GABAA receptor modulators interact with menstrual cycle phase and oral contraceptives to regulate mood in women with bipolar disorder. J Affect Disord 175:108–115, 2015 25601310

Roberts LW (ed): The American Psychiatric Association Publishing Textbook of Psychiatry, 7th Edition. Washington, DC, American Psychiatric Association Publishing, 2019

Rosenblat JD, McIntyre RS: Bipolar disorder and inflammation. Psychiatr Clin North Am 39(1):125–137, 2016 26876323

Ross LE, Murray BJ, Steiner M: Sleep and perinatal mood disorders: a critical review. J Psychiatry Neurosci 30(4):247–256, 2005 16049568

Saunders EF, Fitzgerald KD, Zhang P, et al: Clinical features of bipolar disorder comorbid with anxiety disorders differ between men and women. Depress Anxiety 29(8):739–746, 2012 22461133

Schaffer A, Isometsä ET, Tondo L, et al: Epidemiology, neurobiology and pharmacological interventions related to suicide deaths and suicide attempts in bipolar disorder: part I of a report of the International Society for Bipolar Disorders Task Force on Suicide in Bipolar Disorder. Aust N Z J Psychiatry 49(9):785–802, 2015 26185269

Singh M, Su C: Progesterone and neuroprotection. Horm Behav 63(2):284–290, 2013 22732134

Sit DK, McGowan J, Wiltrout C, et al: Adjunctive bright light therapy for bipolar depression: a randomized double-blind placebo-controlled trial. Am J Psychiatry 175(2):131–139, 2018 28969438

Siu AL, Bibbins-Domingo K, Grossman DC, et al: Screening for depression in adults: US Preventive Services Task Force recommendation statement. JAMA 315(4):380–387, 2016 26813211

Slyepchenko A, Frey BN, Lafer B, et al: Increased illness burden in women with comorbid bipolar and premenstrual dysphoric disorder: data from 1,099 women from STEP-BD study. Acta Psychiatr Scand 136(5):473–482, 2017 28846801

Smithells RW, Sheppard S, Schorah CJ: Vitamin deficiencies and neural tube defects. Arch Dis Child 51(12):944–950, 1976 1015847

Strakowski SM, DelBello MP, Zimmerman ME, et al: Ventricular and periventricular structural volumes in first- versus multiple-episode bipolar disorder. Am J Psychiatry 159(11):1841–1847, 2002 12411217
Task Force on Sudden Infant Death Syndrome: SIDS and other sleep-related infant deaths: updated 2016 recommendations for a safe infant sleeping environment. Pediatrics 138(5):e20162938, 2016 27940804
Teatero ML, Mazmanian D, Sharma V: Effects of the menstrual cycle on bipolar disorder. Bipolar Disord 16(1):22–36, 2014 24467469
Terp IM, Mortensen PB: Post-partum psychoses: clinical diagnoses and relative risk of admission after parturition. Br J Psychiatry 172(6):521–526, 1998 9828994
Thomas AJ, Davis S, Ferrier IN, et al: Elevation of cell adhesion molecule immunoreactivity in the anterior cingulate cortex in bipolar disorder. Biol Psychiatry 55(6):652–655, 2004 15013836
Tomson T, Battino D, Bonizzoni E, et al: Comparative risk of major congenital malformations with eight different antiepileptic drugs: a prospective cohort study of the EURAP registry. Lancet Neurol 17(6):530–538, 2018 29680205
Vajda FJE, O'Brien TJ, Graham J, et al: Is carbamazepine a human teratogen? J Clin Neurosci 23:34–37, 2016 26521756
Vega-Vela NE, Osorio D, Avila-Rodriguez M, et al: L-type calcium channels modulation by estradiol. Mol Neurobiol 54(7):4996–5007, 2017 27525676
Viguera AC, Nonacs R, Cohen LS, et al: Risk of recurrence of bipolar disorder in pregnant and nonpregnant women after discontinuing lithium maintenance. Am J Psychiatry 157(2):179–184, 2000 10671384
Viguera AC, Whitfield T, Baldessarini RJ, et al: Risk of recurrence in women with bipolar disorder during pregnancy: prospective study of mood stabilizer discontinuation. Am J Psychiatry 164(12):1817–1824, quiz 1923, 2007 18056236
Ward HB, Fromson JA, Cooper JJ, et al: Recommendations for the use of ECT in pregnancy: literature review and proposed clinical protocol. Arch Women Ment Health 21(6):715–722, 2018 29796968
Wesseloo R, Kamperman AM, Munk-Olsen T, et al: Risk of postpartum relapse in bipolar disorder and postpartum psychosis: a systematic review and meta-analysis. Am J Psychiatry 173(2):117–127, 2016 26514657
Wesseloo R, Liu X, Clark CT, et al: Risk of postpartum episodes in women with bipolar disorder after lamotrigine or lithium use during pregnancy: a population-based cohort study. J Affect Disord 218:394–397, 2017 28501739
Weston J, Bromley R, Jackson CF, et al: Monotherapy treatment of epilepsy in pregnancy: congenital malformation outcomes in the child. Cochrane Database Syst Rev 11:CD010224, 2016 27819746
Wiens D, DeSoto MC: Is high folic acid intake a risk factor for autism? A review. Brain Sci 7(11):149, 2017 29125540
Wisner KL, Sit DK, McShea MC, et al: Onset timing, thoughts of self-harm, and diagnoses in postpartum women with screen-positive depression findings. JAMA Psychiatry 70(5):490–498, 2013 23487258
Yatham LN, Kennedy SH, Parikh SV, et al: Canadian Network for Mood and Anxiety Treatments (CANMAT) and International Society for Bipolar Disorders (ISBD) 2018 guidelines for the management of patients with bipolar disorder. Bipolar Disord 20(2):97–170, 2018 29536616
Yonkers KA, Wisner KL, Stowe Z, et al: Management of bipolar disorder during pregnancy and the postpartum period. Am J Psychiatry 161(4):608–620, 2004 15056503

# CHAPTER 16

# Postpartum Psychosis

Caitlin Hasser, M.D.
Jovana Martinovic, M.D.
Pooja Lakshmin, M.D.
Mira Zein, M.D.
Melisa Olgun, B.A.
Lucy A. Hutner, M.D.
Sarah M. Nagle-Yang, M.D.
Lauren M. Osborne, M.D.

Postpartum psychosis (PPP) is a rare but severe perinatal psychiatric syndrome that is considered a true psychiatric emergency. Women with PPP typically present with a rapid onset of affective, psychotic, and cognitive symptoms in the early postpartum period. Despite the name, the symptoms of PPP often occur in the setting of known or new-onset bipolar illness or, less often, as a syndrome limited to the postpartum period. Although PPP has been described in the medical literature for hundreds of years, knowledge around its etiology, treatment, and prevention has been slow to accumulate (Osborne 2018). However, recent data suggest important guidelines to inform optimal treatment with the potential to shorten the course of illness and reduce risk of recurrence in subsequent pregnancies (Bergink et al. 2012, 2015).

## Epidemiology

### Rates/Incidence

PPP is rare, with an incidence ranging from 0.9 to 2.6 per 1,000 births according to international data (Osborne 2018; VanderKruik et al. 2017). This incidence is not known to differ substantially in different cultures.

TABLE 16–1. **Risk factors for postpartum psychosis**

| | |
|---|---|
| **Prior history of postpartum psychosis** | Family history of postpartum psychosis |
| **Personal history of bipolar disorder** | Primiparity |
| Family history of bipolar disorder | Discontinuation of maintenance medication |

## Risk Factors

Prior history of PPP and personal or family history of bipolar disorder are the greatest risk factors for PPP (Table 16–1) (Bergink et al. 2016; Jones and Craddock 2001). Primiparity is a risk factor for PPP (Di Florio et al. 2014); if a woman's first delivery is not complicated by PPP, the likelihood of developing PPP in subsequent deliveries is markedly lower (Bergink et al. 2016). Life stressors have not been identified as risk factors, and studies of obstetrical risk are inconsistent (Brockington et al. 1990; Hellerstedt et al. 2013; Meltzer-Brody et al. 2017; Perry et al. 2016). It is important to clarify that many women have no prior risk factors. For example, in a large retrospective study, only 33% of women had an antecedent history of a mood episode (Blackmore et al. 2013). Given the association with personal and family history of bipolar disorder, PPP is often conceptualized as a bipolar spectrum disorder, although somewhere between 20% and 50% of cases appear to be limited to the postpartum (Bergink et al. 2016).

## Screening and Diagnostic Criteria

No screening tools are available for PPP. Although the Edinburgh Postnatal Depression Scale can uncover symptoms of depression or the Young Mania Rating Scale symptoms of mania, neither these nor any other tool is designed for PPP in particular, and neither can capture both the affective and psychotic symptoms. DSM-5 (American Psychiatric Association 2013) does not recognize PPP as a distinct disorder, although the "with postpartum onset" specifier is added to a brief psychotic disorder diagnosis if the onset is during pregnancy or within 4 weeks postpartum. Because PPP is an affective psychosis, this method of classifying it is incomplete. PPP has been categorized in the *International Classification of Diseases* under category F53.1, used to describe severe mental and behavioral disorders associated with the puerperium (Di Florio et al. 2016).

# Clinical Presentation

Among women with PPP, the typical time to onset generally has been 3–10 days, although women with known bipolar disorder may, on average, experience onset more immediately postpartum (Bergink et al. 2016) (Table 16–2). Symptoms last an average of 1 month for women with manic features and 2.5 months for women with mixed or depressed features (Bergink et al. 2011). The onset of symptoms within a period marked by transition and change can make early identification and treatment difficult for first-episode PPP, whereas subsequent episodes are generally more rapidly identified and treated (Blackmore et al. 2013). Early prodromal symptoms may be mild and include insomnia, decreased need for sleep, mood fluctuation, anxiety, and irritability. These signs can be difficult at first to distinguish from normal adjustment after childbirth and postpartum sleep deprivation. With progression, frank mood disturbances

**TABLE 16–2. Clinical presentation of postpartum psychosis**

| |
|---|
| Abnormalities in mood may include manic, mixed, or depressed mood episodes |
| Abnormalities of perception may include auditory hallucinations |
| Abnormalities of thought most commonly include delusions and may include disorganization |
| Delirium-like waxing and waning of cognition and confusion |
| High rates of suicide and infanticide |
| Prodromal period may be marked by sleep disturbances, irritability, and mood fluctuation |
| Rapid onset of symptoms in the first postpartum days to weeks |

(including hypomania, mania, depressive symptoms, or mixed symptoms) may emerge rapidly. Although the syndrome is not delirium, per se, there can be symptom overlap, such as a waxing and waning mental status change and acute disorganization and confusion. Psychotic symptoms most often present as delusions (often but not always involving the infant) but may also include auditory hallucinations. Because symptoms may have a waxing and waning time course, a thorough assessment must include information across multiple time points (Bergink et al. 2016).

A prospective Dutch cohort study showed three distinct subgroups of patients with PPP, with approximately 41% classified as depressed, 34% classified as manic, and 25% classified as "atypical" (Kamperman et al. 2017). Dysphoric mania was more common than euphoria, and all groups had high levels of anxiety and agitation. Only the atypical group demonstrated the classic delirium-like symptoms of disturbance of consciousness, disorientation, or derealization. Visual hallucinations and delusions of childbirth were much more common than other psychotic symptoms, such as thought insertion, broadcasting, withdrawal, or auditory hallucinations with running commentary.

Suicidal ideation and homicidal thoughts are common in PPP, with rates ranging from 8% to 50% (Chandra et al. 2002; Kamperman et al. 2017). Up to 4% of mothers with untreated psychosis in the postpartum period commit infanticide (Brockington 2017). Overall, most maternal filicides (child murder by mothers) are categorized as altruistic and associated with the belief that death would be in the child's best interest or as acutely psychotic with no comprehensible motive. Up to 29% of maternal filicides end in completed suicide by the mother as well (Hatters-Friedman and Resnick 2007). Given these high risks for suicide and infanticide, it is critical to assess directly for suicidal ideation, plans for the children if the mother completed suicide, thoughts or fears of harming the infant, altruistic homicidal ideation, and delusions that are focused on the infant (Bergink et al. 2016; Chandra et al. 2006; Hatters-Friedman and Resnick 2007).

## Course/Prognosis

Even with early treatment, symptoms may persist for up to 1 year postpartum in one-quarter of women, especially if a relapse occurs or an episode of depression follows resolution of acute psychosis (Blackmore et al. 2013; Burgerhout et al. 2017). Up to 20% of marriages will end after an initial episode (Blackmore et al. 2013). However, most women will have functional improvements in work, interpersonal relations, and recreation and will resume premorbid employment and household responsibilities within 9 months (Burgerhout et al. 2017). Among women who experience an incipient PPP episode, most (50%–80%) go on to develop a subsequent serious psychiatric disorder, typically bipolar spectrum disorder (Bergink et al. 2016). A significant minority of women (20%–50%) develop a course of illness with affective psychosis isolated to the postpartum period (Bergink et al. 2016; Blackmore et al. 2013). Many women choose not to have a subsequent pregnancy, but this does not appear to be related to the severity of the postpartum episode (Blackmore et al. 2013). In those who do have a future pregnancy, approximately one-third will have a recurrent episode. The recurrence rate is higher for women with psychosis only in the postpartum period than for those with a diagnosis of bipolar disorder (Wesseloo et al. 2016). Longer duration and severity of the initial PPP episode and more time between pregnancies are other poor prognostic indicators related to recurrence in subsequent pregnancies (Blackmore et al. 2013).

Ms. X is a 26-year-old woman brought into the emergency department by her partner. She is 4 days postpartum after the birth of her first child via spontaneous vaginal delivery at 39 weeks' gestation. Her pregnancy was planned and desired and without medical complication. She has no formal psychiatric history, and family history is notable for a sibling with bipolar disorder.

Per report from her partner, Ms. X was "great" in the first couple of days after delivery. Although she sometimes seemed overwhelmed and short tempered, overall, she was "full of energy" and "captivated" by her infant and caretaking role. In the past 24 hours, however, her behavior has become increasingly odd, unusual, and erratic. He reports that she has become "obsessed" with concerns that their daughter is showing signs of "neurologic damage" despite a reassuring visit to her pediatrician. This morning, Ms. X was found feeding the baby a bottle of water. When the partner asked what she was doing, Ms. X appeared confused and disoriented, but eventually he understood that she was attempting to "flush out the baby's system" because she believed the baby had been fed contaminated breastmilk. She also had set the thermostat to "max heat," stating that the baby had been hypothermic overnight and needed to be "warmed."

On examination, Ms. X appeared guarded, with mild psychomotor agitation. Her thought process was tangential, and her mood was irritable. She became quickly panicked when she was told she would need to stay for further evaluation, stating that her baby was gravely ill, and "I'm the only one who knows what's really going on with her."

## Differential Diagnosis

The differential diagnosis of PPP is broad, especially given the potential overlap with medical complications in the immediate postpartum period. In addition, PPP may have overlap with symptoms of delirium, such as a waxing and waning course and acute confusion; this makes it vital to rule out medical causes of altered mental status. Neuropsychiatric syndromes, such as autoimmune encephalitis, should be considered, particularly when accompanied by neurological symptoms. See Tables 16–3 and 16–4 for a more thorough differential diagnosis and recommended laboratory and radiological investigation in the setting of PPP.

In terms of psychiatric differential diagnosis, multiple psychiatric disorders arise in the postpartum period and should be considered. "Baby blues" is not a psychiatric disorder but a common postpartum experience of transient and self-limited irritability, weepiness, or anxiety that may be distressing but does not significantly impair function. Perinatal depression is characterized by a major depressive episode with onset during pregnancy or within the first 4 weeks postpartum. Women with generalized anxiety disorder or panic disorder commonly experience symptom recurrence in

**TABLE 16–3. Differential diagnosis of postpartum psychosis**

| | |
|---|---|
| Acute infectious process (e.g., endometritis) | Inborn errors of metabolism (e.g., urea cycle disorder) |
| Autoimmune process (e.g., anti-NMDA receptor encephalitis, lupus flare) | Medication induced (e.g., corticosteroid induced) |
| Baby blues | Peripartum blood loss and anemia |
| Embolism | Postpartum depression |
| Generalized anxiety disorder | Postpartum OCD |
| Hormonal abnormality (e.g., primary hyperparathyroidism, thyroid disease, Sheehan's syndrome) | Primary or metastatic malignancy |
| | Substance intoxication or withdrawal |

**TABLE 16–4. Recommended laboratory testing and imaging in the setting of postpartum psychosis**

| | |
|---|---|
| Complete blood count | If neurological symptoms are present, consider |
| Comprehensive metabolic profile | Autoimmune encephalitis and antibody screening |
| Thyroid function tests | Cerebrospinal fluid analysis |
| Urinalysis | Electroencephalogram |
| Urine drug screen | MRI |
| | Serum ammonia concentration |

**TABLE 16–5. Assessing thoughts of harming baby**

| Secondary to obsessions/anxiety | Secondary to PPP/suspected PPP |
|---|---|
| Good insight | Poor insight |
| No psychotic symptoms | Psychotic symptoms |
| Thoughts are intrusive and scary and/or cause anxiety | Delusional beliefs with distortion of reality present |
| Suggests *not* at risk of harming baby | Suggests *is* at risk of harming baby |

PPP=postpartum psychosis.

the postpartum period. OCD may be particularly difficult to differentiate from PPP. Delusional beliefs present during PPP are commonly centered around the child and are easily confused with obsessional thoughts regarding the infant that occur in the setting of postpartum OCD (Table 16–5). Important distinguishing features between these two disorders when assessing thoughts of harming an infant include the level of insight, the degree to which the thoughts or beliefs are ego-syntonic, and other presenting symptoms. In PPP, delusions are likely to be ego-syntonic and with poor insight (Tinkelman et al. 2017).

## Sociodemographic Considerations

No data indicate that either the incidence or the clinical presentation of PPP differs by sociodemographic considerations (Kamperman et al. 2017; Perry et al. 2019). It is worth noting, however, that most of the research on PPP has been done in Europe and the United Kingdom, with largely homogenous populations. This fact, combined with the rarity of the disorder, means that we cannot rule out differences that have not yet been discovered. One group recently found that adverse childhood events, which are a known risk factor for other perinatal mood and anxiety disorders, are not associated with subsequent PPP (Perry et al. 2016).

# Pathophysiology

Childbirth is a clear biological trigger for PPP, but despite this, its etiology is poorly understood. The pathophysiology of PPP is an area of active research that includes genetics, hormonal changes, immune response, and circadian rhythm disruption. Genetic research on first lifetime onset of PPP is scant, but the literature investigating PPP in patients with an underlying bipolar disorder identifies genetic variants of the serotonin transporter gene and potential signal at chromosome 16p13 (Coyle et al. 2000; Jones et al. 2007; Kumar et al. 2007). Genetic polymorphism of *METTL13*, which is involved in estrogen receptor–induced gene transcription, has also been implicated (Thippeswamy et al. 2017). Hormonally, significant changes occur in corticotropin-releasing hormone, adrenocorticotropic hormone, estrogen, and progesterone levels around parturition, leading many to consider particularly the drop in estrogen and its modulation of dopamine as a potential etiology, although evidence for this is not strong (Bergink et al. 2016). Given that peripheral levels of reproductive hormones are not different in affected versus unaffected women, if an association exists, it is more likely that a subset of women is particularly vulnerable to the rapid hormonal changes. Immune activation in the postpartum period has also been considered due to overlap with autoimmune conditions such as encephalitis, thyroiditis, and differences in levels of proinflammatory and immunosuppressive cells in women with histories of PPP (Bergink et al. 2013, 2016; Kumar et al. 2017; Weigelt et al. 2013). One hypothesis posits that dysregulated immune functioning may affect remyelination processes postpartum (Dazzan et al. 2018). Finally, sleep disruption associated with labor, delivery, and the early postpartum period has been implicated, particularly in women with bipolar disorder who have histories of mania triggered by sleep loss (Lewis et al. 2018).

# Psychopharmacology

## Acute Treatment

PPP is a treatable psychiatric emergency and requires immediate evaluation (Figure 16–1). (See Chapter 9, "A Clinical Approach to Psychiatric Diagnosis and Treatment in the Postpartum Period," for further detail on acute assessment and management.) Inpatient psychiatric hospitalization is typically indicated to ensure the safety of the patient and her infant, especially when clinical judgment reveals elevated risk for lethality. Considering safety of the mother and infant, involvement of the mother's family and support for maternal–infant bonding should be important components of care. In the specialized mother–baby psychiatric unit, a model of care that originated in the United Kingdom, the mother and the baby are admitted together to the hospital; these units in-

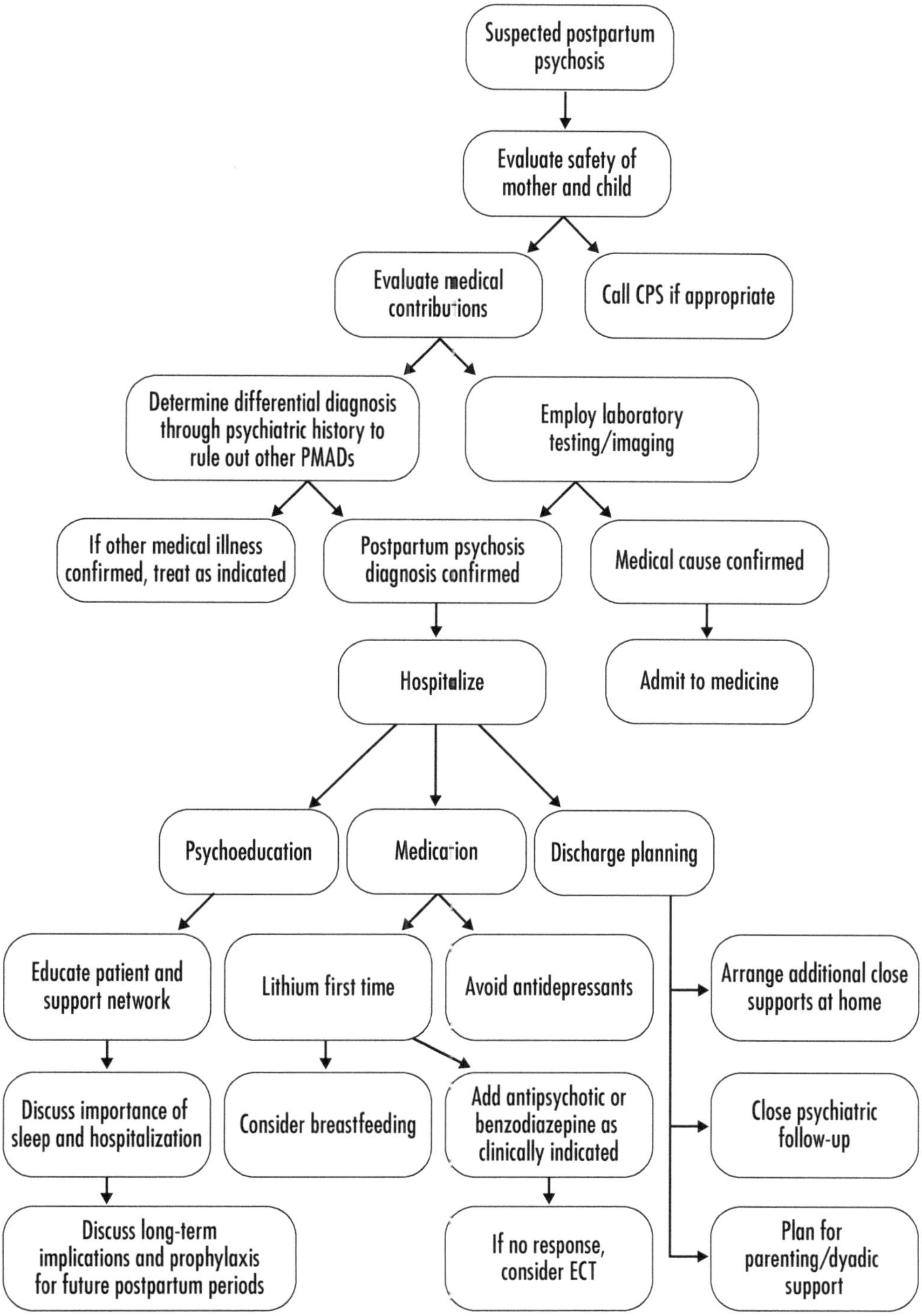


**FIGURE 16–1. Treatment of postpartum psychosis.**
CPS=child protective services; ECT=electroconvulsive therapy; PMADs=postpartum mood and anxiety disorders.

corporate dyadic treatment and enhanced parenting support into the acute psychiatric treatment of the mother (Glangeaud-Freudenthal et al. 2014). The lack of availability of mother–baby units in the United States may affect treatment for postpartum women because a new mother may be reluctant to seek treatment that would require separation from her infant. In the instances in which she is admitted, she may be discharged after acute safety issues have resolved but before complete stabilization to balance the need for bonding and care of the infant (Burgerhout et al. 2017). Whether receiving care in a traditional mental health setting or a mother–baby unit, it is important to develop an individualized treatment plan in collaboration with the family and obstetrical and pediatric teams.

Goals of pharmacological treatment include promoting sleep, improving psychosis, and stabilizing mood. Short-term use of benzodiazepines may be helpful to promote sleep. Case series literature has supported the use of electroconvulsive therapy (ECT), benzodiazepines, lithium monotherapy, adjunctive lithium treatment, and antipsychotic monotherapy (Bergink et al. 2016). ECT has long been used to treat PPP, with a recent large naturalistic study from Sweden demonstrating that ECT in the postpartum period has a significantly higher response rate of 87% in comparison with ECT administered outside the postpartum period (Rundgren et al. 2018). A major expansion from case series literature was a naturalistic cohort study in 64 women who sequentially received benzodiazepines, antipsychotics, and lithium to target each domain (Bergink et al. 2015). Twenty percent of women responded to antipsychotic monotherapy within 2 weeks, with most responding to adjunctive lithium that was then continued as monotherapy after initial remission. In comparison with antipsychotic monotherapy, patients treated with lithium monotherapy had a significantly lower rate of relapse by 9 months postpartum. This evidence supports the many specialists in PPP who argue that the robust response to lithium (as both monotherapy and adjunctive treatment) means that it should be considered the initial intervention unless contraindicated, and antipsychotics and benzodiazepines should be considered adjunctive treatment (Bergink et al. 2016). This is especially applicable in the United States, where psychiatric hospitalizations tend to be far shorter than the several-month stay for the women successfully treated in the study. For women with psychosis limited to the postpartum period, maintenance treatment with lithium should be continued for 9 months after initial stabilization, after which time a gradual and monitored taper can be considered.

In the event of a hospitalization for the acute presentation of PPP, discharge planning requires special consideration. Family involvement in the plan for discharge, including identifying specific supports around nighttime care of the infant, will be critical to continued improvement once outpatient treatment is initiated. Family members or other support persons should be counseled on the early signs of relapse, and close outpatient psychiatric follow-up should be solidified. The inpatient treatment team should carefully consider state requirements around reporting to child protective services. Although most women with successfully treated PPP are unlikely to meet this threshold, child protective services should be notified when there is a reasonable concern for potential child abuse or neglect (Hatters-Friedman et al. 2019).

## Prophylactic Treatment

Prophylactic pharmacological treatment is a powerful tool for preventing PPP in women with known bipolar disorders or who have had a previous episode of PPP. Although women with known bipolar disorder limited to remote and mild symptoms may consider a trial off of medication prior to or during pregnancy, the vast majority of women with bipolar disorder require continuous prophylaxis throughout and after pregnancy to prevent illness recurrence, including PPP. Further information on treatment of bipolar disorder during and after pregnancy can be found in Chapter 13, "Depressive Disorders."

Ms. Y is a 33-year-old, gravida 1, para 1 woman who presents to a reproductive psychiatrist for preconception planning. She has a psychiatric history limited to PPP following the birth of her son, who is now 3 years old. She states that shortly after his birth, she experienced a rapid onset of increased energy, decreased need for sleep, confusion, agitation, anxiety, and paranoid delusions. She recalls fleeting thoughts during that episode that "being in this world" was not safe for her or her baby, although she denies any suicidal or homicidal behaviors or attempts. After an experience at a restaurant in which she was certain the waiters were collaborating to harm her baby, her mother brought Ms. Y into the emergency department. She was admitted to psychiatry and was treated inpatient for 7 days and then discharged into outpatient care. She improved acutely on a regimen of lithium 900 mg/day, quetiapine 300 mg twice daily, and lorazepam 1 mg nightly. Although she has never experienced a symptom recurrence, she has remained on this regimen since that time. She reports that she would very much like to have a second child but is scared to discontinue this regimen that has been so helpful to her: "I know I need this medicine, but my doctor told me it isn't safe during pregnancy. I just need to know what I can take so that I can have a healthy baby and not get sick again."

For women with a history of psychotic illness isolated to the postpartum period, current evidence suggests that the initiation of prophylactic medication immediately after delivery is a highly effective strategy. This treatment strategy has the added benefit of avoiding fetal exposure to medication and should be done in combination with close monitoring throughout pregnancy and anticipatory guidance regarding plans for infant feeding. Lithium has the most evidence to support its efficacy for use in this clinical setting (Bergink et al. 2012; Wesseloo et al. 2016).

For all women at elevated risk for PPP, an individualized and comprehensive postpartum prevention plan can be a useful tool. Components of this plan may include an obstetrical birth plan, as well as a plan for infant monitoring in collaboration with a pediatrician if indicated. Education about warning signs for PPP and appropriate emergency numbers should be provided to both patients and family members. If appropriate, patients can be counseled about the option of providing a release of information for ongoing contact with family members or a psychiatric advanced directive. Direct discussion of strategies to prioritize sleep and maintain a regular circadian rhythm is indicated (Wesseloo et al. 2016).

## Other Management Steps

The patient's breastfeeding status may influence the treatment strategy for PPP. Specifically, while she is acutely psychotic or hospitalized, the mother's contact with the infant may be limited. If she desires to breastfeed, inpatient treatment providers should offer the use of a breast pump unless this is clearly contraindicated by safety concerns. Once stable, however, mothers may wish to return to breastfeeding. Although medication itself is not necessarily a contraindication to breastfeeding, patients should be advised that sleep deprivation due to breastfeeding may negatively affect their recovery and that alternate feeding arrangements—particularly at night—may be a preferred strategy (Lewis et al. 2017; Tinkelman et al. 2017). For specific information on the reproductive safety profiles of commonly used mood stabilizers or antipsychotics, please see the corresponding chapters in this textbook.

### Psychosocial Supports

Despite the severity of PPP and the emphasis on safe and effective emergency interventions, psychosocial support is also a crucial part of management. Involving partners and other loved ones in psychoeducation and approaching treatment with an eye toward family systems is crucially important. Providing support for the mother–infant dyad is critical both in the acute setting and beyond. Last, psychosocial interventions around behavioral management, such as the importance of sleep, are also important interventions (Sharma and Mazmanian 2003).

## Conclusion

PPP is a rare condition that may present with a rapid onset of symptoms early in the postpartum period. PPP presents significantly elevated risk to mother and child if not swiftly diagnosed and treated. Because mothers with PPP most often require inpatient treatment at initial presentation, careful attention to the mother–baby dyad, family system, and maintaining lactation (if desired by the patient) are additional but critical components of care. Women with a prior history of PPP and women with bipolar disorder are at highest risk of developing PPP and should be treated prophylactically in the postpartum period if not already receiving maintenance medication during pregnancy. Although benzodiazepines, antipsychotics, lithium, and ECT all have evidence to support their use in the acute treatment of PPP, lithium has the strongest evidence to support its use in prophylactic treatment.

## Key Points

- Postpartum psychosis (PPP) is a treatable psychiatric emergency that requires immediate evaluation.
- Symptoms include mood fluctuation, alterations of consciousness, and abnormalities of thought and perception arising rapidly within the first days to weeks after childbirth.
- Risk evaluation is critical given high rates of suicide and infanticide.
- A personal history of bipolar disorder is the biggest risk factor for PPP, and many women may eventually be diagnosed with bipolar disorder.
- Lithium, antipsychotics, benzodiazepines and ECT have evidence for treatment of acute PPP.
- Lithium is the recommended medication for prophylaxis.
- Psychosocial support includes psychoeducation for family, attention to sleep, and mother–infant bonding.

## References


American Psychiatric Association: Diagnostic and Statistical Manual of Mental Disorders, 5th Edition. Arlington, VA, American Psychiatric Association, 2013

Bergink V, Kushner SA, Pop V, et al: Prevalence of autoimmune thyroid dysfunction in postpartum psychosis. Br J Psychiatry 198(4):264–268, 2011 21343331

Bergink V, Bouvy PF, Vervoort JS, et al: Prevention of postpartum psychosis and mania in women at high risk. Am J Psychiatry 169(6):609–615, 2012 22407083

Bergink V, Burgerhout KM, Weigelt K, et al: Immune system dysregulation in first-onset postpartum psychosis. Biol Psychiatry 73(10):1000–1007, 2013 23270599

Bergink V, Burgerhout KM, Koorengevel KM, et al: Treatment of psychosis and mania in the postpartum period. Am J Psychiatry 172(2):115–123, 2015 25640930

Bergink V, Rasgon N, Wisner KL: Postpartum psychosis: madness, mania, and melancholia in motherhood. Am J Psychiatry 173(12):1179–1188, 2016 27609245

Blackmore ER, Rubinow DR, O'Connor TG, et al: Reproductive outcomes and risk of subsequent illness in women diagnosed with postpartum psychosis. Bipolar Disord 15(4):394–404, 2013 23651079

Brockington I: Suicide and filicide in postpartum psychosis. Arch Women Ment Health 20(1):63–69, 2017 27778148

Brockington IF, Martin C, Brown GW, et al: Stress and puerperal psychosis. Br J Psychiatry 157(3):331–334, 1990 2245259

Burgerhout KM, Kamperman AM, Roza SJ, et al: Functional recovery after postpartum psychosis: a prospective longitudinal study. J Clin Psychiatry 78(1):122–128, 2017 27631144

Chandra PS, Venkatasubramanian G, Thomas T: Infanticidal ideas and infanticidal behavior in Indian women with severe postpartum psychiatric disorders. J Nerv Ment Dis 190(7):457–461, 2002 12142847

Chandra PS, Bhargavaraman RP, Raghunandan VNGP, et al: Delusions related to infant and their association with mother-infant interactions in postpartum psychotic disorders. Arch Women Ment Health 9(5):285–288, 2006 16937315

Coyle N, Jones I, Robertson E, et al: Variation at the serotonin transporter gene influences susceptibility to bipolar affective puerperal psychosis. Lancet 356(9240):1490–1491, 2000 11081536

Dazzan P, Fusté M, Davies W: Do defective immune system-mediated myelination processes increase postpartum psychosis risk? Trends Mol Med 24(11):942–949, 2018 30348609

Di Florio A, Jones L, Forty L, et al: Mood disorders and parity—a clue to the aetiology of the postpartum trigger. J Affect Disord 152–154:334–339, 2014 24446553

Di Florio A, Munk-Olsen T, Bergink V: The birth of a psychiatric orphan disorder: postpartum psychosis. Lancet Psychiatry 3(6):502, 2016 27262047

Glangeaud-Freudenthal NM, Howard LM, Sutter-Dallay AL: Treatment: mother-infant inpatient units. Best Pract Res Clin Obstet Gynaecol 28(1):147–157, 2014 24054169

Hatters-Friedman S, Resnick PJ: Child murder by mothers: patterns and prevention. World Psychiatry 6(3):137–141, 2007 18188430

Hatters-Friedman S, Prakash C, Nagle-Yang S: Postpartum psychosis: protecting mother and infant: urgent identification and treatment are needed to prevent potentially fatal consequences. Curr Psychiatr 18(4):12–22, 2019

Hellerstedt WL, Phelan SM, Cnattingius S, et al: Are prenatal, obstetric, and infant complications associated with postpartum psychosis among women with pre-conception psychiatric hospitalisations? BJOG 120(4):446–455, 2013 23194279

Jones I, Craddock N: Familiality of the puerperal trigger in bipolar disorder: results of a family study. Am J Psychiatry 158(6):913–917, 2001 11384899

Jones I, Hamshere M, Nangle JM, et al: Bipolar affective puerperal psychosis: genome-wide significant evidence for linkage to chromosome 16. Am J Psychiatry 164(7):1099–1104, 2007 17606662

Kamperman AM, Veldman-Hoek MJ, Wesseloo R, et al: Phenotypical characteristics of postpartum psychosis: a clinical cohort study. Bipolar Disord 19(6):450–457, 2017 28699248

Kumar HB, Purushottam M, Kubendran S, et al: Serotonergic candidate genes and puerperal psychosis: an association study. Psychiatr Genet 17(5):253–260, 2007 17728663

Kumar MM, Venkataswamy MM, Sathyanarayanan G, et al: Immune system aberrations in postpartum psychosis: an immunophenotyping study from a tertiary care neuropsychiatric hospital in India. J Neuroimmunol 310:8–13, 2017 28778450

Lewis KS, Gordon-Smith K, Forty L, et al: Sleep loss as a trigger of mood episodes in bipolar disorder: individual differences based on diagnostic subtype and gender. Br J Psychiatry 211(3):169–174, 2017 28684405

Lewis KJS, Di Florio A, Forty L, et al: Mania triggered by sleep loss and risk of postpartum psychosis in women with bipolar disorder. J Affect Disord 225:624–629, 2018 28889048

Meltzer-Brody S, Maegbaek ML, Medland SE, et al: Obstetrical, pregnancy and socio-economic predictors for new-onset severe postpartum psychiatric disorders in primiparous women. Psychol Med 47(8):1427–1441, 2017 28112056

Osborne LM: Recognizing and managing postpartum psychosis: a clinical guide for obstetric providers. Obstet Gynecol Clin North Am 45(3):455–468, 2018 30092921

Perry A, Gordon-Smith K, Di Florio A, et al: Adverse childhood life events and postpartum psychosis in bipolar disorder. J Affect Disord 205:69–72, 2016 27420133

Perry A, Gordon-Smith K, Webb I, et al: Postpartum psychosis in bipolar disorder: no evidence of association with personality traits, cognitive style or affective temperaments. BMC Psychiatry 19(1):395, 2019 31830938

Rundgren S, Brus O, Båve U, et al: Improvement of postpartum depression and psychosis after electroconvulsive therapy: a population-based study with a matched comparison group. J Affect Disord 235:258–264, 2018 29660641

Sharma V, Mazmanian D: Sleep loss and postpartum psychosis. Bipolar Disord 5(2):98–105, 2003 12680898

Thippeswamy H, Paul P, Purushottam M, et al: Estrogen pathway related genes and their association with risk of postpartum psychosis: a case control study. Asian J Psychiatr 26:82–85, 2017 28483099

Tinkelman A, Hill EA, Deligiannidis KM: Management of new onset psychosis in the postpartum period. J Clin Psychiatry 78(9):1423–1424, 2017 29125722

VanderKruik R, Barreix M, Chou D, et al: The global prevalence of postpartum psychosis: a systematic review. BMC Psychiatry 17(1):272, 2017 28754094

Weigelt K, Bergink V, Burgerhout KM, et al: Down-regulation of inflammation-protective microRNAs 146a and 212 in monocytes of patients with postpartum psychosis. Brain Behav Immun 29:147–155, 2013 23295264

Wesseloo R, Kamperman AM, Munk-Olsen T, et al: Risk of postpartum relapse in bipolar disorder and postpartum psychosis: a systematic review and meta-analysis. Am J Psychiatry 173(2):117–127, 2016 26514657

CHAPTER 17

# Schizophrenia and Related Disorders


Sarah M. Nagle-Yang, M.D.

Susan Hatters Friedman, M.D.

Caitlin Hasser, M.D.

Ashley Mulvihill, M.D.

Andrew M. Novick, M.D., Ph.D.

Allyce K. Jones, DNP, MSN, PMHNP-BC, APRN

Eric Reed, M.D.

Surya Sabhapathy, M.D., M.P.H.


Schizophrenia is a psychiatric illness that requires ongoing treatment throughout the lifespan. It is characterized by abnormalities of perception, thought, behavior, affect, and cognition (American Psychiatric Association 2013). Although the onset for both men and women is typically in early adulthood, women are more likely than men to experience onset in middle age and to have a better overall disease prognosis (Abel et al. 2010). An understanding of the role of estrogen in the disease course of schizophrenia is growing, and emerging data suggest that estrogen plays a protective role against psychosis and that periods of estrogen decline are associated with new onset or exacerbation of psychotic symptoms (Riecher-Rössler et al. 2018).

Historically, women with schizophrenia have had reduced fertility relative to the general population. Deinstitutionalization of persons living with mental illness and advances in psychopharmacology over several decades, however, have contributed to an increase in fertility rates (Vigod et al. 2012). At present, most women with schizophrenia will have at least one pregnancy (Howard et al. 2001). Thus, proficiency in the psychiatric care of women with schizophrenia during the perinatal period is an essential skill for a psychiatric clinician.

**TABLE 17–1. Risk factors for schizophrenia**

| | |
|---|---|
| Cannabis use | Obstetrical complications |
| Genetics | Prenatal exposure to stress or infection |
| Maternal micronutrient deficiency | Trauma exposure |
| Migration | Urbanicity |

This chapter provides an overview of schizophrenia across the female lifespan and an in-depth review of treatment considerations for women with schizophrenia during the perinatal period. For a more detailed review of the clinical approach in reproductive psychiatry or the underlying physiology and pharmacological considerations across the reproductive life cycle, see the corresponding chapters in this text.

# Epidemiology

## Rates/Incidence

Schizophrenia is a relatively uncommon disorder with a lifetime prevalence of 7.2 per 1,000 persons (Jablensky 2017). It is more common in men than women, with a male-to-female incidence ratio of 1.4:1 (Aleman et al. 2003; McGrath et al. 2008). Although some have argued that the reported increased risk for men may be due to methodological limitations of existing research (i.e., studies focused on inpatient settings show a sample bias toward men, who on average have a more severe disease course), the sex ratio appears to persist even when controlling for pertinent factors (Aleman et al. 2003). Because women, on average, show a less severe disease course and a later onset of illness course than men, it remains possible that detection bias is a contributor to the sex ratio. Interestingly, although the peak age of onset for men is in the early 20s, women show a wider distribution in age of onset, with a peak in the early 20s followed by a secondary peak in middle age. Thus, there is a switch from male to female predominance at older ages (Abel et al. 2010).

## Risk Factors

Schizophrenia is a complex neurodevelopmental disorder with molecular, biological, and psychosocial risk factors at specific developmental periods (Table 17–1). It is a highly heritable condition; twin studies show 40%–50% concordance for monozygotic twins and 6%–10% for dizygotic twins (Cardno and Gottesman 2000). Large-scale genome-wide association studies have identified dozens of susceptibility genes, each of which makes a small contribution to illness risk (Foley et al. 2017). Gene/Environment interactions are critical for the conceptualization of schizophrenia risk. Several genes elevate risk potentially through epigenetic mechanisms in the context of specific environmental risk factors, such as prenatal exposure to infection or stress, obstetrical complications, nutrition, cannabis use, migration, urbanicity, and trauma exposure. Acquired brain injury, anti-NMDA receptor encephalitis, and epilepsy are also risk factors for schizophrenia (Clarke et al. 2012).

Perinatal complications of various types have been associated with later development of schizophrenia in population-based cohort studies. These include pregnancy-related (e.g., preeclampsia and gestational diabetes) or delivery complications (e.g., emergency cesarean delivery), and abnormal growth measures (e.g., low birth weight) (Clarke et al. 2012). Although the exact mechanism is unknown, it has been hypothesized that hypoxia experienced during fetal development, labor and delivery, or the neonatal period may interact with genetic vulnerability to increase schizophrenia risk (Cannon et al. 2000). Prenatal infections across a number of pathogens, including influenza and rubella, may increase risk for schizophrenia, particularly with exposure in the first trimester, likely due to an immune-related mechanism (Clarke et al. 2012). Diverse prenatal stress–related exposures, such as war or death of the mother's partner, also elevate risk, although multiple other confounders affect this finding, such as increased risk of infection, fetal hypoxia, or malnourishment (Clarke et al. 2012). Maternal micronutrient deficiencies, such as vitamin D or choline deficiency, may increase risk for schizophrenia (Clarke et al. 2012; McGrath et al. 2010; Ross et al. 2013). Childhood trauma may increase the risk of psychosis up to fourfold (Heins et al. 2011). Cannabis use has an independent risk for development of schizophrenia, particularly in those with specific alleles of the catechol-O-methyltransferase (*COMT*) gene (Clarke et al. 2012). In short, schizophrenia risk is related to a complex synergistic interaction between genetic susceptibility and environmental exposures beginning in the prenatal environment and continuing through adulthood. Given that schizophrenia is based on a stress-diathesis model, there may be sex-specific differences in stress response, neurotransmitter function, or epigenetics that influence the greater risk in men (Remington and Seeman 2015).

## Diagnostic Criteria

Symptoms of psychotic disorders are generally clustered into positive and negative symptoms. Positive symptoms include delusions, hallucinations, and disorganization of thought or behavior. *Delusions* are fixed, false beliefs that persist despite clear evidence to the contrary. They may be bizarre (clearly implausible and not derived from usual life experiences) or nonbizarre and may encompass a wide variety of themes. *Hallucinations* are perception-like experiences, in any sensory modality, that occur in the absence of a true external stimulus. *Disorganized thought* may manifest as tangential, derailed, illogical, or even completely incomprehensible thought processes. *Disorganized behavior* may include odd, nonsensical, or unpredictable behavior; some patients may simply struggle to meaningfully plan or complete goal-oriented tasks. Negative symptoms include decreased emotional expression (e.g., blunted affect, poor eye contact, or impaired prosody of speech), avolition, and anhedonia (Lewis et al. 2017).

Schizophrenia is categorized in DSM-5 in the chapter "Schizophrenia Spectrum and Other Psychotic Disorders" (American Psychiatric Association 2013), which also includes schizoaffective disorder, schizophreniform disorder, brief psychotic disorder, delusional disorder, and substance/medication-induced psychotic disorder. The diagnostic criteria for schizophrenia are summarized in Box 17–1. Although other diagnostic nuances can be found between brief psychotic disorder, schizophreniform disorder, and schizophrenia (e.g., one or two required symptoms, presence of a requirement for functional decline), a primary distinguishing characteristic among these diagnoses is illness duration. Brief psychotic disorder lasts more than 1 day and resolves within 1 month; schizophreniform disorder lasts longer than 1 month but resolves by 6 months; and schizophrenia has a duration of illness longer than 6 months that includes at least 1 month of active-phase symptoms (American Psychiatric Association 2013). Schizoaffective disorder is defined by a major mood episode with concurrent features of active psychosis. It is distinguished from schizophrenia because symptoms meeting criteria for major mood episodes are experienced for most of the illness and from major depressive or bipolar spectrum disorders because psychotic symptoms continue to occur even in the absence of a major mood episode (American Psychiatric Association 2013). Finally, delusional disorder is characterized by the presence of one or more delusions without other features of psychosis or major mood disturbance.

## Box 17–1. DSM-5 Criteria for Schizophrenia

A. Two (or more) of the following, each present for a significant portion of time during a 1-month period (or less if successfully treated). At least one of these must be (1), (2), or (3):

1. Delusions.
2. Hallucinations.
3. Disorganized speech (e.g., frequent derailment or incoherence).
4. Grossly disorganized or catatonic behavior.
5. Negative symptoms (i.e., diminished emotional expression or avolition).

B. For a significant portion of the time since the onset of the disturbance, level of functioning in one or more major areas, such as work, interpersonal relations, or self-care, is markedly below the level achieved prior to the onset (or when the onset is in childhood or adolescence, there is failure to achieve expected level of interpersonal, academic, or occupational functioning).

C. Continuous signs of the disturbance persist for at least 6 months. This 6-month period must include at least 1 month of symptoms (or less if successfully treated) that meet Criterion A (i.e., active-phase symptoms) and may include periods of prodromal or residual symptoms. During these prodromal or residual periods, the signs of the disturbance may be manifested by only negative symptoms or by two or more symptoms listed in Criterion A present in an attenuated form (e.g., odd beliefs, unusual perceptual experiences).

D. Schizoaffective disorder and depressive or bipolar disorder with psychotic features have been ruled out because either 1) no major depressive or manic episodes have occurred concurrently with the active-phase symptoms, or 2) if mood episodes have occurred during active-phase symptoms, they have been present for a minority of the total duration of the active and residual periods of the illness.

E. The disturbance is not attributable to the physiological effects of a substance (e.g., a drug of abuse, a medication) or another medical condition.

F. If there is a history of autism spectrum disorder or a communication disorder of childhood onset, the additional diagnosis of schizophrenia is made only if prominent delusions or hallucinations, in addition to the other required symptoms of schizophrenia, are also present for at least 1 month (or less if successfully treated).

*Specify* if:

The following course specifiers are only to be used after a 1-year duration of the disorder and if they are not in contradiction to the diagnostic course criteria.

**First episode, currently in acute episode:** First manifestation of the disorder meeting the defining diagnostic symptom and time criteria. An *acute episode* is a time period in which the symptom criteria are fulfilled.

**First episode, currently in partial remission:** *Partial remission* is a period of time during which an improvement after a previous episode is maintained and in which the defining criteria of the disorder are only partially fulfilled.

**First episode, currently in full remission:** *Full remission* is a period of time after a previous episode during which no disorder-specific symptoms are present.

**Multiple episodes, currently in acute episode:** Multiple episodes may be determined after a minimum of two episodes (i.e., after a first episode, a remission and a minimum of one relapse).

**Multiple episodes, currently in partial remission**

**Multiple episodes, currently in full remission**

**Continuous:** Symptoms fulfilling the diagnostic symptom criteria of the disorder are remaining for the majority of the illness course, with subthreshold symptom periods being very brief relative to the overall course.

**Unspecified**

*Specify* if:

**With catatonia** (refer to the criteria for catatonia associated with another mental disorder, pp. 119–120, for definition).

**Coding note:** Use additional code 293.89 (F06.1) catatonia associated with schizophrenia to indicate the presence of the comorbid catatonia.

*Specify* current severity:

Severity is rated by a quantitative assessment of the primary symptoms of psychosis, including delusions, hallucinations, disorganized speech, abnormal psychomotor behavior, and negative symptoms. Each of these symptoms may be rated for its current severity (most severe in the last 7 days) on a 5-point scale ranging from 0 (not present) to 4 (present and severe).

**Note:** Diagnosis of schizophrenia can be made without using this severity specifier.

*Source.* Reprinted from American Psychiatric Association: *Diagnostic and Statistical Manual of Mental Disorders*, 5th Edition. Arlington, VA, 2013, pp. 99–100. Copyright © 2013 American Psychiatric Association. Used with permission.

# Clinical Features

## Clinical Presentation

Symptom onset in schizophrenia may be gradual (more common) or precipitous and commonly includes a prodromal period characterized by prominent cognitive and negative symptoms. Although the classic course is one of exacerbations and remissions, a decline in baseline functioning after each relapse is typical. In general, schizophrenia is associated with profound personal, occupational, and social disability. Although approximately one-third of persons living with schizophrenia are able to maintain relatively normative levels of functioning, most patients are significantly impaired by their illness (Sadock et al. 2015). A large majority of patients with schizophrenia are unemployed, and patients with schizophrenia are 13 times more likely to die by suicide than the general population (Saha et al. 2007). Even after accounting for suicide, persons with schizophrenia have a life expectancy of 10–25 years shorter than control subjects (Lambert 2009). Negative symptoms are typically more stable throughout the course of the disease and have a higher negative predictive power relative to positive symptoms for overall disease morbidity (Lewis et al. 2017). Positive prognostic factors include late or acute onset, onset with an obvious precipitating factor, good premorbid functioning, comorbid mood symptoms, marriage, and a strong support system (Sadock et al. 2015).

Significant sex differences exist in the phenomenology of schizophrenia and result in a better overall prognosis for women relative to their male counterparts. In addition to a later average age of onset, women with schizophrenia generally have better premorbid social and occupational functioning, fewer negative symptoms, shorter hospital stays, fewer legal problems, more intimate partnerships, and lower suicide risk compared with men with schizophrenia (Sadock et al. 2015; Yaeger et al. 2006).

Ms. Z is a 28-year-old woman who is brought to the emergency department by the police after she is found wandering on private property, exhibiting disorganized behavior and making vague threats of violence. On interview, she exhibits paranoid delusions, including beliefs that she is being monitored by surveillance equipment across multiple settings. She believes that neighbors are sending her coded messages via benign activities, such as parking their cars on the street or taking out the trash.

After gathering collateral information, the emergency department physician learns that Ms. Z was diagnosed with schizophrenia at the age of 23, following decreased academic and social functioning over a period of months. At the time of initial presentation, she was exhibiting paranoia and experiencing auditory hallucinations. Although initially she had a several-year period of frequent illness recurrence in the context of medication nonadherence, she has more recently had a prolonged period of stability after starting long-acting injectable (LAI) antipsychotic medication.

Ms. Z is surprised but pleased when her pregnancy test is positive. When the emergency physician contacts her treatment provider, she learns that Ms. Z is 3 months overdue for her injection. When the emergency physician approaches Ms. Z about restarting an antipsychotic medication, she adamantly declines, stating "You can't trick me into taking your poison. I'm not going to let you hurt my baby."

## Influence of Reproductive Transitions on Clinical Presentation, Course, and Prognosis

### Estrogen, Menses, and Perimenopause

Sex differences evident in the clinical presentation of schizophrenia have spurred interest in the "estrogen hypothesis of schizophrenia." Riecher-Rössler and Häfner (1993) further described the estrogen hypothesis as two separate but interrelated hypotheses: 1) estrogen protects against psychotic illness and 2) psychosis itself may influence gonadal hormones, resulting in the dysfunction of the hypothalamic-pituitary-gonadal axis. Both hypotheses speak to the current understanding of schizophrenia pathophysiology as it relates to estrogen, which is described in detail later in the "Pathophysiology" section. From a clinical perspective, the estrogen protective hypothesis predicts that women will have increased incidence and severity of psychotic illness when estrogen is lower across the lifespan (Riecher-Rössler and Häfner 1993). Several lines of evidence support this hypothesis (Table 17–2). Regarding incidence, the second peak of onset for schizophrenia occurs among women in the perimenopausal years (coinciding with declining estrogen levels). More than one-quarter of women with schizophrenia experience their first inpatient psychiatric admission after age 45, and twice as many women develop the disease after the age of 40 compared with men (Riecher-

**TABLE 17–2. Differential diagnosis of schizophrenia**

| |
|---|
| Anatomic lesions (e.g., brain tumor, subdural hematoma) |
| Anti-NMDA encephalitis |
| Delirium |
| Endocrine disturbance (e.g., severe hypothyroidism, Cushing syndrome) |
| Epilepsy (e.g., temporal lobe) |
| Heavy metal toxicity |
| Infectious processes (e.g., neurosyphilis, HIV-related opportunistic infections) |
| Medication-induced psychotic disorder (e.g., steroids, chemotherapeutic agents) |
| Metabolic disturbance (e.g., Wilson disease, porphyria) |
| Multiple sclerosis |
| Nutritional deficiency (e.g., thiamine, vitamin $B_{12}$, folate) |
| Paraneoplastic disturbances (e.g., limbic encephalitis) |
| Substance use disorders (e.g., cocaine, organophosphates, or ethanol withdrawal) |
| Other psychiatric disorders |
| Bipolar disorder |
| Borderline personality disorder |
| Delusional disorder |
| Major depressive disorder with psychotic features |
| PTSD, dissociative subtype |
| Schizoaffective disorder |
| Schizophreniform disorder |
| Schizotypal personality disorder |

Rössler et al. 2018). For women with preexisting schizophrenia, perimenopause may bring a worsening of psychotic symptoms (Sajatovic et al. 2003) and longer hospital admissions (Sajatovic et al. 2000). Further suggestive of a relationship between low estrogen and symptom severity, it has been reported that older women with schizophrenia require higher doses of antipsychotic medication to achieve efficacy (Brzezinski et al. 2017; González-Rodríguez et al. 2016). Although, overall, women with schizophrenia have a better prognosis than men, by the third decade of the illness, this trend appears to reverse (Riecher-Rössler et al. 2010; Yaeger et al. 2006).

Additionally, premenopausal women with schizophrenia may be more likely to experience symptom exacerbation in the premenstrual period, coinciding with the point in the menstrual cycle with the lowest estrogen levels. A recent meta-analysis of women with psychotic disorders reported that symptom exacerbation was more common during the premenstrual period as compared with other points in the menstrual cycle. In this study, women with diagnosed psychotic disorders were 1.5 times more likely to experience a psychiatric admission and to report worsening of symptoms on rating scales or other self-report measures in the premenstrual phase (Reilly et al. 2020). Finally, later menarche has been associated with earlier onset of schizophrenia (Cohen et al. 1999; Hayeems and Seeman 2005). One explanation for this might be that earlier exposure to higher levels of estrogen during development may be protective and delay the onset of schizophrenia in vulnerable women. The estrogen hypothesis of schizophrenia (particularly the estrogen protection hypothesis) thus provides a valuable paradigm that helps explain and predict the onset of psychotic illness in women and when women already diagnosed with schizophrenia are likely to be most vulnerable to exacerbation.

## Preconception

Historically, women with schizophrenia were believed to be subfertile. This was likely related to reduced access to sexual encounters during institutionalization of the chronically mentally ill and to hyperprolactinemia commonly induced by first-generation antipsychotics (Smith and Dubovsky 2017). Today, more than half of women with schizophrenia will become pregnant, and the fertility rate of women with schizophrenia approaches that of the general population (Howard et al. 2001; Vigod et al. 2012).

Discussion of family planning goals and sexual practices is an essential aspect of psychiatric care of women with schizophrenia and should occur routinely throughout the reproductive years. In general, women with schizophrenia have higher rates of high-risk sexual activity, including transactional sex, involvement with multiple partners, and lack of contraceptive use (Cournos et al. 1994) compared with healthy control subjects. Rates of unplanned or unwanted pregnancies are higher among women with schizophrenia than in the general population, likely due to inadequate education about contraception and reduced access to care (Miller 1997). The potential for unintended pregnancy should thus be considered for all women of reproductive age, and if the patient does not desire pregnancy, education around contraception should be provided as part of usual psychiatric care. When prescribing medication treatment, the informed consent process with *all* reproductive-age women should necessarily include the known obstetrical, neonatal, and developmental risks of the proposed pharmacological treatment (see Chapter 8, "A Clinical Approach to Psychiatric Diagnosis and Treatment During Pregnancy," and Chapter 9, "A Clinical Approach to Psychiatric Diagnosis and Treatment in the Postpartum Period").

When a woman with schizophrenia does desire pregnancy, proactive preconception planning with the psychiatrist is essential (Table 17–3). A plan should be developed collaboratively and include consideration of risk of the underlying disease and of the recommended treatments. Because women with schizophrenia on average are more likely to experience comorbid medical conditions and substance use disorders, preconception planning should be comprehensive, with a particular focus on modifiable risk factors (e.g., obesity, tobacco use) with known obstetrical and neonatal risk. In the event of hyperprolactinemia-induced infertility, a dose reduction or switch to a prolactin-sparing antipsychotic should be considered in the context of the patient's clinical course and treatment history (Bostwick et al. 2009).

## Pregnancy and Postpartum

Studies investigating the impact of pregnancy on the course of schizophrenia are limited and complicated by the fact that medication discontinuation is common among women with schizophrenia during pregnancy. Petersen et al. (2014) utilized a database of almost 500,000 pregnant women and found that, by the start of the third trimester, only 38% of women prescribed atypical antipsychotics and 19% of women prescribed typical antipsychotics were still receiving treatment. Available evidence does suggest, however, that pregnancy is not protective against chronic psychotic illness and that the severity of illness prior to pregnancy and decisions around mainte-

**TABLE 17–3. Clinical and epidemiological evidence in support of the estrogen hypothesis**

| |
|---|
| Although lower incidence of disease found in women younger than 40 years, incidence after age 40 is higher in women than men. |
| Illness exacerbated during premenstrual period and perimenopause among women with schizophrenia. |
| Later menarche associated with earlier age of onset of schizophrenia. |
| Second peak of illness onset corresponds with average age of menopause. |

nance medication predict the likelihood of relapse. In a recent, large British study of women with serious mental illness during pregnancy, 24% of women with nonaffective psychoses were psychiatrically hospitalized or self-harmed, compared with 12% of pregnant women with affective psychotic or bipolar disorders (Taylor et al. 2018). Recent hospital admission, recent self-harm, substance misuse, smoking, and lack of maintenance medication during the first trimester predicted relapse.

In the postpartum period, women with schizophrenia have an increased risk of relapse, with potentially devastating effects for both the mother and the infant. This increased risk is likely multifactorial in etiology, with multiple contributing factors such as hormonal shifts after delivery, sleep deprivation, and stress (Rochon-Terry et al. 2016). A large population-based cohort study by Munk-Olsen et al. (2006) reported that women with schizophrenia had a fivefold increased risk of first-time hospital admission in the first 30 postpartum days, and this increased risk continued to a lesser degree for the first 6 postpartum months. A follow-up study by the same group looking specifically at readmission rates for women with known preexisting psychiatric diagnoses showed similar results, with a relative risk of approximately fivefold in the first 20 postpartum days and an elevated risk over 6 months (Munk-Olsen et al. 2009). Although both of these population studies reported that women with schizophrenia had a rate of hospitalization that was considerably lower than postpartum women diagnosed with bipolar affective disorders, these findings strongly support the assertion that the postpartum period is a high-risk time for women with schizophrenia. Risk factors for relapse in the postpartum period among women with schizophrenia include acute symptoms during pregnancy, medical or psychiatric comorbidity, higher maternal age, poor social support, lower socioeconomic status, and reduced engagement in antenatal care (Rochon-Terry et al. 2016).

Ms. AA is a 40-year-old woman who is 9 months postpartum. She is referred for an emergency psychiatric evaluation by her daughter's pediatrician. The pediatrician calls ahead to the psychiatrist while the patient is en route and explains that he has been working with Ms. AA on a nutrition plan to address concerns about her daughter's growth; today, however, she became agitated and belligerent during their visit, accusing him of trying to "taint her system." He is unsure of her medical or psychiatric history, although she has always seemed a little "odd" to him.

On initial evaluation, Ms. AA is irritable and guarded but superficially cooperative. She interacts with her daughter in a loving fashion, and her daughter appears clean and appropriately dressed. She reports that this is "all a misunderstanding" and states that the pediatrician just does not like her. She denies any problems with her mood or thoughts of harming herself or others. As the interview progresses, however, the psychiatrist asks Ms. AA to tell her about her daughter: "What kind of baby is she?" She tells him that her daughter is a gift from God, and she goes on to describe a belief that her daughter is, in fact, a representative of God who has been placed on Earth to select the "chosen few" who will survive a coming disaster. She relates that the pediatrician was such an "idiot" that he wanted her to feed her daughter "that chemical milk" (formula) when she knows her daughter should only have "pure" foods, such as water or apple juice.

Limited studies have investigated common delusions during pregnancy and postpartum. Chandra et al. (2006) investigated 108 women with a severe mental illness in the postpartum period who were admitted to an inpatient psychiatric unit in India. They noted that more than half (53%) of the women had delusions related to the infant. When characterizing these mothers further, the authors found that the mothers who had persecutory delusions related to the infant were more likely to demonstrate affectionate behavior and appropriate competency in caring for the basic needs of the infant but were also more likely to be disturbed or agitated if they were separated from the baby. Mothers who had delusions that the baby was ill-fated, a devil, or not their own child were more likely to demonstrate abusive behavior toward the baby. Overall, mothers who had infant-related delusions were more likely to have abusive incidents and to be assessed by staff as unsafe in caring for their baby (Chandra et al. 2006).

Because psychotic mothers with delusions or hallucinations about their infants may be reluctant to share these beliefs, a psychiatric evaluation should include sensitive inquiry into this content. One method is to start by asking the mother about any concerns for the safety of her children and to follow-up with more focused questions as indicated. Careful consideration is required to discern delusional thoughts involving infant harm from obsessional thoughts common in perinatal OCD. Postpartum obsessional thoughts are more likely than delusions to be ego-dystonic in nature and experienced with intact reality testing and good insight. Although postpartum women with obsessional thoughts are at low risk for harming their infants (Abramowitz et al. 2003; Speisman et al. 2011), active psychotic symptoms focused on the fetus or infant may prompt a lower threshold for inpatient hospitalization due to elevated risk (Friedman and Resnick 2007). For further details on the distinction between delusions and obsessions in the perinatal period, as well as a discussion of safety assessment, please see Chapter 20, "Obsessive-Compulsive Disorder."

## Risk of Untreated Illness in the Perinatal Period

When developing a treatment plan for women with schizophrenia during pregnancy, it is important to consider the risks of the underlying disease as a potential exposure. Women with schizophrenia are more likely to receive poor prenatal care, engage in substance misuse, have poor nutrition, and be exposed to intimate partner violence than are healthy control subjects (Møller-Olsen et al. 2018; Yaeger et al. 2006). They also have higher rates of baseline medical comorbidities, such as diabetes, obesity, and hypertension (Liao et al. 2011). Although studies examining the obstetrical outcomes of women with schizophrenia are largely limited by design (e.g., many studies do not control for medication use or multiple confounders), an underlying diagnosis of schizophrenia has been associated with several adverse outcomes, including preterm delivery, low APGAR scores, low birth weight, intrauterine growth restriction, congenital malformation, placental abruption, stillbirth, and infant death (Abel et al. 2014; Friedman et al. 2016; Tosato et al. 2017). Although these associations are reported in general

**TABLE 17–4. Preconception planning considerations for women with schizophrenia**

| |
|---|
| Address potential concern regarding heritability of psychotic disorder and potential referral to genetic counseling. |
| Discuss current substance use patterns (e.g., tobacco, illicit drugs) and their relation to obstetrical risk. |
| Discuss potential risk of underlying illness with consideration of disease severity, time since last acute exacerbation of illness, and family history or personal history of acute episodes in context of childbirth. |
| Discuss risks associated with continuing or ceasing one or all prescribed medications, as well as potential alternative medications. |
| Include routine family planning discussions as part of usual psychiatric care. |
| Provide education regarding benefits of liaison between professionals involved in pregnancy and postpartum care (e.g., obstetricians, psychiatrists, health visitors) and of adhering to routine prenatal care and fetal monitoring. |
| Provide education regarding importance of preconception folic acid supplementation to prevent neural tube defects. |
| Provide education regarding underlying medical risk factors (e.g., metabolic syndrome) and relation to obstetrical risk. |

among women with schizophrenia, women with an acute illness episode during pregnancy appear to be at the greatest risk. In a large, population-based cohort study, Nilsson et al. (2002) showed that although controlling for various maternal factors (e.g., age, education, tobacco use) markedly reduced risk estimates among all women with schizophrenia, those with an acute episode during pregnancy showed approximately double the risk for adverse pregnancy outcomes even after adjusting for these potential confounders. In short, pregnancies among women with schizophrenia should necessarily be considered high risk. Treatment planning should focus on risk reduction, understanding that no zero-risk option is available in this clinical setting.

## Differential Diagnosis and Comorbidities

A full psychiatric evaluation should be performed to diagnose schizophrenia. In some cases, psychotic symptoms may be either completely or partially attributable to substance use (e.g., cocaine, organophosphates, alcohol withdrawal), medications (e.g., steroids, chemotherapeutic agents), or an underlying medical condition (e.g., epilepsy, paraneoplastic syndromes, endocrine disturbance). In the postpartum period, activation of the immune system requires particular consideration because conditions such as postpartum autoimmune thyroiditis and anti-NMDA encephalitis have been associated with postpartum psychotic symptoms (Bergink et al. 2015). Differential diagnoses include other psychiatric disorders with a possible psychotic component, including major depressive disorder, bipolar disorder, schizoaffective disorder, schizophreniform disorder, PTSD dissociative subtype, borderline personality disorder, or schizotypal personality disorder. See Table 17–4 for an expanded list of considerations.

Medical comorbidities are common among women with schizophrenia and include diabetes mellitus, metabolic syndrome, cardiovascular disease, and pulmonary disease, which are believed to contribute to a reduced life expectancy (American Psychiatric Association 2013). At least half of people with schizophrenia use tobacco. Substance misuse and substance use disorders are also common. Tobacco cessation and substance use treatment should be encouraged throughout the lifespan, but especially preconception or during pregnancy due to risk to the fetus. Common psychiatric comorbidities include anxiety, panic disorder, and OCD (American Psychiatric Association 2013).

## Pathophysiology

Despite impressive progress in research, no definitive pathophysiology of schizophrenia has been determined. Instead, multiple biological abnormalities have been identified, from aberrant neurotransmitter function (Howes and Kapur 2009; van Rossum 1966) to inflammation (Mongan et al. 2020) and structural/functional brain changes (Li et al. 2019; Shenton et al. 2001). Not only is it often unclear to what extent these findings are causal but evidence also suggests that individuals may have separate biological mechanisms (Schwarz et al. 2014). It is beyond the scope of this chapter (and book) to provide an overall overview of schizophrenia pathophysiology; this section instead focuses on the relevance of reproductive hormones, particularly estrogen.

As discussed earlier, the estrogen hypothesis of schizophrenia posits both that estrogen is protective and that gonadal dysfunction is inherent in the pathology of schizophrenia (Riecher-Rössler and Häfner 1993). Thus, women with schizophrenia display hypoestrogenism *independent of expected decreases* in estrogen across the lifespan that may increase vulnerability. Compared with control subjects, even antipsychotic-naïve women with schizophrenia demonstrate elevated prolactin levels, decreased estrogen levels, and abnormalities in gonadotropins across the menstrual cycle (González-Blanco et al. 2016; Riecher-Rössler and Kulkarni 2010). Evidence for this gonadal dysfunction in other psychiatric disorders is lacking, which suggests that it is specific to schizophrenia rather than a general consequence of emotional distress (Riecher-Rössler et al. 1998). In addition to decreased estrogen levels, the ability of estrogen to modulate brain function may be altered in schizophrenia. Schizophrenia is also associated with genetic polymorphisms of the estrogen receptor (Wang et al. 2013) and decreased transcription of the estrogen receptor within the dentate gyrus of the brain (Perlman et al. 2005).

There are multiple mechanisms by which low estrogen levels contribute to schizophrenia. Estrogen has a ubiquitous role in the brain, interacting with the neurotransmitters related to schizophrenia and having general procognitive and neuroprotective effects. Neurodegeneration in schizophrenia is associated with declines in gray and white matter and with ventricular enlargement (Hulshoff Pol and Kahn 2008). Estrogen, on the other hand, can increase neurogenesis, synaptic density, and neurotrophic factors (Hara et al. 2015) and offer neuroprotection from free radicals, excitotoxicity, and inflammation (Hara et al. 2015; McEwen and Alves 1999). In all, estrogen has an "antipsychotic" action while buffering against schizophrenia-induced cognitive impairment and neurodegeneration.

Regarding neurotransmitters, dopamine has perhaps the best-known relationship to schizophrenia. Although the dopamine hypothesis, in which schizophrenia is due to excess dopamine activity, has undergone revision, it continues to be supported by various lines of evidence (Howes and Kapur 2009). Estrogen has extensive interaction with the dopamine system but, unfortunately, not in a simple, direct way that fits cleanly within the dopamine hypothesis. If anything, most evidence in animals and humans suggests that estrogen increases dopamine release, as well as tonic dopamine levels in the mesolimbic pathway (Almey et al. 2015; Justice and de Wit 2000; Yoest et al. 2014), which might be expected to exacerbate positive psychotic symptoms. Over time, estrogen does increase levels of mesolimbic dopamine transporters and the density of dopamine type 2 receptors, perhaps in response to increases in dopaminergic tone (Chavez et al. 2010; Sánchez et al. 2012).

Despite evidence for increasing mesolimbic dopamine activity, animal work suggests that estrogen can both act on its own and augment the effects of antipsychotics in behavioral models relevant to psychosis. Prepulse inhibition, a measure of sensory gating that is deficient in schizophrenia, is often used as a model to test antipsychotic drug effects in animals. Estrogen prevents the deficits in sensory gating in rats induced by the dopamine agonist apomorphine (Gogos et al. 2010). Estrogen was also able to reduce amphetamine-induced locomotor sensitization and, when combined with chronic haloperidol, reduce amphetamine-induced dopamine levels in the mesolimbic pathway (Madularu et al. 2014). Such effects are in line with estrogen's ability to augment the efficacy of antipsychotics in humans (see "Estrogen Replacement Therapy" section later). It could be speculated that estrogen regulates mesolimbic dopamine in such a way as to prevent the dopaminergic sensitization that contributes to psychotic symptoms (Glenthøj and Hemmingsen 1997).

Estrogen also increases dopamine in the prefrontal cortex (PFC) in animals (Jacome et al. 2010), probably at least partially due to its ability to decrease activity of the degradation enzyme *COMT* (Schendzielorz et al. 2011). Because schizophrenia (particularly negative symptoms and cognitive deficits) is linked to deficits in frontal cortex dopamine (Howes and Kapur 2009), estrogen-induced increases in PFC dopamine might represent a more direct mechanism for estrogen's therapeutic and protective action.

Besides dopamine, the advent of atypical antipsychotics that antagonize serotonin receptors has emphasized the importance of serotonin in schizophrenia pathology. Estrogen acts to enhance serotonin activity, particularly in the PFC, which might buffer against the cognitive deficits seen in schizophrenia. Specifically, estrogen-treated rats have increased levels of serotonin in the PFC, with concurrent improvement in spatial working memory (Inagaki et al. 2010). A likely mechanism for this effect is the estrogen receptor's ability to act as a transcription factor for the tryptophan hydroxylase gene important in serotonin synthesis (Hiroi and Handa 2013). However, even with tryptophan depletion, estrogen treatment can prevent decreases in PFC activity during a working memory task, suggesting additional pro-serotonergic effects (Epperson et al. 2012).

Like estrogen's behavioral effects on dopamine-induced behavioral models, estrogen treatment in animals and humans can prevent disruption of sensory gating auditory processing via serotonin receptor agonism (Gogos et al. 2006, 2010; Guille et al. 2011). The ability of estradiol to promote serotonergic activity while simultaneously tempering the disruptive effects of direct serotonergic agonism likely speaks to a complex modulatory function. This may be particularly important in schizophrenia, in which both antagonizing serotonin receptors *and* enhancing serotonergic activity are paradoxically therapeutic (Silver 2004).

An additional mechanism by which estrogen might influence schizophrenia pathophysiology is via interactions with the glutamate system. Hypoglutamatergic activity in schizophrenia has been proposed as a mechanism that promotes positive and negative symptoms, and this is supported by the psychomimetic effects of NMDA antagonists such as ketamine and phencyclidine (Balu 2016). Estrogen can enhance glutamate activity under conditions of decreased glutamatergic tone while simultaneously preventing excitotoxicity from excessive glutamate activity (Spampinato et al. 2012). It has also been shown to prevent cognitive deficits (Sutcliffe et al. 2008) and to reduce the sensory gating deficits induced by NMDA antagonists (Gogos et al. 2012).

Finally, although most data have related the gonadal dysfunction in schizophrenia to decreased estrogen, the potential role of progesterone has received less attention. In their review, Sun et al. (2016) pointed out that times of vulnerability to psychosis for women (menstruation, postpartum, and peri-/postmenopause) are also times of decreased progesterone. Progesterone's metabolism into neuroactive steroids such as allopregnanolone plays an important role in GABAergic transmission, which is known to be disrupted in schizophrenia (Marx et al. 2011). On its own, progesterone has effects similar to those of estrogen in preventing the deficits in sensory gating in animals that occur with dopamine agonists (Rupprecht et al. 1999) and NMDA antagonists (van den Buuse et al. 2015). These findings point to a need for additional research in schizophrenia that takes into account the progesterone and progesterone/estrogen interactions.

Other hormones, such as dehydroepiandrosterone, as well as gonadotropins such as luteinizing hormone and follicle-stimulating hormone, may also contribute to the pathophysiology of schizophrenia in women (Hayes et al. 2012). Compared with estrogen, the available evidence on these other hormones is limited. Current evidence does suggest that estrogen interacts with the dopamine, serotonin, and glutamate systems in a way that provides protective and therapeutic action in schizophrenia. When combined with estrogen's general effects on neuroprotection and cognition, this helps explain the pathological role of hypoestrogenism in patients with schizophrenia.

## Treatment

### Pharmacology in Pregnancy

Although various treatment modalities contribute to the comprehensive treatment of psychotic disorders, pharmacotherapy remains at the core of care for both acute and maintenance treatment. In this section, we review safety data for first-generation antipsychotic (FGA) and second-generation antipsychotic (SGA) medications, which are the mainstay of treatment for psychotic disorders, with special consideration given to clozapine and LAI (depot) formulations. Data surrounding antipsychotic exposure in pregnancy and lactation are generally reassuring but are limited in power relative to data concerning other major psychopharmacological agents (e.g., selective serotonin reuptake inhibitors). In addition, available data are plagued by the methodological limitations inherent in studying pregnant or lactating women and are limited to observational case studies, manufacturer reports, registry studies, and, more recently, a select number of larger prospective cohort studies.

When starting a new antipsychotic medication in pregnancy, consider agents with relatively more robust safety information, such as haloperidol, risperidone, olanzapine, aripiprazole, and quetiapine, versus newer agents, such as lurasidone, asenapine, or cariprazine. The unique side effect profile of agents should also be considered. In the context of acute agitation, medications with more sedating qualities may be preferred, whereas in a less acute scenario it may be prudent to avoid these same agents, which may impede the mother's ability to wake overnight for infant care.

Of note, high rates of polypsychopharmacology have been noted in women with schizophrenia during pregnancy (Møller-Olsen et al. 2018; Sadowski et al. 2013), which is of concern due to the risk of negative synergy from various medications. Sadowski et al. (2013) noted an elevated risk of adverse outcomes with the exposure to polypharmacy, including large for gestational age infants, prematurity, neonatal intensive care unit (NICU) admission, neonatal issues with adaptation, and malformations. Thus, when clinically possible, psychiatric clinicians should aim to minimize polypharmacy during pregnancy.

Although all antipsychotic medications are known to cross the placenta, individual agents vary in their placental passage ratio and thus result in varying degrees of fetal exposure. Using maternal and umbilical cord plasma samples collected at delivery, Newport et al. (2007) quantified this ratio for four commonly used antipsychotics across 50 maternal–infant pairs. In this study, the placental passage ratio was highest for olanzapine (72.1%; SD 42%) and the lowest was for quetiapine (23.8%; SD 11.0%). Haloperidol (65.5%; SD 40.3%) and risperidone (49.2%; SD 33.0%) rates were also reported.

Pharmacokinetic changes related to pregnancy are important to consider in the psychiatric care of women with schizophrenia. Pregnancy induces changes in the hepatic cytochrome (CY) P450 system, which may influence the metabolism of antipsychotic medications. There is decreased activity of CYP1A2 (e.g., reduced clearance of olanzapine or clozapine), increased activity of CYP2D6 (e.g., greater clearance of risperidone, haloperidol, and chlorpromazine), and increased activity of CYP3A4 (e.g., greater clearance of lurasidone, aripiprazole, and quetiapine) (Anderson 2005). Because the magnitude of these changes varies considerably among individuals, women maintained on antipsychotics during pregnancy should have close monitoring of clinical symptoms to determine side effect burden and any need for dosage adjustments. LAI antipsychotics bypass first-pass hepatic metabolism; as such, dosing of these may not be affected by pregnancy-related metabolic changes.

Women with psychotic disorders are more likely than their healthy counterparts to smoke (Szatkowski and McNeill 2015). Because smoking induces activity of CYP1A2 (Anderson and Chan 2016), a reduction or cessation in smoking due to pregnancy may lead to an effective increase in levels of olanzapine or clozapine at stable oral dosing. In addition, patients are likely to require higher levels of nicotine replacement therapy in the second and third trimesters due to an increase in CYP2A6 activity (Koren and Pariente 2018; Szatkowski and McNeill 2015).

## First-Generation Antipsychotics

FGAs have been an established treatment for psychotic disorders over decades and historically were also used for treatment of hyperemesis gravidarum. Although data regarding their relative safety in pregnancy have accumulated over several decades, most of these data are limited to case reports and reports of adverse effects compiled by pharmaceutical companies (Abel et al. 2014), yielding information that is limited and often inconsistent in findings.

**Early pregnancy.** Overall, the data on FGAs (including promethazine, chlorpromazine, haloperidol, perphenazine, trifluoperazine, loxapine, thioridazine, flupenthixol, and fluphenazine) suggest that they are not likely to be major teratogens (Diav-Citrin et al. 2005; Einarson and Boskovic 2009). Nonetheless, the association of early exposure to haloperidol with limb abnormalities cannot be definitely ruled out (Gentile 2010), and some studies that have shown an overall increased risk of major malformations are limited by multiple confounders.

**Obstetrical outcomes.** Meta-analyses have shown small but statistically significant increases in earlier delivery and low birth weight, although most of these studies were noted not to be able to separate out drug exposure versus confounders seen in women with severe mental illness (Coughlin et al. 2015; Diav-Citrin et al. 2005). There has been no noted increased risk of spontaneous abortions (Coughlin et al. 2015).

**Delivery effects.** In 2011, the FDA issued a drug safety communication describing a concern about an association between third-trimester exposure to antipsychotic medication (FGAs and SGAs) and extrapyramidal symptoms (EPS) and withdrawal symptoms in the newborn (Kulkarni et al. 2015). This warning was based on 69 cases of infants who had been exposed to antipsychotics and had neonatal symptoms; however, it did not account for multiple confounders (e.g., polypharmacy or underlying illness) present in most of the cases (Kulkarni et al. 2015). EPS have been documented to last up to 10 months, but the vast majority of cases resolve within days, with no long-term adverse sequelae (Galbally et al. 2014).

**Long-term effects.** There have been no differences in IQ or development when FGA-exposed infants were followed up at 5 years of age (Galbally et al. 2014). Prospective studies have shown some delay in gross motor skills at 6 months for some infants, but this effect has been transient and FGA-exposed infants showed no significant differences from control subjects at 12–24 months (Poels et al. 2018).

## Second-Generation Antipsychotics

Use of SGAs has increased dramatically in the general population since their introduction in the 1990s, and recent evidence suggests this trend is seen among pregnant women as well (Epstein et al. 2013). Although SGAs have increasingly replaced FGAs as the mainstay of treatment for schizophrenia, the bulk of this increase cannot be accounted for by use in persons with psychotic illness and is likely due to an increase in prescribing for wider indications (i.e., bipolar disorder) as well as off-label use (i.e., insomnia) (Galbally et al. 2014). With the exception of risperidone and paliperidone, SGAs present less risk for prolactin elevation than the FGAs and may be more favorable for women attempting to conceive. Advantages over FGAs include lower likelihood of EPS and tardive dyskinesia. However, SGAs pose an increased risk for gestational diabetes (Bodén et al. 2012) that can lead to poor outcomes for maternal and fetal health.

**Early pregnancy.** In a large prospective observational cohort study, Habermann et al. (2013) followed the pregnancies of 561 women exposed to SGAs in the first trimester and found that the risk of any malformation was increased in the exposed group relative to nonexposed infants (adjusted OR 2.17; 95% CI 1.20–3.91). When the malformations were analyzed by organ system, the SGAs were associated with an increased incidence of cardiovascular malformations when compared with nonexposure (OR

3.21; 95% CI 1.34–7.67). Because most cardiovascular defects in the SGA group were isolated atrial or ventricular septal defects, the authors noted that detection bias may account for this finding; the exposed group of mother and infants were more likely to have had intensive medical monitoring (Habermann et al. 2013). Furthermore, the comparison group comprised women from the general population who were not taking understudied or teratogenic medications, so it is likely that confounding by indication (i.e., the effect of having underlying illness) or by active illness (i.e., the effect of active symptoms) may also have played a part (some other studies have connected cardiac malformations to schizophrenia itself).

A later and much larger study by Huybrechts et al. (2016) examined the risk of congenital malformations in first-trimester exposure to SGA medications. Using a sample of 1,360,101 pregnant women from a Medicaid database, they examined the pregnancy outcomes of 9,258 women who filled a prescription for an SGA in the first trimester of pregnancy. Analyses were done to compare cumulative data from all exposures to SGAs as well as individual agents (quetiapine, $n$=4,221; aripiprazole, $n$=1,756; risperidone, $n$=1,566; olanzapine, $n$=1,394; and ziprasidone, $n$=697) with women with no antipsychotic exposure. Although the unadjusted analysis did show a small but statistically significant increase in the rate of total major malformations, once the data were adjusted for confounding variables, the rate did not differ significantly from that of the unexposed group (RR 1.05; 95% CI 0.62–1.31) for overall malformations or for cardiac malformations. When this group of SGAs was examined individually, only risperidone was associated with an overall small but statistically significant increased risk of malformations (RR 1.26; 95% CI 1.02–1.56) (Huybrechts et al. 2016).

Cumulatively, the data suggest that, as a class, SGAs do not substantially increase the risk of congenital malformations and should be considered as a treatment option when clinically indicated. Newer SGAs (e.g., lurasidone, iloperidone, and brexpiprazole) have not been adequately represented in these studies to draw any conclusions about their teratogenic potential.

**Obstetrical outcomes.** Because the SGAs have a long-recognized association with metabolic side effects, there has also been concern about their potential to contribute to excess gestational weight gain or gestational diabetes, two complications of pregnancy that are significantly associated with adverse pregnancy outcomes (Oken et al. 2009; Sweeting et al. 2016). Although a registry analysis done by Freeman et al. (2018) did not show a difference in mean weight gain associated with SGA exposure during pregnancy, women in this study who were taking SGAs were more likely to begin pregnancy with a BMI in the obese range ($P$<0.0001) compared with control subjects with similar psychiatric morbidity, illustrating the importance of strategies to address SGA-associated weight gain in women of reproductive age as part of routine practice. In contrast, however, in an analysis of a Medicaid database of 1,543,334 pregnancies, Park et al. (2018) analyzed the risk of developing gestational diabetes among women who continued an SGA medication throughout pregnancy relative to women who had previously been taking an SGA medication but discontinued prior to pregnancy. In this study, women who continued treatment with either olanzapine (absolute risk reduction [aRR] 1.61; 95% CI 1.13–2.29) or quetiapine (aRR 1.28; 95% CI 1.01–1.62) during pregnancy had an increased risk of gestational diabetes. Although some studies have reported a small increase in the risk of miscarriage among women taking quietiapine or aripiprazole, these studies are difficult to interpret because they were not controlled for underlying maternal illness (Damkier and Videbech 2018; Sakai et al. 2017).

**Delivery effects.** There is a paucity of data regarding neonatal outcomes in the setting of SGA exposure during pregnancy, and the studies that have been reported are difficult to interpret due to concomitant exposure to maternal mental illness, comorbidities (e.g., smoking and poor nutrition), and polypharmacy. Although causality cannot be established, SGAs as a class have been associated with EPS, neonatal withdrawal symptoms, and NICU admission (Galbally et al. 2014; Habermann et al. 2013; Kulkarni et al. 2014; Sadowski et al. 2013). As previously discussed, both SGAs and FGAs may be associated with transient EPS after neonatal exposure. Neonatal withdrawal symptoms have also been described, including respiratory distress, feeding difficulties, hypotension, and somnolence (Epstein et al. 2014).

**Long-term effects.** Neurodevelopmental studies of the effects of SGAs in utero are limited. One prospective controlled study compared 22 infants age 6 months who had been exposed to either SGA or FGA medications in utero with 85 nonexposed infants and found that both antipsychotic exposure and underlying maternal mental illness (depression and psychosis) were associated with significantly lower scores on a standard test of neuromotor performance (Johnson et al. 2012). Another study followed 76 infants with in-utero SGA exposure who were matched to 76 unexposed infants born to women without mental illness and found delayed development in cognitive, motor, social-emotional, and adaptive behavior at 2 months of age but not at 12 months. This study suggests transient neurodevelopmental effects among infants born to women taking antipsychotic medications but cannot rule out the contribution of the underlying illness (Peng et al. 2013).

## Clozapine

Although clozapine is categorized as an SGA, it warrants separate mention because it is the gold standard medication for treatment-resistant schizophrenia. Due to potential serious side effects (e.g., seizures, myocarditis, agranulocytosis, weight gain, excess sedation) and the need for routine serum monitoring, its use is reserved for patients for whom other treatments have been ineffective or intolerable (Warnez and Alessi-Severini 2014). Therefore, patients who are appropriate candidates for clozapine are highly likely to require maintenance medication treatment throughout pregnancy to remain at their baseline level of function and symptom control (Friedman and Adityanjee 2003). Reports of clozapine use in pregnancy are very often confounded by polypharmacy, including known teratogens (Friedman and Adityanjee 2003). Mehta and Van Lieshout (2017) noted regarding the current state of the literature, "in the absence of control participants, it is unclear whether these risks are due to clozapine, the experience of serious psychotic illness, previous treatment, or a combination of these" (p. 2). Due to fluctuating clozapine levels during pregnancy, frequent monitoring of serum levels and white blood cell count is recommended regardless of psychiatric stability (Nguyen et al. 2020).

**Early pregnancy.** Clozapine has been used as an FDA-approved medication since 1990 in the United States and for longer in Europe, and no clear pattern of malformations has been noted. The rate of malformations does not appear to be elevated based on available data (Friedman and Adityanjee 2003; Mehta and Van Lieshout 2017). The few studies examining miscarriage rates found no increased risk compared with the general population (Mehta and Van Lieshout 2017).

**Obstetrical outcomes.** Although available data on the obstetrical course of women taking clozapine are limited, it has been reported that pregnant women taking clozapine have elevated rates of obesity and gestational diabetes relative to the general pregnant population (Mehta and Van Lieshout 2017; Nguyen et al. 2020). Side effects of constipation, orthostatic hypotension, and cardiomyopathy have also been noted (Cohen 2017; Ronaldson 2017).

**Delivery effects.** Because the expression of CYP1A2 is underdeveloped during fetal development, clozapine can potentially accumulate in the fetal circulation (Friedman and Adityanjee 2003; Mehta and Van Lieshout 2017). High serum concentrations of clozapine at birth may place the infant at risk of seizures, agranulocytosis, or complications such as floppy infant syndrome (including decreased muscle tone, which is associated with motor developmental delay) (Mehta and Van Lieshout 2017). A case series by Nguyen et al. (2020) also noted fetal nonreactive cardiotocographic recordings and poor neonatal adjustment. They found high rates of adverse neonatal outcomes including requirement for NICU admission and resuscitation at birth.

**Long-term effects.** Data on long-term neurodevelopmental effects of fetal clozapine exposure are lacking, but a recent study indicated that adaptive behavior scores on the Bayley Scales of Infant and Toddler Development were significantly lower in a clozapine-exposed group compared with infants of mothers who were exposed to other antipsychotic agents at both 2 months and 6 months, although they were not different at 12 months (Mehta and Van Lieshout 2017).

## Long-Acting Injections

The literature on LAI antipsychotic use in pregnancy is extremely sparse and limited to a handful of case reports on individual long-acting agents, including haloperidol, fluphenazine, aripiprazole, olanzapine, risperidone, and paliperidone (Ballester-Gracia et al. 2019; Clinebell et al. 2017; Kim et al. 2007; Manouilenko et al. 2018; Özdemir et al. 2015; Sabo et al. 2018; Zamora Rodríguez et al. 2017). Although published cases have not described any reports of major malformations among LAI-exposed infants, there have been reports of adverse obstetrical outcomes and neonatal effects. A case report of a woman taking LAI risperidone in addition to oral risperidone, benztropine, and citalopram reported that her pregnancy was complicated by intrauterine growth restriction and suspected placental insufficiency. The case did not include information about other potential risk factors, such as tobacco or other substance use (Clinebell et al. 2017). Another case report of a patient taking long-acting risperidone reported a healthy outcome and attainment of infant developmental outcomes at 8 months of age (Kim et al. 2007). A report of a woman taking LAI haloperidol noted EPS in the infant that were treated with clonazepam (Collins and Comer 2003).

Because the data on LAI use during pregnancy are insufficient to draw conclusions about safety, many experts recommend switching the patient to the oral formulation of the medication prior to pregnancy or even once pregnancy is diagnosed. Putting this into practice may be difficult, however, because often patients who are prescribed LAIs have a history of nonadherence to oral medication regimens. In addition, LAIs theoretically offer an advantage in pregnancy because they bypass first-pass hepatic metabolism and thus may achieve more stable blood levels throughout the pharmacokinetic changes of pregnancy. As always, an individualized treatment plan should consider the patient's treatment history, disease course, and efficacy of trialed medication. Because switching to an oral agent may increase the risk of relapse in patients who are unlikely to maintain adherence to oral medications, consideration should be given to the continuation of LAIs in select individuals (Clinebell et al. 2017).

## Pharmacology in Lactation

The postpartum period is one of elevated risk of recurrence for women with schizophrenia. Ideally, discussion around infant feeding preferences and treatment planning should occur collaboratively and proactively with the patient early in her pregnancy and regularly as the pregnancy progresses. Psychiatrists should provide available evidence about the risks and benefits of breastfeeding for the patient's specific situation, as well as the associated risks of formula-feeding versus indicated medications.

In the setting of acute psychotic symptoms, suicidality, or homicidality in the postpartum period, an immediate safety assessment should take priority to determine the need for either inpatient hospitalization or measures to address safety while outpatient care is delivered. Women with acute symptoms may not be capable of safely breastfeeding their infants. Furthermore, women with a range of acute or historical symptoms may prefer to formula-feed to allow for more opportunities for consolidated sleep.

The decision of how best to feed an infant is one that should be made in the context of the patient's clinical presentation and history, as well as her personal preferences. When a woman with schizophrenia does choose to breastfeed her infant, the treating psychiatric clinician should proactively discuss a plan for monitoring medication exposure effects on the infant that includes collaboration with the infant's pediatrician and support for adequate sleep. Lactation support services should be part of the treatment plan. When a patient has been treated with an efficacious medication during pregnancy, consideration should be given to continuing that treatment; switching medication during a high-risk period will introduce the infant to multiple exposures and increase the patient's risk of symptom relapse. Discussion of safety assessment in the perinatal period is covered in further detail in Chapter 10, "A Treatment Approach to Psychiatric Emergencies in the Perinatal Period," and further discussion of the general tenets of prescribing during lactation are discussed in Chapter 9.

### First-Generation Antipsychotics

Haloperidol and chlorpromazine have the most robust (although still limited) data regarding use in lactation. Both medications are secreted into breastmilk in small amounts. Limited data suggest no adverse effects in infants exposed to haloperidol monotherapy. Sedation was noted in some infants exposed to chlorpromazine through lactation. Although reports of EPS as a result of lactation exposure are rare, they remain a theoretical risk in infants exposed to FGAs (Iqbal et al. 2005; Smith and Dubovsky 2017).

### Second-Generation Antipsychotics

Olanzapine, quetiapine, and risperidone have the most available data in breastfeeding, with olanzapine and quetiapine being favorable due to the lowest relative infant dose (RID) (Uguz 2016) (Table 17–5). Infant monitoring for sedation is recommended with olanzapine (Uguz 2016). Because lurasidone is highly protein bound (>99%), the

**TABLE 17–5. Relative infant dose and lactation risk category for commonly used antipsychotic medications**

| Medication | Relative infant dose[a] | Hale's lactation risk category[b] |
|---|---|---|
| Aripiprazole | 0.7%–6.44% | L3 |
| Chlorpromazine | 0.3% | L3 |
| Haloperidol | 0.2%–12% | L3 |
| Lurasidone | No data | No data |
| Olanzapine | 0.28%–2.24% | L2 |
| Quetiapine | 0.02%–0.1% | L2 |
| Risperidone | 2.8%–9.1% | L2 |
| Ziprasidone | 0.07%–1.2% | L2 |

[a]Relative infant dose=infant dose via breastmilk (mg/kg/day) divided by maternal dose (mg/kg/day); <10% is generally considered acceptable in breastfeeding.
[b]L1=compatible; L2=probably compatible (medication studied in a limited number of breastfeeding women without evidence of adverse effect); L3=probably compatible, but no controlled studies in breastfeeding women; L4=potentially hazardous; L5=hazardous.

RID is theoretically low (Greenberg and Citrome 2017); however, no data on lurasidone have been published to date, and it is not considered a preferred SGA for breastfeeding mothers (McAllister-Williams et al. 2017). Limited data exist on ziprasidone, but case report data suggest that treatment during lactation results in low levels in breastmilk (Schlotterbeck et al. 2009). Aripiprazole has inconsistent RID levels in available literature, and the potential exists for accumulation in the neonatal period due to its long half-life and the young infant's relative immature hepatic and renal clearance (Uguz 2016; Watanabe et al. 2011). Because aripiprazole is inconsistently reported to decrease prolactin concentrations, it can potentially interfere with the initiation or continuation of lactation (Cuomo et al. 2018). Newer SGAs, such as asenapine and iloperidone, currently have no published data concerning their safety in lactation.

### Clozapine

Clozapine is highly concentrated in breastmilk, with up to triple the concentration found in maternal blood samples (Friedman and Adityanjee 2003). The accumulation of clozapine in breastmilk is likely related to its lipophilic properties (Friedman and Adityanjee 2003; Mehta and Van Lieshout 2017). The Sandoz registry, which included four infants breastfed by mothers taking clozapine, indicated that one infant developed agranulocytosis that spontaneously resolved after termination of breastfeeding and that another infant was excessively tired (Friedman and Adityanjee 2003). Most experts recommend that women taking clozapine not breastfeed (Uguz 2016). If a mother is breastfeeding, monitoring infants for agranulocytosis is recommended (Mehta and Van Lieshout 2017).

## Other Medication Treatments

### Adverse Effect Management in the Perinatal Period

For many patients, antipsychotic choice may be constrained by efficacy, finances, or patient preference. In these situations, the risk of nonadherence to necessary treatment

**TABLE 17–6. Management of adverse effects**

| Adverse effect | Usual management | Considerations in pregnancy/lactation |
|---|---|---|
| Extrapyramidal symptoms (e.g., dystonia, parkinsonism, akathisia) | Benzodiazepines | Early studies suggested increased risk of cleft lip/palate; subsequent research is reassuring. Regular use late in pregnancy may cause neonatal withdrawal, respiratory depression, or floppy baby syndrome (Organization of Teratology Information Specialists 2021). May cause sedation in infant; shorter-acting agents (e.g., lorazepam) are preferred during lactation. |
| | Benztropine | Limited evidence to guide use. |
| | Diphenhydramine | No clear risk of fetal malformation. Rare reports of uterine hyperstimulation in the context of high levels in late pregnancy (Li et al. 2013; Organization of Teratology Information Specialists 2021). Limited evidence for use in lactation; may contribute to somnolence. |
| | Propranolol | Limited information on first-trimester use. Some association with reduced fetal growth (may be confounded by hypertension). Late in pregnancy, may cause neonatal bradycardia and hypoglycemia (Organization of Teratology Information Specialists 2021). Probably compatible with breastfeeding (Hale 2017); relative infant dose of 1%, peak milk concentrations 2–3 hours after oral dose. |
| Metabolic syndrome | Metformin | No clear association with malformations or pregnancy complications. Low breastmilk transmission (Butalia et al. 2017; Organization of Teratology Information Specialists 2021). |
| Tardive dyskinesia | Benzodiazepines | See above as stated in management of extrapyramidal symptoms. |
| | Valbenazine | Limited to no human data. Increased risk of stillbirth and postnatal death in animal studies. Breastfeeding is not recommended either during treatment or for up to 5 days after last dose (Neurocrine Biosciences 2017). |

may significantly outweigh the risk of an additional pharmacological agent. See Table 17–6 for summary of agents commonly used for management of antipsychotic-related side effects. Sedation can be particularly problematic for patients who are breastfeeding or have primary caregiving responsibilities for an infant, especially overnight. Judicious use of split doses may help to reduce sedation while also preserving efficacy.

## Estrogen Replacement Therapy

Although no clear consensus has been found on the role of estrogen replacement therapy in the treatment of women with schizophrenia, data suggest that it has promise as an augmentation strategy to antipsychotics. A 2012 meta-analysis of four randomized, double-blind, placebo-controlled trials totaling 214 patients found that estrogen therapy was more effective than placebo in reducing both positive and negative symptoms (Begemann et al. 2012). Two subsequent randomized controlled trials of 183 (Kulkarni et al. 2015) and 100 (Weiser et al. 2019) women with schizophrenia reported that 200 μg of transdermal estradiol improved mainly positive symptoms, with moderate effect sizes of ~0.4 compared with placebo. Interestingly, Weiser et al. (2019) noted that this improvement was specific for participants who were 38–46 years of age. Although there is much rationale to suggest that estrogen therapy might be most effective in women for whom estrogen levels have already begun to decline, this hypothesis was tempered by the fact that Weiser et al. (2019) found no difference in baseline estrogen levels between younger and older participants.

Other studies have shown improvement in negative and cognitive symptoms and a reduced need for anticholinergic medication in women with schizophrenia taking antipsychotic medication with adjunctive estradiol (Akhondzadeh et al. 2003; Kulkarni et al. 2015). Most data on estrogen augmentation have been in women 45 years of age and younger and thus may not be applicable to postmenopausal women. Among postmenopausal women with schizophrenia, data are sparse and limited by design flaws. Studies in this population have focused on the disease severity and course among women with schizophrenia who are receiving hormone replacement therapy for nonpsychiatric symptoms of menopause compared with age-matched women with schizophrenia not receiving hormonal treatment. Nevertheless, one study showed that women who were taking hormone replacement therapy for menopausal symptoms required lower doses of antipsychotic medication than the control group and that the two groups did not differ significantly in terms of age, ethnicity, education, age of onset, and other factors (Lindamer et al. 2001).

More recent research has focused on raloxifene, a selective estrogen receptor modulator used as a preventive treatment for postmenopausal osteoporosis. Raloxifene has both agonist and antagonist properties on estrogen receptors, with tissue-specific estrogen antagonism in uterine and breast tissue (Sadovsky and Adler 1998). Multiple studies have reported a decrease in both positive and negative symptoms among postmenopausal women with schizophrenia with adjunctive use of raloxifene (Kianimehr et al. 2014; Kulkarni et al. 2010; Usall et al. 2011, 2016). A 2018 meta-analysis of randomized controlled trials confirmed raloxifene's utility in augmentation for improving both positive and negative symptoms in postmenopausal women (Wang et al. 2018). Although some studies have reported a more robust response at higher doses of raloxifene (120 mg vs. 60 mg), it should be noted that 60 mg is generally the recommended dose for prevention of osteoporosis and the dose at which tolerability and safety have been studied.

Kulkarni et al. (2019) have put forth several recommendations for the use of estrogen and selective estrogen receptor modulators in schizophrenia, integrating guidance from the endocrine and menopause literature regarding the use of hormone replacement. Overall, psychiatrists must be familiar with the various forms of hormone treatments, their contraindications, and their side effects. Initial physical health screening prior to initiation, as well as ongoing screening, must occur; this will vary according to the patient's age (Kulkarni et al. 2019).

### Nonpharmacological Somatic Treatment: Electroconvulsive Therapy

Electroconvulsive therapy remains an important and effective option for women who do not respond to or cannot tolerate psychotropics and remain highly symptomatic or suicidal (Smith and Dubovsky 2017). It is considered low risk to both mother and fetus and is more fully discussed in Chapter 13, "Depressive Disorders."

### Psychosocial Interventions

Research into psychosocial interventions for pregnant or postpartum patients with primary psychotic disorders remains quite limited. Several psychosocial treatments show good efficacy for schizophrenia in general and thus may also be useful in the perinatal period. Evidence supports the use of cognitive-behavioral therapy for psychosis, cognitive remediation, illness self-management training, social skills training, assertive community treatment, family psychoeducation, and supported employment (Clark 2016; Mueser et al. 2013; Pharoah et al. 2010). Cook et al. (2014) completed a retrospective multisite study of integrated clinical, rehabilitation, and parenting services for mothers with psychiatric disabilities in general. Their findings suggest that comprehensive integrated programming may improve maternal clinical outcomes, reduce custody loss, and support family reunification (Cook et al. 2014).

## Special Considerations in Psychosis and Reproduction

### Denial of Pregnancy

There are three types of pregnancy denial: pervasive, affective, and psychotic (Miller 2003). In *pervasive denial*, the woman is not aware that she is pregnant. The physical changes of pregnancy, such as weight gain, amenorrhea, and changes in the body, either are not present or are misconstrued (Friedman et al. 2007). The woman may even misinterpret the pain of labor as being abdominal cramping or a need to defecate. In contrast, those with *affective denial* have an intellectual awareness of pregnancy but make little preparation for the delivery, continuing to act as though they are not pregnant. Women with substance use disorders, for example, may experience affective denial that may help to defend against guilt from harming the fetus due to substance use. Finally, in *psychotic denial*, women with a psychotic disorder and often a history of losing custody of older children may experience denial of pregnancy (Miller 1990). Psychotic denial may be intermittent, with women noticing that they are pregnant at some points but not others. For example, a woman with schizophrenia who is hospitalized may believe that she is not pregnant until confronted with her reflection in the mirror, at which point she may briefly acknowledge the pregnancy and then deny it again.

Distinct from denial of pregnancy, *concealment* of pregnancy occurs when a woman knows that she is pregnant and actively hides the pregnancy from family, partners, friends, and coworkers. Risks from denial and concealment of pregnancy include lack of or late prenatal care (Friedman et al. 2009a). Additionally, the risk of neonaticide (murder in the first day of life) is increased in cases of denial or concealment of pregnancy (Friedman and Resnick 2009). Among 211 third-trimester women who presented to the hospital in labor and had received no prenatal care, 29% had experienced some form of pregnancy denial and 9% had concealed their pregnancy (Friedman et al. 2009a). Reasons for presenting to the hospital included having seizures (and being found to be eclamptic) and having back pain that was actually labor pain (Friedman et al. 2009a), among others. Mothers who had denied or concealed their pregnancy often still retained custody. Those with substance use disorders were least likely to retain custody at hospital discharge (Friedman et al. 2009b).

## Delusions of Pregnancy, Simulated Pregnancy, and Pseudocyesis

A woman may present for pregnancy care when she is not actually pregnant for various reasons, including delusions of pregnancy, a simulated pregnancy, or pseudocyesis. Couvade syndrome has also been described among men. Delusions of pregnancy, like delusions at other times in life, involve fixed, false beliefs. They will often occur in the absence of signs and symptoms of pregnancy. Most often, the woman with delusions of pregnancy has an underlying diagnosis of schizophrenia. However, other psychotic disorders, mood disorders, or dementia may also be primary diagnoses (Bera and Sarkar 2015; Uvais 2020). Galactorrhea and amenorrhea are side effects of certain antipsychotic medications and may be misattributed as signs of pregnancy among some women. Delusions of pregnancy may be associated with perceptual experiences of quickening or fetal movements or erotomanic delusions (Bera and Sarkar 2015; Cipriani and Di Fiorino 2015).

In a systematic review of case reports of delusions of pregnancy, Bera and Sarkar (2015) noted 84 cases in the world literature that were published in English. Approximately half of the patients were between the ages of 20 and 40 years, and one-quarter of patients were older than 50 years. Schizophrenia was diagnosed in more than one-third of the cases, followed in frequency by bipolar disorder and depression. Four-fifths of the delusional pregnancy patients reported having a single fetus. Almost half reported they perceived fetal movement. Approximately two-thirds had a good response to treatment (Bera and Sarkar 2015).

In distinction, a *simulated* pregnancy occurs when a woman is aware that she is not pregnant but presents herself as being pregnant for secondary gain. These secondary gains may include getting married or being able to take time away from work or even gains within the legal system when she is the defendant (Bass and Halligan 2014; Bera and Sarkar 2015).

Finally, *pseudocyesis* is a condition described since the time of Hippocrates and is currently included in DSM-5 as an "other specified" somatic symptom disorder. It is defined as a false belief of being pregnant that is associated with *objective signs and reported symptoms of pregnancy*. In pseudocyesis, a patient's conviction *may or may not* be swayed by laboratory testing, ultrasonographic evidence, or physical examination. Classically, the patient has no other signs or symptoms of a psychiatric disorder, and frequent antecedents are pregnancy loss, infertility, isolation, naïveté, and a belief that childbearing is a woman's crucial role. Pseudocyesis is a rare disorder with decreasing incidence; some hypothesize that the development of readily available objective methods of confirming (or ruling out) pregnancy in the earliest weeks of pregnancy (e.g., home pregnancy tests) explains the decrease in prevalence. Although data on its prevalence are lacking, pseudocyesis may be relatively more common in developing countries that place a high cultural value on childbearing (Brockington 1996; Stotland et al. 2005).

When examining any woman who presents with a false belief that she is pregnant, it is important to remember that organic causes and contributors must be included in the differential diagnosis. Secondary amenorrhea can result from dysfunction of the hypothalamus, pituitary gland, or ovaries. Hyperprolactinemia from endocrine abnormalities or antipsychotic medications can clinically present as galactorrhea. Abdominal distention may result from constipation, metabolic or endocrine disorders, or liver disease. Gestational trophoblastic disease may result in multiple symptoms that mimic pregnancy. Astute clinicians will include a thorough history and review of systems in the examination of these beliefs, followed by an appropriate physical examination, laboratory testing, and referral to other physicians when indicated (Bera and Sarkar 2015).

Couvade syndrome also warrants brief mention in this differential. The name comes from the French word *couver*, meaning "to hatch," and it is also known as a *sympathetic pregnancy*. In this syndrome, the partner of a pregnant woman experiences somatic symptoms of pregnancy. Relative to pseudocyesis, the scientific literature on couvade syndrome is scarce and limited to case reports, and no mention of couvade syndrome appears in DSM-5. In the literature that does exist, couvade syndrome is hypothesized to represent a somatic expression of anxiety, identification with the fetus, ambivalence about fatherhood, or parturition envy (Piechowski-Jozwiak and Bogousslavsky 2018). To date, no case reports or other scientific literature on couvade syndrome among same-sex couples were identified in a literature search.

## Ethics and the Treatment of Schizophrenia in the Peripartum

Ethical issues in perinatal psychiatry that merit special consideration when treating women with schizophrenia include the importance of being proactive rather than reactive and the importance of informed consent, enhancing women's decision-making capacities, and relational ethics (Miller 2009). When psychiatrists evaluate and treat any female patient of childbearing age, they should consider that the patient may become pregnant at some point in her treatment. Being proactive in discussions about her desire for pregnancy, contraceptive options, and plans for treatment during pregnancy may allow for a more thoughtful approach than when the potential for pregnancy is unanticipated. Clinical experience indicates that both psychiatrists and patients may make hasty decisions about medications upon recognition of pregnancy, which is best avoided. Treating mental illness throughout pregnancy at the lowest effective dose may prevent the need for polypharmacy and the need for elevated medication doses to stabilize an avoidable acute episode.

When treating a pregnant woman with a psychotic disorder, one should discuss both the risks of the medication treatment and the risks of not treating the mental illness. It is critical that psychiatrists not overlook the risks of failing to treat a psychotic disorder. The benefits of medication, which the woman has likely experienced in the past, also should be discussed. Consideration of obstetrical and fetal risk should be reframed in the context of the mother–infant pair because the overall health and well-being of the mother is in the infant's best interest. Finally, psychiatrists should enhance a woman's decision-making capacity by describing and helping her understand the risks and probabilities of various outcomes, rather than relying on her perceptions, which may be influenced by the experiences of friends or what is reported in the media (Friedman et al. 2018; Miller 2009).

## Considerations of Involuntary Medications

When a pregnant or postpartum woman is acutely psychotic and refuses treatment despite a clear need for that treatment, the psychiatrist should evaluate that patient's capacity for decision-making about psychiatric treatment. This would include whether she can appreciate her diagnosis and the consequences, whether she can understand relevant information about treatment, whether she is able rationally to manipulate this information, and whether she can communicate a clear choice (Friedman et al. 2018). The psychiatrist should also collaborate with obstetrical providers, even in situations in which the patient is on an inpatient psychiatric unit and requiring forced medications.

When completing an evaluation for involuntary treatment in pregnancy, psychiatrists should be aware of the laws in their jurisdiction, the patient's diagnosis, the rationale for treatment, and the reason behind the lack of capacity. It is critical that they collaborate with obstetrical providers and have a clear understanding of rational psychopharmacology in pregnancy. The least restrictive alternatives for appropriate treatment should be determined. When describing the issues to the court, they should clearly identify the risks of no treatment, because courts may only focus on harm from medications rather than on the risks of not treating (Friedman et al. 2018).

## Parenting

Most women with schizophrenia will have at least one pregnancy over a lifetime, and many mothers with schizophrenia parent their own children. Although women with schizophrenia are likely to care deeply about their children and their responsibilities as mothers, as a group they demonstrate significant parenting challenges (Montgomery 2005). On average, women with schizophrenia display less maternal sensitivity toward their infants and are more likely to have infants or toddlers with insecure or disorganized attachment patterns (Wan et al. 2008a) than are healthy control subjects. Multiple factors related to core symptoms of the illness may affect emotional responsiveness, cognition, and ability to interpret accurately the motivations of others.

Consistent with the negative symptom cluster, mothers with schizophrenia are more likely than healthy control subjects to show interactional deficits when with their infants, to display an impaired ability for "mentalization" (or the capacity to appreciate internal states of others) (Brüne et al. 2007), show a more passive or withdrawn parenting style (Shenoy et al. 2019), and engage in less infant-directed speech (Wan et al. 2008b). Women with schizophrenia are also more likely than healthy mothers to struggle with the practical aspects of parenting and to have less knowledge of child development (Abel et al. 2005). Mothers with schizophrenia are additionally more likely than other mothers to lack support and to experience numerous psychosocial stressors. Notably, the barriers to sensitive parenting experienced by women with schizophrenia occur in the context of offspring who already have increased vulnerability for mental illness and cognitive deficits.

Ms. BB is a 33-year-old woman with schizophrenia who presents to her routine psychiatric follow-up visit accompanied by her wife. She discloses that she would like to have a baby and would like to discuss stopping any of her medications that are not safe in pregnancy.

Ms. BB was diagnosed with schizophrenia in her early 20s. Her illness course has consisted of recurrent episodes of psychosis characterized by auditory hallucinations (often command in nature, e.g., telling her not to eat for days at a time) and paranoid delusions. She has had approximately four previous involuntary psychiatric admissions. Since meeting her wife 6 years ago, however, she has remained stable on a regimen of risperidone 6 mg nightly and occasional lorazepam for sleep. Although she has never quite returned to premorbid level of functioning, Ms. BB has been able to maintain this relationship and hold a part-time job at a local grocery store.

Ms. BB discloses that she has been pregnant twice before. Her first pregnancy ended in a miscarriage. Her second pregnancy resulted in a live birth; however, she lost custody of her son at 3 months "because I got put into the hospital." When asked about her menstrual cycles, she reports that she has not menstruated for "years." She expresses a strong desire for pregnancy, stating that she has always wanted to be a mother and cannot wait to have a baby of her own soon. She asks her psychiatrist which medicine she should take so that she can have a healthy baby.

When considering the care of women with schizophrenia during and after pregnancy, it is important to appreciate that temporary or permanent custody loss is common in this population. Overall, approximately half of women with schizophrenia will experience some period of custody loss (Seeman 2012), particularly in times of illness exacerbation. In a study of women admitted to a British inpatient psychiatric mother–baby unit, women with schizophrenia were at highest risk for discharge with some degree of formal child protective services supervision, with more than half of women with this diagnosis (OR 5.16) referred prior to discharge. In this study, mothers with supportive partnerships and mentally well partners had more positive parenting outcomes (Howard et al. 2003).

Support for parenting is an essential component of a treatment plan for mothers with schizophrenia. Because supportive relationships are associated with positive parenting outcomes for these mothers, a focus on building family and other supports is recommended (Abel et al. 2005). Early childhood intervention programs may offer services to high-risk mothers, such as developmental monitoring of the infant and parent coaching. Evidence-based interventions to support parenting among women with schizophrenia are a critical need. In a review of mother–child relational interventions, approximately nine studies were identified that included mothers with a mental disorder, none of which included women with psychotic disorders specifically (Wan et al.

2008a). Inpatient mother–baby units may promote improvements in maternal symptom management and parenting capacity at periods of acute illness exacerbation; however, these time-limited services do not appear to be sufficient to ensure that outcomes are maintained, especially for more vulnerable women (Gearing et al. 2012).

Given the complex needs of this population of mothers, the mother–infant relationship should be an additional clinical focus. Although practical skills training or education around childrearing practices may be useful for women with schizophrenia, these interventions do not directly address the mother–child relationship deficits commonly reported in this population. Dyadic interventions focused on increasing maternal sensitivity and child attachment have shown efficacy in improving maternal sensitivity in women with depression, but it is unclear at present how effective these interventions might be in women with schizophrenia, who may have heightened concerns about custody loss that present a barrier to engagement in such interventions (Gearing et al. 2012; Wan et al. 2008a).

Treating psychiatrists should note their observations about interactions between the mother with schizophrenia and her infant in the record. This may be particularly helpful if concerns about her parenting arise in the future. If appropriate, due to concerns of maltreatment or risk, child protection services should be notified. However, treating psychiatrists should generally refrain from acting as expert witnesses for their own patients, in part because of the potential for bias because of countertransference and the differences between a forensic and treatment evaluation (Strasburger et al. 1997). Parenting capacity evaluations and child abuse reporting are discussed further in Chapter 24 "Forensic Issues in Perinatal Psychiatry."

## Conclusion

Schizophrenia is an uncommon but serious psychiatric illness associated with profound disability across the spheres of personal, social, and occupational functioning. Gender differences in the phenomenology, course, and prognosis of this illness have been described for several decades, and investigations stemming from the estrogen hypothesis of schizophrenia have contributed to the understanding of estrogen's ubiquitous role in the brain and complex interaction with neurotransmitter systems important to cognition, mood, perception, and behavior.

Sociocultural changes and advances in psychopharmacology have contributed to an increase in fertility rates among women with schizophrenia, such that most of these women will have at least one pregnancy. Because they are likely to require pharmacological treatment throughout a pregnancy and may be especially vulnerable to decompensation in the postpartum period, the "general tenet" in reproductive psychiatry of the risk-risk equation is especially pertinent in both preconception planning and treatment planning during and after pregnancy. Finally, because most mothers with schizophrenia do parent their child(ren), psychiatrists must incorporate consideration of the child into safety and risk assessments and proactively consider parenting support as a component of comprehensive care.

## Key Points

- Estrogen likely plays a protective role in the disease course of schizophrenia, and periods of estrogen decline are associated with new onset or exacerbation of psychotic symptoms.
- Most women with schizophrenia will have at least one pregnancy, and discussion of family planning goals and sexual practices is an essential component of psychiatric care.
- Available evidence suggests that pregnancy is not protective against chronic psychotic illness; the postpartum period represents a time of increased risk of relapse for women with schizophrenia.
- Treatment planning for women with schizophrenia during and after pregnancy requires consideration of risk of the untreated illness alongside the risks of efficacious medications, with the goal of risk reduction. It is not possible to eliminate all risk.
- Although evidence on the safety of antipsychotic medications is limited by methodological constraints, available information suggests that these medications are not major teratogens.
- Although many mothers with schizophrenia parent their children, as a group they are at high risk for custody loss. Support for parenting is an essential part of a treatment plan.

## References

Abel KM, Webb RT, Salmon MP, et al: Prevalence and predictors of parenting outcomes in a cohort of mothers with schizophrenia admitted for joint mother and baby psychiatric care in England. J Clin Psychiatry 66(6):781–789, quiz 808–809, 2005 15960575

Abel KM, Drake R, Goldstein JM: Sex differences in schizophrenia. Int Rev Psychiatry 22(5):417–428, 2010 21047156

Abel KM, Au K, Howard LM: Schizophrenia, psychopharmacology, and pregnancy, in Psychopharmacology and Pregnancy: Treatment Efficacy, Risks, and Guidelines. Edited by Galbally M, Snellen M, Lewis A. Berlin, Springer, 2014, pp 119–138

Abramowitz JS, Schwartz SA, Moore KM, et al: Obsessive-compulsive symptoms in pregnancy and the puerperium: a review of the literature. J Anxiety Disord 17(4):461–478, 2003 12826092

Akhondzadeh S, Nejatisafa AA, Amini H, et al: Adjunctive estrogen treatment in women with chronic schizophrenia: a double-blind, randomized, and placebo-controlled trial. Prog Neuropsychopharmacol Biol Psychiatry 27(6):1007–1012, 2003 14499318

Aleman A, Kahn RS, Selten JP: Sex differences in the risk of schizophrenia: evidence from meta-analysis. Arch Gen Psychiatry 60(6):565–571, 2003 12796219

Almey A, Milner TA, Brake WG: Estrogen receptors in the central nervous system and their implication for dopamine-dependent cognition in females. Horm Behav 74:125–138, 2015 26122294

American Psychiatric Association: Diagnostic and Statistical Manual of Mental Disorders, 5th Edition. Arlington, VA, American Psychiatric Association, 2013

Anderson GD: Pregnancy-induced changes in pharmacokinetics: a mechanistic-based approach. Clin Pharmacokinet 44(10):989–1008, 2005 16176115

Anderson GD, Chan LN: Pharmacokinetic drug interactions with tobacco, cannabinoids and smoking cessation products. Clin Pharmacokinet 55(11):1353–1368, 2016 27106177

Avni-Barron O, Gupta R, Miller LJ: Pseudocyesis. UpToDate.com, 2019. Available at: https://www.uptodate.com/contents/pseudocyesis#H990723195. Accessed October 31, 2019.
Ballester-Gracia I, Pérez-Almarcha M, Galvez-Llompart A, et al: Use of long acting injectable aripiprazole before and through pregnancy in bipolar disorder: a case report. BMC Pharmacol Toxicol 20(1):52, 2019 31462311
Balu DT: The NMDA receptor and schizophrenia: from pathophysiology to treatment. Adv Pharmacol 76:351–382, 2016 27288082
Bass C, Halligan P: Factitious disorders and malingering: challenges for clinical assessment and management. Lancet 383(9926):1422–1432, 2014 24612861
Begemann MJ, Dekker CF, van Lunenburg M, et al: Estrogen augmentation in schizophrenia: a quantitative review of current evidence. Schizophr Res 141(2–3):179–184, 2012 22998932
Bera SC, Sarkar S: Delusion of pregnancy: a systematic review of 84 cases in the literature. Indian J Psychol Med 37(2):131–137, 2015 25969595
Bergink V, Armangue T, Titulaer MJ, et al: Autoimmune encephalitis in postpartum psychosis. Am J Psychiatry 172(9):901–908, 2015 26183699
Bodén R, Lundgren M, Brandt L, et al: Antipsychotics during pregnancy: relation to fetal and maternal metabolic effects. Arch Gen Psychiatry 69(7):715–721, 2012 22752236
Bostwick JR, Guthrie SK, Ellingrod VL: Antipsychotic-induced hyperprolactinemia. Pharmacotherapy 29(1):64–73, 2009 19113797
Brockington I: Motherhood and Mental Health. New York, Oxford University Press, 1996, pp 27–34
Brzezinski A, Brzezinski-Sinai NA, Seeman MV: Treating schizophrenia during menopause. Menopause 24(5):582–588, 2017 27824682
Brüne M, Abdel-Hamid M, Lehmkämper C, et al: Mental state attribution, neurocognitive functioning, and psychopathology: what predicts poor social competence in schizophrenia best? Schizophr Res 92(1–3):151–159, 2007 17346931
Butalia S, Gutierrez L, Lodha A, et al: Short- and long-term outcomes of metformin compared with insulin alone in pregnancy: a systematic review and meta-analysis. Diabet Med 34(1):27–36, 2017 27150509
Cannon TD, Rosso IM, Hollister JM, et al: A prospective cohort study of genetic and perinatal influences in the etiology of schizophrenia. Schizophr Bull 26(2):351–366, 2000 10885636
Cardno AG, Gottesman II: Twin studies of schizophrenia: from bow-and-arrow concordances to star wars Mx and functional genomics. Am J Med Genet 97(1):12–17, 2000 10813800
Chandra PS, Bhargavaraman RP, Raghunandan VN, et al: Delusions related to infant and their association with mother-infant interactions in postpartum psychotic disorders. Arch Women Ment Health 9(5):285–288, 2006 16937315
Chavez C, Hollaus M, Scarr E, et al: The effect of estrogen on dopamine and serotonin receptor and transporter levels in the brain: an autoradiography study. Brain Res 1321:51–59, 2010 20079719
Cipriani G, Di Fiorino M: Delusion of pregnancy: an unusual symptom in the context of dementia. Am J Alzheimers Dis Other Demen 30(4):341–345, 2015 25193999
Clark CM: Psychosocial treatments for schizophrenia: an evaluation of theoretically divergent treatment paradigms, and their efficacy. Clin Schizophr Relat Psychoses 10(1):41–50, 2016 23773889
Clarke MC, Kelleher I, Clancy M, et al: Predicting risk and the emergence of schizophrenia. Psychiatr Clin North Am 35(3):585–612, 2012 22929868
Clinebell K, Gannon J, Debrunner S, et al: Long-acting risperidone injections in a pregnant patient with bipolar disorder. Bipolar Disord 19(7):606–607, 2017 29120507
Cohen D: Clozapine and gastrointestinal hypomobility. CNS Drugs 31(12):1083–1091, 2017 29230675
Cohen RZ, Seeman MV, Gotowiec A, et al: Earlier puberty as a predictor of later onset of schizophrenia in women. Am J Psychiatry 156(7):1059–1064, 1999 10401452
Collins KO, Comer JB: Maternal haloperidol therapy associated with dyskinesia in a newborn. Am J Health Syst Pharm 60(21):2253–2255, 2003 14619120
Cook JA, Steigman PJ, Jonikas JA: Outcomes of programs serving mothers with psychiatric disabilities and their young children: a multisite case file abstraction study. Psychiatr Rehabil J 37(3):232–241, 2014 24932997

Coughlin CG, Blackwell KA, Bartley C, et al: Obstetric and neonatal outcomes after antipsychotic medication exposure in pregnancy. Obstet Gynecol 125(5):1224–1235, 2015 25932852
Cournos F, Guido JR, Coomaraswamy S, et al: Sexual activity and risk of HIV infection among patients with schizophrenia. Am J Psychiatry 151(2):228–232, 1994 8296894
Cuomo A, Goracci A, Fagiolini A: Aripiprazole use during pregnancy, peripartum and lactation: a systematic literature search and review to inform clinical practice. J Affect Disord 228:229–237, 2018 29275156
Damkier P, Videbech P: The safety of second-generation antipsychotics during pregnancy: a clinically focused review. CNS Drugs 32(4):351–366, 2018 29637530
Diav-Citrin O, Shechtman S, Ornoy S, et al: Safety of haloperidol and penfluridol in pregnancy: a multicenter, prospective, controlled study. J Clin Psychiatry 66(3):317–322, 2005 15766297
Einarson A, Boskovic R: Use and safety of antipsychotic drugs during pregnancy. J Psychiatr Pract 15(3):183–192, 2009 19461391
Epperson CN, Amin Z, Ruparel K, et al: Interactive effects of estrogen and serotonin on brain activation during working memory and affective processing in menopausal women. Psychoneuroendocrinology 37(3):372–382, 2012 21820247
Epstein RA, Bobo WV, Martin PR, et al: Increasing pregnancy-related use of prescribed opioid analgesics. Ann Epidemiol 23(8):498–503, 2013 23889859
Epstein RA, Moore KM, Bobo WV: Treatment of bipolar disorders during pregnancy: maternal and fetal safety and challenges. Drug Healthc Patient Saf 7:7–29, 2014 25565896
Foley C, Corvin A, Nakagome S: Genetics of schizophrenia: ready to translate? Curr Psychiatry Rep 19(9):61, 2017 28741255
Freeman MP, Sosinsky AZ, Goez-Mogollon L, et al: Gestational weight gain and pre-pregnancy body mass index associated with second-generation antipsychotic drug use during pregnancy. Psychosomatics 59(2):125–134, 2018 29078988
Friedman SH, Adityanjee DR: Use of clozapine in women of childbearing age. Schizophr Res 1(60):355, 2003
Friedman SH, Resnick PJ: Child murder by mothers: patterns and prevention. World Psychiatry 6(3):137–141, 2007 18188430
Friedman SH, Resnick PJ: Neonaticide: Phenomenology and considerations for prevention. Int J Law Psychiatry 32(1):43–47, 2009 19064290
Friedman SH, Heneghan A, Rosenthal M: Characteristics of women who deny or conceal pregnancy. Psychosomatics 48(2):117–122, 2007 17329604
Friedman SH, Heneghan A, Rosenthal M: Characteristics of women who do not seek prenatal care and implications for prevention. J Obstet Gynecol Neonatal Nurs 38(2):174–181, 2009a 19323713
Friedman SH, Heneghan A, Rosenthal M: Disposition and health outcomes among infants born to mothers with no prenatal care. Child Abuse Negl 33(2):116–122, 2009b 19272644
Friedman SH, Moller-Olsen C, Prakash C, et al: Atypical antipsychotic use and outcomes in an urban maternal mental health service. Int J Psychiatry Med 51(6):521–533, 2016 28629296
Friedman SH, Hall RCW, Sorrentino RM: Involuntary treatment of psychosis in pregnancy. J Am Acad Psychiatry Law 46(2):217–223, 2018 30026401
Galbally M, Snellen M, Power J: Antipsychotic drugs in pregnancy: a review of their maternal and fetal effects. Ther Adv Drug Saf 5(2):100–109, 2014 25083265
Gearing RE, Alonzo D, Marinelli C: Maternal schizophrenia: psychosocial treatment for mothers and their children. Clin Schizophr Relat Psychoses 6(1):27–33, 2012 22453867
Gentile S: Antipsychotic therapy during early and late pregnancy: a systematic review. Schizophr Bull 36(3):518–544, 2010 18787227
Glenthøj BY, Hemmingsen R: Dopaminergic sensitization: implications for the pathogenesis of schizophrenia. Prog Neuropsychopharmacol Biol Psychiatry 21(1):23–46, 1997 9075257
Gogos A, Nathan PJ, Guille V, et al: Estrogen prevents 5-HT1A receptor-induced disruptions of prepulse inhibition in healthy women. Neuropsychopharmacology 31(4):885–889, 2006 16237386

Gogos A, Kwek P, Chavez C, et al: Estrogen treatment blocks 8-hydroxy-2-dipropylaminotetralin- and apomorphine-induced disruptions of prepulse inhibition: involvement of dopamine D1 or D2 or serotonin 5-HT1A, 5-HT2A, or 5-HT7 receptors. J Pharmacol Exp Ther 333(1):218–227, 2010 20042529

Gogos A, Kwek P, van den Buuse M: The role of estrogen and testosterone in female rats in behavioral models of relevance to schizophrenia. Psychopharmacology (Berl) 219(1):213–224, 2012 21800043

González-Blanco L, Greenhalgh AMD, Garcia-Rizo C, et al: Prolactin concentrations in antipsychotic-naïve patients with schizophrenia and related disorders: a meta-analysis. Schizophr Res 174(1–3):156–160, 2016 27068570

González-Rodríguez A, Catalán R, Penadés R, et al: Antipsychotic response worsens with postmenopausal duration in women with schizophrenia. J Clin Psychopharmacol 36(6):580–587, 2016 27626286

Greenberg WM, Citrome L: Pharmacokinetics and pharmacodynamics of lurasidone hydrochloride, a second-generation antipsychotic: a systematic review of the published literature. Clin Pharmacokinet 56(5):493–503, 2017 27722855

Guille V, Gogos A, Nathan PJ, et al: Interaction of estrogen with central serotonergic mechanisms in human sensory processing: loudness dependence of the auditory evoked potential and mismatch negativity. J Psychopharmacol 25(12):1614–1622, 2011 20562170

Habermann F, Fritzsche J, Fuhlbrück F, et al: Atypical antipsychotic drugs and pregnancy outcome: a prospective, cohort study. J Clin Psychopharmacol 33(4):453–462, 2013 23764684

Hale TW: Hale's Medications and Mothers' Milk. New York, Springer, 2017

Hara Y, Waters EM, McEwen BS, et al: Estrogen effects on cognitive and synaptic health over the lifecourse. Physiol Rev 95(3):785–807, 2015 26109339

Hayeems RZ, Seeman MV: Puberty and schizophrenia onset, in Estrogen Effects in Psychiatric Disorders. Edited by Riecher-Rössler A, Bergemann N. New York, Springer, 2005, pp 95–106

Hayes E, Gavrilidis E, Kulkarni J: The role of oestrogen and other hormones in the pathophysiology and treatment of schizophrenia. Schizophr Res Treatment 2012:540273, 2012 22966438

Heins M, Simons C, Lataster T, et al: Childhood trauma and psychosis: a case-control and case-sibling comparison across different levels of genetic liability, psychopathology, and type of trauma. Am J Psychiatry 168(12):1286–1294, 2011 21955935

Hiroi R, Handa RJ: Estrogen receptor-β regulates human tryptophan hydroxylase-2 through an estrogen response element in the 5′ untranslated region. J Neurochem 127(4):487–495, 2013 24033289

Howard L, Kumar R, Thornicroft G: Psychosocial characteristics and needs of mothers with psychotic disorders. Br J Psychiatry 178(5):427–432, 2001 11331558

Howard L, Shah N, Salmon M, et al: Predictors of social services supervision of babies of mothers with mental illness after admission to a psychiatric mother and baby unit. Soc Psychiatry Psychiatr Epidemiol 38(8):450–455, 2003 12910341

Howes OD, Kapur S: The dopamine hypothesis of schizophrenia: version III—the final common pathway. Schizophr Bull 35(3):549–562, 2009 19325164

Hulshoff Pol HE, Kahn RS: What happens after the first episode? A review of progressive brain changes in chronically ill patients with schizophrenia. Schizophr Bull 34(2):354–366, 2008 18283048

Huybrechts KF, Hernández-Díaz S, Patorno E, et al: Antipsychotic use in pregnancy and the risk for congenital malformations. JAMA Psychiatry 73(9):938–946, 2016 27540849

Inagaki T, Gautreaux C, Luine V: Acute estrogen treatment facilitates recognition memory consolidation and alters monoamine levels in memory-related brain areas. Horm Behav 58(3):415–426, 2010 20553724

Iqbal MM, Aneja A, Rahman A, et al: The potential risks of commonly prescribed antipsychotics: during pregnancy and lactation. Psychiatry (Edgmont) 2(8):36–44, 2005 21152171

Jablensky A: Worldwide burden of schizophrenia, in Kaplan and Sadock's Comprehensive Textbook of Psychiatry, 10th Edition. Edited by Sadock BL, Sadock VA, Ruiz P. Philadelphia, PA, Lippincott, Williams and Wilkins, 2017, p 1428

Jacome LF, Gautreaux C, Inagaki T, et al: Estradiol and ERβ agonists enhance recognition memory, and DPN, an ERβ agonist, alters brain monoamines. Neurobiol Learn Mem 94(4):488–498, 2010 20828630

Johnson KC, LaPrairie JL, Brennan PA, et al: Prenatal antipsychotic exposure and neuromotor performance during infancy. Arch Gen Psychiatry 69(8):787–794, 2012 22474072

Justice AJ, de Wit H: Acute effects of estradiol pretreatment on the response to d-amphetamine in women. Neuroendocrinology 71(1):51–59, 2000 10644899

Kianimehr G, Fatehi F, Hashempoor S, et al: Raloxifene adjunctive therapy for postmenopausal women suffering from chronic schizophrenia: a randomized double-blind and placebo controlled trial. Daru 22(1):55, 2014 25012765

Kim SW, Kim KM, Kim JM, et al: Use of long-acting injectable risperidone before and throughout pregnancy in schizophrenia. Prog Neuropsychopharmacol Biol Psychiatry 31(2):543–545, 2007 17110011

Koren G, Pariente G: Pregnancy-associated changes in pharmacokinetics and their clinical implications. Pharm Res 35(3):61, 2018 29435666

Kulkarni J, Gurvich C, Lee SJ, et al: Piloting the effective therapeutic dose of adjunctive selective estrogen receptor modulator treatment in postmenopausal women with schizophrenia. Psychoneuroendocrinology 35(8):1142–1147, 2010 20171784

Kulkarni J, Worsley R, Gilbert H, et al: A prospective cohort study of antipsychotic medications in pregnancy: the first 147 pregnancies and 100 one year old babies. PLoS One 9(5):e94788, 2014 24787688

Kulkarni J, Gavrilidis E, Wang W, et al: Estradiol for treatment-resistant schizophrenia: a large-scale randomized-controlled trial in women of child-bearing age. Mol Psychiatry 20(6):695–702, 2015 24732671

Kulkarni J, Butler S, Riecher-Rössler A: Estrogens and SERMS as adjunctive treatments for schizophrenia. Front Neuroendocrinol 53:100743, 2019 30922675

Lambert TJ: The medical care of people with psychosis. Med J Aust 190(4):171–172, 2009 19220177

Lewis S, Escalona R, Keith SJ: Phenomenology of schizophrenia, in Kaplan and Sadock's Comprehensive Textbook of Psychiatry, 10th Edition. Edited by Sadock BL, Sadock VA, Ruiz P. Philadelphia, PA, Lippincott, Williams and Wilkins, 2017, pp 1410–1416

Li S, Hu N, Zhang W, et al: Dysconnectivity of multiple brain networks in schizophrenia: a meta-analysis of resting-state functional connectivity. Front Psychiatry 10:482, 2019 31354545

Liao CH, Chang CS, Wei WC, et al: Schizophrenia patients at higher risk of diabetes, hypertension and hyperlipidemia: a population-based study. Schizophr Res 126(1–3):110–116, 2011 21216567

Lindamer LA, Buse DC, Lohr JB, et al: Hormone replacement therapy in postmenopausal women with schizophrenia: positive effect on negative symptoms? Biol Psychiatry 49(1):47–51, 2001 11163779

Madularu D, Shams WM, Brake WG: Estrogen potentiates the behavioral and nucleus accumbens dopamine response to continuous haloperidol treatment in female rats. Eur J Neurosci 39(2):257–265, 2014 24164675

Manouilenko I, Öhman I, Georgieva J: Long-acting olanzapine injection during pregnancy and breastfeeding: a case report. Arch Women Ment Health 21(5):587–589, 2018 29637404

Marx CE, Bradford DW, Hamer RM, et al: Pregnenolone as a novel therapeutic candidate in schizophrenia: emerging preclinical and clinical evidence. Neuroscience 191:78–90, 2011 21756978

McAllister-Williams RH, Baldwin DS, Cantwell R, et al: British Association for Psychopharmacology consensus guidance on the use of psychotropic medication preconception, in pregnancy and postpartum 2017. J Psychopharmacol 31(5):519–552, 2017 28440103

McEwen BS, Alves SE: Estrogen actions in the central nervous system. Endocr Rev 20(3):279–307, 1999 10368772

McGrath J, Saha S, Chant D, et al: Schizophrenia: a concise overview of incidence, prevalence, and mortality. Epidemiol Rev 30(1):67–76, 2008 18480098

McGrath JJ, Eyles DW, Pedersen CB, et al: Neonatal vitamin D status and risk of schizophrenia: a population-based case-control study. Arch Gen Psychiatry 67(9):889–894, 2010 20819982

Mehta TM, Van Lieshout RJ: A review of the safety of clozapine during pregnancy and lactation. Arch Women Ment Health 20(1):1–9, 2017 27704220
Miller LJ: Psychotic denial of pregnancy: phenomenology and clinical management. Hosp Community Psychiatry 41(11):1233–1237, 1990 2249803
Miller LJ: Sexuality, reproduction, and family planning in women with schizophrenia. Schizophr Bull 23(4):623–635, 1997 9365999
Miller LJ: Denial of pregnancy, in Infanticide: Psychosocial and Legal Perspectives on Mothers Who Kill. Edited by Spinelli MG. Washington, DC, American Psychiatric Publishing, 2003, pp 81–104
Miller LJ: Ethical issues in perinatal mental health. Psychiatr Clin North Am 32(2):259–270, 2009 19486812
Møller-Olsen C, Friedman SH, Prakash C, North A: Clinical characteristics of maternal mental health service users treated with mood stabilizing or antipsychotic medication. Asia-Pac Psychiatry 10(2):e12304, 2018 29226616
Mongan D, Ramesar M, Föcking M, et al: Role of inflammation in the pathogenesis of schizophrenia: a review of the evidence, proposed mechanisms and implications for treatment. Early Interv Psychiatry 14(4):385–397, 2020 31368253
Montgomery P: Mothers with a serious mental illness: a critical review of the literature. Arch Psychiatr Nurs 19(5):226–235, 2005 16226674
Mueser KT, Deavers F, Penn DL, et al: Psychosocial treatments for schizophrenia. Annu Rev Clin Psychol 9:465–497, 2013 23330939
Munk-Olsen T, Laursen TM, Pedersen CB, et al: New parents and mental disorders: a population-based register study. JAMA 296(21):2582–2589, 2006 17148723
Munk-Olsen T, Laursen TM, Mendelson T, et al: Risks and predictors of readmission for a mental disorder during the postpartum period. Arch Gen Psychiatry 66(2):189–195, 2009 19188541
Neurocrine Biosciences: Ingrezza: highlights of prescribing information. April 2017. Available at: https://www.accessdata.fda.gov/drugsatfda_docs/label/2017/209241lbl.pdf. Accessed January 29, 2021.
Newport DJ, Calamaras MR, DeVane CL, et al: Atypical antipsychotic administration during late pregnancy: placental passage and obstetrical outcomes. Am J Psychiatry 164(8):1214–1220, 2007 17671284
Nguyen T, Mordecai J, Watt F, et al: Obstetric and neonatal outcomes of clozapine exposure in pregnancy: a consecutive case series. Arch Women Ment Health 23(3):441–445, 2020 31203441
Nilsson E, Lichtenstein P, Cnattingius S, et al: Women with schizophrenia: pregnancy outcome and infant death among their offspring. Schizophr Res 58(2–3):221–229, 2002 12409162
Oken E, Kleinman KP, Belfort MB, et al: Associations of gestational weight gain with short- and longer-term maternal and child health outcomes. Am J Epidemiol 170(2):173–180, 2009 19439579
Organization of Teratology Information Specialists: Fact sheets. MotherToBaby, 2021. Available at: https://mothertobaby.org/fact-sheets. Accessed January 29, 2021.
Özdemir AK, Pak SC, Canan F, et al: Paliperidone palmitate use in pregnancy in a woman with schizophrenia. Arch Women Ment Health 18(5):739–740, 2015 25599999
Park Y, Hernandez-Diaz S, Bateman BT, et al: Continuation of atypical antipsychotic medication during early pregnancy and the risk of gestational diabetes. Am J Psychiatry 175(6):564–574, 2018 29730938
Peng M, Gao K, Ding Y, et al: Effects of prenatal exposure to atypical antipsychotics on postnatal development and growth of infants: a case-controlled, prospective study. Psychopharmacology (Berl) 228(4):577–584, 2013 23559219
Perlman WR, Tomaskovic-Crook E, Montague DM, et al: Alteration in estrogen receptor alpha mRNA levels in frontal cortex and hippocampus of patients with major mental illness. Biol Psychiatry 58(10):812–824, 2005 16112656
Petersen I, McCrea RL, Osborn DJ, et al: Discontinuation of antipsychotic medication in pregnancy: a cohort study. Schizophr Res 159(1):218–225, 2014 25171856
Pharoah F, Mari J, Rathbone J, et al: Family intervention for schizophrenia. Cochrane Database Syst Rev (12):CD000088, 2010 21154340

Piechowski-Jozwiak B, Bogousslavsky J: Couvade syndrome: custom, behavior or disease? in Neurologic-Psychiatric Syndromes in Focus, Part II, Vol 42. Basel. Switzerland, Karger, 2018, pp 51–58
Poels EMP, Schrijver L, Kamperman AM, et al: Long-term neurodevelopmental consequences of intrauterine exposure to lithium and antipsychotics: a systematic review and meta-analysis. Eur Child Adolesc Psychiatry 27(9):1209–1230, 2018 29948232
Reilly TJ, Sagnay de la Bastida VC, Joyce DW, et al: Exacerbation of psychosis during the perimenstrual phase of the menstrual cycle: systematic review and meta-analysis. Schizophr Bull 46(1):78–90, 2020 31071226
Remington G, Seeman MV: Schizophrenia and the influence of male gender. Clin Pharmacol Ther 98(6):578–581, 2015 26260896
Riecher-Rössler A, Häfner H: Schizophrenia and oestrogens: is there an association? Eur Arch Psychiatry Clin Neurosci 242(6):323–328, 1993 8323981
Riecher-Rössler A, Kulkarni J: Estrogens and gonadal function in schizophrenia and related psychoses, in Biological Basis of Sex Differences in Psychopharmacology, Vol 8. Edited by Neill JC, Kulkarni J. Berlin, Springer, 2010, pp 155–171
Riecher-Rössler A, Häfner H, Dütsch-Strobel A, et al: Gonadal function and its influence on psychopathology. Arch Women Ment Health 1(1):15–26, 1998
Riecher-Rössler A, Pflüger M, Borgwardt S: Schizophrenia in women, in Oxford Textbook of Women and Mental Health. Edited by Kohen D. New York, Oxford University Press, 2010, pp 102–114
Riecher-Rössler A, Butler S, Kulkarni J: Sex and gender differences in schizophrenic psychoses: a critical review. Arch Women Ment Health 21(6):627–648, 2018 29766281
Rochon-Terry G, Gruneir A, Seeman MV, et al: Hospitalizations and emergency department visits for psychiatric illness during and after pregnancy among women with schizophrenia. J Clin Psychiatry 77(4):541–547, 2016 27035409
Ronaldson KJ: Cardiovascular disease in clozapine-treated patients: evidence, mechanisms, and management. CNS Drugs 31(9):777–795, 2017 28808933
Ross RG, Hunter SK, McCarthy L, et al: Perinatal choline effects on neonatal pathophysiology related to later schizophrenia risk. Am J Psychiatry 170(3):290–298, 2013 23318559
Rupprecht R, Koch M, Montkowski A, et al: Assessment of neuroleptic-like properties of progesterone. Psychopharmacology (Berl) 143(1):29–38, 1999 10227077
Sabo T, Bosnjak D, Oreskovic V, et al: Influence of pharmacokinetic features of long-acting injectable aripiprazole in pregnancy. Eur Psychiatry 48S:S359–S566, 2018
Sadock BJ, Sadock VA, Ruiz P (eds): Schizophrenia spectrum and other psychotic disorders, in Kaplan and Sadock's Synopsis of Psychiatry: Behavioral Sciences/Clinical Psychiatry, 11th Edition. Philadelphia, PA, Lippincott, Williams and Wilkins, 2015, pp 317–318
Sadovsky Y, Adler S: Selective modulation of estrogen receptor action. J Clin Endocrinol Metab 83(1):3–5, 1998 9435407
Sadowski A, Todorow M, Yazdani Brojeni P, et al: Pregnancy outcomes following maternal exposure to second-generation antipsychotics given with other psychotropic drugs: a cohort study. BMJ Open 3(7):e003062, 2013 23852139
Saha S, Chant D, McGrath J: A systematic review of mortality in schizophrenia: is the differential mortality gap worsening over time? Arch Gen Psychiatry 64(10):1123–1131, 2007 17909124
Sajatovic M, Donenwirth K, Sultana D, Buckley P: Admissions, length of stay, and medication use among women in an acute care state psychiatric facility. Psychiatr Serv 51(10):1278–1281, 2000
Sajatovic M, Rosenthal MB, Plax MS, et al: Mental illness and menopause: a patient and family perspective. J Gend Specif Med 6(2):31–34, 2003 12814000
Sakai T, Ohtsu F, Mori C, et al: Signal of miscarriage with aripiprazole: a disproportionality analysis of the Japanese Adverse Drug Event Report Database. Drug Saf 40(11):1141–1146, 2017 28664356
Sánchez MG, Morissette M, Di Paolo T: Effect of a chronic treatment with 17β-estradiol on striatal dopamine neurotransmission and the Akt/GSK3 signaling pathway in the brain of ovariectomized monkeys. Psychoneuroendocrinology 37(2):280–291, 2012 21763075

Schendzielorz N, Rysa A, Reenila I, et al: Complex estrogenic regulation of catechol-O-methyl-transferase (COMT) in rats. J Physiol Pharmacol 62(4):483–490, 2011 22100850
Schlotterbeck P, Saur R, Hiemke C, et al: Low concentration of ziprasidone in human milk: a case report. Int J Neuropsychopharmacol 12(3):437–438, 2009 19203410
Schwarz E, van Beveren NJ, Ramsey J, et al: Identification of subgroups of schizophrenia patients with changes in either immune or growth factor and hormonal pathways. Schizophr Bull 40(4):787–795, 2014 23934781
Seeman MV: Intervention to prevent child custody loss in mothers with schizophrenia. Schizophr Res Treatment 2012:796763, 2012 22966446
Shenoy S, Desai G, Venkatasubramanian G, et al: Parenting in mothers with schizophrenia and its relation to facial emotion recognition deficits: a case control study. Asian J Psychiatr 40:55–59, 2019 30738377
Shenton ME, Dickey CC, Frumin M, et al: A review of MRI findings in schizophrenia. Schizophr Res 49(1–2):1–52, 2001 11343862
Silver H: Selective serotonin re-uptake inhibitor augmentation in the treatment of negative symptoms of schizophrenia. Expert Opin Pharmacother 5(10):2053–2058, 2004 15461540
Smith B, Dubovsky SL: Pharmacotherapy of mood disorders and psychosis in pre- and post-natal women. Expert Opin Pharmacother 18(16):1703–1719, 2017 29019422
Spampinato SF, Merlo S, Molinaro G, et al: Dual effect of 17β-estradiol on NMDA-induced neuronal death: involvement of metabotropic glutamate receptor 1. Endocrinology 153(12):5940–5948, 2012 23077075
Speisman BB, Storch EA, Abramowitz JS: Postpartum obsessive-compulsive disorder. J Obstet Gynecol Neonatal Nurs 40(6):680–690, 2011 22092284
Stotland NL, Stewart DE, Munce SE, et al: Obstetrics and gynecology, in The American Psychiatric Association Publishing Textbook of Psychosomatic Medicine. Edited by Levenson JL. Washington, DC, American Psychiatric Association Publishing, 2005, pp 743–744
Strasburger LH, Gutheil TG, Brodsky A: On wearing two hats: role conflict in serving as both psychotherapist and expert witness. Am J Psychiatry 154(4):448–456, 1997 9090330
Sun J, Walker AJ, Dean B, et al: Progesterone: the neglected hormone in schizophrenia? A focus on progesterone-dopamine interactions. Psychoneuroendocrinology 74:126–140, 2016 27608362
Sutcliffe JS, Rhaman F, Marshall KM, et al: Oestradiol attenuates the cognitive deficit induced by acute phencyclidine treatment in mature female hooded-Lister rats. J Psychopharmacol 22(8):918–922, 2008 18208936
Sweeting AN, Ross GP, Hyett J, et al: Gestational diabetes mellitus in early pregnancy: evidence for poor pregnancy outcomes despite treatment. Diabetes Care 39(1):75–81, 2016 26645084
Szatkowski L, McNeill A: Diverging trends in smoking behaviors according to mental health status. Nicotine Tob Res 17(3):356–360, 2015 25180078
Taylor CL, Broadbent M, Khondoker M, et al: Predictors of severe relapse in pregnant women with psychotic or bipolar disorders. J Psychiatr Res 104:100–107, 2018 30015264
Tosato S, Albert U, Tomassi S, et al: A systematized review of atypical antipsychotics in pregnant women: balancing between risks of untreated illness and risks of drug-related adverse effects. J Clin Psychiatry 78(5):e477–e489, 2017 28297592
Uguz F: Second-generation antipsychotics during the lactation period: a comparative systematic review on infant safety. J Clin Psychiatry 36(3):244–252, 2016 27028982
Usall J, Huerta-Ramos E, Iniesta R, et al: Raloxifene as an adjunctive treatment for postmenopausal women with schizophrenia: a double-blind, randomized, placebo-controlled trial. J Clin Psychiatry 72(11):1552–1557, 2011
Usall J, Huerta-Ramos E, Labad J, et al: Raloxifene as an adjunctive treatment for postmenopausal women with schizophrenia: a 24-week double-blind, randomized, parallel, placebo-controlled trial. Schizophr Bull 42(2):309–317, 2016 26591005
Uvais NA: Delusion of pregnancy in a case of dementia. Eur J Geriatr Gerontol 2(1):24–25, 2020
van den Buuse M, Mingon RL, Gogos A: Chronic estrogen and progesterone treatment inhibits ketamine-induced disruption of prepulse inhibition in rats. Neurosci Lett 607:72–76, 2015 26391745

van Rossum JM: The significance of dopamine-receptor blockade for the mechanism of action of neuroleptic drugs. Arch Int Pharmacodyn Ther 160(2):492–494, 1966 5954044
Vigod SN, Seeman MV, Ray JG, et al: Temporal trends in general and age-specific fertility rates among women with schizophrenia (1996–2009): a population-based study in Ontario, Canada. Schizophr Res 139(1–3):169–175, 2012 22658526
Wan MW, Moulton S, Abel KM: A review of mother–child relational interventions and their usefulness for mothers with schizophrenia. Arch Womens Ment Health 11(3):171–179, 2008a 19337701
Wan MW, Penketh V, Salmon MP, et al: Content and style of speech from mothers with schizophrenia towards their infants. Psychiatry Res 159(1–2):109–114, 2008b 18329722
Wang Q, Dong X, Wang Y, et al: Raloxifene as an adjunctive treatment for postmenopausal women with schizophrenia: a meta-analysis of randomized controlled trials. Arch Womens Ment Health 21(1):31–41, 2018 28849318
Wang S, Li W, Zhao J, et al: Association of estrogen receptor alpha gene polymorphism with age at onset, general psychopathology symptoms, and therapeutic effect of schizophrenia. Behav Brain Funct 9:12, 2013 23497414
Warnez S, Alessi-Severini S: Clozapine: a review of clinical practice guidelines and prescribing trends. BMC Psychiatry 14:102, 2014 24708834
Watanabe N, Kasahara M, Sugibayashi R, et al: Perinatal use of aripiprazole: a case report. J Clin Psychopharmacol 31(3):377–379, 2011 21532364
Weiser M, Levi L, Zamora D, et al: Effect of adjunctive estradiol on schizophrenia among women of childbearing age: a randomized clinical trial. JAMA Psychiatry 76(10):1009–1017, 2019 31365044
Yaeger D, Smith HG, Altshuler LL: Atypical antipsychotics in the treatment of schizophrenia during pregnancy and the postpartum. Am J Psychiatry 163(12):2064–2070, 2006 17151155
Yoest K, Cummings J, Becker J: Estradiol, dopamine and motivation Cent Nerv Syst Agents Med Chem 14(2):83–89, 2014 25540977
Zamora Rodríguez FJ, Benitez Vega C, Sanchez-Waisen Hernández MR, et al: Use of paliperidone palmitate throughout a schizoaffective disorder patient's gestation period. Pharmacopsychiatry 50(1):38–40, 2017 27414740

CHAPTER 18

# Trauma and Reproductive Health

Priya Gopalan, M.D.
Elizabeth Albertini, M.D.
Priyanka Amin, M.D.
Maureen Curley, Ph.D.
Jody Glance, M.D.
Saira Kalia, M.D.
Neeta Shenai, M.D.

Understanding the acute and chronic consequences of trauma is a critical aspect of women's mental health care. About 50% of women experience some type of trauma in their lifetime, and women are more likely than men to develop PTSD following a traumatic experience (Tolin and Foa 2006). Early life trauma and adversity have a significant impact on future mental, physical, and sexual health (Centers for Disease Control and Prevention 2020). The greater number of adverse childhood experiences (ACEs) a female child encounters, the more likely she is to grow up to engage in risky sexual behavior, to have a baby in adolescence, to have serious psychiatric illness, and to develop major medical problems, including cancer (Alcalá et al. 2017; Carr et al. 2013; Williams and Finch 2019). With this high prevalence of trauma exposure and its broad clinical impact, it is critical for all providers who treat women to be aware of trauma and its consequences and create a therapeutic environment in which patients can share their trauma histories.

Trauma-informed care (TIC) is a holistic, person-centered approach to treatment that understands and incorporates the biological, psychological, neurological, and social impacts of trauma on an individual and should be used when working with individuals with trauma histories. TIC is a recommended universal clinical approach because physicians and other clinicians often do not know their patients' trauma histories until patients feel safe disclosing details (Substance Abuse and Mental Health Services Administration 2014a, 2014b). The Adverse Childhood Events Study highlighted the high prevalence of trauma in the general population and the need for a sensitive approach to women who have experienced trauma (Felitti et al. 1998). Many of these individuals develop symptoms of PTSD, a trauma- and stressor-related disorder as defined by DSM-5 (American Psychiatric Association 2013).

Pregnancy introduces special considerations around trauma and intimate partner violence (IPV); consequently, major health care organizations such as the American College of Obstetricians and Gynecologists (ACOG) and the U.S. Preventive Services Task Force (USPSTF) encourage universal or widespread screening of individuals for IPV (American College of Obstetricians and Gynecologists 2012; Curry et al. 2018). Interactions with women suspected of being victims of IPV should be approached with empathy; women should be given a forum to discuss their trauma without being interrogated and should be supported through safety planning, appropriate referrals, and documentation. Untreated trauma can adversely affect subsequent pregnancies, intimate and family relationships, and quality of life. Early detection and intervention, increased public awareness, and an environment that validates perinatal trauma can modify and alleviate symptoms.

This chapter focuses on trauma and PTSD as they relate to reproductive health. Traumatic experiences in the context of IPV/sexual trauma, reproductive loss, traumatic delivery, and voluntary termination of pregnancy (VTOP) may lead to the development of PTSD, with sexual trauma leading to higher rates of PTSD than other forms of trauma (Capaldi et al. 2012). Furthermore, a woman's history of childhood adversity and trauma significantly affects her likelihood of developing perinatal PTSD (discussed later) and affective disorders (see Chapter 13, "Depressive Disorders," and Chapter 19, "Anxiety Disorders and Insomnia in the Perinatal Period") in the context of perinatal stress (Smith et al. 2006). This chapter covers evaluation and treatment of PTSD in the context of IPV/sexual trauma, reproductive loss, traumatic delivery, and VTOP.

# Epidemiology

## Rates/Incidence

### Posttraumatic Stress Disorder

Approximately half of all women in the United States will be exposed to at least one traumatic event in their lifetime (Breslau 2002). Research indicates that women are more often victims of sexual assault and childhood sexual abuse than men, and a Centers for Disease Control and Prevention National Intimate Partner and Sexual Violence Survey conducted in 2010 found that one in five women in the United States have been raped at some point in their lives (Smith et al. 2018). Coupled with research indicating women are twice as likely as men to develop PTSD after a traumatic event and to carry this diagnosis across their lifetime (12% of women vs. 6% of men) (Kessler et al. 1995), women as a whole are likely to have higher incidence of PTSD. Women who have a history of childhood abuse are at increased risk of perinatal-onset PTSD, hypothesized to be in part through a heightened likelihood of engaging in abusive or unsupportive relationships or by decreasing the threshold for the emergence of PTSD symptoms related to birth trauma (Smith et al. 2006).

### Intimate Partner Violence

Rates of IPV during pregnancy vary due to differences in screening tools, differing definitions of IPV, and underreporting. Studies have reported rates as low as 1.2% and as high as 28% (García-Moreno et al. 2005). Many incidents of IPV go unreported; thus, the higher number is likely a more accurate estimation of current rates. U.S. rates vary by ethnicity, with higher rates in Alaska Native/non-Hispanic Native Americans and Blacks and lower rates in Asian Americans (Capaldi et al. 2012). Pregnant adolescents and those with <12 years of formal education also are more likely to have experienced IPV during pregnancy compared with women older than 30 years or with ≥16 years of education (Chisholm et al. 2017). Although data are limited, multiple studies report that LGBTQ+ individuals are at equal or higher risk of IPV than cisgender heterosexual individuals (National Coalition Against Domestic Violence 2018; Roberts et al. 2010).

### Reproductive Loss/Traumatic Delivery

Reproductive loss and trauma during pregnancy, such as preeclampsia or traumatic delivery, can also lead to PTSD symptoms in patients. In the United States, 16% of pregnancies end in spontaneous abortion or stillbirth, and about 19% of pregnancies end in elective terminations. Of these losses, approximately 12%–32% lead to symptoms of PTSD (Daugirdaite et al. 2015). Traumatic deliveries also contribute to symptoms of PTSD, with as many as one-third of women rating their delivery as traumatic (Yildiz et al. 2017). However, only approximately 4.6%–6.3% of these women meet criteria for postpartum PTSD (PP-PTSD). Overall, approximately 8% of women have PTSD in pregnancy or postpartum, and fewer (3%) develop new onset of PTSD after a traumatic childbirth (Ross and McLean 2006).

## Risk Factors

### Posttraumatic Stress Disorder

Exposure to a traumatic event does not automatically lead to the development of PTSD. Although most people experience transient PTSD-like symptoms immediately following a traumatic event, these often resolve quickly and without treatment. Conversion to PTSD varies based on intensity and type of trauma. For example, sexual assault is more likely to lead to PTSD than accidents (Capaldi et al. 2012). Gender also seems to play a role; men are more likely than women to develop PTSD after a sexual assault, whereas the reverse is true following a physical assault (Kessler et al. 1995). Common risk factors are listed in Table 18–1.

### Intimate Partner Violence

Women are more likely than men to be physically injured by IPV (Capaldi et al. 2012), and the highest rates of IPV are in women of reproductive age (Hahn et al. 2018). In a study by Silverman et al. (2006), the risk of IPV was greater in the year prior to pregnancy compared to during the pregnancy itself (Silverman et al. 2006); severity of violence may escalate during pregnancy. Risk factors for perinatal IPV are similar to

**TABLE 18–1. Common risk factors for developing PTSD after general trauma exposure**

| | |
|---|---|
| Exposure to interpersonal violence | History of childhood trauma |
| Exposure to more than three traumatic events | Lower level of education |
| Female gender | Premorbid psychiatric diagnoses |

*Source.* Ozer et al. 2003.

**TABLE 18–2. Risk factors associated with developing PTSD following reproductive loss**

| | |
|---|---|
| Demographic and psychosocial risk factors | Younger age, lower level of education, being unpartnered, adversarial or unsupportive relationship with partner, negative circumstances of conception (e.g., rape), concealed pregnancy, poor social support |
| Obstetrical risk factors | Medical complications during pregnancy or labor, previous gynecological complications, advanced gestational age |
| Psychiatric risk factors | Premorbid psychiatric disorders (e.g., mood and anxiety disorders), having a history of other traumatic experiences resulting in PTSD (especially sexual or medical trauma) |

*Source.* Daugirdaite et al. 2015; Vignato et al. 2018.

those published for IPV in the general population: younger age, low education level, unemployment, and low income (Capaldi et al. 2012; Hahn et al. 2018).

### Reproductive Loss/Traumatic Delivery

Risk factors specific to reproductive health include trauma with reproductive loss (Table 18–2) and traumatic birth experiences (Table 18–3). *Reproductive loss* includes miscarriage, stillbirth, and perinatal or neonatal death. Additionally, some women may experience trauma associated with infertility and associated medical procedures, such as in vitro fertilization. *Traumatic birth experiences* include a wide range of medical complications during labor and delivery, poor communication from medical staff, and a lack of privacy or dignity, which can lead the mother to fear for the safety of the infant or herself. People who witness a partner's traumatic birth experience are also at risk of developing PTSD or other psychiatric disorders. As with all forms of potentially traumatic experiences, whether such an event is perceived as a trauma is subjective and depends on a woman's personal experience, including, significantly, her history of earlier adversity and trauma.

## Screening Methods

### Posttraumatic Stress Disorder

Several validated screening tools have been developed for PTSD, including both self-report and interview-based questionnaires. The American Psychological Association's *Clinical Practice Guideline for the Treatment of Posttraumatic Stress Disorder (PTSD) in Adults* was informed by studies utilizing the validated instruments (American Psychological Association 2017) listed in Table 18–4.

**TABLE 18–3. Risk factors associated with developing PTSD following traumatic birth experience**

| | |
|---|---|
| Predisposing | Antenatal psychiatric disorders (especially anxiety, depression, or history of dissociation), previous trauma, high fear of delivery/pain, first delivery |
| Perinatal | Subjective distress during delivery, dissociation, loss of control, emergency cesarean section, neonatal complications |
| Postdelivery | Perception of care received as incompetent/uncaring (likely the greatest predictor of PTSD), rumination on the experience, poor social support |

*Source.* Haagen et al. 2015.

**TABLE 18–4. Validated screening tools for PTSD**

| Interviews | Self-report |
|---|---|
| Clinician Administrated PTSD Scale for DSM-5 (Weathers et al. 2013) | Davidson Trauma Scale (Davidson et al. 1997a) |
| PTSD Symptom Scale Interview (Foa et al. 1993a) | Impact of Event Scale–Revised (Creamer et al. 2003) |
| Structured Clinical Interview, PTSD module (First et al. 1996) | PTSD Symptom Scale Self-Report Version (Foa et al. 1993b) |
| Structured Interview for PTSD (Davidson et al. 1997b) | Short PTSD Rating Interview (Connor and Davidson 2001) |

## Intimate Partner Violence/Sexual Trauma Screening

The ACOG promotes universal screening for IPV at the first prenatal visit, once per trimester, and at postpartum visits (American College of Obstetricians and Gynecologists 2012). All nonpregnant patients should be screened at every routine gynecological visit, as well as at family planning and preconception visits. The USPSTF also recommends universal screening of all women of childbearing age (Curry et al. 2018). Table 18–5 lists groups that are at particularly high risk of IPV and should receive priority for screening.

Screening methods vary based on specific pregnancy and postpartum concerns. Because screening tools rarely account for ethnic or racial differences, the development of more culturally sensitive screening tools may provide better information on racial minorities and PTSD. Black, indigenous, and Hispanic women may not disclose trauma as freely, may not conceptualize what they have experienced chronically as traumatic, and may screen negative on validated instruments that have largely been tested only on white populations. Clinical staff should be educated in principles of TIC to address these limitations in a culturally sensitive way.

Additional considerations in screening include fear of repercussions and retaliation. Racial minorities, who are often unfairly penalized by the child custody system in comparison with white counterparts, may be fearful of accurately answering screening questionnaires (Connell et al. 2007). LGBTQ+ populations may not disclose trauma related to sexual orientation or gender identity for fear of repercussions, in-

**TABLE 18–5. High-risk populations that should be screened for intimate partner violence**

| | |
|---|---|
| Patients who use substances | Women who are socially isolated |
| Pregnant women | Women with a history of physical, sexual, or psychological abuse |
| Same-sex partners/LGBTQ+ population | Women with partners who use substances |
| Women with controlling, angry, or hostile partners | |

cluding rejection by the health care system, family, or employers, or from fear of homophobia and violence (Miller et al. 2016).

Because these considerations may lead to postponement of care or avoidance of medical systems that are fraught with systemic racism and structural stigma, physicians and other clinicians should maintain an even more vigilant stance on creating a welcoming and trauma-informed environment that promotes disclosure and discussions around the physical and mental health implications of trauma.

Many women may feel ashamed or have other reasons to deny IPV. If clinicians are concerned about the potential presence of IPV, verbalizing these concerns to the patient may provide a path for future disclosure. Potential IPV victims should be told that the clinician is always available to talk and that they may call or make another appointment at any time. Multiple inquiries about any instances of IPV should continue across visits. Creating the habit of asking patients on multiple occasions may lead to disclosure with change in circumstances and comfort.

Barriers to asking about IPV often include issues of lack of knowledge and concerns about being intrusive or offensive. Physicians and other providers cite lack of time and resources for screening during routine office visits (Sprague et al. 2012) and may not feel confident in knowing how to address a positive screening (Table 18–6). These barriers may be decreased through education and training modules in IPV for medical students, residents, social workers, therapists, and other mental health and physical health care providers. Physicians and other providers should be trained not to invite the partner into the room during the examination, to make sure patients are fully clothed when discussing IPV, and to assure patients that what they say is confidential (in accordance with state laws). Physicians and other providers should develop strong therapeutic alliances with their patients and ensure a safe environment when asking about IPV. Once physicians and other providers feel comfortable with basic screening options, procedures, and resources, they may be more likely to screen on a regular basis.

## Reproductive Loss and Traumatic Delivery Screening

Ms. CC is a 26-year-old gravida 2 para 1 who presents 5 weeks after an emergency cesarean section at 27 weeks' gestation. She is referred by her obstetrician to a perinatal psychiatrist for evaluation of depression. When asked about her delivery, she shares that she thought her baby would die and continues to experience high fear and anxiety of harm to her baby. She frequently checks her baby to make sure she is breathing, has poor sleep due to the development of debilitating nightmares, avoids hospital settings and physicians, and has frequent thoughts that the worst scenario will occur. She becomes tearful and shares that she is having difficulty bonding with her baby. She also reports that she has experienced this severity of fear twice in the past, once after a pregnancy loss and again after leaving a physically abusive relationship.

**TABLE 18–6. Approach to discussing intimate partner violence (IPV) with patients**

| | |
|---|---|
| Normalize | "We are talking to all of our patients about how safe they feel at home and in their relationships, because intimate partner violence is so common." |
| Assure confidentiality | "Anything we discuss is confidential. I will not tell your partner, child services, or any agencies about what we discuss. The only things I would have to report are if your life (or someone else's life) is in danger or if your children are being harmed." |
| Ask open-ended questions | "How are you feeling about things in your relationship?" |
| | "Would you say it's a healthy relationship?" |
| Obtain details | "How long has this been going on? How frequently does it occur?" |
| | "When was the most recent event?" |
| Access to weapons | "Does your partner own or have access to firearms or other weapons?" |
| Children | "Has your partner ever harmed or threatened to harm the children (including biological, stepchildren, foster children)?" |
| Escalation | "Have the events become more severe or more frequent?" |
| Severity | "What is the most serious event that has occurred?" |
| | "Any use of weapons, choking/strangling, threats to kill you/loved ones or threats of suicide?" |
| Substance use | "Does your partner misuse alcohol or other drugs?" |
| Validate patient | Listen actively and make reflective statements to demonstrate you hear her perspective. |
| | Show empathy and avoid use of words like "alleged" and "supposed." |
| Provide education and support | Assure her that she is not alone and that this is not a rare event. |
| | Inform her that IPV tends to continue and become more severe over time. |
| | Inquire about the common sequelae listed above, including physical and health problems and risky behaviors. |
| | Discuss a safety plan. |
| | Offer resources, including counseling services, hotline numbers, and advocacy resources, and ask her if she would like to schedule another appointment to discuss further. |
| Know legal aspects | Some states require reporting certain acts of violence, such as being hurt with a weapon or firearm or children witnessing IPV. Be sure to check your state's specific laws for reporting. |
| Be aware of resources for IPV reporting laws | www.acf.hhs.gov/sites/default/files/documents/fysb/state_compendium.pdf |
| | www.annemergmed.com/article/S0196-0644(02)75698-9/pdf |

**Table 18–7. Screening questions for reproductive loss/traumatic delivery**

| | |
|---|---|
| Broad screening questions | "How was your pregnancy/delivery?"<br>"During pregnancy/delivery, did you feel your life or your baby's life was in danger?"<br>"How did your pregnancy/delivery differ from what you expected to happen?"<br>"How did you feel about how you were treated during your pregnancy/delivery?"<br>"How well-supported did you feel by hospital staff, family, and friends during your pregnancy/delivery/postpartum?" |
| Symptom-specific questions | "Have you noticed you avoid things that remind you of your pregnancy/delivery (for example, doctors or hospitals)?"<br>"Do you find yourself trying not to think about your pregnancy/delivery because it causes stress or negative emotions?"<br>"Have you or others noticed that you have been checking on your baby more frequently because you worry something bad will happen?"<br>"Are there extra measures you have taken to ensure that your baby and you are safe?"<br>"How do you feel about going to your obstetrician for your postpartum care?" |

Approximately 12%–30% of women may experience PP-PTSD following a reproductive loss or traumatic delivery (American College of Obstetricians and Gynecologists 2018). Diagnosing PP-PTSD is challenging because of the overlap with grief, depression, and anxiety. Although no well-validated instrument is available to test specifically for PP-PTSD, commonly used instruments include

- Perinatal Grief Scale (Toedter et al. 1988)
- Munich Grief Scale (Beutel et al. 1995)
- Perinatal Bereavement Grief Scale (Ritsher and Neugebauer 2002) (validated in Spanish and English)
- Perinatal Grief Intensity Scale (Hutti et al. 1998)

Following a traumatic delivery, the physician or other provider should encourage and facilitate a comprehensive postpartum appointment, with help from family and other supports when possible, to ensure that appropriate screening occurs. This type of trauma may also result in profound grief, shame, or a sense of failure that can decrease the likelihood of the woman scheduling or attending follow-up care, so proactive outreach to screen is imperative (Table 18–7).

## Clinical Features

### Diagnostic Criteria and Clinical Presentation

With each iteration, DSM has revised and expanded the definition of trauma. Initially, only combat was identified as potentially traumatic. DSM-5 recognizes both actual and threatened death, serious injury, and sexual violence, with four mechanisms of exposure (direct exposure, witnessing, trauma to a close loved one, and repeated extreme exposure to aversive details), as criteria for trauma (Box 18–1). Childbirth, childhood neglect, and interpersonal violence are also now considered potentially traumatic. The presence of intrusive symptoms, persistent avoidance of trauma-related stimuli, negative cognitions and mood precipitated by the traumatic event, and hyperarousal lasting more than 1 month with clinically significant functional impairment meets criteria for PTSD. A specifier of dissociative symptoms can be added if the person also has persistent depersonalization or derealization. A subset diagnosis, PP-PTSD, can occur if diagnostic criteria are met during the postpartum period (American Psychiatric Association 2013).

Box 18–1. DSM-5 Criteria for Posttraumatic Stress Disorder

## Posttraumatic Stress Disorder

**Note:** The following criteria apply to adults, adolescents, and children older than 6 years. For children 6 years and younger, see corresponding criteria below.

A. Exposure to actual or threatened death, serious injury, or sexual violence in one (or more) of the following ways:
   1. Directly experiencing the traumatic event(s).
   2. Witnessing, in person, the event(s) as it occurred to others.
   3. Learning that the traumatic event(s) occurred to a close family member or close friend. In cases of actual or threatened death of a family member or friend, the event(s) must have been violent or accidental.
   4. Experiencing repeated or extreme exposure to aversive details of the traumatic event(s) (e.g., first responders collecting human remains; police officers repeatedly exposed to details of child abuse).

      **Note:** Criterion A4 does not apply to exposure through electronic media, television, movies, or pictures, unless this exposure is work related.

B. Presence of one (or more) of the following intrusion symptoms associated with the traumatic event(s), beginning after the traumatic event(s) occurred:
   1. Recurrent, involuntary, and intrusive distressing memories of the traumatic event(s).

      **Note:** In children older than 6 years, repetitive play may occur in which themes or aspects of the traumatic event(s) are expressed.
   2. Recurrent distressing dreams in which the content and/or affect of the dream are related to the traumatic event(s).

      **Note:** In children, there may be frightening dreams without recognizable content.
   3. Dissociative reactions (e.g., flashbacks) in which the individual feels or acts as if the traumatic event(s) were recurring. (Such reactions may occur on a continuum, with the most extreme expression being a complete loss of awareness of present surroundings.)

      **Note:** In children, trauma-specific reenactment may occur in play.
   4. Intense or prolonged psychological distress at exposure to internal or external cues that symbolize or resemble an aspect of the traumatic event(s).
   5. Marked physiological reactions to internal or external cues that symbolize or resemble an aspect of the traumatic event(s).

C. Persistent avoidance of stimuli associated with the traumatic event(s), beginning after the traumatic event(s) occurred, as evidenced by one or both of the following:

1. Avoidance of or efforts to avoid distressing memories, thoughts, or feelings about or closely associated with the traumatic event(s).
2. Avoidance of or efforts to avoid external reminders (people, places, conversations, activities, objects, situations) that arouse distressing memories, thoughts, or feelings about or closely associated with the traumatic event(s).

D. Negative alterations in cognitions and mood associated with the traumatic event(s), beginning or worsening after the traumatic event(s) occurred, as evidenced by two (or more) of the following:

1. Inability to remember an important aspect of the traumatic event(s) (typically due to dissociative amnesia and not to other factors such as head injury, alcohol, or drugs).
2. Persistent and exaggerated negative beliefs or expectations about oneself, others, or the world (e.g., "I am bad," "No one can be trusted," "The world is completely dangerous," "My whole nervous system is permanently ruined").
3. Persistent, distorted cognitions about the cause or consequences of the traumatic event(s) that lead the individual to blame himself/herself or others.
4. Persistent negative emotional state (e.g., fear, horror, anger, guilt, or shame).
5. Markedly diminished interest or participation in significant activities.
6. Feelings of detachment or estrangement from others.
7. Persistent inability to experience positive emotions (e.g., inability to experience happiness, satisfaction, or loving feelings).

E. Marked alterations in arousal and reactivity associated with the traumatic event(s), beginning or worsening after the traumatic event(s) occurred, as evidenced by two (or more) of the following:

1. Irritable behavior and angry outbursts (with little or no provocation) typically expressed as verbal or physical aggression toward people or objects.
2. Reckless or self-destructive behavior.
3. Hypervigilance.
4. Exaggerated startle response.
5. Problems with concentration.
6. Sleep disturbance (e.g., difficulty falling or staying asleep or restless sleep).

F. Duration of the disturbance (Criteria B, C, D, and E) is more than 1 month.

G. The disturbance causes clinically significant distress or impairment in social, occupational, or other important areas of functioning.

H. The disturbance is not attributable to the physiological effects of a substance (e.g., medication, alcohol) or another medical condition.

*Specify* whether:

**With dissociative symptoms:** The individual's symptoms meet the criteria for posttraumatic stress disorder, and in addition, in response to the stressor, the individual experiences persistent or recurrent symptoms of either of the following:

1. **Depersonalization:** Persistent or recurrent experiences of feeling detached from, and as if one were an outside observer of, one's mental processes or body (e.g., feeling as though one were in a dream; feeling a sense of unreality of self or body or of time moving slowly).
2. **Derealization:** Persistent or recurrent experiences of unreality of surroundings (e.g., the world around the individual is experienced as unreal, dreamlike, distant, or distorted).

**Note:** To use this subtype, the dissociative symptoms must not be attributable to the physiological effects of a substance (e.g., blackouts, behavior during alcohol intoxication) or another medical condition (e.g., complex partial seizures).

*Specify* if:

**With delayed expression:** If the full diagnostic criteria are not met until at least 6 months after the event (although the onset and expression of some symptoms may be immediate).

## Posttraumatic Stress Disorder for Children 6 Years and Younger

A. In children 6 years and younger, exposure to actual or threatened death, serious injury, or sexual violence in one (or more) of the following ways:
   1. Directly experiencing the traumatic event(s).
   2. Witnessing, in person, the event(s) as it occurred to others, especially primary caregivers.

      **Note:** Witnessing does not include events that are witnessed only in electronic media, television, movies, or pictures.
   3. Learning that the traumatic event(s) occurred to a parent or caregiving figure.

B. Presence of one (or more) of the following intrusion symptoms associated with the traumatic event(s), beginning after the traumatic event(s) occurred:
   1. Recurrent, involuntary, and intrusive distressing memories of the traumatic event(s).

      **Note:** Spontaneous and intrusive memories may not necessarily appear distressing and may be expressed as play reenactment.
   2. Recurrent distressing dreams in which the content and/or affect of the dream are related to the traumatic event(s).

      **Note:** It may not be possible to ascertain that the frightening content is related to the traumatic event.
   3. Dissociative reactions (e.g., flashbacks) in which the child feels or acts as if the traumatic event(s) were recurring. (Such reactions may occur on a continuum, with the most extreme expression being a complete loss of awareness of present surroundings.) Such trauma-specific reenactment may occur in play.
   4. Intense or prolonged psychological distress at exposure to internal or external cues that symbolize or resemble an aspect of the traumatic event(s).
   5. Marked physiological reactions to reminders of the traumatic event(s).

C. One (or more) of the following symptoms, representing either persistent avoidance of stimuli associated with the traumatic event(s) or negative alterations in cognitions and mood associated with the traumatic event(s), must be present, beginning after the event(s) or worsening after the event(s):

   **Persistent Avoidance of Stimuli**

   1. Avoidance of or efforts to avoid activities, places, or physical reminders that arouse recollections of the traumatic event(s).
   2. Avoidance of or efforts to avoid people, conversations, or interpersonal situations that arouse recollections of the traumatic event(s).

   **Negative Alterations in Cognitions**

   3. Substantially increased frequency of negative emotional states (e.g., fear, guilt, sadness, shame, confusion).
   4. Markedly diminished interest or participation in significant activities, including constriction of play.
   5. Socially withdrawn behavior.
   6. Persistent reduction in expression of positive emotions.

D. Alterations in arousal and reactivity associated with the traumatic event(s), beginning or worsening after the traumatic event(s) occurred, as evidenced by two (or more) of the following:

1. Irritable behavior and angry outbursts (with little or no provocation) typically expressed as verbal or physical aggression toward people or objects (including extreme temper tantrums).
2. Hypervigilance.
3. Exaggerated startle response.
4. Problems with concentration.
5. Sleep disturbance (e.g., difficulty falling or staying asleep or restless sleep).

E. The duration of the disturbance is more than 1 month.

F. The disturbance causes clinically significant distress or impairment in relationships with parents, siblings, peers, or other caregivers or with school behavior.

G. The disturbance is not attributable to the physiological effects of a substance (e.g., medication or alcohol) or another medical condition.

*Specify* whether:

**With dissociative symptoms:** The individual's symptoms meet the criteria for posttraumatic stress disorder, and the individual experiences persistent or recurrent symptoms of either of the following:

1. **Depersonalization:** Persistent or recurrent experiences of feeling detached from, and as if one were an outside observer of, one's mental processes or body (e.g., feeling as though one were in a dream; feeling a sense of unreality of self or body or of time moving slowly).
2. **Derealization:** Persistent or recurrent experiences of unreality of surroundings (e.g., the world around the individual is experienced as unreal, dreamlike, distant, or distorted).

**Note:** To use this subtype, the dissociative symptoms must not be attributable to the physiological effects of a substance (e.g., blackouts) or another medical condition (e.g., complex partial seizures).

*Specify* if:

**With delayed expression:** If the full diagnostic criteria are not met until at least 6 months after the event (although the onset and expression of some symptoms may be immediate).

*Source.* Reprinted from American Psychiatric Association: *Diagnostic and Statistical Manual of Mental Disorders,* 5th Edition. Arlington, VA, 2013, pp. 271–272. Copyright © 2013 American Psychiatric Association. Used with permission.

## Intimate Partner Violence/Sexual Trauma

The symptoms of IPV and sexual trauma manifest within several distinct domains (Chisholm et al. 2017):

- **Physical:** Victim experiences hitting, slapping, punching, shoving, biting, choking, or the use of weapons.
- **Psychological:** Victim experiences threats of violence, intimidation, humiliation, feeling controlled, being socially isolated, being stalked, being forced into illegal activity or into substance use.
- **Sexual:** Victim experiences being forced or coerced into sexual acts in which the person does not want to participate, sabotage of contraception, being coerced into pregnancy or abortion, and intentionally being infected with sexually transmitted infections.

PTSD from IPV and sexual trauma can present with cognitive appraisals, including self-blame, alienation, and fear (Hebenstreit et al. 2015). Dissociation and numbing are frequent symptoms and may serve as a mechanism to cope with recurrent trauma (Braun 1988). Avoidance of intimacy and, conversely, hypersexuality can present with a fluctuating course. Reexperiencing the traumatic event can occur with interpersonal conflict and can lead to hyperarousal in the form of difficulty trusting others. Shame and guilt can result in maladaptive relationship behaviors, anger, and self-injurious behaviors in an attempt to control these cognitions (Foa et al. 1995).

IPV/sexual trauma can also lead to myriad chronic health conditions, including migraines, fibromyalgia, chronic pain, cognitive impairment from brain injury, irritable bowel syndrome, peptic ulcers, chronic abdominal pain, decreased or absent libido, and chronic pelvic pain. Additional sequelae of IPV and sexual trauma include transmission of sexually transmitted infections, unintended pregnancies, urinary tract infections, and acute fractures. The severity of PTSD symptoms has been associated with greater burden of chronic medical conditions (Zoellner et al. 2000). Close collaboration with other medical specialties is essential, given the association of exacerbation of physical symptoms with stress and anxiety.

## Reproductive Loss

Ms. DD is a 36-year-old gravida 4 para 0 who presents when 5 months pregnant, referred by her obstetrician for evaluation of anxiety. She has been trying to get pregnant for 3 years and has had three first-trimester miscarriages. Her medical workup for recurrent miscarriage has been negative. She reports that, when trying to get pregnant, she experiences perseveration about her ovulation schedule, guilt and shame about not being able to keep a pregnancy, and sexual dysfunction. When she became pregnant 5 months ago, her anxiety significantly worsened. She reports feeling terrified "every minute of every day" that she will miscarry, with frequent checking of her underwear for bleeding and constant attention to her body that interferes with normal functioning.

In her prior pregnancy, Ms. DD experienced vaginal bleeding at 8 weeks, and her obstetrician performed a vaginal ultrasound that showed no identifiable abnormalities. She miscarried the following week. She states that she understands that the ultrasound did not cause the miscarriage, but she "can't help feeling like it did," and has avoided obstetrical visits in her current pregnancy. She reports she is no less anxious about miscarriage after completing the first trimester and feels unable to make any preparations for the baby coming "because I feel like it will jinx it." She states that every time she tries to buy something for the baby, she imagines how she will feel holding that object after losing this pregnancy.

The onset of trauma from reproductive loss can occur at any point within the perinatal period where there is an actual or potential threat to the health, life, or viability of the pregnancy or after the loss has occurred. In early pregnancy loss, women often simultaneously learn that they are pregnant and that they are losing the pregnancy, resulting in delayed presentation of trauma symptoms. Data on the trauma of reproductive loss are often limited to spontaneous abortions and stillbirth and often do not include VTOP. All types of reproductive loss or adverse birth outcomes can result in PTSD. Intrusive symptoms can manifest as dreams of babies, flashbacks of abortion procedures, fetal images at varying ages, intense fear of pregnancy, fear of pelvic examinations, intense desire to become pregnant again, and the need or compulsion for a replacement baby (Daugirdaite et al. 2015).

Avoidance of trauma-related stimuli can include direct reminders of the loss or stillbirth experience, including specific people and places, or can escalate to avoidance of pregnancy, intimacy, or of women who are pregnant or have children. Substance use disorders and self-injurious behaviors can emerge to escape reminders of trauma-related stimuli (Daugirdaite et al. 2015). Unique to reproductive loss, negative cognitions typically are exhibited in the form of survivor guilt, which includes guilt about the loss itself and guilt for loving a subsequent healthy baby. Symptoms may intensify around anniversaries of the anticipated date of birth or date of loss or as Mother's Day approaches. The development of panic disorders, anxiety disorders, prolonged grief, and depressive disorders can occur several months to years after a reproductive loss and are highly comorbid (Daugirdaite et al. 2015).

More broadly, trauma associated with infertility may be greater than that associated with an individual pregnancy loss. In the process of undergoing infertility treatments and assisted reproductive technologies, women often experience multiple and repetitive pregnancy losses; each loss has the potential to result in PTSD. As such, women who experience infertility may develop PTSD in addition to suffering prolonged grief (Bartlik et al. 1997).

Gestational trophoblastic disease (GTD), a group of conditions that raise the risk of malignancy and metastasis, includes such etiologies as complete and partial molar pregnancies, choriocarcinomas, and placental site trophoblastic tumors. GTD can develop after pregnancy losses and, as such, may be diagnosed after what was initially expected to be a viable pregnancy. Few studies are available on the psychiatric implications of this kind of experience, but limited data suggest rates of anxiety and depression that exceeded community rates, with more than one-fifth of the study sample reporting GTD-specific traumatic stress symptoms (e.g., avoidance, intrusive thoughts) (Stafford et al. 2011).

## Traumatic Delivery

Manifestation of clinical symptoms following childbirth trauma presents diagnostic challenges (Table 18–8) because symptoms such as hyperarousal and poor sleep are common in early motherhood. Reexperiencing the delivery in the form of intrusive thoughts, images, and nightmares can occur. Typical avoidance of trauma-related stimuli may be centered on medical care and includes avoidance of hospitals, physicians and medical staff, outpatient clinics, and specific procedures, including pelvic examinations (Ayers et al. 2016). Persistence of avoidance can lead to not pursuing future pregnancies or requesting cesarean sections in future pregnancies. A systematic review found scheduled cesarean sections in women with childbirth trauma did not lower antenatal anxiety (Olieman et al. 2017), highlighting the challenges in management of this population. Negative cognitions often carry themes of guilt and shame surrounding motherhood, inability to care for the baby, or fears about the potential for sickness and death in the baby (Ayers et al. 2016). More broadly, chronic PTSD secondary to childbirth trauma has adverse ramifications for maternal health, including mother–infant bonding, relationship with significant other, poorer quality of life, and increased risk of comorbid psychiatric illness (Cook et al. 2018), as well as obstetrical complications in future pregnancies (Hernández-Martínez et al. 2019; Rogal et al. 2007; Seng et al. 2001).

**TABLE 18–8. Clinical presentation of PTSD**

| | |
|---|---|
| Hyperarousal | Difficulty sleeping<br>Heightened startle response<br>Increased irritability or anger |
| Intrusive symptoms | Presence of dissociation, including flashbacks<br>Repeated nightmares<br>Unexpected and reoccurring images or memories of the traumatic event |
| Negative cognitions and mood | Elevated negative evaluations of self or the world<br>Inability to remember important aspects of the trauma<br>Persistent negative emotional state |
| Persistent avoidance | Avoidance of thoughts, people, feelings, places, or physical sensations that are reminders of trauma |

# Course/Prognosis

Trauma as manifested in the perinatal period exists on a spectrum of severity, ranging from adjustment disorders to variants of PTSD and other specified trauma-related disorders. Women may enter the perinatal period with preexisting PTSD or may develop symptoms after exposure to the actual or threatened pregnancy-related event, including the antepartum, labor and delivery, and postpartum phases. In addition to an acute course, trauma symptoms in response to perinatal adverse events can also emerge as delayed or chronic at any point in time across the lifespan (Kim et al. 2015). Psychiatric morbidity may persist beyond the 12-month time frame that typically defines the postpartum period. Perinatal trauma, both preexisting and *de novo*, carries a high incidence of comorbid conditions that complicate the trauma trajectory. Perinatal mood and anxiety disorders (e.g., generalized anxiety disorder and major depressive disorder) and substance use disorders often co-occur with perinatal PTSD (Grekin and O'Hara 2014; Vignato et al. 2018).

The presence of premorbid or comorbid disorders, previous traumatic events, repetitive trauma such as recurrent pregnancy losses, or twin or multiple gestational pregnancies may complicate or prolong the course (Grekin and O'Hara 2014). Additionally, hormonal fluctuations, such as starting or stopping breastfeeding, resuming menses, or introducing contraception, may act to protect against or complicate trauma symptoms (Grekin and O'Hara 2014). Medical complications during the pregnancy, labor, or delivery that threaten the health or welfare of the mother or baby or require neonatal intervention may intensify symptoms (Grekin and O'Hara 2014; Seng et al. 2009). Delayed or inadequate prenatal care and providing childcare to other young children in the home also contribute to a poor prognosis (Grekin and O'Hara 2014).

## Intimate Partner Violence/Sexual Trauma

Unlike other types of trauma, trauma from IPV is typically ongoing and repetitive, often occurring for long periods of time and across multiple partners. The course of IPV trauma is influenced by factors such as the degree of denial on the part of the victim to seek help, the extent of physical or psychological harm the victim may have incurred, and the risks to which she may expose others, although this has the potential to abruptly stop through the involvement of the legal or medical system (Karakurt et al. 2014).

IPV adversely affects not only the woman, as the direct victim, but also her subsequent offspring. IPV during the perinatal period contributes to poor prenatal care and adverse neonatal outcomes, such as low birth weight, infections, substance exposure in utero, miscarriage, and stillbirth (Hellmuth et al. 2014; Holden et al. 2012; Huth-Bocks et al. 2013; Wathen and Macmillan 2013). Children and adolescents exposed to IPV are at higher risk to develop disruptions in maternal attachment and bonding, leading to children with somatic complaints, bedwetting, aggressive behaviors, school problems, early sexual activity, high-risk sexual behaviors, and psychiatric disorders (Wathen and Macmillan 2013). Sexual trauma may be associated with higher rates of endometriosis and other pelvic pain syndromes or may cause disorders in sexual dysfunction (Harris et al. 2018). See Chapter 2, "Gynecological Conditions and Mental Health," and Chapter 3, "Sexual Health and Reproductive Psychiatry," for further details on these conditions.

### Reproductive Loss

The course of trauma-related disorders related to reproductive loss can be complicated by a history of previous losses, the circumstances of the pregnancy, and the degree of support from the partner/father of the baby. Evidence indicates that the length of gestation does not determine the course or intensity of trauma symptoms, and an early gestational loss can be just as distressing as a later one (Leis-Newman 2012). Similarly, losing an unwanted pregnancy can be as distressing as losing a wanted one because the degree of attachment to a pregnancy can change over time, according to circumstances, and across developmental phases within the reproductive lifespan (Leis-Newman 2012).

### Traumatic Delivery

Although longitudinal trajectories for PTSD in the population at large have been well established, data on the clinical course of childbirth-related trauma are limited due to high attrition rates and multiple confounders. A prospective study in the Netherlands enrolled 348 participants, of whom 21% reported delivery as traumatic; however, at 10 months, only 0.35% of the entire sample met criteria for PTSD. Notable limitations include attrition of one-third of the sample and a lack of control for prior trauma and PTSD (Haagen et al. 2015). The largest study to date examined 950 women from a community sample over a 6-month period, 226 of whom identified delivery as traumatic. Four trajectories were identified: resilient (61.9%), recovered (18.5%), chronic PTSD (13.7%), and delayed PTSD (5.8%) (Dikmen-Yildiz et al. 2018). The high rates of recovery implore examination of resilience in addition to risk factors to develop more targeted treatments.

## Differential Diagnosis

The complex presentation of trauma within the perinatal period poses unique diagnostic challenges. For example, normal alterations in mood, anxiety, and behavior as a result of the hormonal influences of pregnancy, lactation, and the postpartum period may compound trauma symptomatology. Pregnancy and the postpartum period present with expected and sometimes dramatic variations in sleep (e.g., inability to sleep, especially within the third trimester) and changes in appetite, both of which may over-

**TABLE 18–9. Differential diagnoses for PTSD in the perinatal period**

| Diagnosis | Symptoms |
|---|---|
| Bipolar disorder I | Easily distracted<br>Irritability, increased arousal<br>Mood lability |
| Depressive disorders | Appetite changes (i.e., marked increase, lack of appetite, nausea)<br>Fatigue, exhaustion, apathy<br>Poor sleep during third trimester of pregnancy or the postpartum period due to normal changes (e.g., infant feeding schedule) vs. insomnia |
| Eating disorders | Anxiety<br>Poor appetite, weight loss |
| Generalized anxiety disorder | Easily annoyed<br>Increased worry, intense fear, helplessness<br>Nightmares<br>On edge, trouble relaxing, hyperarousal<br>Social isolation |
| OCD | Presence of compulsions<br>Recurrent, intrusive thoughts |
| Substance use | Dramatic mood swings<br>Erratic behavior<br>Paranoia, intrusive thoughts, avoidance |

lap with trauma symptoms. Symptoms of increased arousal, feeling on edge, and trouble relaxing may overlap with anxiety disorders or the normal fears of first-time mothers. In addition to normal postpartum changes and anxiety disorders (e.g., generalized anxiety disorder, panic disorder, adjustment disorder with anxiety), the differential diagnosis of trauma and stressor-related disorders also includes an atypical presentation of a depressive disorder, bipolar disorder, obsessive-compulsive disorder, or dissociative disorders. Postpartum delirium should be considered, and nonpsychiatric medical conditions, including postpartum thyroid illness and pulmonary embolism, may mimic the hyperarousal symptoms of PTSD. Table 18–9 reviews a partial psychiatric differential diagnosis for PTSD in the perinatal period.

## Sociodemographic Considerations

Populations who may be predisposed to develop perinatal PTSD include women of younger age; women who lack support from the father of the baby, partner, or family; single parents; women with a preexisting psychiatric disorder; Black women and women of other racial minorities; and LGBTQ+ individuals (Capaldi et al. 2012; Vignato et al. 2018). Psychosocial stressors, such as homelessness, food and financial insecurity, and exposure to violence, can aggravate symptoms of PTSD (Capaldi et al. 2012). Conversely, factors favoring a good prognosis include a shorter duration of trauma symptoms, good premorbid functioning, and strong social supports (Capaldi et al. 2012). Having adequate time to be free from occupational demands during the postpartum period, such as extended maternity or Family Medical Leave, has the potential to alleviate the distress associated with trauma (Meltzer-Brody et al. 2017).

### Economic Considerations

Economic factors play a critical role in the course of perinatal trauma. Having financial security to both care for and provide for the baby and to allow for sufficient time off from work to adjust to the demands of a new infant in the home plays a critical role in the early postpartum course (Meltzer-Brody et al. 2017).

## Pathophysiology

Stress-diathesis models of PTSD include biological, psychological, and social vulnerabilities that are triggered by acute trauma, with the course of illness mediated by risk, vulnerability, and resilience factors (Bomyea et al. 2012). Biological, psychological, and social factors mediate the pathophysiology of trauma and stress-related disorders. No data indicate whether the biological pathways of perinatal PTSD differ from those of PTSD from other causes, so the following discussion on biological factors is drawn from the general literature.

### Biological Factors

The role of hypothalamic-pituitary-adrenal axis suppression by stress hormones is a well-established hallmark of the fear response (Dunlop and Wong 2019), but the relationship between an acute fear response and the prolonged hyperreactivity of PTSD is less well understood. Animal models of extreme chronic stress demonstrate neuronal remodeling, with the most notable changes in the prefrontal cortex and hippocampus. In these areas, prolonged stress produces reductions in synaptic connectivity, disruption in glucocorticoid signaling, increased neuroinflammation, reduced levels of brain-derived neurotrophic factor (BDNF), and deficits in astrocytes (Abdallah et al. 2019; McEwen 2017). Reduced uptake of glutamate in the synapses leads to increased extracellular glutamate and excitotoxicity and ultimately to neuronal atrophy and synaptic loss (Abdallah et al. 2019). In preclinical studies, these neuronal changes are associated with behavioral impairment and anxiety dysregulation. Chronic stress in animal models also results in increased synaptic connectivity and upregulated BDNF in the basolateral amygdala and nucleus accumbens, which is similarly associated with behavioral disturbances (Abdallah et al. 2019; McEwen 2017). Human imaging studies looking at neurobiological findings associated with PTSD have implicated reduced hippocampal volumes and structural differences in the dorsal and rostral anterior cingulate cortices, ventromedial prefrontal cortex, amygdala, and insula (Cirino and Knapp 2019; Fitzgerald et al. 2018). These pathways, and in particular the hypothalamic-pituitary-adrenal axis, are altered in women with chronic PTSD and undergo changes during pregnancy and postpartum, further making women susceptible to peripartum PTSD (Cirino and Knapp 2019).

Genetic studies investigating gene associations with PTSD have found gene variants (e.g., *FKBP5*) that mediate the volume of various brain regions, such as the putamen and amygdala (Kang et al. 2019; van der Merwe et al. 2019). Immune models of PTSD postulate an association of PTSD with proinflammatory states. Studies show that patients with PTSD have increased levels of proinflammatory markers such as interleukin-1β, interleukin-6, tumor necrosis factor-α, and C-reactive protein, suggesting an association and a possible pathogenesis role in PTSD pathophysiology (Hori and Kim 2019). Epigenetic studies suggest allele-specific methylation as a potential association for PTSD and drive intergenerational models of trauma and PTSD (Kang et al. 2019).

### Psychological Factors

Cognitive and affective theories suggest a predisposition to the development of PTSD based on prior cognitive styles and preexisting mental health disorders (Ozer et al. 2003). Other predisposing factors include female gender, family history of psychopathology, and prior trauma exposure (Ozer et al. 2003). The psychological pathophysiology of PTSD is hypothesized to include disruptions in longstanding, firmly held cognitive schema around safety, trust, and self-confidence that lead to a contradictory, conflict-ridden dissonance. This contradictory state with high emotional valence is thought to result in symptoms such as reexperiencing, hyperarousal, avoidance, and dissociation as various methods to reconcile these conflicts (Ford et al. 2015).

### Sociodemographic Considerations

Multiple studies have investigated racial differences in trauma exposure (Alegría et al. 2013; Huth-Bocks et al. 2013; Roberts et al. 2011; Seng et al. 2011). These studies demonstrate that Black individuals have equivalent or higher trauma exposure and likely underreport traumatic events (Seng et al. 2011). They uniformly show a higher lifetime prevalence of PTSD in Black and indigenous women. Black women are at higher risk of being victims of violent crimes, have repeated exposure to racism, and are exposed to toxic stress, making them particularly vulnerable to developing PTSD before or during the perinatal period (Seng et al. 2011).

Although PTSD risk has been shown to be elevated in Black women across sociodemographic groups, race alone is unlikely to be the sole mediator in PTSD pathophysiology. Concomitant risk factors, as determined by social and economic variables and determinants, are likely to contribute as well. Maternal mortality review committee data in recent years indicates higher rates of pregnancy complications for Black women, putting them at a theoretically higher risk of subsequent trauma and stressor-related disorders. Factors related to systemic racism are a driving force in this disparity but are more difficult to identify and study, limiting published studies to data. Social supports, attachment/bonding, and social cognition likely play a mediating role in PTSD pathophysiology, and racial disparities in economics, housing stability, and social constructs may have direct impact on the development of PTSD (Seng et al. 2011).

For LGBTQ+ individuals, who have often faced chronic stress, structural stigma in health care systems have direct implications on both medical comorbidities and all-cause morbidity and mortality (Hatzenbuehler 2009).

## Treatment

Management of PTSD requires comprehensive care, including psychopharmacology, other medical interventions, and psychotherapy. Some guidelines, including those developed by the U.S. Department of Veterans Affairs (VA) and U.S. Department of Defense (DoD), state that psychotherapy and psychopharmacology are equivalent; however, others, including the International Society of Traumatic Stress Studies and the United Kingdom's National Institute for Health and Clinical Excellence, state that psychotherapy is more strongly recommended than psychopharmacology (Forbes et al. 2010). Each case of PTSD is unique in its psychological, biological, and social determinants, and thus has differing treatment implications.

There are five core principles of TIC: safety, trustworthiness, choice, collaboration, and empowerment (Substance Abuse and Mental Health Services Administration 2014a). *Safety* refers to ensuring both physical and emotional security. Physicians and other providers should cultivate a safe space for individuals to discuss trauma and its sequelae. Maintaining appropriate boundaries and making instructions and tasks clear is part of *trustworthiness*, as is following through on commitments. Given the lack of control individuals have had during traumatic experiences, empowering patients to make active *choices* helps to restore their loci of control. Maximizing *collaboration* is also an integral part of TIC, both with patients and with other physicians and providers in their care (Substance Abuse and Mental Health Services Administration 2014a). *Empowerment* also comes through skill building.

## Psychopharmacology

Medications can be used to ameliorate the biological basis for PTSD symptoms along with co-occurring psychiatric diagnoses, and they may indirectly benefit psychological and social symptoms. Clinicians must consider the level of evidence available to support the use of a specific medication and tailor pharmacotherapy to the individual patient. Few studies have specifically investigated medication use for peripartum PTSD or PTSD specific to traumatic delivery, so management is often extrapolated from studies in nonpregnant/postpartum populations.

### First-Line Medications

Evidence for PTSD pharmacology in the general population is strongest for three specific selective serotonin reuptake inhibitors (SSRIs)—sertraline, paroxetine, and fluoxetine—and one serotonin norepinephrine reuptake inhibitor (SNRI)—venlafaxine (U.S. Department of Veterans Affairs and Department of Defense 2017). Currently only sertraline and paroxetine are approved by the FDA for PTSD (Brady et al. 2000; Marshall et al. 2001). Citalopram is a first-line medication option along with sertraline and fluoxetine for child and adolescent patients, as recommended by the American Academy for Child and Adolescent Psychiatry. In PTSD, one mechanism of action of SSRIs might be to stimulate neuronal connections through BDNF, a hypothesis based on animal and clinical studies (Duman et al. 1997; Vermetten et al. 2003). Venlafaxine, a serotonin reuptake inhibitor at lower dosages and a combined SNRI at higher dosages, may work through the same or other mechanisms (Davidson et al. 2006). Data are lacking on other SNRIs. (For a full discussion of the risks of antidepressants vs. risks of no treatment in perinatal populations, please see Chapter 8, "A Clinical Approach to Psychiatric Diagnosis and Treatment During Pregnancy," and Chapter 13.)

### Other Medications

Prazosin is an $\alpha_1$-adrenergic blocker commonly prescribed for posttraumatic nightmares. Prazosin can be helpful for nightmares that cause arousal from sleep due to activation of the sympathetic nervous system, described by patients as waking up in a cold sweat with tachypnea and tachycardia, and has been shown effective in controlled trials (Ahmadpanah et al. 2014; Germain et al. 2012; Raskind et al. 2013; Taylor et al. 2008). However, a 2018 study on military PTSD found that prazosin was no more effective than placebo at treating posttraumatic nightmares (Raskind et al. 2018), which resulted in downgraded recommendations for the use of prazosin by both the VA and the DoD and the American Association of Sleep Medicine (Morgenthaler et al. 2018). Nevertheless, prazosin remains the most evidence-based medication for treatment of posttraumatic nightmares. Pregnancy data for prazosin use are limited, but a small number of human studies investigating prazosin for gestational hypertension raised no major safety concerns (Hong et al. 2018).

Hydroxyzine has been shown to be more effective than placebo at treating posttraumatic nightmares, although it is less effective than prazosin (Ahmadpanah et al. 2014). Like prazosin, pregnancy data for hydroxyzine are limited, but prospective data suggest no teratogenicity risk (Einarson et al. 1997).

β-Blockers provide postsynaptic blockade of norepinephrine at synapses and blockade of adrenaline (epinephrine) at organs such as the heart, sweat glands, and muscles, reducing both the central and peripheral manifestations of hyperarousal. Longstanding interest in using β-blockers to prevent PTSD after a trauma has not been supported by research evidence (Amos et al. 2014). Propranolol has been shown to reduce PTSD symptoms when given before reactivating the traumatic memory, likely through its role in disrupting memory reconsolidation (Brunet et al. 2018). Propranolol has been studied for the management of hypertension in pregnancy and has not been found to be teratogenic; however, some limited data in animal models suggest a small risk of placental insufficiency when used in the third trimester (Schoenfeld et al. 1978).

Benzodiazepines enhance GABA activity at the $GABA_A$ receptor, which produces CNS depression. Evidence is mounting for the harmful effects of chronic benzodiazepine use in patients with PTSD around potential disinhibition, difficulty integrating the traumatic experience, interference with the mental processes needed to benefit from psychotherapy, iatrogenic dependence, and an increase in overall mortality. Two placebo-controlled randomized clinical trials of benzodiazepines for treating PTSD had negative findings: one found that alprazolam did not reduce PTSD symptoms (Braun et al. 1990), and the other found that clonazepam did not improve PTSD-related sleep symptoms (Cates et al. 2004). A 2015 meta-analysis of 18 studies with more than 5,200 participants found benzodiazepines ineffective for PTSD treatment and noted that the risks associated with their use outweigh potential short-term benefits (Guina et al. 2015). As such, benzodiazepines are not recommended for long-term treatment of PTSD. (For a full discussion of the risks of benzodiazepines vs. risks of no treatment in the perinatal period, please see Chapter 19.)

Many other second-line medication options may be used for PTSD, such as trazodone, mirtazapine, monoamine oxidase inhibitors, and tricyclic antidepressants. Buspirone is an agonist at the presynaptic serotonin $5\text{-}HT_{1A}$ receptor and a partial agonist at the postsynaptic serotonin $5\text{-}HT_{1A}$ receptor that case reports suggest might reduce anxiety in PTSD without sedation or dependence, but no randomized trials support its use in PTSD (Wells et al. 1991).

## Other Medical Interventions: Neuromodulation

The most systematically and rigorously studied form of neuromodulation in the treatment of PTSD is repetitive transcranial magnetic stimulation (rTMS) (Koek et al. 2019). rTMS has been shown to be an effective treatment of PTSD in sham-controlled studies for reducing hyperarousal (Osuch et al. 2009; Watts et al. 2012), reexperiencing, intrusive memories, and avoidance and for improving scores on the PTSD Checklist and Clinician-Administered PTSD Scale (Cohen et al. 2004; Kozel et al. 2018; Nam et al. 2013; Watts et al. 2013). Furthermore, a recent study found that rTMS led to more rapid PTSD symptom reduction and more sustained changes immediately preceding cognitive processing therapy (CPT) versus sham transcranial magnetic stimulation prior to CPT (Kozel et al. 2018). rTMS appears to be a safe and well-tolerated treatment during pregnancy (Hizli et al. 2014; Kim et al. 2019).

Electroconvulsive therapy (ECT) as a treatment for PTSD has limited data. A systematic reviewof studies from 1956 to 2016 found that individuals with PTSD who received ECT also had comorbid depression, limiting conclusions on whether PTSD in the absence of comorbid depressive symptoms would respond to ECT (Youssef et al. 2017). Given ECT's potential side effect of retrograde amnesia, harnessing this effect in the treatment of PTSD through having individuals recall the traumatic memory prior to receiving ECT is a theoretical possibility (Misanin et al. 1968). ECT is safe to use during all trimesters of pregnancy (Ward et al. 2018).

## Behavioral Treatments

In 2017, the VA/DoD and American Psychiatric Association (APA) each published a treatment guideline for PTSD. The APA guideline is specifically for treatment of PTSD among adults and strongly recommends cognitive-behavioral therapy, CPT, prolonged exposure (PE), cognitive therapy, brief eclectic psychotherapy, narrative exposure therapy, and written narrative experience. Trauma-focused psychotherapies such as CPT, PE, and eye movement desensitization and reprocessing (EMDR) are found to have greater effect sizes than non-trauma-focused therapies and medications (Chard 2005; Lee et al. 2016; Watts et al. 2013).

There are six tenets that are common to the empirically supported therapies for PTSD (Table 18–10): psychoeducation, emotion regulation, imaginal exposure, cognitive processing, emotions, and memory processing (Schnyder et al. 2015). The goals of psychoeducation are to provide information on the course of PTSD and stress reactions and strategies to manage distress. Emotion regulation skills are taught more implicitly over the course of treatment. Imaginal exposure is a major focus of PE and narrative exposure therapy, although it is still a tenet of all evidence-based psychotherapies for trauma-related disorders (Schnyder et al. 2015). Exposure addresses the challenges of separating the present safety from the past traumatic event(s) (Coventry et al. 2020). Cognitive processing and restructuring (i.e., integration of the lessons from exposure) is another element that can be found in almost all of the empirically supported psychological treatments for PTSD (Diehle et al. 2014; Schnyder et al. 2015).

For the peripartum period, authors have suggested using themes extracted from the perinatal PTSD literature to target psychotherapeutic interventions, such as tailored attention to the nature of the trauma memory, negative appraisal of the trauma and its sequelae, current threats, and strategies intended to control threat/symptoms

**TABLE 18–10. Six core tenets of evidence-based psychotherapies for PTSD**

| Tenet | Application in psychotherapy |
|---|---|
| Cognitive processing | Allow for restructuring or providing meaning to thoughts; key part of integrating lessons from exposure |
| Emotion regulation | Implicitly teach skills; not explicit focus of therapy |
| Emotions | Explore emotions evoked in patient, including anger, grief, guilt, and fear |
| Imaginal exposure | Address challenges of separating the present safe environment from the prior traumatic experience |
| Memory processing | Target encoding, retrieval, consolidation, and storage of memories |
| Psychoeducation | Provide information on the course of PTSD and stress reactions and strategies to manage distress |

(James et al. 2015). For PTSD from traumatic delivery, reexperiencing is one of the most frequently experienced symptoms and may be a treatment target (James et al. 2015). Studies investigating therapy management of perinatal PTSD are similarly limited, although one systematic review suggested that trauma-focused psychotherapies are effective in reducing PTSD symptoms in the early postpartum period (Furuta et al. 2018).

For women who are at higher risk of chronic PTSD and recurrent trauma, especially Black or indigenous women and LGBTQ+ individuals, chronic effects of toxic stress may be a treatment target because these have a direct impact on the mother–baby interaction. Therapies focusing on dyadic treatments are imperative in all women, but especially in these vulnerable subgroups.

## Prolonged Exposure

PE is based on emotional processing theory; patients learn that trauma-related memories are not perilous and experience these memories and feelings. The original intervention protocol was described as 9–12 sessions, each 90–120 minutes in length, with use of both imaginal and in vivo exposure (Foa and Rothbaum 1998). The patient is challenged in a graduated fashion with the goal of achieving success in confronting feared stimuli and coping with evoked affect. PE has been found to be safe and effective in patients with co-occurring dissociation, borderline personality disorder, psychosis, suicidal behavior, nonsuicidal self-injury, substance use disorders, and major depressive disorder (van Minnen et al. 2012). Patients randomly assigned to exposure therapy have significantly greater pre- to posttreatment reductions in PTSD symptoms compared with those who receive supportive counseling, relaxation training, and treatment as usual, including pharmacotherapy (Asukai et al. 2010; Bryant et al. 2003; Schnurr et al. 2007; Taylor et al. 2003). Several meta-analyses have found that exposure therapy is more effective that non-trauma-focused therapies (Bradley et al. 2005; Cusack et al. 2016; Powers et al. 2010; Watts et al. 2013).

## Cognitive Processing Therapy

Trauma affects how individuals perceive themselves and their relation to the world and can create a paralyzing mental state. The main aim of CPT is to shift beliefs toward accommodation of new learning. CPT consists of 12 weekly sessions that can be delivered in either individual or group settings and has been found to have outcomes comparable with those of PE (Resick et al. 2002, 2017). Treatment begins with psychoeducation regarding PTSD, thoughts, and emotions. The patient becomes more aware of the relationship between thoughts and emotions and begins to identify "automatic thoughts" that may be maintaining the PTSD symptoms. Cognitive skills are then introduced, and a connection is established between thoughts, feelings, and behaviors. Distortions and maladaptive cognitions are identified, and cognitive skills are used to challenge the maladaptive beliefs with a focus on new learning.

### Cognitive Therapy

Several studies have investigated specific cognitive therapies in the management of traumatic stress after childbirth. A randomized controlled trial of women after emergent cesarean section found success in the use of an online visuospatial task aimed at reducing intrusive traumatic memories (Horsch et al. 2017). A four-session grief counseling intervention in women who have experienced stillbirths found reduction in PTSD severity (Navidian et al. 2017). An internet-based cognitive-behavioral therapy intervention after childbirth was found to reduce PTSD symptoms in the women randomized to receive the therapy (Nieminen et al. 2016). A recent systematic review and meta-analysis concluded that many trauma-focused psychological interventions can be helpful in reducing symptoms of postpartum PTSD in the short and medium term but that evidence is lacking on whether any particular intervention is more effective than others and on whether these interventions can help women with long-term recovery from clinically significant PTSD (Furuta et al. 2018).

### Eye Movement Desensitization and Reprocessing

EMDR was initially introduced in 1989 as an eight-phase manualized therapy with the objective of assisting patients in accessing and processing traumatic memories while bringing them to an adaptive resolution. Initial focus is on evaluation and planning followed by desensitization and reprocessing, with end goals of installing positive cognitions, replacing negative ones, and releasing associated somatic tension. The novel aspect of EMDR as compared with other trauma-focused therapies for PTSD is its inclusion of eye movements. Although experimental studies have shown that horizontal eye movements are associated with a decrease in the vividness, emotionality, and arousal associated with memories, most of these studies are of healthy participants (van den Hout et al. 2001). Empirical evidence supports EMDR as superior to waitlist controls and comparable with PE and cognitive-based psychotherapies (Davidson and Parker 2001; Powers et al. 2010). Although one meta-analysis found no difference between EMDR and PE, another found PE to be superior to EMDR (Rothbaum et al. 2005; Taylor et al. 2003). One small pilot study of four women that investigated EMDR after childbirth found it to be effective in the reduction of PTSD symptoms (Sandström et al. 2008).

## Treatment Challenges

Treatment challenges fall into three broad categories: physician-/provider-specific, patient-specific, and system barriers. Additional challenges include the lack of studies specific to the management of perinatal PTSD.

## Physician-/Provider-Specific

A qualitative study specific to physicians' perceived barriers for caring for sexual assault survivors found internal barriers to care: fear of a patient disclosing, personal attitudes regarding sexual assault, and the emotional toll of caring for sexual assault survivors (Amin et al. 2017). Physicians and other providers may be unsure about what to do with a positive screen for PTSD. Therapists may lack comfort and competence in providing evidence-based therapies for PTSD. Similarly, physicians may lack knowledge about evidence-based treatment approaches for PTSD, particularly in the peripartum period. Myths continually propagate that trauma-focused therapies will lead to worsening of PTSD symptoms and dropout, a claim not supported by multiple studies (Feeny et al. 2003; Foa et al. 2002).

## Patient-Specific

Individuals with PTSD who have core features of hypervigilance and avoidance may have difficulties with accessing care and trusting physicians and other providers. Using TIC principles can help build therapeutic alliance, especially in individuals who may not wish to disclose trauma when first asked. Universally asking about the core symptoms of PTSD, rather than beginning with more intrusive questioning about specific traumatic events, may help patients discuss posttraumatic stress symptoms more openly. Using a checklist of possible traumatic events without follow-up questions about posttraumatic stress symptoms may lead to underdiagnosis of individuals with PTSD, should a patient choose not to disclose past traumatic events.

## System Barriers

Access to evidence-based treatments for PTSD is limited in many parts of the nation due to inadequate access to mental health services. In a sample of veterans with positive PTSD screens, most men (78.7%) and women (89.5%) would consider treatment for PTSD symptoms, with the largest proportion of both genders preferring counseling over a self-help computer program or phone application (Gutner et al. 2018). A small randomized controlled trial ($N=20$) evaluating the use of the PTSD Coach mobile application with and without clinician support found that both the self-managed and clinician-managed versions led to PTSD symptom reduction based on the PTSD Checklist. The self-managed effect size was 0.41, which increased to 1.4 in the clinician-supported PTSD Coach group, so although this intervention does not necessitate a clinician, which improves access, involving a clinician improved the effectiveness of the intervention (Possemato et al. 2016). Individuals with PTSD stemming from prior medical treatment or discrimination by physicians or other providers may find coming to the clinic or hospital for treatment of PTSD to be retraumatizing. Telemedicine may be a helpful tool for providing evidenced-based trauma-informed treatments to these individuals (Gilmore et al. 2016).

## Special Considerations: Trauma and Psychological Distress Related to Voluntary Terminations of Pregnancy

VTOPs occur when women desire to end pregnancies due to poor timing, lack of resources, fetal anomalies, or fetal reductions. Although many women experience relief after VTOP, some may experience posttraumatic stress syndrome (PTSS) or PTSD. The etiology of PTSS/PTSD after VTOP remains inconclusive. Some studies have concluded that stress after VTOP stems from premorbid or comorbid mental health disorders and not from the termination itself, suggesting that mental health before VTOP predicts mental health afterward (Major et al. 2008; Robinson et al. 2009). Others have found that trauma stems from the unwanted pregnancy and factors surrounding it, such as lack of partner or financial support (Fergusson et al. 2008; Mota et al. 2010). Still others conclude that stress emerges from the termination itself, as well as from a combination of variables (Broen et al. 2005; Coleman et al. 2010; Curley and Johnston 2013). Alternatively, two recent studies found that being denied a VTOP contributed to more psychological distress (Biggs et al. 2017) and worse overall health than undergoing one (Ralph et al. 2019). The etiology of stress disorders after VTOP is considered multifactorial, stemming from any single to a combination of factors.

### Epidemiology

In the United States, about 25% of women have experienced a VTOP. How many of these women go on to experience trauma or stress-related symptoms related to the VTOP is unclear. Some studies find no association between VTOP and PTSS/PTSD (Wallin Lundell et al. 2013). Others find rates of 12%–30% (Fergusson et al. 2008; Hamama et al. 2010).

### Risk and Protective Factors

Adequate information and screening for psychological risks, sufficient time for decision making, resources for alternatives to VTOP, and social support all protect against the development of stress reactions. Conversely, biological vulnerabilities, such as prior mental health problems, substance disorders, and adverse early life events, can increase risk (Table 18–11). Women who are socially isolated, keep the termination and pregnancy secret, or feel pressured or ambivalent about their decision to abort are more vulnerable to develop negative outcomes (Speckhard and Rue 1992). Demographic factors, such as younger age, single status, lack of partner involvement, limited education, and lowered socioeconomic status, have the potential to increase psychological risks. Obstetrical factors, such as prior termination(s), medical complications from the procedure, later gestational age of pregnancy, and viewing the embryo/fetus, can compound risks (Major et al. 2008).

### Screening Methods

Barriers to identifying PTSS/PTSD after a VTOP abound—the assumption that all women experience relief, the lack of consensus on the etiology of termination-related distress, delayed or latent trauma responses, substance use, and limited history tak-

**TABLE 18–11. Risk factors for PTSD after voluntary termination of pregnancy**

| | |
|---|---|
| Ambivalence about decision | Obstetrical risks: |
| Demographic factors: | Later gestational age of pregnancy |
| Single status | Medical complications from the procedure |
| Younger age | Prior termination(s) |
| Early adverse life events | Viewing the embryo/fetus |
| Forced to keep abortion/pregnancy a secret | Pressure to pursue termination |
| Lack of partner involvement | Prior mental health history |
| Limited education | Social isolation |
| Lower socioeconomic status | Substance use disorder |

ing—because clinicians often do not conduct a detailed psychiatric assessment after the procedure (Curley and Johnston 2013). Screening practices vary, and no standard evaluation methods have been developed. The Impact of Event Scale–Revised, Perinatal Grief Scale, Texas Grief Inventory, Primary Care–PTSD Scale, Trauma Symptom Checklist, and Clinician-Administered PTSD Scale have been used to effectively measure symptoms.

## Clinical Features

Often presenting as avoidant symptoms, PTSS/PTSD after VTOP can present with increased substance use (Reardon et al. 2004) or with suicidal and self-injurious behavior (Gissler et al. 1996; Morgan et al. 1997), and high risk-related PTSD can include manifestations of grief and loss, as well as survivor guilt (Speckhard and Rue 1992). Unresolved PTSD after VTOP can lead to disrupted attachment to subsequent pregnancies, babies, and children.

## Course and Prognosis

The onset of PTSS/PTSD after a VTOP ranges from immediately after the procedure to decades later. Times of highest risk include the period between the procedure and the anticipated due date because of the continued physical effects of the pregnancy; anniversary times, such as the date of the procedure, the due date of the anticipated birth, or Mother's Day; and seeing children of similar age as that of the aborted child (Speckhard and Rue 1992). Subsequent pregnancies may also reawaken affect and cognitions associated with a previous VTOP and disrupt the mother's attachment to the target pregnancy. The course of PTSS/PTSD after VTOP waxes and wanes. Symptoms may manifest at vulnerable points across the reproductive lifespan, such as during subsequent pregnancies, subsequent pregnancy losses, problems with infertility or difficulty conceiving, and menopause. Symptoms range from mild distress to severe functional impairment, including high risk of suicidal, self-injurious, and self-destructive behaviors (Gissler et al. 1996; Morgan et al. 1997).

## Sociodemographic Considerations

Women across all sociodemographic strata have the potential to experience stress and trauma disorders after VTOP. Traditional values, membership of a religious faith or culture that opposes abortion, and residing in geographical areas where abortion is not accepted may contribute to negative outcomes (Major et al. 2008). Younger age, single status, and being nulliparous can contribute to abortion trauma as well (Major et al. 2008).

### Research Limitations

Research designs used to examine women's responses to VTOP are limited by

1. The inability to randomize
2. High attrition rates among participants who are lost to follow up
3. Withholding of accurate abortion data among participants who have had abortions, such as number of previous abortions and gestational age at the time of the abortion
4. Use of nonequivalent comparison groups, such as comparing women who have wanted pregnancies (control group; delivery group) with women who have unwanted pregnancies (abortion group, obtained or denied) (Major et al. 2008)
5. Misclassification problems, such as when participants who desire termination later change their minds in favor of parenting (Biggs et al. 2017; Fergusson et al. 2008)

A highly debated diagnosis referred to as *postabortion stress syndrome* is not acknowledged by the American Psychiatric Association or American Psychological Association based on questions about the validity of the research describing this disorder.

### Treatment

Treatment for PTSS/PTSD after VTOP follows principles for treatment of trauma, such as using a phase-oriented approach that includes stabilization, processing, and integration of the trauma narrative. Additionally, supportive readings for grief and loss tailored to the perinatal period can include *On Death and Dying* by Kübler-Ross (1969) and *Grief Counselling and Grief Therapy* by Worden (2013).

## Conclusion

Trauma and PTSD in the perinatal period require consideration of areas that include prior exposure to trauma (especially sexual trauma) and pregnancy factors that may cause trauma, including reproductive loss and traumatic birth experiences. Physicians and other clinicians must remain vigilant in screening carefully for trauma and using TIC principles in managing women with trauma in the perinatal period to ensure sensitive, compassionate, patient-centered care.

## Key Points

- Patients with a history of trauma may face significant challenges in the perinatal period.
- Major health care organizations such as the American College of Obstetricians and Gynecologists and the U.S. Preventive Services Task Force encourage universal or widespread screening of individuals for intimate partner violence.

- Reproductive loss and traumatic birth experiences may lead to the development of PTSD symptoms, and patients who experience these should be evaluated accordingly.
- Populations who may be predisposed to develop perinatal PTSD include women with childhood adversity or trauma; women of younger age; women who lack support from the father of the baby, partner, or family; single parents; and women with comorbid or preexisting psychiatric disorders.
- Trauma-informed care is a holistic approach to treatment that considers the biological, psychological, neurological, and social impact of trauma and is recommended as a universal approach.
- Management options include medications such as selective serotonin reuptake inhibitors and psychotherapy modalities such as cognitive-behavioral therapy, cognitive processing therapy, and eye movement desensitization and reprocessing.

## References

Abdallah CG, Averill LA, Akiki TJ, et al: The neurobiology and pharmacotherapy of posttraumatic stress disorder. Annu Rev Pharmacol Toxicol 59:171–189, 2019 30216745

Ahmadpanah M, Sabzeiee P, Hosseini SM, et al: Comparing the effect of prazosin and hydroxyzine on sleep quality in patients suffering from posttraumatic stress disorder. Neuropsychobiology 69(4):235–242, 2014 24993832

Alcalá HE, Tomiyama AJ, von Ehrenstein OS: Gender differences in the association between adverse childhood experiences and cancer. Womens Health Issues 27(6):625–631, 2017 28774479

Alegría M, Fortuna LR, Lin JY, et al: Prevalence, risk, and correlates of posttraumatic stress disorder across ethnic and racial minority groups in the United States. Med Care 51(12):1114–1123, 2013 24226308

American College of Obstetricians and Gynecologists: ACOG Committee Opinion No. 518: intimate partner violence. Obstet Gynecol 119(2 Pt 1):412–417, 2012 22270317

American College of Obstetricians and Gynecologists: ACOG Committee Opinion No. 736: optimizing postpartum care. Obstet Gynecol 131(5):e140–e150, 2018 29683911

American Psychiatric Association: Diagnostic and Statistical Manual of Mental Disorders, 5th Edition, Arlington, VA, American Psychiatric Association, 2013

American Psychological Association: Clinical Practice Guideline for the Treatment of Posttraumatic Stress Disorder (PTSD) in Adults. Washington, DC, American Psychological Association, 2017. Available at: https://www.apa.org/ptsd-guideline. Accessed July 4, 2020.

Amin P, Buranosky R, Chang JC: Physicians' perceived roles, as well as barriers, toward caring for women sex assault survivors. Womens Health Issues 27(1):43–49, 2017 27863981

Amos T, Stein DJ, Ipser JC: Pharmacological interventions for preventing post-traumatic stress disorder (PTSD). Cochrane Database Syst Rev 7(7):CD006239, 2014 25001071

Asukai N, Saito A, Tsuruta N, et al: Efficacy of exposure therapy for Japanese patients with posttraumatic stress disorder due to mixed traumatic events: a randomized controlled study. J Trauma Stress 23(6):744–750, 2010 21171135

Ayers S, Bond R, Bertullies S, et al: The aetiology of post-traumatic stress following childbirth: a meta-analysis and theoretical framework. Psychol Med 46(6):1121–1134, 2016 26878223

Bartlik B, Greene K, Graf M, et al: Examining PTSD as a complication of infertility. Medscape Womens Health 2(3):1, 1997 9746683

Beutel M, Will H, Völkl K, et al: Assessment of grief exemplified pregnancy loss: development and initial results on the validity of the Munich Grief Scale [in German]. Psychother Psychosom Med Psychol 45(9–10):295–302, 1995 7480585

Biggs MA, Upadhyay UD, McCulloch CE, et al: Women's mental health and well-being 5 years after receiving or being denied an abortion: a prospective, longitudinal cohort study. JAMA Psychiatry 74(2):169–178, 2017 27973641
Bomyea J, Risbrough V, Lang AJ: A consideration of select pre-trauma factors as key vulnerabilities in PTSD. Clin Psychol Rev 32(7):630–641, 2012 22917742
Bradley R, Greene J, Russ E, et al: A multidimensional meta-analysis of psychotherapy for PTSD. Am J Psychiatry 162(2):214–227, 2005 15677582
Brady K, Pearlstein T, Asnis GM, et al: Efficacy and safety of sertraline treatment of posttraumatic stress disorder: a randomized controlled trial. JAMA 283(14):1837–1844, 2000 10770145
Braun BG: The BASK model of dissociation. Dissociation: Progress in the Dissociative Disorders 1(1):4–23, 1988
Braun P, Greenberg D, Dasberg H, et al: Core symptoms of posttraumatic stress disorder unimproved by alprazolam treatment. J Clin Psychiatry 51(6):236–238, 1990 2189869
Breslau N: Gender differences in trauma and posttraumatic stress disorder. J Gend Specif Med 5(1):34–40, 2002 11859685
Broen AN, Moum T, Bødtker AS, et al: The course of mental health after miscarriage and induced abortion: a longitudinal, five-year follow-up study. BMC Med 3:18, 2005 16343341
Brunet A, Saumier D, Liu A, et al: Reduction of PTSD symptoms with pre-reactivation propranolol therapy: a randomized controlled trial. Am J Psychiatry 175(5):427–433, 2018 29325446
Bryant RA, Moulds ML, Guthrie RM, et al: Imaginal exposure alone and imaginal exposure with cognitive restructuring in treatment of posttraumatic stress disorder. J Consult Clin Psychol 71(4):706–712, 2003 12924676
Capaldi DM, Knoble NB, Shortt JW, et al: A systematic review of risk factors for intimate partner violence. Partn Abus 3(2):231–280, 2012 22754606
Carr CP, Martins CM, Stingel AM, et al: The role of early life stress in adult psychiatric disorders: a systematic review according to childhood trauma subtypes. J Nerv Ment Dis 201(12):1007–1020, 2013 24284634
Cates ME, Bishop MH, Davis LL, et al: Clonazepam for treatment of sleep disturbances associated with combat-related posttraumatic stress disorder. Ann Pharmacother 38(9):1395–1399, 2004 15252193
Centers for Disease Control and Prevention: Adverse Childhood Experiences Resources. Atlanta, GA, Centers for Disease Control and Prevention, 2020. Available at: https://www.cdc.gov/violenceprevention/childabuseandneglect/acestudy/journal.html. Accessed July 4, 2020.
Chard KM: An evaluation of cognitive processing therapy for the treatment of posttraumatic stress disorder related to childhood sexual abuse. J Consult Clin Psychol 73(5):965–971, 2005 16287396
Chisholm CA, Bullock L, Ferguson JEJ 2nd: Intimate partner violence and pregnancy: epidemiology and impact. Am J Obstet Gynecol 217(2):141–144, 2017 28551446
Cirino NH, Knapp JM: Perinatal posttraumatic stress disorder: a review of risk factors, diagnosis, and treatment. Obstet Gynecol Surv 74(6):369–376, 2019 31216046
Cohen H, Kaplan Z, Kotler M, et al: Repetitive transcranial magnetic stimulation of the right dorsolateral prefrontal cortex in posttraumatic stress disorder: a double-blind, placebo-controlled study. Am J Psychiatry 161(3):515–524, 2004 14992978
Coleman PK, Coyle CT, Rue VM: Late-term elective abortion and susceptibility to posttraumatic stress symptoms. J Pregnancy 2010:130519, 2010 21490737
Connell CM, Bergeron N, Katz KH, et al: Re-referral to child protective services: the influence of child, family, and case characteristics on risk status. Child Abuse Negl 31(5):573–588, 2007 17537504
Connor KM, Davidson JR: SPRINT: a brief global assessment of post-traumatic stress disorder. Int Clin Psychopharmacol 16(5):279–284, 2001 11552771
Cook N, Ayers S, Horsch A: Maternal posttraumatic stress disorder during the perinatal period and child outcomes: a systematic review. J Affect Disord 225:18–31, 2018 28777972

Coventry PA, Meader N, Melton H, et al: Psychological and pharmacological interventions for posttraumatic stress disorder and comorbid mental health problems following complex traumatic events: systematic review and component network meta-analysis. PLoS Med 17(8):e1003262, 2020 32813696

Creamer M, Bell R, Failla S: Psychometric properties of the Impact of Event Scale—Revised. Behav Res Ther 41(12):1489–1496, 2003 14705607

Curley M, Johnston C: The characteristics and severity of psychological distress after abortion among university students. J Behav Health Serv Res 40(3):279–293, 2013 23576135

Curry SJ, Krist AH, Owens DK, et al: Screening for intimate partner violence, elder abuse, and abuse of vulnerable adults: US Preventive Services Task Force final recommendation statement. JAMA 320(16):1678–1687, 2018 30357305

Cusack K, Jonas DE, Forneris CA, et al: Psychological treatments for adults with posttraumatic stress disorder: a systematic review and meta-analysis. Clin Psychol Rev 43:128–141, 2016 26574151

Daugirdaite V, van den Akker O, Purewal S: Posttraumatic stress and posttraumatic stress disorder after termination of pregnancy and reproductive loss: a systematic review. J Pregnancy 2015:646345, 2015 25734016

Davidson JR, Book SW, Colket JT, et al: Assessment of a new self-rating scale for post-traumatic stress disorder. Psychol Med 27(1):153–160, 1997a 9122295

Davidson JR, Malik MA, Travers J: Structured interview for PTSD (SIP): psychometric validation for DSM-IV criteria. Depress Anxiety 5(3):127–129, 1997b 9323452

Davidson JR, Baldwin D, Stein DJ, et al: Treatment of posttraumatic stress disorder with venlafaxine extended release: a 6-month randomized controlled trial. Arch Gen Psychiatry 63(10):1158–1165, 2006 17015818

Davidson PR, Parker KCH: Eye movement desensitization and reprocessing (EMDR): a meta-analysis. J Consult Clin Psychol 69(2):305–316, 2001 11393607

Diehle J, Schmitt K, Daams JG, et al: Effects of psychotherapy on trauma-related cognitions in posttraumatic stress disorder: a meta-analysis. J Trauma Stress 27(3):257–264, 2014 24852498

Dikmen-Yildiz P, Ayers S, Phillips L: Longitudinal trajectories of post-traumatic stress disorder (PTSD) after birth and associated risk factors. J Affect Disord 229:377–385, 2018 29331697

Duman RS, Heninger GR, Nestler EJ: A molecular and cellular theory of depression. Arch Gen Psychiatry 54(7):597–606, 1997 9236543

Dunlop BW, Wong A: The hypothalamic-pituitary-adrenal axis in PTSD: pathophysiology and treatment interventions. Prog Neuropsychopharmacol Biol Psychiatry 89:361–379, 2019 30342071

Einarson A, Bailey B, Jung G, et al: Prospective controlled study of hydroxyzine and cetirizine in pregnancy. Ann Allergy Asthma Immunol 78(2):183–186, 1997 9048526

Feeny NC, Hembree EA, Zoellner LA: Myths regarding exposure therapy for PTSD. Cognit Behav Pract 10(1):85–90, 2003

Felitti VJ, Anda RF, Nordenberg D, et al: Relationship of childhood abuse and household dysfunction to many of the leading causes of death in adults. The Adverse Childhood Experiences (ACE) Study. Am J Prev Med 14(4):245–258, 1998 9635069

Fergusson DM, Horwood LJ, Boden JML: Abortion and mental health disorders: evidence from a 30-year longitudinal study. Br J Psychiatry 193(6):444–451, 2008 19043144

First MB, Spitzer RL, Gibbon M, et al: Structured Clinical Interview for DSM-IV Axis I Disorders. Washington, DC, American Psychiatric Publishing, 1996

Fitzgerald JM, DiGangi JA, Phan KL: Functional neuroanatomy of emotion and its regulation in PTSD. Harv Rev Psychiatry 26(3):116–128, 2018 29734226

Foa EB, Rothbaum BO: Treating the Trauma of Rape: Cognitive-Behavioral Therapy for PTSD. New York, Guilford, 1998

Foa EB, Riggs DS, Dancu CV, et al: PTSD Symptom Scale–Interview Version (PSS-I). Philadelphia, PA, Edna B. Foa, 1993a

Foa E, Riggs DS, Dancu CV, et al: Reliability and validity of a brief instrument for assessing post-traumatic stress disorder. J Trauma Stress 6(4):459–473, 1993b

Foa EB, Riggs DS, Gershuny BS, et al: Arousal, numbing, and intrusion: symptom structure of PTSD following assault. Am J Psychiatry 152(1):116–120, 1995 7802101
Foa EB, Zoellner LA, Feeny NC, et al: Does imaginal exposure exacerbate PTSD symptoms? J Consult Clin Psychol 70(4):1022–1028, 2002 12182265
Forbes D, Creamer M, Bisson JI, et al: A guide to guidelines for the treatment of PTSD and related conditions. J Trauma Stress 23(5):537–552, 2010 20839310
Ford JD, Grasso DJ, Elhai JD, et al: Etiology of PTSD: What Causes PTSD? Posttraumatic Stress Disorders, 2nd Edition. New York, Academic Press, 2015, pp 81–132
Furuta M, Horsch A, Ng ESW, et al: Effectiveness of trauma-focused psychological therapies for treating post-traumatic stress disorder symptoms in women following childbirth: a systematic review and meta-analysis. Front Psychiatry 9:591, 2018 30515108
García-Moreno C, Jansen HA, Ellsberg M, et al: WHO Multi-Country Study on Women's Health and Domestic Violence Against Women. Geneva, World Health Organization, 2005
Germain A, Richardson R, Moul DE, et al: Placebo-controlled comparison of prazosin and cognitive-behavioral treatments for sleep disturbances in US military veterans. J Psychosom Res 72(2):89–96, 2012 22281448
Gilmore AK, Davis MT, Grubaugh A, et al: "Do you expect me to receive PTSD care in a setting where most of the other patients remind me of the perpetrator?": home-based telemedicine to address barriers to care unique to military sexual trauma and Veterans Affairs hospitals. Contemp Clin Trials 48:59–64, 2016 26992740
Gissler M, Hemminki E, Lönnqvist J: Suicides after pregnancy in Finland, 1987–94: register linkage study. BMJ 313(7070):1431–1434, 1996 8973229
Grekin R, O'Hara MW: Prevalence and risk factors of postpartum posttraumatic stress disorder: a meta-analysis. Clin Psychol Rev 34(5):389–401, 2014 24952134
Guina J, Rossetter SR, DeRhodes BJ, et al: Benzodiazepines for PTSD: a systematic review and meta-analysis. J Psychiatr Pract 21(4):281–303, 2015 26164054
Gutner CA, Pedersen ER, Drummond SPA: Going direct to the consumer: examining treatment preferences for veterans with insomnia, PTSD, and depression. Psychiatry Res 263:108–114, 2018 29524908
Haagen JF, Moerbeek M, Olde E, et al: PTSD after childbirth: a predictive ethological model for symptom development. J Affect Disord 185:135–143, 2015 26172985
Hahn CK, Gilmore AK, Aguayo RO, et al: Perinatal intimate partner violence. Obstet Gynecol Clin North Am 45(3):535–547, 2018 30092927
Hamama L, Rauch SA, Sperlich M, et al: Previous experience of spontaneous or elective abortion and risk for posttraumatic stress and depression during subsequent pregnancy. Depress Anxiety 27(8):699–707, 2010 20577979
Harris HR, Wieser F, Vitonis AF, et al: Early life abuse and risk of endometriosis. Hum Reprod 33(9):1657–1668, 2018 30016439
Hatzenbuehler ML: How does sexual minority stigma "get under the skin"? A psychological mediation framework. Psychol Bull 135(5):707–730, 2009 19702379
Hebenstreit CL, Maguen S, Koo KH, et al: Latent profiles of PTSD symptoms in women exposed to intimate partner violence. J Affect Disord 180:122–128, 2015 25898332
Hellmuth JC, Jaquier V, Swan SC, et al: Elucidating posttraumatic stress symptom profiles and their correlates among women experiencing bidirectional intimate partner violence. J Clin Psychol 70(10):1008–1021, 2014 24752965
Hernández-Martínez A, Rodríguez-Almagro J, Molina-Alarcón M, et al: Postpartum posttraumatic stress disorder: associated perinatal factors and quality of life. J Affect Disord 249:143–150, 2019 30772741
Hizli Sayar G, Ozten E, Tufan E, et al: Transcranial magnetic stimulation during pregnancy. Arch Women Ment Health 17(4):311–315, 2014 24248413
Holden KB, McKenzie R, Pruitt V, et al: Depressive symptoms, substance abuse, and intimate partner violence among pregnant women of diverse ethnicities. J Health Care Poor Underserved 23(1):226–241, 2012 22643473
Hong B, Ding X, Iia H, Zhang J: Combination treatment of captopril and prazosin to treat patients with gestational hypertension. Exp Ther Med 16(4):3694–3702, 2018 30233728

Hori H, Kim Y: Inflammation and post-traumatic stress disorder. Psychiatry Clin Neurosci 73(4):143–153, 2019 30653780

Horsch A, Vial Y, Favrod C, et al: Reducing intrusive traumatic memories after emergency caesarean section: a proof-of-principle randomized controlled study. Behav Res Ther 94:36–47, 2017 28453969

Huth-Bocks AC, Krause K, Ahlfs-Dunn S, et al: Relational trauma and posttraumatic stress symptoms among pregnant women. Psychodyn Psychiatry 41(2):277–301, 2013 23713621

Hutti MH, dePacheco M, Smith M: A study of miscarriage: development and validation of the Perinatal Grief Intensity Scale. J Obstet Gynecol Neonatal Nurs 27(5):547–555, 1998 9773366

James EL, Bonsall MB, Hoppitt L, et al: Computer game play reduces intrusive memories of experimental trauma via reconsolidation-update mechanisms. Psychol Sci 26(8):1201–1215, 2015 26133572

Kang JI, Kim TY, Choi JH, et al: Allele-specific DNA methylation level of FKBP5 is associated with post-traumatic stress disorder. Psychoneuroendocrinology 103:1–7, 2019 30605803

Karakurt G, Smith D, Whiting J: Impact of intimate partner violence on women's mental health. J Fam Violence 29(7):693–702, 2014 25313269

Kessler RC, Sonnega A, Bromet E, et al: Posttraumatic stress disorder in the National Comorbidity Survey. Arch Gen Psychiatry 52(12):1048–1060, 1995 7492257

Kim DR, Wang E, McGeehan B, et al: Randomized controlled trial of transcranial magnetic stimulation in pregnant women with major depressive disorder. Brain Stimul 12(1):96–102, 2019 30249416

Kim WJ, Lee E, Kim KR, et al: Progress of PTSD symptoms following birth: a prospective study in mothers of high-risk infants. J Perinatol 35(8):575–579, 2015 25856762

Koek RJ, Roach J, Athanasiou N, et al: Neuromodulatory treatments for post-traumatic stress disorder (PTSD). Prog Neuropsychopharmacol Biol Psychiatry 92(8):148–160, 2019 30641094

Kozel FA, Motes MA, Didehbani N, et al: Repetitive TMS to augment cognitive processing therapy in combat veterans of recent conflicts with PTSD: a randomized clinical trial. J Affect Disord 229:506–514, 2018 29351885

Kübler-Ross E: On Death and Dying. New York, Macmillan, 1969

Lee DJ, Schnitzlein CW, Wolf JP, et al: Psychotherapy versus pharmacotherapy for posttraumatic stress disorder: systematic review and meta-analyses to determine first-line treatments. Depress Anxiety 33(9):792–806, 2016 27126398

Leis-Newman E: Miscarriage and loss. Monitor on Psychology 43(6):56, 2012

Major B, Applebaum M, Beckman L, et al: American Psychological Association Task Force on Mental Health and Abortion. Washington, DC, American Psychological Association Publishing, 2008

Marshall RD, Beebe KL, Oldham M, et al: Efficacy and safety of paroxetine treatment for chronic PTSD: a fixed-dose, placebo-controlled study. Am J Psychiatry 158(12):1982–1988, 2001 11729013

McEwen BS: Neurobiological and systemic effects of chronic stress. Chronic Stress (Thousand Oaks) 1:1–11, 2017 28856337

Meltzer-Brody S, Maegbaek ML, Medland SE, et al: Obstetrical, pregnancy and socio-economic predictors for new-onset severe postpartum psychiatric disorders in primiparous women. Psychol Med 47(8):1427–1441, 2017 28112056

Miller EC, Goodman LA, Thomas KA, et al: GLBTQDVP Domestic Violence Project: Trauma-Informed Approaches for LGBTQ* Survivors of Intimate Partner Violence: A Review of Literature and a Set of Practice Observations. Boston, MA, The GLBTQ Domestic Violence Project, 2016. Available at: http://www.nationalcenterdvtraumamh.org/wp-content/uploads/2016/09/TIPforLGBQTSurvivors_LitReview.pdf. Accessed February 1, 2021.

Misanin JR, Miller RR, Lewis DJ: Retrograde amnesia produced by electroconvulsive shock after reactivation of a consolidated memory trace. Science 160(3827):554–555, 1968 5689415

Morgan CL, Evans M, Peters JR: Suicides after pregnancy. Mental health may deteriorate as a direct effect of induced abortion. BMJ 314(7084):902, author reply 902–903, 1997 9093118

Morgenthaler TI, Auerbach S, Casey KR, et al: Position paper for the treatment of nightmare disorder in adults: an American Academy of sleep medicine position paper. J Clin Sleep Med 14(6):1041–1055, 2018 29852917

Mota NP, Burnett M, Sareen J: Associations between abortion, mental disorders, and suicidal behaviour in a nationally representative sample. Can J Psychiatry 55(4):239–247, 2010 20416147
Nam DH, Pae CU, Chae JH: Low-frequency, repetitive transcranial magnetic stimulation for the treatment of patients with posttraumatic stress disorder: a double-blind, sham-controlled study. Clin Psychopharmacol Neurosci 11(2):96–102, 2013 24023554
National Coalition Against Domestic Violence: Domestic violence and the LGBTQ community. NCADV.org blog, June 6, 2018. Available at: https://ncadv.org/blog/posts/domestic-violence-and-the-lgbtq-community. Accessed July 4, 2020.
Navidian A, Saravani Z, Shakiba M: Impact of psychological grief counseling on the severity of post-traumatic stress symptoms in mothers after stillbirths. Issues Ment Health Nurs 38(8):650–654, 2017 28745912
Nieminen K, Berg I, Frankenstein K, et al: Internet-provided cognitive behaviour therapy of posttraumatic stress symptoms following childbirth-a randomized controlled trial. Cogn Behav Ther 45(4):287–306, 2016 27152849
Olieman RM, Siemonsma F, Bartens MA, et al: The effect of an elective cesarean section on maternal request on peripartum anxiety and depression in women with childbirth fear: a systematic review. BMC Pregnancy Childbirth 17(1):195, 2017 28629393
Osuch EA, Benson BE, Luckenbaugh DA, et al: Repetitive TMS combined with exposure therapy for PTSD: a preliminary study. J Anxiety Disord 23(1):54–59, 2009 18455908
Ozer EJ, Best SR, Lipsey TL, et al: Predictors of posttraumatic stress disorder and symptoms in adults: a meta-analysis. Psychol Bull 129(1):52–73, 2003 12555794
Possemato K, Kuhn E, Johnson E, et al: Using PTSD Coach in primary care with and without clinician support: a pilot randomized controlled trial. Gen Hosp Psychiatry 38:94–98, 2016 26589765
Powers MB, Halpern JM, Ferenschak MP, et al: A meta-analytic review of prolonged exposure for posttraumatic stress disorder. Clin Psychol Rev 30(6):635–641, 2010 20546985
Ralph LJ, Schwarz EB, Grossman D, et al: Self-reported physical health of women who did and did not terminate pregnancy after seeking abortion services: a cohort study. Ann Intern Med 171(4):238–247, 2019 31181576
Raskind MA, Peterson K, Williams T, et al: A trial of prazosin for combat trauma PTSD with nightmares in active-duty soldiers returned from Iraq and Afghanistan. Am J Psychiatry 170(9):1003–1010, 2013 23846759
Raskind MA, Peskind ER, Chow B, et al: Trial of prazosin for post-traumatic stress disorder in military veterans. N Engl J Med 378(6):507–517, 2018 29414272
Reardon DC, Coleman PK, Cougle JR: Substance use associated with unintended pregnancy outcomes in the National Longitudinal Survey of Youth. Am J Drug Alcohol Abuse 30(2):369–383, 2004 15230081
Resick PA, Nishith P, Weaver TL, et al: A comparison of cognitive-processing therapy with prolonged exposure and a waiting condition for the treatment of chronic posttraumatic stress disorder in female rape victims. J Consult Clin Psychol 70(4):867–879, 2002 12182270
Resick PA, Monson CM, Chard KM: Cognitive Processing Therapy for PTSD: A Comprehensive Manual. New York, Guilford, 2017
Ritsher JB, Neugebauer R: Perinatal Bereavement Grief Scale: distinguishing grief from depression following miscarriage. Assessment 9(1):31–40, 2002 11911232
Roberts AL, Austin SB, Corliss HL, et al: Pervasive trauma exposure among US sexual orientation minority adults and risk of posttraumatic stress disorder. Am J Public Health 100(12):2433–2441, 2010 20395586
Roberts AL, Gilman SE, Breslau J, et al: Race/ethnic differences in exposure to traumatic events, development of post-traumatic stress disorder, and treatment-seeking for post-traumatic stress disorder in the United States. Psychol Med 41(1):71–83, 2011 20346193
Robinson GE, Stotland NL, Russo NF, et al: Is there an "abortion trauma syndrome"? Critiquing the evidence. Harv Rev Psychiatry 17(4):268–290, 2009 19637075
Rogal SS, Poschman K, Belanger K, et al: Effects of posttraumatic stress disorder on pregnancy outcomes. J Affect Disord 102(1–3):137–143, 2007 17291588

Ross LE, McLean LM: Anxiety disorders during pregnancy and the postpartum period: a systematic review. J Clin Psychiatry 67(8):1285–1298, 2006 16965210

Rothbaum BO, Astin MC, Marsteller F: Prolonged exposure versus eye movement desensitization and reprocessing (EMDR) for PTSD rape victims. J Trauma Stress 18(6):607–616, 2005 16382428

Sandström M, Wiberg B, Wikman M, et al: A pilot study of eye movement desensitisation and reprocessing treatment (EMDR) for post-traumatic stress after childbirth. Midwifery 24(1):62–73, 2008 17223232

Schnurr PP, Friedman MJ, Engel CC, et al: Cognitive behavioral therapy for posttraumatic stress disorder in women: a randomized controlled trial. JAMA 297(8):820–830, 2007 17327524

Schnyder U, Ehlers A, Elbert T, et al: Psychotherapies for PTSD: what do they have in common? Eur J Psychotraumatol 6:28186, 2015 26290178

Schoenfeld N, Epstein O, Nemesh L, et al: Effects of propranolol during pregnancy and development of rats. I. Adverse effects during pregnancy. Pediatr Res 12(7):747–750, 1978 693116

Seng JS, Oakley DJ, Sampselle CM, et al: Posttraumatic stress disorder and pregnancy complications. Obstet Gynecol 97(1):17–22, 2001 11152900

Seng JS, Low LK, Sperlich M, et al: Prevalence, trauma history, and risk for posttraumatic stress disorder among nulliparous women in maternity care. Obstet Gynecol 114(4):839–847, 2009 19888043

Seng JS, Kohn-Wood LP, McPherson MD, et al: Disparity in posttraumatic stress disorder diagnosis among African American pregnant women. Arch Women Ment Health 14(4):295–306, 2011 21573930

Silverman JG, Decker MR, Reed E, et al: Intimate partner violence victimization prior to and during pregnancy among women residing in 26 U.S. states: associations with maternal and neonatal health. Am J Obstet Gynecol 195(1):140–148, 2006 16813751

Smith MV, Poschman K, Cavaleri MA, et al: Symptoms of posttraumatic stress disorder in a community sample of low-income pregnant women. Am J Psychiatry 163(5):881–884, 2006 16648330

Smith SG, Zhang X, Basile KC, et al: The National Intimate Partner and Sexual Violence Survey (NISVS): 2015 Data Brief—Updated Release. Atlanta, GA, National Center for Injury Prevention and Control, Centers for Disease Control and Prevention, 2018

Speckhard A, Rue VM: Post abortion syndrome: an emerging public health concern. J Soc Issues 48(3):95–119, 1992

Sprague S, Madden K, Simunovic N, et al: Barriers to screening for intimate partner violence. Women Health 52(6):587–605, 2012 22860705

Stafford L, McNally OM, Gibson P, et al: Long-term psychological morbidity, sexual functioning, and relationship outcomes in women with gestational trophoblastic disease. Int J Gynecol Cancer 21:1256–1263, 2011 21811174

Substance Abuse and Mental Health Services Administration: SAMHSA's Concept of Trauma and Guidance for a Trauma-Informed Care Approach. Washington, DC, U.S. Department of Health and Human Services, 2014a. Available at: https://ncsacw.samhsa.gov/userfiles/files/SAMHSA_Trauma.pdf. Accessed February 1, 2021.

Substance Abuse and Mental Health Services Administration: Treatment Improvement Protocol (TIP) Series No 57: trauma-informed care in behavior health services. Washington, DC, Center for Substance Abuse Treatment, 2014b. Available at: https://store.samhsa.gov/sites/default/files/d7/priv/sma14-4816.pdf. Accessed February 1, 2021.

Taylor FB, Martin P, Thompson C, et al: Prazosin effects on objective sleep measures and clinical symptoms in civilian trauma posttraumatic stress disorder: a placebo-controlled study. Biol Psychiatry 63(6):629–632, 2008 17868655

Taylor S, Thordarson DS, Maxfield L, et al: Comparative efficacy, speed, and adverse effects of three PTSD treatments: exposure therapy, EMDR, and relaxation training. J Consult Clin Psychol 71(2):330–338, 2003 12699027

Toedter LJ, Lasker JN, Alhadeff JM: The Perinatal Grief Scale: development and initial validation. Am J Orthopsychiatry 58(3):435–449, 1988 3407734

Tolin DF, Foa EB: Sex differences in trauma and posttraumatic stress disorder: a quantitative review of 25 years of research. Psychol Bull 132(6):959–992, 2006 17073529

U.S. Department of Veterans Affairs and Department of Defense: VA/DOD clinical practice guideline for the management of posttraumatic stress disorder and acute stress disorder. 2017. Available at: https://www.healthquality.va.gov/guidelines/MH/ptsd/VADoDPTSDCPGFinal012418.pdf. Accessed February 1, 2021.

van den Hout M, Muris P, Salemink E, Kindt M: Autobiographical memories become less vivid and emotional after eye movements. Br J Clin Psychol 40(2):121–130, 2001 11446234

van der Merwe C, Jahanshad N, Cheung JW, et al: Concordance of genetic variation that increases risk for anxiety disorders and posttraumatic stress disorders and that influences their underlying neurocircuitry. J Affect Disord 245:885–896, 2019 30699873

van Minnen A, Harned MS, Zoellner L, et al: Examining potential contraindications for prolonged exposure therapy for PTSD. Eur J Psychotraumatol 3:1, 2012 22893847

Vermetten E, Vythilingam M, Southwick SM, et al: Long-term treatment with paroxetine increases verbal declarative memory and hippocampal volume in posttraumatic stress disorder. Biol Psychiatry 54(7):693–702, 2003 14512209

Vignato J, Connelly CD, Bush RA, et al: Correlates of perinatal post-traumatic stress among culturally diverse women with depressive symptomatology. Issues Ment Health Nurs 39(10):840–849, 2018 30277842

Wallin Lundell I, Georgsson Öhman S, Frans Ö, et al: Posttraumatic stress among women after induced abortion: a Swedish multi-centre cohort study. BMC Womens Health 13(52):52, 2013 24364878

Ward HB, Fromson JA, Cooper JJ, et al: Recommendations for the use of ECT in pregnancy: literature review and proposed clinical protocol. Arch Women Ment Health 21(6):715–722, 2018 29796968

Wathen CN, Macmillan HL: Children's exposure to intimate partner violence: impacts and interventions. Paediatr Child Health 18(8):419–422, 2013 24426794

Watts BV, Landon B, Groft A, et al: A sham controlled study of repetitive transcranial magnetic stimulation for posttraumatic stress disorder. Brain Stimul 5(1):38–43, 2012 22264669

Watts BV, Schnurr PP, Mayo L, et al: Meta-analysis of the efficacy of treatments for posttraumatic stress disorder. J Clin Psychiatry 74(6):e541–e550, 2013 23842024

Weathers FW, Blake DD, Schnurr PP, et al: The Clinician-Administered PTSD Scale for DSM-5 (CAPS-5). Washington, DC, National Center for PTSD, 2013. Available at: https://www.ptsd.va.gov/professional/assessment/adult-int/caps.asp. Accessed February 1, 2021.

Wells BG, Chu CC, Johnson R, et al: Buspirone in the treatment of posttraumatic stress disorder. Pharmacotherapy 11(4):340–343, 1991 1923917

Williams K, Finch BK: Adverse childhood experiences, early and nonmarital fertility, and women's health at midlife. J Health Soc Behav 60(3):309–325, 2019 31526017

Worden JW: Grief Counselling and Grief Therapy: A Handbook for the Mental Health Practitioner, 4th Edition. New York, Springer, 2013

Yildiz PD, Ayers S, Phillips L: The prevalence of posttraumatic stress disorder in pregnancy and after birth: a systematic review and meta-analysis. J Affect Disord 208:634–645, 2017 27865585

Youssef NA, McCall WV, Andrade C: The role of ECT in posttraumatic stress disorder: a systematic review. Ann Clin Psychiatry 29(1):62–70, 2017 28207917

Zoellner LA, Goodwin ML, Foa EB: PTSD severity and health perceptions in female victims of sexual assault. J Trauma Stress 13(4):635–649, 2000 11109236

CHAPTER 19

# Anxiety Disorders and Insomnia in the Perinatal Period

Lucy A. Hutner, M.D.
Joanna V. MacLean, M.D.
Gioia M. Guerrieri, D.O.
Melisa Olgun, B.A.
Julia Frew, M.D.

When it comes to anxiety and reproductive mental health, as a field we still have more questions than answers. On the one hand, anxiety disorders are the most common mental health conditions in women overall (Gregory et al. 2020), and anxiety disorders complicate pregnancy and the postpartum period at a rate higher than depressive disorders—affecting up to one-fifth of all pregnancies (Dennis et al. 2017; Matthey et al. 2003). In addition, perinatal anxiety has been shown to be associated with adverse maternal–infant outcomes, comparable with—and perhaps even exceeding—the impact of perinatal depression (Grigoriadis et al. 2013). Nevertheless, perinatal anxiety is underdiagnosed and undertreated, and understanding of the clinical features, risk factors, pathophysiology, and treatment remains limited (Fallon et al. 2016b; Goodman et al. 2014a; Harrison et al. 2020; Misri et al. 2015). However, clinical and research interest in this area has increased given both its high prevalence and its clear impact on maternal and infant outcomes (Grigoriadis et al. 2018).

---

Dr. Guerrieri contributed to this chapter in her personal capacity. The views expressed are her own and do not necessarily represent the views of the National Institutes of Health or the United States government.

Ms. EE is a 27-year-old gravida 1 para 0 woman at 14 weeks' gestation, with no formal psychiatric history, referred by her obstetrician due to seeming anxious during a prenatal visit. She reports this was a planned pregnancy and that she has been happy when she conceived quickly because she worried that she would have difficulty getting pregnant. She believes she has always been a worrier, but it was not until college that she realized that not everybody "obsessed" about things to the same degree she did. She reports that her mind is constantly ruminating and never really shuts off. She will realize on her drive home from work that she has not even turned the radio on, but it has not felt silent because of all the thoughts going through her mind. She will sometimes get stuck on one worry for an extended period but often is moving among many: situations at work, finances, managing the household, upcoming events.

Since becoming pregnant. Ms. EE has been worried about the health of the baby and about potentially having a miscarriage or birth defect. She has not yet told anybody she is pregnant in case something happens. At the same time, she has wondered how she is going to be able to manage motherhood on top of all her other responsibilities. She has become a lot more nervous when her husband leaves for work or social events, requesting that he let her know once he has arrived safely. She has difficulty falling asleep at night, often taking 2–3 hours due to reviewing her worries. She feels constantly exhausted and has had her doctor complete workups to try and identify the source of her fatigue, which have all come back normal. She frequently has teeth grinding, shoulder tension, and headaches. She is aware of being less efficient at work because her concentration is impaired by her worries, and her boss recently commented on it. In addition, she and her husband have been having increased difficulty because she has been "snapping" at him a lot more about little things, even while she recognizes these things are not important.

It is important to understand the course and treatment of insomnia in pregnancy as a related clinical problem. Insomnia is a common perinatal symptom often assumed to be part of the normal physiology of pregnancy. However, recent evidence has pointed to the detrimental effects of perinatal insomnia itself, such as its relationship to preterm birth (Felder et al. 2017). In addition, perinatal insomnia plays an important role in maternal mental health because it can be both a symptom of an underlying mood or anxiety disorder and a trigger for these conditions. There is a complex interplay between insomnia, depression, and anxiety—making insomnia an important area to address for clinicians who treat women in the perinatal period.

This chapter focuses on the epidemiology, clinical presentation, diagnostic criteria, clinical features, differential diagnosis and assessment, course and prognosis, and treatment of perinatal anxiety disorders in women. We discuss perinatal anxiety disorders both as a group and as distinct DSM-5 (American Psychiatric Association 2013) anxiety disorders; we also discuss related entities cited in the literature, such as pregnancy-specific anxiety. Of note, disorders that contain anxiety symptomatology but are not DSM-5 anxiety disorders, per se, such as OCD and PTSD, are covered comprehensively in other chapters; please see Chapter 18, "Trauma and Reproductive Health," and Chapter 20, "Obsessive-Compulsive Disorder," for details. We also include a summary of insomnia in pregnancy, including its epidemiology, clinical presentation, and treatment options, because this common condition has significant overlap with the symptoms and management of perinatal anxiety disorders.

# Anxiety Disorders in the Perinatal Period

## Epidemiology

### Rates/Incidence

Anxiety disorders are among the most prevalent and consequential health disorders in the United States (Kessler et al. 2012). There are substantial sex differences in the prevalence of anxiety disorders: estimates of the lifetime prevalence of an anxiety disorder in women is 40%, twice that of men (Kessler et al. 2012). A recent meta-analysis estimated that the prevalence of having at least one anxiety disorder in pregnancy was 20.7%, with a trend toward a higher prevalence of anxiety in pregnancy as compared with postpartum (Fawcett et al. 2019). A systematic review found that the prevalence of perinatal anxiety was the same as or higher than that of anxiety in the general population, including generalized anxiety disorder (GAD, 9%) and panic disorder (1%–2%), as well as disorders with anxiety symptomatology, such as OCD (0.2%–4%) and PTSD (0.6%–8%) (Ross and McLean 2006). Many anxiety disorders run a chronic course; thus, many women enter the perinatal period already having an anxiety disorder (O'Hara and Wisner 2014).

Anxiety has extensive comorbidity with other mental health conditions, particularly depression (O'Hara and Wisner 2014). The prevalence of anxiety disorders in adults with comorbid major depressive disorder (MDD) has been estimated to be as high as 56% (Kessler et al. 2003). Anxiety symptoms are more prevalent in depression related to childbirth—specifically postpartum depression (PPD)—than depression that is unrelated to childbirth (Hendrick et al. 2000; Jolley and Betrus 2007). In a large-scale postpartum screening study with diagnostic follow-up, 66% of the women diagnosed with MDD were also diagnosed with an anxiety disorder (Wisner et al. 2013). The converse is also true: Grigoriadis et al. (2011) found that in a cohort of perinatal women, nearly 50% of the sample with GAD had a comorbid major depressive episode (MDE) or another anxiety disorder, and 30% met criteria for both GAD and MDE. They also found significant comorbidity among anxiety-related disorders themselves; in a cohort of perinatal women with GAD, 20% had comorbidity with a specific phobia, 9% with panic disorder, 9% with agoraphobia, and 4% with OCD (Grigoriadis et al. 2011).

### Risk Factors

Biological, mental health, pregnancy-related, and social factors have all been implicated as potential predictors of perinatal anxiety; however, more research is needed to identify factors specific to the perinatal population and to tease apart interrelated factors (Furtado et al. 2018; O'Hara and Wisner 2014). The strongest risk factor for a perinatal anxiety disorder is the presence of a prior anxiety or depressive disorder (O'Hara and Wisner 2014). A recent meta-analysis identified a wide range of risk factors for perinatal onset or exacerbation of anxiety, including comorbid psychiatric disorder, multiparity, family history of psychiatric disorders, comorbid sleep disorder, prenatal oxytocin exposure, hyperemesis gravidarum, lower educational attainment,

**TABLE 19–1. Risk factors for perinatal anxiety**

| | |
|---|---|
| Biological | Comorbid sleep disorders |
| | Elevated perceived stress |
| Mental health | Family history of psychiatric diagnosis |
| | Personal history of psychiatric diagnosis |
| Pregnancy-related | Hyperemesis gravidarum |
| | Multiparity |
| | Past pregnancy loss |
| | Prenatal synthetic oxytocin exposure |
| | Present or past pregnancy complications |
| | Unplanned/Unwanted pregnancy |
| Psychosocial | History of trauma or abuse, including intimate partner violence |
| | Limited social support/lack of partner |
| | Living with extended family members |
| | Lower educational attainment |
| | Presence of adverse life events |

*Source.* Bayrampour et al. 2018; Biaggi et al. 2016; Furtado et al. 2018; Hantsoo and Epperson 2017; Hettema et al. 2004; Mackintosh et al. 2006; O'Hara and Wisner 2014.

and living with extended family members (Furtado et al. 2018). Other factors that have been cited in the literature include high perceived stress, previous or current pregnancy complications, prior pregnancy loss, adverse childhood events/traumatic life experiences, and poor social or partner support (Bayrampour et al. 2018; Biaggi et al. 2016; Hantsoo and Epperson 2017; Hettema et al. 2004; Mackintosh et al. 2006). A recent longitudinal study aimed to identify risk factors for postpartum worsening of anxiety in women with preexisting anxiety disorders; depression symptom severity, antenatal obsessive-compulsive symptoms, and intolerance of uncertainty were significant predictors of postpartum exacerbation (Furtado et al. 2019). Putative risk factors for perinatal anxiety are summarized in Table 19–1.

## Screening

The increasing recognition of the significant impact of anxiety throughout women's lives has resulted in a call for increased screening and resources allocated for diagnosis and treatment (Gregory et al. 2020). In 2020, the Women's Preventive Services Initiative issued a recommendation for widespread screening for anxiety; the age group recommended for screening was broad, from adolescent girls starting at age 13 years through adulthood (Gregory et al. 2020). Given the widespread prevalence and impact of perinatal anxiety, screening specifically in the perinatal period is also recommended. The American College of Obstetricians and Gynecologists (ACOG) issued a recommendation that obstetricians-gynecologists and other obstetrical providers screen at least once during the perinatal period for depression and anxiety using a validated, standardized tool (American College of Obstetricians and Gynecologists 2018). They also recommended that providers conduct a full assessment of emotional and mental well-being in the postpartum period, even if such screening had already been completed during pregnancy (American College of Obstetricians and Gynecologists 2018).

However, effective screening for perinatal anxiety remains limited, in part because many questions remain about the optimal screening tool, starting with which—of many—anxiety symptoms to address (Fairbrother et al. 2019; Matthey et al. 2013a). For example, the Generalized Anxiety Disorder seven-item subscale (Spitzer et al. 2006) identified GAD in perinatal populations with greater accuracy and specificity than the widely used Edinburgh Postnatal Depression Scale (EPDS; Cox et al. 1987). However, the clinical presentation of perinatal anxiety can be highly variable, including symptoms from various DSM-5 disorders, such as panic or intrusive thoughts, making the selection of a single tool difficult (Matthey et al. 2013a; Meades and Ayers 2011). In addition, general anxiety scales may not delineate symptoms of anxiety from the common physical symptoms of pregnancy and postpartum, such as sleep disturbance, which may lead to false positives (Matthey et al. 2013a). Examples include "I feel rested" and "I feel comfortable" in the State-Trait Anxiety Index (STAI; Spielberger et al. 1983) and "I can sit at ease and feel relaxed" in the Hospital Anxiety and Depression Scale (HADS; Zigmond and Snaith 1983). In contrast, the widely used EPDS has the advantage of excluding constitutional symptoms of pregnancy and postpartum (Cox et al. 1987).

In addition, pregnancy and becoming a parent are major life transitions that can feel stressful or overwhelming and can lead to anxiety specific for this distinct period of time, yet general screening tools may not capture anxiety symptoms specific to this population (Fallon et al. 2016b). Many symptoms of perinatal anxiety may not meet DSM-5 criteria for an anxiety disorder but nevertheless may be significant in terms of symptom severity, functional impairment, and impact on maternal and infant outcomes (Phillips et al. 2009). A recent systematic review analyzed the psychometric properties of several generalized anxiety screening tools designed for the general adult population, such as the STAI and the HADS, and concluded that there is a substantial need for further validation of these measures to enable accurate screening and detection in the perinatal population (Meades and Ayers 2011).

On the other hand, several pregnancy-specific self-report questionnaires, such as the Pregnancy Anxiety Scale (Levin 1991), the Pregnancy-Related Anxiety Questionnaire (Van den Bergh 1990), and the Pregnancy-Related Anxiety Scale (Wadhwa et al. 1993) focus on perinatal concerns but may have limited relevance for diagnosable anxiety disorders. Interestingly, although perinatal-specific scales focus on highly specific topics, they may predict adverse maternal–infant outcomes more effectively than general measures of anxiety, and they are distinct from general indices of anxiety and depression (Huizink et al. 2002). It was partly due to results such as these that the concept of pregnancy-specific anxiety—that is, anxiety specific to concerns about pregnancy, delivery, postpartum, and parenthood, and distinct from anxiety experienced at other times of life—was developed (Huizink et al. 2004). For example, a confirmatory factor analysis and a later replication study noted that general anxiety and depression symptoms contributed little to the variance in pregnancy-specific anxiety and that topics specific to the pregnancy itself (e.g., concern about the health of the fetus) were more important factors (Brunton et al. 2019; Huizink et al. 2004).

Yet difficulties in screening also exist with perinatal-specific screening tools. The ACOG cited the EPDS in its recommendation as a screening scale for depression and anxiety, given that it is in widespread use, is a brief self-report scale, is health literacy appropriate, and has been translated into more than 50 languages (American College of Obstetricians and Gynecologists 2018). However, the EPDS was originally developed to identify perinatal depression, and questions regarding anxiety are subsumed within the scale itself. Recent research has suggested that this tool may have multidimensional properties, and it may be able to detect—although perhaps not distinguish—anxiety disorders (Cox et al. 1987; Matthey and Ross-Hamid 2012; Matthey et al. 2013b; Rowe et al. 2008; Tuohy and McVey 2008). However, significant questions remain about the value of scales such as the EPDS in capturing specific symptoms of perinatal anxiety and in delineating whether these anxiety symptoms are part of—or distinct from—depression, and about whether the EPDS is more acceptable and feasible than existing anxiety-specific measures (Matthey et al. 2013a).

Recent advancements have included the development of scales that can both map onto diagnosable anxiety disorders and capture anxiety specific to the perinatal period (Table 19–2); these include the Perinatal Anxiety Screening Scale (PASS; Somerville et al. 2014), the Postpartum Worry Scale–Revised (Moran et al. 2014), and the Postpartum Specific Anxiety Scale (Fallon et al. 2016b). For example, the PASS was specifically developed to detect a broad range of anxiety symptoms, is specific to the perinatal period, and has a four-factor structure including 1) acute anxiety and adjustment, 2) general worry and specific fears, 3) perfectionism and control and trauma, and 4) social anxiety (Somerville et al. 2014, 2015). Preliminary validation of this scale was encouraging—the PASS identified 68% of women with a diagnosable anxiety disorder as compared with the EPDS anxiety subscale, which detected 36% (Somerville et al. 2014).

Screening for perinatal anxiety has the potential to capture a broad population, to lead to earlier diagnosis, and to provide an opportunity for early intervention, which could have important consequences for obstetrical and mental health outcomes for women and their offspring. However, screening is just one aspect of caring for the mental health of women in the perinatal period. Comprehensive health care systems must be in place to pair consistent screening with rigorous assessment, early intervention, and resources for follow-up for women with identified mental health disorders (Kendig et al. 2017). Additionally, future efforts might focus on identifying protective and resilience factors, such as self-efficacy and increased social support, to strengthen psychosocial resources as early as possible and optimize future outcomes (Dunkel Schetter and Tanner 2012).

## Diagnostic Criteria

Anxiety disorders have in common the presence of excessive or uncontrollable worry. In DSM-5, the term *anxiety disorder* refers to a group of distinct but interrelated conditions characterized by excessive fear—the emotional response to a real or perceived current threat—or anxiety—the response to a perceived future threat—and related behavioral disturbances (American Psychiatric Association 2013). Despite the high prevalence of perinatal anxiety, the DSM specifier "with peripartum onset" currently applies solely to mood disorders, not to anxiety disorders (American Psychiatric Association 2013). Some researchers define perinatal GAD if symptoms meet other criteria for a minimum duration of 1 month (vs. 6 months, as per DSM-5 criteria), given the specific time course of excessive worry during pregnancy and postpartum (Buist et al. 2011).

Defining anxiety in the context of reproductive mental health is complex (and confusing). First, perinatal anxiety symptoms, even if they do not fit formal criteria for an anxiety disorder diagnosis (e.g., pregnancy-specific anxiety), are highly prevalent and may cause significant impairment in functioning (O'Hara and Wisner 2014). Second,

**TABLE 19–2. Screening tools for anxiety**

| | |
|---|---|
| Edinburgh Postnatal Depression Scale Anxiety Subscale | Perinatal Anxiety Screening Scale |
| Generalized Anxiety Disorder–7 | Postpartum Specific Anxiety Scale |
| Hospital Anxiety and Depression Scale | Postpartum Worry Scale–Revised |

perinatal anxiety in pregnancy is described in the literature using distinct but interrelated concepts, such as anxiety disorders, pregnancy-specific anxiety, and distress. The following are core features of several of the more commonly described DSM-5 anxiety disorders in the perinatal literature, as well as descriptions of other anxiety-related terms discussed in the literature, including pregnancy-specific anxiety (which has substantial evidence as a distinct clinical entity) and trait anxiety, a little-studied but perhaps impactful subtype.

- *Generalized anxiety disorder*: GAD is the most common perinatal anxiety disorder (Goldfinger et al. 2020). It is characterized by excessive anxiety and worry that occurs for the majority of days and is associated with functional impairment. Worries include a number of events or activities and feel difficult to control (American Psychiatric Association 2013).
- *Panic disorder*: Panic disorder is diagnosed when a person experiences recurrent unexpected panic attacks and persistent worry about additional panic attacks or their consequences (American Psychiatric Association 2013). A *panic attack* is defined by an abrupt surge of intense fear or discomfort, along with symptoms such as accelerated heart rate, feeling dizzy or lightheaded, fear of dying or losing control, and derealization or depersonalization (American Psychiatric Association 2013).
- *Agoraphobia*: Agoraphobia is defined as excessive fear or anxiety about being in a situation in which escape may be difficult or help not available in the event of developing panic-like or embarrassing symptoms. It is often comorbid with panic disorder (American Psychiatric Association 2013).
- *Social anxiety disorder*: Patients with social anxiety disorder experience intense fear or anxiety in social situations in which they may be exposed to possible scrutiny by others (American Psychiatric Association 2013).
- *Specific phobia*: Patients with a specific phobia experience marked fear or anxiety about a specific object or situation (e.g., flying, heights, injections, or seeing blood), and exposure to the object or situation immediately brings about severe fear or anxiety; as a result, these patients will try to avoid the anxiety-provoking stimulus to any extent possible (American Psychiatric Association 2013). Several specific phobias discussed in the perinatal anxiety literature include *emetophobia* (fear of nausea and vomiting) and *tokophobia* (fear of childbirth); of note, fear of childbirth has been further described as fear of childbirth itself (primary) or fear after a prior negative birth experience (secondary) (Dencker et al. 2019).

In addition to the DSM-5 disorders, other perinatal-specific anxiety terms are cited in the literature. *Pregnancy-specific anxiety* describes fears specific to the perinatal period, including about the health of one's baby, the hospital and health care experience (including concerns about the well-being of the pregnancy and oneself), the experience of delivery, and the transition into parenting (Dunkel Schetter 2011; Huizink et al. 2004). It appears to be linked to state anxiety, but it arises out of the specific context of the perinatal period—a series of distinct transitions that can be experienced as stressful and overwhelming (Dunkel Schetter 2011; Fallon et al. 2016b). The prevalence of pregnancy-specific anxiety is virtually equal to that of perinatal GAD, and the symptom severity and functional impairment are also equivalent (Blackmore et al. 2016; Phillips et al. 2009).

Whereas pregnancy-specific anxiety is an example of state anxiety symptoms that are specific to a certain set of external conditions, *trait anxiety* refers to the tendency to report negative emotions such as fears and worries across multiple domains and the stable perception of environmental stimuli as threatening (Dennis et al. 2017). The prevalence of trait anxiety in perinatal populations is high. A recent systematic review and meta-analysis of more than 100 studies and more than 200,000 women noted a prevalence of 29%–33% antenatally and 23% postnatally (Dennis et al. 2017). Lastly, *distress* is a term used in the perinatal literature to describe negative affective states related to stress, such as anxiety or depression symptoms (Rallis et al. 2014b).

# Clinical Features

## Clinical Presentation

Generally, anxiety consists of symptoms in multiple domains, including cognitive (e.g., fear of losing control, frightening thoughts or images), physiological (e.g., increased heart rate, shortness of breath, trembling or shaking), behavioral (e.g., avoidance of threat cues, restlessness, agitation), and affective (e.g., feeling nervous, tense, wound up) (Chand and Marwaha 2020). Perinatal GAD is characterized by excessive, uncontrollable worry that can cause functional impairment (Misri et al. 2015). It is a clinical entity that is distinct from the anxiety associated with PPD, despite extensive comorbidity with it (Misri et al. 2015). The content of the anxiety in perinatal GAD typically revolves around fears about fetal well-being, maternal wellness, partner illness, and parental mortality (Misri et al. 2015). Worry is typically accompanied by physical symptoms of GAD, such as fatigue, irritability, difficulty with concentration, and insomnia; however, these may be mistaken for normal physical symptoms of pregnancy and the postpartum period, making diagnosis challenging (Misri et al. 2015). The symptoms of pregnancy-specific anxiety tend to be focused on core themes of the pregnancy itself, including losing control in or not coping with the pain of labor, fear of the baby being harmed or dying, concerns about changes in physical appearance, and concerns about coping well as a parent (Huizink et al. 2004).

## Course and Prognosis

The severity of symptoms in perinatal anxiety can be variable, and its trajectory over time appears to be dynamic. For example, Matthey and Ross-Hamid (2012) noted a possible difference between transient and enduring perinatal distress; approximately 50% of the women in a cohort study who scored high on either the EPDS or the HADS anxiety subscale at their first prenatal appointment no longer scored "high" 2 weeks later; specific factors related to improvement were reduced morning sickness, reassuring tests from screening ultrasounds, reduced fear of miscarriage, and a reassuring outpatient visit (Matthey and Ross-Hamid 2012).

A recent latent trajectory analysis aimed to define groups in pregnancy through early postpartum (Ahmed et al. 2018). In this cohort, three trajectories were defined for perinatal anxiety: very low-stable (8.9%), low-stable (60.7%), and moderate-stable (30.4%). The risk factors associated with worsening anxiety were past depression, stress level, and income level. A recent large community cohort measured trajectories of perinatal anxiety; multiple distinct groups were noted, ranging from minimal to chronic (Bayrampour et al. 2016). Common risk factors for persistent elevated anxiety symptoms included a history of mental health conditions, a history of abuse/neglect, and low social support.

In addition, the trajectory of perinatal anxiety is interrelated with other factors, such as depression and stress. For example, a recent prospective cohort study noted that levels of depression, anxiety, and stress symptoms all changed over time, with the nadir of distress during the middle of pregnancy (Rallis et al. 2014b). In this study, higher anxiety symptoms early in pregnancy predicted higher anxiety levels throughout the rest of pregnancy; higher depression and stress scores in early and midpregnancy, respectively, predicted higher anxiety scores later in pregnancy (Rallis et al. 2014a).

Perinatal anxiety is associated with a broad range of adverse maternal–infant outcomes. Antenatal anxiety is associated with fewer prenatal visits (Murray et al. 2003), reduced pregnancy weight gain (Dayan et al. 2002), and delayed initiation—and earlier termination—of breastfeeding (Fallon et al. 2016a). Multiple studies have demonstrated an association between antenatal anxiety, particularly pregnancy-specific anxiety, and prematurity and low birth weight (Ding et al. 2014; Dole et al. 2003; Dunkel Schetter 2009; Ibanez et al. 2012; Kramer et al. 2009; Orr et al. 2007; Rose et al. 2016; Sanchez et al. 2013; Staneva et al. 2015). A systematic review and meta-analysis demonstrated additional adverse obstetrical outcomes, including infants who are small for gestational age and infants with reduced head circumference (Grigoriadis et al. 2018). Interestingly, such a robust association between depression and the breadth of these obstetrical outcomes has not been identified in similar meta-analyses, raising the question of whether antenatal anxiety may have a more significant impact on pregnancy outcomes than depression (Grigoriadis et al. 2013).

Comorbid perinatal anxiety and depression have a particularly strong negative impact on prognosis. Comorbid anxiety and depression are linked with more severe symptomatology and with poorer short-term and long-term outcomes, including an increased risk of suicide (Nepon et al. 2010). A recent prospective cohort study of perinatal women with comorbid MDD and GAD demonstrated more severe anxiety symptoms, lower quality of life, and slower symptom remission than perinatal patients with depression who did not have GAD (Misri and Swift 2015). Antenatal anxiety is a strong independent predictor of PPD (Austin et al. 2007; Coelho et al. 2011; Goodman et al. 2014a; Robertson et al. 2004; Sutter-Dallay et al. 2004; Verreault et al. 2014). In addition, there is evidence of a bidirectional relationship; for example, one study of more than 200 perinatal women noted that depressive symptoms earlier in pregnancy predicted higher levels of anxiety in late pregnancy and that anxiety in late pregnancy predicted higher depressive symptomatology in the early postpartum period (Skouteris et al. 2009). Alarmingly, antenatal anxiety in early pregnancy is also associated with suicide risk (Farias et al. 2013).

There is substantial evidence of the negative impact of perinatal stress, depression, and anxiety on fetal neurodevelopment (DiPietro et al. 2002; O'Donnell et al. 2009; Uguz et al. 2013). Proposed mechanisms include alterations in the maternal hypothalamic-pituitary-adrenal (HPA) axis, placental epigenetics, placental mitochondrial dysfunction, maternal immune system activation, and the maternal microbiome (see

Chapter 11, "Stress in Pregnancy"; Chapter 13, "Depressive Disorders"; and Chapter 18 for details of these mechanisms). For example, maternal GAD during pregnancy is associated with lower levels of fetal brain-derived neurotrophic factor in cord blood of newborns, suggesting a potential negative impact on the neurodevelopment of the fetus (Uguz et al. 2013). Perinatal anxiety and depressive disorders can result in infant neurobiological changes similar to chronic stress, such as HPA axis alterations and modifications in brain structures, such as the hippocampus and amygdala (Qiu et al. 2015; Rifkin-Graboi et al. 2015). However, it is uncommon for anxiety to be separated out from the other forms of distress in these studies, so the specific impact of anxiety on fetal and infant neurodevelopment remains unclear.

Perinatal anxiety has a significant and long-lasting adverse impact on children's cognition, social-emotional development, and mental health from infancy through adolescence (Glover 2014; Kingston et al. 2012; Stein et al. 2014; Van den Bergh and Marcoen 2004; Van den Bergh et al. 2005). It has been estimated that approximately 10%–15% of the attributable risk of child behavioral problems are related to antenatal anxiety and stress (Glover 2014). A prospective study in the United States noted that anxiety in pregnant women was associated with less robust maternal–infant bonding (Dubber et al. 2015); less responsive maternal–infant interactions (Stein et al. 2012); withdrawn behavior and blunted emotional tone in the infant (Stein et al. 2012); poor infant cognitive development (Keim et al. 2011); maternal reports of difficult infant temperament (Austin et al. 2005); and negative infant reactivity to novelty (Davis et al. 2004).

A recent large-scale prospective study of more than 1,300 mothers noted that perinatal anxiety—whether antenatal or postnatal—was associated with impaired child social-emotional development at the age of 2 years, even after adjusting for confounding variables (Polte et al. 2019). Children of women with perinatal anxiety have a significantly increased risk of cognitive issues, particularly attentional problems or ADHD, a risk seen independently of postnatal depression (Brouwers et al. 2001; O'Connor et al. 2002; Van Batenburg-Eddes et al. 2013). A recent cohort study of more than 3,500 mother–offspring pairs identified a maternal trajectory of severe depression, stress, and anxiety that later predicted internalizing behaviors in adolescent offspring, despite controlling for important confounding variables such as concurrent maternal depressive and anxious symptoms (Betts et al. 2015).

# Differential Diagnosis and Assessment

## Assessment

An anxiety disorder is a clinical diagnosis. In addition to the use of screening questionnaires, the clinical interview should touch on the cognitive, physical, behavioral, and affective symptoms of anxiety. A basic laboratory workup should include a complete blood count, blood chemistry, thyroid function tests, urinalysis, and urine drug screen (Cosci et al. 2015). If indicated, a more extensive workup may include electroencephalography, brain CT scan, evaluation for infection, or more extensive thyroid function tests (Cosci et al. 2015).

## Differential Diagnosis

Several conditions should be assessed for and ruled out during the evaluation of a patient with perinatal anxiety (Table 19–3). The first is normal worry. Pregnancy and be-

TABLE 19–3. **Differential diagnoses for anxiety disorders**

| | |
|---|---|
| Anemia | Preeclampsia |
| Cardiac dysrhythmia | PTSD |
| Major depressive disorder | Pulmonary embolism |
| OCD | Thyroid dysfunction |
| Postpartum psychosis | |

coming a parent are enormous transitions, and with them come a normal degree of coping with the uncertainties these transitions herald. This is a period of time to which women must adapt. During pregnancy, common topics of worry include body image, health of the baby, their relationship (if present), and logistical issues such as finances (Affonso et al. 1999). In the postpartum period, anxious thoughts often involve mothering skills and the transition to motherhood, breastfeeding, finances, change in partner relationship, physical appearance, and household duties (Wenzel and Stuart 2011).

Intrusive thoughts, particularly of harm coming to the baby, are common in the postpartum period and, although potentially highly distressing, may not be pathological. Thoughts of harm to baby that are ego-dystonic, fleeting, and do not interfere with daily functioning may exist in the context of the normal worrying of new parenthood and must be distinguished from more severe symptomatology that increases the risk of harm (discussed in Chapter 10, "A Treatment Approach to Psychiatric Emergencies in the Perinatal Period," and Chapter 20). It can be difficult to differentiate normal concerns from pathological worry, especially during the first trimester in primiparous women. Clinicians should be alert for the presence of an anxiety disorder if the worries have been present for an extended time, result in functional impairment, consume a lot of time, or have an irrational or intrusive quality (Misri et al. 2015).

Perinatal anxiety, specifically perinatal GAD, can be differentiated from OCD primarily by the nature of the anxious thoughts. OCD is characterized by unwanted, intrusive, repetitive thoughts (obsessions) and ritualistic behaviors (compulsions) (American Psychiatric Association 2013). With GAD, the anxious thoughts are worries about real-life routine matters, which are approached with apprehension and thought distortions (e.g., catastrophizing and generalizing); the content of these tends to shift over time. With OCD, thoughts are intrusive and unrelated to everyday concerns, mostly focused on disastrous outcomes such as harm coming to the infant, and obsessions tend to have stable content over time (Abramowitz et al. 2003). Of note, postpartum psychosis may also contain highly distressing thought content, such as harm coming to the infant; however, the thoughts are ego-syntonic (i.e., delusional) rather than ego-dystonic (i.e., recognized as irrational).

Perinatal anxiety disorders should also be differentiated from trauma-based disorders, such as PTSD. Core clinical features of PTSD include the presence of a trauma; reexperiencing (reliving the traumatic event); emotional numbing; avoidance of thoughts, places, or persons associated with the event; and hyperarousal (Vignato et al. 2017). Delineating anxiety from depression can be challenging in this context, given the extensive comorbidity, and anxious negative ruminations are commonly seen in perinatal depression (Collardeau et al. 2019). The presence of comorbid depression can be identified by the presence of signature depressive symptoms such as low mood, anhedonia, low energy and concentration, poor motivation, and potentially suicidal ideation (American Psychiatric Association 2013). Last, ruling out substance intoxication or withdrawal is also important; although many women reduce or stop substance use when a pregnancy is discovered, a significant number continue to use substances throughout pregnancy, leading to multiple negative maternal–infant outcomes (Ordean et al. 2017).

Many physiological symptoms of pregnancy can mimic anxiety, such as resting elevation of the heart rate. Medical conditions should be ruled out, especially those that are common or life-threatening in pregnancy or postpartum. These include thyroid dysfunction, anemia, and preeclampsia. Medical conditions that should be considered in the differential for new-onset panic attacks include some life-threatening medical disorders, such as pulmonary embolism, cardiac dysrhythmias, or asthma.

# Pathophysiology

Generally, clinically significant anxiety symptoms are thought to arise from a combination of an inherent biological vulnerability and an interaction with a stressful or traumatic environmental situation (Domhardt et al. 2019). Anxiety is not a unitary phenomenon, as evidenced by the multitude of DSM-5 anxiety disorders and the fact that anxiety can be a core feature of other syndromes and disorders, ranging from OCD to alcohol withdrawal to dementia (Robinson et al. 2019). In addition, *fear*—a rapid "flight or fight" behavioral response to an imminent threat—is thought to be distinct from *anxiety*—a lasting state of apprehension about a perceived future threat (Robinson et al. 2019). This suggests that, for example, the pathological fear in specific phobia and the diffuse worry of GAD may have at least somewhat distinct etiologies (Robinson et al. 2019).

In addition, a cogent, concise formulation of the etiology of perinatal anxiety does not yet exist; the pathophysiology of perinatal anxiety disorders is likely multidimensional, with biological, pregnancy-related, and psychosocial factors all implicated. Also, there is a complex relationship among anxiety and stress, mediated by alterations in the maternal HPA axis, epigenetics, mitochondrial dysfunction, and immune system activation (see Chapter 11 for details). A detailed understanding of the etiology of perinatal anxiety, both together with and separate from stress, is evolving. This section highlights several of the most well-described aspects of the pathophysiology of perinatal anxiety as a distinct entity.

## Biological Factors

Neuroanatomical structures that play a role in anxiety include the amygdala, which has efferent projections to the stria terminalis, hippocampus, ventral striatum, orbitofrontal cortex, periaqueductal gray, and hypothalamus (LeDoux 2000). In particular, the bed nucleus of the stria terminalis, an area referred to as the "extended amygdala," appears to regulate anxiety via its GABAergic projections to multiple limbic, hindbrain, and cortical structures (Davis 1998). Other areas thought to be important in the generation or regulation of anxiety include the medial prefrontal cortex and the hippocampus; connectivity between these areas may comprise an anxiety "network" that may be regulated by the dorsolateral prefrontal cortex (Robinson et al. 2019). Most anxiety symptoms are also mediated by the autonomic—particularly the sympathetic—nervous system, and the neurotransmitters thought to be most involved are norepinephrine, serotonin, dopamine, and GABA (Chand and Marwaha 2020).

Many anxiety disorders are at least in part heritable, with a moderate level of familial aggregation; heritability estimates are about 30%–50% (Hettema et al. 2005; Shimada-Sugimoto et al. 2015). Twin studies have noted that genetic architecture is shared among anxiety disorders—consistent with the high clinical comorbidity among them (Hettema et al. 2005). Overall, based on twin studies, both genetic and environmental factors are thought to contribute to anxiety disorder prevalence (Hettema et al. 2005). However, genome-wide association studies have not yet identified genes associated with the diagnosis, leaving open the possibility of a significant role for an environmental impact, potentially mediated through epigenetics (Bartlett et al. 2017).

There is a close—albeit not well understood—relationship between stress and mental health conditions, such as anxiety. For example, from a clinical perspective, a recent study noted that external stress—as measured by number of adverse childhood events—is associated with an increased risk of postpartum psychiatric illness (Meltzer-Brody et al. 2018). Animal models have suggested that early life stress is associated with anxiety behavior, brain volume, neuronal structure, and the plasticity of inhibitory networks (Castillo-Gómez et al. 2017). There has been intense interest in epigenetics to explain the relationship between stress and anxiety; for example, epigenetic control of the HPA axis in stress-responsive brain regions is thought to explain individual variations in anxious behavior (Bartlett et al. 2017). (See Chapters 11 and 18 for details of this relationship.)

Perinatal anxiety—along with perceived stress, regardless of diagnosis—is associated with changes in serum measures of inflammation (e.g., cytokine levels) and immune system function. For example, women with perinatal anxiety have been shown to have increased levels of interleukin (IL)-6, a proinflammatory cytokine (Furtado et al. 2019; Maes et al. 2000; Osborne et al. 2019b). Maes et al. (2000) further posited that the changes identified in immune activation related to the postpartum period, specifically in women with postpartum anxiety, might reflect a lowered anti-inflammatory capacity of the pregnant woman's immune system. A similar pattern (increased IL-6 and reduced levels of IL-10) is seen in pregnant women exposed to psychosocial stressors without perinatal depression or anxiety, suggesting that inflammatory cytokines are risk factors generally for unfavorable outcomes in late pregnancy (Coussons-Read et al. 2007). Additionally, specific changes in inflammatory cytokine profiles were seen in women with severe anxiety without depression as compared with women with comorbid anxiety and depression in late pregnancy, suggesting a specific correlation with anxiety (Leff Gelman et al. 2019).

The well-documented hormone changes in pregnancy (specifically, the rise of estrogen and progesterone during pregnancy and rapid decline within hours of delivery) can predispose some (but not all) pregnant women to the development of perinatal anxiety. Research has shown that levels of hormones measured at a given timepoint are no different between symptomatic women and asymptomatic women across the adult lifespan but that some women experience a differential sensitivity to the changes in hormones as they occur (Schmidt et al. 1998). Thus, it is possible that, in some women, perinatal anxiety is triggered by the hormonal events of pregnancy. For example, one study reported that maternal exposure to synthetic oxytocin conferred an increased risk for the development of perinatal anxiety or depression compared with pregnant women who had no oxytocin exposure (Kroll-Desrosiers et al. 2017). In addition, another study noted that second-trimester allopregnanolone levels predicted postpartum anxiety symptoms in both healthy women and women with mood/anxiety disorders (Osborne et al. 2019a).

There is greater understanding of the relationship between sleep disruption as a precipitant or exacerbating factor for perinatal anxiety disorders. Particularly in socially unfavorable environments, pregnant women lack adequate rest and sleep, which are critical for social functioning and mood. Although the data are still evolving, as expected, sleep deprivation, poor sleep quality, and insomnia confer risk for perinatal anxiety (Furtado et al. 2019; Menke et al. 2019; Osnes et al. 2019; Swanson et al. 2011). The presence of sleep difficulties may also predict a more severe result: a recent study noted that stress-related sleep reactivity—a predictor of insomnia—was associated not only with perinatal insomnia ($P=0.004$), perinatal anxiety ($P=0.30$), and depression ($P<0.001$) but also with suicidal ideation, as measured by a positive answer to item 10 on the EPDS: "The thought of harming myself has occurred to me" ($P=0.025$) (Palagini et al. 2019). See the "Insomnia" section later in this chapter for a detailed discussion of insomnia and its relationship to perinatal anxiety and mood disorders.

Other etiological factors related to perinatal anxiety are starting to be implicated in the pathogenesis of perinatal anxiety disorders, such as alterations in the gut-brain axis and microbiome, immune system deregulation, alterations in glucocorticoid signaling, and insulin resistance (Glendining et al. 2018; Rackers et al. 2018; Sasaki et al. 2013, 2014; Sullivan et al. 2014). However, much remains to be understood in terms of the relationship between these factors and anxiety in the perinatal period.

### Pregnancy-Related and Psychosocial Factors

It would seem intuitively clear that pregnancy complications, independent of previous outcomes, are also associated with the development of perinatal anxiety. Unexpected birth outcomes and previous traumatic events have been shown to contribute to the onset of subsequent perinatal anxiety (Shapiro et al. 2017). For example, women with threatened miscarriage have a greater prevalence of depressive and anxiety symptoms compared with women with physiologically stable pregnancies (Zhu et al. 2018). The Norwegian Mother and Child Cohort Study noted a high degree of anxiety and depressive symptoms in a subsequent pregnancy following a stillbirth, even if the subsequent pregnancy results in a healthy live birth (Gravensteen et al. 2018). Thus, women experiencing pregnancy complications should be appropriately monitored for the onset of anxiety in the perinatal period and referred for appropriate treatment if symptoms of perinatal anxiety are occurring in the context of a complicated pregnancy (Abrar et al. 2020; Fairbrother et al. 2017). (Please see Chapter 5, "Infertility and Perinatal Loss," and Chapter 18 for details.)

Components of the psychological transitions involved in becoming a parent and building a family also may lead to the development of perinatal anxiety. The period surrounding childbirth is one of profound change and is often experienced as stressful and overwhelming (Harrison et al. 2020). For example, a recent study with focus groups identified several key themes of anxiety related to motherhood, including unrealistic expectations of birth and motherhood, stigma, uncertainty, poor maternal confidence, and a lack of mental health support and knowledge. Overall, perinatal women commonly felt undersupported and poorly prepared for motherhood (Harrison et al. 2020). Partner conflict has also been identified as a contributing factor for perinatal anxiety (Bayrampour et al. 2018; Furtado et al. 2019; Hantsoo and Epperson 2017). For example, a recent systematic review and meta-analysis of 120 publications examined the relationship between partner support and perinatal depression and anxiety; emotional closeness and global support were found to be protective against perinatal anxiety (Pilkington et al. 2015). Consensus guidelines are starting to be developed for the facilitation of reciprocal partner support for couples, focusing on topics such as becoming a parent, support through pregnancy and childbirth, communication, and management of conflict (Pilkington et al. 2016).

Last, the process of pregnancy, giving birth, and becoming a parent is embedded within the societal context in which birth occurs, which can play a major role in the etiology of perinatal anxiety. Substantial data link anxiety, depressed mood, and poor sleep with chronic psychosocial stress both during pregnancy and over the course of a woman's lifetime. Commonly cited stressors worldwide include low material resources, poor employment or financial conditions, and heavy family and household responsibilities (Dunkel Schetter and Tanner 2012). Chronic psychosocial stress also includes being a member of a racial minority group that experiences discrimination and systemic racism (Christian 2020; Giscombé and Lobel 2005). Racism and discrimination contribute to negative birth outcomes independent of other types of stress (Dominguez et al. 2008), and several studies have linked these factors to adverse obstetrical outcomes, such as low birth weight (Love et al. 2010). A large population-based study in the United Kingdom concluded that the risk of perinatal anxiety, depression, and serious mental illness was higher in socioeconomically deprived groups and increased with increased maternal age (Ban et al. 2012).

## Treatment

A comprehensive algorithm for a treatment approach to perinatal anxiety does not yet exist. Generally, the approach for perinatal anxiety disorders, such as perinatal GAD, is similar to that for GAD in the general adult population. For mild GAD, nonmedication strategies such as cognitive-behavioral therapy (CBT) are effective; for moderate to severe anxiety, pharmacotherapy is indicated, typically in combination with psychotherapy (Misri et al. 2015). Generally, selective serotonin reuptake inhibitors (SSRIs) and serotonin-norepinephrine reuptake inhibitors (SNRIs) are the first-line agents for addressing perinatal anxiety, and benzodiazepines are effective for short-term use for acute anxiety symptoms; although data on atypical antipsychotics for anxiety are limited, use of these agents may be appropriate for severe manifestations if antidepressants or benzodiazepines have been insufficient to address symptoms (Misri et al. 2015).

As explained in Chapter 8, "A Clinical Approach to Psychiatric Diagnosis and Treatment During Pregnancy," the risk-risk analysis of medications in pregnancy and postpartum is complicated by the limitations of the data, because no gold-standard randomized controlled trials of medications in pregnancy or breastfeeding are available. Instead, data rely on observational studies, which are subject to significant bias and confounding (Howland 2013). In addition, the risks of exposure to a medication in pregnancy and postpartum must be weighed against the known risks of untreated perinatal anxiety.

### Psychopharmacology

SSRIs and SNRIs are the mainstay of pharmacological treatment of anxiety disorders, including during the perinatal period. Overall, SSRIs are the most frequently used class of antidepressant in both the general adult population and in pregnancy (Alwan et al. 2007). If an SSRI/SNRI is going to be started for the first time, it is prudent to select a medication with proven efficacy for perinatal anxiety, a short half-life, low accumulation in breastmilk, and a track record of safety in pregnancy (Misri et al. 2015). SSRIs are extensively discussed in Chapter 13; please see that chapter for details about this medication class in pregnancy and lactation.

Benzodiazepines, a class of antianxiety medications that includes clonazepam, lorazepam, and alprazolam, can be useful in the short-term as either anxiolytics or hypnotics. Benzodiazepines are agonists at the GABA receptor, with inhibitory postsynaptic signaling (D'Hulst et al. 2009). They are commonly prescribed in pregnancy, estimated at 1%–4% of prescriptions, with the highest rate of prescribing in the third trimester (Bais et al. 2020; Hanley and Mintzes 2014; Lacroix et al. 2009; Riska et al. 2014). Lorazepam is the most commonly prescribed benzodiazepine in pregnancy (Bais et al. 2020). Both benzodiazepines and hypnotics cross the placenta, are present in the amniotic fluid, and cross the fetal blood-brain barrier (McElhatton 1994; Vigod and Dennis 2019).

There has been lengthy debate in the literature regarding the reproductive safety of benzodiazepines, especially the risk of congenital malformations. Early studies had suggested an association between benzodiazepines and cleft lip or palate (Dolovich et al. 1998); however, recent data have been reassuring (Ban et al. 2014; Bellantuono et al. 2013; Wikner et al. 2007). A multisite, population-based case-control study raised concerns about malformations associated with benzodiazepine use in pregnancy (e.g., Dandy-Walker malformation, esophageal atresia), although study sizes were small and confidence intervals were wide, emphasizing the need for further data to confirm these results (Tinker et al. 2019). Notably, in this cohort, neither cleft lip/palate nor cardiac malformations were found to be associated with exposure (Tinker et al. 2019).

A large population-based cohort study in the United Kingdom demonstrated no increase in the overall risk of malformations among offspring exposed to diazepam during pregnancy (Ban et al. 2014). However, a study using population-based health data noted that the use of SSRIs and a benzodiazepine in combination was associated with an increase in relative risk of congenital heart defects, even after controlling for confounding variables (Oberlander et al. 2008). A systematic review and meta-analysis appeared to confirm these findings: prenatal benzodiazepine use alone was not associated with an increased risk of congenital malformations with first-trimester exposure, but concurrent use of benzodiazepines and an antidepressant in pregnancy was associated with an increased risk of malformations (Grigoriadis et al. 2019).

Several studies have suggested an association between benzodiazepine use and adverse outcomes early in pregnancy, such as miscarriage (Ban et al. 2012; Sheehy et al. 2019). For example, a nested case-control study that included more than 400,000 pregnancies noted a statistically significant association between the miscarriage rate and benzodiazepine use in the first trimester (Sheehy et al. 2019). However, in this study, the miscarriage rate remained below the baseline rate of 15%–20% of identified pregnancies, and the study could not control for numerous confounding variables, such as the severity of the anxiety, whether the patient actually took the medication, or whether the patient abruptly discontinued the medication when the pregnancy was identified (Sheehy et al. 2019). In addition, a recent cohort study of more than 1.6 million women noted an association between benzodiazepine exposure prior to conception and an increased risk of ectopic pregnancy (Wall-Wieler et al. 2020).

Some concern has been raised that daily or frequent benzodiazepine use in late pregnancy may be associated with symptoms of neonatal intoxication, including respiratory distress or poor tone (Freeman et al. 2018; Iqbal et al. 2002), or with neonatal withdrawal symptoms (Iqbal et al. 2002). In a recent prospective cohort study of almost 800 women, these outcomes were not noted; however, infants did have a higher risk of small head circumference and greater risk of admission to the neonatal intensive care unit (Freeman et al. 2018). A systematic review and meta-analysis focusing on benzodiazepine use and delivery outcomes also noted the increased risk of several adverse outcomes, of which neonatal intensive care admission was the most clinically relevant (Grigoriadis et al. 2020).

There is reassuring information regarding benzodiazepines in breastfeeding. A recent prospectively recruited, retrospectively assessed cohort study at the Motherisk program analyzed data from 124 infants (mean age 11 months) who were exposed to benzodiazepines through breastmilk (Kelly et al. 2012). The most commonly used benzodiazepines were lorazepam (52%), clonazepam (18%), and midazolam (15%). About half of the women ($n=60$) were also taking other medications, typically antidepressants and opioids. Adverse events, including infant sedation, were rare, observed in 2 of the 124 exposed infants (1.6%), and the mothers of both of these infants were taking more than one medication at the time (Kelly et al. 2012). However, avoiding long-acting benzodiazepines, such as diazepam, is recommended given their multiple active metabolites and thus extended presence in breastmilk (Levine et al. 2003).

The impact of benzodiazepines on long-term neurodevelopmental outcomes appears relatively reassuring. For example, a recent large study examined the neurodevelopmental outcomes of the offspring of approximately 40,000 pregnancies up to the age of 5 years (Lupattelli et al. 2019). No difference was found in the main outcomes between the children who were exposed to benzodiazepines and those who were not. There were small but statistically significant differences in subgroups of offspring of women with depression and anxiety (approximately 11% of the cohort) that had late exposure to benzodiazepines or hypnotics. Within these subgroups, exposure to these medications was associated with gross motor deficits in boys only and with communication deficits in children of both sexes (Lupattelli et al. 2019). Of course, even with such a large study, confounding variables (e.g., confounding by indication) remain a concern for these data.

Overall, clinicians should carefully consider whether a benzodiazepine is an optimal choice for a woman's symptoms during the perinatal period because benzodiazepines have several disadvantages. They are not the first-line treatment for anxiety disorders and are meant for short-term use while awaiting the full effect of an evidence-based, first-line treatment such as SSRIs or CBT (Vigod and Dennis 2019). Second, benzodiazepines should be avoided in women with a history of substance abuse given the potential for misuse (Baldwin et al. 2011; see Chapter 21, "Substance Use Disorders"). Third, benzodiazepines have the potential for significant morbidity in addition to any perinatal effects, such as falls and cognitive impairment, especially when administered long-term (Brandt and Leong 2017).

If benzodiazepines are to be prescribed during pregnancy, clinicians should aim to prescribe them sparingly and temporarily, using shorter-acting agents such as lorazepam whenever possible. Women who take benzodiazepines chronically should be counseled regarding the potential risks and benefits of these medications in pregnancy.

Time is of the essence, because abrupt cessation of chronic benzodiazepine use is not recommended due to the risks of withdrawal. Thus, if discontinuation is thought to be appropriate, a gradual taper over a period of months is recommended.

### Other Pharmacological Treatment

Other options include buspirone, antihistamines such as hydroxyzine or diphenhydramine, sedating second-generation antipsychotics such as quetiapine, and sedating antidepressants such as trazodone (Thorsness et al. 2018). Although minimizing polypharmacy is optimal, some women may benefit from the short-term use of additional medications for anxiety or sleep in conjunction with or in place of SSRI or SNRI medications. These are each discussed separately.

Human reproductive safety data regarding buspirone are scarce, although available animal data do not suggest increased risk for malformations (Armstrong 2008). Given this lack of reproductive safety data, other agents may be preferred. Sedating antihistamines, such as diphenhydramine, hydroxyzine, and doxylamine, are commonly used during pregnancy for anxiety and sleep, as well as for pruritis, nausea and vomiting, and allergic symptoms. Reproductive safety data are limited on these agents despite their widespread use; however, they do not appear to be associated with congenital malformations (Li et al. 2013). Second-generation antipsychotic medications, such as quetiapine, may be used at times for anxiety or insomnia; the reproductive safety of these medications is addressed in Chapter 17, "Schizophrenia and Related Disorders." Sedating antidepressants, such as trazodone, are commonly used off-label for insomnia at dosages of 50–200 mg. Reproductive safety data are limited but overall reassuring and do not suggest increased risk of congenital malformations (Einarson et al. 2003, 2009).

## Behavioral and Somatic Treatments

Data regarding specific psychotherapies for perinatal anxiety are evolving. For example, a systematic review of 78 studies of depression, anxiety, and trauma-related disorders noted that although evidence of benefit of both CBT and interpersonal therapy (IPT) for perinatal depression is strong, the evidence for psychotherapy for perinatal anxiety is still quite limited (Nillni et al. 2018). However, several forms of psychotherapy have been studied specifically for anxiety in the perinatal population. Several studies, including a preliminary meta-analysis, have shown benefit of CBT for perinatal anxiety (Green et al. 2015; Maguire et al. 2018). In addition, mindfulness-based CBT has been shown in several studies to have efficacy in reducing pregnancy-related anxiety symptoms and improving the use of adaptive coping strategies and psychological well-being (Goodman et al. 2014b; Zemestani and Fazeli Nikoo 2020). IPT is a time-limited, manualized psychotherapy that focuses on addressing current interpersonal issues related to universal experiences of losses, changes, or conflicts (Stuart 2012). Substantial evidence supports its use in both the prevention and treatment of perinatal depression, and a meta-analysis also supported the use of IPT for the treatment of perinatal anxiety (Sockol 2018). Other psychotherapies currently being studied for their efficacy in perinatal anxiety include acceptance and commitment therapy, which emphasizes mindfulness, acceptance, and recognition of internal values (Bonacquisti et al. 2017). Mobile- and internet-based interventions are also showing some promise in this population, although data are still early and limited (Hussain-Shamsy et al. 2020; Loughnan et al. 2019). Exercise, mindfulness practice, yoga, and other complementary treatments are being evaluated for their efficacy; see Chapter 14, "Integrative Approaches to Perinatal Depression," for details.

# Insomnia

Ms. FF is a 34-year-old woman, gravida 1 para 0, who is currently 36 weeks pregnant. She presents to her reproductive psychiatrist for a routine follow-up visit. She has a history of GAD that, in the past, prior to conception, was well controlled with oral escitalopram 10 mg/day. Prior to conception, she tapered down and off of the escitalopram and initiated CBT to good effect. However, she reports that in the past couple of weeks she has been having a hard time with her sleep. She reports that "no matter what I do, it is impossible to find a comfortable position," and this keeps her awake. Ms. FF also reports that even when she falls asleep, she has to get up several times during the night to go to the bathroom, feeling like "having to go to the bathroom all the time makes it impossible to sleep." She denies snoring or apneic events and states that her wife has not reported anything unusual in her sleep. She feels tired during the day, but because it is so difficult to find a good position, it is hard to take a nap. She asks about whether any medication can help with insomnia and wonders if her sleep difficulties mean that her anxiety is returning.

## Epidemiology

### Rates/Incidence

Insomnia is a major public health problem that affects millions of individuals yearly. Insomnia affects between 10% and 30% of the general adult population (Roth 2007). A recent analysis demonstrated that 50%–80% of patients with a psychiatric diagnosis had difficulty falling or staying asleep in a given year (Smith et al. 2002). Sleep difficulties have been associated with numerous categories of mental health conditions, including MDD, bipolar disorder, anxiety disorders, substance use disorders, PTSD, and primary psychotic disorders (e.g., schizophrenia) (Seow et al. 2016). Overall, insomnia is more common in women than men (Hilty et al. 2009). Women are particularly vulnerable to insomnia during times of reproductive hormonal transitions, such as during pregnancy and perimenopause or menopause (Chaudhry and Susser 2018; Nowakowski and Meers 2019). Questionnaire-based estimates of insomnia in pregnancy range from 30% to 60% (Baker et al. 2009; Bei et al. 2012; Facco et al. 2010; Román-Gálvez et al. 2018). The third trimester in particular tends to be the time of the most marked sleep disturbance, with approximately 60% of women experiencing significant difficulties initiating and maintaining sleep (Sivertsen et al. 2015). Additionally, 25% of perimenopausal women and 30% of postmenopausal women reported getting a good night's sleep only a few nights per month or less (Baker et al. 2009).

### Risk Factors

Risk factors include increasing age, female sex, and comorbid medical conditions (Riemann et al. 2017). In terms of perinatal insomnia, a recent prospective cohort study of nearly 500 pregnant women identified several risk factors for insomnia in pregnancy, including pregestational insomnia, high BMI, and less frequent daily exercise (Román-Gálvez et al. 2018).

## Screening

To our knowledge, screening for insomnia in the general or perinatal population is not common practice. However, several scales have been validated for the clinical assessment of insomnia and are in widespread use. A sleep diary can provide a subjective assessment of bedtime, nighttime awakening, awake time, and sleep quality (Roth 2007). The Pittsburgh Sleep Quality Index (Buysse et al. 1989), although primarily used for research purposes, is a seven-item self-report measure of quality and patterns of sleep that has been validated in pregnant women (Skouteris et al. 2009). The Insomnia Symptoms Questionnaire is a 13-item self-report questionnaire that was validated in more than 100 women at 12 weeks' gestation (Okun et al. 2015).

# Diagnostic Criteria

The diagnostic criteria for insomnia recently underwent major revision with the introduction of DSM-5. In prior editions of DSM, insomnia was characterized as primary or secondary to a mental health condition. However, given the complexity of the relationship, the potential for a bidirectional etiology, and the difficulty in establishing a clear cause and effect pattern, the primary/secondary nomenclature was removed in DSM-5, which recommends that "insomnia disorder" be coded whenever diagnostic criteria for it are met, regardless of a coexisting psychiatric disorder. The diagnostic criteria for insomnia disorder are summarized in Box 19–1.

### Box 19–1. DSM-5 Criteria for Insomnia Disorder

A. A predominant complaint of dissatisfaction with sleep quantity or quality, associated with one (or more) of the following symptoms:
   1. Difficulty initiating sleep. (In children, this may manifest as difficulty initiating sleep without caregiver intervention.)
   2. Difficulty maintaining sleep, characterized by frequent awakenings or problems returning to sleep after awakenings. (In children, this may manifest as difficulty returning to sleep without caregiver intervention.)
   3. Early-morning awakening with inability to return to sleep.

B. The sleep disturbance causes clinically significant distress or impairment in social, occupational, educational, academic, behavioral, or other important areas of functioning.

C. The sleep difficulty occurs at least 3 nights per week.

D. The sleep difficulty is present for at least 3 months.

E. The sleep difficulty occurs despite adequate opportunity for sleep.

F. The insomnia is not better explained by and does not occur exclusively during the course of another sleep-wake disorder (e.g., narcolepsy, a breathing-related sleep disorder, a circadian rhythm sleep-wake disorder, a parasomnia).

G. The insomnia is not attributable to the physiological effects of a substance (e.g., a drug of abuse, a medication).

H. Coexisting mental disorders and medical conditions do not adequately explain the predominant complaint of insomnia.

*Specify* if:

**With non–sleep disorder mental comorbidity,** including substance use disorders
**With other medical comorbidity**
**With other sleep disorder**

**Coding note:** The code 307.42 (F51.01) applies to all three specifiers. Code also the relevant associated mental disorder, medical condition, or other sleep disorder immediately after the code for insomnia disorder in order to indicate the association.

*Specify* if:

**Episodic:** Symptoms last at least 1 month but less than 3 months.

**Persistent:** Symptoms last 3 months or longer.

**Recurrent:** Two (or more) episodes within the space of 1 year.

**Note:** Acute and short-term insomnia (i.e., symptoms lasting less than 3 months but otherwise meeting all criteria with regard to frequency, intensity, distress, and/or impairment) should be coded as an other specified insomnia disorder.

*Source.* Reprinted from American Psychiatric Association: *Diagnostic and Statistical Manual of Mental Disorders,* 5th Edition. Arlington, VA, 2013, pp. 362–363. Copyright © 2013 American Psychiatric Association. Used with permission.

# Clinical Features

## Clinical Presentation

Anyone who has experienced insomnia will immediately recognize the frustrating constellation of symptoms: inability to fall or stay asleep, a subjective sense of poor sleep quality or nonrestorative sleep, daytime sleepiness or functional impairment, and regular or sustained occurrence despite adequate opportunities for sleep (Roth 2007; Schutte-Rodin et al. 2008).

## Course and Prognosis

Insomnia can have profound consequences for physical health, mental health, and quality of life. In the general adult population, chronic insomnia is associated with an increased risk of cardiovascular disease (e.g., hypertension, myocardial infarction), metabolic disorders (e.g., obesity, diabetes mellitus), and all-cause mortality (Ferraro et al. 2014; LeBlanc et al. 2009; Taylor et al. 2003). It is not surprising that sleep disturbance, given its extensive comorbidity and association with psychiatric diagnoses, also affects the severity of mental health conditions. For example, sleep disturbance—independent of the psychiatric syndrome itself—is associated with a negative impact on the course of the mental health condition, including more severe symptoms, higher disorder severity, lower level of functioning, lower quality of life, and less robust response to psychiatric treatment (Kallestad et al. 2012). Quality of life consequences include risk of accidents, decreased work productivity and concentration, increased absenteeism, and impaired daily performance (Roth 2007; Walsh 2004).

Perinatal insomnia is associated with increased rates of gestational diabetes (Facco et al. 2017), higher rates of prolonged labor and operative delivery (Lee and Gay 2004), and preterm birth (Felder et al. 2017; Okun et al. 2011) and has also been linked with near-miss motor vehicle accidents among new parents (Malish et al. 2016). Perinatal sleep disturbances are also associated with perinatal depression and anxiety (Swanson et al. 2011; Wilson et al. 2019), mood changes immediately after birth (Bei et al. 2010), and postpartum psychosis (Sharma and Mazmanian 2003).

## Differential Diagnosis and Assessment

Insomnia is a clinical diagnosis. The assessment of insomnia should include a clinical interview with detailed sleep history, review of sleep questionnaires and any available sleep diaries, review of physical and mental health history, and a physical examination (Riemann et al. 2017). Additional measures such as blood tests, electroencephalography, or electrocardiography should be done as indicated, and polysomnography should be done if another sleep disorder, such as a sleep-related breathing disorder, is suspected (Riemann et al. 2017). In most cases, changes in sleep during pregnancy are physiologically normal, and excessive daytime sleepiness is the predictable result. However, a careful assessment is necessary because insomnia can be a physiologically normal part of pregnancy, a medical complication of pregnancy (e.g., sleep-disordered breathing), a symptom of a mental health condition (e.g., anxiety), a trigger of a mental health condition, or a combination of these (Table 19–4).

Both mood and anxiety disorders can present with sleep disturbances and insomnia and should be carefully evaluated. Mood disorders such as MDD and bipolar disorder can both present with profound disruptions in sleep. In addition, anxiety disorders such as GAD, panic disorder, OCD, and PTSD can all present with perinatal insomnia. At the same time, sleep deprivation can be a profound *trigger* of psychiatric conditions, such as with mood disorders. Substance intoxication or withdrawal can also present with sleep disruption.

Medical diagnoses specific to pregnancy and the postpartum period should be ruled out. Pregnancy may predispose women to sleep-disordered breathing, which is characterized by snoring, gasping, and apneas. Obstructive sleep apnea-hypopnea due to obstruction of airflow in the upper airway is more common in pregnant women than in nonpregnant women, with a prevalence of roughly 10%–25% (Nodine and Matthews 2013). Distinct physiological and hormonal changes in pregnancy, such as weight gain, edema of mucus membranes (from elevated levels of estrogen), and displacement of the diaphragm from an enlarging uterus, can all contribute to breathing-related sleep disorders (Hashmi et al. 2016). Significant predictors of sleep-disordered breathing in pregnancy are age, BMI, and frequent snoring; patients with these risk factors may represent a subpopulation in need of further evaluation (Louis et al. 2018).

Another important diagnosis is restless legs syndrome, which has an increased incidence in pregnancy (estimated to be up to 30%), with symptom severity highest in the third trimester (Manconi et al. 2004). To the relief of sufferers, symptoms typically remit after delivery. Restless legs syndrome can be associated with pregnancy-related iron deficiency, which can be detected by a ferritin level to assess iron stores. Untreated restless legs syndrome increases the risk of depressed mood, and related sleep deprivation is linked with prolonged labor, increased pain perception, higher discomfort during labor, and increased rates of operative delivery (Chang et al. 2010).

## Pathophysiology

To consider the pathophysiology of insomnia, it is helpful to review basic mechanisms of sleep itself. Normal sleep consists of two fundamental neuronal mechanisms. The homeostatic mechanism of sleep induces a pressure to sleep after every hour awake, and the circadian rhythm mechanism drives alertness during the day and sleepiness at night, based on light intensity as the main external "timekeeper" (Anderson 2018).

TABLE 19–4. **Differential diagnoses for insomnia**

| | |
|---|---|
| Generalized anxiety disorder | PTSD |
| Hyperthyroidism | Restless legs syndrome |
| Major depressive disorder | Sleep-related breathing disorders |
| Obstructive sleep apnea-hypopnea | Substance use disorders |
| OCD | |

Both total sleep time and circadian rhythms are subject to significant variations over the course of our lives, including greater fragmentation over time—one of the reasons the prevalence of insomnia tends to increase with age (Ohayon et al. 2004). Short-term insomnia generally arises in association with acute psychosocial stressors, and the sleep disruption tends to resolve when the stressor resolves (Ellis et al. 2012). However, the development of chronic insomnia requires not just the acute stressor but also maladaptive behaviors that can worsen sleep quality and disrupt the homeostatic and circadian rhythm drivers for sleep (Anderson 2018). Paradoxically, some of the most common exacerbating factors are hypervigilant efforts around sleep (e.g., increased attention to and ruminations about sleep), which can lead to hyperarousal, which is a physiological stress response, and to worsened insomnia (Espie et al. 2006).

The relationship between sleep difficulties and mental health conditions overall is complex and may be bidirectional (Krystal 2012). For example, at least 40% of patients with insomnia will eventually be diagnosed with an anxiety disorder, and persistent insomnia is one of the strongest risk factors for depression in the adult population (Anderson 2018; Baglioni et al. 2011). A recent review suggested that sleep disturbance may be a potentially transdiagnostic mechanism across psychiatric diagnoses, and that sleep disturbance and emotion regulation may be neurobiologically linked (Harvey et al. 2011). Emerging evidence implicates autonomic hyperarousal as a pathway to increasing the risk of depression (Fernandez-Mendoza and Vgontzas 2013).

The etiology of perinatal sleep disturbance is also multifactorial. Many dynamic aspects of pregnancy, such as changes in hormone levels, physiology, metabolism, and psychology, likely contribute to sleep disturbances, particularly as pregnancy progresses (Bei et al. 2015; Hashmi et al. 2016). There is also evidence of extensive comorbidity between mental health conditions and insomnia in pregnancy, including anxiety and depressive symptoms; insomnia in pregnancy can be either a sign of a mental health condition, a trigger for one, or both (Chaudhry and Susser 2018; Swanson et al. 2011; Wołynczyk-Gmaj et al. 2017). In the first trimester, sleep changes are most likely related to rapid escalations in reproductive hormone levels, particularly progesterone, which can lead to daytime sleepiness and sleep interruptions at night (Hashmi et al. 2016). Progesterone and its metabolites interact with the $GABA_A$ receptors, which is thought to effect these changes in sleep (Lancel et al. 1996). Sleep in the first trimester is also affected by overall fatigue and the nausea and vomiting familiar to many women who have traversed the first trimester of pregnancy (Lee et al. 2000). By the second trimester, the total amount of sleep time is reduced and subjective reports of interrupted sleep increase, in part due to factors such as nocturnal gastroesophageal reflux (Driver and Shapiro 1992). By the third trimester, <2% of pregnant women report no nocturnal awakenings (Hedman et al. 2002). Common contributing factors include overall discomfort (e.g., backache), frequent trips to the bathroom, fetal movements, reflux, and leg discomfort (Hashmi et al. 2016). In the postpartum period, sleep deprivation is highly prevalent due to nighttime infant feeding and the frequent nocturnal awakenings of the infant (Bei et al. 2015; Hysing et al. 2014).

## Treatment

As with many aspects of perinatal insomnia, the optimal approach to treatment is evolving. This section focuses primarily on CBT for insomnia (CBT-I) and pharmacotherapy for insomnia in pregnancy and postpartum, although other methods are currently under active investigation.

### Cognitive-Behavioral Therapy for Insomnia

In the general adult population, high-quality evidence supports the use of behavioral interventions such as CBT-I as the first-line treatment of insomnia (Benz et al. 2020; Morin et al. 2009; Schutte-Rodin et al. 2008; Trauer et al. 2015). National and international clinical practice guidelines and national organizations have recommended CBT-I as the first-line treatment for insomnia in adults (Baker et al. 2014; National Institutes of Health 2005; Qaseem et al. 2016; Riemann et al. 2017). A recent systematic review found that CBT-I was effective for adults with comorbid psychiatric illnesses, including patients with depression, anxiety, PTSD, and substance abuse disorders (Taylor and Pruiksma 2014). CBT-I is usually delivered over six weekly sessions, typically requiring 4–8 hours of therapy along with weekly sleep diaries to track progress (Anderson 2018).

In addition, evidence supports CBT-I specifically for perinatal insomnia (Bei et al. 2019; Lee et al. 2016; Tomfohr-Madsen et al. 2017). A recent randomized controlled clinical trial revealed greater reduction in insomnia severity and a greater and more rapid insomnia remission (Manber et al. 2019). There was also an improvement in self-reported sleep time above and beyond what was noted with objective measures of sleep; the authors hypothesized that CBT-I may help women feel less distressed about sleep difficulties, including those caused by increased pregnancy-related physical discomfort (Manber et al. 2019). This is important, because self-reported sleep has been shown to be a stronger predictor of maternal mental health than objective measures of sleep itself (Bei et al. 2010). CBT-I is also preferred by pregnant patients, as compared with pharmacotherapy and acupuncture (Sedov et al. 2017). A summary of the steps involved in CBT-I and suggested modifications in pregnancy is provided in Table 19–5.

### Psychopharmacology

**Hypnotic benzodiazepine receptor agonists.** Short-term—fewer than 4 weeks—use of hypnotic benzodiazepine receptor agonists (HBRAs), such as zolpidem, zaleplon, and eszopiclone, is recommended for treatment in the general adult population if CBT-I is not sufficiently effective or is not available (Riemann et al. 2017). However, little is known about the reproductive safety of HBRAs. HBRAs do cross the placenta (Askew 2007; Juric et al. 2009), but little is known about their effects. Data from several small studies suggest that zolpidem does not appear to be associated with an increased risk of congenital malformations (Wikner and Källén 2011; Wikner et al. 2007; Wilton et al. 1998). Several small studies have noted an association between zolpidem use and adverse obstetrical outcomes, such as preterm birth, low birth weight, small for gesta-

TABLE 19–5. **Elements of cognitive-behavioral therapy for insomnia, modified for pregnancy**

| Approach | Focus |
|---|---|
| Cognitive therapy | Address cognitive distortions around sleep |
| | Reduce excessive worry |
| Psychoeducation about sleep in pregnancy | Description of normal sleep/wake cycle |
| | Healthy sleep habits |
| | Infant sleep development |
| | Postpartum sleep recommendations |
| Relaxation training | Progressive muscle relaxation and guided imagery |
| Sleep restriction therapy | Restrict time in bed to achieve high sleep efficiency, modified for pregnancy |
| Stimulus control therapy | Reduce association between bed and insomnia |
| | Strengthen association between bed and sleep |

tional age infant, and operative delivery; however, important confounding variables such as depressive or anxiety symptoms in pregnancy or smoking status may have influenced these outcomes (Wang et al. 2010; Wikner et al. 2007). Of note, HBRAs do have abuse potential, and teratogenic effects have been seen with supratherapeutic doses. For example, a case report made note of a pregnancy complicated by neural tube defects in a patient who was abusing high-dose zolpidem in the first trimester of pregnancy (Sharma et al. 2011). Data regarding HBRAs in lactation are reassuring, albeit scarce. For example, zolpidem has very low rates of transmission into the breastmilk, approximately 0.004%–0.0019% of the maternal dose; the drug was undetectable in the breastmilk 13 hours and 16 hours after the dose (Pons et al. 1989).

Of note, there are sex differences in the use of HBRAs based on variable pharmacokinetics. In 2013, the FDA required the manufacturers of zolpidem to lower the recommended dosage for women from 10 mg to 5 mg (and from 12.5 mg to 6.25 mg for extended release) due to a concern for motor vehicle accidents, excessive daytime sedation, and next-morning functional impairment; women appear to be at higher risk of these adverse effects due to slower rates of elimination of zolpidem as compared with men (Nowakowski and Meers 2019). This is the first and only drug in the United States to have different recommended dosages for women versus men (Greenblatt et al. 2014; Nowakowski and Meers 2019).

Given the limited information for HBRAs, women who require pharmacological intervention for severe sleep disturbance in pregnancy may wish to consider other options. If a sedative-hypnotic is required for sleep during pregnancy, a benzodiazepine may be preferred over an HBRA, especially if anxiety is associated with the sleep disruption. Both trazodone and sedating antihistamines, as discussed earlier (see "Anxiety Disorders in the Perinatal Period"), are options for insomnia as well. Another medication class to consider is sedating tricyclic antidepressants, such as amitriptyline or nortriptyline, especially if depressive symptoms are contributing to the sleep disturbance. Although commonly used for insomnia outside of pregnancy, melatonin is not generally recommended in the perinatal period given the dearth of information about its reproductive safety (Chaudhry and Susser 2018). Tricyclic antidepressants have some advantages in pregnancy despite their significant side effect burden (e.g., orthostasis) and greater risk in overdose (Osborne et al. 2014; Wisner et al. 2009). Multiple studies have been reassuring in terms of lack of evidence of adverse outcomes such as teratogenicity (Wisner et al. 2006), preterm birth or low birth weight (Pearson et al. 2007), persistent pulmonary hypertension of the newborn (Chambers et al. 2006), and long-term developmental outcomes (Nulman et al. 2002). Due to reports of neonatal toxicity, the least cholinergic medications in this class are preferred in pregnancy, such as nortriptyline and desipramine (Suri and Altshuler 2009).

**Management Steps.** Postpartum women prescribed sleep aids should be counseled to have another adult available to care for their infants overnight due to the potential for difficulty waking after taking sedating medication and so that they are able to obtain uninterrupted sleep. Women taking sedating medications should also receive specific counseling regarding safe sleep practices with their infants (Task Force on Sudden Infant Death Syndrome 2016).

## Conclusion

Perinatal anxiety represents a paradox in perinatal mental health. On the one hand, perinatal anxiety disorders are extremely common, affecting more than 20% of all pregnancies—a prevalence higher than that for anxiety in the general population and also higher than for perinatal depression (Dennis et al. 2017; Matthey et al. 2003); moreover, a much larger group of women may have subthreshold symptoms. In addition, perinatal anxiety is associated with known adverse maternal–infant outcomes that are comparable with and perhaps even exceed the impact of perinatal depression (Grigoriadis et al. 2013). On the other hand, perinatal anxiety remains underdiagnosed and undertreated (Misri et al. 2015), and our understanding of its etiology, identification, and optimal treatment is still evolving (Fallon et al. 2016b; Goodman et al. 2014a; Harrison et al. 2020). Research that separates anxiety from depression or distress is minimal.

Perinatal insomnia presents a similar paradox. Insomnia is so common as to be nearly ubiquitous, and sleep disturbance is often considered simply a result of pregnancy itself. However, perinatal insomnia has a significant impact as well, including adverse outcomes such as preterm birth (Felder et al. 2017). It can also be both a trigger for and a symptom of mental health conditions such as depression and anxiety. Therefore, insomnia also represents an important but little-understood area to address for clinicians who treat women in the perinatal period.

There are many unanswered questions and thus future directions for research in perinatal anxiety and insomnia. Basic questions remain, such as the best operative definition for perinatal anxiety, which screening tool best captures this population, understanding the comorbidity between anxiety and depression, and developing optimal treatment for perinatal anxiety specifically. A greater understanding of the physiology of sleep in pregnancy and the nature of sleep disturbances and insomnia will also be of benefit, given both their high prevalence and their clear impact on maternal and infant outcomes (Grigoriadis et al. 2018).

# Key Points

- Anxiety is one of the most common perinatal mental health symptoms.
- Perinatal anxiety is associated with numerous adverse outcomes such as prematurity, low birth weight, and decreased head circumference.
- Perinatal anxiety is an independent risk factor for postpartum depression.
- Anxiety disorders in pregnancy are treatable; psychopharmacology and psychotherapy are both effective.
- Benzodiazepines should be used with caution in pregnancy and postpartum.
- Insomnia in pregnancy is common and should be differentiated from a formal anxiety disorder; the two may co-occur.
- Insomnia is also independently related to adverse outcomes in pregnancy.
- Cognitive-behavioral therapy for insomnia is an effective first-line treatment.

# References

Abramowitz JS, Schwartz SA, Moore KM, et al: Obsessive-compulsive symptoms in pregnancy and the puerperium: a review of the literature. J Anxiety Disord 17(4):461–478, 2003 12826092

Abrar A, Fairbrother N, Smith AP, et al: Anxiety among women experiencing medically complicated pregnancy: a systematic review and meta-analysis. Birth 47(1):13–20, 2020 31222840

Affonso DD, Liu-Chiang CY, Mayberry LJ: Worry: conceptual dimensions and relevance to childbearing women. Health Care Women Int 20(3):227–236, 1999 10633621

Ahmed A, Feng C, Bowen A, et al: Latent trajectory groups of perinatal depressive and anxiety symptoms from pregnancy to early postpartum and their antenatal risk factors. Arch Women Ment Health 21(6):689–698, 2018 29654413

Alwan S, Reefhuis J, Rasmussen SA, et al: Use of selective serotonin-reuptake inhibitors in pregnancy and the risk of birth defects. N Engl J Med 356(26):2684–2692, 2007 17596602

American College of Obstetricians and Gynecologists: ACOG Committee Opinion No. 757: screening for perinatal depression. Obstet Gynecol 132(5):e208–e212, 2018 30629567

American Psychiatric Association: Diagnostic and Statistical Manual of Mental Disorders, 5th Edition. Arlington, VA, American Psychiatric Association, 2013

Anderson KN: Insomnia and cognitive behavioural therapy-how to assess your patient and why it should be a standard part of care. J Thorac Dis 10(suppl 1):S94–S102, 2018 29445533

Armstrong C: ACOG guidelines on psychiatric medication use in pregnancy and lactation. Am Fam Physician 78(6):772–778, 2008

Askew JP: Zolpidem addiction in a pregnant woman with a history of second-trimester bleeding. Pharmacotherapy 27(2):306–308, 2007 17253922

Austin MP, Hadzi-Pavlovic D, Leader L, et al: Maternal trait anxiety, depression and life event stress in pregnancy. Early Hum Dev 81(2):183–190, 2005 15748973

Austin MP, Tully L, Parker G: Examining the relationship between antenatal anxiety and postnatal depression. J Affect Disord 101(1–3):169–174, 2007 17196663

Baglioni C, Battagliese G, Feige B, et al: Insomnia as a predictor of depression: a meta-analytic evaluation of longitudinal epidemiological studies. J Affect Disord 135(1–3):10–19, 2011 21300408

Bais B, Molenaar NM, Bijma HH, et al: Prevalence of benzodiazepines and benzodiazepine-related drugs exposure before, during and after pregnancy: a systematic review and meta-analysis. J Affect Disord 269:18–27, 2020 32217339

Baker FC, Wolfson AR, Lee KA: Association of sociodemographic, lifestyle, and health factors with sleep quality and daytime sleepiness in women: findings from the 2007 National Sleep Foundation "Sleep in America Poll." J Womens Health (Larchmt) 18(6):841–849, 2009 19514826
Baker S, Bhatta S, Bowden E, et al: Clinical guideline for the treatment of primary insomnia in middle-aged and older adults. Agency for Healthcare Research and Quality National Guideline Clearinghouse, Guideline Summary NGC-10414, 2014. Available at: https://www.multiplechronicconditions.org/assets/pdf/Insomnia%20Guidelines/AHRQ_2014_Clinical_guideline_for_the_treatment_of_primary_insomnia_in_middle-aged_and_older_adults.pdf. Accessed February 2, 2021.
Baldwin DS, Waldman S, Allgulander C: Evidence-based pharmacological treatment of generalized anxiety disorder. Int J Neuropsychopharmacol 14(5):697–710, 2011 21211105
Ban L, Gibson JE, West J, et al: Impact of socioeconomic deprivation on maternal perinatal mental illnesses presenting to UK general practice. Br J Gen Pract 62(603):e671–e678, 2012 23265226
Ban L, West J, Gibson JE, et al: First trimester exposure to anxiolytic and hypnotic drugs and the risks of major congenital anomalies: a United Kingdom population-based cohort study. PLoS One 9(6):e100996, 2014 24963627
Bartlett AA, Singh R, Hunter RG: Anxiety and epigenetics. Adv Exp Med Biol 978:145–166, 2017 28523545
Bayrampour H, Tomfohr L, Tough S: Trajectories of perinatal depressive and anxiety symptoms in a community cohort. J Clin Psychiatry 77(11):e1467–e1473, 2016 28076674
Bayrampour H, Vinturache A, Hetherington E, et al: Risk factors for antenatal anxiety: a systematic review of the literature. J Reprod Infant Psychol 36(5):476–503, 2018 30293441
Bei B, Milgrom J, Ericksen J, et al: Subjective perception of sleep, but not its objective quality, is associated with immediate postpartum mood disturbances in healthy women. Sleep 33(4):531–538, 2010 20394323
Bei B, Coo S, Milgrom J, Trinder J: Day-to-day alteration of 24-hour sleep pattern immediately before and after giving birth. Sleep and Biological Rhythms 10:212–221, 2012
Bei B, Coo S, Trinder J: Sleep and mood during pregnancy and the postpartum period. Sleep Med Clin 10(1):25–33, 2015 26055670
Bei B, Pinnington DM, Shen L, et al: A scalable cognitive behavioural program to promote healthy sleep during pregnancy and postpartum periods: protocol of a randomised controlled trial (the SEED project). BMC Pregnancy Childbirth 19(1):254, 2019 31331286
Bellantuono C, Tofani S, Di Sciascio G, et al: Benzodiazepine exposure in pregnancy and risk of major malformations: a critical overview. Gen Hosp Psychiatry 35(1):3–8, 2013 23044244
Benz F, Knoop T, Ballesio A, et al: The efficacy of cognitive and behavior therapies for insomnia on daytime symptoms: a systematic review and network meta-analysis. Clin Psychol Rev 80:101873, 2020 32777632
Betts KS, Williams GM, Najman JM, et al: The relationship between maternal depressive, anxious, and stress symptoms during pregnancy and adult offspring behavioral and emotional problems. Depress Anxiety 32(2):82–90, 2015 24788841
Biaggi A, Conroy S, Pawlby S, et al: Identifying the women at risk of antenatal anxiety and depression: a systematic review. J Affect Disord 191:62–77, 2016 26650969
Blackmore ER, Gustafsson H, Gilchrist M, et al: Pregnancy-related anxiety: evidence of distinct clinical significance from a prospective longitudinal study. J Affect Disord 197:251–258, 2016 26999549
Bonacquisti A, Cohen MJ, Schiller CE: Acceptance and commitment therapy for perinatal mood and anxiety disorders: development of an inpatient group intervention. Arch Women Ment Health 20(5):645–654, 2017 28600645
Brandt J, Leong C: Benzodiazepines and Z-drugs: an updated review of major adverse outcomes reported on in epidemiologic research. Drugs R D 17(4):493–507, 2017 28865038
Brouwers EPM, Baar AL, Van P: Maternal anxiety during pregnancy and subsequent infant development. Infant Behavior and Development 24(1):95–106, 2001
Brunton R, Dryer R, Saliba A, et al: Re-examining pregnancy-related anxiety: a replication study. Women Birth 32(1):e131–e137, 2019 29747955

Buist A, Gotman N, Yonkers KA: Generalized anxiety disorder: course and risk factors in pregnancy. J Affect Disord 131(1–3):277–283, 2011 21269708
Buysse DJ, Reynolds CF 3rd, Monk TH, et al: The Pittsburgh Sleep Quality Index: a new instrument for psychiatric practice and research. Psychiatry Res 28(2):193–213, 1989 2748771
Castillo-Gómez E, Pérez-Rando M, Bellés M, et al: Early social isolation stress and perinatal NMDA receptor antagonist treatment induce changes in the structure and neurochemistry of inhibitory neurons of the adult amygdala and prefrontal cortex. eNeuro 4(2), 2017 28466069
Chambers CD, Hernandez-Diaz S, Van Marter LJ, et al: Selective serotonin-reuptake inhibitors and risk of persistent pulmonary hypertension of the newborn. N Engl J Med 354(6):579–587, 2006 16467545
Chand S, Marwaha R: Anxiety. Treasure Island, FL, StatPearls Publishing, 2020
Chang JJ, Pien GW, Duntley SP, et al: Sleep deprivation during pregnancy and maternal and fetal outcomes: is there a relationship? Sleep Med Rev 14(2):107–114, 2010 19625199
Chaudhry SK, Susser LC: Considerations in treating insomnia during pregnancy: a literature review. Psychosomatics 59(4):341–348, 2018 29706359
Christian LM: At the forefront of psychoneuroimmunology in pregnancy: implications for racial disparities in birth outcomes part 1: behavioral risks factors. Neurosci Biobehav Rev 117:319–326, 2020 31005626
Coelho HF, Murray L, Royal-Lawson M, et al: Antenatal anxiety disorder as a predictor of postnatal depression: a longitudinal study. J Affect Disord 129(1–3):348–353, 2011 20805004
Collardeau F, Corbyn B, Abramowitz J, et al: Maternal unwanted and intrusive thoughts of infant-related harm, obsessive-compulsive disorder and depression in the perinatal period: study protocol. BMC Psychiatry 19(1):94, 2019 30898103
Cosci F, Fava GA, Sonino N: Mood and anxiety disorders as early manifestations of medical illness: a systematic review. Psychother Psychosom 84(1):22–29, 2015 25547421
Coussons-Read ME, Okun ML, Nettles CD: Psychosocial stress increases inflammatory markers and alters cytokine production across pregnancy. Brain Behav Immun 21(3):343–350, 2007 17029703
Cox JL, Holden JM, Sagovsky R: Detection of postnatal depression: development of the 10-item Edinburgh Postnatal Depression Scale. Br J Psychiatry 150:782–786, 1987 3651732
Davis EP, Snidman N, Wadhwa PD, et al: Prenatal maternal anxiety and depression predict negative behavioral reactivity in infancy. Infancy 6(3):319–331, 2004
Davis M: Are different parts of the extended amygdala involved in fear versus anxiety? Biol Psychiatry 44(12):1239–1247, 1998 9861467
Dayan J, Creveuil C, Herlicoviez M, et al: Role of anxiety and depression in the onset of spontaneous preterm labor. Am J Epidemiol 155(4):293–301, 2002 11836191
Dencker A, Nilsson C, Begley C, et al: Causes and outcomes in studies of fear of childbirth: a systematic review. Women Birth 32(2):99–111, 2019 30115515
Dennis CL, Falah-Hassani K, Shiri R: Prevalence of antenatal and postnatal anxiety: systematic review and meta-analysis. Br J Psychiatry 210(5):315–323, 2017 28302701
D'Hulst C, Atack JR, Kooy RF: The complexity of the GABAA receptor shapes unique pharmacological profiles. Drug Discov Today 14(17–18):866–875, 2009 19576998
Ding XX, Wu YL, Xu SJ, et al: Maternal anxiety during pregnancy and adverse birth outcomes: a systematic review and meta-analysis of prospective cohort studies. J Affect Disord 159:103–110, 2014 24679397
DiPietro JA, Hilton SC, Hawkins M, et al: Maternal stress and affect influence fetal neurobehavioral development. Dev Psychol 38(5):659–668, 2002 12220045
Dole N, Savitz DA, Hertz-Picciotto I, et al: Maternal stress and preterm birth. Am J Epidemiol 157(1):14–24, 2003 12505886
Dolovich LR, Addis A, Vaillancourt JMR, et al: Benzodiazepine use in pregnancy and major malformations or oral cleft: meta-analysis of cohort and case-control studies. BMJ 317(7162):839–843, 1998 9748174
Domhardt M, Geßlein H, von Rezori RE, et al: Internet- and mobile-based interventions for anxiety disorders: a meta-analytic review of intervention components. Depress Anxiety 36(3):213–224, 2019 30450811

Dominguez TP, Dunkel-Schetter C, Glynn LM, et al: Racial differences in birth outcomes: the role of general, pregnancy, and racism stress. Health Psychol 27(2):194–203, 2008 18377138
Driver HS, Shapiro CM: A longitudinal study of sleep stages in young women during pregnancy and postpartum. Sleep 15(5):449–453, 1992 1455129
Dubber S, Reck C, Müller M, et al: Postpartum bonding: the role of perinatal depression, anxiety and maternal-fetal bonding during pregnancy. Arch Women Ment Health 18(2):187–195, 2015 25088531
Dunkel Schetter C: Stress processes in pregnancy and preterm birth. Curr Dir Psychol Sci 8:205–209, 2009
Dunkel Schetter C: Psychological science on pregnancy: stress processes, biopsychosocial models, and emerging research issues. Annu Rev Psychol 62:531–558, 2011 21126184
Dunkel Schetter C, Tanner L: Anxiety, depression and stress in pregnancy: implications for mothers, children, research, and practice. Curr Opin Psychiatry 25(2):141–148, 2012 22262028
Einarson A, Bonari L, Voyer-Lavigne S, et al: A multicentre prospective controlled study to determine the safety of trazodone and nefazodone use during pregnancy. Can J Psychiatry 48(2):106–110, 2003 12655908
Einarson A, Choi J, Einarson TR, et al: Incidence of major malformations in infants following antidepressant exposure in pregnancy: results of a large prospective cohort study. Can J Psychiatry 54(4):242–246, 2009 19321030
Ellis JG, Perlis ML, Neale LF, et al: The natural history of insomnia: focus on prevalence and incidence of acute insomnia. J Psychiatr Res 46(10):1278–1285, 2012 22800714
Espie CA, Broomfield NM, MacMahon KM, et al: The attention-intention-effort pathway in the development of psychophysiologic insomnia. Sleep Med Rev 10(4):215–245, 2006 16809056
Facco FL, Kramer J, Ho KH, et al: Sleep disturbances in pregnancy. Obstet Gynecol 115(1):77–83, 2010 20027038
Facco FL, Grobman WA, Reid KJ, et al: Objectively measured short sleep duration and later sleep midpoint in pregnancy are associated with a higher risk of gestational diabetes. Sleep Med Rev 217(4):447.e1–447.e13, 2017 28599896
Fairbrother N, Young AH, Zhang A, et al: The prevalence and incidence of perinatal anxiety disorders among women experiencing a medically complicated pregnancy. Arch Women Ment Health 20(2):311–319, 2017 28032213
Fairbrother N, Corbyn B, Thordarson DS, et al: Screening for perinatal anxiety disorders: room to grow. J Affect Disord 250:363–370, 2019 30877859
Fallon V, Groves R, Halford JC, et al: Postpartum anxiety and infant-feeding outcomes. J Hum Lact 32(4):740–758, 2016a 27565200
Fallon V, Halford JCG, Bennett KM, et al: The Postpartum Specific Anxiety Scale: development and preliminary validation. Arch Women Ment Health 19(6):1079–1090, 2016b 27571782
Farias DR, Pinto TdeJ, Teofilo MMA, et al: Prevalence of psychiatric disorders in the first trimester of pregnancy and factors associated with current suicide risk. Psychiatry Res 210(3):962–968, 2013 24090486
Fawcett EJ, Fairbrother N, Cox ML, et al: The prevalence of anxiety disorders during pregnancy and the postpartum period: a multivariate Bayesian meta-analysis. J Clin Psychiatry 80(4):18r12527, 2019 31347796
Felder JN, Baer RJ, Rand L, et al: Sleep disorder diagnosis during pregnancy and risk of preterm birth. Obstet Gynecol 130(3):573–581, 2017 28796676
Fernandez-Mendoza J, Vgontzas AN: Insomnia and its impact on physical and mental health. Curr Psychiatry Rep 15(12):418, 2013 24189774
Ferraro ZM, Chaput JP, Gruslin A, et al: The potential value of sleep hygiene for a healthy pregnancy: a brief review. ISRN Family Med 2014:928293, 2014 24967333
Freeman MP, Góez-Mogollón L, McInerney KA, et al: Obstetrical and neonatal outcomes after benzodiazepine exposure during pregnancy: results from a prospective registry of women with psychiatric disorders. Gen Hosp Psychiatry 53:73–79, 2018 29958100
Furtado M, Chow CHT, Owais S, et al: Risk factors of new onset anxiety and anxiety exacerbation in the perinatal period: a systematic review and meta-analysis. J Affect Disord 238:626–635, 2018 29957480

Furtado M, Van Lieshout RJ, Van Ameringen M, et al: Biological and psychosocial predictors of anxiety worsening in the postpartum period. J Affect Disord 250:218–225, 2019 30870771
Giscombé CL, Lobel M: Explaining disproportionately high rates of adverse birth outcomes among African Americans: the impact of stress, racism, and related factors in pregnancy. Psychol Bull 131(5):662–683, 2005 16187853
Glendining KA, Fisher LC, Jasoni CL: Maternal high fat diet alters offspring epigenetic regulators, amygdala glutamatergic profile and anxiety. Psychoneuroendocrinology 96:132–141, 2018 29940426
Glover V: Maternal depression, anxiety and stress during pregnancy and child outcome: what needs to be done. Best Pract Res Clin Obstet Gynaecol 28(1):25–35, 2014 24090740
Goldfinger C, Green SM, Furtado M, et al: Characterizing the nature of worry in a sample of perinatal women with generalized anxiety disorder. Clin Psychol Psychother 27(2):136–145, 2020 31746496
Goodman JH, Chenausky KL, Freeman MP: Anxiety disorders during pregnancy: a systematic review. J Clin Psychiatry 75(10):e1153–e1184, 2014a 25373126
Goodman JH, Guarino A, Chenausky K, et al: CALM Pregnancy: results of a pilot study of mindfulness-based cognitive therapy for perinatal anxiety. Arch Women Ment Health 17(5):373–387, 2014b 24449191
Gravensteen IK, Jacobsen EM, Sandset PM, et al: Anxiety, depression and relationship satisfaction in the pregnancy following stillbirth and after the birth of a live-born baby: a prospective study. BMC Pregnancy Childbirth 18(1):41, 2018 29361916
Green SM, Haber E, Frey BN, et al: Cognitive-behavioral group treatment for perinatal anxiety: a pilot study. Arch Women Ment Health 18(4):631–638, 2015 25652951
Greenblatt DJ, Harmatz JS, Singh NN, et al: Gender differences in pharmacokinetics and pharmacodynamics of zolpidem following sublingual administration. J Clin Pharmacol 54(3):282–290, 2014 24203450
Gregory KD, Chelmow D, Nelson HD, et al: Screening for anxiety in adolescent and adult women: a recommendation from the Women's Preventive Services Initiative. Ann Intern Med 173(1):48–56, 2020 32510990
Grigoriadis S, de Camps Meschino D, Barrons E, et al: Mood and anxiety disorders in a sample of Canadian perinatal women referred for psychiatric care. Arch Women Ment Health 14(4):325–333, 2011 21695590
Grigoriadis S, VonderPorten EH, Mamisashvili L, et al: The impact of maternal depression during pregnancy on perinatal outcomes. J Clin Psychiatry 74(4):e321–e341, 2013 23656857
Grigoriadis S, Graves L, Peer M, et al: Maternal anxiety during pregnancy and the association with adverse perinatal outcomes. J Clin Psychiatry 79(5):17r12011, 2018 30192449
Grigoriadis S, Graves L, Peer M, et al: Benzodiazepine use during pregnancy alone or in combination with an antidepressant and congenital malformations: systematic review and meta-analysis. J Clin Psychiatry 80(4):18r12412, 2019 32194935
Grigoriadis S, Graves L, Peer M, et al: Pregnancy and delivery outcomes following benzodiazepine exposure. Can J Psychiatry 65(12):821–834, 2020 32148076
Hanley GE, Mintzes B: Patterns of psychotropic medicine use in pregnancy in the United States from 2006 to 2011 among women with private insurance. BMC Pregnancy Childbirth 14:242, 2014 25048574
Hantsoo L, Epperson CN: Anxiety disorders among women: a female lifespan approach. Focus 15(2):162–172, 2017 28966563
Harrison V, Moore D, Lazard L: Supporting perinatal anxiety in the digital age; a qualitative exploration of stressors and support strategies. BMC Pregnancy Childbirth 20(1):363, 2020 32546131
Harvey AG, Murray G, Chandler RA, et al: Sleep disturbance as transdiagnostic: consideration of neurobiological mechanisms. Clin Psychol Rev 31(2):225–235, 2011 20471738
Hashmi AM, Bhatia SK, Bhatia SK, et al: Insomnia during pregnancy: diagnosis and rational interventions. Pak J Med Sci 32(4):1030–1037, 2016 27648062
Hedman C, Pohjasvaara T, Tolonen U, et al: Effects of pregnancy on mothers' sleep. Sleep Med 3(1):37–42, 2002 14592252

Hendrick V, Altshuler L, Strouse T, et al: Postpartum and nonpostpartum depression: differences in presentation and response to pharmacologic treatment. Depress Anxiety 11(2):66–72, 2000 10812531

Hettema JM, Prescott CA, Kendler KS: Genetic and environmental sources of covariation between generalized anxiety disorder and neuroticism. Am J Psychiatry 161(9):1581–1587, 2004 15337647

Hettema JM, Prescott CA, Myers JM, et al: The structure of genetic and environmental risk factors for anxiety disorders in men and women. Arch Gen Psychiatry 62(2):182–189, 2005

Hilty D, Young JS, Bourgeois JA, et al: Algorithms for the assessment and management of insomnia in primary care. Patient Prefer Adherence 3:9–20, 2009 19936140

Howland RH: Antidepressant medication and pregnancy: time for randomized controlled trials. J Psychosoc Nurs Ment Health Serv 51(2):11–14, 2013 23330797

Huizink AC, de Medina PG, Mulder EJH, et al: Psychological measures of prenatal stress as predictors of infant temperament. J Am Acad Child Adolesc Psychiatry 41(9):1078–1085, 2002

Huizink AC, Mulder EJ, Robles de Medina PG, et al: Is pregnancy anxiety a distinctive syndrome? Early Hum Dev 79(2):81–91, 2004 15324989

Hussain-Shamsy N, Shah A, Vigod SN, et al: Mobile health for perinatal depression and anxiety: scoping review. J Med Internet Res 22(4):e17011, 2020 32281939

Hysing M, Harvey AG, Torgersen L, et al: Trajectories and predictors of nocturnal awakenings and sleep duration in infants. J Dev Behav Pediatr 35(5):309–316, 2014 24906032

Ibanez G, Charles MA, Forhan A, et al: Depression and anxiety in women during pregnancy and neonatal outcome: data from the EDEN mother-child cohort. Early Hum Dev 88(8):643–649, 2012 22361259

Iqbal MM, Sobhan T, Ryals T: Effects of commonly used benzodiazepines on the fetus, the neonate, and the nursing infant. Psychiatr Serv 53(1):39–49, 2002 11773648

Jolley SN, Betrus P: Comparing postpartum depression and major depressive disorder: issues in assessment. Issues Ment Health Nurs 28(7):765–780, 2007 17654110

Juric S, Newport DJ, Ritchie JC, et al: Zolpidem (Ambien) in pregnancy: placental passage and outcome. Arch Women Ment Health 12(6):441–446, 2009 19657707

Kallestad H, Hansen B, Langsrud K, et al: Impact of sleep disturbance on patients in treatment for mental disorders. BMC Psychiatry 12:179, 2012 23107000

Keim SA, Daniels JL, Dole N, et al: A prospective study of maternal anxiety, perceived stress, and depressive symptoms in relation to infant cognitive development. Early Hum Dev 87(5):373–380, 2011 21420261

Kelly LE, Poon S, Madadi P, et al: Neonatal benzodiazepines exposure during breastfeeding. J Pediatr 161(3):448–451, 2012 22504099

Kendig S, Keats JP, Hoffman MC, et al: Consensus bundle on maternal mental health: perinatal depression and anxiety. Obstet Gynecol 129(3):422–430, 2017 28178041

Kessler RC, Berglund P, Demler O, et al: The epidemiology of major depressive disorder: results from the National Comorbidity Survey Replication (NCS-R). JAMA 289(23):3095–3105, 2003 12813115

Kessler RC, Petukhova M, Sampson NA, et al: Twelve-month and lifetime prevalence and lifetime morbid risk of anxiety and mood disorders in the United States. Int J Methods Psychiatr Res 21(3):169–184, 2012 22865617

Kingston D, Tough S, Whitfield H: Prenatal and postpartum maternal psychological distress and infant development: a systematic review. Child Psychiatry Hum Dev 43(5):683–714, 2012

Kramer MS, Lydon J, Séguin L, et al: Stress pathways to spontaneous preterm birth: the role of stressors, psychological distress, and stress hormones. Am J Epidemiol 169(11):1319–1326, 2009 19363098

Kroll-Desrosiers AR, Nephew BC, Babb JA, et al: Association of peripartum synthetic oxytocin administration and depressive and anxiety disorders within the first postpartum year. Depress Anxiety 34(2):137–146, 2017 28133901

Krystal AD: Psychiatric disorders and sleep. Neurol Clin 30(4):1389–1413, 2012 23099143

Lacroix I, Hurault C, Sarramon MF, et al: Prescription of drugs during pregnancy: a study using EFEMERIS, the new French database. Eur J Clin Pharmacol 65(8):839–846, 2009 19365629

Lancel M, Faulhaber J, Holsboer F, et al: Progesterone induces changes in sleep comparable to those of agonistic GABAA receptor modulators. Am J Physiol 271(4 pt 1):e763–e772, 1996 8897866
LeBlanc M, Mérette C, Savard J, et al: Incidence and risk factors of insomnia in a population-based sample. Sleep 32(8):1027–1037, 2009 19725254
LeDoux JE: Emotion circuits in the brain. Annu Rev Neurosci 23:155–184, 2000 10845062
Lee KA, Gay CL: Sleep in late pregnancy predicts length of labor and type of delivery. Am J Obstet Gynecol 191(6):2041–2046, 2004 15592289
Lee KA, Zaffke ME, McEnany G: Parity and sleep patterns during and after pregnancy. Obstet Gynecol 95(1):14–18, 2000 10636494
Lee KA, Gay CL, Alsten CR: Sleep enhancement training for pregnant women. Obstet Gynecol 128(5):964–971, 2016 27741179
Leff Gelman P, Mancilla-Herrera I, Flores-Ramos M, et al: The cytokine profile of women with severe anxiety and depression during pregnancy. BMC Psychiatry 19(1):104, 2019 30943938
Levin JS: The factor structure of the pregnancy anxiety scale. J Health Soc Behav 32(4):368–381, 1991 1765627
Levine RE, Oandasan AP, Primeau LA, et al: Anxiety disorders during pregnancy and postpartum. Am J Perinatol 20(5):239–248, 2003 13680507
Li Q, Mitchell AA, Werler MM, et al: Assessment of antihistamine use in early pregnancy and birth defects. J Allergy Clin Immunol Pract 1(6):666–674, 2013 24565715
Loughnan SA, Joubert AE, Grierson A, et al: Internet-delivered psychological interventions for clinical anxiety and depression in perinatal women: a systematic review and meta-analysis. Arch Women Ment Health 22(6):737–750, 2019 31101993
Louis JM, Koch MA, Reddy UM, et al: Predictors of sleep-disordered breathing in pregnancy. Am J Obstet Gynecol 218(5):521.e1–521.e12, 2018 29523262
Love C, David RJ, Rankin KM, et al: Exploring weathering: effects of lifelong economic environment and maternal age on low birth weight, small for gestational age, and preterm birth in African-American and white women. Am J Epidemiol 172(2):127–134, 2010 20576757
Lupattelli A, Chambers CD, Bandoli G, et al: Association of maternal use of benzodiazepines and Z-hypnotics during pregnancy with motor and communication skills and attention-deficit/hyperactivity disorder symptoms in preschoolers. JAMA Netw Open 2(4):e191435, 2019
Mackintosh MA, Gatz M, Wetherell JL, et al: A twin study of lifetime generalized anxiety disorder (GAD) in older adults: genetic and environmental influences shared by neuroticism and GAD. Twin Res Hum Genet 9(1):30–37, 2006 16611465
Maes M, Lin AH, Ombelet W, et al: Immune activation in the early puerperium is related to postpartum anxiety and depressive symptoms. Psychoneuroendocrinology 25(2):121–137, 2000 10674277
Maguire PN, Clark GI, Wootton BM: The efficacy of cognitive behavior therapy for the treatment of perinatal anxiety symptoms: a preliminary meta-analysis. J Anxiety Disord 60:26–34, 2018 30388545
Malish S, Arastu F, O'Brien LM: A preliminary study of new parents, sleep disruption, and driving: a population at risk? Matern Child Health J 20(2):290–297, 2016 26541593
Manber R, Bei B, Simpson N, et al: Cognitive behavioral therapy for prenatal insomnia: a randomized controlled trial. Obstet Gynecol 133(5):911–919, 2019 30969203
Manconi M, Govoni V, De Vito A, et al: Restless legs syndrome and pregnancy. Neurology 63(6):1065–1069, 2004 15452299
Matthey S, Ross-Hamid C: Repeat testing on the Edinburgh Depression Scale and the HADS-A in pregnancy: differentiating between transient and enduring distress. J Affect Disord 141(2–3):213–221, 2012 22695259
Matthey S, Barnett B, Howie P, et al: Diagnosing postpartum depression in mothers and fathers: whatever happened to anxiety? J Affect Disord 74(2):139–147, 2003 12706515
Matthey S, Fisher J, Rowe H: Using the Edinburgh postnatal depression scale to screen for anxiety disorders: conceptual and methodological considerations. J Affect Disord 146(2):224–230, 2013a 23116811

Matthey S, Valenti B, Souter K, et al: Comparison of four self-report measures and a generic mood question to screen for anxiety during pregnancy in English-speaking women. J Affect Disord 148(2–3):347–351, 2013b 23380518
McElhatton PR: The effects of benzodiazepine use during pregnancy and lactation. Reprod Toxicol 8(6):461–475, 1994 7881198
Meades R, Ayers S: Anxiety measures validated in perinatal populations: a systematic review. J Affect Disord 133(1–2):1–15, 2011 21078523
Meltzer-Brody S, Larsen JT, Petersen L, et al: Adverse life events increase risk for postpartum psychiatric episodes: a population-based epidemiologic study. Depress Anxiety 35(2):160–167, 2018 29172228
Menke RA, Swanson L, Erickson NL, et al: Childhood adversity and sleep are associated with symptom severity in perinatal women presenting for psychiatric care. Arch Women Ment Health 22(4):457–465, 2019 30276477
Misri S, Swift E: Generalized anxiety disorder and major depressive disorder in pregnant and postpartum women: maternal quality of life and treatment outcomes. J Obstet Gynaecol Can 37(9):798–803, 2015 26605449
Misri S, Abizadeh J, Sanders S, et al: Perinatal generalized anxiety disorder: assessment and treatment. J Womens Health (Larchmt) 24(9):762–770, 2015 26125602
Moran TE, Polanin JR, Wenzel A: The Postpartum Worry Scale-Revised: an initial validation of a measure of postpartum worry. Arch Women Ment Health 17(1):41–48, 2014 24026389
Morin CM, Vallières A, Guay B, et al: Cognitive behavioral therapy, singly and combined with medication, for persistent insomnia: a randomized controlled trial. JAMA 301(19):2005–2015, 2009 19454639
Murray L, Woolgar M, Murray J, et al: Self-exclusion from health care in women at high risk for postpartum depression. J Public Health Med 25(2):131–137, 2003 12848402
National Institutes of Health: NIH State-of-the-Science Conference Statement on manifestations and management of chronic insomnia in adults. NIH Consens State Sci Statements 22(2):1–30, 2005 17308547
Nepon J, Belik SL, Bolton J, et al: The relationship between anxiety disorders and suicide attempts: findings from the National Epidemiologic Survey on Alcohol and Related Conditions. Depress Anxiety 27(9):791–798, 2010 20217852
Nillni YI, Mehralizade A, Mayer L, et al: Treatment of depression, anxiety, and trauma-related disorders during the perinatal period: a systematic review. Clin Psychol Rev 66:136–148, 2018
Nodine PM, Matthews EE: Common sleep disorders: management strategies and pregnancy outcomes. J Midwifery Womens Health 58(4):368–377, 2013 23855316
Nowakowski S, Meers JM: Cognitive behavioral therapy for insomnia and women's health: sex as a biological variable. Sleep Med Clin 14(2):185–197, 2019 31029186
Nulman I, Rovet J, Stewart DE, et al: Child development following exposure to tricyclic antidepressants or fluoxetine throughout fetal life: a prospective, controlled study. Am J Psychiatry 159(11):1889–1895, 2002 12411224
Oberlander TF, Weinberg J, Papsdorf M, et al: Prenatal exposure to maternal depression, neonatal methylation of human glucocorticoid receptor gene (NR3C1) and infant cortisol stress responses. Epigenetics 3(2):97–106, 2008 18536531
O'Connor TG, Heron J, Glover V, et al: Antenatal anxiety predicts child behavioral/emotional problems independently of postnatal depression. J Am Acad Child Adolesc Psychiatry 41(12):1470–1477, 2002 12447034
O'Donnell K, O'Connor TG, Glover V: Prenatal stress and neurodevelopment of the child: focus on the HPA axis and role of the placenta. Dev Neurosci 31(4):285–292, 2009 19546565
O'Hara MW, Wisner KL: Perinatal mental illness: definition, description and aetiology. Best Pract Res Clin Obstet Gynaecol 28(1):3–12, 2014 24140480
Ohayon MM, Carskadon MA, Guilleminault C, et al: Meta-analysis of quantitative sleep parameters from childhood to old age in healthy individuals: developing normative sleep values across the human lifespan. Sleep 27(7):1255–1273, 2004 15586779
Okun ML, Schetter CD, Glynn LM: Poor sleep quality is associated with preterm birth. Sleep (Basel) 34(11):1493–1498, 2011 22043120

Okun ML, Buysse DJ, Hall MH: Identifying insomnia in early pregnancy: validation of the Insomnia Symptoms Questionnaire (ISQ) in pregnant women. J Clin Sleep Med 11(6):645–654, 2015
Ordean A, Graves L, Chisamore B, et al: Prevalence and consequences of perinatal substance use-growing worldwide concerns. Subst Abuse 11:1178221817704692, 2017 28634426
Orr ST, Reiter JP, Blazer DG, et al: Maternal prenatal pregnancy-related anxiety and spontaneous preterm birth in Baltimore, Maryland. Psychosom Med 69(6):566–570, 2007 17636150
Osborne LM, Birndorf CA, Szkodny LE, et al: Returning to tricyclic antidepressants for depression during childbearing: clinical and dosing challenges. Arch Women Ment Health 17(3):239–246, 2014 24668283
Osborne LM, Betz JF, Yenokyan G, et al: The role of allopregnanolone in pregnancy in predicting postpartum anxiety symptoms. Front Psychol 10:1033, 2019a 31379633
Osborne LM, Yenokyan G, Fei K, et al: Innate immune activation and depressive and anxious symptoms across the peripartum: an exploratory study. Psychoneuroendocrinology 99:80–86, 2019b 30195110
Osnes RS, Roaldset JO, Follestad T, et al: Insomnia late in pregnancy is associated with perinatal anxiety: a longitudinal cohort study. J Affect Disord 248:155–165, 2019 30735852
Palagini L, Cipollone G, Masci I, et al: Stress-related sleep reactivity is associated with insomnia, psychopathology and suicidality in pregnant women: preliminary results. Sleep Med 56:145–150, 2019 30803833
Pearson KH, Nonacs RM, Viguera AC, et al: Birth outcomes following prenatal exposure to antidepressants. J Clin Psychiatry 68(8):1284–1289, 2007 17854255
Phillips J, Sharpe L, Matthey S, et al: Maternally focused worry. Arch Women Ment Health 12(6):409–418, 2009 19626414
Pilkington PD, Milne LC, Cairns KE, et al: Modifiable partner factors associated with perinatal depression and anxiety: a systematic review and meta-analysis. J Affect Disord 178:165–180, 2015 25837550
Pilkington P, Milne L, Cairns K, et al: Enhancing reciprocal partner support to prevent perinatal depression and anxiety: a Delphi consensus study. BMC Psychiatry 16:23, 2016 26842065
Polte C, Junge C, von Soest T, et al: Impact of maternal perinatal anxiety on social-emotional development of 2-year-olds, a prospective study of Norwegian mothers and their offspring: the impact of perinatal anxiety on child development. Matern Child Health J 23(3):386–396, 2019
Pons G, Francoual C, Guillet P, et al: Zolpidem excretion in breast milk. Eur J Clin Pharmacol 37(3):245–248, 1989 2612539
Qaseem A, Kansagara D, Forciea MA, et al: Management of chronic insomnia disorder in adults: a clinical practice guideline from the American College of Physicians. Ann Intern Med 165(2):125–133, 2016 27136449
Qiu A, Anh TT, Li Y, et al: Prenatal maternal depression alters amygdala functional connectivity in 6-month-old infants. Transl Psychiatry 5(2):e508, 2015 25689569
Rackers HS, Thomas S, Williamson K, et al: Emerging literature in the microbiota-brain axis and perinatal mood and anxiety disorders. Psychoneuroendocrinology 95:86–96, 2018 29807325
Rallis S, Skouteris H, McCabe M, et al: A prospective examination of depression, anxiety and stress throughout pregnancy. Women Birth 27(1):e36–e42, 2014a 25240846
Rallis S, Skouteris H, McCabe M, et al: The transition to motherhood: towards a broader understanding of perinatal distress. Women Birth 27(1):68–71, 2014b 24461688
Riemann D, Baglioni C, Bassetti C, et al: European guideline for the diagnosis and treatment of insomnia. J Sleep Res 26(6):675–700, 2017 28875581
Rifkin-Graboi A, Meaney MJ, Chen H, et al: Antenatal maternal anxiety predicts variations in neural structures implicated in anxiety disorders in newborns. J Am Acad Child Adolesc Psychiatry 54(4):313–321, 2015 25791148
Riska BS, Skurtveit S, Furu K, et al: Dispensing of benzodiazepines and benzodiazepine-related drugs to pregnant women: a population-based cohort study. Eur J Clin Pharmacol 70(11):1367–1374, 2014 25204310
Robertson E, Grace S, Wallington T, et al: Antenatal risk factors for postpartum depression: a synthesis of recent literature. Gen Hosp Psychiatry 26(4):289–295, 2004 15234824

Robinson OJ, Pike AC, Cornwell B, et al: The translational neural circuitry of anxiety. J Neurol Neurosurg Psychiatry 90(12):1353–1360, 2019 31256001
Román-Gálvez RM, Amezcua-Prieto C, Salcedo-Bellido I, et al: Factors associated with insomnia in pregnancy: a prospective cohort study. Eur J Obstet Gynecol Reprod Biol 221:70–75, 2018 29304393
Rose MS, Pana G, Premji S: Prenatal maternal anxiety as a risk factor for preterm birth and the effects of heterogeneity on this relationship: a systematic review and meta-analysis. BioMed Res Int 2016:8312158, 2016 27298829
Ross LE, McLean LM: Anxiety disorders during pregnancy and the postpartum period: a systematic review. J Clin Psychiatry 67(8):1285–1298, 2006 16965210
Roth T: Insomnia: definition, prevalence, etiology, and consequences. J Clin Sleep Med 3(5 suppl):S7–S10, 2007 17824495
Rowe HJ, Fisher JR, Loh WM: The Edinburgh Postnatal Depression Scale detects but does not distinguish anxiety disorders from depression in mothers of infants. Arch Women Ment Health 11(2):103–108, 2008 18463939
Sanchez SE, Puente GC, Atencio G, et al: Risk of spontaneous preterm birth in relation to maternal depressive, anxiety, and stress symptoms. J Reprod Med 58(1–2):25–33, 2013 23447915
Sasaki A, de Vega WC, St-Cyr S, et al: Perinatal high fat diet alters glucocorticoid signaling and anxiety behavior in adulthood. Neuroscience 240:1–12, 2013 23454542
Sasaki A, de Vega W, Sivanathan S, et al: Maternal high-fat diet alters anxiety behavior and glucocorticoid signaling in adolescent offspring. Neuroscience 272:92–101, 2014 24791714
Schmidt PJ, Nieman LK, Danaceau MA, et al: Differential behavioral effects of gonadal steroids in women with and in those without premenstrual syndrome. N Engl J Med 338(4):209–216, 1998 9435325
Schutte-Rodin S, Broch L, Buysse D, et al: Clinical guideline for the evaluation and management of chronic insomnia in adults. J Clin Sleep Med 4(5):487–504, 2008 18853708
Sedov ID, Goodman SH, Tomfohr-Madsen LM: Insomnia treatment preferences during pregnancy. J Obstet Gynecol Neonatal Nurs 46(3):e95–e104, 2017 28343943
Seow LS, Subramaniam M, Abdin E, et al: Sleep disturbance among people with major depressive disorders (MDD) in Singapore. J Ment Health 25(6):492–499, 2016 27935392
Shapiro GD, Séguin JR, Muckle G, et al: Previous pregnancy outcomes and subsequent pregnancy anxiety in a Quebec prospective cohort. J Psychosom Obstet Gynaecol 38(2):121–132, 2017
Sharma A, Sayeed N, Khees CR, et al: High dose zolpidem induced fetal neural tube defects. Curr Drug Saf 6(2):128–129, 2011 21385155
Sharma V, Mazmanian D: Sleep loss and postpartum psychosis. Bipolar Disord 5(2):98–105, 2003
Sheehy O, Zhao JP, Bérard A: Association between incident exposure to benzodiazepines in early pregnancy and risk of spontaneous abortion. JAMA Psychiatry 76(9):948–957, 2019 31090881
Shimada-Sugimoto M, Otowa T, Hettema JM: Genetics of anxiety disorders: genetic epidemiological and molecular studies in humans. Psychiatry Clin Neurosci 69(7):388–401, 2015 25762210
Sivertsen B, Hysing M, Dørheim SK, et al: Trajectories of maternal sleep problems before and after childbirth: a longitudinal population-based study. BMC Pregnancy Childbirth 15(10):129, 2015 26031504
Skouteris H, Wertheim EH, Germano C, et al: Assessing sleep during pregnancy: a study across two time points examining the Pittsburgh Sleep Quality Index and associations with depressive symptoms. Womens Health Issues 19(1):45–51, 2009 19111787
Smith MT, Perlis ML, Park A, et al: Comparative meta-analysis of pharmacotherapy and behavior therapy for persistent insomnia. Am J Psychiatry 159(1):5–11, 2002 11772681
Sockol LE: A systematic review and meta-analysis of interpersonal psychotherapy for perinatal women. J Affect Disord 232:316–328, 2018 29501991
Somerville S, Dedman K, Hagan R, et al: The Perinatal Anxiety Screening Scale: development and preliminary validation. Arch Women Ment Health 17(5):443–454, 2014 24699796
Somerville S, Byrne SL, Dedman K, et al: Detecting the severity of perinatal anxiety with the Perinatal Anxiety Screening Scale (PASS). J Affect Disord 186:18–25, 2015 26226429

Spielberger CD, Gorsuch RL, Lushene R, et al: Manual for the State-Trait Anxiety Inventory. Palo Alto, CA, Consulting Psychologists Press, 1983
Spitzer RL, Kroenke K, Williams JB, et al: A brief measure for assessing generalized anxiety disorder: the GAD-7. Arch Intern Med 166(10):1092–1097, 2006 16717171
Staneva A, Bogossian F, Pritchard M, et al: The effects of maternal depression, anxiety, and perceived stress during pregnancy on preterm birth: a systematic review. Women Birth 28(3):179–193, 2015 25765470
Stein A, Craske MG, Lehtonen A, et al: Maternal cognitions and mother-infant interaction in postnatal depression and generalized anxiety disorder. J Abnorm Psychol 121(4):795–809, 2012
Stein A, Pearson RM, Goodman SH, et al: Effects of perinatal mental disorders on the fetus and child. Lancet 384(9956):1800–1819, 2014 25455250
Stuart S: Interpersonal psychotherapy for postpartum depression. Clin Psychol Psychother 19(2):134–140, 2012 22473762
Sullivan EL, Nousen EK, Chamlou KA: Maternal high fat diet consumption during the perinatal period programs offspring behavior. Physiol Behav 123:236–242, 2014 23085399
Suri R, Altshuler LL: No decision is without risk. J Clin Psychiatry 70(9):1319–1320, 2009 19818253
Sutter-Dallay AL, Giaconne-Marcesche V, Glatigny-Dallay E, et al: Women with anxiety disorders during pregnancy are at increased risk of intense postnatal depressive symptoms: a prospective survey of the MATQUID cohort. Eur Psychiatry 19(8):459–463, 2004 15589703
Swanson LM, Pickett SM, Flynn H, et al: Relationships among depression, anxiety, and insomnia symptoms in perinatal women seeking mental health treatment. J Womens Health (Larchmt) 20(4):553–558, 2011 21417746
Task Force on Sudden Infant Death Syndrome: SIDS and other sleep-related infant deaths: updated 2016 recommendation for a safe infant sleeping environment. Pediatrics 138(5):e20162938, 2016 27940804
Taylor DJ, Pruiksma KE: Cognitive and behavioural therapy for insomnia (CBT-I) in psychiatric populations: a systematic review. Int Rev Psychiatry 26(2):205–213, 2014 24892895
Taylor DJ, Lichstein KL, Durrence HH: Insomnia as a health risk factor. Behav Sleep Med 1(4):227–247, 2003 15600216
Thorsness KR, Watson C, LaRusso EM: Perinatal anxiety: approach to diagnosis and management in the obstetric setting. Am J Obstet Gynecol 219(4):326–345, 2018 29803818
Tinker SC, Reefhuis J, Bitsko RH, et al: Use of benzodiazepine medications during pregnancy and potential risk for birth defects, National Birth Defects Prevention Study, 1997–2011. Birth Defects Res 111(10):613–620, 2019 30891943
Tomfohr-Madsen LM, Clayborne ZM, Rouleau CR, et al: Sleeping for two: an open-pilot study of cognitive behavioral therapy for insomnia in pregnancy. Behav Sleep Med 15(5):377–393, 2017 27124405
Trauer JM, Qian MY, Doyle JS, et al: Cognitive behavioral therapy for chronic insomnia: a systematic review and meta-analysis. Ann Intern Med 163(3):191–204, 2015 26054060
Tuohy A, McVey C: Subscales measuring symptoms of non-specific depression, anhedonia, and anxiety in the Edinburgh Postnatal Depression Scale. Br J Clin Psychol 47(pt 2):153–169, 2008
Uguz F, Sonmez EO, Sahingoz M, et al: Maternal generalized anxiety disorder during pregnancy and fetal brain development: a comparative study on cord blood brain-derived neurotrophic factor levels. J Psychosom Res 75(4):346–350, 2013 24119941
Van Batenburg-Eddes T, Brion MJ, Henrichs J, et al: Parental depressive and anxiety symptoms during pregnancy and attention problems in children: a cross-cohort consistency study. J Child Psychol Psychiatry 54(5):591–600, 2013 23215861
Van den Bergh BR: The influence of maternal emotions during pregnancy on fetal and neonatal behavior. J Prenat Perinat Psychol Health 5(2):119–130, 1990
Van den Bergh BR, Marcoen A: High antenatal maternal anxiety is related to ADHD symptoms, externalizing problems, and anxiety in 8- and 9-year-olds. Child Dev 75(4):1085–1097, 2004
Van den Bergh BR, Mennes M, Oosterlaan J, et al: High antenatal maternal anxiety is related to impulsivity during performance on cognitive tasks in 14- and 15-year-olds. Neurosci Biobehav Rev 29(2):259–269, 2005 15811497

Verreault N, Da Costa D, Marchand A, et al: Rates and risk factors associated with depressive symptoms during pregnancy and with postpartum onset. J Psychosom Obstet Gynaecol 35(3):84–91, 2014 25123985
Vignato J, Georges JM, Bush RA, et al: Post-traumatic stress disorder in the perinatal period: a concept analysis. J Clin Nurs 26(23–24):3859–3868, 2017 28295746
Vigod SN, Dennis CL: Benzodiazepines and the Z-drugs in pregnancy: reasonably reassuring for neurodevelopment but should we really be using them? JAMA Netw Open 2(4):e191430, 2019 30951151
Wadhwa PD, Sandman CA, Porto M, et al: The association between prenatal stress and infant birth weight and gestational age at birth: a prospective investigation. Am J Obstet Gynecol 169(4):858–865, 1993 8238139
Wall-Wieler E, Robakis TK, Lyell DJ, et al: Benzodiazepine use before conception and risk of ectopic pregnancy. Hum Reprod 35(7):1685–1692, 2020 32485732
Walsh JK: Clinical and socioeconomic correlates of insomnia. J Clin Psychiatry 65(suppl 8):13–19, 2004 15153063
Wang LH, Lin HC, Lin CC, et al: Increased risk of adverse pregnancy outcomes in women receiving zolpidem during pregnancy. Clin Pharmacol Ther 88(3):369–374, 2010 20686480
Wenzel A, Stuart SC: Anxiety in Childbearing Women: Diagnosis and Treatment. Washington, DC, American Psychological Association, 2011
Wikner BN, Källén B: Are hypnotic benzodiazepine receptor agonists teratogenic in humans? J Clin Psychopharmacol 31(3):356–359, 2011 21508851
Wikner BN, Stiller CO, Bergman U, et al: Use of benzodiazepines and benzodiazepine receptor agonists during pregnancy: neonatal outcome and congenital malformations. Pharmacoepidemiol Drug Saf 16(11):1203–1210, 2007 17894421
Wilson N, Wynter K, Anderson C, et al: More than depression: a multi-dimensional assessment of postpartum distress symptoms before and after a residential early parenting program. BMC Psychiatry 19(1):48, 2019 30696418
Wilton LV, Pearce GL, Martin RM, et al: The outcomes of pregnancy in women exposed to newly marketed drugs in general practice in England. Br J Obstet Gynaecol 105(8):882–889, 1998
Wisner KL, Hanusa BH, Perel JM, et al: Postpartum depression: a randomized trial of sertraline versus nortriptyline. J Clin Psychopharmacol 26(4):353–360, 2006 16855451
Wisner KL, Sit DK, Hanusa BH, et al: Major depression and antidepressant treatment: impact on pregnancy and neonatal outcomes. Am J Psychiatry 166(5):557–566, 2009 19289451
Wisner KL, Sit DK, McShea MC, et al: Onset timing, thoughts of self-harm, and diagnoses in postpartum women with screen-positive depression findings. JAMA Psychiatry 70(5):490–498, 2013 23487258
Wołynczyk-Gmaj D, Rózanska-Waledziak A, Ziemka S, et al: Insomnia in pregnancy is associated with depressive symptoms and eating at night. J Clin Sleep Med 13(10):1171–1176, 2017 28859715
Zemestani M, Fazeli Nikoo Z: Effectiveness of mindfulness-based cognitive therapy for comorbid depression and anxiety in pregnancy: a randomized controlled trial. Arch Women Ment Health 23(2):207–214, 2020 30982086
Zhu CS, Tan TC, Chen HY, et al: Threatened miscarriage and depressive and anxiety symptoms among women and partners in early pregnancy. J Affect Disord 237:1–9, 2018 29754019
Zigmond AS, Snaith RP: The hospital anxiety and depression scale. Acta Psychiatr Scand 67(6):361–370, 1983 6880820

CHAPTER 20

# Obsessive-Compulsive Disorder

Neha S. Hudepohl, M.D.
Nicole Leistikow, M.D.
Mimi Levine, M.D.
Lauren M. Osborne, M.D.

OCD is a debilitating illness that affects 1.6% of the general population, with a reported range of 0.7%–2.3% across different age demographics (McGuinness et al. 2011). Subthreshold OCD symptoms have been reported in 6% of the primary care population (Chaudron and Nirodi 2010). OCD is consistently reported to be more common in adult women than in adult men (Fontenelle et al. 2006). During times of reproductive transition, the risk of OCD rises above that of the general population. It is hypothesized that changes in gonadal hormone levels and their impact on the serotonin system may play an etiological role in vulnerable populations (Abramowitz et al. 2010a). This, along with genetic factors and the psychological, social, and physical stressors of transitioning to motherhood, leads to an increased risk of obsessive and compulsive symptoms in the perinatal period. Some women meet full criteria for the disorder, but other women have symptoms as part of mood or anxiety disorders. One study of women in a perinatal day hospital found that more than 30% had obsessions, but only 3.9% met criteria for OCD (Schofield et al. 2014).

This chapter focuses on the epidemiology, clinical features, etiology, and treatment of OCD at times of reproductive transition, with particular emphasis on OCD in the perinatal period. Many features of OCD in general apply to the illness during these time periods; although touching on aspects of general OCD is necessary, the content in this chapter largely focuses on the unique aspects of OCD during times of reproductive transition.

# Epidemiology

## Rates/Incidence

OCD has a prevalence of 0.7%–2.3% in the general population, a lifetime prevalence of up to 3.5%, and is the 10th leading cause of disability worldwide (American Psychiatric Association 2013; Kessler et al. 2005; McGuinness et al. 2011; Murray and Lopez 1996; Stein et al. 1997). The illness is likely underdiagnosed, and in the general population, as many as 25% of people experience obsessive and compulsive symptoms that do not rise to the level of diagnosis but can still be clinically significant and impairing (Kessler et al. 2005; Stein et al. 1997). Furthermore, prevalence rates vary based on region, population, and study methodology (McGuinness et al. 2011). OCD is more prevalent in adult women than in adult men (Fontenelle et al. 2006).

Times of reproductive transition, including menarche, perimenopause, and, most commonly, the perinatal period, represent high-risk periods for a subset of women for whom changes in gonadal hormone levels convey increased susceptibility to mood and anxiety symptoms (Abramowitz et al. 2010b). For example, 20%–49% of women with OCD report an exacerbation of symptoms in the premenstrual period (Uguz et al. 2011). Other studies show that 9% of women report onset of OCD symptoms in the perimenopausal period, and 47% of patients with preexisting OCD report exacerbation of symptoms in perimenopause (Labad et al. 2005; Uguz et al. 2007; Vulink et al. 2006). Many women trace the onset of their OCD symptoms to these periods (Abramowitz et al. 2003; Buttolph and Holland 1990; Labad et al. 2005; McGuinness et al. 2011; Neziroglu et al. 1992; Speisman et al. 2011), and the prevalence of OCD at these times is reported in various studies as higher than the prevalence for OCD in the general adult population (Andersson et al. 2003; Labad et al. 2005; McGuinness et al. 2011; Speisman et al. 2011; Sutter-Dallay et al. 2004; Uguz et al. 2007, 2011; Vulink et al. 2006).

In addition to triggering exacerbations, times of major reproductive transition often mark the onset of OCD in female patients. Onset of OCD has classically been associated with puberty, but some studies have shown the association to menarche specifically (Labad et al. 2005). Retrospective studies have shown that 13%–22% of female patients with OCD attribute onset of the illness to menarche (Russell et al. 2013). One study showed that patients with compulsive hoarding behaviors—which can be associated with OCD when the hoarding is a compulsive, compensatory behavior in response to obsessions that are typical of OCD (American Psychiatric Association 2002; Labad et al. 2010; Pertusa et al. 2008)—were more likely to report onset of symptoms within 12 months of menarche (Labad et al. 2010).

There is robust evidence of increased prevalence of both new-onset and exacerbated OCD in the postpartum period. Prevalence rates for pregnancy-related OCD have ranged from 0.2% to 3.5% (Andersson et al. 2003; McGuinness et al. 2011; Sutter-Dallay et al. 2004; Uguz et al. 2007) in various studies, and for postpartum OCD these rates have ranged from 2.3% to 9% (McGuinness et al. 2011; Uguz et al. 2007; Zambaldi et al. 2009). A 2013 meta-analysis showed that OCD prevalence estimates were higher among pregnant and postpartum women compared with the general population, and in this study the prevalence increased linearly from pregnancy to the postpartum period (Russell et al. 2013). Retrospective studies have shown that 2%–39% of female patients attribute the onset of OCD to pregnancy (Russell et al. 2013; Uguz et al. 2011). A larger body of literature examining cases of OCD in the postpartum period revealed that up to 50% of women with OCD have new-onset symptoms during this time (Maina et al. 1999; Russell et al. 2013; Vulink et al. 2006). Women with the onset or exacerbation of OCD during the perinatal period are also more likely to have an exacerbation of symptoms premenstrually, and vice versa (Forray et al. 2010; Russell et al. 2013; Uguz et al. 2011). Patients with a diagnosis of OCD will report pregnancy or the postpartum period as a precipitating stressor for exacerbation of their symptoms; this has been reported in 25%–70% of patients (Labad et al. 2005; Speisman et al. 2011). A 2007 prospective study of 302 women showed that at 6 weeks postpartum, 4% of women showed clinically significant obsessive-compulsive spectrum symptoms (Uguz et al. 2007). Similar results have been seen in other studies around the world (McGuinness et al. 2011).

OCD tends to be highly comorbid with other psychiatric disorders, including mood disorders and other anxiety disorders. Some studies cite the comorbidity with depression at 70.6% and with anxiety disorders at 27.5% (Sharma and Sommerdyk 2015). There are also some reports of comorbidity with bipolar disorder, but this is less well studied in the literature. Obsessive-compulsive symptoms are also more common in women with perinatal mood disorders and have been identified in women with these disorders even in the absence of full criteria for OCD (Abramowitz et al. 2010b).

## Risk Factors

Female sex and times of major reproductive transition are two major risk factors for the development of OCD. Other risk factors have been identified for OCD in general and for perinatal OCD specifically. For general OCD, family and twin studies show increased risk of OCD in families, and thus a genetic component to the illness is suggested (Vasconcelos et al. 2007). Environmental factors also appear to play a role in the development of OCD and are discussed later in this chapter. Gestational factors in pregnancy and parturition can influence the offspring's risk of developing OCD later in life. Obstetrical complications, in particular prolonged labor and edema during pregnancy, can be a risk factor for the development of OCD in the offspring (Vasconcelos et al. 2007). Delivery-related complications, such as the use of forceps, neonatal complications, preterm birth, breech presentation, and delivery by cesarean section, are also associated with an increased risk of OCD in offspring (Brander et al. 2016; Vasconcelos et al. 2007).

In addition, certain risk factors specific to pregnancy may exacerbate the risk of perinatal OCD. Obstetrical complications have been cited as a risk factor, but results vary among studies. Some studies have shown that primiparity, obstetrical complications, and mode of delivery are risk factors for development of postpartum OCD, but others have not shown these findings (Labad et al. 2005; Maina et al. 1999; McGuinness et al. 2011). Having family members with mood and substance use disorders (Sharma and Sommerdyk 2015) is also a risk factor for the development of postpartum OCD. First-time motherhood is a high-risk time for the development of obsessional thinking due to the new responsibilities associated with caring for an infant (Abramowitz et al. 2003; Fairbrother and Abramowitz 2007).

Past psychiatric history can also elevate the risk of perinatal OCD, especially a past history of major depressive disorder (Labad et al. 2005). Certain personality types, such

**TABLE 20–1. Screening methods for perinatal OCD**

| For obsessive-compulsive symptoms | For psychiatric comorbidities |
|---|---|
| Obsessive Compulsive Inventory–Revised | Edinburgh Postnatal Depression Scale |
| Perinatal Obsessive Compulsive Scale | Generalized Anxiety Disorder–7 |
| Yale-Brown Obsessive Compulsive Scale | Patient Health Questionnaire–9 |
| | Perinatal Anxiety Screening Scale |

as avoidant or obsessive-compulsive personality, may also elevate the risk of perinatal OCD (McGuinness et al. 2011; Uguz et al. 2007). The presence of OCD-related dysfunctional beliefs is also thought to be a risk factor in the cognitive-behavioral model of the illness (Abramowitz et al. 2003; Fairbrother and Abramowitz 2007; Sharma and Sommerdyk 2015).

## Screening Methods

Screening for perinatal OCD is similar to that for OCD in the general population, and screening tools are listed in Table 20–1. Commonly used tools include the Yale-Brown Obsessive Compulsive Scale (Y-BOCS; Goodman et al. 1989b, 1989c), Obsessive Compulsive Inventory–Revised (Foa et al. 2002), Dimensional Obsessive-Compulsive Scale (Abramowitz et al. 2010a), and Perinatal Obsessive Compulsive Scale (POCS), which is the only scale specific to obsessive and compulsive symptoms in the perinatal period (Chaudron and Nirodi 2010; Lord et al. 2011b). The Y-BOCS is considered the gold standard for screening and diagnosing OCD due to its psychometric properties (Chaudron and Nirodi 2010; Lord et al. 2011b). It can also be used to measure symptom severity and track treatment response over time (Hudak and Wisner 2012).

The POCS is a self-report scale developed to assess perinatal obsessions and compulsions that was validated in comparison with the Y-BOCS (Lord et al. 2011b). The pilot study revealed good construct validity, high internal consistency, concurrent validity, and discriminative capacity (Lord et al. 2011b; Sharma and Sommerdyk 2015). When compared with the Y-BOCS, the validation study for the POCS showed that perinatal women reported more overall symptoms and higher symptom severity using this instrument. It has both a prenatal and postpartum version, with questions on both thoughts and behaviors (Sharma and Sommerdyk 2015). Additionally, because it is a self-report scale, it allows perinatal women the opportunity to discuss these sensitive topics in an open way with their health care provider (Lord et al. 2011b).

Practitioners screening perinatal or postpartum women for depression should pay close attention to the presence of anxiety symptoms. Studies indicate that perinatal depression and anxiety and obsessive-compulsive symptoms are highly comorbid, yet traditional screening tools for symptoms of depression do not typically evaluate for anxiety symptoms (Abramowitz et al. 2010b). Furthermore, perinatal OCD is often misdiagnosed as depression or is comorbid with depression but not identified and, in both cases, is inadequately treated (Abramowitz et al. 2003; Speisman et al. 2011). If perinatal OCD is identified first, consider screening for comorbid mental illnesses with tools validated in the perinatal population, such as the Edinburgh Postnatal Depression Scale (EPDS) (Cox et al. 1987; Gaynes et al. 2005), the Patient Health Questionnaire–9 (Gjerdingen et al. 2009; Yawn et al. 2009), the Perinatal Anxiety Screening

Scale (Somerville et al. 2014, 2015), the Generalized Anxiety Disorder–7 (Simpson et al. 2014), or others. The EPDS contains questions specific to anxiety and can be used to identify the need for more comprehensive assessment of anxiety and obsessive-compulsive symptoms (Matthey 2008; Simpson et al. 2014). One prospective study, however, has shown that the presence of postpartum OCD can lead to false-positive EPDS scores (Mauri et al. 2010). This may affect potential diagnostic and treatment options for a patient.

# Clinical Features

## Diagnostic Criteria

The diagnostic criteria for OCD from DSM-5 (American Psychiatric Association 2013) are listed in Box 20–1 and are the same as the criteria for perinatal OCD. There is currently no specifier for "with peripartum onset" for the diagnosis of OCD in DSM-5; the manual does, however, discuss the possible onset and exacerbation of OCD symptoms and symptoms that can interfere with the mother–infant relationship in the peripartum period. Perinatal OCD has its onset during pregnancy or within the first postpartum year, with the most common time of within the first 4 weeks following delivery (Sharma and Sommerdyk 2015).

### Box 20–1. DSM-5 Criteria for Obsessive-Compulsive Disorder

A. Presence of obsessions, compulsions, or both:

Obsessions are defined by (1) and (2):

1. Recurrent and persistent thoughts, urges, or images that are experienced, at some time during the disturbance, as intrusive and unwanted, and that in most individuals cause marked anxiety or distress.
2. The individual attempts to ignore or suppress such thoughts, urges, or images, or to neutralize them with some other thought or action (i.e., by performing a compulsion).

Compulsions are defined by (1) and (2):

1. Repetitive behaviors (e.g., hand washing, ordering, checking) or mental acts (e.g., praying, counting, repeating words silently) that the individual feels driven to perform in response to an obsession or according to rules that must be applied rigidly.
2. The behaviors or mental acts are aimed at preventing or reducing anxiety or distress, or preventing some dreaded event or situation; however, these behaviors or mental acts are not connected in a realistic way with what they are designed to neutralize or prevent, or are clearly excessive.

   **Note:** Young children may not be able to articulate the aims of these behaviors or mental acts.

B. The obsessions or compulsions are time-consuming (e.g., take more than 1 hour per day) or cause clinically significant distress or impairment in social, occupational, or other important areas of functioning.

C. The obsessive-compulsive symptoms are not attributable to the physiological effects of a substance (e.g., a drug of abuse, a medication) or another medical condition.

D. The disturbance is not better explained by the symptoms of another mental disorder (e.g., excessive worries, as in generalized anxiety disorder; preoccupation with appearance, as in body dysmorphic disorder; difficulty discarding or parting with possessions, as in hoarding disorder; hair pulling, as in trichotillomania [hair-pulling disorder]; skin picking, as in excoriation [skin-picking] disorder; stereotypies, as in stereotypic movement disorder; ritualized eating behavior, as in eating disorders; preoccupation with substances or gambling, as in substance-related and addictive disorders; preoccupation with having an illness, as in illness anxiety disorder; sexual urges or fantasies, as in paraphilic disorders; impulses, as in disruptive, impulse-control, and conduct disorders; guilty ruminations, as in major depressive disorder; thought insertion or delusional preoccupations, as in schizophrenia spectrum and other psychotic disorders; or repetitive patterns of behavior, as in autism spectrum disorder).

*Specify* if:

**With good or fair insight:** The individual recognizes that obsessive-compulsive disorder beliefs are definitely or probably not true or that they may or may not be true.

**With poor insight:** The individual thinks obsessive-compulsive disorder beliefs are probably true.

**With absent insight/delusional beliefs:** The individual is completely convinced that obsessive-compulsive disorder beliefs are true.

*Specify* if:

**Tic-related:** The individual has a current or past history of a tic disorder.

*Source.* Reprinted from American Psychiatric Association: *Diagnostic and Statistical Manual of Mental Disorders*, 5th Edition. Arlington, VA, 2013, p. 237. 

## Clinical Presentation

OCD is characterized by obsessions (intrusive thoughts, ideas, images, or impulses), compulsions (repetitive or ritualistic behaviors), or a combination of both. Symptoms are time consuming and cause clinically significant distress in important areas of functioning, as well as in family life (Abramowitz et al. 2010b; Albert et al. 2010; Challacombe et al. 2016; Gezginç et al. 2008). OCD can present with variable levels of insight (American Psychiatric Association 2013), but in postpartum women, insight is typically preserved (Hudak and Wisner 2012). The symptoms cannot be better explained by another medical, substance, or psychiatric condition (American Psychiatric Association 2013). OCD with onset at menarche or in the premenstrual period has symptoms similar to those of OCD at other time points in a woman's life or in other populations; no specific studies have yet looked at differences in clinical presentation in this context.

OCD in the peripartum period typically presents with intrusive thoughts and images, often concerning infant harm (Abramowitz et al. 2003; McGuinness et al. 2011; Speisman et al. 2011). Postpartum women with OCD report more aggressive intrusive thoughts than nonpostpartum women with OCD (Hudak and Wisner 2012; Wisner et al. 1999). Typical symptoms with onset during pregnancy can include contamination obsessions, with compulsive cleaning and washing rituals that serve to "neutralize" the obsessions (Forray et al. 2010; McGuinness et al. 2011). In the postpartum period, obsessions often center around ego-dystonic thoughts of infant harm and are accompanied by avoidance and checking compulsions. Thoughts of infant harm can include both thoughts of inadvertent harm to the infant and intrusive thoughts of deliberate harm to the infant (Hudak and Wisner 2012; Sichel et al. 1993b). Obsessions can present as graphic visual images that cause extreme distress in the mother. Content can at times be violent or sexual in nature and can lead to shame and fear in the mother and family (Abramowitz et al. 2003; Forray et al. 2010; Hudak and Wisner 2012). Such thoughts may not be readily disclosed to a psychiatric provider for fear that the infant will be removed or the mother will be placed in involuntary psychiatric hospitalization. These thoughts are distinguished from infanticidal ideation or psychotic delusions by their ego-dystonic nature and preserved insight; they are experienced as unwanted, extremely distressing, and uncomfortable to the patient (Table 20–2) (Abramowitz et al. 2003; Forray et al. 2010; McGuinness et al. 2011; Speisman et al. 2011).

Compulsions in this population typically take the form of contamination-related rituals, such as cleaning or sterilizing baby-related equipment, or of checking and ordering rituals, such as repetitively checking on a sleeping infant (Hudak and Wisner 2012; Speisman et al. 2011). Checking compulsions are the most frequently reported symptom in postpartum women with OCD (Hudak and Wisner 2012). Women frequently check to ensure that they have not harmed the infant (in the case of intrusive thoughts of infant harm), to ensure the infant is still breathing, or to ensure that no harm has befallen the infant. At times, the obsessions can be so extreme as to lead to avoidance of the infant or of common situations or activities that provoke intrusive thoughts, as opposed to true ritualistic behavior (Hudak and Wisner 2012; Koran et al. 2007). Women may avoid such activities as bathing or diapering, avoid objects such as kitchen knives and stairs, or limit contact with the infant in general.

Although acting on urges to harm an infant in perinatal OCD is rare, indirect harm is possible; for example, the patient may avoid or neglect the child, "clean" the child inappropriately with bleach or other harmful substances, or insist on inappropriate neatness (Koran et al. 2007). Rarely, patients can become aggressive when others interfere with their compulsions. In such cases, or any other cases in which the clinician has significant safety concerns, it may be necessary to involve social agencies. Regardless of imminent involvement, a thorough discussion about the role of social agencies is important given the degree to which patients fear legal action and avoid help as a result.

The symptoms and severity of perinatal-onset OCD are time-consuming and distressing. They can often detract from mother–infant bonding and can lead to long-term impairments in attachment patterns (Arnold 1999; Challacombe and Salkovskis 2009). Women with worsening OCD symptoms in the premenstrual or postpartum period frequently have comorbid mood symptoms (Uguz et al. 2011; Wisner et al. 1999) and more frequently report a history of premenstrual worsening of mood symptoms, major depressive disorder, or postpartum depression (PPD) (Labad et al. 2005).

Intrusive thoughts are not specific to perinatal OCD; they have also been reported under normal circumstances and in other perinatal mental health conditions, most specifically PPD (Abramowitz et al. 2003, 2010b; McGuinness et al. 2011; Wisner et al. 1999). Many reports have suggested that such thoughts are common in new parents and do not represent psychopathology when they are experienced as fleeting and momentary. These symptoms can include subthreshold intrusive, distressing, and unwanted thoughts that involve themes of safety, contamination, or harm coming to loved ones (particularly the infant) or even thoughts of harming, shaking, or hitting the infant, especially at times when the infant is difficult to console (McGuinness et al. 2011; Wisner et al. 1999). The thoughts are typically fleeting in nature and do not interfere with normal daily functioning. They have been reported in as many as 34%–

TABLE 20–2. **Risk of postpartum mother harming her infant as determined by assessment of origin, quality, and content of thoughts**

| Secondary to obsessions/anxiety | Secondary to PPP/suspected PPP |
| --- | --- |
| Good insight | Poor insight |
| No psychotic symptoms | Psychotic symptoms |
| Thoughts are intrusive and scary and/or cause anxiety | Delusional beliefs with distortion of reality present |
| Suggests *not* at risk of harming baby | Suggests *is* at risk of harming baby |

PPP=postpartum psychosis.

65% of women after delivery (Abramowitz et al. 2003; Sharma and Sommerdyk 2015). At other times, these symptoms are comorbid with other perinatal mental health disorders, including PPD and other mood disorders (Abramowitz et al. 2010b). Obsessions involving harming the infant have been reported in 57% of women with PPD (Sharma and Sommerdyk 2015).

## Course/Prognosis

The onset of postpartum OCD tends to be variable; approximately half of women experience symptoms abruptly, and the other half have a more gradual onset (Maina et al. 1999; Speisman et al. 2011). OCD tends to have a chronic course over time. Few studies have looked at the course and prognosis of perinatal OCD specifically. A 2011 study showed that women with preexisting OCD who experience worsening symptoms in the perinatal period have a significantly worse course of illness in the presence of comorbid major depressive disorder or an anxiety disorder (Uguz et al. 2011). Depression in particular is associated with a more chronic course of illness and poorer outcomes (Sharma and Sommerdyk 2015; Uguz et al. 2011).

Perinatal OCD is associated with impaired mother–infant relationships and may be associated with impaired attachment patterns and neurodevelopment of infants in extreme cases. Mother–infant interactions have been shown to be affected by early maternal anxiety in several studies (Feldman et al. 2009; Nicol-Harper et al. 2007; Warren et al. 2003). One study comparing postpartum mothers with OCD and their infants with control dyads showed that mothers with OCD were often less confident and reported increased marital distress and less social support than peers (Challacombe et al. 2016), but little research has been done in this area. Breastfeeding rates tend to be lower in postpartum women with OCD. In dyadic observation, mothers with OCD have been rated as less sensitive to infant needs, which is consistent with maternal anxiety disorders in the postpartum period (Challacombe et al. 2016). Mothers with OCD also tend to perceive the quality of their mother–infant relationship as more negative and report finding it difficult to enjoy time with their infant (Challacombe and Salkovskis 2009). One case series showed impairment in mother–infant interactions in 71% of the sample, with the presence of either underinvolvement (avoidance of the infant) or overinvolvement (overprotective care of the infant) (Arnold 1999). Some of these interactions can also be attributed to comorbid PPD.

**TABLE 20–3. Differential diagnosis of perinatal OCD**

| | |
|---|---|
| Generalized anxiety disorder | Normal obsessions, intrusive thoughts, or compulsions in the perinatal period |
| Major depressive disorder with obsessions and compulsions | Obsessive-compulsive personality disorder |
| Medical comorbidity | Postpartum psychosis |

## Evaluation and Differential Diagnosis

In addition to using the screening scales mentioned earlier, psychiatric practitioners must adequately rule out common medical comorbidities that might mimic or exacerbate obsessive and compulsive symptoms in the perinatal patient. In particular, practitioners should conduct a thorough medical history and physical examination, supplemented with laboratory studies when indicated. Referral to the patient's obstetrical provider or other appropriate specialist is indicated with any abnormality in history, physical examination, or laboratory evaluation.

The differential diagnosis of OCD in the perinatal period is listed in Table 20–3 (Sharma and Sommerdyk 2015). OCD in the postpartum period is often misdiagnosed as either generalized anxiety disorder (GAD) or PPD. The primary difference between OCD and GAD is the nature of the thoughts; in GAD, thoughts focus on worry over routine events and are characterized by apprehension and catastrophic thinking. Obsessional thinking is common in PPD. Perinatal depression typically presents with classic depressive symptoms, including sadness or a feeling of being numb or detached; neurovegetative symptoms, such as altered sleep, appetite, and energy; and, at times, the presence of hopelessness or suicidal ideation (see Chapter 13, "Depressive Disorders"). It can also present with high levels of comorbid anxiety that can include panic attacks, anxious rumination, psychomotor agitation, and even obsessions. Perinatal depression with obsessions presents with depressive ruminations, content reflective of real-life circumstances and worries, and typically shifts in content over time; perinatal OCD, on the other hand, presents with senseless intrusive thoughts and concern about disastrous outcomes, with content that is stable over time (Abramowitz et al. 2003; Wisner et al. 1999). Depression is often erroneously diagnosed when OCD is the primary diagnosis (Abramowitz et al. 2010b). The crucial implication of this difference is inadequate treatment choices; depression and OCD are often both treated with selective serotonin reuptake inhibitors (SSRIs), but OCD typically requires more aggressive dosing and exposure therapy (Abramowitz et al. 2010b).

An important distinction must be made between postpartum OCD and postpartum psychosis (PPP), especially in the context of thoughts about harming the infant. Women with perinatal OCD can have intrusive thoughts or obsessions of harm befalling or of harming their infants (Hudak and Wisner 2012). These thoughts can be distinguished from infanticidal ideation, more common in PPP, by their ego-dystonic nature, the level of distress in the woman, and the preservation of insight. Women with perinatal OCD and thoughts of harming their infant typically experience extreme distress from these thoughts, often going to extreme lengths to protect or even avoid their infants (Hudak and Wisner 2012). Insight is typically preserved. In contrast, thoughts of harming the infant in PPP are characterized by delusional beliefs and absent insight. PPP is most commonly a manifestation of bipolar disorder, but a postpartum-only variant is increasingly being recognized (Bergink et al. 2016). Perceptual disturbances are typically not present in perinatal OCD, whereas they are common in PPP. In the case of ego-dystonic, intrusive thoughts of infant harm, it is not recommended to separate mother and infant but, rather, to treat the mother using evidence-based treatment options for OCD, such as exposure and response prevention (ERP) in a higher level of care (i.e., partial hospitalization or inpatient hospitalization when indicated) (Challacombe and Salkovskis 2009; Howard et al. 2006). Nonetheless, evaluating psychiatrists must screen carefully for infanticidal ideation and take the necessary precautions to ensure the safety of both mother and infant.

### Sociodemographic Considerations

OCD in general has a similar age of onset, gender distribution, and psychiatric comorbidity across the world, and the general symptom structure tends to be consistent (American Psychiatric Association 2013). Cultural and religious variation exists, however, in the subjective experience, course, and outcome of OCD across differing contexts (Stein and Rapoport 1996). The literature regarding sociodemographic considerations of OCD at times of reproductive transition is insufficient. Studies looking at populations outside of the United States show similar patterns of OCD in pregnancy and the postpartum period, as well as higher rates of onset and exacerbation of OCD symptoms at other times of reproductive transition (McGuinness et al. 2011). Few data have been published on racial, socioeconomic, or other characteristics specific to perinatal OCD. More research is needed into these important considerations to facilitate improved understanding, detection, and treatment of these illnesses.

## Pathophysiology

### Biological

There are few published studies about the biological contributors to the pathophysiology of perinatal OCD (Lord et al. 2011a; Serati et al. 2015). However, numerous studies have linked various biological systems to obsessions and compulsions in the general population, and others have linked biological systems to mood and anxiety symptoms in the perinatal period. By examining these two related types of symptoms, we may arrive at some hypotheses concerning the biological etiology of perinatal OCD.

#### Genetic Factors

No large-scale studies of genetic factors in perinatal OCD have yet been published. One case report of a woman with new-onset OCD in the postpartum period reported an incidentally found deletion (9q33.1) in genes affecting systemic inflammation and glial-guided neuronal migration; the same deletion has been associated with general OCD and with autism, ADHD, and other psychiatric problems (Serati et al. 2015). A substantial body of literature connects genetic factors in general OCD, with the most consistent findings for serotonin transporter polymorphism *5-HTTLPR* and *HTR2A*

**TABLE 20–4. Genes with potential application to perinatal OCD**

| Genes implicated in both OCD and postpartum depression | Strength of evidence |
|---|---|
| *BDNF* | Weak |
| *COMT* | Weak |
| *ESR1* | Weak |
| *5-HTTLPR* | Medium |
| *MAOA* | Weak |
| *OXTR* | Weak |

polymorphism rs6311 (or rs6313) (Corregiari et al. 2012; Mak et al. 2015; Sinopoli et al. 2017). (For a complete review, see Standeven et al. 2020). The most promising avenue for future genetic research on perinatal OCD may lie in those genes that are overlapping in research on general OCD and on perinatal mood and anxiety disorders. The National Institute of Mental Health Genetics Initiative Bipolar Disorder project and the Genetics of Recurrent Early Onset Depression study found maximum linkage peaks for postpartum depressive symptoms on chromosomes 1q21.3–q32.1 and 9p24.3–p22.3, which have also been implicated in general OCD (Mahon et al. 2009). The *5-HTTLPR* polymorphisms implicated in general OCD have also been implicated in PPD with onset within 6–8 weeks after delivery (McEvoy et al. 2017). Polymorphisms in the gene for catechol-*O*-methyltransferase (*COMT*), the enzyme that breaks down catecholamines, have been noted and replicated in general OCD and have been noted in PPD (Pooley et al. 2007; Taylor 2013). Some studies have implicated a polymorphism in the monoamine oxidase A (*MAOA*) gene in both OCD (with possible differences by sex) and PPD, but other studies have not found this association, and no consensus has yet been reached (Camarena et al. 2001; Lochner et al. 2004; McEvoy et al. 2017). Similarly, brain-derived neurotrophic factor (*BDNF*) (Hall et al. 2003; Katerberg et al. 2009; McEvoy et al. 2017), the estrogen receptor α (*ESR1*) (Alonso et al. 2011; McEvoy et al. 2017), and the oxytocin receptor (*OXTR*) (Kang et al. 2017) have all been studied in both general OCD and PPD, but with contradictory results and no clear application to the genetics of perinatal OCD (Table 20–4).

## Neurotransmitters and the Cortico-Striato-Thalamo-Cortical Circuitry

Gene polymorphisms in the serotonin transporter are not the only evidence linking the serotonin system to general OCD—although again, direct evidence for the perinatal period is lacking. Animal research has shown decreases in serotonin levels in the medial prefrontal cortex in mice with a compulsive phenotype as compared with healthy mice (Winter et al. 2018), and human research has shown abnormalities in the serotonin transporter system in patients with OCD, both through peripheral markers (Delorme et al. 2005) and through PET studies of transporter binding (Spies et al. 2015). Some studies have also found higher concentrations of 5-HIAA, serotonin's chief metabolite, in subjects with OCD, but this finding has been inconsistent and cannot be relied on to support a causal role for serotonin (Winter et al. 2018). Perhaps the most compelling evidence comes from studies showing that antidepressants that affect the serotonin system are more efficacious than those that do not (Stein et al. 2012)—a finding that is also known in reproductive mood disorders, such as premenstrual dysphoric disorder (Sepede et al. 2016).

Most evidence shows that the serotonergic deficit affects chiefly the cortico-striato-thalamo-cortical circuitry, with studies implicating both markers of the serotonin system (e.g., auditory evoked potentials) (Mavorgiorgou et al. 2010) and imaging of transporter availability (Pogarell et al. 2003). Other studies targeting the same brain circuitry have shown a possible role for other neurotransmitters, including glutamate (Pittenger et al. 2011) and GABA (Wang et al. 2014; Winter et al. 2018). Recent studies have shown altered levels of GABA in the anterior cingulate cortex (Li et al. 2019 and orbitofrontal cortex (Zhang et al. 2016) of subjects with OCD compared with healthy subjects, but studies to date are contradictory (some higher, some lower), so the most we can say at this point is that GABA dysregulation may be at work. The role of GABA is especially intriguing in the perinatal context because of the substantial evidence that allopregnanolone, a progesterone metabolite that is a potent allosteric modulator of the $GABA_A$ receptor, may play an important role in perinatal mood and anxiety disorders (McEvoy and Osborne 2019; Meltzer-Brody et al. 2018; Osborne et al. 2017).

## Stress Response System

Several studies have examined dysregulation of the stress response system in general OCD, with mixed results. There is some consensus that the circadian pattern is unchanged, but people with OCD exhibit a higher basal level of cortisol than healthy control subjects (Kluge et al. 2007; Monteleone et al. 1994). In a small pilot study, Lord et al. (2011a) compared the response to a psychological stressor (cold pressor test) between women with postpartum OCD and healthy postpartum control subjects and found that women with OCD had higher basal salivary levels. Although their levels remained higher throughout the stressor, they did not as a group show a greater stress response than the healthy women (either by cortisol or by salivary alpha amylase), indicating that perhaps *some* women with postpartum OCD have a delayed or exaggerated stress response. Women with OCD were also more stressed and anxious overall and rated the stressor test higher in subjective stress than did healthy control subjects. Thus, evidence does not now exist for an overall altered stress response system in perinatal OCD but, rather, for an alteration that may affect only a subset of women.

## Thyroid Hormone and Oxytocin

No studies have examined the role of thyroid dysregulation in perinatal OCD. There is evidence of thyroid dysfunction in children and adolescents with general OCD (McCracken and Hanna 2005), in individuals with anxiety and trauma-related disorders (Friedman et al. 2005; Ittermann et al. 2015), and in PPD and PPP (Bergink et al. 2011, 2018; Dama et al. 2016; Pedersen et al. 2016; Wesseloo et al. 2018), making this a ripe area for research in perinatal OCD. Some studies have looked at the role of oxytocin, but the data are limited, and results are mixed. Some animal studies have associated elevated oxytocin with fewer compulsive-like behaviors (Mitra et al. 2017), and one human study found that OCD subjects had higher overall oxytocin levels than healthy control subjects (but that within the OCD group, lower oxytocin was associated with more severe symptoms) (Marazziti et al. 2012). Another group found that baseline oxytocin levels were positively correlated with obsessive-compulsive symptoms in people with OCD but only among those who would go on to respond to SSRIs (Humble et al. 2013), indicating interplay between the oxytocin and serotonin systems and possible different endophenotypes in subjects with OCD. No human studies have looked specifically at the role of oxytocin in perinatal OCD.

## Reproductive Hormones

The dramatic shift that occurs in reproductive hormones across pregnancy and especially at childbirth may also be related to the biology of perinatal OCD. As mentioned, some evidence supports a role for estrogen through polymorphisms in the *ESR1* gene that have been linked to contamination and cleaning symptoms in patients with OCD (Labad et al. 2011) and to symptoms of both premenstrual dysphoric disorder and PPD (McEvoy and Osborne 2019). Animal literature supports a role for estrogen, with studies linking estradiol withdrawal or lack of estradiol to anxiety-like and compulsive-like behaviors (Flaisher-Grinberg et al. 2009; Hill et al. 2007; Mitra et al. 2016). Because estrogen increases serotonin synthesis, it is possible that estrogen withdrawal at delivery could lead to a drop in serotonin. Progesterone also changes rapidly across the peripartum, and although there is no evidence that progesterone levels themselves are implicated in peripartum OCD, considerable evidence has shown dysregulation of its metabolite, allopregnanolone, in perinatal mood and anxiety symptoms (McEvoy and Osborne 2019).

## Immune System

The final biological area that may plausibly be related to perinatal OCD is the immune system. The peripartum is a time of substantial changes in the immune system, with innate immune barriers enhanced but some aspects of adaptive immunity weakened; this changes across the peripartum to allow for necessary changes in inflammatory status that permit implantation early on, retention of the fetus throughout, and parturition. Although no studies have focused on the contribution of the immune system to perinatal OCD, there is substantial evidence for its contribution to both perinatal mood and anxiety disorders and to general OCD. This research covers autoantibodies and other markers of autoimmune illness (Cosco et al. 2019; Pearlman et al. 2014; Sharma et al. 2011); peripheral inflammatory markers, including tumor necrosis factor (TNF)-$\alpha$, interleukin (IL)-6, C-C motif chemokine 3, IL-8, soluble TNF receptors 1 and 2, and IL-1$\beta$, with the strongest evidence for IL-6 (Fluitman et al. 2010; Gray and Bloch 2012; Osborne and Monk 2013; Osborne et al. 2019b); leukocyte subpopulations (Kant et al. 2018; Marazziti et al. 1999, 2009; Osborne et al. 2019a; Ravindran et al. 1999); and effects of treatment on immune functioning (Marazziti et al. 2009). The evidence overall is mixed, in part due to a lack of coordination among studies, which use different markers of immune functioning and of psychiatric symptoms, making comparisons challenging.

Thus, although there are promising areas of research for the biological origins of perinatal OCD, including genetic factors, the stress response system, hormonal factors, and the immune system, the data at this point are too few to be able to point to a cause or set of causes. In most cases, we have not even established an association yet in the perinatal period, so it will be many years before we can greatly advance our understanding of the biological etiology of perinatal OCD.

# Psychosocial Precipitants

In addition to biological factors, several psychological, behavioral, cultural, and medical factors may contribute to the perinatal onset or exacerbation of OCD. These include overvaluing fears pertaining to the infant, performing repetitive behaviors to protect the infant that exacerbate fears, sleep deprivation (which also has biological consequences), and coping with medical comorbidities such as autoimmune diseases (Maina et al. 1999).

## Fear of Infant Harm

Mild obsessive-compulsive symptoms are widespread and normative among new parents, with both fathers and mothers in several studies reporting unwanted intrusive thoughts about causing harm, both accidental and intentional, to their baby and trying strategies to get rid of these thoughts (Abramowitz et al. 2003, 2006; Collardeau et al. 2019; Fairbrother and Woody 2008). The ubiquity of postpartum intrusive fears of infant harm and preventative behaviors, as well as their genetic and biological basis, has led theorists to hypothesize that such thoughts may have conferred evolutionary survival value in the past, perhaps by increasing vigilance to danger or protective behaviors in settings that were more threatening than are typical in modern times (Ross and McLean 2006). Unfortunately, in a vulnerable subset of women, intrusive thoughts around fear of infant harm can grow out of control, becoming more frequent, lasting, and severe.

Thoughts of intentional harm to the infant are universally more distressing than thoughts of accidental harm (Fairbrother and Woody 2008). In addition to other risk factors already discussed, psychologists following a cognitive-behavioral model have identified several dysfunctional attitudes or beliefs that may contribute to intrusive thoughts becoming obsessions. Studies suggest that those who are more at risk of developing worse symptoms have tendencies toward perfectionism or hyperresponsibility, overestimate the importance of their thoughts and interpret them as dangerous threats, and feel a need to control or extinguish these thoughts (Abramowitz et al. 2006; Fairbrother and Woody 2008). One prospective study of first-time parents found that negative interpretations of unwanted intrusive thoughts within the first month postpartum was predictive of worse obsessive-compulsive symptoms at 12 weeks postpartum (Abramowitz et al. 2007).

## Repetitive Behaviors

As intrusive thoughts grow more distressing, women commonly take protective measure in response to these thoughts, a tendency that is natural yet maladaptive, exacerbating rather than ameliorating symptoms. Typical repetitive behaviors to protect the baby can include avoiding spending time with the baby, checking on a sleeping baby more often than necessary, taking unnecessary precautions with the baby, and developing time-consuming cleaning rituals. Both avoidance and other compulsive behaviors contribute to the cycle of intrusive thoughts: they result in a short-term reduction in anxiety caused by the thought, reinforce the thought's significance by deeming it worth acting on (negatively interpreting a harmless thought as a threat), and trigger the thought to recur, which in turn triggers a compensatory or neutralizing behavior, renewing the cycle. Psychotherapy treatments, discussed later, focus on preventing ritualized responses or avoidance when distressing thoughts arise in order to decrease the significance accorded them. Therapy also focuses on attempting to reduce the need to control or extinguish the thoughts (Timpano et al. 2011). Shame or fear and concealment around sharing these thoughts with others is also thought to contribute to their maintenance (Newth and Rachman 2001).

## Sleep Deprivation

In addition to dysfunctional beliefs and behaviors, sleep deprivation postpartum (whether via modulation of hormonal or immunological factors or via separate mechanisms) is likely a strong risk factor for obsessive-compulsive symptoms in vulnerable women. At least one study has shown that most women with OCD onset or exacerbation postpartum also have concomitant anxiety or mood disorders, which may drive sleep disturbances or be exacerbated by them (Arnold 1999; Miller et al. 2013). OCD, outside of the postpartum period, has been associated with reduced sleep duration, more frequent sleep interruptions, delayed sleep phase disorder, and rapid eye movement sleep disturbances, potentially making postpartum women who are vulnerable to OCD even more sensitive to the typical sleep impairment that comes from participating in overnight infant care and lactation (Nordahl et al. 2018; Paterson et al. 2013; Sharma 2019).

Protecting healthy sleep behaviors from postpartum obsessive-compulsive symptoms is an added challenge. Extrapolating from research on general OCD, which has found that both obsessions and compulsions can compete with sleep, postpartum obsessions involving worry about the baby may make it hard to resume sleep after interruptions for overnight care, and compulsive behaviors common to postpartum OCD, such as checking on an infant while sleeping or cleaning to avoid contamination, may decrease the hours available to sleep by using up time (Sharma 2019; Timpano et al. 2014). Cultural expectations around a woman's role as primary caregiver, especially overnight, may make it harder for women to ask for assistance in protecting their own sleep. In cultures that prioritize work outside of the home, women staying home with the baby in the immediate postpartum may err in protecting the sleep of their partners leaving for jobs; arguably the prioritization should be flipped in the postpartum period to preserve sleep as much as possible for women at risk for mental illness. Regardless of its cause, sleep deprivation can both trigger and sustain obsessive-compulsive symptoms (Sharma 2019).

Coping with medical comorbidities, such as autoimmune diseases, and their treatment may also ignite flares of OCD in the postpartum. A large registry-based study found that women with OCD are more likely to have any autoimmune disease, with the top five associations being found for Sjogren's syndrome, celiac disease, Guillain-Barré syndrome, Crohn's disease, and Hashimoto's thyroiditis (Mataix-Cols et al. 2018). During pregnancy, many autoimmune diseases abate in intensity, with subsequent flares postpartum or with postpartum status increasing the risk for developing a new autoimmune disease (Adams Waldorf and Nelson 2008). Some proinflammatory cytokines have been found to be elevated in the immediate postpartum period (Cheng and Pickler 2014; Osborne and Monk 2013). Thus, after delivery, when OCD risk is highest, inflammatory factors may play a role in triggering OCD, and symptoms (e.g., pain or discomfort) or treatments (e.g., steroids) may contribute to insomnia or depression and drive OCD exacerbations via sleep deprivation and mood dysregulation (Sharma 2019). Many pathways increase the risk for obsessive-compulsive symptoms in the perinatal period: genetic, biological, psychological, behavioral, and others. However, each also comes with opportunities for intervention, prevention, and further research.

## Treatment

The treatment of perinatal OCD has not been studied extensively; therefore, treatment is conducted in the same manner as for general OCD, with adaptations appropriate to the perinatal context (Hudak and Wisner 2012). Treatment is indicated when OCD symptoms interfere with functioning or cause significant distress (Koran et al. 2007). Given the negative impact on the entire family system, including the infant, perinatal OCD should be treated aggressively (Brandes et al. 2004). Psychiatric management consists of an array of therapeutic modalities, most of which fall under the categories of pharmacotherapy (mainly serotonin reuptake inhibitors [SRIs]) and cognitive-behavioral therapy (CBT) (Figure 20–1). Presently, there does not seem to be any theoretical basis for predicting that perinatal OCD would respond differently to these interventions than does general OCD (Abramowitz et al. 2003).

The selection of which intervention to use in the perinatal population depends on a host of factors, including severity of illness, co-occurring psychiatric and medical conditions, past psychiatric and treatment history, current safety concerns, degree of impairment in functioning, patient preferences, cultural and personal values, motivation for treatment, family/caregiver involvement in symptoms and role in support, and risk profile of both available treatments and no treatment (Koran et al. 2007). Given this complexity, allotting extra time and support in the decision-making process, to the extent that is reasonable and not compromising safety, is key when working with perinatal patients (see Chapter 8, "A Clinical Approach to Psychiatric Diagnosis and Treatment During Pregnancy").

An important first step is to establish and maintain a strong therapeutic alliance, because this facilitates sharing of goals and eventual treatment adherence. Key features of alliance-building with patients with OCD include instilling hope, listening attentively, repeating explanations (given the excessive doubting characteristic of OCD), and exploring patients' explanatory model of their symptoms (Koran et al. 2007; Sadock et al. 2000). Regarding the latter, patients can often blend symptoms with aspects of their inner selves (Nikodijevic et al. 2015), leading to confusion and overall marked distress. This is especially true in perinatal cases, when intrusive thoughts involving harm to the baby raise feelings of guilt, shame, and fear (Fairbrother and Woody 2008)—so much so that patients are often reluctant to share their symptoms with others, including providers. Providing reassurance and making use of psychoeducation are therefore critical.

Many patients are relieved to learn basic facts about OCD, including its prevalence, the shame that many patients experience, that it is not due to "bad mothering," and that treatments can be effective (Koran et al. 2007). For patients who are particularly distressed by intrusive thoughts of infant harm, an explanation that such symptoms are common in perinatal OCD and do not typically reflect true desires or inner character especially resonates. Of course, this should be accompanied by a thorough safety evaluation, with an extensive discussion about potential infant harm, if indicated. Educa-

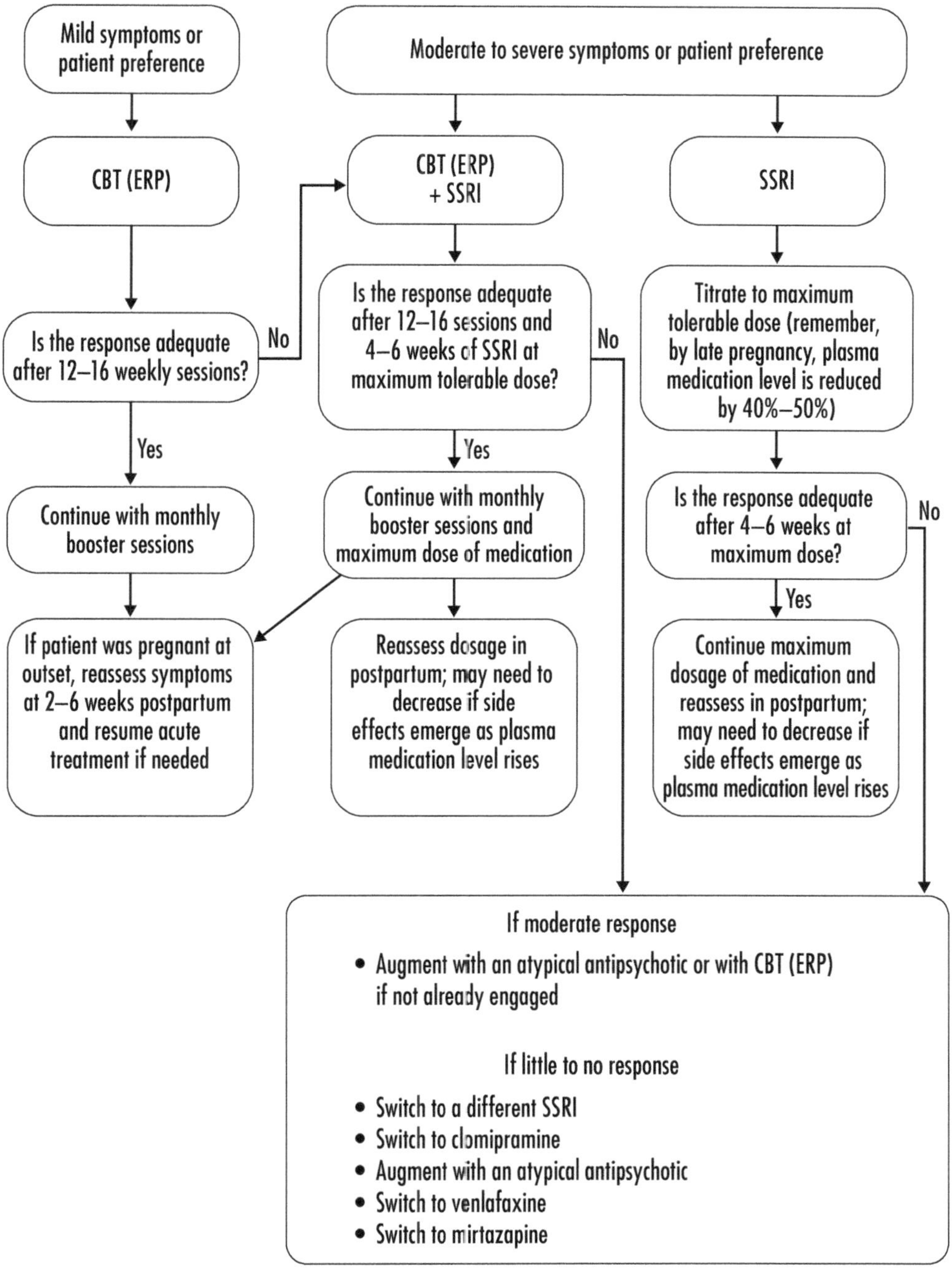


**FIGURE 20–1. Treatment of perinatal OCD.**
CBT=cognitive-behavioral therapy; ERP=exposure and response prevention; SSRI=selective serotonin reuptake inhibitor.

tion should also be offered to involved family members, especially in perinatal cases, because the entire family system can be negatively affected. In addition, family members can unknowingly collude in the patient's OCD symptoms, sometimes leading to harmful effects on the family (e.g., job loss due to a partner's or family's accommodation of avoidance behaviors) (Jennings et al. 1999). Informational materials, including those provided by consumer advocacy organizations, such as the International OCD Foundation (www.iocdf.org), as well as perinatal-specific sources, such as the MGH Center for Women's Mental Health (www.womensmentalhealth.org), can be very helpful for those who seek additional help outside of formal treatment settings.

As with any psychiatric assessment, a complete history and mental status examination are necessary. Key features include assessment for co-occurring conditions, particularly those with higher incidence in OCD populations (e.g., mood disorders, anxiety disorders, tics, and Tourette syndrome); a thorough review of past psychiatric and treatment history, including medication and psychotherapy trials; a general medical history (especially in the rare event that OCD is a manifestation of a medical illness); family history; and social history—with a particular focus on the patient's social support system and her overall level of functioning in the home and work/school domains. Family members can be important allies in treatment efforts (Koran et al. 2007); they also may need help themselves, in which case family therapy may be indicated.

As described earlier in the "Clinical Features" section, it is critical to differentiate OCD symptoms from delusions, which represent a psychotic process and, if involving infant harm, are more strongly associated with actual risk to the infant (Abramowitz et al. 2003; Sharma and Sommerdyk 2015). Such symptom evaluation can be part of the overall safety assessment indicated in all psychiatric evaluations; it should also involve inquiry into self-harm and suicidality and may rely on collateral information from family members. This is also an opportunity for psychoeducation because many patients are reluctant to share their disturbing intrusive thoughts out of fear of legal action and fear that their children will be taken from their care (Brandes et al. 2004; Jennings et al. 1999).

Also as described earlier, symptom evaluation should distinguish obsessions and compulsions from other disorders and should also involve a systematic approach to symptom severity. If no rating scale is used, quantification of the number of hours per day spent in obsessing and in performing compulsions, and the degree of effort applied to trying to escape the obsessions and resist the behaviors, is recommended (Koran et al. 2007). Such information will inform treatment goals, which should be modest at the start given the extended period needed for marked clinical improvement. Reasonable goals include <1 hour per day spent obsessing and performing compulsive behaviors, mild OCD-related anxiety, and little to no interference of OCD with tasks of ordinary living, including childcare (Koran et al. 2007).

In general, patients should be cared for in the least restrictive setting that is able to provide safe and effective treatment (Koran et al. 2007). Most OCD can be managed in the outpatient setting; hospital or partial hospitalization may be indicated, however, when the patient is not able to care for herself or if there is significant risk for harm to self or others, including a child. Even if outpatient, treatment intensity can be rigorous, including daily psychotherapy. Regardless of setting, treatment should be coordinated with physicians treating co-occurring medical conditions, other clinicians, and social agencies. In prenatal cases, coordination with the patient's obstetrician is critical not only to discuss the risks of treatments versus no treatment but also to share information on the patient's overall well-being and ability to function because these can impact obstetrical outcomes.

No randomized controlled trials of treatments for perinatal OCD have been published. As such, clinical guidelines for the treatment of OCD in general populations largely inform treatment options and decisions, with important adaptations relevant to the perinatal period, such as the risk profile of medications in pregnancy and risks to the pregnancy of untreated illness. In general populations, CBT and SRIs (SSRIs and clomipramine) are recommended on the basis of clinical trial results as safe and effective first-line treatments for OCD (Bandelow et al. 2008). Each of these treatments, along with others, is discussed in the following sections.

## Psychopharmacology

Both treatment and psychiatric illness in the perinatal period carry risks. Because the medications used for OCD are by and large the same used for other disorders (particularly depression), we do not repeat the discussion of risks here. Please see Chapter 8 and Chapter 9, "A Clinical Approach to Psychiatric Diagnosis and Treatment in the Postpartum Period," for an overview of the perinatal treatment approach and Chapter 13 for specific risk information about antidepressants. Fluoxetine, fluvoxamine, paroxetine, and sertraline are approved by the FDA for treatment of OCD and are recommended pharmacological agents (American Psychiatric Association 2013; Bergeron et al. 2002; Bisserbe et al. 1997; Denys et al. 2003, 2004; Goodman et al. 1989a, 1996; Greist 1995; Hoehn-Saric et al. 2000; Hollander et al. 2003; Jenike et al. 1997; Joffe and Swinson 1987; Koran et al. 2007; Smeraldi et al. 1992; Tollefson et al. 1994). Escitalopram and citalopram, although they lack FDA approval for this indication, are also recommended agents on the basis of recent evidence (Dougherty et al. 2009; Montgomery et al. 2001; Pampaloni et al. 2010; Stein et al. 2007). Clomipramine, a mixed serotonin-norepinephrine reuptake inhibitor, as well as a cholinergic and histaminic blocking agent, also has FDA approval for treatment of OCD. Meta-analyses of placebo-controlled trials suggest greater efficacy for clomipramine, but the results of head-to-head trials comparing clomipramine with SSRIs do not support this. As such, all of the aforementioned agents are considered equally effective in treatment of OCD (Vulink et al. 2005), although an individual patient may respond better to one over another. Regarding tolerability, SSRIs are routinely better tolerated given their more benign side effect profile (Mundo et al. 2000) and, as such, are recommended as first-line agents. In general populations, an SSRI alone is recommended for a patient who is not able to cooperate with CBT, has previously responded well to a given drug, or prefers treatment with an SSRI alone. SSRI monotherapy can also be considered in cases of severe OCD because the medication may diminish symptom severity sufficiently to allow the patient to engage in CBT (Koran et al. 2007).

Second-line approaches include the use of antipsychotics, which are used as augmentation for SSRIs; modest evidence supports the use of haloperidol, risperidone, quetiapine, olanzapine, and aripiprazole (Bystritsky et al. 2004; Denys et al. 2004; Erzegovesi et al. 2005; Hollander et al. 2003; McDougle et al. 1994, 2000; Selvi et al. 2011). Modest evidence also supports the use of venlafaxine monotherapy (Denys et al. 2003, 2004) and mirtazapine monotherapy. Third-line approaches, supported mostly by open-label studies, case series, and reports, include augmentation with buspirone (Jenike and Baer 1988; Pigott et al. 1992), lithium (American Psychiatric Association 2002), pindolol (Dannon et al. 2000), riluzole (Coric et al. 2005), and oral morphine sulfate (Koran et al. 2005), as well as monotherapy with D-amphetamine (Insel et al. 1983; Joffe et al. 1991), tramadol (Shapira et al. 1997), monoamine oxidase inhibitors (Jenike et al. 1997), anticonvulsants (Jenike and Brotman 1984; Joffe and Swinson 1987), L-tryptophan (Yaryura-Tobias and Bhagavan 1977), and transdermal nicotine (Koran et al. 2007; Lundberg et al. 2004).

The extant literature on the pharmacotherapy of OCD in perinatal populations includes only open-label studies (Sharma and Sommerdyk 2015). In one case series, two-thirds of patients with postpartum OCD treated with fluvoxamine showed a positive response, defined as 30% or greater decrease in total Y-BOCS score (Arnold 1999). In another case series, 15 patients with postpartum OCD treated with fluoxetine, clomipramine, desipramine, or a combination of these drugs showed significant responsiveness to SSRIs following 12 weeks of treatment, with improvement maintained with continued treatment over a 1-year period (Sichel et al. 1993a). In another case series, 64.7% (11/17) of patients with treatment-resistant postpartum OCD treated with quetiapine as augmentation for SSRIs (paroxetine, fluoxetine, sertraline) and SNRIs (venlafaxine) showed responsiveness to this regimen, with a mean dose of 112.5 mg/day and a mean reduction of 59.6% in Y-BOCS scores (Misri et al. 2004). In a case series of four women with postpartum OCD, symptoms improved with fluoxetine (Buttolph and Holland 1990).

In general populations, successful medication treatment should be continued for 1–2 years before being gradually tapered by 10%–25% every 1–2 months while observing for symptom return or exacerbation (Koran et al. 2007). This is also recommended for perinatal cases, although changes to the regimen may be indicated in certain contexts, such as breastfeeding. In general, for breastfeeding patients who are taking SSRIs, the relatively benign side effect profile of SSRIs in lactation (including almost negligible secretion into breastmilk in some cases, such as sertraline) favors the use of pharmacological approaches.

## Nonpharmacological Somatic Treatments

Somatic therapies used in the treatment of adult OCD include deep brain stimulation and other forms of neurosurgery, transcranial magnetic stimulation (TMS), and electroconvulsive therapy (ECT). None of these therapies is considered a first-line treatment for OCD because most of the evidence for them exists in the form of case reports/series and unblinded studies (Greenberg et al. 2003, 2005; Jenike et al. 1991). The risk for significant morbidity associated with neurosurgical techniques renders them indicated only for treatment-refractory cases. Similarly, given the limited evidence base of ECT as an OCD treatment strategy in general populations, ECT is reserved only for those cases in which there is a co-occurring disorder for which ECT is a known effective treatment. A recent randomized controlled trial of deep TMS for OCD suggested positive results, but more research is needed (Carmi et al. 2019). None of these strategies has been investigated in perinatal OCD cases.

## Behavioral Treatments

CBT is the only form of psychotherapy for OCD whose effectiveness is supported by controlled trials (Koran et al. 2007). No controlled studies demonstrate effectiveness of dynamic psychotherapy or psychoanalysis in dealing with the core symptoms of OCD, although these modalities could be useful in certain contexts—for example, helping a patient overcome her resistance to starting treatment. Motivational interviewing can also be helpful in this regard (Koran et al. 2007). Family therapy may be indicated in the context of family tensions due to OCD symptoms or to ameliorate family collusion with symptoms. Supportive therapy can be helpful (Brandes et al. 2004), especially in perinatal cases when initial treatment decision-making is particularly difficult. No controlled trials have evaluated other psychosocial methods, mindfulness approaches, or acceptance and commitment therapy (Koran et al. 2007).

In general populations, CBT that relies on behavioral techniques, such as ERP, is recommended because it has the most evidentiary support (Cordioli et al. 2003; Eddy et al. 2004; Fals-Stewart et al. 1993; Fisher and Wells 2005; Foa et al. 2005; Franklin et al. 2000; Greist et al. 2002; Lindsay et al. 1997; McLean et al. 2001; Nakatani et al. 2005; Rothbaum and Shahar 2000; Warren and Thomas 2001). In this modality, patients are taught to confront feared situations and objects and to refrain from performing rituals. Exposures may include in-vivo and imaginal confrontations of feared consequences. Exposures are graded from mildly to more intensely anxiety provoking. Patients must face their fears for a prolonged period while refraining from indulging in their usual ritualizing. The goal is to weaken the connections between the feared stimuli causing distress and the performance of rituals bringing relief from distress (Koran et al. 2007).

There is also some, although relatively less, data on use of CBT that, while incorporating behavioral techniques, focuses on cognitive approaches aimed at identifying, challenging, and modifying dysfunctional beliefs (Ellis 1962; Emmelkamp and Beens 1991; Emmelkamp et al. 1988; Jones and Menzies 1998; van Oppen et al. 1995). Such dysfunctional beliefs include magical thinking, an inflated sense of responsibility for unwanted events, overestimations of the probability of feared events, the assumption that thoughts are morally equivalent to actions or inevitably lead to action (thought-action fusion), perfectionism, the belief that anxiety/discomfort will persist forever, and the need for control (Koran et al. 2007; Wilhelm et al. 2005).

Although some randomized trials have investigated the efficacy of combined treatment (CBT consisting of ERP+SRI) compared with either SRI or CBT alone, limitations in their design prevent definitive conclusions (Cottraux et al. 1990; Foa et al. 2005; Hohagen et al. 1998; Koran et al. 2007; Marks et al. 1980, 1988; van Balkom et al. 1998). In the absence of definitive data, combined treatment is reasonable in cases involving treatment of a co-occurring disorder that is SSRI responsive, to augment a partial response to monotherapy (Tenneij et al. 2005), and to reduce the chance of relapse when medication is discontinued (Simpson et al. 2004). Combined treatment may also be considered in cases of severe OCD because the medication may diminish symptom severity enough to allow the patient to engage in CBT (Koran et al. 2007). In general populations, CBT alone (consisting of ERP) is recommended for patients who are not too depressed, anxious, or severely ill to cooperate with this treatment modality or who prefer not to take medications and are willing to do the work that CBT requires (American Psychiatric Association 2007). Although many perinatal patients may prefer this approach to minimize potential exposures in pregnancy, a thorough risk-risk discussion is required first, with thoughtful consideration of medication options (see "Treatment Challenges" section).

In perinatal populations, the extant literature on psychotherapy-based treatments for OCD is limited to observational studies. In one study, six patients with postpartum OCD underwent CBT over 2 weeks and demonstrated improvement on self-report and clinician-rated measures that was sustained over a 3- to 5-month period (Challacombe and Salkovskis 2009). In another case study, a woman with postpartum OCD demonstrated significant improvement and clinical remission after eight CBT sessions (Christian and Storch 2009). A cognitive-behavioral prevention program incorporated into a childbirth education class appeared effective in reducing postpartum obsessive-compulsive symptoms (Timpano et al. 2011). In a study of postpartum women with depression and anxiety disorders including OCD, both paroxetine and combined treatment were found effective, although one was not superior to the other (Misri et al. 2004).

Given the limited data in perinatal populations, it is recommended to follow CBT treatment guidelines for nonperinatal OCD: 13–20 weekly sessions for most patients, with "booster" sessions for 3–6 months afterward for more severely ill patients, those with a history of relapse, or those showing signs of early relapse (Koran et al. 2007; Sharma and Sommerdyk 2015). Session length can vary from 45 minutes to 2 hours, and treatment can be delivered in individual, group, or family therapy contexts. In the absence of available CBT, providers can rely on self-help treatment guides and are also recommended to direct patients to OCD support groups. With perinatal patients, whose schedules are often limited due to childcare responsibilities, work responsibilities, or the physical burdens of pregnancy, it is important to have a realistic discussion about what frequency of therapy sessions is reasonable given each woman's circumstances.

## Treatment Challenges

Although treatment strategies in perinatal OCD are largely informed by guidelines developed for nonperinatal populations, there are important modifications to note. In general populations, the selection of CBT, an SSRI, or combined treatment depends on the nature and severity of the patient's symptoms, nature of co-occurring psychiatric and medical conditions, the availability of CBT, the patient's past treatment history, current medications that the patient is taking, and the patient's preferences (Koran et al. 2007). Indeed, these all come into play in perinatal cases; however, the risk-risk analysis, as described in detail in Chapter 8, is expanded to include potential risks to a fetus—both as a result of the treatments themselves and from lack of (or under-) treatment. Once the risks of treatment and the risks of no treatment/undertreatment are clarified (Spinelli 2012), initial steps in decision-making can be more easily taken. Cases in which medication (an SSRI) would be heavily considered include high severity of symptoms (especially leading to safety concerns or marked impairment of functioning), a history of prior good response to an SSRI, and a history of prior ineffective trial of CBT alone. Because many cases do not necessarily include these elements, and often fall in a "gray zone" of severity, other factors to consider include the patient's preference, willingness and ability to engage in close follow-up, presence or absence of family and social support, and time/financial resources (with regard to pursuing psychotherapy). Given the potential for CBT to decrease relapse rates when medication is discontinued (which is always a possibility in perinatal cases), it is generally recommended that patients who are proceeding with SSRI treatment also pursue CBT if possible.

As is the case with perinatal depression and anxiety disorders, all SSRIs are reasonable options with regard to risk profile in pregnancy and lactation (Table 20–5), with the possible exception of paroxetine, which had been linked with cardiac malformations in earlier epidemiological studies. Recent data have not supported this finding,

**TABLE 20–5. Recommended first-line agents for perinatal OCD**

| | |
|---|---|
| Citalopram | Fluvoxamine* |
| Escitalopram | Sertraline* |
| Fluoxetine* | |

*FDA-approved for treatment of OCD.

however (Huybrechts et al. 2014). As is the case in general populations, clomipramine is a second-line approach in perinatal cases given its relatively less benign side effect profile compared with SSRIs. Exceptions to this include prior history of successful response to clomipramine in the past.

Once the decision is made to pursue medication treatment in perinatal OCD, following guidelines for nonperinatal OCD is generally recommended, with some modifications. Because the prospect of starting medication in pregnancy or postpartum is worrisome to many perinatal patients, it is not unreasonable to start at half doses to minimize side effects and provide reassurance. At the start, it is important to set the patient's expectations appropriately, with the knowledge that substantial symptom improvement often does not occur until 4–6 weeks after initiation of medication, and many patients may need up to 10–12 weeks. Medication doses can be titrated up every 5–7 days or as indicated by the manufacturer. Although careful avoidance of overmedication is important in perinatal cases, undermedication also carries risks because the patient and her baby would be exposed to the double risk of the disease process and the medication itself, without reaping benefits of the treatment. It is thus important to pursue the minimum *effective* dose, which is likely to equate to higher SSRI doses (as would be the case for nonperinatal populations). Compared with nonperinatal patients, perinatal patients would benefit from more frequent follow-up visits and monitoring during this uptitration process. This is especially the case for pregnant patients as they enter their third trimester, when plasma drug levels can drop due to increased metabolism, thereby necessitating higher doses for symptom control (Sit et al. 2006). It is also critical to closely monitor for side effects and to explain these fully to the patient ahead of time. Pharmacotherapy-based approaches to address side effect complaints such as insomnia and fatigue may be considered, but these should be pursued with caution given the general preference to avoid polypharmacy in perinatal cases and the unknown risk profile of many of these agents in pregnancy and lactation.

As would be the case in nonperinatal populations, an alternative treatment should be considered when good response is not achieved after 13–20 weeks of weekly outpatient CBT in perinatal cases. Strategies at this point include increasing to daily CBT or adding an SSRI (combined treatment). For perinatal patients taking SSRIs who have not achieved a good response after 8–12 weeks (including 4–6 weeks at the highest comfortably tolerated dose), the following factors, which could be contributing to low or negligible treatment response, should be addressed first, if relevant: interference by co-occurring conditions, inadequate patient adherence, presence of psychosocial stressors, family members' accommodation or reinforcing of symptoms, inability to tolerate medication (Koran et al. 2007), and decreased therapeutic efficacy of medication due to physiological changes of pregnancy. If such factors have already been addressed, or are not relevant, then the following strategies can be considered: switch to a different

SSRI, switch to clomipramine, augment with antipsychotic medications, switch to venlafaxine, or switch to mirtazapine. Given the limited evidence base for mirtazapine with regard to efficacy, the more robust data regarding the risk profile of SSRIs as compared with venlafaxine and antipsychotics, and the general preference to avoid polypharmacy in perinatal cases (American College of Obstetricians and Gynecologists 2008), it is recommended to switch to a different SSRI first (assuming that the patient has not already done so).

Augmentation with antipsychotics may be preferred if the patient has already demonstrated a partial response to an SSRI. The selection of an antipsychotic must consider known risks in pregnancy and side effect profile, notably metabolic side effects with second-generation antipsychotics and associated pregnancy complications, such as gestational diabetes. It is reassuring, however, that antipsychotics do not appear to be linked with teratogenic risk (Damkier and Videbech 2018). For a detailed discussion of the risks of antipsychotics versus the risks of no treatment, please see Chapter 15, "Bipolar Disorder and Related Disorders," and Chapter 17, "Schizophrenia and Related Disorders." Venlafaxine carries a similar risk profile as SSRIs, although with less supporting data; one study showed a possible increased risk for postpartum hemorrhage, but conclusions could not be drawn (Palmsten et al. 2013). For cases that do not respond to any of these approaches, third-line agents or other somatic therapies can be considered, in consultation with specialists (maternal-fetal medicine specialist and reproductive psychiatrist), given the concerning risk profiles of these treatments in pregnancy and lactation.

## Conclusion

In summary, the clinical guidelines for perinatal OCD are similar to those for nonperinatal populations. In cases of mild to moderate OCD, nonpharmacological treatments such as CBT (incorporating ERP) can be used. In more severe cases, or those cases in which the patient responded well to a medication in the past, pharmacological strategies are recommended, with SSRIs as first-line options. Tricyclic (e.g., clomipramine) and other antidepressants are second-line strategies if SSRI trials are not effective. Reasonable adjunctive agents include second-generation antipsychotics. Other somatic treatments could be considered for treatment-refractory cases, but the evidence base in perinatal populations to support these interventions is very limited.

## Key Points

- Obsessions are common in the perinatal period.
- Perinatal obsessions can include intrusive thoughts of harm coming to the child, *but having such thoughts does not necessarily mean the mother is at risk of harming her child.*
- Distinguishing between ego-syntonic and ego-dystonic thoughts is the key to understanding the risk of harm.

- Cognitive-behavioral therapy with exposure and response prevention remains the gold standard for treating OCD in the perinatal period.
- Selective serotonin reuptake inhibitors and tricyclic antidepressants can be effective but generally require higher doses for OCD than for depression.

# References

Abramowitz JS, Schwartz SA, Moore KM, et al: Obsessive-compulsive symptoms in pregnancy and the puerperium: a review of the literature. J Anxiety Disord 17(4):461–478, 2003 12826092

Abramowitz JS, Khandker M, Nelson CA, et al: The role of cognitive factors in the pathogenesis of obsessive-compulsive symptoms: a prospective study. Behav Res Ther 44(9):1361–1374, 2006 16352291

Abramowitz JS, Nelson CA, Rygwall R, et al: The cognitive mediation of obsessive-compulsive symptoms: a longitudinal study. J Anxiety Disord 21(1):91–104, 2007 16806800

Abramowitz JS, Deacon BJ, Olatunji BO, et al: Assessment of obsessive-compulsive symptom dimensions: development and evaluation of the Dimensional Obsessive-Compulsive Scale. Psychol Assess 22(1):180–198, 2010a 20230164

Abramowitz JS, Meltzer-Brody S, Leserman J, et al: Obsessional thoughts and compulsive behaviors in a sample of women with postpartum mood symptoms. Arch Women Ment Health 13(6):523–530, 2010b 20607572

Adams Waldorf KM, Nelson JL: Autoimmune disease during pregnancy and the microchimerism legacy of pregnancy. Immunol Invest 37(5):631–644, 2008 18716941

Albert U, Maina G, Bogetto F, et al: Clinical predictors of health-related quality of life in obsessive-compulsive disorder. Compr Psychiatry 51(2):193–200, 2010 20152302

Alonso P, Gratacòs M, Segalàs C, et al: Variants in estrogen receptor alpha gene are associated with phenotypical expression of obsessive-compulsive disorder. Psychoneuroendocrinology 36(4):473–483, 2011 20850223

American College of Obstetricians and Gynecologists: ACOG Practice Bulletin: clinical management guidelines for obstetrician-gynecologists number 92, April 2008 (replaces practice bulletin number 87, November 2007). Use of psychiatric medications during pregnancy and lactation. Obstet Gynecol 111(4):1001–1020, 2008 18378767

American Psychiatric Association: Practice guideline for the treatment of patients with bipolar disorder (revision). Am J Psychiatry 159(4 suppl):1–50, 2002 11958165

American Psychiatric Association: Practice Guideline for the Treatment of Patients With Obsessive-Compulsive Disorder. Arlington, VA, American Psychiatric Association, 2007

American Psychiatric Association: Diagnostic and Statistical Manual of Mental Disorders, 5th Edition. Arlington, VA, American Psychiatric Association, 2013

Andersson L, Sundström-Poromaa I, Bixo M, et al: Point prevalence of psychiatric disorders during the second trimester of pregnancy: a population-based study. Am J Obstet Gynecol 189(1):148–154, 2003 12861154

Arnold LM: A case series of women with postpartum-onset obsessive-compulsive disorder. Prim Care Companion J Clin Psychiatry 1(4):103–108, 1999 15014682

Bandelow B, Zohar J, Hollander E, et al: World Federation of Societies of Biological Psychiatry (WFSBP) guidelines for the pharmacological treatment of anxiety, obsessive-compulsive and post-traumatic stress disorders—first revision. World J Biol Psychiatry 9(4):248–312, 2008 18949648

Bergeron R, Ravindran AV, Chaput Y, et al: Sertraline and fluoxetine treatment of obsessive-compulsive disorder: results of a double-blind, 6-month treatment study. J Clin Psychopharmacol 22(2):148–154, 2002 11910259

Bergink V, Kushner SA, Pop V, et al: Prevalence of autoimmune thyroid dysfunction in postpartum psychosis. Br J Psychiatry 198(4):264–268, 2011 21343331

Bergink V, Rasgon N, Wisner KL: Postpartum psychosis: madness, mania, and melancholia in motherhood. Am J Psychiatry 173(12):1179–1188, 2016 27609245

Bergink V, Pop VJM, Nielsen PR, et al: Comorbidity of autoimmune thyroid disorders and psychiatric disorders during the postpartum period: a Danish nationwide register-based cohort study. Psychol Med 48(8):1291–1298, 2018 28929982

Bisserbe J, Lane R, Flament M, et al: A double-blind comparison of sertraline and clomipramine in outpatients with obsessive-compulsive disorder. Eur Psychiatry 12(2):82–93, 1997 19698511

Brander G, Rydell M, Kuja-Halkola R, et al: Association of perinatal risk factors with obsessive-compulsive disorder: a population-based birth cohort, sibling control study. JAMA Psychiatry 73(11):1135–1144, 2016 27706475

Brandes M, Soares CN, Cohen LS: Postpartum onset obsessive-compulsive disorder: diagnosis and management. Arch Women Ment Health 7(2):99–110, 2004 15083345

Buttolph M, Holland A: Obsessive-compulsive disorders in pregnancy and childbirth, in Obsessive-Compulsive Disorder: Theory and Management, 2nd Edition. Edited by Jenike MA, Baer L, Minchiello WE. Chicago, IL, Yearbook Medical Publishers, 1990, pp 89–95

Bystritsky A, Ackerman DL, Rosen RM, et al: Augmentation of serotonin reuptake inhibitors in refractory obsessive-compulsive disorder using adjunctive olanzapine: a placebo-controlled trial. J Clin Psychiatry 65(4):565–568, 2004 15119922

Camarena B, Rinetti G, Cruz C, et al: Additional evidence that genetic variation of MAO-A gene supports a gender subtype in obsessive-compulsive disorder. Am J Med Genet 105(3):279–282, 2001 11353450

Carmi L, Tendler A, Bystritsky A, et al: Efficacy and safety of deep transcranial magnetic stimulation for obsessive-compulsive disorder: a prospective multicenter randomized double-blind placebo-controlled trial. Am J Psychiatry 176(11):931–938, 2019 31109199

Challacombe F, Salkovskis P: A preliminary investigation of the impact of maternal obsessive-compulsive disorder and panic disorder on parenting and children. J Anxiety Disord 23(7):848–857, 2009 19464141

Challacombe FL, Salkovskis PM, Woolgar M, et al: Parenting and mother-infant interactions in the context of maternal postpartum obsessive-compulsive disorder: effects of obsessional symptoms and mood. Infant Behav Dev 44:11–20, 2016 27259042

Chaudron LH, Nirodi N: The obsessive-compulsive spectrum in the perinatal period: a prospective pilot study. Arch Women Ment Health 13(5):403–410, 2010 20221779

Cheng CY, Pickler RH: Perinatal stress, fatigue, depressive symptoms, and immune modulation in late pregnancy and one month postpartum. ScientificWorldJournal 2014:652630, 2014 24587741

Christian LM, Storch EA: Cognitive behavioral treatment of postpartum onset: obsessive compulsive disorder with aggressive obsessions. Clin Case Stud 8(1):72–83, 2009

Collardeau F, Corbyn B, Abramowitz J, et al: Maternal unwanted and intrusive thoughts of infant-related harm, obsessive-compulsive disorder and depression in the perinatal period: study protocol. BMC Psychiatry 19(1):94, 2019 30898103

Cordioli AV, Basso de Sousa M, Bochi DB: Intravenous clomipramine in severe and refractory obsessive-compulsive disorder. J Clin Psychopharmacol 23(6):665–666, 2003 14624197

Coric V, Taskiran S, Pittenger C, et al: Riluzole augmentation in treatment-resistant obsessive-compulsive disorder: an open-label trial. Biol Psychiatry 58(5):424–428, 2005 15993857

Corregiari FM, Bernik M, Cordeiro Q, et al: Endophenotypes and serotonergic polymorphisms associated with treatment response in obsessive-compulsive disorder. Clinics (São Paulo) 67(4):335–340, 2012 22522758

Cosco TD, Pillinger T, Emam H, et al: Immune aberrations in obsessive-compulsive disorder: a systematic review and meta-analysis. Mol Neurobiol 56(7):4751–4759, 2019 30382535

Cottraux J, Mollard E, Bouvard M, et al: A controlled study of fluvoxamine and exposure in obsessive-compulsive disorder. Int Clin Psychopharmacol 5(1):17–30, 1990 2110206

Cox JL, Holden JM, Sagovsky R: Detection of postnatal depression: development of the 10-item Edinburgh Postnatal Depression Scale. Br J Psychiatry 150:782–786, 1987 3651732

Dama M, Steiner M, Lieshout RV: Thyroid peroxidase autoantibodies and perinatal depression risk: a systematic review. J Affect Disord 198:108–121, 2016 27011366
Damkier P, Videbech P: The safety of second-generation antipsychotics during pregnancy: a clinically focused review. CNS Drugs 32(4):351–366, 2018 29637530
Dannon PN, Sasson Y, Hirschmann S, et al: Pindolol augmentation in treatment-resistant obsessive compulsive disorder: a double-blind placebo controlled trial. Eur Neuropsychopharmacol 10(3):165–169, 2000 10793318
Delorme R, Betancur C, Callebert J, et al: Platelet serotonergic markers as endophenotypes for obsessive-compulsive disorder. Neuropsychopharmacology 30(8):1539–1547, 2005 15886722
Denys D, van der Wee N, van Megen HJ, et al: A double blind comparison of venlafaxine and paroxetine in obsessive-compulsive disorder. J Clin Psychopharmacol 23(6):568–575, 2003 14624187
Denys D, van Megen HJ, van der Wee N, et al: A double-blind switch study of paroxetine and venlafaxine in obsessive-compulsive disorder. J Clin Psychiatry 65(1):37–43, 2004 14744166
Dougherty DD, Jameson M, Deckersbach T, et al: Open-label study of high (30 mg) and moderate (20 mg) dose escitalopram for the treatment of obsessive-compulsive disorder. Int Clin Psychopharmacol 24(6):306–311, 2009 19730388
Eddy KT, Dutra L, Bradley R, et al: A multidimensional meta-analysis of psychotherapy and pharmacotherapy for obsessive-compulsive disorder. Clin Psychol Rev 24(8):1011–1030, 2004 15533282
Ellis A: Reason and Emotion in Psychotherapy. New York, Lyle Stuart, 1962
Emmelkamp PM, Beens H: Cognitive therapy with obsessive-compulsive disorder: a comparative evaluation. Behav Res Ther 29(3):293–300, 1991 1679324
Emmelkamp P, Visser S, Hoekstra R: Cognitive therapy vs exposure in vivo in the treatment of obsessive-compulsives. Cognitive Therapy and Research 12(1):103–114, 1988
Erzegovesi S, Guglielmo E, Siliprandi F, et al: Low-dose risperidone augmentation of fluvoxamine treatment in obsessive-compulsive disorder: a double-blind, placebo-controlled study. Eur Neuropsychopharmacol 15(1):69–74, 2005 15572275
Fairbrother N, Abramowitz JS: New parenthood as a risk factor for the development of obsessional problems. Behav Res Ther 45(9):2155–2163, 2007 17084810
Fairbrother N, Woody SR: New mothers' thoughts of harm related to the newborn. Arch Women Ment Health 11(3):221–229, 2008 18463941
Fals-Stewart W, Marks AP, Schafer J: A comparison of behavioral group therapy and individual behavior therapy in treating obsessive-compulsive disorder. J Nerv Ment Dis 181(3):189–193, 1993 8445378
Feldman R, Granat A, Pariente C, et al: Maternal depression and anxiety across the postpartum year and infant social engagement, fear regulation, and stress reactivity. J Am Acad Child Adolesc Psychiatry 48(9):919–927, 2009 19625979
Fisher PL, Wells A: How effective are cognitive and behavioral treatments for obsessive-compulsive disorder? A clinical significance analysis. Behav Res Ther 43(12):1543–1558, 2005 16239151
Flaisher-Grinberg S, Albelda N, Gitter L, et al: Ovarian hormones modulate "compulsive" lever-pressing in female rats. Horm Behav 55(2) 356–365, 2009 18996389
Fluitman S, Denys D, Vulink N, et al: Lipopolysaccharide-induced cytokine production in obsessive-compulsive disorder and generalized social anxiety disorder. Psychiatry Res 178(2):313–316, 2010 20452055
Foa EB, Huppert JD, Leiberg S, et al: The Obsessive-Compulsive Inventory: development and validation of a short version. Psychol Assess 14(4):485–496, 2002 12501574
Foa EB, Liebowitz MR, Kozak MJ, et al: Randomized, placebo-controlled trial of exposure and ritual prevention, clomipramine, and their combination in the treatment of obsessive-compulsive disorder. Am J Psychiatry 162(1):151–161, 2005 15625214
Fontenelle LF, Mendlowicz MV, Versiani M: The descriptive epidemiology of obsessive-compulsive disorder. Prog Neuropsychopharmacol Biol Psychiatry 30(3):327–337, 2006 16412548
Forray A, Focseneanu M, Pittman B, et al: Onset and exacerbation of obsessive-compulsive disorder in pregnancy and the postpartum period. J Clin Psychiatry 71(8):1061–1068, 2010 20492843

Franklin ME, Abramowitz JS, Kozak MJ, et al: Effectiveness of exposure and ritual prevention for obsessive-compulsive disorder: randomized compared with nonrandomized samples. J Consult Clin Psychol 68(4):594–602, 2000 10965635
Friedman MJ, Wang S, Jalowiec JE, et al: Thyroid hormone alterations among women with posttraumatic stress disorder due to childhood sexual abuse. Biol Psychiatry 57(10):1186–1192, 2005 15866559
Gaynes BN, Gavin N, Meltzer-Brody S, et al: Perinatal depression: prevalence, screening accuracy, and screening outcomes. Evid Rep Technol Assess (Summ) (119):1–8, 2005 15760246
Gezginç K, Uguz F, Karatayli S, et al: The impact of obsessive-compulsive disorder in pregnancy on quality of life. Int J Psychiatry Clin Pract 12(2):134–137, 2008 24916624
Gjerdingen D, Crow S, McGovern P, et al: Postpartum depression screening at well-child visits: validity of a 2-question screen and the PHQ-9. Ann Fam Med 7(1):63–70, 2009 19139451
Goodman WK, Price LH, Rasmussen SA, et al: Efficacy of fluvoxamine in obsessive-compulsive disorder: a double-blind comparison with placebo. Arch Gen Psychiatry 46(1):36–44, 1989a
Goodman WK, Price LH, Rasmussen SA, et al: The Yale-Brown Obsessive Compulsive Scale. I. Development, use, and reliability. Arch Gen Psychiatry 46(11):1006–1011, 1989b 2684084
Goodman WK, Price LH, Rasmussen SA, et al: The Yale-Brown Obsessive Compulsive Scale. II. Validity. Arch Gen Psychiatry 46(11):1012–1016, 1989c 2510699
Goodman WK, Kozak MJ, Liebowitz M, et al: Treatment of obsessive-compulsive disorder with fluvoxamine: a multicentre, double-blind, placebo-controlled trial. Int Clin Psychopharmacol 11(1):21–29, 1996 8732310
Gray SM, Bloch MH: Systematic review of proinflammatory cytokines in obsessive-compulsive disorder. Curr Psychiatry Rep 14(3):220–228, 2012 22477442
Greenberg BD, Price LH, Rauch SL, et al: Neurosurgery for intractable obsessive-compulsive disorder and depression: critical issues. Neurosurg Clin N Am 14(2):199–212, 2003 12856488
Greenberg BD, Nahas Z, Carpenter LL: Current status of deep brain stimulation. Primary Psychiatry 12(10):59–64, 2005
Greist J: Efficacy of fluvoxamine in obsessive-compulsive disorder: results of a multicentre, double blind, placebo-controlled trial. Eur J Clin Res 7:195–204, 1995
Greist JH, Marks IM, Baer L, et al: Behavior therapy for obsessive-compulsive disorder guided by a computer or by a clinician compared with relaxation as a control. J Clin Psychiatry 63(2):138–145, 2002 11874215
Hall D, Dhilla A, Charalambous A, et al: Sequence variants of the brain-derived neurotrophic factor (BDNF) gene are strongly associated with obsessive-compulsive disorder. Am J Hum Genet 73(2):370–376, 2003 12836135
Hill RA, McInnes KJ, Gong EC, et al: Estrogen deficient male mice develop compulsive behavior. Biol Psychiatry 61(3):359–366, 2007 16566897
Hoehn-Saric R, Ninan P, Black DW, et al: Multicenter double-blind comparison of sertraline and desipramine for concurrent obsessive-compulsive and major depressive disorders. Arch Gen Psychiatry 57(1):76–82, 2000 10632236
Hohagen F, Winkelmann G, Rasche-Rüchle H, et al: Combination of behaviour therapy with fluvoxamine in comparison with behaviour therapy and placebo: results of a multicentre study. Br J Psychiatry Suppl (35):71–78, 1998 9829029
Hollander E, Baldini Rossi N, Sood E, et al: Risperidone augmentation in treatment-resistant obsessive-compulsive disorder: a double-blind, placebo-controlled study. Int J Neuropsychopharmacol 6(4):397–401, 2003 14604454
Howard M, Battle CL, Pearlstein T, et al: A psychiatric mother-baby day hospital for pregnant and postpartum women. Arch Women Ment Health 9(4):213–218, 2006 16718517
Hudak R, Wisner KL: Diagnosis and treatment of postpartum obsessions and compulsions that involve infant harm. Am J Psychiatry 169(4):360–363, 2012 22476676
Humble MB, Uvnäs-Moberg K, Engström I, et al: Plasma oxytocin changes and anti-obsessive response during serotonin reuptake inhibitor treatment: a placebo controlled study. BMC Psychiatry 13:344, 2013 24359174
Huybrechts KF, Hernández-Díaz S, Avorn J: Antidepressant use in pregnancy and the risk of cardiac defects. N Engl J Med 371(12):1168–1169, 2014 25229932

Insel TR, Hamilton JA, Guttmacher LB, et al: D-amphetamine in obsessive-compulsive disorder. Psychopharmacology (Berl) 80(3):231–235, 1983 6412267

Ittermann T, Völzke H, Baumeister SE, et al: Diagnosed thyroid disorders are associated with depression and anxiety. Soc Psychiatry Psychiatr Epidemiol 50(9):1417–1425, 2015 25777685

Jenike MA, Baer L: An open trial of buspirone in obsessive-compulsive disorder. Am J Psychiatry 145(10):1285–1286, 1988 3048120

Jenike MA, Brotman AW: The EEG in obsessive-compulsive disorder. J Clin Psychiatry 45(3):122–124, 1984 6698944

Jenike MA, Baer L, Ballantine T, et al: Cingulotomy for refractory obsessive-compulsive disorder: a long-term follow-up of 33 patients. Arch Gen Psychiatry 48(6):548–555, 1991 2039338

Jenike MA, Baer L, Minichiello WE, et al: Placebo-controlled trial of fluoxetine and phenelzine for obsessive-compulsive disorder. Am J Psychiatry 154(9):1261–1264, 1997 9286186

Jennings KD, Ross S, Popper S, et al: Thoughts of harming infants in depressed and nondepressed mothers. J Affect Disord 54(1–2):21–28, 1999 10403143

Joffe RT, Swinson RP: Carbamazepine in obsessive-compulsive disorder. Biol Psychiatry 22(9):1169–1171, 1987 3651536

Joffe RT, Swinson RP, Levitt AJ: Acute psychostimulant challenge in primary obsessive-compulsive disorder. J Clin Psychopharmacol 11(4):237–241, 1991 1680885

Jones MK, Menzies RG: Danger ideation reduction therapy (DIRT) for obsessive-compulsive washers. A controlled trial. Behav Res Ther 36(10):959–970, 1998 9714946

Kang JI, Kim HW, Kim CH, et al: Oxytocin receptor gene polymorphisms exert a modulating effect on the onset age in patients with obsessive-compulsive disorder. Psychoneuroendocrinology 86:45–52, 2017 28915380

Kant R, Pasi S, Surolia A: Auto-reactive Th17-cells trigger obsessive-compulsive-disorder like behavior in mice with experimental autoimmune encephalomyelitis. Front Immunol 9:2508, 2018 30429853

Katerberg H, Lochner C, Cath DC, et al: The role of the brain-derived neurotrophic factor (BDNF) val66met variant in the phenotypic expression of obsessive-compulsive disorder (OCD). Am J Med Genet B Neuropsychiatr Genet 150B(8):1050–1062, 2009 19219856

Kessler RC, Berglund P, Demler O, et al: Lifetime prevalence and age-of-onset distributions of DSM-IV disorders in the National Comorbidity Survey Replication. Arch Gen Psychiatry 62(6):593–602, 2005 15939837

Kluge M, Schüssler P, Künzel HE, et al: Increased nocturnal secretion of ACTH and cortisol in obsessive compulsive disorder. J Psychiatr Res 41(11):928–933, 2007 17049559

Koran LM, Aboujaoude E, Bullock KD, et al: Double-blind treatment with oral morphine in treatment-resistant obsessive-compulsive disorder. J Clin Psychiatry 66(3):353–359, 2005 15766302

Koran LM, Hanna GL, Hollander E, et al: Practice guideline for the treatment of patients with obsessive-compulsive disorder. Am J Psychiatry 164(7 suppl):5–53, 2007 17849776

Labad J, Menchón JM, Alonso P, et al: Female reproductive cycle and obsessive-compulsive disorder. J Clin Psychiatry 66(4):428–435, quiz 546, 2005 15816784

Labad J, Alonso P, Segalas C, et al: Distinct correlates of hoarding and cleaning symptom dimensions in relation to onset of obsessive-compulsive disorder at menarche or the perinatal period. Arch Women Ment Health 13(1):75–81, 2010 19657706

Labad J, Alonso P, Segalàs C, et al: Reproductive hormone sensitivity and obsessive-compulsive disorder: are there differences in the genetic predisposition between symptom dimensions? J Clin Psychiatry 72(3):417–418, 2011 21450163

Li Y, Zhang CC, Kathrin Weidacker, et al: Investigation of anterior cingulate cortex gamma-aminobutyric acid and glutamate-glutamine levels in obsessive-compulsive disorder using magnetic resonance spectroscopy. BMC Psychiatry 19(1):164, 2019 31146727

Lindsay M, Crino R, Andrews G: Controlled trial of exposure and response prevention in obsessive-compulsive disorder. Br J Psychiatry 171:135–139, 1997 9337948

Lochner C, Hemmings SM, Kinnear CJ, et al: Gender in obsessive-compulsive disorder: clinical and genetic findings. Eur Neuropsychopharmacol 14(2):105–113, 2004 15013025

Lord C, Hall G, Soares CN, et al: Physiological stress response in postpartum women with obsessive-compulsive disorder: a pilot study. Psychoneuroendocrinology 36(1):133–138, 2011a 20537805
Lord C, Rieder A, Hall GB, et al: Piloting the perinatal obsessive-compulsive scale (POCS): development and validation. J Anxiety Disord 25(8):1079–1084, 2011b 21824744
Lundberg S, Carlsson A, Norfeldt P, et al: Nicotine treatment of obsessive-compulsive disorder. Prog Neuropsychopharmacol Biol Psychiatry 28(7):1195–1199, 2004 15610934
Mahon PB, Payne JL, MacKinnon DF, et al: Genome-wide linkage and follow-up association study of postpartum mood symptoms. Am J Psychiatry 166(11):1229–1237, 2009 19755578
Maina G, Albert U, Bogetto F, et al: Recent life events and obsessive-compulsive disorder (OCD): the role of pregnancy/delivery. Psychiatry Res 89(1):49–58, 1999 10643877
Mak L, Streiner DL, Steiner M: Is serotonin transporter polymorphism (5-HTTLPR) allele status a predictor for obsessive-compulsive disorder? A meta-analysis. Arch Women Ment Health 18(3):435–445, 2015 25896187
Marazziti D, Presta S, Pfanner C, et al: Immunological alterations in adult obsessive-compulsive disorder. Biol Psychiatry 46(6):810–814, 1999 10494449
Marazziti D, Mungai F, Masala I, et al: Normalisation of immune cell imbalance after pharmacological treatments of patients suffering from obsessive-compulsive disorder. J Psychopharmacol 23(5):567–573, 2009 18755814
Marazziti D, Baroni S, Giannaccini G, et al: A link between oxytocin and serotonin in humans: supporting evidence from peripheral markers. Eur Neuropsychopharmacol 22(8):578–583, 2012 22297159
Marks IM, Stern RS, Mawson D, et al: Clomipramine and exposure for obsessive-compulsive rituals: 1. Br J Psychiatry 136:1–25, 1980 6986939
Marks IM, Lelliott P, Basoglu M, et al: Clomipramine, self-exposure and therapist-aided exposure for obsessive-compulsive rituals. Br J Psychiatry 152:522–534, 1988 3167404
Mataix-Cols D, Frans E, Pérez-Vigil A, et al: A total-population multigenerational family clustering study of autoimmune diseases in obsessive-compulsive disorder and Tourette's/chronic tic disorders. Mol Psychiatry 23(7):1652–1658, 2018 29133949
Matthey S: Using the Edinburgh Postnatal Depression Scale to screen for anxiety disorders. Depress Anxiety 25(11):926–931, 2008 18041072
Mauri M, Oppo A, Montagnani MS, et al: Beyond "postpartum depressions": specific anxiety diagnoses during pregnancy predict different outcomes: results from PND-ReScU. J Affect Disord 127(1–3):177–184, 2010 20554326
Mavorgiorgou P, Gohle D, Winter C, et al: Low serotonergic function and its normalization by treatment with sertraline in obsessive-compulsive disorder—an auditory evoked potential study. J Clin Psychopharmacol 30(3):341–343, 2010 20473079
McCracken JT, Hanna GL: Elevated thyroid indices in children and adolescents with obsessive-compulsive disorder: effects of clomipramine treatment. J Child Adolesc Psychopharmacol 15(4):581–587, 2005 16190790
McDougle CJ, Goodman WK, Leckman JF, et al: Haloperidol addition in fluvoxamine-refractory obsessive-compulsive disorder: a double-blind, placebo-controlled study in patients with and without tics. Arch Gen Psychiatry 51(4):302–308, 1994 8161290
McDougle CJ, Epperson CN, Pelton GH, et al: A double-blind, placebo-controlled study of risperidone addition in serotonin reuptake inhibitor-refractory obsessive-compulsive disorder. Arch Gen Psychiatry 57(8):794–801, 2000 10920469
McEvoy K, Osborne LM: Allopregnanolone and reproductive psychiatry: an overview. Int Rev Psychiatry 31(3):237–244, 2019 30701996
McEvoy K, Osborne LM, Nanavati J, et al: Reproductive affective disorders: a review of the genetic evidence for premenstrual dysphoric disorder and postpartum depression. Curr Psychiatry Rep 19(12):94, 2017 29082433
McGuinness M, Blissett J, Jones C: OCD in the perinatal period: is postpartum OCD (ppOCD) a distinct subtype? A review of the literature. Behav Cogn Psychother 39(3):285–310, 2011
McLean PD, Whittal ML, Thordarson DS, et al: Cognitive versus behavior therapy in the group treatment of obsessive-compulsive disorder. J Consult Clin Psychol 69(2):205–214, 2001

Meltzer-Brody S, Colquhoun H, Riesenberg R, et al: Brexanolone injection in post-partum depression: two multicentre, double-blind, randomised, placebo-controlled, phase 3 trials. Lancet 392(10152):1058–1070, 2018 30177236
Miller ES, Chu C, Gollan J, et al: Obsessive-compulsive symptoms during the postpartum period. A prospective cohort. J Reprod Med 58(3–4):115–122, 2013 23539879
Misri S, Reebye P, Corral M, et al: The use of paroxetine and cognitive-behavioral therapy in postpartum depression and anxiety: a randomized controlled trial. J Clin Psychiatry 65(9):1236–1241, 2004 15367052
Mitra S, Bastos CP, Bates K, et al: Ovarian sex hormones modulate compulsive, affective and cognitive functions in a non-induced mouse model of obsessive-compulsive disorder. Front Behav Neurosci 10:215, 2016 27881956
Mitra S, Mucha M, Owen S, et al: Postpartum lactation-mediated behavioral outcomes and drug responses in a spontaneous mouse model of obsessive-compulsive disorder. ACS Chem Neurosci 8(12):2683–2697, 2017 28945961
Monteleone P, Catapano F, Del Buono G, et al: Circadian rhythms of melatonin, cortisol and prolactin in patients with obsessive-compulsive disorder. Acta Psychiatr Scand 89(6):411–415, 1994 8085472
Montgomery SA, Kasper S, Stein DJ, et al: Citalopram 20 mg, 40 mg and 60 mg are all effective and well tolerated compared with placebo in obsessive-compulsive disorder. Int Clin Psychopharmacol 16(2):75–86, 2001 11236072
Mundo E, Maina G, Uslenghi C: Multicentre, double-blind, comparison of fluvoxamine and clomipramine in the treatment of obsessive-compulsive disorder. Int Clin Psychopharmacol 15(2):69–76, 2000 10759337
Murray CJ, Lopez AD: The Global Burden of Disease: A Comprehensive Assessment of Mortality and Disability From Diseases, Injuries, and Risk Factors in 1990 and Projected to 2020: Summary. Geneva, World Health Organization, 1996
Nakatani E, Nakagawa A, Nakao T, et al: A randomized controlled trial of Japanese patients with obsessive-compulsive disorder: effectiveness of behavior therapy and fluvoxamine. Psychother Psychosom 74(5):269–276, 2005 16088264
Newth S, Rachman S: The concealment of obsessions. Behav Res Ther 39(4):457–464, 2001 11280343
Neziroglu F, Anemone R, Yaryura-Tobias JA: Onset of obsessive-compulsive disorder in pregnancy. Am J Psychiatry 149(7):947–950, 1992 1609876
Nicol-Harper R, Harvey AG, Stein A: Interactions between mothers and infants: impact of maternal anxiety. Infant Behav Dev 30(1):161–167, 2007 17292789
Nikodijevic A, Moulding R, Anglim J, et al: Fear of self, doubt and obsessive compulsive symptoms. J Behav Ther Exp Psychiatry 49(Pt B):164–172, 2015 25748202
Nordahl H, Havnen A, Hansen B, et al: Sleep disturbances in treatment-seeking OCD-patients: changes after concentrated exposure treatment. Scand J Psychol 59(2):186–191, 2018 29244201
Osborne LM, Monk C: Perinatal depression: the fourth inflammatory morbidity of pregnancy? Theory and literature review. Psychoneuroendocrinology 38(10):1929–1952, 2013 23608136
Osborne LM, Gispen F, Sanyal A, et al: Lower allopregnanolone during pregnancy predicts postpartum depression: an exploratory study. Psychoneuroendocrinology 79:116–121, 2017 28278440
Osborne LM, Brar A, Klein SL: The role of Th17 cells in the pathophysiology of pregnancy and perinatal mood and anxiety disorders. Brain Behav Immun 76:7–16, 2019a 30465878
Osborne LM, Yenokyan G, Fei K, et al: Innate immune activation and depressive and anxious symptoms across the peripartum: an exploratory study. Psychoneuroendocrinology 99:80–86, 2019b 30195110
Palmsten K, Huybrechts KF, Michels KB, et al: Antidepressant use and risk for preeclampsia. Epidemiology 24(5):682–691, 2013 23873072
Pampaloni I, Sivakumaran T, Hawley CJ, et al: High-dose selective serotonin reuptake inhibitors in OCD: a systematic retrospective case notes survey. J Psychopharmacol 24(10):1439–1445, 2010 19351803
Paterson JL, Reynolds AC, Ferguson SA, et al: Sleep and obsessive-compulsive disorder (OCD). Sleep Med Rev 17(6):465–474, 2013 23499210

Pearlman DM, Vora HS, Marquis BG, et al: Anti-basal ganglia antibodies in primary obsessive-compulsive disorder: systematic review and meta-analysis. Br J Psychiatry 205(1):8–16, 2014 24986387

Pedersen C, Leserman J, Garcia N, et al: Late pregnancy thyroid-binding globulin predicts perinatal depression. Psychoneuroendocrinology 65:84–93, 2016 26731573

Pertusa A, Fullana MA, Singh S, et al: Compulsive hoarding: OCD symptom, distinct clinical syndrome, or both? Am J Psychiatry 165(10):1289–1298, 2008 18483134

Pigott TA, L'Heureux F, Hill JL, et al: A double-blind study of adjuvant buspirone hydrochloride in clomipramine-treated patients with obsessive-compulsive disorder. J Clin Psychopharmacol 12(1):11–18, 1992 1552034

Pittenger C, Bloch MH, Williams K: Glutamate abnormalities in obsessive compulsive disorder: neurobiology, pathophysiology, and treatment. Pharmacol Ther 132(3):314–332, 2011 21963369

Pogarell O, Hamann C, Pöpperl G, et al: Elevated brain serotonin transporter availability in patients with obsessive-compulsive disorder. Biol Psychiatry 54(12):1406–1413, 2003 14675805

Pooley EC, Fineberg N, Harrison PJ: The met(158) allele of catechol-O-methyltransferase (COMT) is associated with obsessive-compulsive disorder in men: case-control study and meta-analysis. Mol Psychiatry 12(6):556–561, 2007 17264842

Ravindran AV, Griffiths J, Merali Z, et al: Circulating lymphocyte subsets in obsessive compulsive disorder, major depression and normal controls. J Affect Disord 52(1–3):1–10, 1999 10357012

Ross LE, McLean LM: Anxiety disorders during pregnancy and the postpartum period: a systematic review. J Clin Psychiatry 67(8):1285–1298, 2006 16965210

Rothbaum BO, Shahar F: Behavioral treatment of obsessive-compulsive disorder in a naturalistic setting. Cognitive and Behavioral Practice 7(3):262–270, 2000

Russell EJ, Fawcett JM, Mazmanian D: Risk of obsessive-compulsive disorder in pregnant and postpartum women: a meta-analysis. J Clin Psychiatry 74(4):377–385, 2013 23656845

Sadock BJ, Sadock VA, Ruiz P (eds): Comprehensive Textbook of Psychiatry, Vol 1. Philadelphia, PA, Lippincott Williams & Wilkins, 2000

Schofield CA, Battle CL, Howard M, et al: Symptoms of the anxiety disorders in a perinatal psychiatric sample: a chart review. J Nerv Ment Dis 202(2):154–160, 2014 24469528

Selvi Y, Atli A, Aydin A, et al: The comparison of aripiprazole and risperidone augmentation in selective serotonin reuptake inhibitor-refractory obsessive-compulsive disorder: a single-blind, randomised study. Hum Psychopharmacol 26(1):51–57, 2011 21308781

Sepede G, Sarchione F, Matarazzo I, et al: Premenstrual dysphoric disorder without comorbid psychiatric conditions: a systematic review of therapeutic options. Clin Neuropharmacol 39(5):241–261, 2016 27454391

Serati M, Benatti B, Buoli M, et al: Post-partum obsessive-compulsive disorder associated with 9q33.1 deletion. Aust N Z J Psychiatry 49(10):943–944, 2015 25922355

Shapira NA, Keck PE Jr, Goldsmith TD, et al: Open-label pilot study of tramadol hydrochloride in treatment-refractory obsessive-compulsive disorder. Depress Anxiety 6(4):170–173, 1997 9559288

Sharma TR, Kline DB, Shreeve DF, et al: Psychiatric comorbidities in patients with celiac disease: is there any concrete biological association? Asian J Psychiatr 4(2):150–151, 2011 23051084

Sharma V: Role of sleep deprivation in the causation of postpartum obsessive-compulsive disorder. Med Hypotheses 122:58–61, 2019 30593425

Sharma V, Sommerdyk C: Obsessive-compulsive disorder in the postpartum period: diagnosis, differential diagnosis and management. Womens Health (Lond) 11(4):543–552, 2015 26246310

Sichel DA, Cohen LS, Dimmock JA, et al: Postpartum obsessive compulsive disorder: a case series. J Clin Psychiatry 54(4):156–159, 1993a 8486594

Sichel DA, Cohen LS, Rosenbaum JF, et al: Postpartum onset of obsessive-compulsive disorder. Psychosomatics 34(3):277–279, 1993b 8493313

Simpson HB, Liebowitz MR, Foa EB, et al: Post-treatment effects of exposure therapy and clomipramine in obsessive-compulsive disorder. Depress Anxiety 19(4):225–233, 2004 15274171

Simpson W, Glazer M, Michalski N, et al: Comparative efficacy of the generalized anxiety disorder 7-item scale and the Edinburgh Postnatal Depression Scale as screening tools for generalized anxiety disorder in pregnancy and the postpartum period. Can J Psychiatry 59(8):434–440, 2014 25161068

Sinopoli VM, Burton CL, Kronenberg S, et al: A review of the role of serotonin system genes in obsessive-compulsive disorder. Neurosci Biobehav Rev 80:372–381, 2017 28576508

Sit D, Rothschild AJ, Wisner KL: A review of postpartum psychosis. J Womens Health (Larchmt) 15(4):352–368, 2006 16724884

Smeraldi E, Erzegovesi S, Bianchi I, Pasquali L: Fluvoxamine vs clomipramine treatment in obsessive-compulsive disorder: a preliminary study. New Trends in Experimental and Clinical Psychiatry 8(2):63–65, 1992

Somerville S, Dedman K, Hagan R, et al: The Perinatal Anxiety Screening Scale: development and preliminary validation. Arch Women Ment Health 17(5):443–454, 2014 24699796

Somerville S, Byrne SL, Dedman K, et al: Detecting the severity of perinatal anxiety with the Perinatal Anxiety Screening Scale (PASS). J Affect Disord 186:18–25, 2015 26226429

Speisman BB, Storch EA, Abramowitz JS: Postpartum obsessive-compulsive disorder. J Obstet Gynecol Neonatal Nurs 40(6):680–690, 2011 22092284

Spies M, Knudsen GM, Lanzenberger R, et al: The serotonin transporter in psychiatric disorders: insights from PET imaging. Lancet Psychiatry 2(8):743–755, 2015 26249305

Spinelli M: Antidepressant treatment during pregnancy. Am J Psychiatry 169(2):121–124, 2012 22318792

Standeven LR, Nestadt G, Samuels J: Genetics of perinatal obsessive-compulsive disorder, in Biomarkers of Postpartum Psychiatric Disorders. Edited by Payne JL, Osborne LM. New York, Academic Press, 2020, pp 95–110

Stein DJ, Rapoport JL: Cross-cultural studies and obsessive-compulsive disorder. CNS Spectrums 1(1):42–46, 1996

Stein DJ, Andersen EW, Tonnoir B, et al: Escitalopram in obsessive-compulsive disorder: a randomized, placebo-controlled, paroxetine-referenced, fixed-dose, 24-week study. Curr Med Res Opin 23(4):701–711, 2007 17407626

Stein DJ, Koen N, Fineberg N, et al: A 2012 evidence-based algorithm for the pharmacotherapy for obsessive-compulsive disorder. Curr Psychiatry Rep 14(3):211–219, 2012 22527872

Stein MB, Forde DR, Anderson G, et al: Obsessive-compulsive disorder in the community: an epidemiologic survey with clinical reappraisal. Am J Psychiatry 154(8):1120–1126, 1997

Sutter-Dallay AL, Giaconne-Marcesche V, Glatigny-Dallay E, et al: Women with anxiety disorders during pregnancy are at increased risk of intense postnatal depressive symptoms: a prospective survey of the MATQUID cohort. Eur Psychiatry 19(8):459–463, 2004 15589703

Taylor S: Molecular genetics of obsessive-compulsive disorder: a comprehensive meta-analysis of genetic association studies. Mol Psychiatry 18(7):799–805, 2013 22665263

Tenneij NH, van Megen HJ, Denys DA, et al: Behavior therapy augments response of patients with obsessive-compulsive disorder responding to drug treatment. J Clin Psychiatry 66(9):1169–1175, 2005 16187776

Timpano KR, Abramowitz JS, Mahaffey BL, et al: Efficacy of a prevention program for postpartum obsessive-compulsive symptoms. J Psychiatr Res 45(11):1511–1517, 2011 21764404

Timpano KR, Carbonella JY, Bernert RA, et al: Obsessive compulsive symptoms and sleep difficulties: exploring the unique relationship between insomnia and obsessions. J Psychiatr Res 57:101–107, 2014 25038630

Tollefson GD, Rampey AH Jr, Potvin JH, et al: A multicenter investigation of fixed-dose fluoxetine in the treatment of obsessive-compulsive disorder. Arch Gen Psychiatry 51(7):559–567, 1994 8031229

Uguz F, Akman C, Kaya N, et al: Postpartum-onset obsessive-compulsive disorder: incidence, clinical features, and related factors. J Clin Psychiatry 68(1):132–138, 2007 17284141

Uguz F, Kaya V, Gezginc K, et al: Clinical correlates of worsening in obsessive-compulsive symptoms during pregnancy. Gen Hosp Psychiatry 33(2):197–199, 2011 21596214

van Balkom AJ, de Haan E, van Oppen P, et al: Cognitive and behavioral therapies alone versus in combination with fluvoxamine in the treatment of obsessive compulsive disorder. J Nerv Ment Dis 186(8):492–499, 1998 9717867
van Oppen P, de Haan E, van Balkom AJ, et al: Cognitive therapy and exposure in vivo in the treatment of obsessive compulsive disorder. Behav Res Ther 33(4):379–390, 1995 7755525
Vasconcelos MS, Sampaio AS, Hounie AG, et al: Prenatal, perinatal, and postnatal risk factors in obsessive-compulsive disorder. Biol Psychiatry 61(3):301–307, 2007 17123475
Vulink NC, Denys D, Westenberg HG: Bupropion for patients with obsessive-compulsive disorder: an open-label, fixed-dose study. J Clin Psychiatry 66(2):228–230, 2005 15705009
Vulink NC, Denys D, Bus L, et al: Female hormones affect symptom severity in obsessive-compulsive disorder. Int Clin Psychopharmacol 21(3):171–175, 2006 16528139
Wang HR, Woo YS, Bahk WM: Potential role of anticonvulsants in the treatment of obsessive-compulsive and related disorders. Psychiatry Clin Neurosci 68(10):723–732, 2014 24735021
Warren R, Thomas JC: Cognitive-behavior therapy of obsessive-compulsive disorder in private practice: an effectiveness study. J Anxiety Disord 15(4):277–285, 2001 11474814
Warren SL, Gunnar MR, Kagan J, et al: Maternal panic disorder: infant temperament, neurophysiology, and parenting behaviors. J Am Acad Child Adolesc Psychiatry 42(7):814–825, 2003
Wesseloo R, Kamperman AM, Bergink V, et al: Thyroid peroxidase antibodies during early gestation and the subsequent risk of first-onset postpartum depression: a prospective cohort study. J Affect Disord 225:399–403, 2018 28850854
Wilhelm S, Steketee G, Reilly Harrington NA, et al: Effectiveness of cognitive therapy for obsessive-compulsive disorder: an open trial. Journal of Cognitive Psychotherapy 19(2):173–179, 2005
Winter C, Greene DM, Mavrogiorgou P, et al: Altered serotonergic and GABAergic neurotransmission in a mice model of obsessive-compulsive disorder. Behav Brain Res 337:240–245, 2018 28916503
Wisner KL, Peindl KS, Gigliotti T, et al: Obsessions and compulsions in women with postpartum depression. J Clin Psychiatry 60(3):176–180, 1999 10192593
Yaryura-Tobias JA, Bhagavan HN: L-tryptophan in obsessive-compulsive disorders. Am J Psychiatry 134(11):1298–1299, 1977 333953
Yawn BP, Pace W, Wollan PC, et al: Concordance of Edinburgh Postnatal Depression Scale (EPDS) and Patient Health Questionnaire (PHQ-9) to assess increased risk of depression among postpartum women. J Am Board Fam Med 22(5):483–491, 2009 19734393
Zambaldi CF, Cantilino A, Montenegro AC, et al: Postpartum obsessive-compulsive disorder: prevalence and clinical characteristics. Compr Psychiatry 50(6):503–509, 2009 19840587
Zhang Z, Fan Q, Bai Y, et al: Brain gamma-aminobutyric acid (GABA) concentration of the prefrontal lobe in unmedicated patients with obsessive-compulsive disorder: a research of magnetic resonance spectroscopy. Shanghai Jingshen Yixue 28(5):263–270, 2016 28638200

# CHAPTER 21

# Substance Use Disorders

Julia Frew, M.D.
Lauren Augello, M.D.
Marley Doyle, M.D.
Constance Guille, M.D.
Susan Karabell, M.D.
Lulu Zhao, M.D.

Substance use disorders (SUDs) generate special concerns for women and their health care providers, particularly in the perinatal period. Considerations include the teratogenicity of substances of abuse, the potential for neonatal substance withdrawal, the stigma related to substance use in pregnancy, and concerns about child protection reporting in cases of maternal substance use. Integrated care models that provide coordinated SUD treatment and obstetrical care show promise for improving outcomes for women with SUDs and their children. This chapter reviews the epidemiology, clinical features, pathophysiology, and treatment of SUDs in women generally, with a particular focus on the perinatal period.

## Epidemiology

### Rates/Incidence

The development and prognosis of SUDs are gendered. In the United States, 45% of people age 12 years or older who use illicit drugs are women. Women are most at risk of substance use between the ages of 18 and 29 years, coinciding with their reproductive years. In the United States, tobacco, alcohol, and cannabis are the three substances used most commonly during pregnancy. Notably, polysubstance use is common, with up to 50% of women endorsing use of more than one substance (Forray 2016).

**TABLE 21–1. Estimates of perinatal substance use**

| Substance | Subjects using substances during pregnancy, % | Subjects resuming use postpartum, % |
|---|---|---|
| Alcohol | 35 | 51% |
| Cannabis | 10–43 | 41% |
| Opioids | 14–22 | >50% |
| Sedative-hypnotics (i.e., benzodiazepines, barbiturates) | Unknown | Unknown |
| Stimulants | Cocaine: 1–10<br>Methamphetamines: 1–5 | Cocaine: 27% |
| Tobacco | 12–25 | 16% |

*Source.* Forray et al. 2015; Haight et al. 2018; McLafferty et al. 2016; Rodriguez and Smith 2019.

Reported rates of substance use vary depending on the methodology of the study. The figures listed in Table 21–1 indicate use of each substance and do not distinguish between indicated substance use, substance misuse, or SUDs. Using opioids as an example, a study of publicly insured women in Tennessee showed that 28% filled a prescription for an opioid prenatally (Patrick et al. 2015). However, the estimated risk for opioid use disorder in pregnancy ranges from 0.4% to 0.8% (Patrick et al. 2012). Moreover, certain substances such as methamphetamine and benzodiazepines have extremely limited epidemiological data because they are frequently used in conjunction with other illicit substances and are rarely studied alone. Finally, certain substances have much higher rates of polysubstance misuse compared with others. Data from the National Survey on Drug Use and Health, for example, found that 96% of heroin users also used at least one other substance in the past year, and 61% used at least three different drugs (Jones et al. 2015). Meanwhile, pregnant women reporting cannabis use were unlikely to use other substances unless they were also involved with the criminal justice system (Washio et al. 2018).

In general, women endorse lower levels of substance use during pregnancy compared with pre-pregnancy (Forray et al. 2015). This may result from a combination of advice from clinicians concerning the negative consequences of substance use in pregnancy, negative messages regarding substance use from society and health care professionals, increased access to treatment services during pregnancy, and maternal concern about the impact of substances on the fetus. Postpartum, however, these same forces become less pronounced, and a significant proportion of women resume substance use. One study found that by 3 months postpartum, 58% of women had resumed smoking, 41% had resumed cannabis use, and 27% had resumed cocaine use (Forray et al. 2015). Because of the high risk of recurrent drug use postpartum, mortality is also heightened during this period. A study of women in Massachusetts found that overdose deaths from opioids were particularly heightened 7–12 months postpartum, nearly four times the overdose rate in the third trimester (Schiff et al. 2018). Meanwhile, a study of maternal deaths in Colorado from the years 2004–2012 found that most women who died from self-harm (either suicide or overdose) had comorbid substance use and affective psychiatric disorders (Metz et al. 2016).

## Tobacco

Tobacco is the most common substance used during pregnancy. Women who smoke cigarettes are less likely to abstain from all substances during pregnancy and have a higher prevalence of polysubstance use, with comorbid alcohol and cannabis use being the most common. Feelings of depression may contribute to continued smoking during pregnancy; in an observational study, women who continued to smoke cigarettes during pregnancy reported significantly more depressive symptoms than recent ex-smokers and nonsmokers (Munafò et al. 2008). Within 1 year postpartum, 80% of women who quit smoking in pregnancy had resumed smoking (Forray and Foster 2015). Women who smoke prior to pregnancy are more likely to cease breastfeeding to resume smoking (Forray and Foster 2015). Limited data are available regarding the use of alternative forms of tobacco during the perinatal period, although the rates of electronic cigarette use are increasing among women of reproductive age (Forray and Foster 2015).

## Alcohol

Among pregnant women in the United States, the prevalence of any alcohol use ranges from 10% to 80% and is 3% for binge drinking (Dejong et al. 2019). Among women who reported drinking before pregnancy, 87% achieved remission during pregnancy, 6.6% reduced their intake, and 6.4% did not reduce their intake (Dejong et al. 2019). According to the 2013 Substance Abuse and Mental Health Services Administration National Survey on Drug Use and Health (NSDUH), risk factors for continued alcohol use during pregnancy include age between 35 and 44 years, having college degree, being employed, or being of American Indian, Alaskan Native, or non-Hispanic Black ethnicity (Dejong et al. 2019). Of women drinking in late pregnancy, the highest prevalence of alcohol use was in non-Hispanic college graduates older than 35 years (Dejong et al. 2019). Social stressors were associated with higher likelihood of continuing alcohol use during the third trimester. Limited data exist regarding alcohol use in breastfeeding, but one study found that 24%–80% of women consume alcohol while breastfeeding (Dejong et al. 2019).

## Cannabis

According to the NSDUH, the self-reported prevalence of cannabis use in pregnancy increased between 2002 and 2017. Women reporting any cannabis use during the first trimester of pregnancy rose from 5.7% in 2002–2003 to 12.1% in 2016–2017. Daily or near-daily use during the first trimester was reported by 1.8% of women in 2002–2003 and by 5.3% in 2016–2017. Use of cannabis daily or near-daily in later trimesters increased from 0.6% to 2.5% (second trimester) and from 0.5% to 2.5% (third trimester) between 2002–2003 and 2016–2017. These data suggest not only increased overall use of cannabis among reproductive-age women but also a possible perception of lower risk of cannabis in pregnancy in 2016–2017 compared with 2002–2003 (Volkow et al. 2019).

## Stimulant Drugs of Abuse

The prevalence of cocaine use in pregnancy is estimated to be 1.1% (Forray and Foster 2015). Women with cocaine use disorder tend to use higher amounts of other drugs, including tobacco, marijuana, and alcohol, during pregnancy. The most common pattern of cocaine use during pregnancy is periods of binges followed by forced abstinence and withdrawal (Ait-Daoud et al. 2019).

Prevalence rates of methamphetamine use during pregnancy range from 1% to 5% (Forray and Foster 2015). Hospitalization of pregnant women for amphetamine abuse doubled from 1988 to 2004, and methamphetamines were the primary substance for which pregnant women sought treatment in that period (Smid et al. 2019). Women who use methamphetamine during pregnancy are more likely to have co-occurring psychiatric disorders, use other substances, and have limited engagement in prenatal care (Forray and Foster 2015; Smid et al. 2019).

### Opioids

The prevalence of maternal opioid use in pregnancy increased nearly fivefold from 1.19 per 1,000 live hospital births in 2000 to 5.63 per 1,000 live births in 2009 (Patrick et al. 2012). Studies of Medicaid-enrolled women have found that 18.5%–29% filled an opioid prescription during pregnancy (Yazdy et al. 2015). Pregnancy-related deaths due to opioid misuse more than doubled between 2007 and 2016, increasing from 4% to 10% (Gemmill et al. 2019). Psychiatric comorbidity is common among perinatal women with opioid use disorder, particularly mood and anxiety disorders (Arnaudo et al. 2017). Most women with opioid use disorder also use other substances: 77%–95% of women also smoke cigarettes (Forray and Foster 2015), about 26.6%report cocaine use, 56.6% report regular alcohol use, and 73.5% report regular cannabis use in one study (Brogly et al. 2018).

## Risk Factors

Overall, the risk factors for SUDs during pregnancy (except alcohol use) include age <25 years, low education level (less than high school), lower socioeconomic status, comorbid psychiatric disorders, polysubstance use prior to pregnancy, social stressors, family history of substance use disorders, and trauma history, including adult or childhood sexual abuse and intimate partner violence (Ait-Daoud et al. 2019; Cook et al. 2017). Risk factors are summarized in Table 21–2.

## Screening Methods

All women should be screened for substance use. Screening allows providers to identify patients at risk, stratify severity, and intervene based on level of acuity. Universal screening is also recommended by professional organizations such as the American Academy of Pediatrics, American College of Obstetricians and Gynecologists, American Medical Association, American Psychiatric Association, Centers for Disease Control and Prevention, and World Health Organization. In the peripartum period, screening is recommended at the initial prenatal visit and should be repeated every trimester for women who screened positive initially for past or current use (Wright et al. 2016). Reporting mandates vary widely per state, and physicians should be familiar with the laws in their area of practice. To the extent allowed by law, physicians should strive to maintain patient confidentiality, autonomy, and dignity (American College of Obstetricians and Gynecologists 2017a). The application of legal statutes by physicians to enforce substance use treatment disrupts the trust necessary to establish a therapeutic physician–patient relationship (American College of Obstetricians and Gynecologists 2011).

TABLE 21–2. **Risk factors for substance use disorders and alcohol use in pregnancy**

| Substance use disorders | Alcohol use |
|---|---|
| Age < 25 years | Age between 35 and 44 years |
| Comorbid psychiatric disorders | Alaskan Native |
| Family history of substance use disorders | American Indian |
| Intimate partner violence | College degree |
| Low education level (less than high school) | Non-Hispanic Black |
| Lower socioeconomic status | |
| Polysubstance use prior to pregnancy | |
| Social stressors | |
| Trauma history (adult or childhood sexual abuse) | |

TABLE 21–3. **Validated perinatal substance use screening questionnaires**

| Questionnaire | Description |
|---|---|
| 4P's (parents, partner, past use, present pregnancy), 4P's Plus, 5P's (peers, partner, parents, past use, present use) | Four- to six-question screener exploring past and recent exposure to substances |
| Substance Use Risk Profile–Pregnancy | Three brief questions; classifies respondents into low, medium, and high risk for problematic drug and alcohol use |
| T-ACE (tolerance, annoyed, cut down, eye-opener) | Four-question screener for problematic alcohol use in pregnant women |

*Source.* World Health Organization 2014.

Table 21–3 lists options for validated substance abuse screening tools developed specifically for the peripartum population. Other screens, such as the Drug Abuse Screening Test or the National Institute on Drug Abuse Quick Screen, may also be appropriate because these are validated in general medical settings. They may all be administered in person or remotely by a medical staff member or by the patient. Urine and blood drug testing may be used to confirm or monitor substance use but should not be used as a population-level screening method, due to methodological concerns.

Many of the perinatal screening tools are highly sensitive but less specific because they are brief and ask broad questions about at-risk exposures or behaviors. In short, they are designed to facilitate conversations about substance use. A positive screen should prompt further evaluation, with the goal of defining factors such as the time period, frequency, and amount of use and severity of functional impairment.

Providers should screen patients for substance use in an open-ended, empathetic, and nonjudgmental manner, provide education on the harmful effects of substance use, assess and support motivation to change, and refer to specialty or a higher level of care as indicated (Wright et al. 2016). This process is formally known as screening, brief intervention, and referral to treatment (SBIRT). SBIRT is recognized as the standard of care based on expert opinion and the recommendation of professional organizations (Centers for Disease Control and Prevention; U.S. Preventive Services Task

Force [USPSTF]; Wright et al. 2015). In addition to screening, doctors should compile a list of resources and providers in their community that can help patients with transitions of care and to bolster support.

## Diagnostic Criteria

DSM-5 (American Psychiatric Association 2013) defines SUD as a pathological pattern of behaviors related to the use of the substance. One key feature of SUDs is the underlying alteration in brain reward circuitry that persists beyond intoxication and detoxification. Ten separate classes of drugs are included in the SUDs: alcohol; caffeine; cannabis; hallucinogens; inhalants; opioids; sedatives, hypnotics, and anxiolytics; stimulants; tobacco; and other or unknown substances. Each of these substances has the potential to activate the brain reward pathway, although the mechanism of action may differ. See Boxes 21–1 through 21–4 for the DSM-5 diagnostic criteria for various SUDs. Specifiers may be applied to the diagnostic criteria to indicate severity, ranging from mild to moderate or severe. DSM-5 also includes the specifier "with peripartum onset" for mood disorders to indicate onset of mood symptoms during pregnancy or the first 4 weeks postpartum. However, this specifier should not be applied to SUDs (American Psychiatric Association 2013).

### Box 21–1. DSM-5 Criteria for Alcohol Use Disorder

A. A problematic pattern of alcohol use leading to clinically significant impairment or distress, as manifested by at least two of the following, occurring within a 12-month period:

1. Alcohol is often taken in larger amounts or over a longer period than was intended.
2. There is a persistent desire or unsuccessful efforts to cut down or control alcohol use.
3. A great deal of time is spent in activities necessary to obtain alcohol, use alcohol, or recover from its effects.
4. Craving, or a strong desire or urge to use alcohol.
5. Recurrent alcohol use resulting in a failure to fulfill major role obligations at work, school, or home.
6. Continued alcohol use despite having persistent or recurrent social or interpersonal problems caused or exacerbated by the effects of alcohol.
7. Important social, occupational, or recreational activities are given up or reduced because of alcohol use.
8. Recurrent alcohol use in situations in which it is physically hazardous.
9. Alcohol use is continued despite knowledge of having a persistent or recurrent physical or psychological problem that is likely to have been caused or exacerbated by alcohol.
10. Tolerance, as defined by either of the following:
    a. A need for markedly increased amounts of alcohol to achieve intoxication or desired effect.
    b. A markedly diminished effect with continued use of the same amount of alcohol.
11. Withdrawal, as manifested by either of the following:
    a. The characteristic withdrawal syndrome for alcohol (refer to Criteria A and B of the criteria set for alcohol withdrawal, pp. 499–500).

b. Alcohol (or a closely related substance, such as a benzodiazepine) is taken to relieve or avoid withdrawal symptoms.

*Specify* if:

**In early remission:** After full criteria for alcohol use disorder were previously met, none of the criteria for alcohol use disorder have been met for at least 3 months but for less than 12 months (with the exception that Criterion A4, "Craving, or a strong desire or urge to use alcohol," may be met).

**In sustained remission:** After full criteria for alcohol use disorder were previously met, none of the criteria for alcohol use disorder have been met at any time during a period of 12 months or longer (with the exception that Criterion A4, "Craving, or a strong desire or urge to use alcohol," may be met).

*Specify* if:

**In a controlled environment:** This additional specifier is used if the individual is in an environment where access to alcohol is restricted.

**Code based on current severity:** Note for ICD-10-CM codes: If an alcohol intoxication, alcohol withdrawal, or another alcohol-induced mental disorder is also present, do not use the codes below for alcohol use disorder. Instead, the comorbid alcohol use disorder is indicated in the 4th character of the alcohol-induced disorder code (see the coding note for alcohol intoxication, alcohol withdrawal, or a specific alcohol-induced mental disorder). For example, if there is comorbid alcohol intoxication and alcohol use disorder, only the alcohol intoxication code is given, with the 4th character indicating whether the comorbid alcohol use disorder is mild, moderate, or severe: F10.129 for mild alcohol use disorder with alcohol intoxication or F10.229 for a moderate or severe alcohol use disorder with alcohol intoxication.

*Specify* current severity:

**305.00 (F10.10) Mild:** Presence of 2–3 symptoms.
**303.90 (F10.20) Moderate:** Presence of 4–5 symptoms.
**303.90 (F10.20) Severe:** Presence of 6 or more symptoms.

*Source.* Reprinted from American Psychiatric Association: *Diagnostic and Statistical Manual of Mental Disorders,* 5th Edition. Arlington, VA, 2013, pp. 490–491. Copyright © 2013 American Psychiatric Association. Used with permission.

## Box 21–2. DSM-5 Criteria for Cannabis Use Disorder

A. A problematic pattern of cannabis use leading to clinically significant impairment or distress, as manifested by at least two of the following, occurring within a 12-month period:

1. Cannabis is often taken in larger amounts or over a longer period than was intended.
2. There is a persistent desire or unsuccessful efforts to cut down or control cannabis use.
3. A great deal of time is spent in activities necessary to obtain cannabis, use cannabis, or recover from its effects.
4. Craving, or a strong desire or urge to use cannabis.
5. Recurrent cannabis use resulting in a failure to fulfill major role obligations at work, school, or home.
6. Continued cannabis use despite having persistent or recurrent social or interpersonal problems caused or exacerbated by the effects of cannabis.
7. Important social, occupational, or recreational activities are given up or reduced because of cannabis use.
8. Recurrent cannabis use in situations in which it is physically hazardous.

9. Cannabis use is continued despite knowledge of having a persistent or recurrent physical or psychological problem that is likely to have been caused or exacerbated by cannabis.
10. Tolerance, as defined by either of the following:
    a. A need for markedly increased amounts of cannabis to achieve intoxication or desired effect.
    b. Markedly diminished effect with continued use of the same amount of cannabis.
11. Withdrawal, as manifested by either of the following:
    a. The characteristic withdrawal syndrome for cannabis (refer to Criteria A and B of the criteria set for cannabis withdrawal).
    b. Cannabis (or a closely related substance) is taken to relieve or avoid withdrawal symptoms.

*Specify* if:

**In early remission:** After full criteria for cannabis use disorder were previously met, none of the criteria for cannabis use disorder have been met for at least 3 months but for less than 12 months (with the exception that Criterion A4, "Craving, or a strong desire or urge to use cannabis," may be met).

**In sustained remission:** After full criteria for cannabis use disorder were previously met, none of the criteria for cannabis use disorder have been met at any time during a period of 12 months or longer (with the exception that Criterion A4, "Craving, or a strong desire or urge to use cannabis," may be present).

*Specify* if:

**In a controlled environment:** This additional specifier is used if the individual is in an environment where access to cannabis is restricted.

**Code based on current severity:** Note for ICD-10-CM codes: If a cannabis intoxication, cannabis withdrawal, or another cannabis-induced mental disorder is also present, do not use the codes below for cannabis use disorder. Instead, the comorbid cannabis use disorder is indicated in the 4th character of the cannabis-induced disorder code (see the coding note for cannabis intoxication, cannabis withdrawal, or a specific cannabis-induced mental disorder). For example, if there is comorbid cannabis-induced anxiety disorder and cannabis use disorder, only the cannabis-induced anxiety disorder code is given, with the 4th character indicating whether the comorbid cannabis use disorder is mild, moderate, or severe: F12.180 for mild cannabis use disorder with cannabis-induced anxiety disorder or F12.280 for a moderate or severe cannabis use disorder with cannabis-induced anxiety disorder.

*Specify* current severity:

**305.20 (F12.10) Mild:** Presence of 2–3 symptoms.

**304.30 (F12.20) Moderate:** Presence of 4–5 symptoms.

**304.30 (F12.20) Severe:** Presence of 6 or more symptoms.

*Source.* Reprinted from American Psychiatric Association: *Diagnostic and Statistical Manual of Mental Disorders,* 5th Edition. Arlington, VA, 2013, pp. 509–510. 

## Box 21–3. DSM-5 Criteria for Opioid Use Disorder

A. A problematic pattern of opioid use leading to clinically significant impairment or distress, as manifested by at least two of the following, occurring within a 12-month period:
    1. Opioids are often taken in larger amounts or over a longer period than was intended.

2. There is a persistent desire or unsuccessful efforts to cut down or control opioid use.
3. A great deal of time is spent in activities necessary to obtain the opioid, use the opioid, or recover from its effects.
4. Craving, or a strong desire or urge to use opioids.
5. Recurrent opioid use resulting in a failure to fulfill major role obligations at work, school, or home.
6. Continued opioid use despite having persistent or recurrent social or interpersonal problems caused or exacerbated by the effects of opioids.
7. Important social, occupational, or recreational activities are given up or reduced because of opioid use.
8. Recurrent opioid use in situations in which it is physically hazardous.
9. Continued opioid use despite knowledge of having a persistent or recurrent physical or psychological problem that is likely to have been caused or exacerbated by the substance.
10. Tolerance, as defined by either of the following:
    a. A need for markedly increased amounts of opioids to achieve intoxication or desired effect.
    b. A markedly diminished effect with continued use of the same amount of an opioid.

    **Note:** This criterion is not considered to be met for those taking opioids solely under appropriate medical supervision.
11. Withdrawal, as manifested by either of the following:
    a. The characteristic opioid withdrawal syndrome (refer to Criteria A and B of the criteria set for opioid withdrawal, pp. 547–548).
    b. Opioids (or a closely related substance) are taken to relieve or avoid withdrawal symptoms.

    **Note:** This criterion is not considered to be met for those individuals taking opioids solely under appropriate medical supervision.

*Specify* if:

**In early remission:** After full criteria for opioid use disorder were previously met, none of the criteria for opioid use disorder have been met for at least 3 months but for less than 12 months (with the exception that Criterion A4, "Craving, or a strong desire or urge to use opioids," may be met).

**In sustained remission:** After full criteria for opioid use disorder were previously met, none of the criteria for opioid use disorder have been met at any time during a period of 12 months or longer (with the exception that Criterion A4, "Craving, or a strong desire or urge to use opioids," may be met).

*Specify* if:

**On maintenance therapy:** This additional specifier is used if the individual is taking a prescribed agonist medication such as methadone or buprenorphine and none of the criteria for opioid use disorder have been met for that class of medication (except tolerance to, or withdrawal from, the agonist). This category also applies to those individuals being maintained on a partial agonist, an agonist/antagonist, or a full antagonist such as oral naltrexone or depot naltrexone.

**In a controlled environment:** This additional specifier is used if the individual is in an environment where access to opioids is restricted.

**Coding based on current severity:** Note for ICD-10-CM codes: If an opioid intoxication, opioid withdrawal, or another opioid-induced mental disorder is also present, do not use the codes below for opioid use disorder. Instead, the comorbid opioid use disorder is indicated in the 4th character of the opioid-induced disorder code (see the coding note for opioid intoxication, opioid withdrawal, or a specific opioid-induced mental disorder). For example, if there is comorbid opioid-induced depressive disorder and opioid use disorder, only the opioid-induced depressive disorder code is given, with the 4th character indicating whether the comorbid opioid use disorder is mild, moderate, or severe: F11.14 for mild opioid use disorder with opioid-induced depressive disorder or F11.24 for a moderate or severe opioid use disorder with opioid-induced depressive disorder.

*Specify* current severity:

**305.50 (F11.10) Mild:** Presence of 2–3 symptoms.
**304.00 (F11.20) Moderate:** Presence of 4–5 symptoms.
**304.00 (F11.20) Severe:** Presence of 6 or more symptoms.

*Source.* Reprinted from American Psychiatric Association: *Diagnostic and Statistical Manual of Mental Disorders,* 5th Edition. Arlington, VA, 2013, pp. 541–542. 

## Box 21–4. DSM-5 Criteria for Tobacco Use Disorder

A. A problematic pattern of tobacco use leading to clinically significant impairment or distress, as manifested by at least two of the following, occurring within a 12-month period:

1. Tobacco is often taken in larger amounts or over a longer period than was intended.
2. There is a persistent desire or unsuccessful efforts to cut down or control tobacco use.
3. A great deal of time is spent in activities necessary to obtain or use tobacco.
4. Craving, or a strong desire or urge to use tobacco.
5. Recurrent tobacco use resulting in a failure to fulfill major role obligations at work, school, or home (e.g., interference with work).
6. Continued tobacco use despite having persistent or recurrent social or interpersonal problems caused or exacerbated by the effects of tobacco (e.g., arguments with others about tobacco use).
7. Important social, occupational, or recreational activities are given up or reduced because of tobacco use.
8. Recurrent tobacco use in situations in which it is physically hazardous (e.g., smoking in bed).
9. Tobacco use is continued despite knowledge of having a persistent or recurrent physical or psychological problem that is likely to have been caused or exacerbated by tobacco.
10. Tolerance, as defined by either of the following:
    a. A need for markedly increased amounts of tobacco to achieve the desired effect.
    b. A markedly diminished effect with continued use of the same amount of tobacco.
11. Withdrawal, as manifested by either of the following:
    a. The characteristic withdrawal syndrome for tobacco (refer to Criteria A and B of the criteria set for tobacco withdrawal).
    b. Tobacco (or a closely related substance, such as nicotine) is taken to relieve or avoid withdrawal symptoms.

*Specify* if:

**In early remission:** After full criteria for tobacco use disorder were previously met, none of the criteria for tobacco use disorder have been met for at least 3 months but for less than 12 months (with the exception that Criterion A4, "Craving, or a strong desire or urge to use tobacco," may be met).

**In sustained remission:** After full criteria for tobacco use disorder were previously met, none of the criteria for tobacco use disorder have been met at any time during a period of 12 months or longer (with the exception that Criterion A4, "Craving, or a strong desire or urge to use tobacco," may be met).

*Specify* if:

**On maintenance therapy:** The individual is taking a long-term maintenance medication, such as nicotine replacement medication, and no criteria for tobacco use disorder have been met for that class of medication (except tolerance to, or withdrawal from, the nicotine replacement medication).

**In a controlled environment:** This additional specifier is used if the individual is in an environment where access to tobacco is restricted.

**Coding based on current severity:** Note for ICD-10-CM codes: If a tobacco withdrawal or tobacco-induced sleep disorder is also present, do not use the codes below for tobacco use disorder. Instead, the comorbid tobacco use disorder is indicated in the 4th character of the tobacco-induced disorder code (see the coding note for tobacco withdrawal or tobacco-induced sleep disorder). For example, if there is comorbid tobacco-induced sleep disorder and tobacco use disorder, only the tobacco-induced sleep disorder code is given, with the 4th character indicating whether the comorbid tobacco use disorder is moderate or severe: F17.208 for moderate or severe tobacco use disorder with tobacco-induced sleep disorder. It is not permissible to code a comorbid mild tobacco use disorder with a tobacco-induced sleep disorder.

*Specify* current severity:

**305.1 (Z72.0) Mild:** Presence of 2–3 symptoms.

**305.1 (F17.200) Moderate:** Presence of 4–5 symptoms.

**305.1 (F17.200) Severe:** Presence of 6 or more symptoms.

*Source.* Reprinted from American Psychiatric Association: *Diagnostic and Statistical Manual of Mental Disorders*, 5th Edition. Arlington, VA, 2013, pp. 571–572. 

The American Society of Addiction Medicine defines *addiction* as a primary, chronic disease of brain reward, motivation, memory, and related circuitry, including dysfunction in these circuits leading to characteristic biological, psychosocial, and spiritual manifestations. This is reflected in an individual's pathological pursuit of reward or relief through substance use and other behaviors.*The ICD-10 Classification of Mental and Behavioural Disorders* (World Health Organization 1992) includes a section on SUDs categorized by substance. Regardless of the diagnostic criteria used, the perinatal period does not alter the diagnosis, nor is a specific specifier required.

## Clinical Features

Sex and gender differences in psychological and physiological responses to drugs of abuse have been well documented and affect the clinical presentation of women with SUDs. Women progress through the stages of addiction differently than men; they transition from casual drug use to addiction faster (known as "telescoping"), are more reactive to stimuli that trigger relapse, and have higher rates of relapse than men (Bobzean et al. 2014). Women often initiate substance use with a partner and, once initiated, increase their rate of drug use more rapidly. Women are more likely to share injecting equipment, a fact that may explain why 40%–75% of pregnant women who inject intravenous drugs have hepatitis C antibodies (Krans et al. 2016). Importantly, women with SUDs during pregnancy are often marginalized or disadvantaged, and most endorse a history of trauma. Two-thirds of women with SUDs have experienced sexual abuse, and just as many have experienced interpersonal violence (Burns et al. 2016). When women enter substance abuse treatment programs, they typically present with more severe addiction and higher prevalence of co-occurring mental health disorders (Greenfield et al. 2010). For details on the clinical presentation of substance intoxication in the perinatal period, please see Chapter 10,"A Treatment Approach to Psychiatric Emergencies in the Perinatal Period."

# Course/Prognosis

## Obstetrical Outcomes

Women with SUDs are more likely to experience poor nutrition, inadequate prenatal care, poverty, chronic medical problems such as HIV and hepatitis C, and higher rates of intimate partner violence (Cook et al. 2017; Forray and Foster 2015). Medical complications of drug use, such as bacteremia, cardiac disease, cellulitis, diabetes, sexually transmitted infections, urinary tract infections, and vitamin deficiencies are common. Use of alcohol and drugs impairs absorption of micronutrients, which can lead to fetal abnormalities such as intrauterine growth restriction and fetal alcohol spectrum disorder. Depending on the specific drug exposure, other obstetrical complications can occur, such as placental abruption, placenta previa, intrauterine demise, spontaneous abortion, preterm labor and delivery, and premature rupture of membranes (Forray and Foster 2015).

## Maternal Mental Health

Women with SUDs commonly experience co-occurring mental health disorders and report more severe functional impairment compared with men (McHugh et al. 2018). More than half (and in some studies nearly all) of treatment-seeking women with co-occurring mental health and SUDs have a history of trauma (Greenfield et al. 2010). Women are more likely to be referred to substance use treatment by community agencies, mental health providers, and physical health care providers rather than by the legal system, which is a more common referral pathway for men (Greenfield et al. 2010). Women may seek treatment for SUDs earlier in the course of illness than men, but they may require accommodations to stay in treatment due to social factors, including family obligations and childcare needs (McHugh et al. 2018). For individual substances, overlap with maternal mental health conditions are common. For example, smoking tobacco during pregnancy is more than four times more common among pregnant women with a major depressive episode (Goodwin et al. 2017).

## Mother–Child Dyad

Substance use, especially illicit substance use, has far reaching implications for the mother–child dyad. Substance use can also lead to disrupted parental care and dysfunctional mother–infant bonding, which can potentiate the negative effects of prenatal drug exposure (Forray and Foster 2015). Nationally, parental substance use is the single largest predictor of child out-of-home placement, and parental drug use as the primary reason for child removal doubled between 2000 and 2016 (National Center on Substance Abuse and Child Welfare 2021). For mothers, losing custody of a child is associated with significantly worse maternal mental health outcomes than experiencing the death of a child (Wall-Wieler et al. 2018). Data also suggest that loss of child custody increases the risk of continued maternal drug use, as well as criminal involvement, among disadvantaged women (Harp and Oser 2018). Therefore, a dyadic care model must carefully balance the need to protect child safety with the goal of family reunification. Please see Chapter 24, "Forensic Issues in Perinatal Psychiatry," for a detailed discussion of child safety.

## Tobacco

Tobacco and nicotine exposure are associated with adverse pregnancy outcomes, including damage to the umbilical cord structure, miscarriage, increased risk of ectopic pregnancy, placental abruption, preterm birth, low birth weight, small for gestational age infants, and increased infant mortality (Forray 2016; Horne et al. 2014). Prenatal nicotine exposure in humans is associated with greater risk of orofacial clefts and potentially a range of other congenital anomalies (Holbrook 2016). Postnatal morbidities, such as sudden infant death syndrome, have been associated with both prenatal maternal smoking and secondhand exposure. Both intrauterine and passive tobacco smoke exposure have also been associated with an increased risk of asthma, ear infections, and respiratory illnesses (Forray 2016). Nicotine transfers in relatively high quantity in breastmilk; higher amounts of nicotine are passed through breastmilk than through the placenta prenatally. Smoking more than 10 cigarettes per day may decrease milk production. Exposure to tobacco in breastmilk may also alter babies' sleep patterns (McLafferty et al. 2016).

## Alcohol

Alcohol use during pregnancy is associated with the most well-established adverse fetal and child health effects of all prenatal substance exposures (Pruett et al. 2013). Alcohol consumed during pregnancy is concentrated in the amniotic fluid, metabolized away at 3%–4% of maternal metabolic rates, and readily absorbed into fetal blood (Burd et al. 2012). Consequently, the fetus is exposed to the same blood alcohol level as the mother, resulting in fetal toxicity and potential teratogenicity (McLafferty et al. 2016). *Fetal alcohol syndrome*, first described in 1973, refers to a pattern of craniofacial, limb, and cardiovascular defects associated with prenatal-onset growth deficiency and developmental delay. The term *fetal alcohol spectrum disorder* (FASD) is now used to describe a broader range of pathologies, including low birth weight, small for gestational age infant, preterm birth, spontaneous abortions, behavioral problems, developmental delay, and cognitive deficits (DeVido et al. 2015). FASD is the most common and preventable cause of intellectual disability in the United States. No amount of alcohol use is recommended during pregnancy; evidence for the safety of even low to moderate alcohol use during pregnancy is inconclusive (Henderson et al. 2007).

Literature examining the effects of alcohol use during lactation is limited. Alcohol readily diffuses in and out of breastmilk, and human milk levels generally parallel maternal blood alcohol levels. Milk levels typically peak at about 30–60 minutes after ingestion and fall rapidly if no additional alcohol is ingested (Reece-Stremtan and Marinelli 2015). Studies evaluating infant effects of maternal alcohol consumption have been mixed, with some mild effects noted in infant sleep patterns, amount of milk consumed during breastfeeding sessions, and early psychomotor development (Reece-Stremtan and Marinelli 2015). It has been reported that alcohol consumption decreases milk supply (decreased prolactin response to infant suckling) and may negatively affect infant motor development (D'Apolito 2013). The current recommendation of the American Academy of Pediatrics (2021) is for cautious and limited use during lactation.

## Cannabis

The endocannabinoid system is present early in fetal development, and it plays a key role in mediating neuronal maturation and development of key neurotransmitter systems in the CNS. Cannabis exposure in pregnancy during critical periods of brain development can induce subtle and long-lasting alterations in neurodevelopment (Jaques et al. 2014). Current evidence does not support an association between marijuana exposure and any specific congenital birth defects (Metz and Stickrath 2015). Cannabis exposure in pregnancy has been associated with stillbirth, preterm birth, fetal growth restriction, and lower birth weight, but these findings have been inconsistent and confounded by frequent co-use with tobacco and other substances and sociodemographic factors (Metz and Stickrath 2015). Also noteworthy is that the potency of marijuana has been steadily increasing, from about 3% in the 1980s to 12% in 2012, so data from previous studies may no longer be relevant (Volkow et al. 2014). Cannabis is lipophilic; therefore, it readily crosses the placental barrier and passes into breastmilk; breastmilk levels of delta-tetrahydrocannabinol can accumulate up to eightfold in comparison with plasma levels and can be found in breastmilk for up to 6 days following maternal use (Ordean and Kim 2020).

Three long-term prospective longitudinal human studies followed offspring from the neonatal period into childhood and adolescence. Subtle neurobehavioral disturbances have been demonstrated in cannabis-exposed neonates, such as exaggerated and prolonged startle responses and sleep-cycle problems (Jaques et al. 2014). Greater externalizing behaviors, including impulsivity and hyperactivity, were reported in children, as well as impairments in early executive function, abstract and visual reasoning, and visuoperceptual functioning in adolescents (Huizink 2014). It is not possible to determine the degree to which these effects were directly related to prenatal cannabis exposure or to potential confounding variables. In addition, a large retrospective analysis of all live births in Ontario, Canada, over a 5-year period recently found an increased rate of autism in the children of mothers who used cannabis in pregnancy (Corsi et al. 2020).

## Sedative-Hypnotics

Research regarding benzodiazepine exposure in pregnancy is limited to prescribed benzodiazepines. The data regarding fetal risks associated with in-utero exposure to benzodiazepines are mixed and inconclusive (McLafferty et al. 2016). In addition to the potential risks of direct exposure, there are concerns about the effects of benzodiazepine withdrawal on the fetus, as discussed later in the "Treatment" section. For further detail on the uses and risks of benzodiazepines in pregnancy and lactation, please see Chapter 19, "Anxiety Disorders and Insomnia in the Perinatal Period."

## Stimulant Drugs of Abuse

Prenatal cocaine exposure results in vasoconstriction that can affect the fetus at any stage of pregnancy (McLafferty et al. 2016). Several large studies have consistently identified several adverse outcomes associated with cocaine use during pregnancy, including premature rupture of membranes, placental abruption, preterm birth, low birth weight, and small for gestational age infants (Forray 2016; Gouin et al. 2011). The long-term effects of prenatal cocaine exposure on cognitive, motor, and language development have been inconsistent, with some studies reporting positive findings, and some studies finding small or no effects (Frank et al. 2001). This inconsistency is likely related to the confounding effects of the postnatal environment, including dysfunctional parenting, unstable home environments, and frequent rates of polysubstance abuse (Forray 2016). Its high lipid solubility and bioavailability allow cocaine to cross readily into maternal plasma and into the breastmilk. Case reports and case series are available of infants developing cocaine intoxication through breastmilk exposure (D'Apolito 2013).

Like cocaine use in pregnancy, methamphetamine use has been linked with shorter gestational ages, lower birth weight, fetal loss, developmental effects, preeclampsia, gestational hypertension, and intrauterine fetal death (Forray 2016). Infants who were exposed to methamphetamines in utero may display trouble feeding, sleep disruption, and abnormalities of muscle tone, which resolve spontaneously within several weeks (McLafferty et al. 2016). Amphetamines can inhibit prolactin release and may reduce breastmilk supply. Case reports show maternal serum to breastmilk ratios ranging from 1:1 to 1:7.5, with no clinical correlation regarding effect (McLafferty et al. 2016).

## Opioids

Although prescription and illicit opioids are not known to be directly teratogenic to the fetus (McLafferty et al. 2016), significant risks are associated with untreated maternal opioid use disorder. Obstetrical complications can include preeclampsia, intrauterine growth restriction, placental insufficiency and abruption, premature rupture of membranes, postpartum hemorrhage, low Apgar scores, preterm labor, and fetal demise (McLafferty et al. 2016). The exact mechanism by which opioid use has these effects is unclear, but it is hypothesized that the poor outcomes are related to repeated peaks and troughs in serum levels, intermittent exposure to opioid withdrawal, and concurrent lifestyle factors (McLafferty et al. 2016). Neonatal risks associated with maternal opioid use disorder include postnatal growth deficiency, microcephaly, neurobehavioral problems associated with neonatal abstinence syndrome, and sudden infant death syndrome. Neonatal abstinence syndrome, also known as neonatal opioid withdrawal syndrome, is a postnatal withdrawal syndrome that can occur in about 70% of neonates exposed to opioids in utero and is characterized by irritability, feeding difficulties, tremors, hypertonia, emesis, loose stools, seizures, and respiratory distress (Kocherlakota 2014). Breastfeeding has been shown to reduce neonatal abstinence syndrome severity in opioid-exposed newborns and should be encouraged (Reece-Stremtan and Marinelli 2015). Some infants will require treatment with opioid agonist medications if symptoms cannot be managed through nonpharmacological means.

Recent longitudinal studies comparing demographically matched groups of infants exposed and not exposed to methadone in utero showed some cognitive and motor delays in the exposed infants, but this is likely influenced by environmental risk factors and the fact that infants were exposed to methadone prenatally (Reece-Stremtan and Marinelli 2015).

# Differential Diagnosis

Not all substance use in pregnancy constitutes an SUD; therefore, clinicians must assess carefully to determine whether DSM-5 criteria for SUDs are met, incorporating patient self-report, available laboratory data, and external information (e.g., legal charges related to substance use) when available.

## Sociodemographic Considerations

### Gender and Racial Disparities

Significant and widespread gender and racial disparities exist in the legal treatment of SUDs. For example, women, especially women of color, are disproportionately incarcerated for nonviolent drug offenses compared with men (Malinowska-Sempruch and Rychkova 2015). The commonly held but erroneous assumption that people of color are more likely to use drugs affects how people of color are treated by medical providers. For example, in Pinellas County, Florida, one study found that Black women with a positive drug screen were reported to authorities at 10 times the rate of white women (Chasnoff et al. 1990). Another example is demonstrated in the legal consequences for use of crack cocaine—commonly associated with Black Americans—as compared with powder cocaine, more commonly used by white individuals. In the 1980s, substance use in pregnancy gained widespread attention with the media reporting an explosion of "crack babies," mostly in the Black community (Chira 1990; Winerip 2013).

In the 1980s, President Reagan signed the Anti-Drug Abuse Act of 1986 into law, enacting harsh punishments for drug crimes, such as mandatory minimum sentences for the distribution of cocaine and severe punishment for the distribution of crack cocaine. Over time, attitudes in the United States have shifted over how harshly drug offenders should be punished, resulting in changes in the law. In 2010, the Fair Sentencing Act was passed, which tried to address the disparity in punishment between crack cocaine and powder cocaine offenders, and the First Step Act, signed by President Trump in 2018, gave judges more leeway to cut down mandatory minimum sentences and made the Fair Sentencing Act retroactive to apply to people sentenced prior to its passage (Fair Sentencing Act 2010; First Step Act 2018).

### Legal Considerations

Pregnant women with SUDs continue to face a range of legal consequences, from criminal to civil, with the most extreme consequences resulting in incarceration and termination of parental rights (Angelotta et al. 2016). Although no state currently has a law that explicitly defines substance use in pregnancy as a criminal offense, women have been charged under a range of criminal offenses for using substances while pregnant, including criminal child endangerment (*Reyes v. Superior Court of the State of California* 1977), delivery of a controlled substance to a minor via the umbilical cord (*Johnson v. State of Florida* 1992), and manslaughter (*State of Hawaii v. Aiwohi* 2005) and had convictions upheld of criminal child neglect and homicide (*Whitner v. South Carolina* 1997;

*McKnight v. South Carolina* 2008) and chemical endangerment of a child (*Ankrom v. State of Alabama* 2011) (Angelotta et al. 2016). Twenty-three states and the District of Columbia consider substance use during pregnancy to be child abuse, and three consider it grounds for civil commitment.

Under the federal Child Abuse Prevention and Treatment Act, health care providers are required to notify state agencies about substance-exposed infants under their care (Keeping Children and Families Safe Act 2003). Methods for detecting substance use and indications for reporting vary based on state interpretation: 25 states and the District of Columbia require health care professionals to report suspected prenatal drug use, and 8 states require them to test for prenatal drug exposure if there is high suspicion for use (Guttmacher Institute 2021). Although this legislation is intended to protect children, it can also deter women from engaging in care and can interfere with the relationship between health care providers and patients (Angelotta et al. 2016; Poland et al. 1993). One study found that women using cocaine or opiates were more than six times more likely to have received little to no prenatal care, with fear of reporting to police or child welfare authorities cited as one of the greatest barriers to engagement (Schempf and Strobino 2009).

We know that engagement in prenatal care can reduce harmful effects of substance use in pregnancy. Engagement in prenatal care alone reduces risk of low birth weight and prematurity, factors strongly associated with neonatal mortality (El-Mohandes et al. 2003). Multiple professional organizations such as the American Academy of Pediatrics, American College of Obstetricians and Gynecologists, American Medical Association, and American Psychiatric Association have called for universal access, early intervention, and timely initiation of care for women with SUDs in the perinatal period and caution against discrimination and social or legal measures that may thwart these efforts (American Psychiatric Association 2021). Thus, we have an opportunity in pregnancy because women may be more motivated to seek treatment and abstain from substance use in this period (Forray et al. 2015). This contrasts with high postpartum relapse rates, when stressors potentially increase and support often diminishes (Forray et al. 2015).

Evidence consistently demonstrates support for low-barrier access to comprehensive prenatal care and addictions treatment (El-Mohandes et al. 2003; Lester et al. 2004) in improving both neonatal and maternal outcomes. Conversely, the deleterious effects of punitive policies have been shown to deter women from seeking treatment and to interfere with the therapeutic relationship between doctor and patient (Angelotta et al. 2016; Paltrow et al. 2000; Poland et al. 1993; Schempf and Strobino 2009). The following case example describes management of SUDs in pregnancy and postpartum.

> Ms. GG is a 25-year-old woman, gravida 4 para 1021 with opioid use disorder who presents for her initial prenatal appointment at 24 weeks' gestation. She is tearful and describes feeling very worried about her pregnancy. She elaborates that her daughter, who is now 3 years old, was removed from her custody immediately after delivery because of her positive urine drug screen. She feared engaging in care earlier in this pregnancy because she was afraid of people judging her and fearful of child protective services (CPS) becoming involved in her life again. She had planned to stop using opiates on her own by purchasing illicit buprenorphine on the street and tapering, but she notes that it has been too difficult to stop. She describes wanting to engage in both prenatal care

and treatment for her opioid use disorder but is fearful that "they'll take my baby away." She notes that after her daughter was removed from her care, she felt so depressed and hopeless that she immediately returned to using drugs. "I can't go through that again," she says.

Using best practices, Ms. GG's doctor expresses empathy for her challenging situation and validates how difficult yet brave it is that she came in, highlighting her goals of having a healthy pregnancy with the hope of parenting. She asks Ms. GG to fill out a screening tool, explaining that she asks all patients to fill it out on their first visit and often a few more times throughout pregnancy and even postpartum. Ms. GG completes her 5P's screen in the clinic, answering "yes" to all five questions. The doctor thanks her for her honesty and takes a more detailed substance use history. Together, they review the substances she has been using and how they might affect both her and the baby. The doctor describes that based on her acuity, it would be best for Ms. GG to be managed in an integrated obstetrical and addictions program, adding that she might even benefit from a higher level of care given her current instability and limited support. The doctor listens to Ms. GG describe her goals and nonjudgmentally explores her ambivalence around engagement. She also provides Ms. GG with a list of community resources that could help her.

Given Ms. GG's anxiety about CPS, the doctor reviews the state's reporting requirements, highlighting the shared goals between Ms. GG and her treatment team and the future support that will be provided regardless of whether a CPS investigation is opened. Together, they develop a treatment plan to help Ms. GG to work toward her goals while respecting her autonomy to choose which recommendations to accept at this time.

# Pathophysiology

## Biological Factors

It is well established that estrogen's effects on dopamine systems may contribute to sex differences in addiction. Estrogen facilitates release of dopamine (Bobzean et al. 2014). Studies of the menstrual cycle in rodents and humans have found that the follicular phase is associated with greater positive subjective effects of cocaine, relative to the luteal phase. Administration of progesterone attenuates the subjective response to cocaine (Evans and Foltin 2010). Among postpartum women, progesterone treatment has been associated with lower rates of cocaine relapse (McHugh et al. 2018).

Neuroimaging research has identified sex differences in brain volume and function in response to several substances. For example, both females and males with cocaine use disorder exhibited lower gray matter volume relative to control subjects, but the regions exhibiting these volumetric differences varied (McHugh et al. 2018). Hypothalamic-pituitary-adrenocortical dysregulation in women may play a role in vulnerability to substance use relapse in the context of negative affect, such as in times of emotional stress (Greenfield et al. 2010). The possible neurobiological effects of pregnancy on reward circuitry and substance use are largely unknown, so it is unclear whether reductions in substance use during pregnancy are mediated by psychosocial factors or whether biology may also play a role. One study found that gray matter cortical volume was reduced in postpartum mothers who had used substances during pregnancy compared with mothers who had not used substances, particularly in frontal brain regions, and that gray matter volume was negatively correlated with levels of behavioral activation in substance-using mothers (Rutherford et al. 2015).

## Psychological Factors

Mood and anxiety disorders are common among women with SUDs. In a national epidemiological survey conducted in 2009, 12-month prevalence rates of mood and anxiety disorders in women with SUDs were 29.7% and 26.2%, respectively (Greenfield et al. 2010). A comprehensive psychiatric assessment is crucial to differentiate substance-induced, transient symptoms from a separate, non-drug-related disorder.

Many women who use substances in pregnancy have significant trauma histories, including physical and sexual abuse. Among treatment-seeking women with SUDs, rates of physical and sexual abuse are as high as 55%–99% (Greenfield et al. 2010). It has been reported that one-third to one-half of substance-abusing women had experienced some kind of sexual abuse during childhood (Hans 1999). Women with SUDs are more likely to have been raised by parents with SUDs. Although the intergenerational patterns of substance use may have some genetic basis, ample evidence also suggests problematic relationships in families with a parent with SUD that raises concerns about intergenerational transmission of problematic parenting behavior (Hans 1999).

## Social Considerations

Social risk factors for problematic substance use in pregnancy include unintended pregnancy, lower level of education, unemployment, younger age, environmental stress, intimate partner violence, easy access to substances, and lack of knowledge of the impact of substances on fetal development (Louw 2018). Women with SUDs tend to live more chaotic lives. They are often involved with men who also use drugs (Hans 1999). The common perception of substance abuse as a problem of poor women of color is inaccurate, and this perception may be acted on by medical providers in a prejudicial manner (Hans 1999).

# Treatment

## Overview

Despite the high prevalence of use, women only account for one in five individuals in substance use treatment, indicating barriers to access unique to women (Meyer et al. 2019). Pregnancy may present a window of opportunity for the treatment of SUDs. During this time, women are more likely to have access to health insurance and are often motivated toward positive health behaviors. Health care providers have multiple points of contact with pregnant women and can work with women to improve their health, potentially preventing the generational transmission of this chronic disease. However, during pregnancy, women may avoid substance use treatment due to fear of legal and social ramifications; fewer than 10% of pregnant patients with SUDs receive any treatment for those disorders (Ait-Daoud et al. 2019; Cook et al. 2017; Ryan 2019).

## Nicotine Use Disorders

The maternal, fetal, and newborn harms of smoking are well established (Forray 2016). Pharmacotherapies evaluated for nicotine cessation for pregnant women include nicotine replacement therapy and bupropion. To date, no published studies have examined the efficacy of varenicline or electronic nicotine delivery system for pregnant women with nicotine use disorders. A total of eight randomized controlled trials including 2,199 women have been conducted with nicotine replacement therapy, and one trial including 11 women has been conducted with bupropion as an adjunct to cognitive-behavioral therapy for perinatal smoking cessation (Coleman et al. 2015). Overall, nicotine replacement therapy appears to increase the rate of perinatal smoking cessation by 40%, but when nonplacebo randomized controlled trials are excluded from analyses, it is no more effective than placebo for smoking cessation in pregnant women (Coleman et al. 2015). Compliance in the randomized controlled trials was low and may explain the lack of efficacy of nicotine replacement therapy for perinatal smoking cessation. The rates of poor obstetrical outcomes (e.g., miscarriage, stillbirth, premature birth, low birth weight, admission to neonatal intensive care, cesarean section, congenital abnormalities, neonatal death) among women assigned to nicotine replacement therapy, compared with women assigned to placebo or a control group, appear to be similar, and the long-term impact of nicotine replacement therapy on child development is unknown. Due to its lack of efficacy for perinatal smoking cessation, nicotine replacement therapy is not routinely recommended. However, it may be considered in a woman who has a history of successful smoking cessation with the use of this therapy in the past, after carefully weighing the risks of continued nicotine use compared with the use of nicotine replacement therapy.

The primary treatment for perinatal nicotine use disorders includes behavioral interventions, such as motivational interviewing or contingency management, which have shown modest success in reducing smoking or relapse to nicotine use in pregnant women (Chamberlain et al. 2013; Heckman et al. 2010). Contingency management with financial incentives appears to be the most effective for smoking cessation during pregnancy (Chamberlain et al. 2013; Lerfino et al. 2015); however, implementation of financial incentives can be challenging for treatment programs. Treatments aimed at relapse prevention in the postpartum period have included psychoeducation and motivational interviewing and have demonstrated modest success (Levitt et al. 2007).

## Alcohol Use Disorders

No known studies have evaluated the efficacy of FDA-approved pharmacological interventions for the treatment of alcohol use disorder (i.e., naltrexone, disulfiram, acamprosate) among pregnant women in general or pregnant women with alcohol use disorder (Zagon et al. 1998). However, clinical data using naltrexone for the treatment of opioid use disorder during pregnancy are available, and, overall, naltrexone does not appear to be associated with poor birth outcomes (Wachman et al. 2019). Interpretation of these data is limited by small sample sizes, lack of control groups, minimal control for confounding variables, and lack of long-term follow-up. Pharmacological treatments for perinatal alcohol use disorder are not routinely recommended due to the paucity of efficacy and safety data. However, patients and providers need to carefully weigh the well-known risks of alcohol use in pregnancy against the potential benefits and both known and unknown risks of pharmacotherapy.

No studies to our knowledge have systematically examined the effects of perinatal alcohol withdrawal or benzodiazepine treatment for perinatal alcohol withdrawal.

The use of benzodiazepines for perinatal alcohol withdrawal, however, would pose less risk than untreated alcohol withdrawal or continued use of alcohol during pregnancy (Thibaut et al. 2019). Historical studies examining the risks of benzodiazepine use during pregnancy have shown inconsistent associations with fetal malformations (DeVido et al. 2015). Recent data in this area, however, are more reassuring and show that prospective cohort studies are less likely than case control studies to show an association between fetal malformations and benzodiazepine use (Bellantuono et al. 2013). Recent studies have raised concerns about possible associations between benzodiazepine use and ectopic pregnancy and spontaneous abortion, but thus far these results have not been replicated (Sheehy et al. 2019; Wall-Wieler et al. 2020). Chronic use of benzodiazepines during pregnancy is associated with benzodiazepine withdrawal in the newborn, particularly with higher doses (DeVido et al. 2015). Clinicians and their patients must weigh the risks of benzodiazepine exposure against the risks of alcohol withdrawal or continued alcohol use during pregnancy. Although benzodiazepine use is justified for the treatment of alcohol withdrawal, ongoing benzodiazepine maintenance treatment for alcohol use disorder is not supported by evidence.

Behavioral interventions evaluated for the reduction of alcohol use in pregnancy include motivational enhancement therapy, brief psychodynamic psychotherapy, interpersonal psychotherapy, educational interventions, family-focused therapy, professional group education, self-help, and cognitive-behavioral therapy (DeVido et al. 2015; Stade et al. 2009). Most treatments have shown some benefit in increasing abstinence or reducing alcohol consumption among pregnant women. Given the limited number of studies with small sample sizes and a high risk of bias, however, it is unclear if one intervention type is superior (Stade et al. 2009).

## Cannabis

To date, no pharmacological treatments are available for cannabis use disorders. Motivational interviewing, cognitive-behavioral therapy, and contingency management demonstrate some success in the reduction of cannabis use among adult women, but these interventions have not specifically been evaluated among pregnant women (Forray 2016). Providers are encouraged to screen for cannabis use in pregnancy, inform women of the known risks associated with marijuana use, and provide evidence-based psychotherapy to support the reduction of perinatal cannabis use (American College of Obstetricians and Gynecologists 2017b).

## Stimulants

Pharmacological interventions are not available at this time for the treatment of cocaine or methamphetamine use disorders. Motivational interviewing, cognitive-behavioral therapy, and contingency management have shown benefit in reducing cocaine use, with contingency management having the greatest benefit for the reduction of perinatal cocaine use (Terplan et al. 2015). Fewer studies have examined interventions to reduce perinatal methamphetamine use, but one small pilot study demonstrated the feasibility of reinforcement-based treatment, which includes a combination of motivational interviewing, highly individualized treatment planning, and case management (Jones et al. 2014).

# Opioids

The standard of care for the treatment of perinatal opioid use disorder includes pharmacotherapy with either methadone or buprenorphine (Substance Abuse and Mental Health Services Administration 2018) as part of a comprehensive treatment program including prenatal care, psychological and pharmacological treatment interventions for relapse prevention, psychological and pharmacological treatment interventions to address comorbid trauma or other mental health problems, and social services to address the myriad psychosocial stressors that commonly occur in women with opioid use disorder. Buprenorphine (including monotherapy and buprenorphine + naloxone formulations) and methadone are considered first-line treatment for opioid use disorder in pregnancy and are recommended by major organizations including the American College of Obstetricians and Gynecologists, American Society for Addiction Medicine, United Nations, and World Health Organization as the optimal approach to treatment of opioid use disorder during pregnancy (Jones and Kraft 2019).

Although maternal and delivery outcomes are similar for women treated with buprenorphine or methadone, infants exposed to buprenorphine are less likely to require medication for treatment of neonatal opioid withdrawal syndrome, require less medication for treatment of this syndrome if medication is required, and have shorter hospital stays postdelivery (Jones and Kraft 2019). Fetuses exposed to buprenorphine appear to have higher levels of heart rate variability, more heart rate accelerations, greater coupling between heart rate and movement, less motor activity suppression, and lower likelihood of a nonreactive nonstress test than those exposed to methadone (Klaman et al. 2017). Some data suggest a greater incidence of intrauterine growth restriction in fetuses exposed to methadone (Klaman et al. 2017). Current literature does not indicate an increased risk for birth defects in infants exposed to maternal buprenorphine or methadone treatment (Klaman et al. 2017); thus, no compelling evidence suggests that methadone is either superior or inferior to buprenorphine for the treatment of opioid use disorder (Minozzi et al. 2013), and the decision to choose methadone or buprenorphine is largely driven by patient preference, feasibility, and prior treatment response.

Pregnant women with opioid use disorder should be prescribed naloxone, and partners and family members should be educated on the administration of this drug in the context of a life-threatening overdose, as well as the risks associated with perinatal withdrawal after the administration of naloxone. Opioid taper or opioid detoxification, also known as medication-assisted withdrawal, is not recommended during pregnancy due to the high risk for relapse to substance use and the maternal, fetal, and newborn consequences associated with return to drug use (Guille et al. 2017; Terplan et al. 2018). Additionally, the risks of maternal, obstetrical, fetal, and newborn complications associated with opioid withdrawal during pregnancy are largely unknown (Terplan et al. 2018).

Despite the recommendation against medication-assisted withdrawal and lack of evidence to support its use in reducing the risk of newborn opioid withdrawal syndrome, women may want to pursue this treatment approach. It is important that providers and patients have a balanced, evidence-based discussion with respect to the risks of medications used to treat opioid use disorder in pregnancy and the risks of untreated illness. A shared decision-making tool is available to provide information about these risks and to help patients and providers make well-informed decisions that are in line with patient preferences and values (Guille et al. 2019).

Among behavioral treatments, contingency management has the greatest evidence for the reduction of opioid use in pregnant women (Jones et al. 2001; Terplan et al. 2015). However, implementation of reinforcements, particularly financial incentives, can be challenging for treatment programs.

## Conclusion

Pregnancy represents an important window of opportunity for engagement in treatment of SUDs. Comprehensive treatment programs that provide coordinated prenatal care, addiction treatment, behavioral health treatment, and help addressing social determinants of health show promise for improving pregnancy and birth outcomes, as well as long-term outcomes for women and their children.

## Key Points

- Alcohol is a known teratogen. Fetal alcohol spectrum disorders are the most common and preventable cause of intellectual disability in the United States.
- Aside from the use of benzodiazepines for management of alcohol withdrawal, medications for alcohol use disorder (disulfiram, acamprosate, naltrexone) are not commonly used in pregnancy due to lack of data regarding reproductive safety.
- Tobacco use in pregnancy is associated with adverse pregnancy and birth outcomes. Women with major depressive disorder are more likely to smoke.
- Data supporting the efficacy of most smoking cessation treatments in pregnant women are as yet limited, but the harms of tobacco use are such that nicotine replacement therapy and bupropion are reasonable to consider in conjunction with behavioral interventions for smoking cessation.
- Cannabis use in pregnancy has been associated with adverse pregnancy and birth outcomes and adverse neurobehavioral outcomes in children, although causality is difficult to determine due to risks of confounding in observational studies.
- Women should be encouraged to avoid cannabis during pregnancy and while breastfeeding and should be offered other treatment options if they indicate using cannabis to address common pregnancy-related symptoms, such as nausea or insomnia.
- The standard of care for opioid use disorder during pregnancy is medication-assisted treatment with either buprenorphine (in buprenorphine or buprenorphine/naloxone formulations) or methadone; opioid detoxification during pregnancy is not recommended.

- Although neonatal opioid withdrawal can occur in infants exposed to medication-assisted treatment in utero, these neonatal symptoms can be managed both nonpharmacologically and through medication treatment.
- Use of stimulants such as methamphetamine or cocaine in pregnancy is associated with adverse pregnancy and birth outcomes. Pharmacological treatments are not yet available, so comprehensive behavioral treatment and psychosocial supports are recommended for pregnant women with cocaine or methamphetamine use disorders.
- Negative stereotypes about women of color and their likelihood of substance use affect how clinicians assess and respond to substance use disorders in different racial/ethnic groups, with Black women referred to the criminal justice system at much higher rates. Clinicians must be vigilant about these biases.

## References


Ait-Daoud N, Blevins D, Khanna S, et al: Women and addiction: an update. Med Clin North Am 103(4):699–711, 2019 31078201

American Academy of Pediatrics: Fetal Alcohol Spectrum Disorders Program: Frequently Asked Questions. Ithaca, NY, American Academy of Pediatrics, 2021. Available at: Substance Abuse and Mental Health Services Administration: https://www.aap.org/en-us/advocacy-and-policy/aap-health-initiatives/fetal-alcohol-spectrum-disorders-toolkit/Pages/Frequently-Asked-Questions.aspx. Accessed February 3, 2021.

American College of Obstetricians and Gynecologists: ACOG Committee opinion No 473: substance abuse reporting and pregnancy: the role of the obstetrician-gynecologist. Obstet Gynecol 117(1):200–201, 2011 21173672

American College of Obstetricians and Gynecologists: Committee opinion No 711: opioid use and opioid use disorder in pregnancy. Obstet Gynecol 130(2):e81–e94, 2017a 28742676

American College of Obstetricians and Gynecologists: Marijuana use during pregnancy and lactation. Committee Opinion No. 722. Obstet Gynecol 130(4):e205–e209, 2017b 28937574

American Psychiatric Association: Diagnostic and Statistical Manual of Mental Disorders, 5th Edition. Arlington, VA, American Psychiatric Association, 2013

American Psychiatric Association: Health Insurance Coverage and Access to Care: Opioid Epidemic. Washington, DC, American Psychiatric Association, 2021. Available at: https://www.psychiatry.org/psychiatrists/advocacy/federal-affairs/health-insurance-coverage-access-to-care/opioid-epidemic. Accessed June 2021.

Ankrom v. State of Alabama, 152 So.3d 373 (2011)

Angelotta C, Weiss CJ, Angelotta JW, et al: A moral or medical problem? The relationship between legal penalties and treatment practices for opioid use disorders in pregnant women. Womens Health Issues 26(6):595–601, 2016 27773527

Arnaudo CL, Andraka-Christou B, Allgood K: Psychiatric co-morbidities in pregnant women with opioid use disorders: prevalence, impact, and implications for treatment. Curr Addict Rep 4(1):1–13, 2017 28357191

Bellantuono C, Tofani S, Di Sciascio G, et al: Benzodiazepine exposure in pregnancy and risk of major malformations: a critical overview. Gen Hosp Psychiatry 35(1):3–8, 2013 23044244

Bobzean SAM, DeNobrega AK, Perrotti LI: Sex differences in the neurobiology of drug addiction. Exp Neurol 259:64–74, 2014 24508560

Brogly SB, Saia KE, Werler MM, et al: Prenatal treatment and outcomes of women with opioid use disorder. Obstet Gynecol 132(4):916–922, 2018 30204704

Burd L, Blair J, Dropps K: Prenatal alcohol exposure, blood alcohol concentrations and alcohol elimination rates for the mother, fetus and newborn. J Perinatol 32(9):652–659, 2012 22595965

Burns L, Coleman-Cowger VH, Breen C: Managing maternal substance use in the perinatal period: current concerns and treatment approaches in the United States and Australia. Subst Abuse 10(1 suppl 1):55–61, 2016 27980414
Chamberlain C, O'Mara-Eves A, Oliver S, et al: Psychosocial interventions for supporting women to stop smoking in pregnancy. Cochrane Database Syst Rev 10(10):CD001055, 2013 24154953
Chasnoff IJ, Landress HJ, Barrett ME: The prevalence of illicit-drug or alcohol use during pregnancy and discrepancies in mandatory reporting in Pinellas County, Florida. N Engl J Med 322(17):1202–1206, 1990 2325711
Chira S: Children of crack: are the schools ready? New York Times, May 25, 1990. Available at: https://www.nytimes.com/1990/05/25/us/children-crack-are-schools-ready-special-report-crack-babies-turn-5-schools.html. Accessed August 19, 2019.
Coleman T, Chamberlain C, Davey MA, et al: Pharmacological interventions for promoting smoking cessation during pregnancy. Cochrane Database Syst Rev 12(12):CD010078, 2015 26690977
Cook JL, Green CR, de la Ronde S, et al: Epidemiology and effects of substance use in pregnancy. J Obstet Gynaecol Can 39(10):906–915, 2017 28935056
Corsi DJ, Donelle J, Sucha E, et al: Maternal cannabis use in pregnancy and child neurodevelopmental outcomes. Nat Med 26(10):1536–1540, 2020 32778828
D'Apolito K: Breastfeeding and substance abuse. Clin Obstet Gynecol 56(1):202–211, 2013 23337847
Dejong K, Olyaei A, Lo JO: Alcohol use in pregnancy. Clin Obstet Gynecol 62(1):142–155, 2019 30575614
DeVido J, Bogunovic O, Weiss RD: Alcohol use disorders in pregnancy. Harv Rev Psychiatry 23(2):112–121, 2015 25747924
El-Mohandes A, Herman AA, Nabil El-Khorazaty M, et al: Prenatal care reduces the impact of illicit drug use on perinatal outcomes. J Perinatol 23(5):354–360, 2003 12847528
Evans SM, Foltin RW: Does the response to cocaine differ as a function of sex or hormonal status in human and non-human primates? Horm Behav 58(1):13–21, 2010 19733571
Ex Parte Hope Elisabeth Ankrom v. State of Alabama, 2013 WL 135748 (Ala.)
Fair Sentencing Act, S.1789, Pub.L. No. 111-220, 124 Stat. 2372, 2010
First Step Act. H.R. 5682, 115th Cong., 2d Sess., (2017–2018). May 23, 2018
Forray A: Substance use during pregnancy. F1000Res 5:F1000 Faculty Rev-887, 2016 27239283
Forray A, Foster D: Substance use in the perinatal period. Curr Psychiatry Rep 17(11):91, 2015
Forray A, Merry B, Lin H, et al: Perinatal substance use: a prospective evaluation of abstinence and relapse. Drug Alcohol Depend 150:147–155, 2015 25772437
Frank DA, Augustyn M, Knight WG, et al: Growth, development, and behavior in early childhood following prenatal cocaine exposure: a systematic review. JAMA 285(12):1613–1625, 2001
Gemmill A, Kiang MV, Alexander MJ: Trends in pregnancy-associated mortality involving opioids in the United States, 2007–2016. Am J Obstet Gynecol 220(1):115–116, 2019 30273587
Goodwin RD, Cheslack-Postava K, Nelson DB, et al: Smoking during pregnancy in the United States, 2005–2014: the role of depression. Drug Alcohol Depend 179:159–166, 2017 28783546
Gouin K, Murphy K, Shah PS: Knowledge synthesis group on determinants of low birth weight and preterm births: effects of cocaine use during pregnancy on low birthweight and preterm birth: systematic review and meta analyses. Am J Obstet Gynecol 204:340.e1–340.e12, 2011
Greenfield SF, Back SE, Lawson K, et al: Substance abuse in women. Psychiatr Clin North Am 33(2):339–355, 2010 20385341
Guille C, Barth K, Mateus Nino JF, et al: Treatment of pregnant women with prescription opioid use disorder. Am J Psychiatry 174(3):208–214, 2017 28245688
Guille C, Jones H, Abuhamad A, et al: A shared decision-making tool for the treatment of perinatal opioid use disorder. Psychiatric Research and Clinical Practice 1(1):27–31, 2019
Guttmacher Institute: Substance use during pregnancy. Guttmacher Institute, February 21, 2021. Available at: https://www.guttmacher.org/state-policy/explore/substance-use-during-pregnancy. Accessed February 3, 2021.
Haight SC, Ko JY, Tong VT, et al: Opioid use disorder documented at delivery hospitalization—United States, 1999–2014. MMWR Morb Mortal Wkly Rep 67(31):845–849, 2018 30091969
Hans SL: Demographic and psychosocial characteristics of substance-abusing pregnant women. Clin Perinatol 26(1):55–74, 1999 10214543

Harp KLH, Oser CB: A longitudinal analysis of the impact of child custody loss on drug use and crime among a sample of African American mothers. Child Abuse Negl 77:1–12, 2018 29287167
Heckman CJ, Egleston BL, Hofmann MT: Efficacy of motivational interviewing for smoking cessation: a systematic review and meta-analysis. Tob Control 19(5):410–416, 2010 20675688
Henderson J, Gray R, Brocklehurst P: Systematic review of effects of low-moderate prenatal alcohol exposure on pregnancy outcome. BJOG 114(3):243–252, 2007 17233797
Holbrook BD: The effects of nicotine on human fetal development. Birth Defects Res C Embryo Today 108(2):181–192, 2016 27297020
Horne AW, Brown JK, Nio-Kobayashi J, et al: The association between smoking and ectopic pregnancy: why nicotine is BAD for your fallopian tube. PLoS One 9(2):e89400, 2014 24586750
Huizink AC: Prenatal cannabis exposure and infant outcomes: overview of studies. Prog Neuropsychopharmacol Biol Psychiatry 52:45–52, 2014 24075896
Jaques SC, Kingsbury A, Henshcke P, et al: Cannabis, the pregnant woman and her child: weeding out the myths. J Perinatol 34(6):417–424, 2014 24457255
Johnson v. State of Florida, 602 So. 2d 1288 (Fla. Sup. Ct. 1992)
Jones CM, Logan J, Gladden RM, et al: Vital signs: demographic and substance use trends among heroin users—United States, 2002–2013. MMWR Morb Mortal Wkly Rep 64(26):719–725, 2015 26158353
Jones HE, Kraft WK: Analgesia, opioids, and other drug use during pregnancy and neonatal abstinence syndrome. Clin Perinatol 46(2):349–366, 2019 31010564
Jones HE, Haug N, Silverman K, et al: The effectiveness of incentives in enhancing treatment attendance and drug abstinence in methadone-maintained pregnant women. Drug Alcohol Depend 61(3):297–306, 2001 11164694
Jones HE, Deppen K, Hudak ML, et al: Clinical care for opioid-using pregnant and postpartum women: the role of obstetric providers. Am J Obstet Gynecol 210(4):302–310, 2014 24120973
Keeping Children and Families Safe Act, S. 342. 108th Congress (2003–2004), 2003
Kocherlakota P: Neonatal abstinence syndrome. Pediatrics 134(2):e547–e561, 2014 25070299
Klaman SL, Isaacs K, Leopold A, et al: Treating women who are pregnant and parenting for opioid use disorder and the concurrent care of their infants and children: literature review to support national guidance. J Addict Med 11(3):178–190, 2017 28406856
Krans EE, Zickmund SL, Rustgi VK, et al: Screening and evaluation of hepatitis C virus infection in pregnant women on opioid maintenance therapy: a retrospective cohort study. Subst Abus 37(1):88–95, 2016 26569631
Lerfino D, Mantzari E, Hirst J, et al: Financial incentives for smoking cessation in pregnancy: a single-arm intervention study assessing cessation and gaming. Addiction 110(4):680–688, 2015 25727238
Lester BM, Andreozzi L, Appiah L: Substance use during pregnancy: time for policy to catch up with research. Harm Reduct J 1(1):5, 2004 15169566
Levitt C, Shaw E, Wong S, et al: Systematic review of the literature on postpartum care: effectiveness of interventions for smoking relapse prevention, cessation, and reduction in postpartum women. Birth 34(4):341–347, 2007 18021150
Louw KA: Substance use in pregnancy: the medical challenge. Obstet Med 11(2):54–66, 2018 29997687
Malinowska-Sempruch K, Rychkova O: The impact of drug policy on women. Open Society Foundations, 2015. Available at: https://www.opensocietyfoundations.org/publications/impact-drug-policy-women. Accessed August 19, 2019.
McHugh RK, Votaw VR, Sugarman DE, et al: Sex and gender differences in substance use disorders. Clin Psychol Rev 66:12–23, 2018 29174306
McKnight v. State, 661 S.E.2d 354 (S.C. 2008)
McLafferty LP, Becker M, Dresner N, et al: Guidelines for the management of pregnant women with substance use disorders. Psychosomatics 57(2):115–130, 2016 26880374
Metz TD, Stickrath EH: Marijuana use in pregnancy and lactation: a review of the evidence. Am J Obstet Gynecol 213(6):761–778, 2015 25986032
Metz TD, Rovner P, Hoffman MC, et al: Maternal deaths from suicide and overdose in Colorado, 2004–2012. Obstet Gynecol 128(6):1233–1240, 2016 27824771

Meyer JP, Isaacs K, El-Shahawy O, et al: Research on women with substance use disorders: reviewing progress and developing a research and implementation roadmap. Drug Alcohol Depend 197:158–163, 2019 30826625
Minozzi S, Amato L, Vecchi S, et al: Maintenance agonist treatments for opiate-dependent pregnant women. Cochrane Database Syst Rev (12):CD006318, 2013 24366859
Munafò MR, Heron J, Araya R: Smoking patterns during pregnancy and postnatal period and depressive symptoms. Nicotine Tob Res 10(11):1609–1620, 2008 18988073
National Center on Substance Abuse and Child Welfare: Child welfare and treatment statistics. Substance Abuse and Mental Health Services Administration, 2021. Available at: https://ncsacw.samhsa.gov/research/child-welfare-and-treatment-statistics.aspx. Accessed February 3, 2021.
Ordean A, Kim G: Cannabis use during lactation: literature review and clinical recommendations. J Obstet Gynaecol Can 42(10):1248–1253, 2020 31992503
Paltrow LM, Cohen DS, Carey CA: Year 2000 overview: governmental responses to pregnant women who use alcohol or other drugs. Women's Law Project and the National Advocates for Pregnant Women 1:8, 2000
Patrick SW, Schumacher RE, Benneyworth BD, et al: Neonatal abstinence syndrome and associated health care expenditures: United States, 2000–2009. JAMA 307(18):1934–1940, 2012 22546608
Patrick SW, Dudley J, Martin PR, et al: Prescription opioid epidemic and infant outcomes. Pediatrics 135(5):842–850, 2015 25869370
Poland ML, Dombrowski MP, Ager JW, et al: Punishing pregnant drug users: enhancing the flight from care. Drug Alcohol Depend 31(3):199–203, 1993 8462410
Pruett D, Waterman EH, Caughey AB: Fetal alcohol exposure: consequences, diagnosis, and treatment. Obstet Gynecol Surv 68(1):62–69, 2013 23322082
Reece-Stremtan S, Marinelli KA: ABM clinical protocol #21: guidelines for breastfeeding and substance use or substance use disorder, revised 2015. Breastfeed Med 10(3):135–141, 2015
Reyes v. Superior Court of the State of California, 75 Cal.App.3d 214, 219 [141 Cal.Rptr. 912] (1977)
Rodriguez JJ, Smith VC: Epidemiology of perinatal substance use: exploring trends in maternal substance use. Semin Fetal Neonatal Med 24(2):86–89, 2019 30777708
Rutherford HJ, Gerig G, Gouttard S, et al: Investigating maternal brain structure and its relationship to substance use and motivational systems. Yale J Biol Med 88(3):211–217, 2015 26339203
Ryan SA: Substance abuse in pregnancy. Clin Obstet Gynecol 62(1):112–117, 2019 30664586
Schempf AH, Strobino DM: Drug use and limited prenatal care: an examination of responsible barriers. Am J Obstet Gynecol 200(4):412.e1–412.e10, 2009 19217591
Schiff DM, Nielsen T, Terplan M, et al: Fatal and nonfatal overdose among pregnant and postpartum women in Massachusetts. Obstet Gynecol 132(2):466–474, 2018 29995730
Sheehy O, Zhao JP, Bérard A: Association between incident exposure to benzodiazepines in early pregnancy and risk of spontaneous abortion. JAMA Psychiatry 76(9):948–957, 2019 31090881
Smid MC, Metz TD, Gordon AJ: Stimulant use in pregnancy: an under-recognized epidemic among pregnant women. Clin Obstet Gynecol 62(1):168–184, 2019 30601144
Stade BC, Bailey C, Dzendoletas D, et al: Psychological and/or educational interventions for reducing alcohol consumption in pregnant women and women planning pregnancy. Cochrane Database Syst Rev 2(2):CD004228, 2009 19370597
State of Hawaii v. Aiwohi, 123 P.3d 1210 (Hawaii 2005)
Substance Abuse and Mental Health Services Administration: Clinical Guidance for Treating Pregnant and Parenting Women With Opioid Use Disorder and Their Infants. HHS Publ No (SMA) 18-5054. Rockville, MD, Substance Abuse and Mental Health Services Administration, 2018
Terplan M, Ramanadhan S, Locke A, et al: Psychosocial interventions for pregnant women in outpatient illicit drug treatment programs compared to other interventions. Cochrane Database Syst Rev 4(4):CD006037, 2015 25835053
Terplan M, Laird HJ, Hand DJ, et al: Opioid detoxification during pregnancy: a systematic review. Obstet Gynecol 131(5):803–814, 2018 29630016

Thibaut F, Chagraoui A, Buckley L, et al: WFSBP and IAWMH guidelines for the treatment of alcohol use disorders in pregnant women. World J Biol Psychiatry 20(1):17–50, 2019 30632868
Volkow ND, Baler RD, Compton WM, et al: Adverse health effects of marijuana use. N Engl J Med 370(23):2219–2227, 2014 24897085
Volkow ND, Han B, Compton WM, et al: Self-reported medical and nonmedical cannabis use among pregnant women in the United States. JAMA 322(2):167–169, 2019 31211824
Wachman EM, Saia K, Miller M, et al: Naltrexone treatment for pregnant women with opioid use disorder compared to matched buprenorphine controls. Clin Ther 41(9):1681–1689, 2019 31358302
Wall-Wieler E, Roos LL, Bolton J, et al: Maternal mental health after custody loss and death of a child: a retrospective cohort study using linkable administrative data. Can J Psychiatry 63(5):322–328, 2018 29082774
Wall-Wieler E, Robakis TK, Lyell DJ, et al: Benzodiazepine use before conception and risk of ectopic pregnancy. Hum Reprod 35(7):1685–1692, 2020 32485732
Washio Y, Mark K, Terplan M: Characteristics of pregnant women reporting cannabis use disorder at substance use treatment entry. J Addict Med 12(5):395–400, 2018 29864087
Whitner v. South Carolina, 492 S.E.2d 777 (1997)
Winerip M: Revisiting the "crack babies" epidemic that was not. New York Times, May 20, 2013. Available at: https://www.nytimes.com/2013/05/20/booming/revisiting-the-crack-babies-epidemic-that-was-not.html. Accessed August 19, 2019.
World Health Organization: The ICD-10 Classification of Mental and Behavioural Disorders: Clinical Descriptions and Diagnostic Guidelines. Geneva, World Health Organization, 1992
World Health Organization: Guidelines for the Identification and Management of Substance Use and Substance Use Disorders in Pregnancy. Geneva, Switzerland, 2014
Wright TE, Schuetter R, Tellei J, et al: Methamphetamines and pregnancy outcomes. J Addict Med 9(2):111–117, 2015 25599434
Wright TE, Terplan M, Ondersma SJ, et al: The role of screening, brief intervention, and referral to treatment in the perinatal period. Am J Obstet Gynecol 215(5):539–547, 2016 27373599
Yazdy MM, Desai RJ, Brogly SB: Prescription opioids in pregnancy and birth outcomes: a review of the literature. J Pediatr Genet 4(2):56–70, 2015 26998394
Zagon IS, Tobias SW, Hytrek SD, et al: Opioid receptor blockade throughout prenatal life confers long-term insensitivity to morphine and alters mu opioid receptors. Pharmacol Biochem Behav 59(1):201–207, 1998 9443556

CHAPTER 22

# Eating Disorders

Robin Valpey, M.D.
Jyoti Sachdeva, M.D.
Joy E. Moel, Ph.D.

Eating disorders (EDs) are a group of diagnoses characterized by disturbance in eating that leads to impairment in health and psychosocial functioning (American Psychiatric Association 2013). Disordered eating can lead to numerous medical sequelae across many organ systems, including reproductive pathways. Although most of these pathophysiological sequelae are reversible with treatment of the disorder and accompanying decrease in disordered eating behavior and weight restoration, some can be life threatening (Treasure et al. 2010). Given the high risk of mortality in this population, providers must be aware of the diagnostic criteria and potential medical complications associated with EDs.

Overall, EDs are more common among women than men, with large sex differences seen in both anorexia nervosa (AN) and bulimia nervosa (BN). Because they most commonly present in the reproductive years, the interplay between EDs and the reproductive cycle is an important component of this diagnosis. In this chapter, we review the common presentations and complications of EDs, risk factors, etiologies, and treatment options, with particular focus on presentation in the perinatal period and implications for reproductive function.

## Epidemiology

### Rates/Incidence

The most common forms of ED during a woman's reproductive years include AN, BN, and binge eating disorder (BED), and these disorders are associated with decreased quality of life, increased health care costs, and high mortality rates (Arcelus et al. 2011).

Although their onset is highest during adolescence and young adulthood, the prevalence of recurring ED later in life highlights the need for attention to symptoms at older ages as well (Ward et al. 2019). Binge eating, rather than restrictive patterns, and increased medical morbidity characterize midlife or perimenopausal EDs (Mangweth-Matzek and Hoek 2017). EDs at any age are highly comorbid with medical and other psychiatric conditions, most notably anxiety disorders (up to 80%), depressive disorders (up to 80%), and substance use disorders (up to 40%) (Erskine and Whiteford 2018; Grilo et al. 2009; Kaye et al. 2004).

AN has a peak incidence for women between ages 15 and 19 years (Attia and Walsh 2009). The lifetime prevalence is 0.4% for women, and AN occurs much more frequently in women than men, at a ratio of 10:1 (Hoek 2006). Approximately 20% of women with AN have a chronic course, whereas 33% improve with partial or residual features, and 46% go on to fully recover (Steinhausen et al. 2009). Although relatively rare, AN must be taken seriously because weight loss and malnutrition can lead to medical comorbidities and life-threatening conditions (Westmoreland et al. 2016). In fact, the mortality rate is approximately 5% for AN, and the standardized mortality ratio (SMR; observed deaths in population) is 5.9, which is higher than most other psychiatric disorders and the general population (Arcelus et al. 2011). Medical complications from limited nutritional intake and suicide are the most frequent causes of death (Arcelus et al. 2011).

BN is a more common diagnosis than AN, with a lifetime prevalence rate estimated between 1.5% and 3% (Hoek 2006). This disorder also occurs much more commonly for women than men, again at a ratio of 10:1. Peak incidence in women occurs between the ages of 16 and 20 years, and although recovery rates for the short-term success of treatment are good (50%–70%), relapse rates are high and have been shown to range from 30% to 85% at 6 months to 6 years posttreatment. The SMR is 1.9, with approximately 20% of these deaths due to suicide (Arcelus et al. 2011).

BED is somewhat more common in women than AN or BN, with a lifetime prevalence of approximately 3%. Peak incidence for women occurs between ages 18 and 20 years (Stice 2016). Sex differences in BED appear smaller than those observed in AN and BN, and BED is more likely to be associated with obesity (Javaras et al. 2008).

## Racial, Cultural, and Socioeconomic Considerations

A 2018 U.S. study using a nationally representative sample of more than 36,000 subjects indicated race/ethnicity differences among those with an ED diagnosis (Coffino et al. 2019). Hispanic and non-Hispanic Black respondents had a significantly lower lifetime risk of AN compared with non-Hispanic whites; lifetime risk of BN was similar across racial/ethnicity groups. Lifetime risk of BED was also lower among non-Hispanic Black respondents compared with non-Hispanic white subjects, although this was not found in the 12-month data and was also not seen in Hispanic respondents. In addition, higher income was associated with greater odds of having an ED diagnosis. However, an Australian study found that symptoms of EDs distributed equally across socioeconomic status (Mulders-Jones et al. 2017).

Some of the reasons for these differences may be related to disparities in screening, diagnosis, and treatment among different populations. Studies indicate that individuals of color are less likely than their white counterparts to be asked by a doctor about ED symptoms (Becker et al. 2003), receive an ED diagnosis (Sonneville and Lipson

2018), obtain recommendation for further evaluation or care (Becker et al. 2003), or seek care for their disordered eating symptoms (Cachelin et al. 2001; Coffino et al. 2019). In addition, less affluent individuals are less likely to perceive a need for treatment or to receive care, and treatment of EDs is often concentrated in more affluent areas (Sonneville and Lipson 2018), thus contributing to the disparity noted.

The evidence also indicates that, in adolescence, LGBTQ+ individuals may be at higher risk for EDs than the general population. Some studies indicate that sexual-minority males have greater body dissatisfaction and may engage in more disordered eating than their sexual-majority peers (McClain and Peebles 2016). The data on transgender individuals are much more limited, with some studies showing the presence of EDs in this population (one focusing in particular on male-to-female transgender individuals) but little data to show whether either prevalence or presentation differs from that of the cisgender population (Jones et al. 2016; Khoosal et al. 2009).

## Special Considerations in the Peripartum Period

The peripartum can be a high-risk time for the onset or a relapse of eating-disordered behavior, but it can also be an opportunity for recovery because women are often motivated to make changes to benefit the health of the baby. In fact, remission rates during pregnancy have been shown to range anywhere from 29% to 78% (Micali et al. 2007). These women have decreased concern for weight and shape and decreased restricting or purging behaviors. However, pregnancy can also trigger a relapse of symptoms in a subset of patients, and at least 5% of women still meet criteria for an ED during pregnancy (Easter et al. 2013). Physiological changes during pregnancy, such as increased food cravings or morning sickness, can be a trigger for BN or BED. Hyperemesis gravidarum, a severe type of nausea and vomiting during pregnancy, has also been associated with a worsening of ED symptoms during the peripartum period (Lingam and McCluskey 1996). In the postpartum period, stress related to the transition to motherhood and body changes may contribute to increased EDs (Andersen and Ryan 2009).

Pica is generally a rare ED, but it must also be considered during the peripartum period because it is the most common ED to occur during pregnancy. Pica is the craving and chewing of substances that have no nutritional value, such as ice, clay, soil, or paper. A recent meta-analysis estimated the prevalence of pica during pregnancy to be 27.8% (Fawcett et al. 2016).

Like during other times of a woman's life, EDs in the peripartum period are associated with additional mental health concerns (Santos et al. 2017). Significant comorbidity exists between EDs and perinatal depression, generalized anxiety disorder, OCD, and PTSD during the peripartum period (Andersen and Ryan 2009).

Ms. HH is a 34-year-old married woman currently struggling with infertility. She expresses contentment in her marriage and enjoys her career in health care. She denies psychiatric history, but when asked more about her patterns with eating and exercise, she notes a pattern change about 10 years prior. Although Ms. HH had always been focused on health and exercise, she began to have excessive exercise and thought that she had to exercise in order to take in any food. She denies any other compensatory behaviors, including any purging or laxative use, as well as any conscious restricting. Her weight had dropped to its lowest, 107 lb, a few years prior, but at time of evaluation, she weighs 118.5 lb. She had normal menses since puberty until 10 years ago and has not had spontaneous menses since. Ms. HH initially sought help with a fertility specialist about 2 years ago and successfully completed in vitro fertilization, and she now has a healthy 18-month-old daughter. However, she is now trying for her second child and has had two unsuccessful rounds of in vitro fertilization. She is struggling more with mood and anxiety surrounding fertility issues and feels increased stress at home in her relationship and with her child.

# Risk Factors

Risk factors for EDs are multifactorial and include various biological, psychological, environmental, and sociocultural factors, as outlined in Table 22–1. Biological risk factors include genetics and hormonal factors, type I diabetes mellitus, and a family history of ED or other mental health diagnoses (Culbert et al. 2015). Psychological risk factors include body image dissatisfaction, internalization of the "thin ideal," and a personal history of depression, anxiety, and substance use disorder (Ulfvebrand et al. 2015), as well as personality traits and disorders including neuroticism, perfectionism, impulsivity, obsessive-compulsive personality disorder, and borderline personality disorder (Culbert et al. 2015; Mazzeo et al. 2006). Anxiety disorders have been found to have an onset in childhood prior to the onset of AN or BN (Kaye et al. 2004). Environmental risk factors include family and social factors, such as family discord, family dieting, and parental criticism (Fairburn and Harrison 2003). Sexual, physical, or emotional abuse puts women at risk for an ED, and sexual abuse has been identified as a specific risk factor for BN (Fairburn and Harrison 2003; Sanci et al. 2008). Sociocultural risk factors include media exposure to the thin ideal, weight stigma, and societal endorsement of weight loss and dieting (Culbert et al. 2015; Martínez-González et al. 2003). Clearly, the etiology of ED is complex and involves a multitude of individual and environmental risk factors.

## Special Considerations in the Peripartum Period

EDs may be triggered in at-risk women during times of profound body changes and significant life change, both of which occur during the peripartum period (Andersen and Ryan 2009). It is also important to note that the risk factors for pica appear to be somewhat different from those for AN, BN, and BED. Stress and nutritional deficiencies, such as iron deficiency, are primary considerations that may increase risk for pica during pregnancy (Fawcett et al. 2016). In addition, geographical region, socioeconomic status, and education also appear to impact pica prevalence, because rates were higher in Africa and among those of lower education attainment and socioeconomic status (Fawcett et al. 2016).

# Screening Methods

The medical and psychiatric risks associated with an ED diagnosis warrant increased awareness and recognition of the signs and symptoms in order to ensure timely identification and adequate treatment. Providers should have a low threshold to initiate a screening and should incorporate a formal screening process into their clinical practice due to the severity of the consequences of an ED diagnosis and the secrecy and denial that often surround ED behaviors (Andersen and Ryan 2009). Providers have numerous screening tools they can use to identify patients with a possible ED. The SCOFF (sick, control, one, fat, food; Morgan et al. 1999) and the Eating Disorder

TABLE 22–1. **Risk factors for eating disorders**

| | |
|---|---|
| Biological | Genetics, hormonal changes, type I diabetes, family history of eating disorder or other mental health disorder |
| Environmental | Family discord, parental criticism, family dieting, history of abuse |
| Psychological | Personal history of mental health disorder, body image dissatisfaction, neuroticism, perfectionism, impulsivity, cognitive inflexibility |
| Sociocultural | Media exposure to thin ideal, weight stigma, societal endorsement of dieting |

Screen for Primary Care (Cotton et al. 2003) are brief screening measures ideally suited for most settings, including primary care. Both include five clinician-administered questions, and two or more positive responses on either measure is strongly associated with an ED diagnosis. The Eating Disorder Examination Questionnaire (Fairburn and Beglin 1994) is a widely used and more extensive 28-item self-report questionnaire. Each of these instruments is available in many languages and can greatly increase the odds of detecting an ED in women. Screening should be targeted to high-risk times over the course of a woman's lifespan, beginning after puberty, into young adulthood, during peripartum transitions, and through the perimenopausal period. When a positive screen is identified, a referral or care coordination with specialists in the ED field is recommended. Hospitalization may need to be initiated when suicidality or serious medical complications are identified during the screening process (Andersen and Ryan 2009).

### Special Considerations in the Peripartum Period

Weight and eating habits are closely monitored during pregnancy, yet recognizing ED symptoms can still be difficult during the peripartum period. In addition to the typical risk factors listed in the previous section, warning signs of an ED during the peripartum period may include a lack of weight gain over two consecutive prenatal visits in the second trimester, unexplained hyperkalemia or other electrolyte abnormalities, hyperemesis gravidarum, gastrointestinal problems, abnormally low BMI, low bone density, sexual dysfunction, subfertility, miscarriage, preterm delivery, or low birth weight in offspring (Andersen and Ryan 2009).

## Diagnostic Criteria

The ED diagnoses are characterized by disordered eating behaviors accompanied by psychological reactions to these behaviors, body image, or weight. The DSM-5 diagnostic criteria for AN, BN, and BED are outlined in Boxes 22–1, 22–2, and 22–3 (American Psychiatric Association 2013). Although weight changes can be seen in all EDs, AN specifically has low weight as a component of the diagnostic criteria. Low weight can be obtained via restricting behaviors or compensatory behaviors, including bingeing and purging. BED is distinguished from BN by its lack of compensatory behaviors after a binge, although many patients with BED may have some restricting behaviors between binge episodes (not part of diagnostic criteria).

## Box 22–1. DSM-5 Criteria for Anorexia Nervosa

A. Restriction of energy intake relative to requirements, leading to a significantly low body weight in the context of age, sex, developmental trajectory, and physical health. *Significantly low weight* is defined as a weight that is less than minimally normal or, for children and adolescents, less than that minimally expected.
B. Intense fear of gaining weight or of becoming fat, or persistent behavior that interferes with weight gain, even though at a significantly low weight.
C. Disturbance in the way in which one's body weight or shape is experienced, undue influence of body weight or shape on self-evaluation, or persistent lack of recognition of the seriousness of the current low body weight.

**Coding note:** The ICD-9-CM code for anorexia nervosa is **307.1,** which is assigned regardless of the subtype. The ICD-10-CM code depends on the subtype (see below).

*Specify* whether:

**(F50.01) Restricting type:** During the last 3 months, the individual has not engaged in recurrent episodes of binge eating or purging behavior (i.e., self-induced vomiting or the misuse of laxatives, diuretics, or enemas). This subtype describes presentations in which weight loss is accomplished primarily through dieting, fasting, and/or excessive exercise.

**(F50.02) Binge-eating/purging type:** During the last 3 months, the individual has engaged in recurrent episodes of binge eating or purging behavior (i.e., self-induced vomiting or the misuse of laxatives, diuretics, or enemas).

*Specify* if:

**In partial remission:** After full criteria for anorexia nervosa were previously met, Criterion A (low body weight) has not been met for a sustained period, but either Criterion B (intense fear of gaining weight or becoming fat or behavior that interferes with weight gain) or Criterion C (disturbances in self-perception of weight and shape) is still met.

**In full remission:** After full criteria for anorexia nervosa were previously met, none of the criteria have been met for a sustained period of time.

*Specify* current severity:

The minimum level of severity is based, for adults, on current body mass index (BMI) (see below) or, for children and adolescents, on BMI percentile. The ranges below are derived from World Health Organization categories for thinness in adults; for children and adolescents, corresponding BMI percentiles should be used. The level of severity may be increased to reflect clinical symptoms, the degree of functional disability, and the need for supervision.

**Mild:** BMI $\geq 17$ kg/m$^2$
**Moderate:** BMI 16–16.99 kg/m$^2$
**Severe:** BMI 15–15.99 kg/m$^2$
**Extreme:** BMI $< 15$ kg/m$^2$

*Source.* Reprinted from American Psychiatric Association: *Diagnostic and Statistical Manual of Mental Disorders,* 5th Edition. Arlington, VA, 2013, pp. 338–339. 

## Box 22–2. DSM-5 Criteria for Bulimia Nervosa

A. Recurrent episodes of binge eating. An episode of binge eating is characterized by both of the following:
   1. Eating, in a discrete period of time (e.g., within any 2-hour period), an amount of food that is definitely larger than what most individuals would eat in a similar period of time under similar circumstances.

2. A sense of lack of control over eating during the episode (e.g., a feeling that one cannot stop eating or control what or how much one is eating).

B. Recurrent inappropriate compensatory behaviors in order to prevent weight gain, such as self-induced vomiting; misuse of laxatives, diuretics, or other medications; fasting; or excessive exercise.
C. The binge eating and inappropriate compensatory behaviors both occur, on average, at least once a week for 3 months.
D. Self-evaluation is unduly influenced by body shape and weight.
E. The disturbance does not occur exclusively during episodes of anorexia nervosa.

*Specify* if:

**In partial remission:** After full criteria for bulimia nervosa were previously met, some, but not all, of the criteria have been met for a sustained period of time.

**In full remission:** After full criteria for bulimia nervosa were previously met, none of the criteria have been met for a sustained period of time.

*Specify* current severity:

The minimum level of severity is based on the frequency of inappropriate compensatory behaviors (see below). The level of severity may be increased to reflect other symptoms and the degree of functional disability.

**Mild:** Average of 1–3 episodes of inappropriate compensatory behaviors per week.

**Moderate:** Average of 4–7 episodes of inappropriate compensatory behaviors per week.

**Severe:** Average of 8–13 episodes of inappropriate compensatory behaviors per week.

**Extreme:** Average of 14 or more episodes of inappropriate compensatory behaviors per week.

*Source.* Reprinted from American Psychiatric Association: *Diagnostic and Statistical Manual of Mental Disorders,* 5th Edition. Arlington, VA, 2013, p. 345. 

## Box 22–3. DSM-5 Criteria for Binge-Eating Disorder

A. Recurrent episodes of binge eating. An episode of binge eating is characterized by both of the following:
   1. Eating, in a discrete period of time (e.g., within any 2-hour period), an amount of food that is definitely larger than what most people would eat in a similar period of time under similar circumstances.
   2. A sense of lack of control over eating during the episode (e.g., a feeling that one cannot stop eating or control what or how much one is eating).
B. The binge-eating episodes are associated with three (or more) of the following:
   1. Eating much more rapidly than normal.
   2. Eating until feeling uncomfortably full.
   3. Eating large amounts of food when not feeling physically hungry.
   4. Eating alone because of feeling embarrassed by how much one is eating.
   5. Feeling disgusted with oneself, depressed, or very guilty afterward.
C. Marked distress regarding binge eating is present.
D. The binge eating occurs, on average, at least once a week for 3 months.
E. The binge eating is not associated with the recurrent use of inappropriate compensatory behavior as in bulimia nervosa and does not occur exclusively during the course of bulimia nervosa or anorexia nervosa.

*Specify* if:

**In partial remission:** After full criteria for binge-eating disorder were previously met, binge eating occurs at an average frequency of less than one episode per week for a sustained period of time.

**In full remission:** After full criteria for binge-eating disorder were previously met, none of the criteria have been met for a sustained period of time.

*Specify* current severity:

The minimum level of severity is based on the frequency of episodes of binge eating (see below). The level of severity may be increased to reflect other symptoms and the degree of functional disability.

**Mild:** 1–3 binge-eating episodes per week.

**Moderate:** 4–7 binge-eating episodes per week.

**Severe:** 8–13 binge-eating episodes per week.

**Extreme:** 14 or more binge-eating episodes per week.

*Source.* Reprinted from American Psychiatric Association: *Diagnostic and Statistical Manual of Mental Disorders*, 5th Edition. Arlington, VA, 2013, p. 350. 

Outside of the most common forms of EDs, additional diagnoses exist for alternative disordered eating behaviors, as briefly described in Table 22–2. For individuals who have ED behaviors without meeting full criteria for a specific diagnosis, the most likely diagnosis is other specified feeding and eating disorder. Specific patterns are often named, including atypical AN, purging disorder, and night eating syndrome.

# Clinical Features

## Clinical Presentation

Although the diagnostic criteria for EDs focus mainly on the behaviors and psychological symptoms surrounding these behaviors, weight, and body image, EDs are also associated with medical symptoms and complications. These physical characteristics are sometimes more apparent to others and can be the trigger to providers to evaluate for an ED. Table 22–3 outlines the symptoms associated with the three most common ED diagnoses.

### Anorexia Nervosa

As detailed in DSM-5, AN is characterized by the hallmark symptom of energy restriction resulting in significantly low body weight, intense fear of gaining weight, and faulty perception of body shape and weight. Patients show intense preoccupation with food and peculiar behaviors around it, for example, collecting recipes, preparing elaborate meals for others, cutting food into small pieces, hiding food, frequently monitoring their weight, checking appearance in mirrors, measuring body parts for fat, and more (Sadock and Sadock 2007). Additional symptoms are driven by starvation-related medical symptomatology. Patients may develop dehydration, renal damage, electrolyte imbalances, hypoglycemic episodes, abnormal lipid profiles, hypothermia, dependent edema, bradycardia, hypotension, and lanugo (appearance of neonatal-like hair) (Sadock and Sadock 2007). Nutritional insufficiency driven by hypothalamic-pi-

**TABLE 22–2. Other feeding and eating disorders**

| Disorder | Diagnostic criteria/symptoms |
|---|---|
| Pica | 1. Persistent eating of nonnutritive nonfood substances over a period of at least 1 month<br>2. The eating of these substances is inappropriate to developmental level<br>3. Not culturally supported or socially normative<br>4. If in context of another mental disorder (e.g., intellectual disability), condition is severe enough to warrant clinical attention |
| Rumination disorder | 1. Repeated regurgitation (rechewed, reswallowed, or spit out) of food for >1 month<br>2. Not attributed to other gastrointestinal issue<br>3. If in context of another mental disorder (e.g., intellectual disability), condition is severe enough to warrant clinical attention |
| Other specified feeding and eating disorder | Symptoms characteristic of a feeding and eating disorder that cause clinically significant distress or impairment but do not meet full criteria for any of the disorders; clinician must communicate reason presentation does not meet criteria |
| Atypical anorexia nervosa | Criteria for anorexia nervosa are met, but individual's weight is within or above normal range |
| Bulimia nervosa or binge eating disorder of low frequency or limited duration | Criteria for disorder are met, but behaviors occur less than once a week and/or less than 3 months |
| Night eating syndrome | Recurrent episodes of night eating as manifested by eating after awakening from sleep or by excessive food consumption after evening meal; patient has awareness and recall |
| Purging disorder | Recurrent purging behavior to influence weight or shape in the absence of binge eating |
| Additional diagnoses not included | Avoidant restrictive food intake disorder<br>Unspecified eating disorder |

*Source.* American Psychiatric Association 2013.

**TABLE 22–3. Predominant eating disorder symptoms and reproductive sequelae**

| Symptoms | Anorexia nervosa | Bulimia nervosa | Binge eating disorder |
|---|---|---|---|
| Main characteristic | Intense fear of gaining weight<br>Low body weight<br>Misperception of body weight<br>Restriction of energy intake | Binge eating<br>Normal or overweight<br>Purging behaviors | Binge eating<br>No purging<br>Overweight/Obese |
| Associated physical symptoms | Abnormal lipids<br>Bradycardia<br>Brittle nails<br>Dehydration<br>Edema<br>Electrolyte imbalance<br>Hypoglycemia<br>Hypotension<br>Hypothermia<br>Lanugo<br>Liver damage<br>Osteoporosis<br>Renal damage | Dental caries<br>Edema<br>Electrolyte imbalances<br>Esophageal tears<br>Gastric problems<br>Hypotension<br>Russell's sign (scarring on back of hand due to induction of vomiting) | Obesity related illnesses:<br>Diabetes<br>Heart disease<br>Hypertension<br>Obstructive sleep apnea |
| Mental health symptoms | Anxiety<br>Denial<br>Depression<br>High suicide risk | Anxiety<br>Depression<br>Impulse-control disorders | Anxiety<br>Depression<br>Impulse-control disorders<br>Guilt |
| Menstrual dysfunction | Primary and secondary amenorrhea | Menstrual irregularity<br>Polycystic ovary syndrome | Irregular periods<br>Polycystic ovary syndrome |
| Reproductive health issues | Higher risk of cesarean-section delivery<br>Infertility<br>Lower gestational weight gain<br>Perinatal and postpartum depression<br>Preterm labor<br>Substance exposure<br>Unplanned pregnancy | Excessive gestational weight gain<br>Higher risk of cesarean-section delivery<br>Infertility<br>Preterm labor<br>Unplanned pregnancy | Excessive gestational weight gain<br>Gestational diabetes<br>Large for gestational age infant<br>Maternal hypertension<br>Perinatal depression<br>Prolonged labor |

tuitary-gonadal (HPG) axis dysregulation causes amenorrhea, infertility, sexual dysfunction, and osteoporosis (Boisseau 2016). Psychological factors complicating illness include depression, anxiety, severe denial of low body weight, traits of perfectionism, and overcontrol (Cardwell 2013).

### Bulimia Nervosa

BN is characterized by episodes of binge eating and compensatory purging behaviors (American Psychiatric Association 2013). Purging behaviors may include self-induced vomiting, laxative abuse, diuretic or emetic abuse, fasting, or excessive exercise. Patients with BN are usually in the normal and overweight range, are less likely to have disruption of the HPG axis, and tend to have preserved sexual function (Cardwell 2013). Given the recurrent purging, these patients are at risk of dental erosion, caries, fractures, gastric or esophageal tears, vomiting-related hypokalemia, and hypochloremic alkalosis (Sadock and Sadock 2007). In contrast to women with AN, these women are characterized by impulsivity and lack of control (Cardwell 2013) and have high comorbidity of mood and impulse-control disorders (Sadock and Sadock 2007).

## Course and Prognosis Across the Female Reproductive Lifespan

Given the close association among weight, body fat, and the HPG axis, EDs can have a major impact on women throughout the reproductive cycle. As shown in Table 22–3, these effects on reproduction vary by diagnosis and can change over time.

### Effect on Menstrual Cycle and Fertility

Menstrual cycle irregularity, including primary and secondary amenorrhea, is a common symptom of major EDs (Boisseau 2016). Although most women with AN have amenorrhea as a presenting symptom, it is not pathognomonic of the disorder and is no longer included in the diagnostic criteria (American Psychiatric Association 2013). The strongest predictors of amenorrhea in women with EDs include low BMI, low caloric intake, and higher level of exercise (Kimmel et al. 2016). Menstrual irregularity is also common in patients with BN and BED (Poyastro Pinheiro et al. 2007). There is a noteworthy association of BN and BED with polycystic ovary syndrome (PCOS). More than 75% of patients with BN have PCOS, and one in four patients with PCOS meet criteria for BN (McCluskey et al. 1992). Menstrual and sexual dysfunction in EDs also contribute to fertility difficulties in this population (Linna et al. 2013).

### Eating Disorders and Pregnancy

Pregnancy in patients with EDs is often unplanned. Women with AN are at twofold risk of unplanned pregnancy, and those with BN are at 30-fold increased risk, compared with women in the general population (Claydon et al. 2018; Micali et al. 2014). Unplanned pregnancy puts the woman and fetus at risk through delayed prenatal care, unintended substance exposures, and inadequate nourishment, because maladaptive eating may continue while the patient is unaware of the pregnancy (Kimmel et al. 2016). Pregnancy in these women is often associated with negative effects as they struggle with changing body image in the face of pregnancy-related weight gain, poor sense of self-worth, worry about the baby's health, and the dilemma of discussing their ED with a health care provider (Tierney et al. 2011). Many patients conceal their ED,

TABLE 22–4. **Maternal and infant risks associated with eating disorders in pregnancy**

| Maternal | Fetal/Obstetrical |
|---|---|
| Anemia, nutritional disorders | Developmental delays |
| Comorbidity with depression | Intrauterine growth retardation |
| Earlier breastfeeding cessation | Lower birth weight |
| Hyperemesis gravidarum | Perinatal death |
| Poor mother–infant bonding | Premature birth |
| Poor prenatal care | Small (anorexia) or large (bulimia/binge eating) for gestational age infant |
| Preeclampsia | |
| Substance use disorders | |

pregnancy, or both, which puts the pregnancy at high risk (Cardwell 2013). Women with AN tend to have lower gestational weight gain, whereas those with BN and BED may have excessive weight gain (Koubaa et al. 2005). Women with EDs tend to have a higher incidence of gestational hypertension, preeclampsia, and hyperemesis gravidarum (Koubaa et al. 2005).

## Maternal and Infant Risks Associated With Eating Disorders in Pregnancy

Adequate maternal nutrition and weight gain are crucial for a healthy pregnancy and fetal development, so an active ED puts both the mother and the fetus at high risk (Table 22–4). Suboptimal nutrition in pregnancy may contribute to the risk of nutritional disorders, such as anemia, Korsakoff psychosis, Wernicke's syndrome, and scurvy (Cardwell 2013). Severe calorie restriction increases the likelihood of intrauterine growth restriction, low birth weight, small head circumference, microcephaly, and small for gestational age infants (Koubaa et al. 2005). Additionally, these infants do not catch up with peers, and developmental delays persist throughout life (Park et al. 2003). Per several studies, gestational age was lowest among children of women with AN and highest among children of women with BED. Children of women with AN are at increased risk of very premature birth and have a fourfold increased risk of perinatal death (Linna et al. 2014). An especially challenging pregnancy is that of women with BN and gestational diabetes, in which the patient may use insulin injection as a purging method (Cardwell 2013).

Ms. II is a 28-year-old married female, gravida 1 para 0, currently at 25 weeks' gestation, with concerns about weight gain in pregnancy. She shares her history of emotional abuse and parental marital discord in childhood, as well as high pressure in both academics and cross-country sports. Around age 13, Ms. II began to restrict certain foods to help enhance performance in her sport, but this gradually spiraled out of control over the next year to the point of escalating restriction, calorie counting, and overexercise that led to ongoing weight loss. Her menarche was delayed until age 16, and her disordered eating persisted until she began treatment with intensive psychotherapy and work with a dietician. She was doing well for about 3 years prior to her pregnancy, which was unplanned; her pre-pregnancy weight was 104 lb, with a height of 5 ft, 1 in. She had significant hyperemesis in the first trimester and rapidly lost 10 lb. Nausea has since improved, and she now weighs 105 lb but without further weight gain. Ms. II struggles with the

TABLE 22–5. **Differential diagnosis of eating disorders**

| | |
|---|---|
| Endocrine | Hyperthyroidism, glucocorticoid insufficiency, diabetes |
| Gastrointestinal | Inflammatory bowel disease, celiac or other malabsorptive disease, peptic ulcer disease, gastroparesis, gastric outlet obstruction, gastroesophageal reflux, eosinophilic gastroenteritis, chronic idiopathic intestinal pseudo-obstruction |
| Infectious | Chronic infections (e.g., tuberculosis), HIV |
| Neoplastic | CNS tumors or other malignancies |
| Psychiatric | Major depressive disorder, bipolar disorder, OCD, social phobia, body dysmorphic disorder, psychotic disorders, ADHD |

changes in her body, feeling as though she is "waking up in someone else's body" and says that this pregnancy is emotionally traumatic. She also shares anxiety that her clothes are feeling tighter and significant anxiety about visits with her obstetrician due to fears that the doctor will continue to push her to gain weight. Ms. II notes that at her last obstetrical visit, she was instructed to increase her calories to 2,000 per day; this caused a feeling of panic, and she was unable to eat anything the rest of the day.

### Postpartum Concerns

Studies show that mothers with EDs are at risk of early cessation of breastfeeding. These women are also at greater risk of depression and anxiety during pregnancy and in the postpartum period (Franko et al. 2001). For many women with ED, the postpartum period is particularly challenging because they struggle to adjust to a new body and motherhood, and this often leads to an exacerbation of symptoms (Zerwas et al. 2014). A neonatal complication seen in mothers with BN is "slimming," in which they project their body image onto the baby and perceive the baby as "fat." This mother then may restrict feedings for or induce vomiting in the baby (Cardwell 2013).

### Menopause and Eating Disorders

Research shows that the prevalence of EDs in midlife has been increasing, and up to 4.6% of midlife women ages 40–60 years may meet full criteria for diagnosis of an ED (Mangweth-Matzek et al. 2014). Perimenopause can be a window of vulnerability for the development or exacerbation of EDs due to reproductive hormone changes (Baker and Runfola 2016). The prevalence of BED is higher in the older population, whereas the incidence of AN seems to decrease (Baker and Runfola 2016).

## Differential Diagnosis

When evaluating someone for a possible ED, consider other medical and psychiatric conditions that could be contributing to symptoms. Among pregnant women, peripartum nausea and appetite changes, as well as hyperemesis gravidarum, should be considered. Other medical diagnoses can also mimic symptoms of EDs, as documented in Table 22–5.

Regarding psychiatric diagnosis, appetite and eating patterns are also often affected by mood disorders, including both unipolar depression and bipolar spectrum illnesses. In addition, the highly structured eating patterns seen in many EDs are akin to the obsessions and compulsions seen in OCD, and similar thoughts and actions related to nonfood items and tasks need to be fully assessed. The impulsivity seen in ADHD and some personality disorders (e.g., borderline personality disorder) may also mimic the seemingly impulsive eating patterns seen in BN and BED, and overemphasized beliefs and delusions seen in body dysmorphic and psychotic disorders also have similarities with EDs.

# Pathophysiology

## Biological, Psychological, and Social Contributions

The genetic basis of EDs has been well documented, most notably in twin studies showing greater concordance in monozygotic twins compared with dizygotic twins (Mazzeo et al. 2009, 2010; Mitchell et al. 2010), and meta-analyses have shown moderate to high heritability (Culbert et al. 2015). More recent studies into the specific heritability of AN have identified genetic loci on chromosome 12 (Duncan et al. 2017). Neuroimaging also supports biological contribution to the development of EDs, with studies identifying structural changes in gray matter volume (particularly in the limbic system) and in ventricle and sulci size in AN (Phillipou et al. 2014) and changes in the frontal and temporoparietal areas in BN (Donnelly et al. 2018). Functional changes have also been identified in the corticolimbic, dorsostriatal, and corticostriatal circuits, with particular differences noted in insular and cingulate cortex activity, which are highly involved in motivation, goal-directed behavior, and emotional processes (Phillipou et al. 2014). Some of these changes appear to reverse with weight restoration, suggesting that differences may be consequences of the disorder rather than etiological contributors (Phillipou et al. 2014).

Sociocultural factors are not only risk factors but also likely at play in the development of EDs. Although these disorders have been identified across time and cultures, increased adoption of the idealization of thinness in the 20th century and exposure to Western cultural values have both been associated with increased rates of EDs (Culbert et al. 2015). Internalization of the social ideal is likely a key variable because not all individuals exposed to thin ideal media develop an ED (Culbert et al. 2015; Martínez-González et al. 2003). Twin studies have identified individual differences in both genetic and environmental factors for thin ideal internalization, indicating the complexity of this vulnerability (Culbert et al. 2015).

As mentioned, personality traits have also been purported as part of the etiological model, with specific association of EDs with negative emotionality/neuroticism, perfectionism, and impulsivity/negative urgency (Culbert et al. 2015). Individuals with AN and BN also have decreased cognitive flexibility, as evidenced by impaired performance on cognitive flexibility tasks (Wu et al. 2014); these deficits may even persist into recovery and weight restoration (Culbert et al. 2015).

## Connection With Reproductive Hormones

As evidenced by the prior inclusion of amenorrhea as a diagnostic criterion, the connection between EDs and reproductive hormones and function has been well established. The concept that a critical level of stored energy or fat mass was required for initiation and maintenance of menstrual function was developed in the 1960s, with later identification of leptin as a key hormone (Andersen and Ryan 2009). Produced in the adipose cells, leptin is a mediator between stored energy balance and hypothalamic-pituitary-ovarian (HPO) axis function. Women with low body weight (whether from an ED or other etiology) have characteristically low leptin levels, and studies suggest that a threshold level exists that permits menstruation (Andersen and Ryan 2009). Ghrelin produced by cells in the stomach is also an important metabolic fuel detector, with elevated ghrelin levels suppressing the HPO axis and resulting in amenorrhea. Insulin and peptide YY are also required for normal reproductive function, and these, along with the other peripheral metabolic mediators, communicate both directly and indirectly to the gonadotropin-releasing hormone–producing neurons in the hypothalamus (Andersen and Ryan 2009).

Hormonal changes occur in women with EDs, with resulting alterations in reproductive function. Specific changes include inhibition of normal pulsatile gonadotropin-releasing hormone release and low levels of luteinizing hormone, follicle-stimulating hormone, and estradiol. This leads to ovarian changes, with characteristically smaller volumes and rare dominant follicles. These alterations present clinically in ovulatory dysfunction and impairment in luteolysis, endometrial development, fertility, menstruation, and bone growth (Andersen and Ryan 2009).

## Treatment

Treatment of EDs often involves a multidisciplinary approach, including elements of dietary changes and weight restoration, psychotherapy, and pharmacotherapy. Management of EDs during pregnancy offers different opportunities and challenges compared with that for women in other parts of the reproductive cycle. Treatment of pregnant women with an ED should focus on weight restoration and adequate nutrition, with early referral to a nutritionist and vitamin supplementation (Andersen and Ryan 2009). Weight gain should be monitored closely, with understanding that necessary weight gain may be greater for those at lower weights compared with the general population. Women should be educated about the risks for both mother and baby that are associated with disordered eating behaviors during pregnancy (Andersen and Ryan 2009).

For women with EDs who are not yet pregnant, the time of trying to conceive can be another potential window for intervention. Education should be provided on the association between infertility and ED symptoms (discussed later), and women should be encouraged to seek ED treatment prior to conception (Andersen and Ryan 2009).

### Psychopharmacology

Pharmacotherapy options for EDs vary by diagnosis. Medications are not considered first-line or primary treatment for AN, whereas they are more often indicated as a component of treatment in BN and BED. Nutritional rehabilitation (including weight restoration when necessary) and psychotherapy, with emphasis on an interdisciplinary team approach, are the mainstays of treatment for all individuals with EDs.

#### Antidepressants

Selective serotonin reuptake inhibitors (SSRIs) are among the most commonly prescribed medications for those with EDs. When these are used during the perinatal period, a risk-risk analysis is an important part of decision making. (Please see Chapter 8,

"A Clinical Approach to Psychiatric Diagnosis and Treatment During Pregnancy," and Chapter 13, "Depressive Disorders," for further details.) Antidepressants have been found to reduce binge-purge episodes in individuals with BN, even after controlling for comorbid depression (Davis and Attia 2017). They have similarly been associated with a decrease in binge eating with BED, although they have not been associated with weight loss. Fluoxetine is the only FDA-approved medication for BN, although sertraline, fluvoxamine, and citalopram have also been studied in both BN and BED and can be utilized (Davis and Attia 2017). Because a key study demonstrated superior response to higher-dose fluoxetine (60 mg) compared with both lower-dose fluoxetine (20 mg) and placebo (Levine et al. 1992), higher doses of antidepressants are often used when treating BN (Davis and Attia 2017).

In AN, antidepressants have not been shown to improve either weight gain or weight maintenance in weight-restored individuals (Davis and Attia 2017). Theories posit that the lack of response may be related to underlying malnutrition or neurotransmitter deficits. Despite this, antidepressants are often prescribed for individuals with AN as part of their treatment plan. This is likely related to the high rates of comorbidity with depression and anxiety, whose symptoms can affect and potentially interfere with ED treatment. Because these comorbid diagnoses are treated primarily with antidepressants, addition of these agents could provide additional benefit for those with EDs.

SSRIs are often considered first-line due to their favorable side effect profile, and their lower risk of weight gain (compared with other classes of antidepressants) may make them more palatable to patients. Other classes of antidepressants have also been studied, including tricyclic antidepressants (TCAs; e.g., imipramine, desipramine, and amitriptyline) and monoamine oxidase inhibitors (MAOIs; e.g., phenelzine) in BN and serotonin-norepinephrine reuptake inhibitors (duloxetine) in BED (Davis and Attia 2017). TCAs and MAOIs tend to be used less frequently due to their side effect profiles, with notable concerns for sedation and constipation, which are both common baseline symptoms of those with EDs. In contrast, bupropion is often avoided for individuals with EDs due to the potential for decreased appetite and the increased risk of seizures in those with BN, whose purging behavior and attendant electrolyte abnormalities lower the seizure threshold (Horne et al. 1988).

## Antipsychotics

Antipsychotics are considered another treatment option for EDs, largely due to their potential for anxiolysis and to mitigate the rigid or obsessional thinking often seen within these disorders; their frequent association with weight gain may also make them appealing for clinicians, although evidence to support that approach is mixed (Davis and Attia 2017, 2019). For a full discussion of the risks of using these medications in the perinatal period, please see Chapter 17, "Schizophrenia and Related Disorders." Although studies of first-generation antipsychotics have not shown positive results, a recent study of olanzapine showed a statistically significant increase in BMI over time compared with placebo (Attia et al. 2019). Despite improvement in weight, olanzapine had no significant impact on cognitions and psychological symptoms, and no group differences were found in Yale-Brown Obsessive Compulsive Scale, Center for Epidemiologic Studies Depression Scale, Eating Disorders Examination, or Zung Anxiety Inventory scores (Attia et al. 2019; Davis and Attia 2019).

Studies of other second-generation antipsychotics, including risperidone, quetiapine, and aripiprazole, have shown mixed results, with olanzapine remaining the agent with the most consistent evidence for efficacy in AN (Davis and Attia 2017). Case reports have also described the use of aripiprazole in BN (Trunko et al. 2011), although other second-generation antipsychotics may be avoided by clinicians due to concerns that the side effect of appetite induction could contribute to binge episodes.

## Antiepileptics

Topiramate has been shown to reduce both bingeing and purging in individuals with BN (Hoopes et al. 2003), although its association with weight loss can inhibit its use in some individuals for whom weight loss may be contraindicated. Topiramate can also be used as treatment for BED, with demonstrated reductions in binge eating frequency and weight that appear to sustain with longer-term use (McElroy et al. 2004). It has also been trialed in combination with phentermine in treatment of BED, with limited studies showing cessation of binge eating and significant weight loss (Davis and Attia 2017). However, initiation of these medications during pregnancy requires a risk-risk discussion given the potential impact on both mother and fetus, particularly given the association with malformations seen with topiramate and concerns for weight loss with phentermine. For a full discussion of the potential risks in the perinatal period, please see Table 22–6.

Zonisamide has also been studied for BED, showing benefits in both weight loss and reducing binge episodes. In one study in which zonisamide was added to cognitive-behavioral therapy (CBT), patients with zonisamide augmentation had reduced BMI and reduced binge eating frequency 1 year after treatment (Ricca et al. 2009).

## Other Medications

Stimulants and other weight/appetite-impacting medications have also been studied in BED. A full discussion of risks associated with use of stimulants in the perinatal period can be found in Chapter 23, "Attention-Deficit/Hyperactivity Disorder." Lisdexamfetamine is the first medication to receive an FDA indication for BED, with supporting studies demonstrating significant reductions in binge eating frequency and improvement in Clinical Global Impressions scores (McElroy et al. 2015). Although it does not have specific indications, lisdexamfetamine is also associated with decreasing weight, BMI, and triglyceride levels (Davis and Attia 2019). The lipase inhibitor orlistat has been studied in BED, showing benefit in weight loss and reducing Eating Disorder Inventory–2 scores, although not for reducing binge-eating frequency. Chromium has also been studied in BED, with moderate doses demonstrating improved glycemic control (not seen with placebo or high-dose groups), although further study is needed (Davis and Attia 2017). The risks associated with these nonstimulant appetite-impacting medications are described in Table 22–6.

Used as an adjunct for some anxiety disorders, D-cycloserine has shown mixed results in the treatment of AN when combined with exposure therapy (Davis and Attia 2017). The synthetic cannabinoid agonist dronabinol has shown some benefit in weight gain compared with placebo for women with AN, although it was also associated with increased energy expenditure (Davis and Attia 2017). Information for risk-risk discussion in the perinatal period for these supplements is also found in Table 22–6.

TABLE 22–6. **Medication risk discussion in pregnancy**

| | Early pregnancy | Other pregnancy | Obstetrical and neonatal outcomes | Long-term effects | Lactation |
|---|---|---|---|---|---|
| **Antiepileptics** | | | | | |
| Phentermine | Abnormalities in phospholipid storage found in rat/guinea pig studies[1] but not human studies<br>No finding of increased rate of congenital anomalies[2]<br>Weight loss possibly associated with neural tube defects[3] | ND | Possibly associated with maternal hypertension, placental abruption, and mild preeclampsia[4] | ND | ND |
| Topiramate | One pregnancy registry[5] indicated incidence of cleft/lip palate (2.2%) and hypospadias (5.1%) (higher than background population), although mothers may have been on other antiepileptics<br>Another registry[11] showed OR 3.8 for malformations in exposed infants vs. unexposed and incidence of 1.4% for cleft palate<br>Two other registries[6,12] showed no increase in risk of malformations | Increased rate of SGA infants, lower mean BW and length, decrease in mean head circumference, higher risk of microcephaly[6,7] | Possible increase in fetal distress at birth and CS deliveries, but insufficient for conclusions[8] | Exposure in first or second trimester not associated with decrements in offspring verbal/nonverbal abilities, processing speed, or IQ[9] | Ratio of milk to maternal plasma 0.83<br>Concentrations in breastfed infants detectable but below quantification limit with no AE[10] |
| Zonisamide | Cases of malformation taken in combination with other antiepileptic(s)[13]; case reports of successful pregnancies with monotherapy[14] | Lower mean BW and length[7] | ND | ND | Ratio of milk to plasma 0.93; no AE |

**TABLE 22–6. Medication risk discussion in pregnancy *(continued)***

| | Early pregnancy | Other pregnancy | Obstetrical and neonatal outcomes | Long-term effects | Lactation |
|---|---|---|---|---|---|
| **Other medications** | | | | | |
| Chromium | No association found with neural tube defects or malformations[15] | Increased risk of low BW[16] | Increased risk of preterm birth[16]<br>Levels found in cord blood but no AE in infants[17] | ND | Excreted in milk; not impacted when chromium intake increased[18] |
| D-Cycloserine | ND | ND | ND | ND | ND |
| Dronabinol | No consistent association with malformations; increased risk of miscarriage and stillbirth (after controlling for cigarette smoking)[19] | Possible dose-dependent relationship with risk of low BW/SGA (data inconsistent)[20,21] | Some data on increased risk of preterm birth[21]<br>Increased risk of NICU admission[21]<br>Neonates can have increased tremulousness, altered visual response to light, withdrawal-like crying, alterations in sleep patterns (diminish within 30 days)[22] | Two cohorts found impulsivity in early childhood; hyperactivity and inattention and decrease in executive functioning in later childhood and adolescence; and increase in adult recreational drug use[23,24] | THC and metabolites concentrated in milk and absorbed by infant; estimated infant dose 2.5% of maternal dose[25] |
| Orlistat | Findings do not suggest an increased rate of malformation[26,27] | ND | ND | ND | ND |

AE=adverse effects; BW=birth weight; CS=cesarean-section; ND=no data found; NICU=neonatal intensive care unit; OR=odds ratio; SGA=small for gestational age; THC=tetrahydrocannabinol

*Source.* [1]Thoma-Laurie et al. 1983; [2]Jones et al. 2002; [3]Robert et al. 1995; [4]Sands 1962; [5]Hunt et al. 2008; [6]Veiby et al. 2014; [7]Hernández-Díaz et al. 2014; [8]Rihtman et al. 2012; [9]Bromley et al. 2016; [10]Ohman et al. 2002; [11]Hernández-Díaz et al. 2012; [12]Vajda et al. 2016; [13]Kondo et al. 1996; [14]Shimoyama et al. 1999; [15]Eizaguirre-Garcia et al. 2000; [16]Xia et al. 2016; [17]deSouza et al. 2012; [18]Kumpulainen et al. 1980; [19]Coleman-Cowger et al. 2018; [20]English et al. 1997; [21]Hayatbakhsh et al. 2012; [22]Cook et al. 1990; [23]Fried and Smith 2001; [24]Goldschmidt et al. 2012; [25]Baker et al. 2018; [26]Perrio et al. 2007; [27]Källén 2014.

### Special Considerations in Pharmacotherapy

When prescribing for low-weight individuals, dosage adjustments should be considered due to an increased risk of side effects in the setting of decreased volume of distribution. Depleted protein stores can also increase the percentage of unbound or free drug in the serum, further supporting the recommendation to start at low initial doses and titrate slowly to effect.

## Weight Restoration and Medical Interventions

Weight restoration and nutritional rehabilitation are the cornerstone of treatment in individuals with EDs, particularly when at low weight. Goals of nutritional rehabilitation are to stabilize the patient medically, reverse medical complications that occur in the low-weight state, and restore weight and normal eating patterns. This improved nutritional state can also lead to improved cognitive function and emotional regulation and stability (Attia and Walsh 2009). Nutritional rehabilitation is best provided in a multidisciplinary approach, including behavioral management, nutritional counseling, and medical monitoring. A key component is often the introduction of regular, structured meals, with additional monitoring of patients to ensure appropriate intake without the use of disordered eating behaviors, including compensatory behaviors such as exercise or purging.

During the time of initial weight restoration, patients should be closely monitored given the risk of refeeding syndrome. Refeeding syndrome is a potentially fatal complication of nutritional rehabilitation and occurs rarely in moderately severe cases (~6%) and more commonly in mildly severe cases (>20%) (Ornstein et al. 2003). This syndrome is marked by numerous electrolyte derangements and clinical sequelae, including hypophosphatemia, hypokalemia, hypomagnesemia, thiamine deficiency, peripheral edema, rhabdomyolysis, and hemolysis. More severe medical complications have also been reported, including congestive heart failure, seizures, delirium, cardiac dysrhythmia, and even sudden death (Fuentebella and Kerner 2009; Ornstein et al. 2003). Of most import is phosphorus level because hypophosphatemia is considered the hallmark and predominant cause of refeeding syndrome. The pathogenesis of this relates to increased cellular uptake of phosphorus (along with potassium and magnesium) when insulin is released in the body in response to glucose upon refeeding. Risk of this syndrome is increased in more severely malnourished individuals (i.e., those who begin refeeding at lower weight/percent of ideal body weight), those not fed/underfed for at least 10–14 days, and those with recent significant weight loss (>10% in last 1–2 months) (Fuentebella and Kerner 2009).

Refeeding syndrome is avoided and mitigated through appropriate introduction of nourishment and close monitoring physically and biochemically. Initial caloric intake should approximate or be less than estimated energy expenditure, with slow increase in caloric intake during early refeeding. Fluid intake should also be monitored and restricted as necessary to prevent fluid overload, particularly in those at risk of cardiac dysfunction. Electrolytes should be closely monitored and deficiencies immediately corrected, with particular focus on phosphorus, potassium, and magnesium by daily measurement until stability is met (Fuentebella and Kerner 2009). In addition, thiamine, vitamin B complex, and multivitamins should be started with refeeding because thiamine deficiency is a frequent complication of malnourishment and can have severe consequences (including Wernicke's encephalopathy) (Mehanna et al. 2009).

Recent studies have looked at higher initial caloric intake with more rapid increases that have not shown worsening in medical complications and refeeding syndrome when electrolytes have been appropriately monitored and abnormalities corrected (Garber et al. 2016). Current recommendations now opt for more aggressive caloric values for those with mild to moderate malnutrition in the setting of close electrolyte monitoring.

## Behavioral Treatments

Patients with EDs can be treated at various levels of care, and many require more intensive treatment beyond typical outpatient care given the medical risks and complexities of the disorder. Recommendations remain to offer outpatient treatment to those with EDs, with inpatient intervention reserved for those at greatest medical (e.g., high risk of refeeding syndrome) or psychiatric (e.g., comorbid depression with suicidality) risk (Treasure et al. 2010). Descriptions of the varied levels of care are found in Table 22–7. Universal across treatment modalities is the involvement of a multidisciplinary team, often including a psychiatrist, psychologist/therapist, dietician, nurses, and a general medical provider.

Psychotherapy is the preferred evidence-based intervention for most EDs. CBT has been well studied in the treatment of EDs and has been found to be a superior treatment modality for BN and BED (Davis and Attia 2019; Treasure et al. 2010). Due to its efficacy, CBT techniques have been adapted for group environment, telemedicine services, and self-help modalities, including an internet-based manualized CBT group therapy delivered via group chat (Davis and Attia 2019). Interpersonal psychotherapy is also an effective treatment for EDs, although treatment response appears to be slower and potentially less robust compared with CBT (Davis and Attia 2019; Treasure et al. 2010). Given the high prevalence of emotional dysregulation in EDs, dialectical behavioral therapy has also been proposed as a treatment, and data support its use in BN and BED, although evidence in AN is limited (Davis and Attia 2019). Acceptance and commitment therapy has also been considered as a treatment to target the underlying maladaptive cognitions and behaviors in EDs, although data remain limited (Davis and Attia 2019).

For children and adolescents with EDs, first-line treatment involves family-based therapy, in which responsibility for refeeding the child is placed back on the parents. Recommendations are for early and aggressive treatment, given that early response to treatment and initial weight gain are likely the greatest predictors of treatment outcomes, including posttreatment remission (Davis and Attia 2019).

## Treatment Challenges

One challenge to the treatment of EDs is their changing presentation over time. Patients may initially present with certain disordered eating symptoms (e.g., predominant restricting behaviors) and later progress to other symptoms (e.g., binge/purge behaviors). This can lead to treatment challenges, particularly when certain treatments are less effective or even contraindicated when behaviors change. Most important to consider are medications associated with appetite reduction and weight loss; although individuals with BN may be of normal to high weight initially, they may develop more severe symptoms that result in low weight and a subsequent diagnosis of AN. Such factors should be considered in the initial selection of pharmacotherapy.

**TABLE 22–7. Eating disorder levels of care**

| Level of care | Typical clinical format | Patient criteria |
|---|---|---|
| Inpatient | Group therapy<br>Meals and snacks supervised<br>Medical specialties for consultation<br>Nutritional consultations<br>Psychiatric hospitalization (often locked unit)<br>Psychiatric management by physician daily<br>24/7 Nursing and support staff<br>24/7 Supervision with close observation (including around mealtimes and in bathroom) | Blood pressure <90/60 mm Hg<br>Cardiovascular abnormalities other than bradycardia<br>Dehydration<br>Heart rate <40 bpm<br>Lack of improvement or rapid worsening while in outpatient treatment<br>Potassium <3 mmol/L<br>Rapid weight loss of several kilograms within 1 week<br>Symptomatic hypoglycemia<br>Temperature <36.1°C (97.0°F)<br>Weight <75% of expected weight |
| Residential | Daily programming (individual, group, and family treatment)<br>Can be a step down from inpatient or treatment step up from outpatient<br>Housing provided so patients can stay overnight with some level of supervision (less than inpatient psychiatric hospitalization, not locked unit) | Medically stable (typically does not have level of medical care that can be provided during inpatient admission)<br>Needs greater length of time in treatment than provided on inpatient unit<br>Requires close monitoring and supervised meals in a structured and supervised setting for most of the day (e.g., can control behaviors while in program but engages in behavior when unsupervised) |
| Partial hospitalization | 5 days a week, 6–8 hours per day<br>Two supervised meals and one snack daily<br>Includes:<br>Nutritional counseling<br>Close medical monitoring<br>Group therapy<br>Individual therapy (2–3 hours/week)<br>Psychiatric management by physician weekly | Requires close monitoring and supervised meals<br>Has failed to benefit from less intensive care<br>Is acutely ill but does not require inpatient hospitalization<br>Needs step-down care after inpatient hospitalization |

TABLE 22–7. **Eating disorder levels of care *(continued)***

| Level of care | Typical clinical format | Patient criteria |
|---|---|---|
| Intensive outpatient | 3 days a week, 3 hours per day<br>One supervised meal<br>Includes<br>Nutritional counseling<br>Close medical monitoring<br>Group therapy<br>Individual therapy (1–2 hours/ week)<br>Psychiatric management by physician every 1–2 weeks | Would benefit from structure of a program but does not require partial level of care<br>Would benefit from support in continued recovery after returning to work or school |
| Outpatient | Frequency determined by clinician and patient (weekly to monthly)<br>Individual therapy and/or group work<br>Often in conjunction with outpatient dietician, primary care team | Overall stable eating disorder behaviors with little or no medical complications |

Another challenge is managing patients with severe and enduring EDs (SEEDs). For those who have persistent symptoms that are not responding to highly aggressive treatment, referral to a higher level of care may not be indicated despite serious symptoms. Intensive treatment focuses on amelioration of ED symptoms, which might not be a realistic goal for those with SEED symptoms. Individuals with SEEDs may also remain symptomatic at discharge, which could be a reflection of external limitations on length of treatment, and patient factors related to ambivalence about change and inability to fully address the complex functions of disordered eating symptoms and their associations with comorbid psychopathology. Valuing a patient's autonomy by assessing readiness for change and identifying specific goals of care is an important component of treatment in SEED cases.

# Conclusion

EDs are a group of psychiatric diagnoses associated with numerous medical comorbidities and risk of severe complications and mortality. Care must be taken to identify individuals with disordered eating symptoms, including application of screening methods across various medical settings. Treatment should be focused initially on weight restoration and safe nutritional rehabilitation, with particular focus on avoiding complications of refeeding, most notably refeeding syndrome. Further treatment should address underlying cognitive distortions related to food and body image and underlying psychosocial contributors to the development of the disease.

Due to the associated changes in the HPO axis, most women struggling with disordered eating have associated changes in reproductive functioning. The experience and symptoms associated with pregnancy may also affect the course of an ED. Providers caring for women with ED symptoms should be aware of these potential alterations throughout the reproductive life cycle, including effects on puberty, menstruation, conception/fertility, and pregnancy. Women with EDs should understand the risks to both mother and baby when symptoms are active during pregnancy, and treatment should focus on a multidisciplinary approach including psychiatry, psychology, nutrition, and obstetrical care to ensure care throughout the perinatal period.

## Key Points

- Eating disorders (EDs) are a group of diagnoses characterized by disturbance in eating that lead to functional impairment and are associated with numerous potentially severe medical comorbidities.
- In addition to strong genetic correlation, risk factors for the development of EDs include cultural influences of the thin ideal, specific psychological traits, psychosocial factors, and comorbid psychiatric disorders.
- The perinatal period can be a high-risk time for onset or relapse of disordered eating behaviors in some, whereas for others it can be a time of motivation for recovery.
- Given the connection with reproductive hormones, EDs can be associated with effects on puberty, menstruation, fertility, and pregnancy.
- Active ED symptoms during pregnancy carry risk for both mother and baby.
- Initial treatment of EDs is focused on weight restoration and nutritional rehabilitation, with focus on medical monitoring given risk of negative sequelae from refeeding syndrome.
- Treatment most often requires a multidisciplinary team approach, including behavioral medicine, physical medicine, and nutrition, with the major focus on psychotherapy approaches to address ED cognitions and behaviors.
- Data on use of psychopharmacology in EDs are somewhat limited, although antidepressants (particularly for bulimia nervosa), antipsychotics (for anorexia nervosa), and psychostimulants (for binge eating disorder) have been studied, with some FDA approvals.
- Treatment of EDs often requires varied levels of care, including inpatient, partial hospitalization, intensive outpatient, and outpatient options.

## References

American Psychiatric Association: Diagnostic and Statistical Manual of Mental Disorders, 5th Edition. Arlington, VA, American Psychiatric Association, 2013

Andersen AE, Ryan GL: Eating disorders in the obstetric and gynecologic patient population. Obstet Gynecol 114(6):1353–1367, 2009 19935043

Arcelus J, Mitchell AJ, Wales J, et al: Mortality rates in patients with anorexia nervosa and other eating disorders: a meta-analysis of 36 studies. Arch Gen Psychiatry 68(7):724–731, 2011 21727255

Attia E, Walsh BT: Behavioral management for anorexia nervosa. N Engl J Med 360(5):500–506, 2009 19179317

Attia E, Steinglass JE, Walsh BT, et al: Olanzapine versus placebo in adult outpatients with anorexia nervosa: a randomized clinical trial. Am J Psychiatry 176(6):449–456, 2019 30654643

Baker JH, Runfola CD: Eating disorders in midlife women: a perimenopausal eating disorder? Maturitas 85:112–116, 2016 26857889

Baker T, Datta P, Rewers-Felkins K, et al: Transfer of inhaled cannabis into human breast milk. Obstet Gynecol 131(5):783–788, 2018 29630019

Becker AE, Franko DL, Speck A, et al: Ethnicity and differential access to care for eating disorder symptoms. Int J Eat Disord 33(2):205–212, 2003 12616587

Boisseau CL: Identification and management of eating disorders in gynecology: menstrual health as an underutilized screening tool. Am J Obstet Gynecol 215(5):572–578, 2016 27422054

Bromley RL, Calderbank R, Cheyne CP, et al: Cognition in school-age children exposed to levetiracetam, topiramate, or sodium valproate. Neurology 87(18):1943–1953, 2016 27581218

Cachelin FM, Rebeck R, Veisel C, et al: Barriers to treatment for eating disorders among ethnically diverse women. Int J Eat Disord 30(3):269–278, 2001 11746286

Cardwell MS: Eating disorders during pregnancy. Obstet Gynecol Surv 68(4):312–323, 2013

Claydon EA, Davidov DM, Zullig KJ, et al: Waking up every day in a body that is not yours: a qualitative research inquiry into the intersection between eating disorders and pregnancy. BMC Pregnancy Childbirth 18(1):463–476, 2018 30497443

Coffino JA, Udo T, Grilo CM: Rates of help-seeking in US adults with lifetime DSM-5 eating disorders: prevalence across diagnoses and differences by sex and ethnicity/race. Mayo Clin Proc 94(8):1415–1426, 2019 31324401

Coleman-Cowger VH, Oga EA, Peters EN, et al: Prevalence and associated birth outcomes of co-use of cannabis and tobacco cigarettes during pregnancy. Neurotoxicol Teratol 68:84–90, 2018

Cook PS, Peterson RC, Moore DT: Alcohol, Tobacco, and Other Drugs May Harm the Unborn. Edited by Haase TB. Rockville, MD, U.S. Department of Health and Human Services, 1990

Cotton MA, Ball C, Robinson P: Four simple questions can help screen for eating disorders. J Gen Intern Med 18(1):53–56, 2003 12534764

Culbert KM, Racine SE, Klump KL: Research review: what we have learned about the causes of eating disorders—a synthesis of sociocultural, psychological, and biological research. J Child Psychol Psychiatry 56(11):1141–1164, 2015 26095891

Davis H, Attia E: Pharmacotherapy of eating disorders. Curr Opin Psychiatry 30(6):452–457, 2017 28806268

Davis LE, Attia E: Recent advances in therapies for eating disorders. F1000 Res 8:1693, 2019

deSouza RM, Wallace D, Costa ML, et al: Transplacental passage of metal ions in women with hip resurfacing: no teratogenic effects observed. Hip Int 22(1):96–99, 2012 22383325

Donnelly B, Touyz S, Hay P, et al: Neuroimaging in bulimia nervosa and binge eating disorder: a systematic review. J Eat Disord 6:3, 2018 29468065

Duncan L, Yilmaz Z, Gaspar H, et al: Significant locus and metabolic genetic correlations revealed in genome-wide association study of anorexia nervosa. Am J Psychiatry 174(9):850–858, 2017 28494655

Easter A, Bye A, Taborelli E, et al: Recognising the symptoms: how common are eating disorders in pregnancy? Eur Eat Disord Rev 21(4):340–344, 2013 23495197

Eizaguirre-Garcia D, Rodriquez-Andres D, Watt GC: Congenital anomalies in Glasgow between 1982 and 1989 and chromium waste. J Public Health Med 22(1):54–58, 2000

English DR, Hulse GK, Milne E, et al: Maternal cannabis use and birth weight: a meta-analysis. Addiction 92(11):1553–1560, 1997 9519497

Erskine HE, Whiteford HA: Epidemiology of binge eating disorder. Curr Opin Psychiatry 31(6):462–470, 2018 30113324

Fairburn CG, Beglin SJ: Assessment of eating disorders: interview or self-report questionnaire? Int J Eat Disord 16(4):363–370, 1994 7866415

Fairburn CG, Harrison PJ: Eating disorders. Lancet 361(9355):407–416, 2003 12573387

Fawcett EJ, Fawcett JM, Mazmanian D: A meta-analysis of the worldwide prevalence of pica during pregnancy and the postpartum period. Int J Gynaecol Obstet 133(3):277–283, 2016 26892693

Franko DL, Blais MA, Becker AE, et al: Pregnancy complications and neonatal outcomes in women with eating disorders. Am J Psychiatry 158(9):1461–1466, 2001 11532732
Fried PA, Smith AM: A literature review of the consequences of prenatal marihuana exposure: an emerging theme of a deficiency in aspects of executive function. Neurotoxicol Teratol 23(1):1–11, 2001
Fuentebella J, Kerner JA: Refeeding syndrome. Pediatr Clin North Am 56(5):1201–1210, 2009
Garber AK, Sawyer SM, Golden NH, et al: A systematic review of approaches to refeeding in patients with anorexia nervosa. Int J Eat Disord 49(3):293–310, 2016 26661289
Goldschmidt L, Richardson GA, Willford JA, et al: School achievement in 14-year-old youths prenatally exposed to marijuana. Neurotoxicol Teratol 34(1):161–167, 2012 21884785
Grilo CM, White MA, Masheb RM: DSM-IV psychiatric disorder comorbidity and its correlates in binge eating disorder. Int J Eat Disord 42(3):228–234, 2009 18951458
Hayatbakhsh MR, Flenady VJ, Gibbons KS, et al: Birth outcomes associated with cannabis use before and during pregnancy. Pediatr Res 71(2):215–219, 2012 22258135
Hernández-Díaz S, Smith CR, Shen A, et al: Comparative safety of antiepileptic drugs during pregnancy. Neurology 78(21):1692–1699, 2012 22551726
Hernández-Díaz S, Mittendorf R, Smith CR, et al: Association between topiramate and zonisamide use during pregnancy and low birth weight. Obstet Gynecol 123(1):21–28, 2014 24463659
Hoek HW: Incidence, prevalence and mortality of anorexia nervosa and other eating disorders. Curr Opin Psychiatry 19(4):389–394, 2006 16721169
Hoopes SP, Reimherr FW, Hedges DW, et al: Treatment of bulimia nervosa with topiramate in a randomized, double-blind, placebo-controlled trial, part 1: improvement in binge and purge measures. J Clin Psychiatry 64(11):1335–1341, 2003 14658948
Horne RL, Ferguson JM, Pope HG Jr, et al: Treatment of bulimia with bupropion: a multicenter controlled trial. J Clin Psychiatry 49(7):262–266, 1988 3134343
Hunt S, Russell A, Smithson WH, et al: Topiramate in pregnancy: preliminary experience from the UK Epilepsy and Pregnancy Register. Neurology 71(4):272–276, 2008 18645165
Javaras KN, Pope HG, Lalonde JK, et al: Co-occurrence of binge eating disorder with psychiatric and medical disorders. J Clin Psychiatry 69(2):266–273, 2008 18348600
Jones BA, Haycraft E, Murjan S, Arcelus J: Body dissatisfaction and disordered eating in trans people: a systematic review of the literature. Int Rev Psychiatry 28(1):81–94, 2016 26618239
Jones KL, Johnson KA, Dick LM, et al: Pregnancy outcomes after first trimester exposure to phentermine/fenfluramine. Teratology 65(3):125–130, 2002 11877776
Källén BAJ: Antiobesity drugs in early pregnancy and congenital malformations in the offspring. Obes Res Clin Pract 8(6):e571–e576, 2014 25434912
Kaye WH, Bulik CM, Thornton L, et al: Comorbidity of anxiety disorders with anorexia and bulimia nervosa. Am J Psychiatry 161(12):2215–2221, 2004 15569892
Khoosal D, Langham C, Palmer B, et al: Features of eating disorder among male-to-female transsexuals. Sexual and Relationship Therapy 24(2):217–229, 2009
Kimmel MC, Ferguson EH, Zerwas S, et al: Obstetric and gynecologic problems associated with eating disorders. Int J Eat Disord 49(3):260–275, 2016 26711005
Kondo T, Kaneko S, Amano Y, et al: Preliminary report on teratogenic effects of zonisamide in the offspring of treated women with epilepsy. Epilepsia 37(12):1242–1244, 1996 8956859
Koubaa S, Hällström T, Lindholm C, et al: Pregnancy and neonatal outcomes in women with eating disorders. Obstet Gynecol 105(2):255–260, 2005 15684148
Kumpulainen J, Vuori E, Mäkinen S, et al: Dietary chromium intake of lactating Finnish mothers: effect on the Cr content of their breast milk. Br J Nutr 44(3):257–263, 1980 7437410
Levine LR, Pope HG, Enas GG, et al: Fluoxetine in the treatment of bulimia nervosa: a multicenter, placebo-controlled, double-blind trial. Arch Gen Psychiatry 49(2):139–147, 1992 1550466
Lingam R, McCluskey S: Eating disorders associated with hyperemesis gravidarum. J Psychosom Res 40(3):231–234, 1996 8861118
Linna MS, Raevuori A, Haukka J, et al: Reproductive health outcomes in eating disorders. Int J Eat Disord 46(8):826–833, 2013 23996114
Linna MS, Raevuori A, Haukka J, et al: Pregnancy, obstetric, and perinatal health outcomes in eating disorders. Am J Obstet Gynecol 211(4):392.e1–392.e8, 2014 24705128

Mangweth-Matzek B, Hoek HW: Epidemiology and treatment of eating disorders in men and women of middle and older age. Curr Opin Psychiatry 30(6):446–451, 2017 28825955

Mangweth-Matzek B, Hoek HW, Pope HG Jr: Pathological eating and body dissatisfaction in middle-aged and older women. Curr Opin Psychiatry 27(6):431–435, 2014 25247455

Martínez-González MA, Gual P, Lahortiga F, et al: Parental factors, mass media influences, and the onset of eating disorders in a prospective population-based cohort. Pediatrics 111(2):315–320, 2003 12563057

Mazzeo SE, Slof-Op't Landt MC, Jones I, et al: Associations among postpartum depression, eating disorders, and perfectionism in a population-based sample of adult women. Int J Eat Disord 39(3):202–211, 2006 16498586

Mazzeo SE, Mitchell KS, Bulik CM, et al: Assessing the heritability of anorexia nervosa symptoms using a marginal maximal likelihood approach. Psychol Med 39(3):463–473, 2009 18485259

Mazzeo SE, Mitchell KS, Bulik CM, et al: A twin study of specific bulimia nervosa symptoms. Psychol Med 40(7):1203–1213, 2010 19818201

McClain Z, Peebles R: Body image and eating disorders among lesbian, gay, bisexual, and transgender youth. Pediatr Clin North Am 63(6):1079–1090, 2016 27865334

McCluskey SE, Lacey JH, Pearce JM: Binge-eating and polycystic ovaries. Lancet 340(8821):723, 1992 1355813

McElroy SL, Shapira NA, Arnold LM, et al: Topiramate in the long-term treatment of binge-eating disorder associated with obesity. J Clin Psychiatry 65(11):1463–1469, 2004 15554757

McElroy SL, Hudson JI, Mitchell JE, et al: Efficacy and safety of lisdexamfetamine for treatment of adults with moderate to severe binge-eating disorder: a randomized clinical trial. JAMA Psychiatry 72(3):235–246, 2015 25587645

Mehanna H, Nankivell PC, Moledina J, et al: Refeeding syndrome: awareness, prevention and management. Head Neck Oncol 1:4, 2009 19284691

Micali N, Treasure J, Simonoff E: Eating disorders symptoms in pregnancy: a longitudinal study of women with recent and past eating disorders and obesity. J Psychosom Res 63(3):297–303, 2007 17719368

Micali N, dos-Santos-Silva I, De Stavola B, et al: Fertility treatment, twin births, and unplanned pregnancies in women with eating disorders: findings from a population-based birth cohort. BJOG 121(4):408–416, 2014 24206173

Mitchell KS, Neale MC, Bulik CM, et al: Binge eating disorder: a symptom-level investigation of genetic and environmental influences on liability. Psychol Med 40(11):1899–1906, 2010 20132584

Morgan JF, Reid F, Lacey JH: The SCOFF questionnaire: assessment of a new screening tool for eating disorders. BMJ 319(7223):1467–1468, 1999 10582927

Mulders-Jones B, Mitchison D, Girosi F, et al: Socioeconomic correlates of eating disorder symptoms in an Australian population-based sample. PLoS One 12(1):e0170603, 2017 28141807

Ohman I, Vitols S, Luef G, et al: Topiramate kinetics during delivery, lactation, and in the neonate: preliminary observations. Epilepsia 43(10):1157–1160, 2002 12366729

Ornstein RM, Golden NH, Jacobson MS, et al: Hypophosphatemia during nutritional rehabilitation in anorexia nervosa: implications for refeeding and monitoring. J Adolesc Health 32(1):83–88, 2003 12507806

Park RJ, Senior R, Stein A: The offspring of mothers with eating disorders. Eur Child Adolesc Psychiatry 12(suppl 1):I110–I119, 2003 12567222

Perrio MJ, Wilton LV, Shakir SA: The safety profiles of orlistat and sibutramine: results of prescription-event monitoring studies in England. Obesity (Silver Spring) 15(11):2712–2722, 2007 18070762

Phillipou A, Rossell SL, Castle DJ: The neurobiology of anorexia nervosa: a systematic review. Aust N Z J Psychiatry 48(2):128–152, 2014 24194589

Poyastro Pinheiro A, Thornton LM, Plotonicov KH, et al: Patterns of menstrual disturbance in eating disorders. Int J Eat Disord 40(5):424–434, 2007 17497704

Rihtman T, Parush S, Ornoy A: Preliminary findings of the developmental effects of in utero exposure to topiramate. Reprod Toxicol 34(3):308–311, 2012 22659273

Ricca V, Castellini G, Lo Sauro C, et al: Zonisamide combined with cognitive behavioral therapy in binge eating disorder: a one-year follow-up study. Psychiatry (Edgmont) 6(11):23–28, 2009 20049147
Robert E, Francannet C, Shaw G: Neural tube defects and maternal weight reduction in early pregnancy. Reprod Toxicol 9(1):57–59, 1995 8520132
Sadock BJ, Sadock VA: Eating disorders, in Kaplan and Sadock's Synopsis of Psychiatry: Behavioral Sciences/Clinical Psychiatry, 10th Edition. Philadelphia, PA, Lippincott Williams & Wilkins, 2007, pp 727–748
Sanci L, Coffey C, Olsson C, et al: Childhood sexual abuse and eating disorders in females: findings from the Victorian Adolescent Health Cohort Study. Arch Pediatr Adolesc Med 162(3):261–267, 2008 18316664
Sands RX: Obesity and pregnancy: weight control with a resinate. Am J Obstet Gynecol 83:1617–1621, 1962 14496899
Santos AMD, Benute GRG, Santos NOD, et al: Presence of eating disorders and its relationship to anxiety and depression in pregnant women. Midwifery 51:12–15, 2017 28500866
Shimoyama R, Ohkubo T, Sugawara K: Monitoring of zonisamide in human breast milk and maternal plasma by solid-phase extraction HPLC method. Biomed Chromatogr 13(5):370–372, 1999 10425030
Sonneville KR, Lipson SK: Disparities in eating disorder diagnosis and treatment according to weight status, race/ethnicity, socioeconomic background, and sex among college students. Int J Eat Disord 51(6):518–526, 2018 29500865
Steinhausen HC, Grigoroiu-Serbanescu M, Boyadjieva S, et al: The relevance of body weight in the medium-term to long-term course of adolescent anorexia nervosa: findings from a multisite study. Int J Eat Disord 42(1):19–25, 2009 18683885
Stice E: Interactive and mediational etiologic models of eating disorder onset: evidence from prospective studies. Annu Rev Clin Psychol 12:359–381, 2016 26651521
Thoma-Laurie DL, Walker ER, Reasor MJ: Chlorphentermine-induced neonatal and maternal pulmonary phospholipidosis in rats. Exp Mol Pathol 38(3):310–321, 1983 6852205
Tierney S, Fox JR, Butterfield C, et al: Treading the tightrope between motherhood and an eating disorder: a qualitative study. Int J Nurs Stud 48(10):1223–1233, 2011 21176902
Treasure J, Claudino AM, Zucker N: Eating disorders. Lancet 375(9714):583–593, 2010 19931176
Trunko ME, Schwartz TA, Duvvuri V, et al: Aripiprazole in anorexia nervosa and low-weight bulimia nervosa: case reports. Int J Eat Disord 44(3):269–275, 2011 20186719
Ulfvebrand S, Birgegård A, Norring C, et al: Psychiatric comorbidity in women and men with eating disorders: results from a large clinical database. Psychiatry Res 230(2):294–299, 2015 26416590
Vajda FJE, O'Brien TJ, Graham J, et al: Is carbamazepine a human teratogen? J Clin Neurosci 23:34–37, 2016 26521756
Veiby G, Daltveit AK, Engelsen BA, et al: Fetal growth restriction and birth defects with newer and older antiepileptic drugs during pregnancy. J Neurol 261(3):579–588, 2014 24449062
Ward ZJ, Rodriguez P, Wright DR, et al: Estimation of eating disorders prevalence by age and associations with mortality in a simulated nationally representative US cohort. JAMA Netw Open 2(10):e1912925, 2019 31596495
Westmoreland P, Krantz MJ, Mehler PS: Medical complications of anorexia nervosa and bulimia. Am J Med 129(1):30–37, 2016 26169883
Wu M, Brockmeyer T, Hartmann M, et al: Set-shifting ability across the spectrum of eating disorders and in overweight and obesity: a systematic review and meta-analysis. Psychol Med 44(16):3365–3385, 2014 25066267
Xia W, Hu J, Zhang B, et al: A case-control study of maternal exposure to chromium and infant low birth weight in China. Chemosphere 144:1484–1489, 2016 26498095
Zerwas SC, Von Holle A, Perrin EM, et al: Gestational and postpartum weight change patterns in mothers with eating disorders. Eur Eat Disord Rev 22(6):397–404, 2014 25201473

CHAPTER 23

# Attention-Deficit/ Hyperactivity Disorder

Lucy A. Hutner, M.D.
Jaina Amin, M.D.
Jeanne Coulehan, C.N.M., M.P.H.
Madhumathi Rao, M.D.
Melisa Olgun, B.A.
Mimi Levine, M.D.

ADHD is an early onset, highly prevalent neurobehavioral disorder characterized by significant deficits in two major domains: inattention and hyperactivity/impulsivity (American Psychiatric Association 2013; Kooij et al. 2010; Spencer et al. 2007). ADHD is typically diagnosed in childhood, but it often persists into adulthood, leading to functional impairment in school, work, and social settings throughout the person's life (Agnew-Blais et al. 2016; Asherson 2010; Barbaresi et al. 2013; Faraone et al. 2015). ADHD in adults was recognized relatively recently (McCarthy et al. 2009), thus a comprehensive understanding is still evolving (Kooij et al. 2010); in turn, there are many more questions than answers regarding ADHD in women and in the perinatal period.

Despite the lack of comprehensive information, ADHD is an important condition to address in the setting of reproductive mental health. An increasing number of women of reproductive age are diagnosed with ADHD (Leong et al. 2017; Louik et al. 2015), and they are at substantially increased risk of comorbidities such as depression, anxiety, self-injury, and substance use disorders (Owens et al. 2017). They are likely to face significant difficulties with work, school, interpersonal relationships, and everyday functioning (Corbisiero et al. 2017; Eddy et al. 2019). Although this hypothesis has yet to be examined rigorously, pregnancy and new motherhood may represent a time of additional significant psychosocial stress related to the large number of tasks associated with the transition to motherhood (Freeman 2014). An increasing number of women of reproductive age are taking prescribed stimulant medications for the treatment of ADHD (Haervig et al. 2014; Louik et al. 2015; Renoux et al. 2016). Yet our understanding of the reproductive safety profile of medications prescribed for ADHD is limited and has been complicated by significant confounding variables, such as the effects of ADHD itself and of stimulant misuse (Bro et al. 2015; Diav-Citrin et al. 2016; Haervig et al. 2014; Källén et al. 2013; Newport et al. 2016; Wright et al. 2015).

This chapter summarizes the epidemiology, diagnostic criteria, clinical features, differential diagnosis and assessment, course/prognosis, and treatment of ADHD, with a focus on its relationship to reproductive mental health. Of note, although ADHD is considered a lifespan disorder beginning in childhood, this chapter primarily focuses on ADHD in adults, specifically in women and in the perinatal period.

Ms. JJ is a 32-year-old woman who presents to a reproductive psychiatrist inquiring about whether she can take her stimulants during pregnancy. She has been taking stimulant medication on and off since she was 12, when teachers noticed she was unable to sit still and was "daydreaming all the time" and recommended neuropsychological testing, which was consistent with an ADHD diagnosis. She also had testing and deadline accommodations all throughout high school and college. Ms. JJ has used several different stimulants, and she states that dexamphetamine and methylphenidate have both been effective. She is now stable on a dose of Vyvanse, 40 mg/day orally, which is effective. She is very worried about her job as an attorney during a future pregnancy and about completing her work effectively if she stops her stimulants. She is also worried about pregnancy-related fatigue and "brain fog" and how to manage that along with her demanding work. Ms. JJ is "worried because no matter what I do, it's all a risk, and I feel like I have to choose between a healthy pregnancy and being able to work at all." She reports that she put herself through college and law school and is the primary breadwinner between herself and her partner. She also financially supports her widowed mother, who is disabled with a chronic medical condition.

# Epidemiology

## Rates/Incidence

ADHD is common neurodevelopmental disorder with a high prevalence throughout the lifespan (Cho et al. 2017; Kessler et al. 2006; Kooij et al. 2010). The prevalence in children and adolescents is approximately 3%–7% (Thomas et al. 2015), and in adults it ranges from 2% to 5% (Fayyad et al. 2007; Kessler et al. 2005; Kooij et al. 2005; Simon et al. 2009). Adult ADHD is underdiagnosed and undertreated due to its relatively recent recognition as a disorder (McCarthy et al. 2009), the presence of mental health comorbidities that may "mask" it (Kooij et al. 2010), shifting symptomatology from childhood to adulthood (Biederman et al. 2000), and stigma about the condition itself, particularly around the use of stimulant medication (Buitelaar 2001; Biederman et al. 1993). ADHD is commonly seen in women, with an estimated prevalence of 3.2% (Kessler et al. 2006). In childhood, the male to female sex ratio is approximately 3:1, but in adults it is closer to 1:1 (Cortese et al. 2016; Rösler et al. 2006). It is unclear what drives the change in ratio over time; it has been hypothesized that at least one factor may be detection failure, leading to an underdiagnosis of female ADHD in childhood (Davies 2014; Young et al. 2020).

**TABLE 23–1. Risk factors for progression from childhood to adult ADHD**

| | |
|---|---|
| Combined subtype of ADHD in childhood | Increased symptom severity of ADHD in childhood |
| Comorbid depression or other mental health conditions | Parental psychopathology |
| Family history of ADHD | Social adversity |

The impact of ADHD on affected individuals and their loved ones is enormous. The direct health care expenditures for the treatment of ADHD, as well as the indirect economic deficits (e.g., loss of working hours), are also substantial. A recent study estimated that the total excess cost of ADHD in the United States in 2000 was $31.6 billion, including treatment of ADHD, other health care costs for patients and their family members, and loss of work time (Birnbaum et al. 2005). A recent study examining a claims database of more than 3,000 adult patients with ADHD noted that they were significantly more likely than the comparison cohort without ADHD to have psychiatric and medical comorbidities, higher outpatient and inpatient costs, and higher prescription drug and total medical costs (Secnik et al. 2005).

## Risk Factors

Risk factors for perinatal ADHD have not yet been clearly delineated. Childhood predictors of adult ADHD include family history of ADHD, the combined subtype of ADHD in childhood, increased symptom severity, comorbid depression or other mental health conditions, social adversity, and parental psychopathology (Table 23–1) (Biederman et al. 1996; Lara et al. 2009). The prevalence does not appear to differ by race or ethnicity or in response to treatment, but Black and Hispanic children are diagnosed with ADHD at much lower rates than white children (Alvarado and Modesto-Lowe 2017). Although less is known about these differences in adult ADHD, it is clear that rates of detection are substantially lower among racial and ethnic minority groups (Chung et al. 2019).

## Screening

Screening for adult or perinatal ADHD is not in widespread practice, although there have been calls for increasing recognition and detection of ADHD given its significant impact on functioning and on physical and mental health across the lifespan (Ebert et al. 2003; National Institute for Health and Care Excellence 2008; Nutt et al. 2007). Several validated rating scales are in clinical use for the assessment of ADHD (Rösler et al. 2006); rating scales specific to the perinatal population have yet to be established. Rating scales applicable for adults include the Wender-Utah Rating Scale (Ward et al. 1993) and the Childhood Symptoms Scale (Barkley and Murphy 1998), which retrospectively address childhood symptoms consistent with ADHD; self-report scales that mainly focus on the DSM criteria, such as the Connors Adult ADHD Rating Scale (Conners et al. 1999) and the Adult Self Report Scale (Adler et al. 2003); and observer scales that can be used by clinicians or family members, such as the Brown Attention-Deficit Disorder Rating Scale (Brown 1996). Both the self-report and the observer scales use Likert scales to quantify the severity symptoms, ranging from 0 to 3, making these scales useful for

**TABLE 23–2. Selected rating scales used in the diagnosis of ADHD in adults**

| | |
|---|---|
| Adult ADHD Rating Scale–IV | Connors Adult ADHD Rating Scales |
| Adult ADHD Self-Report Scale Symptom Checklist v1.1 | Current Symptoms Scale |
| Brown Attention-Deficit Disorder Rating Scale and Diagnostic Form | Wender-Reimherr Adult Attention Deficit Disorder Scale |
| Childhood Symptom Scale (retrospective) | Wender Utah Rating Scale (retrospective) |

following the course of ADHD quantitatively (Rösler et al. 2006). Commonly used rating scales in clinical practice are summarized in Table 23–2.

Comprehensive diagnostic interviews have also been developed for adult ADHD, both to evaluate diagnostic criteria and to assess various psychopathological syndrome scores, functional impairment, indices of pervasiveness, quality of life, and comorbidities (Rösler et al. 2006), such as the Brown Attention-Deficit Disorder Diagnostic Form (Brown 1996). The Wender-Reimherr Adult Attention Deficit Disorder Scale (Wender 1995) is a clinician-rated scale designed to detect ADHD in adults (Marchant et al. 2013). Several scales have been specifically designed to assess gender-specific symptoms in ADHD, including the ADHD Self-Rating Scale for Women (Nadeau and Quinn 2005). However, few empirical data exist that would allow for understanding of their utility in clinical practice, and no rating scales are specific to the perinatal period.

# Diagnostic Criteria

The DSM-5 (American Psychiatric Association 2013) diagnostic criteria for ADHD apply to both childhood and adult ADHD, with no specifier for the perinatal period. Three primary subtypes have been identified: predominantly inattentive, hyperactive-impulsive, and combined presentations (Young et al. 2020). Please see Box 23–1 for the DSM-5 diagnostic criteria for ADHD.

### Box 23–1. DSM-5 Criteria for Attention-Deficit/Hyperactivity Disorder

A. A persistent pattern of inattention and/or hyperactivity-impulsivity that interferes with functioning or development, as characterized by (1) and/or (2):

1. **Inattention:** Six (or more) of the following symptoms have persisted for at least 6 months to a degree that is inconsistent with developmental level and that negatively impacts directly on social and academic/occupational activities:

   **Note:** The symptoms are not solely a manifestation of oppositional behavior, defiance, hostility, or failure to understand tasks or instructions. For older adolescents and adults (age 17 and older), at least five symptoms are required.

   a. Often fails to give close attention to details or makes careless mistakes in schoolwork, at work, or during other activities (e.g., overlooks or misses details, work is inaccurate).

   b. Often has difficulty sustaining attention in tasks or play activities (e.g., has difficulty remaining focused during lectures, conversations, or lengthy reading).

   c. Often does not seem to listen when spoken to directly (e.g., mind seems elsewhere, even in the absence of any obvious distraction).

d. Often does not follow through on instructions and fails to finish schoolwork, chores, or duties in the workplace (e.g., starts tasks but quickly loses focus and is easily sidetracked).
e. Often has difficulty organizing tasks and activities (e.g., difficulty managing sequential tasks; difficulty keeping materials and belongings in order; messy, disorganized work; has poor time management; fails to meet deadlines).
f. Often avoids, dislikes, or is reluctant to engage in tasks that require sustained mental effort (e.g., schoolwork or homework; for older adolescents and adults, preparing reports, completing forms, reviewing lengthy papers).
g. Often loses things necessary for tasks or activities (e.g., school materials, pencils, books, tools, wallets, keys, paperwork, eyeglasses, mobile telephones).
h. Is often easily distracted by extraneous stimuli (for older adolescents and adults, may include unrelated thoughts).
i. Is often forgetful in daily activities (e.g., doing chores, running errands; for older adolescents and adults, returning calls, paying bills, keeping appointments).

2. **Hyperactivity and impulsivity:** Six (or more) of the following symptoms have persisted for at least 6 months to a degree that is inconsistent with developmental level and that negatively impacts directly on social and academic/occupational activities:
**Note:** The symptoms are not solely a manifestation of oppositional behavior, defiance, hostility, or a failure to understand tasks or instructions. For older adolescents and adults (age 17 and older), at least five symptoms are required.
a. Often fidgets with or taps hands or feet or squirms in seat.
b. Often leaves seat in situations when remaining seated is expected (e.g., leaves his or her place in the classroom, in the office or other workplace, or in other situations that require remaining in place).
c. Often runs about or climbs in situations where it is inappropriate. (**Note:** In adolescents or adults, may be limited to feeling restless.)
d. Often unable to play or engage in leisure activities quietly.
e. Is often "on the go," acting as if "driven by a motor" (e.g., is unable to be or uncomfortable being still for extended time, as in restaurants, meetings; may be experienced by others as being restless or difficult to keep up with).
f. Often talks excessively.
g. Often blurts out an answer before a question has been completed (e.g., completes people's sentences; cannot wait for turn in conversation).
h. Often has difficulty waiting his or her turn (e.g., while waiting in line).
i. Often interrupts or intrudes on others (e.g., butts into conversations, games, or activities; may start using other people's things without asking or receiving permission; for adolescents and adults, may intrude into or take over what others are doing).

B. Several inattentive or hyperactive-impulsive symptoms were present prior to age 12 years.
C. Several inattentive or hyperactive-impulsive symptoms are present in two or more settings (e.g., at home, school, or work; with friends or relatives; in other activities).
D. There is clear evidence that the symptoms interfere with, or reduce the quality of, social, academic, or occupational functioning.
E. The symptoms do not occur exclusively during the course of schizophrenia or another psychotic disorder and are not better explained by another mental disorder (e.g., mood disorder, anxiety disorder, dissociative disorder, personality disorder, substance intoxication or withdrawal).

*Specify* whether:

**314.01 (F90.2) Combined presentation:** If both Criterion A1 (inattention) and Criterion A2 (hyperactivity-impulsivity) are met for the past 6 months.

**314.00 (F90.0) Predominantly inattentive presentation:** If Criterion A1 (inattention) is met but Criterion A2 (hyperactivity-impulsivity) is not met for the past 6 months.

**314.01 (F90.1) Predominantly hyperactive/impulsive presentation:** If Criterion A2 (hyperactivity-impulsivity) is met and Criterion A1 (inattention) is not met for the past 6 months.

*Specify* if:

**In partial remission:** When full criteria were previously met, fewer than the full criteria have been met for the past 6 months, and the symptoms still result in impairment in social, academic, or occupational functioning.

*Specify* current severity:

**Mild:** Few, if any, symptoms in excess of those required to make the diagnosis are present, and symptoms result in no more than minor impairments in social or occupational functioning.

**Moderate:** Symptoms or functional impairment between "mild" and "severe" are present.

**Severe:** Many symptoms in excess of those required to make the diagnosis, or several symptoms that are particularly severe, are present, or the symptoms result in marked impairment in social or occupational functioning.

*Source.* Reprinted from American Psychiatric Association: *Diagnostic and Statistical Manual of Mental Disorders,* 5th Edition. Arlington, VA, 2013, pp. 59–61. 

Numerous changes to the diagnostic criteria of ADHD were made with the publication of DSM-5, including an increase in age of onset from 7 to 12 years, allowance of the concurrent diagnosis of ADHD and autism spectrum disorder, and reduction of the cut point from six symptoms to five symptoms in adults (Matthews et al. 2014). Even with these changes, the diagnosis of ADHD as it applies to adults has been a matter of evolution—and some controversy—over time because uncertainties remain about how well diagnostic criteria meet the complexity of the adult clinical phenotype (Matte et al. 2012). A recent large cohort study of more than 3,500 adults aimed to describe the phenotype of adult ADHD and assess the psychometric validity of the DSM-5 diagnosis (Vitola et al. 2017). In this study, the adult ADHD prevalence with the use of DSM-5 criteria was significantly higher when compared with that obtained using DSM-IV criteria (American Psychiatric Association 1994) and increased almost threefold when the age-of-onset criterion was removed (Vitola et al. 2017). In addition, latent class analysis noted that adult ADHD comprises mainly inattentive and not hyperactive/impulsive symptoms, that inattention was the symptom cluster most highly correlated with functional impairment, and that even the best cutoff for diagnosis (four or more symptoms) yielded low sensitivity and specificity (Vitola et al. 2017). This suggests that both construct and discriminant validity challenges remain for the ADHD diagnostic criteria as applied to adults, despite recent modifications in DSM-5 (Vitola et al. 2017).

Other models have been proposed for the diagnostic criteria for ADHD that focus on specific features of the disorder in adults. For example, the Utah criteria developed by Wender consist of the requirement of a long-standing and consistent history of symptoms (dating back to at least age 7) and adult symptoms consisting of hyperactivity and poor concentration, with at least two of the following five associated symptoms: affective lability, "hot" temper, inability to complete tasks and disorganization, stress intolerance, and impulsivity (Wender 1995). These diagnostic criteria take into account the affective lability—most often, the brief, intense affective outbursts—commonly seen in adult ADHD; this affective liability in turn serves to increase cognitive disorganization and distractibility (Wender 1995). Other suggested diagnostic models include affective lability and other aspects of adult ADHD, including specific cognitive functions and its functional impact on adult life. For example, the Brown criteria consist of five core dimensions, including activation and organization, sustained attention, sustained energy and effort, managing affective interference, and working memory and recall (Brown 1996); the Copeland criteria consist of eight dimensions, including inattention and distractibility, impulsivity, activity level problems, noncompliance, underachievement, disorganization and learning difficulties, emotional difficulties, and poor peer relations and impaired family relationships (Copeland 1991).

# Clinical Features

## Clinical Presentation

The classic clinical presentation of ADHD includes two major symptom domains: inattention and hyperactivity/impulsivity. Examples of inattention symptoms include failing to pay close attention to details, making careless mistakes in tasks, appearing not to listen or hold attention, failing to finish tasks, not following through, and having difficulty with organization. The domain of hyperactivity/impulsivity includes symptoms such as fidgeting, squirming in seat, being "on the go," talking excessively, blurting out an answer, having trouble waiting their turn, and interrupting others (American Psychiatric Association 2013).

Despite having the same DSM diagnostic criteria, adult ADHD symptoms can present differently than in childhood. The more overtly impairing symptoms (hyperactivity and impulsivity) that may be particularly prominent in childhood seem to become less obvious over time (Kooij et al. 2010). More subtle—yet still impairing—symptoms such as inattention, disorganization, and inner restlessness tend to predominate in adulthood, as well as significant problems with executive functioning (Adler et al. 2017; Biederman et al. 2000; Fischer et al. 2005; Hart et al. 1995; Kooij et al. 2001; Wender et al. 2001). This cluster of symptoms leaves a footprint in the pragmatic aspects of adult life; adult patients often struggle with time management and procrastination, a feeling of internal restlessness, feeling overwhelmed or distracted, and starting but not finishing tasks (Fredriksen et al. 2014; Halmøy et al. 2009; Minde et al. 2003; Young et al. 2020). Anxiety, insomnia, and demoralization follow (Agarwal et al. 2012; Piñeiro-Dieguez et al. 2016; Seo et al. 2014), and the impulsivity inherent to ADHD often leads to comorbid substance misuse (Capusan et al. 2016; Piñeiro-Dieguez et al. 2016) or binge eating (Brunault et al. 2019).

Other domains also appear to play an important role in adult ADHD, including difficulties with cognitive impairment and emotional regulation. Most adults with ADHD have measurable cognitive dysfunction (Holst and Thorell 2017), although the degree of impairment can be highly variable; patients with significant executive dysfunction, working memory difficulties, or impulsivity tend to have the highest degree of functional impairment in their daily lives (Mostert et al. 2015; Skodzik et al. 2017; Theiling and Petermann 2016). Cognitive impairment in ADHD is underappreciated yet important (Holst and Thorell 2017; Mostert et al. 2015; Skodzik et al. 2017; Theiling and

Petermann 2016) because it can have an enormous impact on educational attainment, work mastery, and interpersonal functioning (Geffen and Forster 2018).

Emotional dysregulation is also highly common in ADHD (Gallo and Posner 2016); a recent review estimated the prevalence in adults is 30%–70% (Shaw et al. 2014). Emotional dysregulation may take the form of aggressive behavior, emotional lability, poor frustration tolerance, and excessive excitability, and this component appears to have significant long-term consequences throughout the lifespan (Shaw et al. 2014). Alterations in motivation and processing of reinforcement, which might underlie some of the emotional dysregulation symptoms, have also been reported in ADHD (Shaw et al. 2014).

Gender-based differences are also apparent in ADHD symptomatology. Although girls and women can present with both inattention and hyperactive-impulsive symptoms, the severity may be lower overall, particularly for the hyperactive-impulsive domain (Young et al. 2020). Inattention may present as being easily distracted, forgetful, disorganized, overwhelmed, or lacking motivation (Quinn 2005; Young et al. 2020); hypertalkativeness and emotional reactivity are seen more often than excessive motor activity (Quinn 2005). Girls are more likely to present with internalizing symptoms and to become anxious, depressed, and socially withdrawn (Quinn 2005). The emotional lability and dysregulation commonly seen in ADHD, such as irritability, low frustration tolerance, and mood alterations, may occur more commonly and severely in women (Cortese 2012; Hollingdale et al. 2014; Shaw et al. 2014). Whether there are differences in clinical presentation in women in the perinatal period is unknown. For girls and women, however, ADHD is often a hidden disorder that is ignored or misdiagnosed, which causes them to suffer in silence. Without proper treatment, many females who have ADHD experience psychological and academic impairments. In addition, most report low self-esteem, impaired social relationships, and a general demoralization.

Delineating the symptoms of ADHD from the (putative) physiological cognitive changes of pregnancy can be difficult, and the two may overlap. Early observations suggested that certain cognitive functions, such as memory, were negatively impacted by pregnancy and that pregnant women were more likely than nonpregnant women to subjectively report memory changes (Poser et al. 1986; Sharp et al. 1993). The informal (and unfortunate) term *pregnancy brain* likely refers to this widely cited phenomenon of hormonal changes impacting cognition; however, objective studies of this hypothesis have had mixed results (Freeman 2014). For example, one small study showed that pregnant women performed better on verbal cognitive tasks after delivery than before, and no associations were noted between sex hormone levels and cognitive performance (Buckwalter et al. 1999). However, a subsequent study demonstrated that verbal memory declined and processing speed slowed in third-trimester pregnant women compared with nonpregnant women; similar results were seen in the postpartum period (Henry and Sherwin 2012). In this study, cognitive changes were associated with hormonal changes; for example, estrogen and cortisol levels were negatively associated with attention scores postpartum (Henry and Sherwin 2012).

A recent meta-analysis attempted to shed light on this issue; although the results were inconsistent, there were two major findings: 1) pregnant women were found to be impaired on some but not all selective measures of memory—specifically, memory functions that place relatively high demands on executive cognitive control, and

2) similar changes were noted both in pregnancy and the postpartum period (Henry and Rendell 2007). However, inconsistencies persist throughout the data. For example, animal studies have shown that higher progesterone and estrogen levels (as seen in pregnancy) improve memory—pregnant rats outperform nonpregnant rats on tests of memory and cognition (Paris and Frye 2008). Other animal studies have noted structural brain changes in pregnancy even in the absence of functional memory impairment (Galea et al. 2000). Overall, given the inconsistencies in the data, one tentative conclusion may be that cognitive impairments, if they occur in pregnancy or postpartum, are subtle and may not be experienced universally; given the impairment in memory and executive function in ADHD, it is possible that women with preexisting ADHD are a vulnerable subgroup for cognitive worsening in pregnancy (Freeman 2014).

## Course/Prognosis

It is now understood that ADHD persists throughout the lifespan (Young et al. 2020). Evidence indicates that ADHD persists into adulthood in approximately two-thirds of cases (Barkley et al. 2002; Gittelman et al. 1985; Lara et al. 2009; Lie 1992; Mannuzza et al. 1991, 1993; Weiss et al. 1985); more recent estimates have been even higher, estimating the persistence of symptoms to be approximately 80% (Cheung et al. 2016; van Lieshout et al. 2016). A recent meta-analysis demonstrated that, of the cases that persist, most patients have residual symptomatology with functional impairment, whereas a minority continue to exhibit the full-blown disorder (Faraone et al. 2006). Symptoms tend to decline over time from childhood to adulthood (Faraone et al. 2006; Willcutt 2012), particularly those in the hyperactive/impulsive domain; data regarding the trajectory of the inattentive symptoms are more mixed (Larsson et al. 2011). This trajectory appears similar in both sexes (Hinshaw et al. 2006; Lapalme et al. 2018; Monuteaux et al. 2010).

Some have speculated about the existence of an adult-onset variant of ADHD (Alexander and Farrelly 2018; Faraone and Biederman 2016; Moffitt et al. 2015). Evidence supporting this is offered by studies that have examined the continuity of ADHD in birth cohorts and found little overlap between those who met DSM-5 criteria in adulthood and those who had met it in childhood (Castellanos 2015). If adult-onset ADHD is a disorder with biology distinct from that of childhood-onset ADHD, perhaps a distinct biology also exists in the perinatal period, making this an intriguing area for future research.

Adult ADHD has profound negative consequences in everyday life. Studies of patients with untreated ADHD have found numerous long-term adverse consequences, including poor physical health, impaired quality of life (Agarwal et al. 2012; Seo et al. 2014), impaired relationships and higher rates of divorce (Minde et al. 2003), difficulties with education and employment (Fredriksen et al. 2014; Halmøy et al. 2009), financial distress (Brook et al. 2013), impaired driving safety (Biederman et al. 2012; Fuermaier et al. 2017), premature death from accidents (Dalsgaard et al. 2015), and higher rates of imprisonment (Wilens et al. 2004). Evidence suggested an increased mortality in women with ADHD relative to men, which persists after controlling for comorbidities, such as substance use disorders, and is driven by accidents. It is hypothesized that underdiagnosis and thus undertreatment in women leads to a greater risk of accidental death (Dalsgaard et al. 2015).

ADHD is highly comorbid with other mental health conditions. ADHD alone is uncommon in the adult population, and it may co-occur with other disorders as much as 75% of the time (Faraone and Biederman 1998; Rösler et al. 2006). Common comorbidities with adult ADHD include autism spectrum disorder, depressive disorders, bipolar disorder, anxiety disorders, OCD, eating disorders (i.e., anorexia nervosa, bulimia nervosa, binge eating disorder), PTSD, learning disorders, personality disorders, and impulse-control disorders (Capusan et al. 2016; Huntley and Young 2014; Kessler et al. 2006; Nazar et al. 2016; Pliszka 1998; Sobanski 2006).

Of particular importance is the relationship between ADHD and substance use disorders. In adulthood, patients with ADHD are more likely to use tobacco (Brassett-Grundy and Butler 2004), to engage in higher rates of substance use (Huntley and Young 2014), and to develop alcohol and substance use disorders (Charach et al. 2011). Notably, evidence has shown at least equal—if not higher—risk of alcohol and cannabis use disorders in women with ADHD compared with men (Ottosen et al. 2016). In addition, the presence of comorbid ADHD may portend a less favorable prognosis; for example, comorbid ADHD and bipolar disorder is associated with earlier onset of symptoms and a more chronic and disabling course than bipolar disorder alone (Brus et al. 2014). A recent systematic review also showed an association between ADHD and suicidality in all age groups and in both sexes that was mediated by the presence of psychiatric comorbidities (Furczyk and Thome 2014).

There appear to be significant sex differences in the course and prognosis of ADHD throughout the lifespan (Young et al. 2020). Internalizing disorders, such as anxiety and depression, are more often reported in women than in men with ADHD (Cortese et al. 2016; Edvinsson et al. 2013; Gershon 2002), as are borderline personality disorder traits (Stepp et al. 2012) and self-harming behaviors (Hollingdale et al. 2014), likely prompted by impulsivity. The impulsivity inherent in ADHD can lead to an increase in risk-taking behavior and undesired consequences in women (Quinn and Madhoo 2014). For example, adolescent girls with undiagnosed ADHD may engage in at-risk behaviors such as early sexual activity, have an increased number of sexual partners, and experience a greater frequency of sexually transmitted infections (Barkley et al. 2006; Quinn 2005). Women with ADHD also have a higher risk of teenage, early, or unplanned pregnancies (Skoglund et al. 2019). They may be vulnerable to sexual harassment, exploitation, and abusive relationships; the Adult Psychiatric Morbidity survey in the United Kingdom found that 27% of women who experienced extensive physical or sexual abuse had ADHD traits (McManus et al. 2009). Along with the other mental health comorbidities, such as depression and PTSD, alcohol and other substance use disorders are highly comorbid with ADHD in women, often beginning at an early age (Wilens et al. 1995).

No systematic studies have yet been published on the course of ADHD through the perinatal period (Baker and Freeman 2018). Women with ADHD who are pregnant have a higher risk of continued tobacco use and of being obese or underweight (Skoglund et al. 2019). Women with undiagnosed ADHD are hypothesized to struggle more with parenting, balancing work with household management, and maintaining partnerships and interpersonal relationships (Nadeau and Quinn 2002; Young et al. 2020), although empirical data on this topic are scarce. It has also been hypothesized that, in the perinatal period, women may experience significant psychosocial stress related to the large number of tasks associated with the transition to motherhood; however, this has not yet been examined rigorously (Freeman 2014; Young et al. 2020).

Given concerns regarding the risks of stimulant use in pregnancy, many women elect to discontinue stimulant treatment during pregnancy and breastfeeding; however, little is known about the impact of treatment (or lack thereof) on occupational functioning, quality of interpersonal relationships, impact on comorbid mental health conditions, and quality of life in women with ADHD in the perinatal period (Freeman 2014). Untreated ADHD increases the risk of tobacco dependence (Kollins et al. 2005), yet there are clear recommendations regarding the importance of smoking cessation in pregnancy given the substantial evidence of adverse outcomes (Siu and U.S. Preventive Services Task Force 2015). Similarly, stimulant treatment for ADHD reduces the risk of maternal substance use disorders and tobacco dependence (Groenman et al. 2013), a factor that should be considered in the risk-risk discussion of stimulant exposure in pregnancy. Of course, because prenatal factors are thought to be environmental risk factors for ADHD in the offspring, a robust understanding of ADHD of women in the perinatal period would serve to address the mental health needs of their infants and children in an intergenerational manner.

# Differential Diagnosis and Assessment

## Assessment

ADHD is a clinical diagnosis. In adults, that diagnosis requires a detailed clinical interview and assessment, including retrospective assessment of childhood ADHD symptoms by patient recall or collateral information; evidence of ADHD prior to the age of 12 (e.g., by school records, childhood health assessments, or family observations); an enduring pattern of difficulties that impair social functioning and limit school or occupational attainment; and current adult ADHD symptomatology, including symptom severity and pervasiveness, functional impairment, quality of life issues, and psychiatric comorbidity (Geffen and Forster 2018; Rösler et al. 2006). The assessment of ADHD should include a review of screening questionnaires, a review of physical and mental health history, and a physical examination (Geffen and Forster 2018). Weight and cardiovascular fitness, particularly blood pressure, are particularly important data points because ADHD treatments may influence these parameters. A personal or family history of cardiac ischemia or cardiac arrhythmias should be elicited because this may preclude treatment with stimulants (Geffen and Forster 2018). Additional measures, such as blood tests, electroencephalogram, CT scan, or MRI scan, should be considered as indicated (Rösler et al. 2006).

## Differential Diagnosis

Table 23–3 summarizes the differential diagnosis of ADHD, including both medical and psychiatric disorders. Both mood and anxiety disorders can present with attentional difficulties and should be carefully evaluated. Major depressive disorder can be identified by the presence of signature depressive symptoms such as low mood, anhedonia, low energy and concentration, poor motivation, and potentially suicidal ideation (American Psychiatric Association 2013). Bipolar disorder is a particularly important diagnostic consideration given the morbidity (and potential mortality) that accompanies this disorder in the perinatal period. Please see Chapter 15, "Bipolar Disorder and

**TABLE 23–3. Differential diagnosis of ADHD**

| | |
|---|---|
| Borderline personality disorder | Obstructive sleep apnea |
| Generalized anxiety disorder | PTSD |
| Major depressive episode | Substance use disorder (e.g., caffeine, nicotine) |
| Manic or mixed episode | Traumatic brain injury |
| Medication-induced (e.g., thyroxine, corticosteroids) | |
| Neurological conditions (e.g., epilepsy, Tourette's syndrome) | |

Related Disorders," for details of this diagnosis in the perinatal period. There is overlapping symptomatology, and substantial comorbidity, between adult ADHD and bipolar disorder, such as the presence of distractibility or impulsivity; however, there are also key differences. Adult ADHD has a higher prevalence, an earlier age of symptom onset, and a chronic as opposed to cyclic course.

Although mood symptoms can sometimes be present with ADHD, mood episodes of adequate duration for diagnosis are the hallmark of bipolar disorder. Psychotic symptoms are not a diagnostic component of ADHD (Brus et al. 2014). In addition, anxiety disorders, such as generalized anxiety disorder, panic disorder, and PTSD, can all present with difficulties with concentration and distractibility. Last, ruling out substance intoxication or withdrawal is critical; although many women reduce or stop substance use when a pregnancy is discovered, a significant number continue to use substances throughout pregnancy, leading to multiple negative maternal–infant outcomes (Ordean et al. 2017). The presence of significant impulsivity and affective lability can raise the question of borderline personality disorder; however, the two can be distinguished by the presence of other symptoms specific to borderline personality disorder, including frantic efforts to avoid abandonment, identity disturbance, and recurrent suicidal behavior (American Psychiatric Association 2013).

Medical conditions that should be ruled out include thyroid disease, systemic disease such as hepatic failure, obstructive sleep apnea, and neurological disorders such as Tourette's syndrome and epilepsy (Geffen and Forster 2018; Post and Kurlansik 2012). Side effects of commonly prescribed medications and substances, such as steroids, antihistamines, caffeine, and nicotine, can also mimic ADHD symptoms (Post and Kurlansik 2012).

## Pathophysiology

ADHD is a clinically heterogeneous disorder that has a wide range of clinical presentations. These include substantial variations in neurocognitive impact, structural and functional brain abnormalities, behavioral patterns, psychiatric comorbidities, and trajectories over time (Faraone et al. 2015). Given this level of heterogeneity, it is perhaps not surprising that no single etiology nor core set of etiologies of ADHD has been identified, despite extensive analysis. Alternatively, it has been proposed that a combination of several genetic and environmental risk factors interact together to increase susceptibility to ADHD (Faraone et al. 2015) and that ADHD itself may comprise a heterogeneous cluster of distinct syndromes (Matthews et al. 2014).

Extensive analysis from neurocognitive, neurophysiological, and neuroimaging studies supports the idea that brain dysfunction plays a central role in ADHD in both children and adults (Bekker et al. 2005a, 2005b; Seidman et al. 2004a, 2004b, 2005). Functional MRI studies have demonstrated brain dysfunction with cognitive tasks specific to ADHD (Makris et al. 2008; Paloyelis et al. 2007; Pliszka et al. 2006; Rubia et al. 2005; Suskauer et al. 2008). A consistent set of neural circuits involved in executive functioning, reward processing, and attention has been associated with ADHD, including the frontoparietal, dorsal frontostriatal, and mesocorticolimbic circuits, as well as the default mode and cognitive control networks (Alexander and Farrelly 2018; Gallo and Posner 2016).

In terms of brain structural findings, MRI studies have demonstrated smaller volumes in the right frontal areas, cerebellum, corpus callosum, and caudate, as well as cortical thinning (Castellanos 2002; Castellanos et al. 1996, 2001; Durston 2008; Durston et al. 2004; Makris et al. 2007; Seidman et al. 2006; Semrud-Clikeman et al. 1994; Valera et al. 2007). Recent studies have also demonstrated brain volume differences in the bilateral amygdala, nucleus accumbens, and hippocampus (Hoogman et al. 2017). PET scanning demonstrates abnormal glucose metabolism in the prefrontal and premotor areas of the frontal lobe in adults (Ernst et al. 1998; Zametkin et al. 1990, 1993), and single photon emission computed tomography studies demonstrate hypoperfusion/hypofunctioning in the prefrontal and striatal regions in both children and older adults (Amen et al. 2008; Lou et al. 1989). Alterations in neurotransmitter systems, including the dopaminergic, serotonergic, and glutamatergic systems, are observed in ADHD populations (Dunn et al. 2019).

Evidence from family, twin, and adoption studies strongly supports a genetic basis of ADHD (Alberts-Corush et al. 1986; Biederman et al. 1990a; Faraone et al. 2000; Sprich et al. 2000) and high heritability (Faraone et al. 2005; Larsson et al. 2014). Twin studies estimate its heritability to be 70%–80% (Burt 2009) and have shown that this heritability extends from childhood through adulthood (Chang et al. 2013). Family studies show that the parents and siblings of a child with ADHD have a twofold to eightfold increased risk of ADHD themselves (Biederman et al. 1990b, 1992). There is also evidence of genetic factors in the distinct dimensions of ADHD; for example, one twin study noted that heritability of inattention was 0.39, whereas the heritability of impulsivity-hyperactivity was 0.69 (Sherman et al. 1997).

However, researchers have yet to find the needle in the haystack—that is, which (if any) genetic contribution is the most significant. Even though twin studies have estimated that additive genetic effects are thought to explain up to 80% of the variance in the ADHD phenotype (Albayrak et al. 2008; Thapar et al. 1999), each gene marker identified thus far has had too small an effect to explain the totality of the heritability of ADHD (Durston 2008; Faraone et al. 2005). Genome-wide scans have identified evidence of linkage in several chromosomal regions, including 5p12, 10q26, 12q23, and 16p13 (Fisher et al. 2002; Smalley et al. 2002), and in one region proximal to the dopamine transporter gene (Bakker et al. 2003; Hebebrand et al. 2006; Ogdie et al. 2003); however, a recent meta-analysis found no significant genome-wide associations, suggesting that the contribution of these markers is low (Neale et al. 2010).

In terms of specific genes, evidence supports the role of neurotransmitter involvement with markers in or near the relevant receptor genes; examples include dopamine transporter-1 (*DAT1*), dopamine D4 and D5 receptors (*DRD4*, *DRD5*), the serotonin-transporter-linked polymorphic region (*5HTTPLR*), 5-hydroxytryptamine receptor 1B (*HTR1B*), synaptosomal-associated protein 25 (*SNAP25*), and the $\alpha_2$ receptor (Barr et al. 2001; Cook et al. 1995; Gizer et al. 2009; Rivero et al. 2013). The seven-repeat allele of *DRD4* has attracted particular interest, given substantial evidence that dopamine functioning is involved in the pathogenesis of ADHD (Faraone et al. 2001). However, given the gap between high heritability and the fact that candidate genes account for only about 5% of the genetic variation in ADHD, it is thought that gene-environment interactions, gene-gene interactions, or the presence of rare genetic variants may also play a role (Faraone et al. 2015; Matthews et al. 2014; Neale et al. 2010; Nijmeijer et al. 2010; Williams et al. 2012).

Other biological factors are areas of active interest (Dunn et al. 2019). Evidence supporting the role of inflammation includes the relationship between ADHD and autoimmune disorders (Instanes et al. 2017; Liao et al. 2016; Lin et al. 2016), an association of ADHD with increased serum cytokines (Anand et al. 2017), and evidence of antibodies against relevant targets in ADHD, such as the dopamine transporter polymorphisms associated with inflammatory pathways and ADHD (Giana et al. 2015). In addition, early evidence suggests that prenatal exposure to inflammation is associated with changes in offspring brain development, such as reductions in cortical gray matter volume (Short et al. 2010) and alterations in neurotransmitter function (Luchicchi et al. 2016). Other biological factors that have been proposed to play a role in the pathogenesis of ADHD include sex hormones, particularly in women. For example, a growing body of evidence demonstrates that sex hormones can regulate intracellular signaling systems thought to be abnormal in ADHD. This functional interaction between sex hormones and neurotransmitter systems may be associated with the clinical features of ADHD in women (Haimov-Kochman and Berger 2014); however, little is known about the role of sex hormones in the pathophysiology of ADHD (Gross-Tsur et al. 2006).

There has been extensive research into environmental factors that play a role in the pathogenesis of ADHD (Banerjee et al. 2007). However, recent studies have noted the complexity of determining causality and of delineating environmental effects from genetic and familial confounding variables (Sciberras et al. 2017). Despite the complexity, several prenatal exposures have been hypothesized to be related to ADHD in the offspring. Of the putative environmental factors, preterm birth and low birth weight appear to have the strongest relationship with the pathogenesis of ADHD in offspring (Botting et al. 1997; Milberger et al. 1997b; Sciberras et al. 2017; Stevens et al. 2008). Other cited exposures include prenatal exposure to alcohol, nicotine, illicit substances, hypertension, maternal stress, and severe early life deprivation such as prolonged childhood separation (Banerjee et al. 2007; Milberger et al. 1997a). Tobacco use in pregnancy has often been cited as a strong risk factor for ADHD in the offspring; however, genetic and familial factors may play a stronger role than previously thought (Sciberras et al. 2017). In addition, prenatal exposure to nicotine may be related to genetic effects rather than the direct toxic effects of nicotine or other tobacco components (Thapar et al. 2009). Other factors, including maternal medical conditions, such as autoimmune illness (Xiang et al. 2018); medication exposures, such as acetaminophen (Liew et al. 2014); and environmental toxins, such as lead (Nigg et al. 2010), have been proposed, but the limited evidence available is difficult to interpret, and further well-designed studies are required (Sciberras et al. 2017).

# Treatment

## Psychopharmacology

### Stimulants

The gold standard of ADHD treatment is psychopharmacology, typically with psychostimulants such as methylphenidate or amphetamine, in combination with behavioral psychotherapy (Baker and Freeman 2018; Thapar and Cooper 2016). There is clear evidence that maximum therapeutic efficacy is obtained when psychosocial support is delivered in addition to pharmacotherapy, rather than with pharmacotherapy alone (Cherkasova et al. 2020; Philipsen et al. 2015; Young et al. 2017). Stimulants are generally thought to have higher efficacy for adult ADHD than nonstimulants (Faraone and Glatt 2010; Peterson et al. 2008; Mészáros et al. 2009). The use of stimulant medication to treat ADHD in women has risen dramatically in recent years, leading to more women becoming pregnant while taking stimulant medications. The Centers for Disease Control and Prevention recently used a commercial database to estimate the percentage of reproductive-aged women who filled prescriptions for ADHD medications each year; from 2003 to 2015, the percentage rose by an astounding 344% to an overall prevalence of 4% of women (Anderson et al. 2018). Current estimates are that approximately 1% of pregnant women in the United States use medications for the treatment of ADHD, making these medications one of the most commonly prescribed in pregnancy overall (Anderson et al. 2018; Louik et al. 2015). Although discontinuation of pharmacological treatment during pregnancy may be a viable option for women with mild symptoms, those with severe symptoms may require continued use in order to maintain psychological, social, and occupational functioning throughout pregnancy.

Several systematic studies have examined the risks of perinatal exposure to stimulants (Dideriksen et al. 2013; Pottegård et al. 2014; Wajnberg et al. 2011); however, many of these studies are derived from data with significant confounding variables, such as illicit stimulant use/misuse, use of stimulants as an anorectic drug, and comorbid substance abuse, tobacco use, or polypharmacy (Besag 2014; Bolea-Alamanac et al. 2014; Humphreys et al. 2007; Nörby et al. 2017). In addition, some studies have yielded outcomes that are either inconsistent or could also be attributed to untreated maternal ADHD (Bro et al. 2015; Diav-Citrin et al. 2016; Haervig et al. 2014; Källén et al. 2013; Newport et al. 2016; Wright et al. 2015). Clinical discussions regarding the risks of exposure to stimulants in pregnancy must be balanced against the substantial risks of untreated perinatal ADHD, including driving hazards and major functional impairment in both work and home life (Freeman 2014).

**Early pregnancy.** Data are mostly reassuring regarding the risk of birth defects and stimulant exposure (Aktepe et al. 2009; Debooy et al.1993; Diav-Citrin et al. 2016; Dideriksen et al. 2013; Källén et al. 2013; Milkovich and van der Berg 1977; Nörby et al. 2017; Pottegård et al. 2014), although a few human studies have noted an association of stimulant exposure with cardiac (Jiang et al. 2019; Levin 1971; Nora et al. 1970), gastrointestinal (Anderson et al. 2020; Elliott et al. 2009), and limb malformations (Anderson et al. 2020). Several studies have noted an association between stimulant exposure and miscarriage (Haervig et al. 2014), although at least some of these data were complicated by significant confounding variables, such as a prior history of miscarriage (Diav-Citrin et al. 2016) or confounding by indication (Bro et al. 2015).

**Obstetrical outcomes.** Adverse pregnancy outcomes associated with stimulant medications are likely to be related to their vasoconstrictive effects, which may impair placental perfusion. A number of studies have demonstrated an association between stimulant exposure and adverse pregnancy outcomes, such as low birth weight, small for gestational age infant, infant withdrawal, and premature birth; however, these studies were also complicated by confounders, including stimulant misuse and tobacco dependence (Debooy et al. 1993; Ladhani et al. 2011; Smith et al. 2003; Wright et al. 2015). More recent studies have focused on women taking prescribed doses of stimulant medications. Bro et al. (2015) utilized birth registry data to examine information from 989,932 pregnancies, of which 186 of the pregnant women had used methylphenidate or atomoxetine. They found that, as compared with unexposed infants, those exposed to one of these medications during pregnancy were at increased risk for Apgar scores <10 (adjusted relative risk 2.06; 95% CI 1.11–3.82) (Bro et al. 2015).

In a later cohort study, Nörby et al. (2017) analyzed birth registry data of 964,734 infants, of whom 1,591 were exposed to ADHD medications during pregnancy. Analysis of these data concluded that infants exposed to ADHD medications were at elevated risk for admission to a neonatal intensive care unit (adjusted OR 1.5; 95% CI 1.3–1.7), CNS-related disorders (adjusted OR 1.9; 95% CI 1.1–3.1), and moderate preterm birth (adjusted OR 1.3; 95% CI 1.1–1.6) (Nörby et al. 2017). Both studies (Bro et al. 2015; Nörby et al. 2017) were limited by the fundamental differences between participants in the exposed versus unexposed groups. Cohen et al. (2017) conducted a population-based cohort study of more than 3,000 pregnancies exposed to prescribed psychostimulants. After controlling for multiple confounders, they noted a small increased relative risk of preeclampsia (RR 1.29; 95% CI 1.11–1.49) in women exposed to stimulants versus unexposed women and a small increased relative risk of preterm birth for women who continued to use stimulants into the second half of pregnancy (RR 1.30; 95% CI 1.10–1.55) relative to those with only early pregnancy exposure (Cohen et al. 2017). Cumulatively, these data suggest a small increased risk for adverse obstetrical outcomes with psychostimulant use during pregnancy.

**Long-term effects.** Data regarding fetal neurodevelopment and long-term offspring outcomes are limited. Data from animal models have demonstrated alterations in dopamine receptor expression and transmission in rodents (Flores et al. 2011), as well as decreased motor activity in postpubertal zebrafish (Levin et al. 2011), but it is unclear how that may relate to clinical relevance in humans. Human studies are limited, although one large, population-based, prospective cohort study found that prescribed stimulant exposure was associated with an increased risk of neonatal CNS disorders, such as seizures (Nörby et al. 2017).

**Lactation.** In addition, information is scarce regarding stimulant use in breastfeeding to help guide clinical decision making in the postpartum period. Given the potential negative effects in utero, it is theoretically possible that stimulant exposure via breastmilk could negatively affect infant growth and appetite or sleep patterns; however, the limited data thus far have suggested that these agents are compatible with breastfeeding. One small case series of mother–infant nursing pairs in which the mother was taking dextroamphetamine reported no adverse effects in the nurslings, and the serum levels of dextroamphetamine in the infants ranged from low to undetectable (Ilett et al. 2007). Estimates of maternal transmission of stimulant medication in breastmilk have ranged from 0.16% to 5.7% (Hackett et al. 2006; Ilett et al. 2007; Spigset et al. 2007), below the 10% relative infant dose figure often cited as the threshold for safety in breastfeeding (Hale and Rowe 2014). Please see Chapter 1, "The Reproductive Life Cycle," for details on maternal transmission thresholds in breastmilk.

## Bupropion

Although bupropion is not considered as effective as stimulants for the symptoms of ADHD, it may be a suitable alternative for some women (Faraone and Glatt 2010; Mészáros et al. 2009; Peterson et al. 2008), and it may have specific advantages, particularly for women with comorbid depression or women who desire pharmacological support for smoking cessation (Baker and Freeman 2018; Freeman 2014).

**Early pregnancy.** Overall, more data support the reproductive safety of bupropion in pregnancy than support stimulants, although there is less information as compared with, for example, selective serotonin reuptake inhibitors. There has been concern about an association with bupropion exposure and cardiovascular malformations; for example, one retrospective case control study using data from a birth defect registry noted a small increase in the relative risk of cardiovascular left ventricular outflow defects (with an absolute risk calculated to be 2 out of 1,000 pregnancies) (Alwan et al. 2010). However, overall studies have been reassuring. For example, prospective registry data found that the birth defect rate with bupropion exposure in the first trimester was 3.6%, similar to that found in the unexposed population, and there was no clear pattern of birth defects (Bupropion Pregnancy Registry 2008).

Another prospective study found no evidence of a higher rate of malformations with bupropion exposure as compared with groups with other antidepressant exposure or no exposure (Chun-Fai-Chan et al. 2005). Furthermore, a large epidemiological study of more than 150,000 women compared women with bupropion exposure in the first trimester with bupropion exposure in the second trimester and exposure to another antidepressant in the first trimester; no increase in birth defects with first trimester bupropion exposure was noted (Cole et al. 2007). A recent systematic review aimed to consolidate these findings; this review supported the finding of a small increase in relative risk of cardiac malformations, although the absolute risk was low, and confounders such as the indication for smoking cessation may have contributed (Hendrick et al. 2017). One small study noted an elevated risk of miscarriage with bupropion exposure as compared with a control group; however, the rate remained within that of the general population (Chun-Fai-Chan et al. 2005; Hendrick et al. 2017).

**Obstetrical outcomes.** Data about other pregnancy or delivery outcomes with bupropion exposure are scarce. One small study of 30 pregnant women taking bupropion for smoking cessation showed no statistical differences in birth weight, Apgar score, or length of gestation in exposed infants (Nanovskaya et al. 2017).

**Long-term effects.** There is a paucity of data regarding the long-term neurodevelopmental effects of bupropion. Although one study analyzing insurance claims–based data reported an association between bupropion exposure in utero and ADHD diagnosed by the age of 5, many potential confounders may contribute to this association (Figueroa 2010).

**Lactation.** Data regarding bupropion exposure through breastfeeding is also limited, but small case series have noted low to undetectable levels of bupropion in infant serum (Baab et al. 2002; Briggs et al. 1993), and the relative infant dose has been estimated to be a reassuring 5.7% (Davis et al. 2009). There was a single case report of a nursing infant whose mother observed a possible seizure after exposure to bupropion in breastmilk; this raises a plausible concern because bupropion is known to lower the seizure threshold (Chaudron and Schoenecker 2004).

## Other Medications

Scant reproductive safety information is available about other medications sometimes used for the treatment of ADHD, including atomoxetine and guanfacine. To our knowledge, no systematic studies in human pregnancy are available that have examined the safety of these medications (Freeman 2014). A few case reports and a registry analysis show no specific malformations or adverse pregnancy outcomes for either agent thus far (Alessi and Spalding 2003; Källén et al. 2013; Philipp 1980).

## Behavioral and Somatic Treatments

No known perinatal-specific psychotherapies have been developed for the management of ADHD. However, data are accumulating regarding nonpharmacological approaches in the general adult population, specifically cognitive-behavioral therapy (CBT) (Mongia and Hechtman 2012). CBT tailored for adult ADHD typically focuses on a combination of building organizational skills, such as prioritization and time management, and challenging self-defeating cognitions (Jensen et al. 2016; Morgensterns et al. 2016; Solanto et al. 2010; Vidal-Estrada et al. 2012). A recent meta-analysis examining CBT for ADHD in adults demonstrated effect sizes comparable with those of well-established behavioral therapies for children with ADHD (Knouse et al. 2017). Further work remains, however, for identifying the core principles of treatment-related change in adults so that more tailored treatments can be developed and applied to both the adult and the perinatal population (Knouse et al. 2017). Last, executive function coaching (Prevatt and Yelland 2015) and exercise (Den Heijer et al. 2017; Vysniauske et al. 2020) also have some evidence of benefit in adult ADHD.

Specific attention may be required to address the complex situations faced by women with ADHD in the perinatal period and early parenting, as they aim to balance multiple occupational demands, home management, and family/parenting responsibilities (Young et al. 2020), especially because household and parenting duties tend to be disproportionately borne by women (Treas and Tai 2016). Solutions have been cited in the literature, such as reducing the workload if possible and taking public transportation instead of driving (Baker and Freeman 2018). Comprehensive programs of support have yet to be developed, but suggested interventions cited include the development of targeted support to manage feelings of stress and distress, manage and regulate emotions, support sexual health and safety, cope with rejection and isolation, manage interpersonal conflict, learn assertiveness skills, and develop compromise and negotiation strategies in order to improve occupational and social outcomes and women's ability to cope with everyday stressors (Young et al. 2020).

## Conclusion

ADHD is a common, lifelong neurodevelopmental disorder that has a significant impact on functioning in daily life in school, work, and social settings and on physical and mental health throughout the lifespan (Agnew-Blais et al. 2016; Barbaresi et al. 2013; Faraone et al. 2015). Contrary to a prior understanding of ADHD solely as a childhood disorder, it is now clear that ADHD persists through the lifespan (Asherson 2010) and that there may be a distinct adult-onset version. However, a comprehensive understanding of ADHD in adulthood, in women specifically, and in the perinatal period is just beginning to be elucidated (Freeman 2014; Kooij et al. 2010).

Because of its high prevalence and significant impact, ADHD is an important condition to address in the setting of reproductive mental health. Women of reproductive age are increasingly diagnosed with ADHD (Leong et al. 2017; Louik et al. 2015), and they are at substantially increased risk of comorbidities, including depression, anxiety, and substance use disorders (Owens et al. 2017) in addition to significant difficulties with work, school, interpersonal relationships, and everyday functioning (Corbisiero et al. 2017; Eddy et al. 2019). When women with ADHD enter pregnancy and new motherhood, they may be under increased psychosocial stress, although data regarding this time period are very limited (Freeman 2014). The use of stimulant medications by women of reproductive age has increased significantly, and in turn these medications are among the most commonly prescribed in pregnancy (Anderson et al. 2018; Haervig et al. 2014; Louik et al. 2015; Renoux et al. 2016). Yet our understanding of the reproductive safety profile of prescribed medications is limited and is complicated by significant confounding variables (Bro et al. 2015; Diav-Citrin et al. 2016; Haervig et al. 2014; Källén et al. 2013; Newport et al. 2016; Wright et al. 2015). Because prenatal factors are thought to be environmental risk factors for ADHD in the offspring, a robust understanding of ADHD in women in the perinatal period would serve to address the mental health needs of their children in an intergenerational manner.

A great deal remains to be discovered regarding the epidemiology, diagnosis, clinical presentation, diagnostic criteria, screening and assessment, and treatment of adults with ADHD generally, and women with ADHD specifically—both within and outside of the perinatal period. Future directions for an understanding of ADHD and reproductive mental health remain a wide-open field, and a greater understanding of this highly prevalent and impairing disorder could improve the mental and physical health of women and their offspring for multiple generations.

## Key Points

- ADHD is a common neurodevelopmental disorder that has a lifelong impact. It is associated with major functional impairment in multiple arenas, such as work, school, and social life.
- Adult ADHD is highly comorbid with other mental health conditions, including depression, anxiety, and substance use disorders.

- Optimal treatment of ADHD includes a combination of medication and psychosocial support.
- Stimulants are one of the most commonly prescribed medication in pregnancy. An increasing number of women of reproductive age have been diagnosed with ADHD and prescribed stimulants for this condition.
- Data regarding the risks of stimulant exposure in pregnancy and breastfeeding historically have contained significant confounding variables, such as the impact of ADHD itself and substance misuse.
- Data are still evolving regarding the reproductive safety profile of stimulants; much of their effect appears to be related to fetal growth and placental function.

## References


Adler LA, Faraone SV, Spencer TJ, et al: The structure of adult ADHD. Int J Methods Psychiatr Res 26(1):e1555, 2017 28211596

Adler L, Kessler R, Spencer T: Adult ADHD Self-Report Scale–V1.1 (ASRS-V1.1) Screener: From WHO Composite International Diagnostic Interview. Geneva, World Health Organization, 2003. Available at: https://www.hcp.med.harvard.edu/ncs/ftpdir/adhd/6Q_ASRS_English.pdf. Accessed February 5, 2021.

Agarwal R, Goldenberg M, Perry R, et al: The quality of life of adults with attention deficit hyperactivity disorder: a systematic review. Innov Clin Neurosci 9(5–6):10–21, 2012 22808445

Agnew-Blais JC, Polanczyk GV, Danese A, et al: Evaluation of the persistence, remission, and emergence of attention-deficit/hyperactivity disorder in young adulthood. JAMA Psychiatry 73(7):713–720, 2016 27192174

Aktepe E, Ozkorumak E, Tanriöver-Kandil S: Pregnancy and delivery complications and treatment approach in attention deficit hyperactivity disorder. Turk J Pediatr 51(5):478–484, 2009 20112604

Albayrak O, Friedel S, Schimmelmann BG, et al: Genetic aspects in attention-deficit/hyperactivity disorder. J Neural Transm (Vienna) 115(2):305–315, 2008 18200432

Alberts-Corush J, Firestone P, Goodman JT: Attention and impulsivity characteristics of the biological and adoptive parents of hyperactive and normal control children. Am J Orthopsychiatry 56(3):413–423, 1986 3740224

Alessi NE, Spalding S: Atomoxetine and pregnancy (comment). J Am Acad Child Adolesc Psychiatry 42(8):883–884, author reply 884–885, 2003 12874488

Alexander L, Farrelly N: Attending to adult ADHD: a review of the neurobiology behind adult ADHD. Ir J Psychol Med 35(3):237–244, 2018 30124185

Alvarado C, Modesto-Lowe V: Improving treatment in minority children with attention deficit/hyperactivity disorder. Clin Pediatr (Phila) 56(2):171–176, 2017 27113035

Alwan S, Reefhuis J, Botto LD, et al: Maternal use of bupropion and risk for congenital heart defects. Am J Obstet Gynecol 203:52.e1–52.e6, 2010

Amen DG, Hanks C, Prunella J: Preliminary evidence differentiating ADHD using brain SPECT imaging in older patients. J Psychoactive Drugs 40(2):139–146, 2008 18720662

American Psychiatric Association: Diagnostic and Statistical Manual of Mental Disorders, 4th Edition. Washington, DC, American Psychiatric Association, 1994

American Psychiatric Association: Diagnostic and Statistical Manual of Mental Disorders, 5th Edition. Arlington, VA, American Psychiatric Association, 2013

Anand D, Colpo GD, Zeni G, et al: Attention-deficit/hyperactivity disorder and inflammation: what does current knowledge tell us? A systematic review. Front Psychiatry 8:228, 2017 29170646

Anderson KN, Ailes EC, Danielson M, et al: Attention-deficit/hyperactivity disorder medication prescription claims among privately insured women aged 15–44 years—United States, 2003–2015. MMWR Morb Mortal Wkly Rep 67(2):66–70, 2018 29346342

Anderson KN, Dutton AC, Broussard CS, et al: ADHD medication use during pregnancy and risk for selected birth defects: National Birth Defects Prevention Study, 1998–2011. J Atten Disord 24(3):479–489, 2020 29519207
Asherson P: ADHD across the lifespan. Medicine (Baltimore) 40:623–627, 2010
Baab SW, Peindl KS, Piontek CM, et al: Serum bupropion levels in 2 breastfeeding mother-infant pairs. J Clin Psychiatry 63(10):910–911, 2002 12416600
Baker AS, Freeman MP: Management of attention deficit hyperactivity disorder during pregnancy. Obstet Gynecol Clin North Am 45(3):495–509, 2018 30092924
Bakker SC, van der Meulen EM, Buitelaar JK, et al: A whole-genome scan in 164 Dutch sib pairs with attention-deficit/hyperactivity disorder: suggestive evidence for linkage on chromosomes 7p and 15q. Am J Hum Genet 72(5):1251–1260, 2003 12679898
Banerjee TD, Middleton F, Faraone SV: Environmental risk factors for attention-deficit hyperactivity disorder. Acta Paediatr 96(9):1269–1274, 2007 17718779
Barbaresi WJ, Colligan RC, Weaver AL, et al: Mortality, ADHD, and psychosocial adversity in adults with childhood ADHD: a prospective study. Pediatrics 131(4):637–644, 2013 23460687
Barkley RA, Murphy KR: Attention-Deficit Hyperactivity Disorder: A Clinical Workbook. New York, Guilford, 1998
Barkley RA, Fischer M, Smallish L, et al: The persistence of attention-deficit/hyperactivity disorder into young adulthood as a function of reporting source and definition of disorder. J Abnorm Psychol 111(2):279–289, 2002 12003449
Barkley RA, Fischer M, Smallish L, et al: Young adult outcome of hyperactive children: adaptive functioning in major life activities. J Am Acad Child Adolesc Psychiatry 45(2):192–202, 2006 16429090
Barr CL, Xu C, Kroft J, et al: Haplotype study of three polymorphisms at the dopamine transporter locus confirm linkage to attention-deficit/hyperactivity disorder. Biol Psychiatry 49(4):333–339, 2001 11239904
Bekker EM, Kenemans JL, Hoeksma MR, et al: The pure electrophysiology of stopping. Int J Psychophysiol 55(2):191–198, 2005a 15649550
Bekker EM, Overtoom CC, Kenemans JL, et al: Stopping and changing in adults with ADHD. Psychol Med 35(6):807–816, 2005b 15997601
Besag FM: ADHD treatment and pregnancy. Drug Saf 37(6):397–408, 2014 24794209
Biederman J, Faraone SV, Keenan K, et al: Family genetic and psychosocial risk factors in DSM-III attention deficit disorder. J Am Acad Child Adolesc Psychiatry 29(4):526–533, 1990a 2387786
Biederman J, Keenan K, Faraone SV: Parent-based diagnosis of attention deficit disorder predicts a diagnosis based on teacher report. J Am Acad Child Adolesc Psychiatry 29(5):698–701, 1990b 2228921
Biederman J, Faraone SV, Keenan K, et al: Further evidence for family genetic risk factors in attention deficit hyperactivity disorder. Patterns of comorbidity in probands and relatives psychiatrically and pediatrically referred samples. Arch Gen Psychiatry 49(9):728–738, 1992 1514878
Biederman J, Faraone SV, Spencer T, et al: Patterns of psychiatric comorbidity, cognition, and psychosocial functioning in adults with attention deficit hyperactivity disorder. Am J Psychiatry 150(12):1792–1798, 1993 8238632
Biederman J, Faraone S, Milberger S, et al: Predictors of persistence and remission of ADHD into adolescence: results from a four-year prospective follow-up study. J Am Acad Child Adolesc Psychiatry 35(3):343–351, 1996 8714323
Biederman J, Mick E, Faraone SV: Age-dependent decline of symptoms of attention deficit hyperactivity disorder: impact of remission definition and symptom type. Am J Psychiatry 157(5):816–818, 2000 10784477
Biederman J, Fried R, Hammerness P, et al: The effects of lisdexamfetamine dimesylate on driving behaviors in young adults with ADHD assessed with the Manchester driving behavior questionnaire. J Adolesc Health 51(6):601–607, 2012 23174471
Birnbaum HG, Kessler RC, Lowe SW, et al: Costs of attention deficit-hyperactivity disorder (ADHD) in the US: excess costs of persons with ADHD and their family members in 2000. Curr Med Res Opin 21(2):195–206, 2005 15801990

Bolea-Alamanac BM, Green A, Verma G, et al: Methylphenidate use in pregnancy and lactation: a systematic review of evidence. Br J Clin Pharmacol 77(1):96–101, 2014 23593966

Botting N, Powls A, Cooke RW, Marlow N: Attention deficit hyperactivity disorders and other psychiatric outcomes in very low birthweight children at 12 years. J Child Psychol Psychiatry 38(8):931–941, 1997 9413793

Brassett-Grundy A, Butler NR: Prevalence and adult outcomes of Attention-Deficit/Hyperactivity Disorder: evidence from a 30-year prospective longitudinal study. Bedford Group Occasional Paper No 2. London, Bedford Group, 2004. Available at: https://cls.ucl.ac.uk/wp-content/uploads/2017/07/BG_OccPaper2_ADHD_outcomes_2004.pdf. Accessed February 5, 2021.

Briggs GG, Samson JH, Ambrose PJ, et al: Excretion of bupropion in breast milk. Ann Pharmacother 27(4):431–433, 1993 8477117

Bro SP, Kjaersgaard MI, Parner ET, et al: Adverse pregnancy outcomes after exposure to methylphenidate or atomoxetine during pregnancy. Clin Epidemiol 7:139–147, 2015 25657597

Brook JS, Brook DW, Zhang C, et al: Adolescent ADHD and adult physical and mental health, work performance, and financial stress. Pediatrics 131(1):5–13, 2013 23230074

Brown TE: Brown Attention-Deficit Disorder Scales for Adolescents and Adults: Manual. San Antonio, TX, The Psychological Corporation, 1996

Brunault P, Frammery J, Montaudon P, et al: Adulthood and childhood ADHD in patients consulting for obesity is associated with food addiction and binge eating, but not sleep apnea syndrome. Appetite 136:25–32, 2019 30641157

Brus MJ, Solanto MV, Goldberg JF: Adult ADHD vs. bipolar disorder in the DSM-5 era: a challenging differentiation for clinicians. J Psychiatr Pract 20(6):428–437, 2014 25406047

Buckwalter JG, Stanczyk FZ, McCleary CA, et al: Pregnancy, the postpartum, and steroid hormones: effects on cognition and mood. Psychoneuroendocrinology 24(1):69–84, 1999 10098220

Buitelaar JK: Discussion of attention deficit-hyperactivity disorder (ADHD): facts, opinions and emotions [in Dutch]. Ned Tijdschr Geneeskd 145(31):1485–1489, 2001 11512418

Bupropion Pregnancy Registry: Final report: 1 September 1997 through 31 March 2008. Wilmington, NC, Kendle International (for GlaxoSmithKline), 2008. Available at: http://pregnancyregistry.gsk.com/documents/bup_report_final_2008.pdf. Accessed September 30, 2020.

Burt SA: Rethinking environmental contributions to child and adolescent psychopathology: a meta-analysis of shared environmental influences. Psychol Bull 135(4):608–637, 2009 19586164

Capusan AJ, Kuja-Halkola R, Bendtsen P, et al: Childhood maltreatment and attention deficit hyperactivity disorder symptoms in adults: a large twin study. Psychol Med 46(12):2637–2646, 2016 27376862

Castellanos FX: Anatomic magnetic resonance imaging studies of attention-deficit/hyperactivity disorder. Dialogues Clin Neurosci 4(4):444–448, 2002 22034444

Castellanos FX: Is adult-onset ADHD a distinct entity? Am J Psychiatry 172(10):929–931, 2015 26423474

Castellanos FX, Giedd JN, Marsh WL, et al: Quantitative brain magnetic resonance imaging in attention-deficit hyperactivity disorder. Arch Gen Psychiatry 53(7):607–616, 1996 8660127

Castellanos FX, Giedd JN, Berquin PC, et al: Quantitative brain magnetic resonance imaging in girls with attention-deficit/hyperactivity disorder. Arch Gen Psychiatry 58(3):289–295, 2001 11231836

Chang Z, Lichtenstein P, Asherson PJ, et al: Developmental twin study of attention problems: high heritabilities throughout development. JAMA Psychiatry 70(3):311–318, 2013 23303526

Charach A, Yeung E, Climans T, et al: Childhood attention-deficit/hyperactivity disorder and future substance use disorders: comparative meta-analyses. J Am Acad Child Adolesc Psychiatry 50(1):9–21, 2011 21156266

Chaudron LH, Schoenecker CJ: Bupropion and breastfeeding: a case of a possible infant seizure. J Clin Psychiatry 65(6):881–882, 2004 15291673

Cherkasova MV, French LR, Syer CA, et al: Efficacy of cognitive behavioral therapy with and without medication for adults with ADHD: a randomized clinical trial. J Atten Disord 24(6):889–903, 2020 28413900

Cheung CHM, Rijsdijk F, McLoughlin G, et al: Cognitive and neurophysiological markers of ADHD persistence and remission. Br J Psychiatry 208(6):548–555, 2016 26250744
Cho SW, Lee YJ, Lee SA, et al: Comparison of adults with attention-deficit hyperactivity disorder depending on the age of being diagnosed in childhood and adulthood: based on retrospective review in one university hospital. Journal of Korean Academy of Child and Adolescent Psychiatry 28(3):183–189, 2017
Chun-Fai-Chan B, Koren G, Fayez I, et al: Pregnancy outcome of women exposed to bupropion during pregnancy: a prospective comparative study. Am J Obstet Gynecol 192(3):932–936, 2005 15746694
Chung W, Jiang SF, Paksarian D, et al: Trends in the prevalence and incidence of attention-deficit/hyperactivity disorder among adults and children of different racial and ethnic groups. JAMA Netw Open 2(11):e1914344, 2019 31675080
Cohen JM, Hernández-Díaz S, Bateman BT, et al: Placental complications associated with psychostimulant use in pregnancy. Obstet Gynecol 130(6):1192–1201, 2017 29112657
Cole JA, Modell JG, Haight BR, et al: Bupropion in pregnancy and the prevalence of congenital malformations. Pharmacoepidemiol Drug Saf 16(5):474–484, 2007 16897811
Conners CK, Ehrhard D, Sparrow D: CAARS Adult ADHD Rating Scales. New York, Multi-health Systems, 1999
Cook EH Jr, Stein MA, Krasowski MD, et al: Association of attention-deficit disorder and the dopamine transporter gene. Am J Hum Genet 56(4):993–998, 1995 7717410
Copeland ED: Medications for Attention Disorders (ADHD/ADD) and Related Medical Problems (Tourette's Syndrome, Sleep Apnea, Seizure Disorders). Atlanta, GA, SPI Press, 1991
Corbisiero S, Hartmann-Schorro RM, Riecher-Rössler A, et al: Screening for adult attention-deficit/hyperactivity disorder in a psychiatric outpatient population with specific focus on sex differences. Front Psychiatry 8:115, 2017 28713294
Cortese S: The neurobiology and genetics of attention-deficit/hyperactivity disorder (ADHD): what every clinician should know. Eur J Paediatr Neurol 16(5):422–433, 2012 22306277
Cortese S, Faraone SV, Bernardi S, et al: Gender differences in adult attention-deficit/hyperactivity disorder: results from the National Epidemiologic Survey on Alcohol and Related Conditions (NESARC). J Clin Psychiatry 77(4):e421–e428, 2016 27137426
Dalsgaard S, Østergaard SD, Leckman JF, et al: Mortality in children, adolescents, and adults with attention deficit hyperactivity disorder: a nationwide cohort study. Lancet 385(9983):2190–2196, 2015 25726514
Davies W: Sex differences in attention deficit hyperactivity disorder: candidate genetic and endocrine mechanisms. Front Neuroendocrinol 35(3):331–346, 2014 24680800
Davis MF, Miller HS, Nolan PE Jr: Bupropion levels in breast milk for 4 mother-infant pairs: more answers to lingering questions. J Clin Psychiatry 70(2):297–298, 2009 19265649
Debooy VD, Seshia MM, Tenenbein M, et al: Intravenous pentazocine and methylphenidate abuse during pregnancy: maternal lifestyle and infant outcome. Am J Dis Child 147(10):1062–1065, 1993 7692723
Den Heijer AE, Groen Y, Tucha L, et al: Sweat it out? The effects of physical exercise on cognition and behavior in children and adults with ADHD: a systematic literature review. J Neural Transm (Vienna) 124(suppl 1):3–26, 2017 27400928
Diav-Citrin O, Shechtman S, Arnon J, et al: Methylphenidate in pregnancy: a multicenter, prospective, comparative, observational study. J Clin Psychiatry 77(9):1176–1181, 2016 27232650
Dideriksen D, Pottegård A, Hallas J, et al: First trimester in utero exposure to methylphenidate. Basic Clin Pharmacol Toxicol 112(2):73–76, 2013 23136875
Dunn GA, Nigg JT, Sullivan EL: Neuroinflammation as a risk factor for attention deficit hyperactivity disorder. Pharmacol Biochem Behav 182:22–34, 2019 31103523
Durston S: Converging methods in studying attention-deficit/hyperactivity disorder: what can we learn from neuroimaging and genetics? Dev Psychopathol 20(4):1133–1143, 2008 18838034
Durston S, Hulshoff Pol HE, Schnack HG, et al: Magnetic resonance imaging of boys with attention-deficit/hyperactivity disorder and their unaffected siblings. J Am Acad Child Adolesc Psychiatry 43(3):332–340, 2004 15076267

Ebert D, Krause J, Roth-Sackenheim C: [ADHD in adulthood—guidelines based on expert consensus with DGPPN support] [in German]. Nervenarzt 74(10):939–946, 2003 14655655
Eddy LD, Jones HA, Snipes D, et al: Associations between ADHD symptoms and occupational, interpersonal, and daily life impairments among pregnant women. J Atten Disord 23(9):976–984, 2019 28043206
Edvinsson D, Lindström E, Bingefors K, et al: Gender differences of axis I and II comorbidity in subjects diagnosed with attention-deficit hyperactivity disorder as adults. Acta Neuropsychiatr 25(3):165–174, 2013 25287470
Elliott L, Loomis D, Lottritz L, et al: Case-control study of a gastroschisis cluster in Nevada. Arch Pediatr Adolesc Med 163(11):1000–1006, 2009 19884590
Ernst M, Zametkin AJ, Matochik JA, et al: DOPA decarboxylase activity in attention deficit hyperactivity disorder adults: a [fluorine-18]fluorodopa positron emission tomographic study. J Neurosci 18(15):5901–5907, 1998 9671677
Faraone SV, Biederman J: Neurobiology of attention-deficit hyperactivity disorder. Biol Psychiatry 44(10):951–958, 1998 9821559
Faraone SV, Biederman J: Can attention-deficit/hyperactivity disorder onset occur in adulthood? JAMA Psychiatry 73(7):655–656, 2016 27191055
Faraone SV, Glatt SJ: A comparison of the efficacy of medications for adult attention-deficit/hyperactivity disorder using meta-analysis of effect sizes. J Clin Psychiatry 71(6):754–763, 2010
Faraone SV, Biederman J, Mick E, et al: Family study of girls with attention deficit hyperactivity disorder. Am J Psychiatry 157(7):1077–1083, 2000 10873914
Faraone SV, Doyle AE, Mick E, et al: Meta-analysis of the association between the 7-repeat allele of the dopamine D(4) receptor gene and attention deficit hyperactivity disorder. Am J Psychiatry 158(7):1052–1057, 2001 11431226
Faraone SV, Perlis RH, Doyle AE, et al: Molecular genetics of attention-deficit/hyperactivity disorder. Biol Psychiatry 57(11):1313–1323, 2005 15950004
Faraone SV, Biederman J, Mick E: The age-dependent decline of attention deficit hyperactivity disorder: a meta-analysis of follow-up studies. Psychol Med 36(2):159–165, 2006 16420712
Faraone SV, Asherson P, Banaschewski T, et al: Attention-deficit/hyperactivity disorder. Nat Rev Dis Primers 1:15020, 2015 27189265
Fayyad J, De Graaf R, Kessler R, et al: Cross-national prevalence and correlates of adult attention-deficit hyperactivity disorder. Br J Psychiatry 190:402–409, 2007 17470954
Figueroa R: Use of antidepressants during pregnancy and risk of attention-deficit/hyperactivity disorder in the offspring. J Dev Behav Pediatr 31(8):641–648, 2010 20613624
Fischer M, Barkley RA, Smallish L, et al: Executive functioning in hyperactive children as young adults: attention, inhibition, response perseveration, and the impact of comorbidity. Dev Neuropsychol 27(1):107–133, 2005 15737944
Fisher SE, Francks C, McCracken JT, et al: A genomewide scan for loci involved in attention-deficit/hyperactivity disorder. Am J Hum Genet 70(5):1183–1196, 2002 11923911
Flores G, de Jesús Gómez-Villalobos M, Rodríguez-Sosa L: Prenatal amphetamine exposure effects on dopaminergic receptors and transporter in postnatal rats. Neurochem Res 36(10):1740–1749, 2011 21611835
Fredriksen M, Dahl AA, Martinsen EW, et al: Childhood and persistent ADHD symptoms associated with educational failure and long-term occupational disability in adult ADHD. Atten Defic Hyperact Disord 6(2):87–99, 2014 24497125
Freeman MP: ADHD and pregnancy. Am J Psychiatry 171(7):723–728, 2014 24980168
Fuermaier AB, Tucha L, Evans BL, et al: Driving and attention deficit hyperactivity disorder. J Neural Transm (Vienna) 124(suppl 1):55–67, 2017 26419597
Furczyk K, Thome J: Adult ADHD and suicide. Atten Defic Hyperact Disord 6(3):153–158, 2014 25063344
Galea LA, Ormerod BK, Sampath S, et al: Spatial working memory and hippocampal size across pregnancy in rats. Horm Behav 37(1):86–95, 2000 10712861
Gallo EF, Posner J: Moving towards causality in attention-deficit hyperactivity disorder: overview of neural and genetic mechanisms. Lancet Psychiatry 3(6):555–567, 2016 27183902

Geffen J, Forster K: Treatment of adult ADHD: a clinical perspective. Ther Adv Psychopharmacol 8(1):25–32, 2018 29344341

Gershon J: A meta-analytic review of gender differences in ADHD. J Atten Disord 5(3):143–154, 2002 11911007

Giana G, Romano E, Porfirio MC, et al: Detection of auto-antibodies to DAT in the serum: interactions with DAT genotype and psycho-stimulant therapy for ADHD. J Neuroimmunol 278:212–222, 2015 25468771

Gittelman R, Mannuzza S, Shenker R, et al: Hyperactive boys almost grown up. I. Psychiatric status. Arch Gen Psychiatry 42(10):937–947, 1985 4037987

Gizer IR, Ficks C, Waldman ID: Candidate gene studies of ADHD: a meta-analytic review. Hum Genet 126(1):51–90, 2009 19506906

Groenman AP, Oosterlaan J, Rommelse NN, et al: Stimulant treatment for attention-deficit hyperactivity disorder and risk of developing substance use disorder. Br J Psychiatry 203(2):112–119, 2013 23846996

Gross-Tsur V, Goldzweig G, Landau YE, et al: The impact of sex and subtypes on cognitive and psychosocial aspects of ADHD. Dev Med Child Neurol 48(11):901–905, 2006 17044958

Hackett LP, Kristensen JH, Hale TW, et al: Methylphenidate and breast-feeding. Ann Pharmacother 40(10):1890–1891, 2006 16940409

Haervig KB, Mortensen LH, Hansen AV, et al: Use of ADHD medication during pregnancy from 1999 to 2010: a Danish register-based study. Pharmacoepidemiol Drug Saf 23(5):526–533, 2014 24590619

Haimov-Kochman R, Berger I: Cognitive functions of regularly cycling women may differ throughout the month, depending on sex hormone status; a possible explanation to conflicting results of studies of ADHD in females. Front Hum Neurosci 8:191, 2014 24744721

Hale TW, Rowe HE: Medications and Mothers' Milk, 16th Edition. Amarillo, TX, Hale, 2014

Halmøy A, Fasmer OB, Gillberg C, et al: Occupational outcome in adult ADHD: impact of symptom profile, comorbid psychiatric problems, and treatment: a cross-sectional study of 414 clinically diagnosed adult ADHD patients. J Atten Disord 13(2):175–187, 2009 19372500

Hart EL, Lahey BB, Loeber R, et al: Developmental change in attention-deficit hyperactivity disorder in boys: a four-year longitudinal study. J Abnorm Child Psychol 23(6):729–749, 1995 8609310

Hebebrand J, Dempfle A, Saar K, et al: A genome-wide scan for attention-deficit/hyperactivity disorder in 155 German sib-pairs. Mol Psychiatry 11(2):196–205, 2006 16222334

Hendrick V, Suri R, Gitlin MJ, et al: Bupropion use during pregnancy: a systematic review. Prim Care Companion CNS Disord 19(5):17r02160, 2017 28973846

Henry JD, Rendell PG: A review of the impact of pregnancy on memory function. J Clin Exp Neuropsychol 29(8):793–803, 2007 18030631

Henry JF, Sherwin BB: Hormones and cognitive functioning during late pregnancy and postpartum: a longitudinal study. Behav Neurosci 126(1):73–85, 2012 21928875

Hinshaw SP, Owens EB, Sami N, et al: Prospective follow-up of girls with attention-deficit/hyperactivity disorder into adolescence: evidence for continuing cross-domain impairment. J Consult Clin Psychol 74(3):489–499, 2006 16822106

Hollingdale J, Woodhouse E, Asherson P, et al: A pilot study examining ADHD and behavioural disturbance in female mentally disordered offenders. AIMS Public Health 1(2):100–108, 2014

Holst Y, Thorell LB: Neuropsychological functioning in adults with ADHD and adults with other psychiatric disorders. J Atten Disord 21(2):137–148, 2017 24134875

Hoogman M, Bralten J, Hibar DP, et al: Subcortical brain volume differences in participants with attention deficit hyperactivity disorder in children and adults: a cross-sectional mega-analysis. Lancet Psychiatry 4(4):310–319, 2017 28219628

Humphreys C, Garcia-Bournissen F, Ito S, et al: Exposure to attention deficit hyperactivity disorder medications during pregnancy. Can Fam Physician 53(7):1153–1155, 2007 17872810

Huntley Z, Young S: Alcohol and substance use history among ADHD adults: the relationship with persistent and remitting symptoms, personality, employment, and history of service use. J Atten Disord 18(1):82–90, 2014 22653809

Ilett KF, Hackett LP, Kristensen JH, et al: Transfer of dexamphetamine into breast milk during treatment for attention deficit hyperactivity disorder. Br J Clin Pharmacol 63(3):371–375, 2007 17380592

Instanes JT, Halmøy A, Engeland A, et al: Attention-deficit/hyperactivity disorder in offspring of mothers with inflammatory and immune system diseases. Biol Psychiatry 81(5):452–459, 2017 26809250

Jensen CM, Amdisen BL, Jørgensen KJ, et al: Cognitive behavioural therapy for ADHD in adults: systematic review and meta-analyses. Atten Defic Hyperact Disord 8(1):3–11, 2016 26801998

Jiang HY, Zhang X, Jiang CM, et al: Maternal and neonatal outcomes after exposure to ADHD medication during pregnancy: a systematic review and meta-analysis. Pharmacoepidemiol Drug Saf 28(3):288–295, 2019 30585374

Källén B, Borg N, Reis M: The use of central nervous system active drugs during pregnancy. Pharmaceuticals (Basel) 6(10):1221–1286, 2013 24275849

Kessler RC, Adler L, Ames M, et al: The prevalence and effects of adult attention deficit/hyperactivity disorder on work performance in a nationally representative sample of workers. J Occup Environ Med 47(6):565–572, 2005 15951716

Kessler RC, Adler L, Barkley R, et al: The prevalence and correlates of adult ADHD in the United States: results from the National Comorbidity Survey Replication. Am J Psychiatry 163(4):716–723, 2006 16585449

Knouse LE, Teller J, Brooks MA: Meta-analysis of cognitive-behavioral treatments for adult ADHD. J Consult Clin Psychol 85(7):737–750, 2017 28504540

Kollins SH, McClernon FJ, Fuemmeler BF: Association between smoking and attention-deficit/hyperactivity disorder symptoms in a population-based sample of young adults. Arch Gen Psychiatry 62(10):1142–1147, 2005 16203959

Kooij JJS, Aeckerlin LP, Buitelaar JK: [Functioning, comorbidity and treatment of 141 adults with attention deficit hyperactivity disorder (ADHD) at a psychiatric outpatient department] (in Dutch). Ned Tijdschr Geneeskd 145(31):1498–1501, 2001 11512422

Kooij JJS, Buitelaar JK, van den Oord EJ, et al: Internal and external validity of attention-deficit hyperactivity disorder in a population-based sample of adults. Psychol Med 35(6):817–827, 2005 15997602

Kooij SJ, Bejerot S, Blackwell A, et al: European consensus statement on diagnosis and treatment of adult ADHD: the European Network Adult ADHD. BMC Psychiatry 10:67, 2010 20815868

Ladhani NN, Shah PS, Murphy KE, et al: Prenatal amphetamine exposure and birth outcomes: a systematic review and metaanalysis. Am J Obstet Gynecol 205(3):219.e1–219.e7, 2011 21658669

Lapalme M, Déry M, Dubé M, et al: Developmental course of ADHD symptoms based on multi-rater report in girls and boys with or without a disruptive behavior disorder. J Emot Behav Disord 26(2):106–118, 2018

Lara C, Fayyad J, de Graaf R, et al: Childhood predictors of adult attention-deficit/hyperactivity disorder: results from the World Health Organization World Mental Health Survey Initiative. Biol Psychiatry 65(1):46–54, 2009 19006789

Larsson H, Dilshad R, Lichtenstein P, et al: Developmental trajectories of DSM-IV symptoms of attention-deficit/hyperactivity disorder: genetic effects, family risk and associated psychopathology. J Child Psychol Psychiatry 52(9):954–963, 2011 21434915

Larsson H, Chang Z, D'Onofrio BM, et al: The heritability of clinically diagnosed attention deficit hyperactivity disorder across the lifespan. Psychol Med 44(10):2223–2229, 2014 24107258

Leong C, Raymond C, Château D, et al: Psychotropic drug use before, during, and after pregnancy: a population-based study in a Canadian cohort (2001–2013). Can J Psychiatry 62(8):543–550, 2017 28545329

Levin JN: Amphetamine ingestion with biliary atresia. J Pediatr 79(1):130–131, 1971 5091254

Levin ED, Sledge D, Roach S, et al: Persistent behavioral impairment caused by embryonic methylphenidate exposure in zebrafish. Neurotoxicol Teratol 33(6):668–673, 2011 21741476

Liao TC, Lien YT, Wang S, et al: Comorbidity of atopic disorders with autism spectrum disorder and attention deficit/hyperactivity disorder. J Pediatr 171:248–255, 2016 26846570

Lie N: Follow-ups of children with attention deficit hyperactivity disorder (ADHD): review of literature. Acta Psychiatr Scand Suppl 368:1–40, 1992 1642137

Liew Z, Ritz B, Rebordosa C, et al: Acetaminophen use during pregnancy, behavioral problems, and hyperkinetic disorders. JAMA Pediatr 168(4):313–320, 2014 24566677
Lin YT, Chen YC, Gau SS, et al: Associations between allergic diseases and attention deficit hyperactivity/oppositional defiant disorders in children. Pediatr Res 80(4):480–485, 2016 27356086
Lou HC, Henriksen L, Bruhn P, et al: Striatal dysfunction in attention deficit and hyperkinetic disorder. Arch Neurol 46(1):48–52, 1989 2783366
Louik C, Kerr S, Kelley KE, et al: Increasing use of ADHD medications in pregnancy. Pharmacoepidemiol Drug Saf 24(2):218–220, 2015 25630904
Luchicchi A, Lecca S, Melis M, et al: Maternal immune activation disrupts dopamine system in the offspring. Int J Neuropsychopharmacol 19(7):pyw007, 2016 26819283
Makris N, Biederman J, Valera EM, et al: Cortical thinning of the attention and executive function networks in adults with attention-deficit/hyperactivity disorder. Cereb Cortex 17(6):1364–1375, 2007 16920883
Makris N, Buka SL, Biederman J, et al: Attention and executive systems abnormalities in adults with childhood ADHD: a DT-MRI study of connections. Cereb Cortex 18(5):1210–1220, 2008 17906338
Mannuzza S, Klein RG, Addalli KA: Young adult mental status of hyperactive boys and their brothers: a prospective follow-up study. J Am Acad Child Adolesc Psychiatry 30(5):743–751, 1991 1938789
Mannuzza S, Klein RG, Bessler A, et al: Adult outcome of hyperactive boys: educational achievement, occupational rank, and psychiatric status. Arch Gen Psychiatry 50(7):565–576, 1993 8317950
Marchant BK, Reimherr FW, Robison D, et al: Psychometric properties of the Wender-Reimherr Adult Attention Deficit Disorder Scale. Psychol Assess 25(3):942–950, 2013 23647041
Matte B, Rohde LA, Grevet EH: ADHD in adults: a concept in evolution. Atten Defic Hyperact Disord 4(2):53–62, 2012 22588789
Matthews M, Nigg JT, Fair DA: Attention deficit hyperactivity disorder. Curr Top Behav Neurosci 16:235–266, 2014 24214656
McCarthy S, Asherson P, Coghill D, et al: Attention-deficit hyperactivity disorder: treatment discontinuation in adolescents and young adults. Br J Psychiatry 194(3):273–277, 2009 19252159
McManus S, Meltzer H, Brugha T, et al: Adult Psychiatric Morbidity in England 2007: Results of a Household Survey. Leeds, UK, The NHS Information Centre, 2009
Mészáros A, Czobor P, Bálint S, et al: Pharmacotherapy of adult attention deficit hyperactivity disorder (ADHD): a meta-analysis. Int J Neuropsychopharmacol 12(8):1137–1147, 2009 19580697
Milberger S, Biederman J, Faraone SV, et al: Further evidence of an association between attention-deficit/hyperactivity disorder and cigarette smoking. Findings from a high-risk sample of siblings. Am J Addict 6(3):205–217, 1997a 9256986
Milberger S, Biederman J, Faraone SV, et al: Pregnancy, delivery and infancy complications and attention deficit hyperactivity disorder: issues of gene-environment interaction. Biol Psychiatry 41(1):65–75, 1997b 8988797
Milkovich L, van der Berg BJ: Effects of antenatal exposure to anorectic drugs. Am J Obstet Gynecol 129(6):637–642, 1977 920764
Minde K, Eakin L, Hechtman L, et al: The psychosocial functioning of children and spouses of adults with ADHD. J Child Psychol Psychiatry 44(4):637–646, 2003 12751853
Moffitt TE, Houts R, Asherson P, et al: Is adult ADHD a childhood-onset neurodevelopmental disorder? Evidence from a four-decade longitudinal cohort study. Am J Psychiatry 172(10):967–977, 2015 25998281
Mongia M, Hechtman L: Cognitive behavior therapy for adults with attention-deficit/hyperactivity disorder: a review of recent randomized controlled trials. Curr Psychiatry Rep 14(5):561–567, 2012 22878974
Monuteaux MC, Mick E, Faraone SV, et al: The influence of sex on the course and psychiatric correlates of ADHD from childhood to adolescence: a longitudinal study. J Child Psychol Psychiatry 51(3):233–241, 2010 19769586

Morgensterns E, Alfredsson J, Hirvikoski T: Structured skills training for adults with ADHD in an outpatient psychiatric context: an open feasibility trial. Atten Defic Hyperact Disord 8(2):101–111, 2016 26410823

Mostert JC, Onnink AMH, Klein M, et al: Cognitive heterogeneity in adult attention deficit/hyperactivity disorder: a systematic analysis of neuropsychological measurements. Eur Neuropsychopharmacol 25(11):2062–2074, 2015 26336867

Nadeau KG, Quinn P: Women's AD/HD Self-Assessment Symptom Inventory (SASI). Washington, DC, Advantage Books, 2002. Available at: http://www.merkercounseling.com/ADHDSelfAssessmentWomen.pdf. Accessed February 4, 2021.

Nanovskaya TN, Oncken C, Fokina VM, et al: Bupropion sustained release for pregnant smokers: a randomized, placebo-controlled trial. Am J Obstet Gynecol 216(4):e1–e9, 2017 27890648

National Institute for Health and Care Excellence: Attention Deficit Hyperactivity Disorder: The NICE Guideline on Diagnosis and Management of ADHD in Children, Young People, and Adults. Leicester, UK, The British Psychological Society and The Royal College of Psychiatrists, 2008

Nazar BP, Bernardes C, Peachey G, et al: The risk of eating disorders comorbid with attention-deficit/hyperactivity disorder: a systematic review and meta-analysis. Int J Eat Disord 49(12):1045–1057, 2016 27859581

Neale BM, Medland SE, Ripke S, et al: Meta-analysis of genome-wide association studies of attention-deficit/hyperactivity disorder. J Am Acad Child Adolesc Psychiatry 49(9):884–897, 2010 20732625

Newport DJ, Hostetter AL, Juul SH, et al: Prenatal psychostimulant and antidepressant exposure and risk of hypertensive disorders of pregnancy. J Clin Psychiatry 77(11):1538–1545, 2016 28076672

Nigg JT, Nikolas M, Mark Knottnerus G, et al: Confirmation and extension of association of blood lead with attention-deficit/hyperactivity disorder (ADHD) and ADHD symptom domains at population-typical exposure levels. J Child Psychol Psychiatry 51(1):58–65, 2010 19941632

Nijmeijer JS, Hartman CA, Rommelse NN, et al: Perinatal risk factors interacting with catechol O-methyltransferase and the serotonin transporter gene predict ASD symptoms in children with ADHD. J Child Psychol Psychiatry 51(11):1242–1250, 2010 20868372

Nora JJ, Vargo TA, Nora AH, et al: Dexamphetamine: a possible environmental trigger in cardiovascular malformations. Lancet 1(7659):1290–1291, 1970 4192516

Nörby U, Winbladh B, Källén K: Perinatal outcomes after treatment with ADHD medication during pregnancy. Pediatrics 140(6):e20170747, 2017 29127207

Nutt DJ, Fone K, Asherson P, et al: Evidence-based guidelines for management of attention-deficit/hyperactivity disorder in adolescents in transition to adult services and in adults: recommendations from the British Association for Psychopharmacology. J Psychopharmacol 21(1):10–41, 2007 17092962

Ogdie MN, Macphie IL, Minassian SL, et al: A genomewide scan for attention-deficit/hyperactivity disorder in an extended sample: suggestive linkage on 17p11. Am J Hum Genet 72(5):1268–1279, 2003 12687500

Ordean A, Wong S, Graves L: No. 349-substance use in pregnancy. J Obstet Gynaecol Can 39(10):922.e2–937.e2, 2017 28935057

Ottosen C, Petersen L, Larsen JT, et al: Gender differences in associations between attention-deficit/hyperactivity disorder and substance use disorder. J Am Acad Child Adolesc Psychiatry 55(3):227–34.e4, 2016 26903256

Owens EB, Zalecki C, Gillette P, et al: Girls with childhood ADHD as adults: cross-domain outcomes by diagnostic persistence. J Consult Clin Psychol 85(7):723–736, 2017 28414486

Paloyelis Y, Mehta MA, Kuntsi J, et al: Functional MRI in ADHD: a systematic literature review. Expert Rev Neurother 7(10):1337–1356, 2007 17939771

Paris JJ, Frye CA: Estrous cycle, pregnancy, and parity enhance performance of rats in object recognition or object placement tasks. Reproduction 136(1):105–115, 2008 18390689

Peterson K, McDonagh MS, Fu R: Comparative benefits and harms of competing medications for adults with attention-deficit hyperactivity disorder: a systematic review and indirect comparison meta-analysis. Psychopharmacology (Berl) 197(1):1–11, 2008 18026719

Philipp E: Guanfacine in the treatment of hypertension due to pre-eclamptic toxaemia in thirty women. Br J Clin Pharmacol 10(suppl 1):137S–140S, 1980 6994768
Philipsen A, Jans T, Graf E, et al: Effects of group psychotherapy, individual counseling, methylphenidate, and placebo in the treatment of adult attention-deficit/hyperactivity disorder: a randomized clinical trial. JAMA Psychiatry 72(12):1199–1210, 2015 26536057
Piñeiro-Dieguez B, Balanzá-Martínez V, García-García P, et al: Psychiatric comorbidity at the time of diagnosis in adults with ADHD: the CAT Study. J Atten Disord 20(12):1066–1075, 2016 24464326
Pliszka SR: Comorbidity of attention-deficit/hyperactivity disorder with psychiatric disorder: an overview. J Clin Psychiatry 59(suppl 7):50–58, 1998 9680053
Pliszka SR, Glahn DC, Semrud-Clikeman M, et al: Neuroimaging of inhibitory control areas in children with attention deficit hyperactivity disorder who were treatment naive or in long-term treatment. Am J Psychiatry 163(6):1052–1060, 2006 16741206
Poser CM, Kassirer MR, Peyser JM: Benign encephalopathy of pregnancy: preliminary clinical observations. Acta Neurol Scand 73(1):39–43, 1986 3953258
Post RE, Kurlansik SL: Diagnosis and management of adult attention-deficit/hyperactivity disorder. Am Fam Physician 85(9):890–896, 2012 22612184
Pottegård A, Hallas J, Andersen JT, et al: First-trimester exposure to methylphenidate: a population-based cohort study. J Clin Psychiatry 75(1):e88–e93, 2014 24502866
Prevatt F, Yelland S: An empirical evaluation of ADHD coaching in college students. J Atten Disord 19(8):666–677, 2015 23509112
Quinn PO: Treating adolescent girls and women with ADHD: gender-specific issues. J Clin Psychol 61(5):579–587, 2005 15723425
Quinn PO, Madhoo M: A review of attention-deficit/hyperactivity disorder in women and girls: uncovering this hidden diagnosis. Prim Care Companion CNS Disord 16(3):10, 2014 25317366
Renoux C, Shin JY, Dell'Aniello S, et al: Prescribing trends of attention-deficit hyperactivity disorder (ADHD) medications in UK primary care, 1995–2015. Br J Clin Pharmacol 82(3):858–868, 2016 27145886
Rivero O, Sich S, Popp S, et al: Impact of the ADHD-susceptibility gene CDH13 on development and function of brain networks. Eur Neuropsychopharmacol 23(6):492–507, 2013 22795700
Rösler M, Retz W, Thome J, et al: Psychopathological rating scales for diagnostic use in adults with attention-deficit/hyperactivity disorder (ADHD). Eur Arch Psychiatry Clin Neurosci 256(suppl 1):i3–i11, 2006 16977549
Rubia K, Smith AB, Brammer MJ, et al: Abnormal brain activation during inhibition and error detection in medication-naive adolescents with ADHD. Am J Psychiatry 162(6):1067–1075, 2005 15930054
Sciberras E, Mulraney M, Silva D, et al: Prenatal risk factors and the etiology of ADHD: review of existing evidence. Curr Psychiatry Rep 19(1):1, 2017 28091799
Secnik K, Swensen A, Lage MJ: Comorbidities and costs of adult patients diagnosed with attention-deficit hyperactivity disorder. Pharmacoeconomics 23(1):93–102, 2005 15693731
Seidman LJ, Doyle A, Fried R, et al: Neuropsychological function in adults with attention-deficit/hyperactivity disorder. Psychiatr Clin North Am 27(2):261–282, 2004a 15063997
Seidman LJ, Valera EM, Bush G: Brain function and structure in adults with attention-deficit/hyperactivity disorder. Psychiatr Clin North Am 27(2):323–347, 2004b 15064000
Seidman LJ, Valera EM, Makris N: Structural brain imaging of attention-deficit/hyperactivity disorder. Biol Psychiatry 57(11):1263–1272, 2005 15949998
Seidman LJ, Valera EM, Makris N, et al: Dorsolateral prefrontal and anterior cingulate cortex volumetric abnormalities in adults with attention-deficit/hyperactivity disorder identified by magnetic resonance imaging. Biol Psychiatry 60(10):1071–1080, 2006 16876137
Semrud-Clikeman M, Filipek PA, Biederman J, et al: Attention-deficit hyperactivity disorder: magnetic resonance imaging morphometric analysis of the corpus callosum. J Am Acad Child Adolesc Psychiatry 33(6):875–881, 1994 8083145
Seo JY, Lee CS, Park CS, et al: Mediating effect of depressive symptoms on the relationship between adult attention deficit hyperactivity disorder and quality of life. Psychiatry Investig 11(2):131–136, 2014 24843367

Sharp K, Brindle PM, Brown MW, et al: Memory loss during pregnancy. Br J Obstet Gynaecol 100(3):209–215, 1993 8476824
Shaw P, Stringaris A, Nigg J, et al: Emotion dysregulation in attention deficit hyperactivity disorder. Am J Psychiatry 171(3):276–293, 2014 24480998
Sherman DK, Iacono WG, McGue MK: Attention-deficit hyperactivity disorder dimensions: a twin study of inattention and impulsivity-hyperactivity. J Am Acad Child Adolesc Psychiatry 36(6):745–753, 1997 9183128
Short SJ, Lubach GR, Karasin AI, et al: Maternal influenza infection during pregnancy impacts postnatal brain development in the rhesus monkey. Biol Psychiatry 67(10):965–973, 2010 20079486
Simon V, Czobor P, Bálint S, et al: Prevalence and correlates of adult attention-deficit hyperactivity disorder: meta-analysis. Br J Psychiatry 194(3):204–211, 2009 19252145
Siu AL, U.S. Preventive Services Task Force: Behavioral and pharmacotherapy interventions for tobacco smoking cessation in adults, including pregnant women: U.S. Preventive Services Task Force Recommendation Statement. Ann Intern Med 163(8):622–634, 2015 26389730
Skodzik T, Holling H, Pedersen A: Long-term memory performance in adult ADHD. J Atten Disord 21(4):267–283, 2017 24232170
Skoglund C, Kopp Kallner H, Skalkidou A, et al: Association of attention-deficit/hyperactivity disorder with teenage birth among women and girls in Sweden. JAMA Netw Open 2(10):e1912463, 2019 31577361
Smalley SL, Kustanovich V, Minassian SL, et al: Genetic linkage of attention-deficit/hyperactivity disorder on chromosome 16p13, in a region implicated in autism. Am J Hum Genet 71(4):959–963, 2002 12187510
Smith L, Yonekura ML, Wallace T, et al: Effects of prenatal methamphetamine exposure on fetal growth and drug withdrawal symptoms in infants born at term. J Dev Behav Pediatr 24(1):17–23, 2003 12584481
Sobanski E: Psychiatric comorbidity in adults with attention-deficit/hyperactivity disorder (ADHD). Eur Arch Psychiatry Clin Neurosci 256(suppl 1):i26–i31, 2006 16977548
Solanto MV, Marks DJ, Wasserstein J, et al: Efficacy of meta-cognitive therapy for adult ADHD. Am J Psychiatry 167(8):958–968, 2010 20231319
Spencer TJ, Biederman J, Mick E: Attention-deficit/hyperactivity disorder: diagnosis, lifespan, comorbidities, and neurobiology. Ambul Pediatr 7(1 suppl):73–81, 2007 17261486
Spigset O, Brede WR, Zahlsen K: Excretion of methylphenidate in breast milk. Am J Psychiatry 164(2):348, 2007 17267805
Sprich S, Biederman J, Crawford MH, et al: Adoptive and biological families of children and adolescents with ADHD. J Am Acad Child Adolesc Psychiatry 39(11):1432–1437, 2000 11068899
Stepp SD, Burke JD, Hipwell AE, et al: Trajectories of attention deficit hyperactivity disorder and oppositional defiant disorder symptoms as precursors of borderline personality disorder symptoms in adolescent girls. J Abnorm Child Psychol 40(1):7–20, 2012 21671009
Stevens SE, Sonuga-Barke EJ, Kreppner JM, et al: Inattention/overactivity following early severe institutional deprivation: presentation and associations in early adolescence. J Abnorm Child Psychol 36(3):385–398, 2008 17965931
Suskauer SJ, Simmonds DJ, Fotedar S, et al: Functional magnetic resonance imaging evidence for abnormalities in response selection in attention deficit hyperactivity disorder: differences in activation associated with response inhibition but not habitual motor response. J Cogn Neurosci 20(3):478–493, 2008 18004945
Thapar A, Cooper M: Attention deficit hyperactivity disorder. Lancet 387(10024):1240–1250, 2016 26386541
Thapar A, Holmes J, Poulton K, et al: Genetic basis of attention deficit and hyperactivity. Br J Psychiatry 174:105–111, 1999 10211163
Thapar A, Rice F, Hay D, et al: Prenatal smoking might not cause attention-deficit/hyperactivity disorder: evidence from a novel design. Biol Psychiatry 66(8):722–727, 2009 19596120
Theiling J, Petermann F: Neuropsychological profiles on the WAIS-IV of adults with ADHD. J Atten Disord 20(11):913–924, 2016 24448224

Thomas R, Sanders S, Doust J, et al: Prevalence of attention-deficit/hyperactivity disorder: a systematic review and meta-analysis. Pediatrics 135(4):e994–e1001, 2015 25733754

Treas J, Tai T: Gender inequality in housework across 20 European nations: lessons from gender stratification theories. Sex Roles 74:495–511, 2016

Valera EM, Faraone SV, Murray KE, et al: Meta-analysis of structural imaging findings in attention-deficit/hyperactivity disorder. Biol Psychiatry 61(12):1361–1369, 2007 16950217

van Lieshout M, Luman M, Twisk JWR, et al: A 6-year follow-up of a large European cohort of children with attention-deficit/hyperactivity disorder-combined subtype: outcomes in late adolescence and young adulthood. Eur Child Adolesc Psychiatry 25(9):1007–1017, 2016 26837866

Vidal-Estrada R, Bosch-Munso R, Nogueira-Morais M, et al: Psychological treatment of attention deficit hyperactivity disorder in adults: a systematic review. Actas Esp Psiquiatr 40(3):147–154, 2012 22723133

Vitola ES, Bau CH, Salum GA, et al: Exploring DSM-5 ADHD criteria beyond young adulthood: phenomenology, psychometric properties and prevalence in a large three-decade birth cohort. Psychol Med 47(4):744–754, 2017 27866484

Vysniauske R, Verburgh L, Oosterlaan J, et al: The effects of physical exercise on functional outcomes in the treatment of ADHD: a meta-analysis. J Atten Disord 24(5):644–654, 2020 26861158

Wajnberg R, Diav-Citrin O, Shechtman S, et al: Pregnancy outcome after in utero exposure to methylphenidate: a prospective comparative cohort study. Reprod Toxicol 31(2):267, 2011

Ward MF, Wender PH, Reimherr FW: The Wender Utah Rating Scale: an aid in the retrospective diagnosis of childhood attention deficit hyperactivity disorder. Am J Psychiatry 150(6):885–890, 1993 8494063

Weiss G, Hechtman L, Milroy T, et al: Psychiatric status of hyperactives as adults: a controlled prospective 15-year follow-up of 63 hyperactive children. J Am Acad Child Psychiatry 24(2):211–220, 1985 3989165

Wender PH: Attention-Deficit Hyperactivity Disorder in Adults. New York, Oxford University Press, 1995

Wender PH, Wolf LE, Wasserstein J: Adults with ADHD: an overview. Ann N Y Acad Sci 931:1–16, 2001 11462736

Wilens TE, Spencer TJ, Biederman J: Are attention-deficit hyperactivity disorder and the psychoactive substance use disorders really related? Harv Rev Psychiatry 3(3):160–162, 1995 9384944

Wilens TE, Faraone SV, Biederman J: Attention-deficit/hyperactivity disorder in adults. JAMA 292(5):619–623, 2004 15292088

Willcutt EG: The prevalence of DSM-IV attention-deficit/hyperactivity disorder: a meta-analytic review. Neurotherapeutics 9(3):490–499, 2012 22976615

Williams NM, Franke B, Mick E, et al: Genome-wide analysis of copy number variants in attention deficit hyperactivity disorder: the role of rare variants and duplications at 15q13.3. Am J Psychiatry 169(2):195–204, 2012 22420048

Wright TE, Schuetter R, Tellei J, Sauvage L: Methamphetamines and pregnancy outcomes. J Addict Med 9(2):111–117, 2015 25599434

Xiang AH, Wang X, Martinez MP, et al: Maternal gestational diabetes mellitus, Type 1 Diabetes, and Type 2 Diabetes during pregnancy and risk of ADHD in offspring. Diabetes Care 41(12):2502–2508, 2018 30373735

Young S, Emilsson B, Sigurdsson JF, et al: A randomized controlled trial reporting functional outcomes of cognitive-behavioural therapy in medication-treated adults with ADHD and comorbid psychopathology. Eur Arch Psychiatry Clin Neurosci 267(3):267–276, 2017 27752827

Young S, Adamo N, Ásgeirsdóttir BB, et al: Females with ADHD: an expert consensus statement taking a lifespan approach providing guidance for the identification and treatment of attention-deficit/ hyperactivity disorder in girls and women. BMC Psychiatry 20(1):404, 2020 32787804

Zametkin AJ, Nordahl TE, Gross M, et al: Cerebral glucose metabolism in adults with hyperactivity of childhood onset. N Engl J Med 323(20):1361–1366, 1990 2233902

Zametkin AJ, Liebenauer LL, Fitzgerald GA, et al: Brain metabolism in teenagers with attention-deficit hyperactivity disorder. Arch Gen Psychiatry 50(5):333–340, 1993 8489322

# CHAPTER 24

# Forensic Issues in Perinatal Psychiatry

Susan Hatters Friedman, M.D.
Aimee Kaempf, M.D.
Jacqueline Landess, M.D., J.D.
Sarah M. Kauffman, M.D.

Reproductive psychiatry has many intersections with forensic psychiatry and the legal system. Issues of informed consent for treatment or voluntary termination of pregnancy (VTOP), mothering and risk, reproductive psychiatry in corrections, and infertility are areas for which an understanding of forensic and legal issues is invaluable for the reproductive psychiatrist. This chapter provides an overview of these intersections for the practicing psychiatrist.

When women obtain a VTOP, their capacity to provide informed consent must be considered. Additional hurdles include recent U.S. laws requiring state-generated "informed consent" information, which is distinct from the process of obtaining informed consent. Informed consent is also critical in pregnancy and postpartum. Psychiatrists often have worries about malpractice risk from prescribing medications in pregnancy. However, it is critical for the psychiatrist not to fail to treat the pregnant woman, which can also precipitate bad outcomes and malpractice risk. Proactive discussions with women of childbearing age, mothers, and families are paramount. Rarely, psychiatrists may need to assess pregnant women for involuntary treatment (i.e., treatment over objection) and testify regarding this assessment.

Capacity and risk are similarly at issue in parenting capacity evaluations. As mandated reporters, reproductive psychiatrists must consider the risk of child maltreatment among their patients. They need to consider not only the risk of peripartum suicide but also the risk of infanticide. Another specific population is women who are incarcerated, who are often of childbearing age. Women may experience pregnancy and delivery while incarcerated, and most incarcerated women have children. Finally, gestational surrogacy may present legal and psychiatric issues for both the gestational carrier and the intended mother.

## Voluntary Termination of Pregnancy and Informed Consent

Approximately half of all pregnancies in the United States are unintended, with about 40% of unintended pregnancies ending in VTOP (Finer and Zolna 2016). Rates of unintended pregnancies in America are highest among women who are younger in age (18–24 years), who are of low income, who have not completed high school, who are non-Hispanic Black, and who are cohabiting with a partner but never married (Finer and Zolna 2016).

The Centers for Disease Control and Prevention (CDC) has collected data regarding VTOPs in the United States since 1969. The latest available data (from 2015) indicated a rate of 11.8 terminations per 1,000 women ages 15–44 years, and a ratio of 188 terminations per 1,000 live births. In the United States, women in their 20s account for most terminations. Approximately 91% of terminations occurred in the first trimester, with only 1.3% occurring after 21 weeks' gestation. Approximately one-quarter were described as early medical terminations (nonsurgical termination of pregnancy at ≤8 weeks' gestation). Since 2006, the number, rate, and ratio of terminations reported to the CDC have steadily declined, with a growing percentage classified as early medical terminations (Jatlaoui et al. 2018).

In the landmark case *Roe v. Wade* (1973), the U.S. Supreme Court ruled that unduly restrictive state regulation of VTOP is unconstitutional, thereby effectively legalizing the procedure. Since *Roe v. Wade,* states have created various laws aimed at regulating the circumstances under which VTOPs can be obtained. Common legislative provisions include hospital requirements for terminations, limits on public funding, restrictions on private insurance coverage, gestational age limits, bans on "partial birth" terminations, allowing health care providers or institutions to refuse termination services, state-mandated counseling, waiting periods, and mandated parental involvement in a minor's decision to have a termination (Guttmacher Institute 2019a). The most common of such provisions are "informed consent" laws requiring that women seeking VTOPs be presented with state-created informational materials before a termination can be performed (Daniels et al. 2016).

Informed consent (separate from the provisions required by various states, which are described later) is the process whereby communication between a patient and physician results in a patient's ability to make a knowledgeable decision to consent to or decline a specific medical intervention. Informed consent is an ethical and legal requirement and stems from an individual's right to determine what happens to her body. Informed consent requires three fundamental elements: 1) competency of the patient (or surrogate) to make decisions, 2) disclosure to the patient of relevant information, and 3) lack of coercion (or voluntariness) in decision-making (Gossman et al. 2019). Standards for what information needs to be disclosed by clinicians to meet informed consent requirements vary by state but generally include

1. The diagnosis or medical condition,
2. The nature and purpose of the proposed intervention,
3. The risks and benefits of the proposed intervention, and

4. The risks and benefits of other treatment options, including forgoing treatment (Gossman et al. 2019).

As with all medical decisions requiring informed consent, there can be complexity in determining a patient's capacity to make decisions regarding VTOP. Historically, women with intellectual or mental disabilities have been denied reproductive freedoms. In 2006, the Convention on the Rights of Persons with Disabilities sought to change these attitudes and provide women with reproductive autonomy by tailoring decision making to the needs of the specific individual (Ngwena 2018). In women with severe mental illness, this tailored approach can take the form of assisted or surrogate decision-making depending on the patient's decision-making capacity (Coverdale et al. 2004).

It is important to note that most women with mental illness are able to demonstrate the cognitive understanding and appreciation of the consequences of a VTOP for themselves and their fetus and to use this to communicate a voluntary decision. There are cases, however, in which this ability may be acutely or chronically impaired. The restricted time window in which decisions about termination must be made can be particularly challenging. In women who have impaired capacity during this crucial period, various strategies can be implemented to assist in decision-making. The first step in this process involves determining whether the patient has a guardian and, if so, determining whether the guardian has the authority to make decisions concerning pregnancy (Zalpuri et al. 2015). If such a guardian does exist, a substituted judgment should take into consideration the patient's long-standing values and preferences. If such a guardian does not exist, assisted decision-making may be utilized. Assisted decision-making can involve strategies such as discussing with the woman her past preferences regarding pregnancy and motherhood and then helping to guide her decision-making based on any previously stated preferences.

Since 2010, more and more states have adopted termination "informed consent" statutes that, as noted earlier, require women seeking terminations be presented with state-authored informational materials prior to the procedure (Daniels et al. 2016). These statutes have little to do with standard informed consent. Instead, they involve giving women seeking VTOPs state-authored information about the alternatives and risks to termination and about embryological and fetal development (Daniels et al. 2016). Of the 37 states identified by 2013 as having these laws, 23 states had made their material available to the public. These were included in an analysis that found that 31% of the statements in the "informed consent" material were medically inaccurate (with inaccurate statements ranging from 15% to 46% of the material for individual states). Examples of medically inaccurate information included statements such as the head being formed by 2 weeks and the ability to record brain activity at 4 weeks. These inaccurate statements call into question the constitutionality of these laws. Although "informed consent" laws were upheld by the Supreme Court in *Planned Parenthood of Southeastern Pennsylvania v. Casey* (1992), it is noted that information should be "truthful" and "nonmisleading" and help the woman to make a "thoughtful and informed" decision (Daniels et al. 2016). This mandatory dissemination of inaccurate information is particularly concerning given that two-thirds of women seeking VTOP live in states with these mandates (Daniels et al. 2016).

In addition to inaccurate information regarding embryological development, the mandated counseling in eight states includes statements about adverse psychological responses to termination, and some cite an increased risk of suicidality after termination (Guttmacher Institute 2019b). Although studies have shown an increased rate of mental disorders and suicide attempts in women who undergo VTOP, these studies often have serious methodological problems, including not controlling for factors leading to the choice of termination or using inappropriate control groups (i.e., comparing women who have VTOPs with women who have never had a VTOP or who chose to give birth) (Biggs et al. 2018). This comparison is problematic because there may be significant differences among these groups, such as in financial resources or access to VTOP, that may be independently related to mental disorders. Data from the Turnaway Study (in which mothers who were refused VTOPs were compared with those granted VTOPs during a similar time period) showed that over a 5-year follow-up period, women who terminated a pregnancy were not at higher risk of suicidal ideation compared with women who were denied access to VTOPs. Additionally, the overall rates of suicidal ideation were low in both groups when compared with studies of pregnant and postpartum women (Biggs et al. 2018). Thus, "informed consent" for VTOP should not necessarily include the risk of increased suicidality secondary to having one.

Judicial bypass of parental consent for VTOP, in which a pregnant minor can obtain a VTOP with judicial consent as opposed to parental consent, occurs in most states (Friedman et al. 2015). These teenagers may legally be referred to as Jane Does. A metropolitan Ohio study considering the characteristics of Jane Does found that their mean age was 16.4 years and that they usually had long-term boyfriends. They had often shared that they were pregnant with trusted adults but not with their parents, out of concern of being kicked out of the house or of family violence. The vast majority (95%) were eventually granted the judicial bypass. Mental health professionals may be involved in these evaluations and, depending on the state, may be asked to opine whether the teenager is sufficiently mature or whether notification of her parents is against her best interests. In completing such evaluations, one must consider general principles of informed consent and determine whether the decision is being made knowingly, voluntarily, and with appropriate decision-making capacity (Friedman et al. 2015).

## Legal and Malpractice Concerns Regarding Medications in Pregnancy

Regarding the use of psychotropic medications in pregnancy, studies have predominantly been retrospective and therefore are prone to bias and limitations. In evaluating studies, readers must consider the risks associated with the mental illness itself, associated comorbidities such as substance use, and effects of poor prenatal care and of additional medications (Friedman and Hall 2013). For a detailed discussion of risk-risk analysis in treatment decisions, please see Chapter 8, "A Clinical Approach to Psychiatric Diagnosis and Treatment During Pregnancy." Some studies are based on whether women filled prescriptions, without querying whether the medication was ingested. Some studies fail to have an *a priori* hypothesis while running data about prescriptions across a wide range of potential outcomes. Other studies suffer from small sample sizes. Studies also conflict: whereas some studies have implicated selective serotonin reuptake inhibitors in adverse birth outcomes, others have found a lack of increase in birth defects (Friedman and Hall 2013).

Clinicians treating pregnant women must make rational decisions about medication, discuss this decision-making with the patient (who is the ultimate decision-maker), and document the encounter carefully. The clinician should educate the patient about the risk of untreated illness and the risk of medications. It is critical that the patient understand that a lack of medication use does not ensure a safe pregnancy. Family or significant others should also be involved in these discussions whenever possible (Friedman and Hall 2013). Informed consent forms are appropriate for electroconvulsive therapy, as in the nonpregnant population; however, informed consent documents are not necessary for pregnant women regarding medications in general. Rather, it is the discussion and shared decision-making that are crucial.

Psychiatrists should be aware that unplanned pregnancy is more common among women with mental illness, and many women become pregnant while being treated with psychotropic medications. Thus, it is important to discuss the potential for pregnancy and options for birth control with all women of childbearing age who enter psychiatric treatment, regardless of whether they report being sexually active. Medications known to be relatively safe in pregnancy should be considered when prescribing for women of childbearing age—even when women report no current plans for pregnancy. If a patient becomes pregnant unintentionally, she should know to be in contact with the psychiatrist, and the psychiatrist should not make knee-jerk decisions in these cases. Consultation with colleagues is invaluable in lawsuit prevention.

Lawsuits may occur related to negative birth outcomes. One must remember, however, that lawsuits can also occur because of wrongful death by suicide or infanticide because appropriate treatment was not given in the perinatal period (Friedman and Hall 2013). A bias toward failure to treat occurs when physicians are concerned only about acts of commission, in which the treatment provided by the doctor leads to a negative outcome, rather than acts of omission—that is, the lack of treatment of the illness (Friedman 2015; Miller 2009). One should be aware of this possible bias and ensure that, in discussions with patients, one considers and carefully describes both the risks of treating and the risks of not treating.

## Involuntary Treatment and Treating Over Objection

Antipsychotic medication may be necessary on an involuntary basis if an acutely psychotic patient refuses medication despite a clear need for treatment. This may occur during pregnancy. For a detailed discussion of emergency management of patients in pregnancy, please see Chapter 10, "A Treatment Approach to Psychiatric Emergencies in the Perinatal Period." As discussed earlier, the psychiatrist should assess the patient's capacity to provide informed consent. In some cases, she will have misconceptions about the use of medications in pregnancy. When completing evaluations and preparing potential testimony for involuntary treatment and pregnancy, the psychiatrist should consider diagnosis, treatment rationale, why capacity is lacking, and any less restrictive alternatives. In these cases, psychiatrists should provide clear descriptions regarding the risk of forgoing treatment in addition to any concerns about the harms that may arise from treatment (Friedman et al. 2018). The psychiatrist should also communicate with the obstetrical team to ensure coordination of care.

## Parenting Capacity Evaluations

Parenting capacity involves the ability of parents to care for and meet the needs of their children appropriately. Assessment of parenting capacity may arise in various legal contexts, including termination of parental rights proceedings, custody disputes, and allegations of child abuse or neglect (Grisso 2003). Mental health professionals may be asked to provide an opinion regarding an individual's ability to parent. Determining fitness to parent is an inherently difficult task because there is no clear consensus regarding what constitutes minimal parental fitness (Budd 2005). Furthermore, future behaviors, such as child abuse and violence, are difficult to predict, and parenting values and childrearing styles differ across families and cultures (Grisso 2003). Complicating matters, parenting capacity evaluations typically occur within the legal arena, which has its own set of challenges (Budd 2005).

Assessment of parenting capacity should focus on an individual's ability to parent, the parent–child relationship, and whether parenting is sufficient to meet the child's basic safety and emotional needs (Budd 2005). Additionally, parenting skills should be evaluated with respect to the specific developmental needs of the children involved. Risk factors that may be linked to child maltreatment include active psychiatric symptoms or substance abuse, childhood history of abuse, social isolation, unrealistic expectations, failure to appropriately interpret and respond to the child's cues, parental stress, unsafe home environment, and a history of violence. Protective factors include good social support, attunement to the child's needs, positive parental role models, insight into mental health difficulties, treatment adherence, and the ability to recognize how the parent's mental illness or history of abuse may impact the child (Jacobsen et al. 1997). In addition, the psychiatric evaluator should be aware that socioeconomic factors may represent "equal or greater risk to children than the individual risk of parental mental illness" (Benjet et al. 2003). Evaluators tend to advocate for "optimal family environments for children" rather than focus on what is simply adequate (Benjet et al. 2003). Further complicating psychiatric assessment, courts may ask evaluators to comment on what constitutes minimally adequate care for the child or if a child is at imminent risk of harm, both conditions that an evaluator may have difficulty determining (Benjet et al. 2003).

Although no definitive data have linked mental illness with parental unfitness, per se, courts may explicitly or implicitly presume unfitness based on a parent's substance use disorder, intellectual disability, or other psychiatric illness (Melton et al. 2007). Some laws explicitly identify conditions that are grounds for termination of parental rights. For instance, Nebraska law states that termination may occur if a parent is unfit due to "habitual use of intoxicating liquor or narcotic drugs" (Nebraska Rev Stat 43-292 2020). Missouri law presumes unfitness if a parent has pled guilty or been convicted of a drug felony within the previous 3 years and has at least one other child who has been found to be abused or neglected or if the parent has failed to complete recommended treatment (Mo Ann. Stat. 211.447 2011). Other states list factors for the court to consider in determining fitness rather than listing strict conditions. Under Massachusetts law, for example, courts must consider whether a parent has a psychiatric condition that is "likely to continue for a prolonged, indeterminate period" and makes the parent "unlikely to provide minimally acceptable care for the child" (Mass Ann. Laws 2021). In summary, jurisdictions vary in how mental illness is defined, determined, and applied in parental fitness assessments. Psychiatric evaluators are in a unique position to provide education to legal professionals and to dispel stereotypes of mental illness.

Evaluation of parenting capacity for the courts is a forensic assessment. The forensic evaluation differs from a clinical evaluation in that the traditional doctor–patient relationship does not apply. Various clinical, legal, and ethical dilemmas arise when a mental health professional attempts to serve as both treating clinician and forensic evaluator. Forensic and clinical roles are fundamentally different and conflicting with regard to the overall goal of the work, the nature of the relationship between evaluator and evaluee, assessment strategies, and ethical principles entailed (Strasburger et al. 1997). Clinicians not trained in forensic assessment should be wary of performing parenting capacity assessments for legal purposes. Mistakes commonly seen in parental fitness evaluations include failure to disclose the purpose of the evaluation and limitations of confidentiality, overreliance on a single source of information, and overstated conclusions and recommendations (Budd 2005). Such deficiencies may have significant ramifications in the lives of parents and children, resulting in crucial decisions regarding custody and parental rights being based on incomplete, invalid, or misleading information (Jacobsen et al. 1997). Given the inherent role of conflicts and important consequences in parenting capacity cases, mental health professionals should avoid acting as both treating clinician and forensic evaluator when questions of parental fitness arise (Strasburger et al. 1997).

## Child Abuse Risk and Duty to Report

Child maltreatment is usually conceptualized as including physical abuse, neglect, sexual abuse, and emotional abuse. Child maltreatment is usually defined by state law. *Physical abuse* includes intentional use of force against a child that may result in injury; *neglect* includes a caregiver's failure to meet the child's basic physical, medical, educational, and emotional needs; *sexual abuse* involves attempted sexual acts or exploitation; and *emotional abuse* involves behavior conveying to the child that he or she is worthless or valued only to meet the caregiver's needs (McEwan and Friedman 2016). There is an approximately tenfold difference between the prevalence of child maltreatment self-report and the reports to child protection agencies (McEwan and Friedman 2016). Approximately one-quarter of reported cases are substantiated in the United States (McEwan and Friedman 2016). In the cases not substantiated, there may be a lack of evidence, poor cooperation, investigatory issues, or a lack of maltreatment.

Although psychiatrists are mandated reporters of child maltreatment, they often have concerns about breaking confidentiality. However, completing the compulsory reporting may contribute in a positive way to the therapeutic process, especially if the professional discusses the need to report with the parent. Clinicians should keep in mind, however, that parents may be reluctant to seek treatment or to disclose symptoms for fear of being reported to child protective services (CPS) and losing custody. Even though treated mental illness is not specifically linked with child maltreatment, approximately one-quarter of mothers with serious mental illness will lose custody of their children, including approximately half of mothers with schizophrenia (McEwan and Friedman 2016).

Although parental mental illness is often asserted as a risk factor for child abuse, literature supporting this claim is limited. In reality, most parents who abuse children are not mentally ill (McEwan and Friedman 2016). Methodological issues often exist in studies that purport to demonstrate a higher risk of child maltreatment in parents with a history of mental illness. The psychiatrist should consider that mental illness that is appropriately treated would not be expected to lead to an increased violence risk in general. Friedman and McEwan (2018) found that parents with psychiatric symptoms who were treated at a psychiatric hospital were at lower risk of violence toward children than other parents in their same communities. Mental illness, then, should be considered a dynamic, rather than static, risk factor regarding violence risk toward children. Considering specific symptoms of a mental illness that may lead to child maltreatment is of utility; for example, disorganized thinking in schizophrenia may lead to neglect, whereas hallucinations could lead to violence (McEwan and Friedman 2016). Substance use and personality disorders are considered additional risk factors for violence against children and in general.

Physicians working with children and families should have basic knowledge of their statutory duty to report suspected abuse or neglect. Mandated reporting laws began to appear across the United States during the 1960s. The federal Child Abuse Prevention and Treatment Act, which was enacted in 1974, further formalized these statutes by requiring states, contingent on federal funding, to identify processes and procedures by which certain individuals were required to report suspicions of child maltreatment. Today, all states have mandated reporting statutes, but these laws vary in terms of the individuals or entities named as mandated reporters, the standards for making the report, the type of harm that is reportable, and whether the reporter's identity is disclosed (Child Welfare Information Gateway 2019a). Not surprisingly, many states designate professionals such as social workers, physicians, police, teachers, or others who have routine contact with children as mandated reporters; however, 18 states require universal mandated reporting regardless of profession (Child Welfare Information Gateway 2019a). State laws may also state that a designated professional must generally report "abuse or neglect" or more specifically define the prohibited harm. For instance, the District of Columbia requires reporting of suspicion of fetal alcohol spectrum disorder in infants younger than 12 months. Multiple states require film processors to report photographs or other media depicting child pornography, and other states specifically require reporting of child victims of human trafficking (McTavish et al. 2019).

Although the specific language varies, statutory standards generally require reporting from mandated reporters (e.g., physicians) when they suspect or have reason to suspect that a child has been abused or neglected (Landess and Friedman 2018). This is a relatively low standard, intended to overinclude cases of potential child maltreatment, which conceivably results in high numbers of false positives. Despite this low standard, existing literature confirms that physicians tend to underidentify and underreport abuse (Flaherty and Sege 2005). Professionals may not report because they do not believe the information received is reportable, perceive problems with CPS, or fear malpractice suits or retaliation or due to other personal bias (Badger 1989; Lindberg et al. 2015). Physicians may feel that reporting to CPS leads to no action or, worse, to an adverse outcome for the child or family. In terms of penalties, professionals who knowingly or willfully fail to make a report can be charged with a misdemeanor in most states. In some states, such as Florida, failure to report is a felony (Child Welfare Information Gateway 2019b). However, critics have pointed out that professionals often are not convicted or do not face stiff penalties for failing to report child maltreatment; for example, between 2004 and 2014 in Colorado, charges were filed in 65 cases for a failure to report, with only five resulting in convictions (Steffen 2014).

## Infanticide and Violence Risk Assessment

In analyzing the world literature, Friedman and Resnick (2007) found that although many cases of maternal infanticide occurred in the context of child abuse, some mothers made suicide attempts at the same time. Studies of maternal infanticide found that the mothers were often unemployed caregivers of their children in their early 20s who experienced psychiatric disorders. Among mothers who committed filicide (killing one's child who is younger than 18 years) in the general population, mothers were often socially isolated, of lower socioeconomic status, and full-time caregivers who had relationship problems or had been victimized by intimate partner violence. In some cases, crying or other child factors were identified as precipitants. Some mothers had previously maltreated their children, whereas others were devoted mothers with mental illness. Substance abuse was also seen in this population, as were psychosis and depression (Friedman and Resnick 2007). When specifically considering psychiatric samples of maternal filicide, these mothers had often experienced depression, psychosis, and suicidal thinking. Some had personality disorders. Significant stressors in life were often found. It was recommended that psychiatrists assess for risk of filicide systematically, such as they do for suicide, first entertaining the possibility that such an act could occur (Friedman and Resnick 2007).

Motives for maternal filicide initially described by Resnick (1969) and further described by Friedman and Resnick (2007) include *altruistic* (murder out of love), which may be part of an extended suicide or may occur for psychotic or nonpsychotic reasons (e.g., a child's debilitating illness); *acutely psychotic* (with no comprehensible motive, e.g., responding to command auditory hallucinations); *fatal maltreatment* (the final outcome of chronic neglect or abuse); *unwanted child*; and *partner revenge* (e.g., in the midst of a custody battle). Among the motives for filicide, altruistic filicide is often related to postpartum psychosis (PPP) or postpartum depression (PPD), and acutely psychotic filicide is often related to PPP (Friedman et al. 2019a). However, partner revenge, unwanted child, and fatal maltreatment cases are rarely related to PPP, although a mother with this diagnosis may experience difficulty providing for the infant's needs because of her psychosis. Specifically, in PPP, a mother may be at risk of child maltreatment due to delusional thinking, irritable mood state, or confusion. PPP itself elevates the risk of both infanticide and suicide (Friedman et al. 2019a). For a complete discussion of PPP, please see Chapter 16, "Postpartum Psychosis"; for suicide, please see Chapter 10.

Suicide is noted to be the cause of up to one-fifth of deaths in the postpartum period. If women with PPD are experiencing suicidal thoughts, the risk of infanticide must also be considered. Jennings et al. (1999) found that 41% of mothers with PPD experienced thoughts of harming their child. However, psychiatrists often still do not ask about thoughts of child harm (Friedman et al. 2008). Although many mothers may experience these thoughts, obviously only a small fraction ever act on them, but these thoughts should be queried and considered in the risk assessment. Specifically, mothers who report they are thinking about suicide should be directly asked about plans for their children should they commit suicide. Psychiatrists should also ask about hallucinations or delusions about the children, which may elevate the risk (Friedman and Resnick 2007). Overvalued or delusional beliefs about the infant should particularly be queried (Landess and Friedman 2018).

If thoughts of harming a child are present, one should consider whether they are related to OCD or due to psychosis. OCD occurring alone has not been demonstrated to increase risk of infanticide (Booth et al. 2014). In fact, intrusive thoughts about child harm are not uncommon in the postpartum period, and it is crucial that clinicians be able to distinguish between intrusive thoughts of harm that are ego-dystonic and horrifying to the mother (i.e., obsessions) and those that are ego-syntonic (i.e., delusions). For a complete discussion of OCD, please see Chapter 20, "Obsessive-Compulsive Disorder." Stigma against mental illness and media emphasis on cases of child killing have resulted in a culture in which most women are unaware of how common intrusive thoughts are in the postpartum period and are ashamed to reveal such thoughts. This shame can often lead to mothers being unwilling to seek care because of fear that health care professionals will report them to CPS. When evaluating a mother with infanticidal thoughts, therefore, clinicians should consider the child's risk and the need for notification of CPS and should carefully document their thinking, being careful to normalize the idea of obsessive intrusive thoughts and approach the topic without judgment so that women are more willing to share their experiences without fear of repercussion.

Approximately one-fifth to one-quarter of mothers who commit filicide commit suicide at the same time. Many mothers make a serious suicide attempt conjointly with the filicide but do not die (Friedman et al. 2008). In considering the difference between maternal filicide cases and maternal filicide-suicide cases, the traditional predictors of suicide were not able to distinguish between the mothers who attempted suicide and the mothers who did not. Mothers who committed suicide along with the filicide often had altruistic motives and were more likely to use firearms. Owning a firearm has been described as a risk factor for lethal acts in general but should also be considered among this population of mothers.

In general, marriage is considered a protective factor against suicide, as is being a mother to a child under 18. However, one must still consider the risk of both infanticide and suicide. Suggestions for prevention of filicide-suicide include appropriate treatment of mental illness, with careful evaluations of mothers regarding parenting and any suicidal or filicidal thoughts. Community education about symptoms of postpartum mental illness may also help mothers appropriately seek psychiatric treatment. Parents who have suicidal thinking or who have delusions involving their children should be further evaluated regarding their risk (Friedman et al. 2007).

Data concerning neonaticide are somewhat different from those concerning filicide. *Neonaticide* is a unique act of child murder that occurs in the first day of the child's life and has its own specific circumstances (Friedman 2019; Resnick 1970). Neonaticide is almost always an act of the mother alone. She has often not bonded with her fetus and may have experienced either denial or concealment of the pregnancy throughout. She often no longer has a relationship with the father of the baby and is often from a disadvantaged background. If she lives with her parents, she may have been afraid of being kicked out of her home or of being shunned by her cultural or religious community. Women who commit neonaticide often did not obtain prenatal care. The motive for neonaticide is commonly that the child is unwanted (Friedman 2019). Denial of pregnancy was described by Miller (2003) as including pervasive denial, affective denial, and psychotic denial. In *pervasive denial*, a woman may be totally unaware of her pregnancy, and her body may behave as though she were not pregnant, such as continuing to experience cyclical vaginal bleeding. Alternatively, in *affective denial*, the woman may be aware cognitively of her pregnancy but continue to act as though she were not pregnant. In these cases, she may have planned to get a VTOP but did not go through with it, hoping rather that the pregnancy would disappear (Friedman et al. 2007). Finally, in the rarer *psychotic denial*, a woman with a psychotic disorder and sometimes a history of custody loss denies that she could be pregnant. *Concealment of pregnancy*, alternatively, occurs when a woman consciously hides her pregnancy from others (Friedman and Resnick 2009).

Reproductive psychiatrists who are considering testifying as expert witnesses in child murder cases would be well advised to review literature regarding writing forensic reports and testifying in court, as well as understanding the legal standard for not guilty by reason of insanity or factors that mitigate the offense (Friedman et al. 2021).

## Pregnancy and Mothering in Corrections

Women are the fastest growing population in the U.S. correctional system, and most incarcerated women are of reproductive age, with 6%–10% of incarcerated women being pregnant (American Civil Liberties Union 2021; Clarke and Simon 2013). As in other areas of U.S. society, there are racial and ethnic disparities in the imprisoned population. Black women are more than twice as likely, and Hispanic women 1.3 times as likely, to be imprisoned as white women. The rate for Black women has been declining since 2000, whereas those for white and Hispanic women have been increasing (The Sentencing Project 2020).

Although the standards of perinatal care within the correctional system are the same as those in the community, providing an equivalent level of care during incarceration is difficult for a number of reasons, including higher rates of obstetrical risk factors among inmates and operational restrictions inherent to institutions. Compared with community samples, incarcerated women are more likely to have unplanned pregnancies complicated by lack of prenatal care, poor nutrition, trauma, substance abuse, mental illness, chronic medical problems, lack of social support, and low socioeconomic status (Clarke and Adashi 2011). Institutional barriers to providing prenatal care include the process of transferring women to outside medical facilities, coordination of care among correctional and community providers, delays in accessing emergency obstetrical services, and inmates' lack of control over living conditions, including sleep schedules, food choices, timing of meals, and activity levels (Clarke and Adashi 2011; Friedman et al. 2019b).

Several organizations, including the American College of Obstetricians and Gynecologists, the Federal Bureau of Prisons, and the National Commission on Correctional Health Care, have proposed standards for perinatal care in correctional settings, including pregnancy testing; access to pregnancy counseling and VTOP services, assessment and treatment for substance abuse and depression, delivery in a licensed hospital with facilities for high-risk pregnancies, and postpartum contraception (Committee on Health Care for Underserved Women of American College of Obstetricians and Gynecologists 2011). In practice, policies regarding pregnancy and the provision of perinatal care vary, with many states lacking prenatal care policies regarding routine medical examinations, treatment for women with high-risk pregnancies, and pregnancy outcomes reporting (National Women's Law Center 2010).

Correctional systems are increasingly faced with challenges centered around providing care to pregnant inmates. Pregnancy testing is not routine in institutions, which often rely on inmate self-report, with confirmation testing performed as needed (Committee on Health Care for Underserved Women of American College of Obstetricians and Gynecologists 2011; Kelsey et al. 2017). Although incarceration does not preclude a woman's right to access VTOP, inconsistent practices have led to unreliable access to VTOP services for inmates (Roth 2011). The routine use of restraints among pregnant inmates is controversial (Hall et al. 2015) and should be limited to absolute necessity involving an imminent risk of escape or harm that cannot be managed with other interventions (National Task Force on the Use of Restraints With Pregnant Women Under Correctional Custody 2012). Pregnancy-related education is especially important for this population, with perinatal education and doula programs showing positive results (Ferszt and Erickson-Owens 2008).

Despite the many challenges involved in providing care to pregnant inmates, studies show improved outcomes for pregnancies managed during incarceration than for women with similar risk factors whose pregnancies are managed in the community, with higher birth weights and lower rates of stillbirth (Knight and Plugge 2005; Sufrin et al. 2019). This suggests that certain aspects of confinement, such as access to prenatal care, stable housing, reduced exposure to violence, and restricted access to alcohol, tobacco, and illicit drugs, may promote perinatal outcomes among high-risk women (Friedman et al. 2020; Knight and Plugge 2005; Sufrin et al. 2019). Breastfeeding is not usually feasible in prison due to barriers such as physical separation from the infant and lack of access to breast pumping and storage equipment (Shlafer et al. 2018).

Less than one-quarter of American states have mother–baby units where infants can reside in an incarcerated setting with their mothers; most incarcerated women are separated from their infants shortly after birth (Friedman et al. 2020). These children are generally either placed in kinship care (i.e., care of children by relatives or, in some jurisdictions, close family friends) or in foster care. For children placed in kinship care, grandparents are the most common caregiver (Glaze and Maruschak 2010). Notably, children of incarcerated mothers are more likely to be placed in foster care than children of incarcerated fathers, which highlights the particularly devastating impact on a family when a mother is incarcerated (Glaze and Maruschak 2010).

In the United States, this separation can lead to termination of parental rights for the incarcerated mother. For children placed in foster care for longer than 15 months (including because their parent is in prison), the Adoption and Safe Families Act (1997) seeks to place them into permanent adoption, which necessitates termination of parental rights (Clarke and Simon 2013; Warner 2015). When a child is placed in foster care, it can be particularly hard for a mother to reunify with her child, with one study finding that incarcerated mothers were half as likely to regain custody of children in foster care compared with nonincarcerated women (Christian 2009).

Most female correctional facilities offer a parenting program, but most of these programs do not include visitation (Miller et al. 2014), despite contact during incarceration being an important predictor of reunification (Gilham 2012). However, most incarcerated women keep in some form of regular contact with their children. Even for those mothers who are afforded in-person visits, many factors such as geographical distance, a physical environment that is not child-friendly, security procedures, restrictions on physical contact, and short length of visitation can be problematic (O'Malley and Devaney 2016; Schubert et al. 2016). To address these challenges, some prisons have tried videoconferencing, with limited success (Cramer et al. 2017), and others have tried having the parent record bedtime stories and sending the recordings to their children (Poehlmann et al. 2010). Encouraging communication between incarcerated mothers and their children is important because prolonged separation has a significant impact on psychological outcomes for the children. Children of incarcerated mothers have been noted to be at increased risk for sleep disorders, depression, anger, and anxiety (Mignon and Ransford 2012).

## Infertility and the Law

The increasing use of reproductive technologies has led to complex ethical and legal considerations. (For a complete discussion of infertility and assisted reproductive technologies, please see Chapter 5, "Infertility and Perinatal Loss.") As an example, gestational surrogacy is increasingly used as a form of assisted reproduction, particularly for individuals who cannot or choose not to carry a child because of medical problems, age, marital status, male same-sex couples, transgender couples, or other reasons. In the United States, 18,400 infants were born from gestational carriers between 1999 and 2013, and most of these children were born after 2010 (Centers for Disease Control and Prevention 2016). *Gestational carriers* are women who become pregnant and give birth to a child with the intention of relinquishing the child to the intended parents. The surrogacy can be traditional, in which the gestational carrier's eggs are used, or gestational, in which an embryo is transferred into the gestational carrier's uterus. However, only gestational surrogacy is widely practiced today (Söderström-Anttila et al. 2016). Gestational carriers are typically paid for their medical costs and other reasonable pregnancy-related expenses. This arrangement is known as "altruistic surrogacy," and a relative is often the gestational carrier in these arrangements. In contrast, in commercial arrangements, gestational carriers are paid for their services in addition to these typical reimbursements.

Commercial surrogacy tends to be controversial because of concerns that the gestational carrier may be coerced or exploited, whereas altruistic arrangements are more broadly accepted. Commercial surrogacy is not allowed in some countries. For instance, both India and Cambodia ban commercial surrogacy. In Cambodia, a surrogate can be charged with human trafficking and may face up to 20 years in prison (Blomberg 2019). Other countries, such as Canada and New Zealand, allow only altruistic arrangements (Cornell Law School 2017). Still others, such as Iceland, Germany, and France, ban surrogacy altogether. In the United States, no federal law governs surrogacy, leaving individual states to delineate appropriate parameters. Legal scholars note that consequently no clear and consistent regulatory framework guides surrogates and intended parents

(Feldman 2018), but many states do allow some form of surrogacy. States that do not allow surrogacy may subject offenders to civil or even criminal sanctions. For instance, until the passage of the Child-Parent Security Act in April 2020, participants in a commercial surrogacy arrangement in New York were subject to civil fines (Family Equality 2020). Prior to the passage of this Act, agencies or individuals who assisted in these arrangements were also potentially subject to felony prosecution. Surrogacy contracts were also viewed as void or unenforceable, meaning that the gestational carrier, rather than the intended parent, could potentially be viewed as the legal parent (Cornell Law School 2017).

Various restrictions on surrogacy have led intended parents to seek surrogacy in foreign countries, a practice known as "gestational tourism" (Deonandan 2015). This practice is not without its risks. A recent example is that of Aki Mukai, a media personality in Japan who, along with her husband, sought out a surrogate in Nevada given Japan's prohibition of surrogacy. Even though Mukai's own embryos were used, the Japanese government refused to recognize her as the legal mother of the twin children, resulting in a protracted legal battle that ultimately led to Mukai adopting her own biological children (Sanchanta 2011). Another example that made recent headlines is the stranding of hundreds of babies born to gestational surrogates in Ukraine when international borders closed during the COVID-19 pandemic (Varenikova 2020; Widdicombe 2020).

Medical guidelines regarding the eligibility of surrogates exist, but it is at a clinic or agency's discretion to choose to follow these standards. The American Society of Reproductive Medicine (ASRM) recommends that a gestational carrier be between the ages of 21 and 45 years, have at least one child, have had full-term and uncomplicated previous pregnancies, and ideally have had no more than five total previous deliveries, at most three of which were via cesarean section. Potential gestational carriers should also have psychosocial consultations with a mental health professional, who is also often the ethical gatekeeper determining whether a woman is psychologically fit to be a surrogate (Braverman 2015). In contrast, standards regarding eligibility of intended parents are poorly defined. When mental health professionals are involved with intended parents, it is in three primary roles—psychoeducator, evaluator, and ethical gatekeeper—similar to the roles they play for potential surrogates (Braverman 2015). However, mental health professionals are often not involved with intended parents at all. For instance, in a 2005 survey, only 18% of ASRM clinics consistently had intended parents meet with mental health professionals (Braverman 2015).

Sometimes questions arise regarding the medical provider's ethical and legal obligations to the surrogate in light of the competing interests of the intended parents. For instance, what if a surrogate discloses that she has been drinking alcohol, not taking her vitamins, or engaging in behavior that might put the fetus at risk? Although the ASRM supports disclosure to the intended parents in limited circumstances, others have asserted that a surrogate's physician does not have a medical or legal relationship with the intended parents, and thus the ongoing duty to preserve confidentiality remains with the surrogate (Horner and Burcher 2018).

Other legal questions may arise regarding the custody of the child. Rarely, a surrogate refuses to relinquish the baby to the intended parents. Courts have come down on either side of this issue, but in general, in cases in which the intended parents are the genetic parents, it is likely that the court will find them to also be the legal parents. In the landmark California case of *Johnson v. Calvert* (1993), the parental rights of the intended, and genetic, parents were upheld over those of the surrogate mother. Complex challenges arise, however, in cases in which donor sperm or eggs are used or the surrogate is the genetic mother.

A systematic review of studies exploring the psychological outcomes for surrogate mothers did not reveal serious psychopathologies attributed to the surrogacy process. Several of the included studies noted that some of the surrogate mothers endorsed moderate difficulties relinquishing the child (Söderström-Anttila et al. 2016). This same review also looked at psychological outcomes for mothers of children who were the product of surrogacies and found there were no major differences in psychological outcomes for these mothers compared with those who conceived naturally. Importantly, it has been noted that the quality of evidence for both outcomes was low and more research is needed (Söderström-Anttila et al. 2016).

## Conclusion

In summary, there is much overlap between legal and forensic issues and reproductive psychiatry with regard to informed consent and decision-making capacity for VTOP and for medication treatment in the peripartum, as well as involuntary treatment in the peripartum. Parenting capacity is a specific capacity that the expert witness may be asked to evaluate. Child maltreatment risk and infanticide risk should be considered by the treating psychiatrist, as well as risk of suicide. The reproductive psychiatrist may also be involved in correctional mental health care of women, who often have children but limited interaction with them unless they are in a mother–baby unit. Finally, surrogate mothers and intended parents require special ethical and legal consideration for the reproductive psychiatrist.

## Key Points

- Informed consent for voluntary termination of pregnancy (VTOP) may be complicated by impaired decision-making capacity and mandated "informed consent" laws in many states, which may include misinformation regarding VTOP.
- Concerns about malpractice lawsuits in pregnancy should not prevent appropriate care. The discussion with the patient about the risks and benefits of medication, alternatives, and no treatment should be carefully documented.
- Treatment over a patient's objection may be necessary in severe cases of mania or psychosis, and the psychiatrist should be able to explain the risks and benefits to the court.
- Mental health professionals may become involved in cases relating to parenting capacity. Serving as both treating clinician and forensic expert should be avoided in such cases due to issues related to dual agency.
- Psychiatrists are mandated reporters of child abuse in U.S. jurisdictions. Physicians should be aware of the statutory standards for reporting child abuse, which in most states is suspicion or reason to suspect that abuse is occurring.

- When a mother experiences perinatal mental illness, not only should a suicide risk assessment be performed but infanticide and violence risk must also be considered.
- Pregnancy and mothering during incarceration are becoming more common in the United States as more women enter the criminal justice system. Despite the many challenges involved in caring for incarcerated pregnant women, pregnancy outcomes overall are positive, likely due to certain beneficial aspects of confinement, such as access to prenatal care, stable housing, reduced exposure to violence, and restricted access to alcohol, tobacco, and illicit drugs.
- Although most children of incarcerated mothers are placed in either kinship care or foster care, most mothers are able to maintain some form of contact with their children while incarcerated.
- Surrogacy is banned in many countries, and although it is allowed in the United States, laws vary by state regarding the legality of surrogacy, how the surrogate may be compensated, and the parental rights of the surrogate.

## References


Adoption and Safe Families Act, P.L. 105-89, 1997

American Civil Liberties Union: ACLU Briefing Paper: The Shackling of Pregnant Women and Girls in U.S. Prisons, Jails and Youth Detention Centers. New York, American Civil Liberties Union, 2021. Available at: https://www.aclu.org/other/aclu-briefing-paper-shackling-pregnant-women-girls-us-prisons-jails-youth-detention-centers. Accessed June 14, 2019.

Badger LW: Reporting of child abuse: influence of characteristics of physician, practice, and community. South Med J 82(3):281–286, 1989 2922618

Benjet C, Azar ST, Kuersten-Hogan R: Evaluating the parental fitness of psychiatrically diagnosed individuals: advocating a functional-contextual analysis of parenting. J Fam Psychol 17(2):238–251, 2003 12828020

Biggs MA, Gould H, Barar RE, et al: Five-year suicidal ideation trajectories among women receiving or being denied an abortion. Am J Psychiatry 175(9):845–852, 2018 29792049

Blomberg M: Cambodia urged not to criminalize surrogate mothers with new law. Reuters, May 17, 2019

Booth BD, Friedman SH, Curry S, et al: Obsessions of child murder: underrecognized manifestations of obsessive-compulsive disorder. J Am Acad Psychiatry Law 42(1):66–74, 2014 24618521

Braverman AM: Mental health counseling in third-party reproduction in the United States: evaluation, psychoeducation, or ethical gatekeeping? Fertil Steril 104(3):501–506, 2015 26171997

Budd KS: Assessing parenting capacity in a child welfare context. Children and Youth Services Review 27(4):429–444, 2005

Centers for Disease Control and Prevention: ART and Gestational Carriers (online). Atlanta, GA, Centers for Disease Control and Prevention, August 5, 2016. Available at: https://www.cdc.gov/art/key-findings/gestational-carriers.html. Accessed November 2, 2019.

Child Abuse Prevention and Treatment Act, 42 U.S.C. § 5106a[b][2][B][i] 1974

Child-Parent Security Act, Senate bill S2071B (N.Y.), 2020

Child Welfare Information Gateway: Mandatory Reporters of Child Abuse and Neglect. Washington, DC, U.S. Department of Health and Human Services, Children's Bureau, 2019a

Child Welfare Information Gateway: Penalties for Failure to Report and False Reporting of Child Abuse and Neglect. Washington, DC, U.S. Department of Health and Human Services, Children's Bureau, 2019b

Christian SM: Children of Incarcerated Parents. Washington, DC, National Conference of State Legislatures, March 2009. Available at: https://www.ncsl.org/documents/cyf/childrenofincarceratedparents.pdf. Accessed June 8, 2019.
Clarke JG, Adashi EY: Perinatal care for incarcerated patients: a 25-year-old woman pregnant in jail. JAMA 305(9):923–929, 2011 21304069
Clarke JG, Simon RE: Shackling and separation: motherhood in prison. Virtual Mentor 15(9):779–785, 2013 24021108
Committee on Health Care for Underserved Women of American College of Obstetricians and Gynecologists: ACOG Committee Opinion No. 511: health care for pregnant and postpartum incarcerated women and adolescent females. Obstet Gynecol 118(5):1198–1202, 2011 22015908
Cornell Law School, International Human Rights Policy Advocacy Clinic, National Law University, Delhi: Should Compensated Surrogacy Be Permitted or Prohibited? Ithaca, NY, Cornell Law Faculty, 2017. Available at: https://scholarship.law.cornell.edu/facpub/1551. Accessed November 22, 2019.
Coverdale JH, McCullough LB, Chervenak FA: Assisted and surrogate decision making for pregnant patients who have schizophrenia. Schizophr Bull 30(3):659–664, 2004 15631258
Cramer L, Goff M, Peterson B, et al: Parent-Child Visiting Practices in Prisons and Jails. Washington, DC, Urban Institute, 2017. Available at: https://www.urban.org/sites/default/files/publication/89601/parent-child_visiting_practices_in_prisons_and_jails.pdf. Accessed June 14, 2019.
Daniels CR, Ferguson J, Howard G, et al: Informed or misinformed consent? Abortion policy in the United States. J Health Polit Policy Law 41(2):181–209, 2016 26732319
Deonandan R: Recent trends in reproductive tourism and international surrogacy: ethical considerations and challenges for policy. Risk Manag Healthc Policy 8:111–119, 2015 26316832
Family Equality: The Child-Parent Security Act in New York. April 2020. Available at: http://www.familyequality.org/resources/child-parent-security-act-new-york. Accessed May 25, 2020.
Feldman EA: Baby M turns 30: the law and policy of surrogate motherhood. Am J Law Med 44(1):7–22, 2018 29764324
Ferszt GG, Erickson-Owens DA: Development of an educational/support group for pregnant women in prison. J Forensic Nurs 4(2):55–60, 2008 18522603
Finer LB, Zolna MR: Declines in unintended pregnancy in the United States, 2008–2011. N Engl J Med 374(9):843–852, 2016 26962904
Flaherty EG, Sege R: Barriers to physician identification and reporting of child abuse. Pediatr Ann 34(5):349–356, 2005 15948346
Friedman SH: The ethics of treating depression in pregnancy. J Prim Health Care 7(1):81–83, 2015 25770721
Friedman SH: Neonaticide, in Family Murder: Pathologies of Love. Edited by Friedman SH. Washington, DC, American Psychiatric Association Publishing, 2019, pp 53–67
Friedman SH, Hall RCW: Antidepressant use during pregnancy: how to avoid clinical and legal pitfalls. Curr Psychiatr 12(2):10–16, 2013
Friedman SH, Resnick PJ: Child murder by mothers: patterns and prevention. World Psychiatry 6(3):137–141, 2007 18188430
Friedman SH, McEwan MV: Treated mental illness in parents and risk of child abuse perpetration. Psychiatr Serv 69(2):211–216, 2018 29089007
Friedman SH, Resnick PJ: Neonaticide: phenomenology and considerations for prevention. Int J Law Psychiatry 32(1):43–47, 2009 19064290
Friedman SH, Heneghan A, Rosenthal M: Characteristics of women who deny or conceal pregnancy. Psychosomatics 48(2):117–122, 2007 17329604
Friedman SH, Sorrentino RM, Stankowski JE, et al: Psychiatrists' knowledge about maternal filicidal thoughts. Compr Psychiatry 49(1):106–110, 2008 18063049
Friedman SH, Hendrix T, Haberman J, et al: Judicial bypass of parental consent for abortion: characteristics of pregnant minor "Jane Doe's." J Nerv Ment Dis 203(6):401–405, 2015 26034870

Friedman SH, Hall RCW, Sorrentino RM: Involuntary treatment of psychosis in pregnancy. J Am Acad Psychiatry Law 46(2):217–223, 2018 30026401
Friedman SH, Prakash C, Nagle-Yang S: Postpartum psychosis: protecting mother and infant. Curr Psychiatr 18(4):12–21, 2019a
Friedman SH, Tamburello AC, Kaempf A, Hall RCW: Prescribing for women in corrections. J Am Acad Psychiatry Law 47(4):476–485, 2019b 31519733
Friedman SH, Kaempf A, Kauffman S: The realities of pregnancy and mothering while incarcerated. J Am Acad Psychiatry Law 48(3):365–375, 2020 32404363
Friedman SH, Riordan D, Short J: Writing the report: pearls of wisdom for the expert witness, in Infanticide and Filicide: Foundations in Maternal Mental Health Forensics. Edited by Wong G, Parnham G. Arlington, VA, American Psychiatric Association Publishing, 2021, pp 217–264
Gilham JJM: A qualitative study of incarcerated mothers' perceptions of the impact of separation on their children. Soc Work Public Health 27(1–2):89–103, 2012 22239380
Glaze LE, Maruschak LM: Parents in prison and their minor children. Bureau of Justice Statistics Special Report, March 30, 2010. Available at: https://www.bjs.gov/content/pub/pdf/pptmc.pdf. Accessed November 22, 2019.
Gossman W, Thornton I, Hipskind JE: Informed consent, in StatPearls. Treasure Island, FL, StatPearls Publishing, 2019. Available at: https://www.ncbi.nlm.nih.gov/books/NBK430827. Accessed October 2, 2019.
Grisso T: Evaluating Competencies: Forensic Assessments and Instruments, 2nd Edition. New York, Academic/Plenum, 2003
Guttmacher Institute: Counseling and waiting periods for abortion. Guttmacher.org, October 2019a. Available at: https://www.guttmacher.org/state-policy/explore/counseling-and-waiting-periods-abortion. Accessed November 22, 2019
Guttmacher Institute: An overview of abortion laws. Guttmacher.org, 2019b. Available at: https://www.guttmacher.org/state-policy/explore/overview-abortion-laws. Accessed on October 2, 2019.
Hall RCW, Friedman SH, Jain A: Pregnant women and the use of correction restraints and substance use commitment. J Am Acad Psychiatry Law 43(3):359–368, 2015 26438814
Horner C, Burcher P: A surrogate's secrets are(n't) safe with me: patient confidentiality in the care of a gestational surrogate. J Med Ethics 2018 29899014 Epub ahead of print
Jacobsen T, Miller LJ, Kirkwood KP: Assessing parenting competency in individuals with severe mental illness: a comprehensive service. J Ment Health Adm 24(2):189–199, 1997 9110522
Jatlaoui TC, Boutot ME, Mandel MG, et al: Abortion surveillance—United States, 2015. MMWR Surveill Summ 67(13):1–45, 2018 30462632
Jennings KD, Ross S, Popper S, et al: Thoughts of harming infants in depressed and nondepressed mothers. J Affect Disord 54(1–2):21–28, 1999 10403143
Johnson v Calvert, 5 Cal. 4th 84, 851 P.2d 776, 19 Cal. Rptr. 2d 494, 1993 Cal. LEXIS 2474, 93 Cal. Daily Op. Service 3739, 93 Daily Journal DAR 6409 (Cal. May 20, 1993)
Kelsey CM, Medel N, Mullins C, et al: An examination of care practices of pregnant women incarcerated in jail facilities in the United States. Matern Child Health J 21(6):1260–1266, 2017 28236159
Knight M, Plugge E: The outcomes of pregnancy among imprisoned women: a systematic review. BJOG 112(11):1467–1474, 2005 16225564
Landess J, Friedman SH: Case challenge: a 28-year-old new mother with insomnia and anxiety. Psychiatr Ann 48(2):71–74, 2018
Lindberg DM, Beaty B, Juarez-Colunga E, et al: Testing for abuse in children with sentinel injuries. Pediatrics 136(5):831–838, 2015 26438705
Mass Ann. Laws Ch. 210, § 3, 2021
McEwan M, Friedman SH: Violence by parents against their children: reporting of maltreatment suspicions, child protection, and risk in mental illness. Psychiatr Clin North Am 39(4):691–700, 2016 27836161
McTavish JR, Kimber M, Devries K, et al: Children's and caregivers' perspectives about mandatory reporting of child maltreatment: a meta-synthesis of qualitative studies. BMJ Open 9(4):e025741, 2019 30948587

Melton GB, Petrila J, Poythress NG, et al: Psychological Evaluations for the Courts, 3rd Edition. New York, Guilford, 2007
Mignon SI, Ransford P: Mothers in prison: maintaining connections with children. Soc Work Public Health 27(1–2):69–88, 2012 22239379
Miller AL, Weston LE, Perryman J, et al: Parenting while incarcerated: tailoring the strengthening families program for use with jailed mothers. Child Youth Serv Rev 44:163–170, 2014 26612963
Miller LJ: Denial of pregnancy, in Infanticide: Psychosocial and Legal Perspectives on Mothers Who Kill. Edited by Spinelli MG. Washington DC, American Psychiatric Publishing, 2003, pp 81–104
Miller LJ: Ethical issues in perinatal mental health. Psychiatr Clin North Am 32(2):259–270, 2009
Mo Ann. Stat. 211.44, 2011
National Task Force on the Use of Restraints With Pregnant Women Under Correctional Custody: Best Practices in the Use of Restraints With Pregnant Women and Girls Under Correctional Custody (Department of Justice grant No 2010-DJ-BX-K080). Washington, DC, U.S. Department of Health and Human Services, 2012. Available at: https://www.nasmhpd.org/sites/default/files/Best_Practices_Use_of_Restraints_Pregnant%282%29.pdf. Accessed February 5, 2021.
National Women's Law Center: Mothers Behind Bars: A State-By-State Report Card and Analysis of Federal Policies on Conditions of Confinement for Pregnant and Parenting Women and the Effect on Their Children. Washington, DC, The Rebecca Project for Human Rights/National Women's Law Center, 2010. Available at: https://www.nwlc.org/sites/default/files/pdfs/mothersbehindbars2010.pdf. Accessed May 3, 2019.
Nebraska Revised Statute 43-292, 2020. Available at: https://nebraskalegislature.gov/laws/statutes.php?statute=43-292. Accessed on November 22, 2019.
Ngwena CG: Reproductive autonomy of women and girls under the Convention on the Rights of Persons With Disabilities. Int J Gynaecol Obstet 140(1):128–133, 2018 29034953
O'Malley S, Devaney C: Maintaining the mother child relationship within the Irish prison system: the practitioner perspective. Child Care Pract 22(1):20–34, 2016
Planned Parenthood of Southeastern Pennsylvania v. Casey, 505 US 833 (1992)
Poehlmann J, Dallaire D, Loper AB, et al: Children's contact with their incarcerated parents: research findings and recommendations. Am Psychol 65(6):575–598, 2010 20822198
Resnick PJ: Child murder by parents: a psychiatric review of filicide. Am J Psychiatry 126(3):325–334, 1969 5801251
Resnick PJ: Murder of the newborn: a psychiatric review of neonaticide. Am J Psychiatry 126(10):1414–1420, 1970 5434623
Roe v. Wade, 410 US 113 (1973)
Roth R: Abortion access for imprisoned women: marginalized medical care for a marginalized group. Womens Health Issues 21(3 suppl):S14–S15, 2011 21530831
Sanchanta M: A debate arrives with Japan politician's baby. Wall Street Journal, January 6, 2011. Available at: https://www.wsj.com/articles/SB10001424052748704415104576065253692270070. Accessed November 4, 2019.
Schubert EC, Duininck M, Shlafer RJ: Visiting Mom: a pilot evaluation of a prison-based visiting program serving incarcerated mothers and their minor children. J Offender Rehabil 55(4):213–234, 2016 27867281
The Sentencing Project: Incarcerated Women and Girls. Washington, DC, The Sentencing Project, November 24, 2020. Available at: https://www.sentencingproject.org/publications/incarcerated-women-and-girls. Accessed November 22, 2020.
Shlafer RJ, Davis L, Hindt LA, et al: Intention and initiation of breastfeeding among women who are incarcerated. Nurs Womens Health 22(1):64–78, 2018 29433701
Söderström-Anttila V, Wennerholm UB, Loft A, et al: Surrogacy: outcomes for surrogate mothers, children and the resulting families: a systematic review. Hum Reprod Update 22(2):260–276, 2016 26454266
Steffen J: Few punishments for those who fail to report abuse. The Denver Post, July 4, 2014. Available at: https://www.denverpost.com/2014/07/04/few-punishments-for-those-who-fail-to-report-abuse. Accessed October 21, 2019.

Strasburger LH, Gutheil TG, Brodsky A: On wearing two hats: role conflict in serving as both psychotherapist and expert witness. Am J Psychiatry 154(4):448–456, 1997 9090330

Sufrin C, Beal L, Clarke J, et al: Pregnancy outcomes in US prisons 2016–2017. Am J Public Health 109(5):799–805, 2019 30897003

Varenikova M: Ukraine's backlog of babies born to surrogates begins to ease. New York Times, June 10, 2020. Available at: https://www.nytimes.com/2020/06/10/world/europe/ukraine-coronavirus-surrogate-babies.html. Accessed September 1, 2020.

Warner J: Infants in orange: an international model-based approach prison nurseries. Hastings Womens Law J 26(1):65–92, 2015

Widdicombe L: The stranded babies of the coronavirus disaster. The New Yorker, July 20, 2020. Available at: https://www.newyorker.com/news/news-desk/the-stranded-babies-of-the-coronavirus-disaster. Accessed September 1, 2020.

Zalpuri I, Byatt N, Gramann SB, et al: Decisional capacity in pregnancy: a complex case of pregnancy termination. Psychosomatics 56(3):292–297, 2015 25591494

APPENDIX

# Pregnancy and Lactation Considerations for Psychotropic Medications

| Medication | Dosage, *mg/day** | Pregnancy considerations | Lactation considerations |
|---|---|---|---|
| **Selective serotonin reuptake inhibitors (SSRIs)** (Chapters 6, 7, 13, 19) | | Pharmacokinetics of pregnancy lead to plasma concentration drop of 40%–50% by end of pregnancy. No guidelines on how to factor this into dosing. Associated with small increased risk of preterm birth (as is depression); possible association with small absolute risk of persistent pulmonary hypertension; risk of poor neonatal adaptation syndrome. | Considered compatible with BF, with infant serum levels <10% of maternal levels (10% being the threshold set for safety by the AAP); all can cause increased prolactin and galactorrhea; see additional comments on individual drugs. |
| Citalopram (Celexa) | Starting: 10–20<br>Typical: 20–60 (FDA maximum 40) | Relatively well studied; evidence does not support teratogenicity; see SSRI class risks above. | Infant serum levels 0.7%– 5.9% of maternal level; no contraindications. |
| Escitalopram (Lexapro) | Starting: 5–10<br>Typical: 10–30 (FDA maximum 20) | Limited data, but no known teratogenicity; see SSRI class risks above. | Infant serum levels range from 0.7% to 6.7% of maternal levels; no contraindications. |
| Fluoxetine (Prozac, Prozac Weekly, Selfemra, Sarafem) | Starting: 10–20<br>Typical: 20–80 | Well studied in pregnancy trials and neurodevelopmental trials in children. Evidence supports no teratogenicity; increased half-life may make it less desirable for pregnancy or breastfeeding if other choices are possible. See SSRI class risks above. | Average amount of drug in breastmilk higher than with other SSRIs, with active metabolite measurable in infant serum; agents with lower excretion may be preferred UNLESS mother is already taking or has history of response to fluoxetine. |
| Fluvoxamine (Faverin, Luvox, Luvox CR) | Starting: 25–50<br>Typical: 100–300 | Limited data, but no known teratogenicity. Metabolization by numerous CYP450 enzymes may mean heightened risk of drug–drug interactions. See SSRI class risks above. | Most studies show infant serum levels <10% of maternal levels, but one study reported >10% for one in three infants; no known adverse effects on infants beyond case reports. |

| Medication | Dosage, *mg/day** | Pregnancy considerations | Lactation considerations |
|---|---|---|---|
| **SSRIs *(continued)*** | | | |
| Paroxetine (Paxil, Paxil CR, Pexeva) | Starting: 10–20<br>Typical: 20–60 | Relatively well studied. Some evidence of a small increase in cardiovascular defects in early literature, but this is not supported by recent studies. See SSRI class risks above. | Most studies show infant serum levels <5% of maternal levels; no known adverse effects on infants beyond case reports. |
| Sertraline (Zoloft) | Starting: 25–50<br>Typical: 150–250 | Well studied in pregnant women, with no known teratogenicity. See SSRI class risks above. | Has most evidence for safety in BF with lowest passage into breastmilk (one study showing infant levels=0.5% of maternal levels). |
| Vilazodone (Viibryd) | Starting: 10<br>Typical: 10–40 | No data in pregnant women. | No data in lactation. |
| Vortioxetine (Brintellix) | Starting: 10<br>Typical: 10–20 | No data in pregnant women. | No data in lactation. |
| **Serotonin-norepinephrine reuptake inhibitors (SNRIs)** (Chapters 6, 7, 13, 19) | | Less well studied than SSRIs. Pharmacokinetics of pregnancy lead to plasma concentration drop of 40%–50% by end of pregnancy. No guidelines on how to factor this into dosing. Associated with small increased risk of preterm birth (as is depression); possible association with small absolute risk of persistent pulmonary hypertension; risk of poor neonatal adaptation syndrome. | Less well studied than the SSRIs, but likely compatible with BF, with infant serum levels <10% of maternal levels (10% being the threshold set for safety by the AAP). All can cause increased prolactin and galactorrhea. See additional comments on individual drugs. |
| Desvenlafaxine (Pristiq) | Starting: 50<br>Typical: 50–100, but dosages up to 400 have been used | No systematic studies in human pregnancy. No teratogenicity found in animal data; close relationship to venlafaxine makes it likely that effects would be similar. | Infant serum levels <10% of maternal levels; much lower drug exposure for infant than those using equivalent dose of venlafaxine. |

| Medication | Dosage, *mg/day** | Pregnancy considerations | Lactation considerations |
|---|---|---|---|
| **SNRIs** ***(continued)*** | | | |
| Duloxetine (Cymbalta) | Starting: 20–30<br>Typical: 30–120 | Limited data in humans, but bulk of evidence supports no teratogenicity in either humans or animals. | Not very well studied, but in existing data infant serum levels quite low (<1% of maternal level). |
| Venlafaxine (Effexor) | Starting: 37.5–75<br>Typical: 75–350 | Can be associated with hypertension, so monitor blood pressure closely across pregnancy, especially for women with risk factors for preeclampsia. Bulk of evidence supports no known teratogenicity; recent large population study that found evidence for congenital defects did not control for underlying illness. | Metabolized to desvenlafaxine, and both are found in milk and infant serum. Infant serum levels in most studies are low, but in one study concentration of venlafaxine + desvenlafaxine was 37% of maternal level. No known adverse effects in infants. |
| **Tricyclic antidepressants (TCAs)**<br>(Chapters 13, 19) | | More side effects than SSRIs; orthostatic hypotension can be particularly difficult in pregnancy. No known teratogenicity based on human and animal data. All have great advantage of dosing by serum level, so can easily monitor pharmacokinetic changes across pregnancy for dosage adjustment. | Limited studies, but data are reassuring. Considered compatible with BF. |
| Amitriptyline (Elavil) | Starting: 25 qhs<br>Typical: 75–300; may be increased by 25 mg every 3–7 days. Monitor plasma levels. | Animal studies indicate possible interference with embryo development. Human studies have not confirmed increased risk of birth defects. | Limited studies indicate undetectable infant serum concentration. |

| Medication | Dosage, *mg/day** | Pregnancy considerations | Lactation considerations |
|---|---|---|---|
| **TCAs *(continued)*** | | | |
| Clomipramine (Anafranil) | Starting: 25 qhs<br>Typical: 150–250; may be increased by 25 mg every 3–7 days. Monitor plasma levels. | Animal and human data indicate no known teratogenicity based on animal data. Limited human data show possible risk of cardiac malformations. | Limited studies indicate undetectable infant serum concentration. |
| Desipramine (Norpramin) | Starting: 25 qhs<br>Typical: 150–300; may be increased by 25 mg every 3–7 days. Monitor plasma levels. | Animal and human data indicate no known teratogenicity (studies mostly involved imipramine, a closely related agent). | Limited studies indicate undetectable infant serum concentration. |
| Doxepin (Sinequan) | Starting: 25 qhs<br>Typical: 75–150; 3–6 for insomnia. May be increased by 25 mg every 3–7 days (other than for insomnia). Monitor plasma levels. | Animal data and limited human reports indicate no expected increase in teratogenicity. | Limited data. One study indicates infant's simultaneous serum concentration is 15% of maternal serum level of metabolite *N*-desmethyldoxepin. |
| Imipramine (Tofranil) | Starting: 25 qhs<br>Typical: 150–300; may be increased by 25 mg every 3–7 days. Monitor plasma levels. | Animal and human data indicate no known teratogenicity. | Limited studies indicate undetectable infant serum concentration. |
| Nortriptyline (Pamelor) | Starting: 10–25 qhs<br>Typical: 75–150; may be increased by 25 mg every 3–7 days. Monitor plasma levels. | Lower burden of adverse side effects and more safety data available than for other TCAs. No evidence of increase in congenital malformations; no evidence of effects on child neurobehavior or development. Preferred in pregnancy because of the quantity of data and lower side effect burden. | No known adverse effects in BF; limited studies indicate barely detectable infant serum concentration. |

| Medication | Dosage, *mg/day** | Pregnancy considerations | Lactation considerations |
|---|---|---|---|
| **Other antidepressants** | | | |
| Bupropion (Wellbutrin SR or Wellbutrin XL) (Chapter 13) | Starting: 100 (SR), 150 (XL)<br>Typical: 200–450 (SR), 300–450 (XL) | Limited human data, mostly registry. No known teratogenicity. Lack of sexual side effects and weight gain makes it appealing to many postpartum women. Also useful for smoking cessation. Decreases seizure threshold and should thus not be used in patients with preeclampsia. | Low levels in breast milk, in most case studies undetectable. Bulk of evidence shows no adverse effects. Case report of seizure in infant whose mother also took other drugs. |
| Mirtazapine (Remeron) (Chapters 13, 19) | Starting: 10–15<br>Typical: 15–60 | Limited human data (case reports only). No known teratogenicity from animal data. Fewer sexual side effects than many other antidepressants; works as an antiemetic, so useful in hyperemesis gravidarum (although research base is limited) or in patients in need of weight restoration. | Low levels in breast milk, ranging from undetectable to <1% of maternal dose. Adverse effects unlikely, but data are limited; some case reports of galactorrhea and elevated prolactin. |

| Medication | Dosage, *mg/day** | Pregnancy considerations | Lactation considerations |
|---|---|---|---|
| **Mood stabilizers** | | | |
| Lithium (Chapters 15, 16) | Starting: 300<br>Typical: 900–1,200 for maintenance; 1,800 for treatment of an acute episode | Recent data suggest lithium may have an association with cardiac or overall malformations, but this risk occurs at a much lower magnitude than previously postulated (cumulatively reported at OR <2) and is likely dose dependent, with those taking >900 mg at higher risk. Some risk of infant diabetes insipidus leading to polyhydramnios. Rare association with newborn decreased muscle tone and initial difficulty breathing and feeding. Clearance of lithium may increase by 30%–50% during pregnancy. Lithium levels should be checked regularly throughout pregnancy, proximate to delivery, and anytime the patient is at risk for dehydration (e.g., hyperemesis gravidarum, prolonged labor) or has impaired renal function (e.g., preeclampsia). Regular monitoring of kidney and thyroid function is recommended. In the event of incremental increases during pregnancy, lithium should be restarted at pre-pregnancy dosage after delivery. High-resolution ultrasound and fetal cardiography recommended at 16–20 weeks' gestation. | Breastfeeding complicated by risk of lithium toxicity in dehydrated infants but can be managed with pediatrician vigilance and guidance. Serum lithium levels in the breastfed infants of mothers taking lithium have ranged from 10% to 50% of simultaneous maternal serum lithium levels. One systematic review recommended monitoring of infant lithium, thyroid stimulating hormone, and renal function tests if clinically indicated. |

| Medication | Dosage, *mg/day** | Pregnancy considerations | Lactation considerations |
|---|---|---|---|
| **Mood stabilizers** ***(continued)*** | | | |
| Carbamazepine (Tegretol) (Chapter 15) | Starting: 200 mg bid<br>Typical: 400–1,200 mg bid | Risk of neural tube defects. Some studies show craniofacial abnormalities and developmental delay. If used during pregnancy, AAN recommends folate supplementation (4–5 mg/day); limited evidence supports vitamin K supplementation near delivery to prevent neonatal bleeding. | Considered compatible with BF at moderate doses. In limited studies, infant carbamazepine serum levels quite variable, especially when other drugs also being used (5%–44% of maternal level). No evidence of adverse effects. |
| Gabapentin (Neurontin) (Chapters 7, 15) | Starting: 300; should be increased to 300 mg bid over 3 days<br>Typical: 1,200–3,600 mg in two or three divided doses per day | Limited evidence. Animal studies show evidence of fetal growth impairment and developmental delay; few small studies in humans show no increased risk of malformations. Limited evidence of efficacy in patients with bipolar disorder or psychosis. Risks may outweigh therapeutic benefits. | Considered compatible with BF at moderate doses. Infants' serum levels average 7% (range 4%–12%) of mother's serum levels, but no evidence of adverse effects. |

| Medication | Dosage, *mg/day** | Pregnancy considerations | Lactation considerations |
|---|---|---|---|
| **Mood stabilizers *(continued)*** | | | |
| Lamotrigine (Lamictal) (Chapter 15) | Starting: 25 for 2 weeks, then 50 for 2 weeks, then 100<br>Typical: 100–400 | Older data reporting oral cleft defects have not been confirmed. No other congenital malformations. Titrate slowly due to risk for SJS (not a good choice for acute symptoms); earlier recommendations for high-dose folate supplementation to reduce the risk of malformations have recently been revised down to typical 1 mg/day. Clearance of lamotrigine increases up to 300% during pregnancy. Some experts recommend obtaining a baseline lamotrigine level and regular monitoring of lamotrigine levels throughout pregnancy. In the event of incremental increases during pregnancy, lamotrigine should be decreased in incrementally every 3–4 days until pre-pregnancy dose is resumed. | Considered compatible with BF, but infants display high serum levels and should be monitored carefully for adverse effects, especially rash. In one study, infant serum concentration averaged 32.5% (range 18%–46%) of maternal serum concentration. Other studies indicate range of 30%–50% of maternal serum concentration. |
| Oxcarbazepine (Trileptal) (Chapter 15) | Starting: 300 mg bid<br>Typical: 1,200–2,400 in divided doses | No human data; animal data suggest same risks as closely related carbamazepine. If used in pregnancy, high-dose folate supplementation (4–5 mg/day) is required. | Infant serum concentration of active metabolite 5% of mothers' serum concentrations. Limited data indicate no adverse effects for infants. |
| Topiramate (Topamax) (Chapter 15) | Starting: 25<br>Typical: 50–300 | Developmental toxicity in animal studies. Limited human studies show an association with oral cleft defects. Limited evidence of efficacy in patients with bipolar disorder; risks may outweigh therapeutic benefits. | One study found infant serum levels 15% of mother's simultaneous serum level 3 hours after dose. Limited data indicate no adverse effects for infants. |

| Medication | Dosage, *mg/day** | Pregnancy considerations | Lactation considerations |
|---|---|---|---|
| **Mood stabilizers** ***(continued)*** | | | |
| Valproic acid (Depakote) (Chapter 15) | Starting: 250–500<br>Typical: 1,200–1,500 in patients with mania | Discontinue in pregnancy if possible. Risk of major malformations has been reported from 5% to 11% with first-trimester valproate monotherapy and includes neural tube defects, craniofacial defects, cardiovascular anomalies, skeletal and limb malformations, and genitourinary defects. Risk has been found to be dose dependent, rising significantly (up to 20-fold) with daily doses >1,000 mg. Also associated with neurodevelopmental delay, decreased IQ, and increased cognitive defects. If used in pregnancy, high-dose folate supplementation (4–5 mg/day) is required. | Considered compatible with BF. Mean ratio of maternal-to-infant serum level 0.12; no correlation observed between simultaneous maternal serum and infant serum concentration. No adverse effects in infants. |
| **Benzodiazepines (BZDs)** (Chapters 10, 19) | | No known association with congenital defects. Caution is warranted to avoid neonatal withdrawal and respiratory depression. | Considered compatible with BF. Infrequent small doses of shorter half-life agents preferred. |
| Alprazolam (Xanax) | Starting: 0.75–1.5 in divided doses<br>Typical: 1–4 (immediate release) for anxiety; 5–6 (immediate release) for panic disorder; 2–6 (extended release) for panic disorder | No known teratogenicity in animals except at very high dose-level exposure. Limited human data; in utero exposure may lead to transient withdrawal symptoms in fetus. | Withdrawal symptoms may occur from lactation exposure to BZDs. Infant–maternal serum level ratio not available. |

| Medication | Dosage, *mg/day** | Pregnancy considerations | Lactation considerations |
|---|---|---|---|
| **BZDs *(continued)*** | | | |
| Clonazepam (Klonopin) | Starting: 0.5–1 in divided doses<br>Typical: 0.5–2 in divided doses | No known teratogenicity in animal or human studies. Withdrawal effects possible in the fetus. When combined with SRIs, increased risk of mild transient neonatal complications. | Other agents preferred for BF women due to observed infant sedation (long half-life). Infant–maternal serum level ratio not available. |
| Diazepam (Valium) | Starting: 2–10 in divided doses<br>Typical: 4–40 in divided doses | Causes oral cleft defects in mice; limited human data show no increase in congenital malformations. Withdrawal symptoms possible in neonates. More likely than some other BZDs to accumulate in the fetus (not preferred in pregnancy). | Other agents preferred in BF women because of long half-life. Studies have shown infant's diazepam serum level was 0.7 μg/L and nordiazepam was 46 μg/L when mother's simultaneous serum levels were 100 and 200 μg/L for the drug and metabolite, respectively. |
| Lorazepam (Ativan) | Starting: 0.5–1.5 in divided doses<br>Typical: 2–6 in divided doses | No increase in congenital anomalies in animal or human data. May cause sedation and hypotonia in newborns when used near delivery. | Low levels in infant serum during BF, no reports of adverse effects, and shorter half-life make this the preferred BZD. Infant–maternal serum level ratio not available. |
| Temazepam (Restoril) | Starting: 15 qhs<br>Typical: 15–30 qhs | No increase in congenital malformations in animal data. No systematic human studies, but one case report of fetal death when combined with diphenhydramine. | Low levels in serum of breastfed infants and considered compatible. Infant–maternal serum level ratio not available. |
| **Other antianxiety agents** | | | |
| Buspirone (Buspar) (Chapter 19) | Starting: 20 mg bid<br>Typical: 15–60 daily in divided doses | Animal data reveal no known increase in congenital malformations. Human data extremely limited. | Limited data in BF; low serum levels for infants, but not systematically studied. |

| Medication | Dosage, *mg/day** | Pregnancy considerations | Lactation considerations |
|---|---|---|---|
| **Other antianxiety agents *(continued)*** | | | |
| Hydroxyzine (Vistaril, Atarax) (Chapter 19) | Starting: 25 mg up to four times daily<br>Typical: 50–100 mg up to four times daily | Malformations of palate and skeleton in rodent data. Human data quite limited. In humans, case reports indicate no consistent pattern of congenital defects or long-term effects, but data extremely limited. Decreases fetal heart response, but unclear what effect this may have. | No data specific to hydroxyzine. For other antihistamines, limited data are largely reassuring, with some reports of irritability and drowsiness. In theory, anticholinergic effects could decrease milk supply, but no known data. |
| **First-generation antipsychotics (FGAs)** (Chapters 10, 15, 16, 17) | | No evidence of congenital defects, but some reports of EPS for both mother and child. | Largely considered compatible with BF, but data available for only some drugs. |
| Chlorpromazine (Thorazine) | Starting: 50–100<br>Typical: 200–800 | Abnormal embryo development in animal data, but no increase in congenital malformations in limited human data. Some reports of EPS following third-trimester use. | Drowsiness and lethargy have been noted. Very limited data indicate no adverse developmental effects when used alone. Milk levels do not correlate well with maternal serum or dose. Infant–maternal level ratio not available. |
| Haloperidol (Haldol) | Starting: 1–5<br>Typical: 2–40 | More human data than for other FGAs. Abnormal embryo development in animal data, but no increase in congenital malformations in human data. Some reports of EPS following third-trimester use. | Doses ≤10 mg produce low levels in infant. No adverse effects on development noted when used alone. Monitor for drowsiness. Infant–maternal level ratio not available. |
| Fluphenazine (Prolixin) | Starting: 0.5–10 in divided doses<br>Typical: 2–40 in divided doses | Has been associated with cleft palate and other congenital defects in mice. Limited human data do not indicate an increase in congenital malformations. Transient neonatal complications have been observed. | No published data. Limited long-term data from other similar drugs show no long-term developmental effects. |

| Medication | Dosage, *mg/day** | Pregnancy considerations | Lactation considerations |
|---|---|---|---|
| **FGAs *(continued)*** | | | |
| Perphenazine (Trilafon) | Starting: 2–4 mg tid<br>Typical: 12–24 in divided doses | High doses have caused congenital malformations in animals, but limited human data do not indicate an increase in congenital malformations. | Limited data show low levels in breast milk. No evidence of long-term developmental effects in limited data. Monitor for drowsiness. Infant–maternal level ratio not available. |
| **Second-generation antipsychotics (SGAs)** (Chapters 10, 15, 16, 17) | | Increasing data show no evidence of congenital defects for most; metabolic effects in infant possible. Third-trimester exposure may increase neonatal complications including EPS, withdrawal, toxicity from residual exposure. | Largely considered compatible with BF except for clozapine, although data limited for some drugs. Many will increase prolactin and thus may affect milk supply. |
| Aripiprazole (Abilify) | Starting: 2–5 as augmentation for depression or anxiety; 5–10 for mood stabilization; 10–15 for psychosis<br>Typical: 5–10 as augmentation for depression or anxiety; 10–20 for mood stabilization; 15–30 for psychosis | Limited data. Recent registry data indicate no increased incidence of birth defects. Animal studies demonstrated developmental toxicity including teratogenic effects at doses higher than the maximum recommended. Patients should be monitored for macrosomia. | Limited data show that doses ≤15 mg produce low levels in milk. No evidence of adverse infant effects in limited data. Least likely to affect prolactin. Infant-maternal serum level ratio not available. |
| Asenapine (Sycrest, Saphris) | Starting: 10 in two divided doses<br>Typical: 20 in two divided doses | Animal data show no increase in congenital malformations. No human data. | No data. |

| Medication | Dosage, *mg/day** | Pregnancy considerations | Lactation considerations |
|---|---|---|---|
| SGAs *(continued)* | | | |
| Clozapine (Clozaril) | Starting: 25 qhs; increase by 25–50 mg/day as tolerated<br>Typical: Determined by plasma level; need trough level of 350 ng/L for response | Animal data show no increase in congenital malformations. Human data, including registry data and some controlled studies, indicate no increase in malformations and no long-term developmental effects. | Few published data. Sedation and hematological effects noted in infants. BF contraindicated for most women due to risk for agranulocytosis in infant. |
| Lurasidone (Latuda) | Starting: 20–40<br>Typical: 40–120 | Animal data indicate no increase in congenital anomalies. No human data available. | No human data available. |
| Olanzapine (Zyprexa) | Starting: 2.5–5 as augmentation for depression; 5–10 for mood stabilization or psychosis<br>Typical: 10–15 for mood stabilization; 20–30 for acute psychosis | Animal and human data, including recent registry data, indicate no increased incidence of congenital defects. Patients should be monitored for macrosomia and gestational diabetes mellitus. | More data available during BF (no adverse effects reported, including developmental data in infants—a preferred atypical agent in lactation). Infants should be monitored for sedation. Serum concentrations in breastfed (extent not stated) infants were less than the limit of detection in multiple samples. |

| Medication | Dosage, *mg/day** | Pregnancy considerations | Lactation considerations |
|---|---|---|---|
| SGAs *(continued)* | | | |
| Quetiapine (Seroquel) | Starting: 25 mg bid; increase by 25–50 mg/day until effective dosage<br>Typical: 200–300 for bipolar disorder; 100–400 for mood stabilization; 400–800 for acute mania or psychosis | Animal and human data, including recent registry data, indicate no increase in congenital defects. Patients should be monitored for macrosomia and gestational diabetes mellitus. | Low levels in infant serum and no reports of adverse effects in infants; preferred agent. Simulations of infant exposure indicate expected infant serum concentrations <0.6% of maternal serum concentration. |
| Risperidone (Risperdal) | Starting: 1 in divided doses<br>Typical: 2–8 for acute mania or psychosis; not generally used as augmentation for depression or anxiety or as a primary mood stabilizer | Limited data. Recent registry data, animal studies, and other human experience indicate no increased incidence of birth defects. Patients should be monitored for macrosomia. One recent large study with good adjustment for confounding found a slight increase in cardiac defects for risperidone alone among all atypical agents. | Relatively high passage into breastmilk makes this a second-line agent in BF. Higher incidence of hyperprolactinemia than for other atypical drugs. Simultaneous infant–maternal serum ratio not available. |
| Ziprasidone (Geodon) | Starting: 20 mg bid<br>Typical: 40–200 in divided doses | Animal data indicate effects on embryo development. Human data limited but do not indicate an increase in congenital malformations. | Limited data. No adverse effects noted in few case reports. Hyperprolactinemia may be transient, less severe than some other agents. Infant–maternal serum ratio not available. |

| Medication | Dosage, *mg/day** | Pregnancy considerations | Lactation considerations |
|---|---|---|---|
| **Alternative/Complementary** | | | |
| Black cohosh (Chapters 7, 14) | Starting: Usual dosage (varies by preparation)<br>Typical: 20–40 mg bid. Used for PMS and perimenopausal symptoms. Evidence limited; not FDA regulated. Different brands may have very different preparations. | No animal or human data in pregnancy. Preparations vary; not regulated by FDA. | Lack of safety data and possible estrogenicity are potential concerns during lactation. |
| Omega-3 fatty acids (Chapters 13, 14) | Starting: 1,000–2,000<br>Typical: 2,000–4,000 | Normal component of healthy diet. Not expected to cause adverse effects. Limited data for supplementation, but neither adverse effects nor benefits observed. Preparations vary; not regulated by FDA. | Normal component of healthy diet. Not expected to cause adverse effects. Some animal and human literature has raised concerns for adverse effects of supplementation on infant growth and cognition, but findings have not been replicated. |
| Phytoestrogens and soy (Chapters 13, 14) | Starting: Varies by preparation<br>Typical: Varies by preparation | Limited data indicate that consumption of isoflavones in food is not expected to increase congenital anomalies. Preparations vary; not regulated by FDA. | No data. |
| *S*-adenosyl-L-methionine (Chapters 13, 14) | Starting: 200<br>Typical: 800–1,600 | No data. Preparations vary; not regulated by FDA. | No data. |
| St. John's wort (Chapter 14) | Starting: Varies; 300 mg tid frequently used, may start as low as 20 mg<br>Typical: For anxiety, 900 mg bid; for depression, 20–1,800 mg bid | Animal data show no known increase in malformations. Little human data in pregnancy. Preparations vary; not regulated by FDA. | Limited data. One lactation study showed some increase in colic and lethargy, but others have not. Infant–maternal serum ratio not available. |

| Medication | Dosage, *mg/day** | Pregnancy considerations | Lactation considerations |
|---|---|---|---|
| **Alternative/Complementary** *(continued)* | | | |
| Vitex agnus castus (Chasteberry) (Chapters 6, 7, 14) | Starting: Usual dosage (varies by preparation)<br>Typical: 35–60 mg of dried supplement in divided doses or 40 drops of liquid extract in the morning | Limited data indicate no increase in malformations. Should be avoided in pregnancy because it is a uterine stimulant. Preparations vary; not regulated by FDA. | No data on use in BF. Demonstrated to reduce prolactin concentrations. |
| **Sleep aids** | | | |
| Melatonin (Chapter 19) | Starting: 0.5 qhs<br>Typical: 1–3 qhs | Limited data on administration of exogenous melatonin in pregnancy. No known teratogenicity. | Exogenous administration has no specific use in BF; no safety data. |
| Trazodone (Desyrel) (Chapters 13, 19) | Starting: 25–50<br>Typical: 50–200 in patients with sleep disorders; 150–400 in patients with major depressive disorder | Limited data. No known teratogenicity from animal data, but no systematic human data exist. | Studies of milk indicate infant levels likely very low, but no published studies of infant serum levels confirm this. Limited data, but no known adverse effects in infants. |
| Zolpidem (Chapter 19) | Starting: 5 mg qhs (6.25 if controlled release)<br>Typical: 10 mg qhs (12.5 if controlled release) | Limited data. | Limited data. Produces low levels in milk and has short half-life, so unlikely to produce adverse effects. Data on infant–maternal serum ratio not available. |

AAN=American Academy of Neurology; AAP=American Academy of Pediatrics; BF=breastfeeding; EPS=extrapyramidal symptoms; PMS=premenstrual syndrome; SJS=Stevens-Johnson syndrome; SRI=serotonin reuptake inhibitor.
*Unless otherwise noted.

*Source.* Data from National Library of Medicine 2006; Osborne and Payne 2017; Reprotox.org; Sachs and Committee on Drugs 2013; Stahl 2017.

## References

National Library of Medicine: Drugs and lactation database (LactMed). 2006. Available at: www.ncbi.nlm.nih.gov/books/NBK501922. Accessed February 5, 2021.

Osborne LM, Payne JL: Clinical updates in women's health care: mood and anxiety disorders. Obstet Gynecol 16(5):674, 2017 28832483

Sachs HC, Committee on Drugs: The transfer of drugs and therapeutics into human breast milk: an update on selected topics. Pediatrics 132(3):e769–e809, 2013 23979084

Stahl SM: Prescriber's Guide, 6th Edition. Cambridge, UK, Cambridge University Press, 2017

# Index

Page numbers printed in **boldface** type refer to tables or figures.

www.ingramcontent.com/pod-product-compliance
Ingram Content Group UK Ltd.
Pitfield, Milton Keynes, MK11 3LW, UK
UKHW060959120926
8556IPUK00033B/907

9 781615 373062